Saunders Review for NCLEX-RN

2nd Edition

Esther Matassarin-Jacobs, RN, PhD, OCN
Associate Professor
Niehoff School of Nursing
Loyola University of Chicago
Chicago, Illinois

W.B. SAUNDERS COMPANY
Harcourt Brace & Company
Philadelphia   London   Toronto   Montreal   Sydney   Tokyo

W.B. Saunders Company
A Division of Harcourt Brace & Company

The Curtis Center
Independence Square West
Philadelphia, Pennsylvania 19106

Library of Congress Cataloging-in-Publication Data

Matassarin-Jacobs, Esther.
    Saunders review for NCLEX-RN / Esther Matassarin-Jacobs. —2nd
ed.
       p.   cm.
    Includes bibliographical references and index.
    ISBN 0–7216–4993–9
    1. Nursing—Examinations, questions, etc. 2. Nursing—Outlines,
syllabi, etc.   I. Title. II. Title: Review for NCLEX-RN.
    [DNLM: 1. Licensure, Nursing—examination questions. 2. Nursing—
examination questions.   WY 18 M4245sb 1994]
RT55.M27   1994
610.73′076—dc20
DNLM/DLC   93-22879

Saunders Review for NCLEX-RN   ISBN 0–7216–4993–9

Printed in the United States of America

Last digit is the print number: 10   9   8   7   6   5   4   3   2   1

To Rachel, our niece,
the newest member of the household.
I hope your time with us
is a happy and productive one.
To my husband, Philip,
for everything.

Contributors

Maureen B. Barrett, RN, MSN, C
Instructor
Aurora University
Aurora, Illinois

Carol Ann Birch, RN, MSN, CCRN
Instructor
South Dakota State University
College of Nursing
Rapid City, South Dakota

Joyce M. Black, RN, MSN, C
Assistant Professor of Adult Health Nursing
University of Nebraska Medical Center
Omaha, Nebraska

Karen J. Egenes, RN, EdD
Assistant Professor
Niehoff School of Nursing
Loyola University of Chicago
Chicago, Illinois

Frank D. Hicks, RN, MS, CCRN
Assistant Professor
Medical—Surgical Nursing
Niehoff School of Nursing
Loyola University of Chicago
Chicago, Illinois

Susan Rowen James, RN, MSN
Pediatric Ambulatory Care Nurse
Pediatric/Adolescent Medical Association
Falmouth, Massachusetts
Clinical Instructor
University of Massachusetts—Dartmouth
N. Dartmouth, Massachusetts

Judith A. Jennrich, RN, PhD, CCRN
Assistant Professor
Medical—Surgical Nursing
Niehoff School of Nursing
Loyola University of Chicago
Chicago, Illinois

Virginia McMahon Keatley, RN, MSN
Lecturer
Widener University
Chester, Pennsylvania

Mary Ann Noonan, RN, MSN
Assistant Professor
Medical—Surgical Nursing
Niehoff School of Nursing
Loyola University of Chicago
Chicago, Illinois

Jo Ann Petty, RN, MSN, OCN
Oncology Clinical Nurse Specialist
La Grange Memorial Hospital
La Grange, Illinois

Nancy Spector, RN, DNSc, MSN, BSN
Assistant Professor
Loyola University of Chicago
Chicago, Illinois

Donna Starsiak, RN, MSN, C
Assistant Professor
Medical—Surgical Nursing
Loyola University of Chicago
Chicago, Illinois

Mary Szyszka, RN, MSN, OCN
Oncology Clinical Nurse Specialist
Ambulatory Programs
Loyola University Medical Center
Maywood, Illinois

Marianne G. Zelewsky, RN, MSN, C
Assistant Professor
Community Nursing
Loyola University of Chicago
Chicago, Illinois

Preface

I have spent most of my professional career working with undergraduate students, teaching them nursing and helping them prepare for the State Board Licensing Examination. I have also spent most of this time learning everything possible about the NCLEX-RN. Recently I have been studying the new examination format, the NCLEX/CAT-RN, in order to help graduates prepared for this new, computerized examination. I have also taught review courses throughout the country to help graduates pass the examination. All of this experience has gone into the preparation of this review text.

Remember, no review text can replace the education you have received, but this book should help you pull it all together so that you can be successful on the licensure examination.

Use this book as a tool to guide your studying. Pay particular attention to the first two chapters, which contain important information on the test itself. These chapters will give you the latest information on the examination and the practical information to help you prepare to take the examination. The overall pre-test that follows Chapter 2 is a 93-question test that gives you a lot of test-taking hints. This will help you not only with content but with testing in general.

I wish you all well on the achievement of your goal—licensure as a registered nurse. If you work hard and prepare well, I am certain you will be successful.

ESTHER MATASSARIN-JACOBS, RN, PhD, OCN

Acknowledgments

I want to thank all my contributors to this wonderful edition, but also those who contributed to the first edition. A special thanks to Ilze Rader, who helped a great deal with this edition so I could complete it and my other commitments.

Contents

UNIT IV

The Childbearing Family

Chapter 15

Prenatal Period   567

Chapter 16

Intrapartum Period   599

Chapter 17

Postpartum Period   623

Chapter 18

The Newborn   637

UNIT V

The Mental Health Client

Chapter 19

Treatment Modalities   657

UNIT I

Preparation for the NCLEX/CAT-RN

1

NCLEX/CAT-RN
Test Plan

GENERAL INFORMATION AND TEST DESCRIPTION

The NCLEX/CAT-RN is a 1-day, potentially 5-hour examination designed by the National Council of State Boards of Nursing (NCSBN) to test the graduate's ability to practice entry-level registered nursing in a safe and effective manner. This is done by testing the graduate's knowledge of entry-level nursing practice through the application of that knowledge to health care situations that require interventions by the beginning nurse. What should be covered on the examination was identified in a study by Kane et al. (1986) in *A Study of Nursing Practice and Role Delineation, and Job Analysis of Entry-Level Performance of Registered Nurses,* which analyzed the activities of the entry-level registered nurse. This study established a framework of entry-level performance that incorporated the nursing process and specific client needs. Using the test plan, "each NCLEX/CAT-RN examination reflects the knowledge, skills, and abilities essential for application of the phases of the nursing process to meet the needs of clients with commonly occurring health problems" (NCSBN, 1987, p. 1).

The examination itself consists of one test of up to 265 questions. The computer-adaptive testing (CAT) model allows for a varying number of questions, based on the student's ability. The examination is given in a single sitting. The questions are written by faculty members who teach registered nurse students, as well as clinical practitioners from a wide variety of settings who supervise new registered nurse graduates. The examination may be taken twice yearly, the first time no sooner than 30 days after the student has completed a nursing program.

CAT is a new form of testing for the NCLEX/CAT-RN. This form of testing is scheduled to begin in 1994. CAT refers to a way of predicting success or failure on the examination using a limited number of questions of varying levels of difficulty. CAT uses a statistical model to analyze your responses and then gives you either an easier question if you have not mastered the level or a more difficult one if you have. The examination can be completed in 75 questions for students who are either clear passes or clear failures, or may take up to 265 questions for a clear decision on pass or fail to be made. The examination may last for up to 5 hours, less if a clear pass–fail decision is obvious.

You may take the examination any time after 30 days from the date you complete your basic nursing program. You apply to your State Board of Nursing, providing the documentation of your successful completion of a basic nursing program. The State Board then notifies the Educational Testing Service (ETS) of your eligibility. The ETS sends you a registration form; when this is completed and processed, the ETS

3

sends you a ticket of examination eligibility. You will then call your local Sylvan Key Center and request an appointment. Be ready to give several possible times and dates, because only 10 candidates can be tested at any one time. The centers will probably have two or three 5-hour sessions a day, 6 days a week. When you go to take the examination, you will not be allowed to take anything into the testing room with you. After 2 hours of testing, you will be given a mandatory 10-minute break; then after another 1½ hours, you will be given an optional 10-minute break. These breaks will not be counted against your 5-hour testing time, although any other breaks you take will be counted.

There is a nationwide passing score, which means that if you pass the examination in one state, you can seek reciprocity to practice in any other state in the United States. Your score is reported as simply a pass or fail. You will receive this report after the examination, not at the testing site, although the score is reported to the ETS within 48 hours of your testing. The ETS then reports your results to your State Board of Nurse Examiners, which notifies you. The time this takes varies by state. Your goal is to do as well as possible in order to demonstrate your mastery of the required knowledge. A passing score should be thought of as the same level of competency that you have had to exhibit throughout your educational preparation for nursing practice—approximately a "C" level, or about 75%. If you can achieve this level,

you should have no difficulty passing the NCLEX/CAT-RN.

The examination is composed of multiple-choice questions with only one correct answer. Figure 1–1 shows you what the questions will look like on the computer screen. There are two types of questions. Some consist of a case study on the screen with a question (Fig. 1–1A), and some consist of a question without a case study (Fig. 1–1B). A running total of items appears at the top of the screen. The same case study appears on the screen each time a related question is asked. The questions with a given case study, however, may not be presented consecutively. There is no penalty for guessing an answer—if you can make a reasonable guess, go ahead. Strategies for testing are discussed later.

The test is given on the computer, although the graduate will not have to be computer-literate. Only two keys will work on the computer (Fig. 1–2), the space bar (Fig. 1–2A) and the enter or return ↵ key (Fig. 1–2B). The examination begins with a keyboard tutorial. If you are unable to complete this successfully, Sylvan personnel will give you additional information.

The test is mixed in content—that is, pediatric, maternity, medical/surgical, and mental health nursing are all presented in the examination. The distribution of content is given below. Knowing about the test can make it less threatening for you.

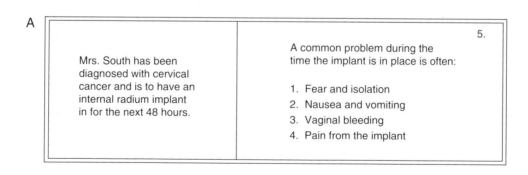

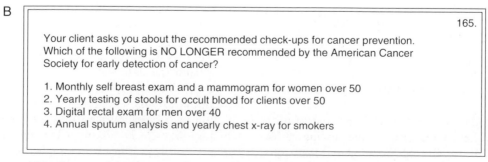

FIGURE 1–1. *A* and *B*, Example of how test questions look on the computer screen.

FIGURE 1–2. Functional keys. *A*, Spacebar. *B*, Enter key (return ⏎).

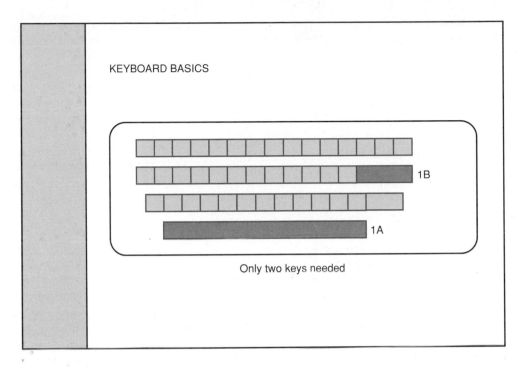

Although the test plan may seem somewhat complicated, it is important for the graduate nurse to be familiar with it so that preparation for the examination can be systematic and complete. By becoming familiar with the areas tested, you can be ready for the examination.

COMPONENTS OF THE TEST PLAN

Levels of Cognitive Ability

The levels of cognitive ability of the items on the NCLEX/CAT-RN are knowledge, comprehension, application, and analysis. The majority of the questions are of the application or analysis level. This means that you will not be able to simply answer with facts on most items. This higher level requires that you take a fact—such as the normal white blood cell count—and apply this knowledge of normal to a specific question. For example:

Martha has a white blood cell count of 17,000/mm³. Which of the following is an appropriate nursing intervention in the care of Martha?
　① Administer antibiotics as ordered
　② Maintain protective isolation
　③ Warn her to avoid people with colds
　④ Nothing; this is a normal count

The correct answer is choice 1, because the white blood count (WBC) is elevated, which indicates that there is an infection and that the proper therapy is antibiotics. You have to take several steps to answer this question. First, you must know the normal WBC, a simple fact; second, you must know what an elevated WBC means; and third, you must know what the usual treatment is for this problem. You are applying your knowledge to a specific situation.

Nursing Process

The five phases of the nursing process are the major divisions of the test plan. The categories are Assessment, Analysis, Planning, Implementation, and Evaluation. Each phase receives equal weight on the examination. This means that there are approximately equal numbers of questions from each phase. The phases can be defined as:

1. Assessment: setting data base
   a. Objective and subjective data about the client
   b. Collection and verification of data from all available sources
   c. Clinical manifestations
   d. Client's ability for self-care
   e. Health care team member's ability to provide care
   f. Environment
   g. Own and other health care team members' reactions to client
   h. Communicating data to other members of the health care team
2. Analysis: using assessment data to establish actual and potential health problems
   a. Interpretation, validation, and organization of data

b. Reassessment as needed

c. Formulation and communication of nursing diagnoses

3. Planning: setting and prioritizing goals and expected outcomes

a. Setting and prioritizing goals of care with assistance of all involved

b. Anticipation of needs based on priorities

c. Establishment and modification of plan of care, using all pertinent data and involving all persons needed to plan care

d. Establishment of expected outcomes

4. Implementation: the actions needed to meet established goals

a. Teaching/learning activities

b. Provision of care based on established goals

c. Organization, supervision, management, and evaluation of ongoing care

d. Levels of prevention

e. Safe, effective administration of medication and other treatments

f. Individualizing and prioritizing all care

g. Recording and reporting all information correctly

h. Health promotion activities

i. Activities to return client to maximal functioning

j. Establishment of therapeutic environment

5. Evaluation: determination of degree to which goals and expected outcomes have been met

a. Evaluation of expected and unexpected outcomes

b. Comparison of outcomes with expected outcomes

c. Planning for needed changes in goals based on evaluation

d. Verification of diagnostic data

e. Evaluation of client's understanding of teaching and therapeutic regimen

Categories of Client Needs

In order to categorize the health needs of individuals into some logical structure, the NCSBN, based on the results of its job analysis survey, devised four categories of client needs. These categories are weighted so that they, rather than the traditional subject matter areas, become the means by which the test is divided. The division is:

I.	Safe, effective care environment	25%–31%
II.	Physiological integrity	42%–48%
III.	Psychosocial integrity	9%–15%
IV.	Health promotion and maintenance	12%–18%

Under each of these areas, specific nursing content is identified.

I. *Safe, effective care environment* includes content such as knowledge of biological, psychological, and social principles; management principles; therapeutic communication; expected outcome of therapeutic interventions; protective and safety functions; client rights and confidentiality; quality assurance; implementation of treatments; cultural and religious influences; continuity of care; and infectious diseases.

II. *Physiological integrity* includes content such as normal anatomy and physiology; pathophysiology; pharmacology; nutrition; invasive treatments; routine nursing interventions; documentation; emergency care; expected and unexpected response to treatment; body mechanics; effects of immobility; activities of daily living; comfort; and special equipment.

III. *Psychosocial integrity* includes mental health content such as therapeutic communication; behavior; treatments; pharmacology; pathology; teaching/learning; documentation and accountability; and community resources.

IV. *Health promotion and maintenance* includes content related to health promotion such as communication; teaching/learning; documentation; community resources; family; wellness; adaptation; growth and development, including birth, parenting, sexuality, and death and dying; and immunity.

PREPARING FOR THE EXAMINATION

The NCLEX/CAT-RN contains 265 questions. You will have up to 5 hours to complete the examination. This is an important point to note, because it means that you will have only about 1 minute to answer each question. Time can be one of the most difficult things to manage in the testing situation; the next section offers suggestions on how to handle this potential problem.

The examination is composed entirely of multiple-choice questions. For each question, there are only four possible answers given. This type of question tests your knowledge without unnecessarily confusing you, as the older multiple-choice questions often did. You can practice with this type of question by marking your answers in the practice tests in each chapter or at the end of this book.

There is no penalty for guessing on this examination, but you should be careful not to start "wild guessing." If you guess, make it an educated guess by eliminating one or two of the possible responses. This can double your chances of being correct.

You should begin to prepare for the examination well in advance of the actual test. The best preparation is the course of study you have taken to prepare you as a nurse; nothing can replace this. If you were successful in your course of study, then, with proper and adequate preparation, you should be able to successfully complete the NCLEX/CAT-RN. Your notes and your textbooks will provide you with a great deal of material for your preparation. This review text can help you to organize and focus your study if it is used correctly.

If your program offered assessment tests, such as the many standardized commercial tests, use the results of these tests to help you identify areas of strength and weakness. If you scored low on those tests, usually below the 50th percentile, you should identify those as areas of content you must review in order to succeed on the NCLEX/CAT-RN.

Preparation is also a mental process. You must continually visualize yourself as being knowledgeable and successful. It is not uncommon for individuals to fail simply because they have mentally prepared themselves for failure. You need to approach the entire process with an attitude of success and preparation. Adequately preparing for the test will help you form this attitude of self-assurance and self-confidence. Visualize yourself as passing the NCLEX/CAT-RN and practicing as a registered nurse.

USING THIS TEXT

This text is designed to help you approach your preparation in a systematic and logical manner. By carefully identifying the specific areas in which you possess less knowledge, you can remedy the situation and improve your chances for success.

How should you use this text to help you successfully prepare for the NCLEX/CAT-RN? You have already started by reading the first section, which describes the content of the NCLEX/CAT-RN. A knowledge of this should improve your self-confidence when you see the examination itself.

Of course, a simple list of the material to be covered is not the only thing you will need to know. Chapter 2 is directed toward helping you improve your skills in answering test questions correctly. By learning a better way of taking multiple-choice tests, you can help improve your testing ability. Many people lose needless points because they are simply not "test-wise." Application of the information given to you in that section can help you avoid this.

With proper use, this review text can help you prepare for the examination itself. There are at least two ways to actually use the review material. First, you can simply review the sections containing material that you feel uncomfortable with. In this way, if you have already identified your own learning deficits, you can progress quickly through the material. The only problem with this is that most people tend to either try to go through everything or spend unnecessary time reviewing material they have already mastered.

Sometimes it is really hard to identify just what you do not know.

Second, this text is designed to help you assess your knowledge and then immediately review the material you were less familiar with. Before each major section there is a pre-test so that you can judge your knowledge of that section. Take the pre-test. If you are able to answer all or most of the questions, then this is an area of content that does not need much study. If you simply want to scan the material, do so. If you did not do well on the pre-test, then carefully review the section for content. Once you feel comfortable with this material, take the post-test that is available at the end of each major section. This pre-test/post-test format allows you to progress successfully through the content and to be well prepared for the examination.

There is a simulated practice test at the end of the text that can be used before and after your preparation. A score of at least 200 correct answers is roughly equivalent to a passing score on the NCLEX/CAT-RN. You can take these practice tests in a "real-life" situation. Set an alarm clock for 5 hours and try to finish the test within the actual time limit. When you are done, check your answers carefully, read all the rationales and codes, and write down those areas that are still giving you trouble. Go back and study those areas. The practice test can be a great confidence builder. When you see how much you actually know, you will feel better able to handle the material that you do not know as well.

There is also a 93-question practice test at the beginning of the text. This can also be treated as a simulated examination; however, the rationales in this test contain test-taking strategies to help you better understand how to best take this test.

No review text can teach you everything you should have learned in your nursing program. This is a review text. If you find an area that you really do not understand and the review book does not seem to provide enough information that you fully understand it, go back to your textbooks or class notes to cover that one area in greater detail. Remember, this is a review book, so use it as such and it can help you to be successful on the NCLEX/CAT-RN.

BIBLIOGRAPHY

Kane, M., Kingsbury, C., Colton, D., and Estes, C. (1986). *A study of nursing practice and role delineation, and job analysis of entry-level performance of registered nurses.* Chicago: National Council of State Boards of Nursing, Inc.
National Council of State Boards of Nursing. (1987). *NCLEX-RN: Test plan for the national council licensure examination for registered nurses.* Chicago: National Council of State Boards of Nursing, Inc.

2

Test-Taking Strategies

UNDERSTANDING THE TEST QUESTIONS

How do you successfully take a multiple-choice examination? The answer to this question is fairly long, but as your understanding of multiple-choice test items increases, so do your chances of successfully answering them. Successful test-taking can be learned, and it can improve your ability to answer multiple-choice questions.

First, the most important point is to focus on *reading* and understanding the question. Reading may seem like a simple matter, but most mistakes are made because the test-taker does not read the question carefully and completely. Along with reading the question, it is vital that you carefully read each response that follows the stem of the question. Test-takers often read quickly and choose the first response that looks good. Sometimes they do not even read all the possible responses. When a question is asking for priorities, all four responses will probably be correct, but only one will be the priority answer.

When you read the question, pay close attention to any specific information within the case study or stem of the question that can direct you to the correct answer. Sometimes the stem will contain a key statement: "your first action"; "which would be appropriate"; "an inappropriate intervention for this client"; "an important assessment"; "the best goal"; or "the most appropriate response." Phrases such as these can help you focus your response. For example:

UNSUCCESSFUL adaptation to the middle years would be characterized by:

①　Reassessment of role within the home
②　Achievement of career goals
③　Increased involvement in community activities
④　Acceptance of retirement

This type of question, which asks for the one thing that is incorrect, can be easy to answer. The best way to approach this question is to treat each response as a true–false item. In the above question, look at each response. Choice 1 is true; the middle years are a time to reassess the roles within the family. Choice 2 is true; this is a time when most persons achieve their career goals. Choice 3 is also true; this is a time when adults focus more on their role in the community. Choice 4 in this case is false and is the correct answer for this question. The middle years are a time not of accepting retirement, but only of beginning to prepare for it. By focusing on the important part of the question—UNSUCCESSFUL—and treating each response as a separate item, you should be able to find the one false response. This technique is appropriate any time the question contains a negative such as "least" or "inappropriate." Even if you can narrow down the possibilities to two responses, you have doubled your chances of guessing correctly.

Time control is another important factor. You will have slightly more than 1 minute per question. Speed and accuracy are skills that can be improved. Take

8

one of the pre-tests or post-tests and block out 10 items. Set an alarm for 10 minutes and begin. Practicing this way several times will help to improve your speed. During the actual test situation, you can do two important things to help improve your speed. First, take a watch and set limits and checks for yourself, such as by 30 minutes you should be on at least question 30. If you are not, then you must speed up. Do not wait until the end of the test period to notice that you have fallen behind. The other thing to do is to guess at the answer. If an item takes you more than 1 minute, simply make the best guess you can and go on.

Understanding the focus of the question can also help direct your response to it. A question that asks for an assessment requires an answer that provides more data. One that asks for a goal would require you to focus on the specific problem addressed and find a measurable, realistic goal. To give you practice with focusing on each step of the nursing process and each area of client need, examples of each are presented. Each rationale also has a code following it, so that you are able to identify the specific content areas each question represents. *The code is as follows: 1 to 5, phase of the nursing process; I to IV, area of client need; then the specific content area is stated.*

Examples of questions from each of these categories follow so that you can better understand the foci and to help you learn more about test taking. To provide you with more help, a general pre-test is provided immediately following this chapter. The rationales for this test include test-taking strategies.

PHASES OF THE NURSING PROCESS

1. Assessment

Which of the following assessments should the nurse make when the client returns from having a long leg cast applied to a newly broken tibia?
1. Circulation and sensation proximal to the cast
2. Temperature of the cast
3. Capillary refill of the toes
4. Presence of Homans' sign in the opposite leg

This item focuses on assessment. The correct answer is choice 3; the most important assessment for the nurse to make is the circulation and sensation distal to the cast. Choice 1 is incorrect because it states proximal, not distal. Choice 2 is not important on a fresh cast, because "hot" spots of infection would not appear this soon. Choice 4 is an important assessment at any time, but a fresh fracture client would probably not have developed a thrombophlebitis yet. At the end of the rationales in this text, you will see a code like the following: 1, II. Fractures/Casts.

2. Analysis

Mr. Jones is not performing leg exercises and coughing and deep-breathing exercises postoperatively. Which of the following is the most appropriate nursing diagnosis?
1. Noncompliance related to lack of interest in healing
2. Fear related to possible wound dehiscence
3. Knowledge deficit related to inadequate preoperative teaching
4. Pain related to postoperative incision

There are no data to support choices 1 and 4, which leaves choices 2 and 3 as possibilities. If you knew nothing else, it would be worthwhile to simply guess between the two. If we closely examine the two, however, we must ask why he would fear wound disruption. It is probably the same reason why he will not cough and deep breathe: inadequate teaching. Choice 3 is best answer, because you know that lack of knowledge is one of the main causes of nonperformance. 2, I. Surgical Intervention.

3. Planning

Which of the following is an appropriate goal for a primigravida on her first postpartum day? Mother will be able to:
1. Bathe infant without help
2. Provide complete care of newborn
3. Hold and interact with newborn
4. Feed newborn without assistance

This question asks the nurse to set an achievable goal for a new mother with her first baby. Choices 1, 2, and 4 are probably unrealistic goals for a new mother on the first day after birth. Choice 3 is not only realistic but also the most desirable goal, because mother–infant bonding is one of the most important goals to achieve. 3, IV. Postpartal Care.

4. Implementation

You have difficulty inserting the rectal catheter for an enema. Your best action is to:
1. Wait a few minutes for the lubricant to take effect
2. Tell the client to calm down
3. Wait a few seconds until the sphincter relaxes
4. Chart that you were unable to give the enema

The best answer for this item is choice 3. The nurse knows that temporarily waiting often allows the sphincter to relax. The other answers are not appropriate actions and would do nothing to ease insertion of the catheter. 4, II. Lower GI.

5. Evaluation

Which of the following would indicate successful learning by your client, whom you have been teaching about an 1800 calorie diabetic diet?

(1) Client eats all food on tray
(2) Client states understanding of diet
(3) Client's wife understands dietary restrictions
(4) Client correctly marks menu for 1800 calorie ADA diet

In order to evaluate learning, the nurse must have measurable data. The only answer that provides this is choice 4. Choice 1 does not reflect learning. Choice 2 is not measurable; how do you know that the client understands? Choice 3 is also not measurable and does not address the client directly. 5, II. Diabetes Mellitus.

CATEGORIES OF CLIENT NEEDS

I. Safe, Effective Care Environment

The client at greatest risk for postoperative bleeding would be an arthritic who has been taking:

(1) Aspirin
(2) Maalox
(3) Prednisone
(4) Acetaminophen

This item focuses on client safety and expected outcomes of treatment. In order to answer it, you also need some knowledge of medication side effects. Choice 1 is the answer, because aspirin has an anticoagulant effect on the blood and could predispose to postoperative bleeding. A question like this could be followed by one or two related questions such as "Precautions to take to decrease the risk of bleeding include" or even "In order to prevent the bleeding risk in the above question, the nurse should." Questions often come in a series, so it is important to be sure of your first answer and then follow through along that same line to answer them all correctly. 2, I. Surgical Intervention.

II. Physiological Integrity

Mr. Wilson is admitted with COPD. He tells you that his breathing treatments leave him unable to eat because of all the mucus he brings up. To decrease this anorexia and improve his nutritional intake, the nurse should:

(1) Schedule the treatments for right after meals
(2) Administer frequent mouth care, especially before meals
(3) Request a change to a liquid diet
(4) Ask the physician to start hyperalimentation

This item focuses on a physiological need for adequate nutrition and an expected result of treatment. Choice 1 makes no sense, because it is likely to increase vomiting. Choices 3 and 4 take away the normal diet, an important part of preventing debilitation in the chronically ill client. Only choice 2 would be appropriate. This also offers an example of an instance in which the test-taker often wants another answer: choice 5, "Schedule the treatments between meals." It can be frustrating when the answer you want is not there. Forget it and go with the best answer available. You are not allowed to write in your choice! 4, II. COPD.

III. Psychosocial Integrity

Mary had a very bad day at work and is very angry with her supervisor. When she comes home from work, she punishes her daughter by grounding her for a week for not taking out the trash. This is an example of what defense mechanism?

(1) Projection
(2) Denial
(3) Displacement
(4) Sublimation

This is a fairly simple comprehension level question. You should be able to recognize the description of choice 3, displacement. The items from this section test your knowledge of mental health concepts. There are fewer of these questions on the examination than in any other category. The other responses are other defense mechanisms. 2, III. Defense Mechanisms.

IV. Health Promotion and Maintenance

Discharge instructions for Mr. Wilson, who has COPD, should NOT include which of the following?

(1) Smoking cessation
(2) Avoidance of temperature extremes
(3) Avoidance of industrial air pollution
(4) Avoidance of humidified air

This item asks for the one thing you would *not* teach Mr. Wilson about health promotion. Using the true–false approach, choices 1 and 3 are easily apparent as being true. Again, if you don't know at this point, guess. Looking at the other two, we know that the COPD client has thick, tenacious sputum, so humidity should help, making choice 4 the false answer, which is the correct answer in this case. Do not make the mistake of reading too fast and missing the "avoidance." 4, IV. COPD.

COMMON TEST-TAKING MISTAKES

There are some other common mistakes that test-takers often make. Have you ever found yourself changing answers a lot? Many people continue to re-hash a question in their minds and convince themselves that there is a hidden meaning or some trick. **STOP.** There are no trick questions on this examination, and the items have been examined closely to make sure that there are no hidden meanings. They are straightforward questions, so do not try to second-guess anyone.

It is rarely correct to change an answer. Your odds of changing it to a correct response are very low, your first instinct usually being correct. Change an answer *only* if you have truly seen some missed information or suddenly remembered an important fact. Once you have answered a question and verified that the answer is your chosen one, you will not be allowed to come back to that question. You are also not allowed to skip questions, but do not let this bother you; simply give it your best guess and go on. Do not let yourself become upset. Stop, take a deep breath, and simply go to the next item.

This brings us to another important area, your state of mind. Many people have what is called "test anxiety." This means that the simple thought of the test makes you tense and you are liable to freeze up or become very nervous during the test. If this happens to you, there are a number of things you can do ahead of time to prepare. First, practice some sort of relaxation exercises, just like the ones you teach mothers to use for delivery. Practice those slow deep breaths and imagine yourself blowing away all your tension. If you become comfortable with this technique before the test, it can be very useful during the test.

People also tend to experience anger and frustration over certain test items, a feeling guaranteed to break your concentration. If you find this happening to you because you think an item is dumb or unlikely to happen, laugh at it, do not get angry. Put all that emotion away until after the test. This also happens when the response you want just is not listed. You get angry and frustrated. Stop; your only choices are those listed there, so choose the best one.

Should you guess? Yes, but make those guesses educated ones. What does that mean? It means that you should first try to decrease the number of possible responses. With four responses, you have a 1 in 4 or 25% chance; with three responses, a 1 in 3 or 33% chance; with two responses, you have a 50% chance of guessing correctly. Even on very difficult items, taking a little time to eliminate even one answer improves your odds. Do not just wild guess recklessly. This can decrease your confidence. When you reach

that dilemma—is it choice 1 or 3?—then just guess and go on. Do not spend time going back and forth between the two. Simply choose one, go on, and forget it!

Another tension breaker is *not* studying the night before the examination. It is a terrible temptation to do so, but it will not help. It will only serve to increase your anxiety. Keep imagining yourself having successfully completed the test and on being a successful registered nurse.

Another way to decrease your tension and anxiety is to plan for comfort. Be on time! One of the worst things you can do is arrive late and risk not even being allowed to sit for the examination, or rushing in at the last minute so that your concentration is off. If the site is far away and you anticipate traffic, stay at a place closer to the site or leave with plenty of time and a plan of alternate routes. Eat a good meal before the exam; 5 hours of testing is a long time. Bring some hard candy for during the test. Carry extra tissues and anything else you might need to ensure your comfort so that all your concentration can be on the test.

Will these tips improve your test-taking skills? They should. Combined with a proper planned review, they should help you do better on the licensure examination and help you to achieve your goal—licensure as a registered nurse.

HINTS FOR REPEAT TEST-TAKERS

What if this is not the first time you have taken the test? You can still benefit from this review text. You received a report from the testing company reporting simple FAIL. The sheet along with it identified your weaknesses according to the categories listed earlier. You can use this as a guide to help you study.

The best way to study, however, is to simply use the pre- and post-tests provided in this text and review whatever areas are indicated. Work on your reading and comprehension. Graduates often report that they had difficulty with the reading level on the test. If this was your problem, a reading comprehension course may be of benefit.

If you did not pass the test the first time, do not give up on yourself. You can take the examination any time after you receive your report and reapply. You are not a failure; you have simply failed one examination. You have another chance, and it is up to you to make the most of it. See if your school provides any support or if there are other persons where you work who also did not pass. Often you can form study groups or just provide support for each other. The important thing is to prepare this time and to be successful.

Practice Test Pre-Test

1. Mr. Joseph is experiencing paresthesia in his right arm following a car accident. Which of the following is the most appropriate way for the nurse to assess the progress of his condition?
   1. Test for proprioception
   2. Test for discrimination sense
   3. Test for touch and pain sensation
   4. Test for extinction

2. Mr. Francis is experiencing clumsiness and has fallen three times during the past week. He reports that his right leg feels "weak." Which of the following assessments of his motor system is most appropriate?
   1. Tests for cerebellar function
   2. Tests for brain stem lesions
   3. Dermatome identification of the legs
   4. Tests for cutaneous reflexes

Ann Grant is a 50-year-old woman who is seen by the doctor for the possibility of breast cancer.

---

3. Which of the following is a risk factor for breast cancer?
   1. Jewish women of European descent
   2. Multiparity
   3. Japanese women in Japan
   4. Early artificial menopause

4. Which of the following is a low-risk factor for breast cancer?
   1. Family history of breast cancer
   2. First child before age 25
   3. No children
   4. Early menarche, late menopause

5. Which of the following are clinical manifestations of breast cancer Mrs. Grant might have noticed?
   1. Mobile, encapsulated lump
   2. Elevation of the nipple
   3. Painful regular lump
   4. Absence of nipple discharge

6. A mammogram is a screening test for breast cancer. Which of the following is the American Cancer Society's recommendation for mammography?
   1. Women under age 50 should have one every 5 years
   2. Women over age 60 should have them yearly
   3. All women should have a baseline study around age 40
   4. They should be done only as recommended by the woman's physician

7. Mrs. Grant had a breast biopsy that was positive for cancer. She is scheduled for a modified radical mastectomy tomorrow morning. Which of the following is a priority goal of preoperative teaching for Mrs. Grant?
   1. Client will be prepared for a skin graft

② Client will understand range-of-motion exercises

③ Client will express her sense of loss

④ Client will understand the symptoms of menopause

Mrs. Grant has a modified radical mastectomy. She returns from surgery with a Hemovac in place.

---

8. Which of the following would be appropriate nursing care for the client with a Hemovac?
   ① Irrigate the tubing needed
   ② Avoid emptying the Hemovac
   ③ Prevent kinks in the tubing
   ④ Pin the Hemovac to the back of her gown

9. In order to decrease the postoperative lymphedema of the affected arm, which of the following should Mrs. Grant perform?
   ① Elevate her arm on pillows above heart level
   ② Keep the arm fixed over the surgical site
   ③ Apply a warm pad over the affected arm
   ④ Use only the unaffected arm for all activities

10. On the first postoperative day, the nurse recommends that Mrs. Grant begin arm exercises. Which of the following is the best exercise for Mrs. Grant at this time?
   ① Abducting the affected arm and flexing the elbow
   ② "Wall walking" exercises every 4 hours
   ③ Using a rope pulley to extend her shoulder
   ④ Washing her face with the affected arm

11. Which of the following is a realistic goal for Mrs. Grant 3 days after surgery?
   ① Client will be able to use affected arm in normal manner
   ② Client will be able to tolerate full liquid diet
   ③ Client will be able to perform care of own Hemovac
   ④ Client will cope effectively with loss of breast

Mrs. Grant seems depressed about her loss at times and happy about the positive outcome of her surgery at other times.

---

12. The nurse realizes that this behavior on the part of Mrs. Grant indicates which of the following?
   ① Mrs. Grant is neurotic and should see the social worker
   ② Clients often require a great deal of time adjusting to this loss
   ③ Mrs. Grant is simply vain and needs time to adjust
   ④ Clients often need some time alone after a loss such as this

13. Mrs. Grant asks if she still has to do a monthly breast self-examinations. Which of the following would be the best response by the nurse?
   ① "Yes, the cancer is likely to spread to the other breast."
   ② "No, there is no further risk of breast cancer."
   ③ "No, the doctor will do it every 3 months."
   ④ "Yes, there is an increased risk of a new cancer in the other breast."

Mr. Hilliard has COPD after a history of smoking three packs of cigarettes per day for 20 years. His arterial blood gas results are a PaO_2 of 85, a $PaCO_2$ of 40, and an HCO_3 of 24.

---

14. Which of the following should be initiated by the nurse?
   ① Administer oxygen at 2 L as ordered
   ② Provide for assisted ventilation
   ③ Administer $NaHCO_3$ as ordered
   ④ No action is needed; this is normal

15. Mr. Hilliard finds that after smoking or exercise he experiences difficulty breathing, headaches, and nausea. The nurse recognizes that these are clinical manifestations of which of the following?
   ① Hypoxia
   ② Hypercapnia
   ③ Hypocapnia
   ④ Hyperventilation

16. Mr. Hilliard's mobility is limited because he experiences dyspnea with minimal exertion. Which of the following pulmonary function findings should the nurse expect to observe?
   ① Decreased vital capacity
   ② Normal expiratory time
   ③ Normal forced expiratory volume
   ④ Decreased residual volume

17. Mr. Hilliard is started on a course of corticosteroids. Which of the following nursing assessments is most important in connection with this therapy?
    1. The need for more oxygen therapy
    2. The need for improved nutrition
    3. Whether he is still smoking
    4. Any indications of infection

18. Which of the following techniques should the nurse teach Mr. Hilliard to encourage proper breathing exercises?
    1. High chest breathing
    2. Inhalation should be two to three times longer than exhalation
    3. Pursed lip-breathing
    4. Inhalation through the mouth and exhalation through the nose

19. In which of the following positions should the nurse place Mr. Hilliard to perform percussion and postural drainage to the apical segments of his lungs?
    1. Sitting
    2. Trendelenburg
    3. Side-lying
    4. Prone

20. Which of the following nursing interventions will help prevent the complication of hypoxia during deep tracheal suctioning of Mr. Hilliard?
    1. Suction once per hour
    2. Use sterile technique
    3. Hyperventilate the lungs before suctioning
    4. Use 100% oxygen that has been humidified

21. Which of the following would be an appropriate goal for Mr. Hilliard?
    1. Client will maintain $PaCO_2$ of less than 50 mm Hg
    2. Client will have a PaO_2 above 90 mm Hg
    3. Client will have an O_2 saturation of greater than 95%
    4. Client will have an HCO_3 of less than 23

22. Mr. Freed has thick, tenacious tracheal secretions that he has difficulty bringing up through his tracheostomy. Which of the following nursing measures will aid in liquefying these secretions prior to suctioning?
    1. Hyperventilate the lungs with oxygen before suctioning
    2. Instill normal saline directly into the trachea
    3. Encourage him to cough and deep breathe more often
    4. Use postural drainage to mobilize the secretions

Mr. John Bass, age 58, has a lengthy history of cigarette smoking. He has been coughing up blood. He is undergoing a diagnostic work-up. The CEA (carcinoembryonic antigen) level is low.

23. Mr. Bass tells the nurse that he is relieved that he does not have lung cancer. Which of the following would be the most appropriate response for the nurse to make?
    1. "It must be very reassuring to know you don't have cancer."
    2. "You must remember that you are in a high-risk category and bleeding is a warning."
    3. "Let's talk about what the CEA level means."
    4. "Would you like to think about stopping smoking?"

24. If Mr. Bass is diagnosed with lung cancer, the nurse determines that an appropriate nursing diagnosis is high risk for ineffective airway clearance due to obstructing tumor. Which of the following is the most appropriate goal?
    1. Client will not suffer pain when coughing
    2. Client will not develop impaired gas exchange
    3. Client will be able to ambulate without any evidence of dyspnea
    4. Client will cough effectively by splinting his chest

Nick Barker, 55 years old, had a lobectomy yesterday for lung cancer. He has chest tubes in place and is complaining of pain.

25. When observing the chest tube drainage system, the nurse notes a slight up-and-down movement of the fluid in the water-seal chamber. Based on this observation, which is the most appropriate nursing intervention?
    1. Milk the chest tube
    2. Reposition Mr. Barker
    3. Continue to monitor the system
    4. Notify the physician immediately

26. Intermittent bubbling is noted in the water-seal chamber. Which of the following is the most appropriate nursing intervention for this?
    1. Clamp the chest tube and notify the physician
    2. Encourage Mr. Barker to continue deep breathing

③ Change the drainage unit

④ Check the tubes closely for an air leak

27. The physician decides to increase the suction for Mr. Barker from 15 to 20 cm of water. In order to accomplish this, the nurse should:

① Add water to the suction-control chamber

② Increase the setting on the wall suction

③ Lower the chest drainage unit

④ Remove water from the suction control chamber

28. Mr. Barker is having the chest tube removed. Which of the following is most appropriate nursing intervention before this procedure?

① Assist the client into a prone position

② Administer pain medications one half hour prior to the removal

③ Encourage him to deep breathe while the tubes are removed

④ Empty the collection chambers completely before removal

29. Mr. Jason, a 40-year-old sedentary executive, has a positive family history of heart disease. He asks the nurse about lifestyle changes that will prevent a heart attack. The nurse should counsel him that:

① Relaxation techniques are the best means of prevention

② A low-sodium, low-cholesterol diet will dramatically lower his risk

③ Sex, age, and family history are nonmodifiable risk factors

④ If he stops alcohol and nicotine consumption, he will prevent a heart attack

30. Ms. Hays, 69 years old, has had a cardiac catheterization procedure. After the examination, the nurse must carefully monitor the catheter site for:

① Hematoma formation

② Local reaction to the dye

③ Circulatory collapse

④ Heparin effects

David Jacobs, age 76, has a long history of congestive heart failure. He is admitted to the intensive care unit with severe dyspnea, orthopnea, fear, wheezing, sweating, bubbling respirations, and cyanosis.

---

31. The nurse knows that Mr. Jacobs' symptoms probably indicate the development of:

① Chronic congestive heart failure

② Acute pulmonary edema

③ Acute myocardial infarction

④ Chronic bronchitis

32. Rotating tourniquets are ordered for Mr. Jacobs. Which of the following goals describes the purpose of this intervention?

① To strengthen the myocardial beat

② To decrease venous pooling in the extremities

③ To slow venous return to the right ventricle

④ To prevent cardiac arrhythmias

33. Which of the following clinical manifestations should the nurse assess to determine if the rotating tourniquets have been applied with enough force?

① Presence of a peripheral pulse on the uncuffed extremity

② Presence of a pulse proximal to each tourniquet

③ No blanching of nail beds of each extremity

④ Presence of a peripheral pulse distal to each tourniquet

34. Cardiac compensation occurs as a part of the sequela of congestive heart failure. Which of the following are considered to be cardiac compensatory mechanisms?

① Ventricular dilation, ventricular hypertrophy, and tachycardia

② Hepatomegaly, splenomegaly, and right ventricular hypertrophy

③ Headache, drowsiness, and confusion

④ Bradycardia, restlessness, and hyperventilation

35. Martin Smith, 73 years old, has just returned from the operating room, where he had a permanent pacemaker inserted. The primary nurse must assess for possible postoperative complications. Which of the following assessments would lead the nurse to notify the physicians immediately?

① The site around his incision is slightly reddened

② His pulse rate has increased from a preoperative rate of 45 to a postoperative rate of 65

③ He experiences a slight temperature elevation, 99.5° F, 24 hours postoperatively

④ He complains of not being able to stop his hiccoughs

36. Which of the following clients is at the highest risk for the development of coronary heart disease?

① An African-American man, age 37

② A Caucasian man, age 45

③ An African-American woman, age 45

④ A Caucasian woman, age 37

Mr. Carter, 56 years old, is admitted to the hospital with a diagnosis of stable angina.

37. Which of the following statements made by Mr. Carter to the nurse would indicate the need for further teaching about his condition?
    ① "My chest pain can occur again if I overexert myself."
    ② "If I rest, the chest pain should lessen."
    ③ "I need to try to be less emotional about things."
    ④ "Each time I have chest pain my heart is damaged."

38. The nurse instructs Mr. Carter in the proper administration of nitroglycerin (NTG). Which of the following would NOT be included in the teaching plan?
    ① When the angina begins, place one tablet under your tongue and allow it to dissolve
    ② Always carry fresh NTG tablets in an air-tight, light-resistant bottle, because their potency is lost after 6 months
    ③ Repeat the dosage every 5 to 10 minutes times 3 or until the pain is relieved; if the pain is not relieved, notify the physician
    ④ NTG becomes less effective over time, so it should be used sparingly, only if absolutely needed

39. The nurse is helping Mr. Carter fill out his menu. Which of the following breakfast choices, if selected by Mr. Carter, would indicate that he understands his dietary prescription?
    ① Bran flakes with skim milk, apple slices, orange juice
    ② Scrambled eggs, whole wheat toast, prune juice
    ③ Oatmeal with cream, stewed prunes, hot tea
    ④ French toast with syrup, grapefruit half, skim milk

Ms. Amis, 55 years old, is diagnosed with moderate hypertension. Her current treatment includes chlorothiazide (Diuril) and methyldopa (Aldomet), a diet low in salt, cholesterol, calories, and saturated fat, and an exercise regimen.

40. Which of the following statements by Ms. Amis indicates the need for further diet teaching?
    ① "I can eat frozen fruit and vegetables."
    ② "I'll buy water-packed, canned tuna."
    ③ "I'll stop putting catsup on my meat."
    ④ "I'm going to eat more Chinese foods."

41. The doctor recommends that Ms. Amis increase her dietary calcium. Which of the following food choices is NOT high in calcium?
    ① Lentil soup
    ② Citrus fruit salad
    ③ Baked squash
    ④ Sardine sandwich

42. Ms. Amis asks if she can take her own blood pressure at home. Which of the following would be the most appropriate response for the nurse to give?
    ① "Taking blood pressure at home is difficult to do."
    ② "Generally, this is not suggested."
    ③ "Let's discuss this. It is a good idea."
    ④ "You will need someone at home to take it for you."

Mrs. Mason, 70 years old, has a long history of diabetes and peripheral vascular disease. She is admitted for a below-the-knee amputation as a result of gangrene of the right foot.

43. Which of the following emotional responses on the part of Mrs. Mason should the nurse expect in the preoperative period?
    ① Relief that the procedure will remove the infection
    ② Grief over the anticipated loss of her limb
    ③ Anger at the health care team for taking away her leg
    ④ Fear that she will lose the other leg later

44. Which of the following nursing interventions would best meet Mrs. Mason's mobility needs after a below-the-knee amputation?
    ① Assisting Mrs. Mason to stay out of bed as long as possible
    ② Elevating the residual right limb on a pillow continuously
    ③ Teaching her to lift 5-pound weights with her arms
    ④ Providing passive range-of-motion exercises to the unaffected leg

45. Mrs. Mason is participating in stump wrapping, because she has a goal of complete

independence in all activities of daily living. The nurse should inform her that the goal of this activity is to:

1. Provide range of motion for the upper extremities as well as the residual limb
2. Keep the residual limb clean and dry
3. Improve the muscle tone in the residual limb
4. Shape the stump for the prosthesis

46. The nurse recognizes that meeting Mrs. Mason's safety needs is important to her long-term rehabilitation. Which of the following nursing interventions best meets these needs?
1. Encourage her always to use her walker to ambulate
2. Provide her with a wheelchair
3. Assist her with ambulation standing by her affected side
4. Encourage her to avoid walking at all until her prosthesis is fitted

47. Which of the following conditions would NOT be a contraindication to fitting Mrs. Mason with a prosthesis?
1. Her current age
2. Peripheral neuropathy
3. COPD and chronic CHF
4. Lack of cooperation

48. Which of the following clients would probably NOT be a candidate for intermittent catheterization?
1. A 15 year old who cannot understand sterile technique
2. A 26 year old quadriplegic
3. A woman with an active sex life
4. A man who refuses to follow any schedule

Ms. Green, 68 years old, has a recurrent urinary tract infections. An acid-ash diet is prescribed.

---

49. Which of the following foods should the nurse advise Ms. Green to eliminate from her diet?
1. Carbonated beverages
2. Dairy products
3. Eggs
4. Whole grains

50. Ms. Green is successful in acidification of her urine. This change in pH should prompt the nurse to consult with the physician regarding an adjustment in the administration of:
1. Aminoglycosides

2. Methoxamine hippurate
3. Mandelate
4. All antibiotics

51. Which of the following findings during the nurse's assessment would suggest that a client has developed end-stage renal failure?
1. Sudden decrease in serum creatinine and proportional rise in the BUN
2. Slow decrease in glomerular filtration rate as measured by creatinine clearance
3. Stable or slowly rising creatinine clearance with anemia and bone disease
4. Rapidly decreasing serum creatinine with anemia; small, contracted kidneys; and bone disease

52. Mrs. Wilkes, 55 years old, is scheduled for her first hemodialysis treatment this morning. The nurse plans to withhold her breakfast and her morning doses of methyldopa (Aldomet) and hydralazine (Apresoline). What is the primary reason for withholding these medications?
1. To prevent nausea and vomiting because she did not eat breakfast
2. To prevent an unpredictable dosage, because the medications will be dialyzed off during the treatment
3. Ultrafiltration during dialysis will act as a substitute for the medications
4. The medications could cause severe hypotension during dialysis

53. Mr. Foster, 60 years old, is on a regular diet during his hospitalization for severe alcoholic cirrhosis. The nurse observes that he appears to become drowsy after each meal. Which of the following nursing interventions is most appropriate?
1. Administer stimulants as ordered
2. Assess him for signs of asterixis
3. Order stat blood work
4. Administer sedatives at night to let him sleep more

54. Which of the following is usually the first clinical manifestation of tumors of the head of the pancreas that the nurse might assess?
1. Jaundice
2. Gas and belching
3. Severe weight loss
4. High fevers

55. Which of the following complications of myxedema might the nurse assess in a client with severe hypothyroidism?
1. Coronary heart disease
2. Altered liver function
3. Hyperglycemia
4. Hypertension

56. Mrs. Collier, 27 years old, is pregnant for the first time. She asks the nurse what effect her diet will have on her baby. The nurse should explain to her that:
    ① Poor nutrition is associated with low–birth-weight infants
    ② Infant obesity is related to excess dietary intake during pregnancy
    ③ Brain growth will be severely retarded unless the mother's diet meets the minimum daily requirements
    ④ Excessive eating will adversely affect fetal growth

57. A new mother tells the nurse that she read that she should not feed her infant large amounts of starch because the infant will develop diarrhea. She asks why this is the case. The nurse explains that starch causes diarrhea in infants under 4 months old because:
    ① Glycogen storage is decreased in the liver and muscle
    ② Essential amino acids are absent
    ③ Water imbalances occur
    ④ Intestinal amylase is present in reduced amounts

58. Nutritional counseling is necessary for the family of which of the following children?
    ① Sam, whose family incorporates cultural food preferences into the diet.
    ② Aimee, whose weight is above the 75th percentile for her age group
    ③ Ben, whose growth occurs in spurts, rather than on a continuum
    ④ Mike, whose height is below the 10th percentile for his age group

59. The nurse is conducting a nutritional assessment on Tad, age 7, with his mother. Based on the data, the nurse determines that Tad is experiencing an alteration in nutrition: less than body requirements related to decreased appetite. Which of the following goals should the nurse recommend to Tad's mother?
    ① Tad will eat dessert first to ensure adequate calorie intake
    ② Tad's mother will not purchase "junk food" and sweets for snacks
    ③ Tad's mother will control portion sizes and insist that he finish all his meal
    ④ Tad will eat desired foods first and least desired foods last

60. Mrs. Marder calls the clinic because her 1 month old child has been running a fever of 102°F for the last 24 hours. She asks the nurse what she should do about this. The nurse should tell Mrs. Marder to:
    ① Give the baby a tepid sponge bath to reduce the fever
    ② Give the baby acetaminophen infant drops every 4 hours based on the infant's weight
    ③ Bring the baby into the clinic today to be seen by the physician
    ④ Increase the baby's fluid intake and watch the baby for another 24 hours

61. When a muscle relaxant or narcotic has been administered to a child as part of an anesthetic, for which of the following manifestations should the recovery room nurse particularly be alert?
    ① Shock
    ② Postintubation croup
    ③ Delirium
    ④ Respiratory depression

62. Which of the following is the first thing the nurse should do when a young child returns to the pediatric unit following a surgical procedure?
    ① Review the postoperative orders with the recovery room nurse just outside the child's door
    ② Administer pain medication before transferring the child to the bed
    ③ Complete a general assessment of the child's condition
    ④ Increase the rate of the IV to promote the child's urination

63. Which of the following age-related differences causes delayed absorption of orally administered drugs in neonates and young infants?
    ① Highly acidic gastric pH
    ② Immature blood flow to muscles and peripheral tissues
    ③ Larger portion of body water
    ④ Reduced gastric motility and irregular peristalsis

64. The recommended dose of a drug is 60 to 90 mg per Kg daily in five to six divided doses. The nurse has an order to administer 120 mg of the drug every 4 hours to a child who weighs 10 Kg. The nurse's most appropriate action should be to:
    ① Look at the drug container to determine how many mg are contained in each mL.
    ② Check whether the dose exceeds the maximum allowed in 24 hours
    ③ Locate the correct drug in the correct preparation
    ④ Perform the necessary calculations to obtain the amount desired in equivalent mL dosage

65. To facilitate the administration of oral

medication to a preschool-age child, the nurse should:

1. Dilute the medication in a favorite liquid and allow the child to hold the cup
2. Mix the medication in a small amount of ice cream and make sure the child swallows all of the medication
3. Explain the purpose of the medication and allow the child time to express resistance before giving the medication
4. Set limits about the need to take medication and offer praise immediately after the task is accomplished

66. Rachel, age 8, has an infection in her external ear canal. When teaching Rachel and her mother how to administer ear drops, the nurse should:
    1. Demonstrate for the mother how to pull the pinna of Rachel's ear up and back while instilling the ear drops
    2. Instruct them to keep the medication in the refrigerator until just before administration
    3. Explain to Rachel that she should remain seated with her head tilted back for several minutes after instillation
    4. Show the mother how to place and secure a cotton ball into Rachel's ear canal using nonallergenic tape after instillation

67. Cerebral palsy is a disorder in which individuals have difficulty with voluntary muscle control. Which of the following would be a realistic goal for the child with cerebral palsy?
    1. The child will have normal intelligence
    2. The child's brain damage will not progress
    3. The child will be able to function independently
    4. The child's muscle coordination will improve with age

Marge, 16 years old, is pregnant. The nurse sees her in the prenatal clinic for the first time when she is 7 months pregnant.

---

68. Research has shown that, in comparison to children of older mothers, the offspring of adolescent mothers experience:
    1. Poorer self-esteem
    2. More academic difficulties
    3. Fewer physical problems during childhood
    4. Greater opportunities for mother–child interactions

69. Each time Marge comes into the clinic after the first visit, she only talks about herself, not about her unborn child. As a result of this behavior, the nurse recognizes that:
    1. Marge's use of denial is very strong
    2. This is a normal response because adolescents are egocentric
    3. Marge probably wishes that she had gotten an abortion
    4. Marge should be referred for counseling

70. Personal fable is a normal component of adolescent thinking. Which statement made by Marge illustrates this developmental factor in relation to adolescent pregnancy?
    1. "Everyone says you should douche after intercourse so you don't get pregnant."
    2. "I didn't want to get pregnant, so it couldn't happen to me."
    3. "But he said he loved me."
    4. "All of my friends are having intercourse, so why shouldn't I?"

71. Which response by the nurse is most appropriate when Marge asks whether she should keep her baby after delivery?
    1. "What do your parents and friends think you should do?"
    2. "It's going to be hard for you to go out with your friends with a new baby to care for."
    3. "Let's consider what this new baby will mean to you in terms of time and energy."
    4. "If I were you and I had my whole life ahead, I would try to have the baby adopted."

72. Primary prevention strategies associated with adolescent pregnancy focus on:
    1. Identifying available support systems for pregnant adolescents
    2. Assessing the risk status of a pregnant adolescent
    3. Advising pregnant adolescents on how to tell their parents about their pregnancy
    4. Providing adolescents with information about birth control clinics

73. The school health nurse incorporates the concept of secondary prevention into practice with teenagers by:
    1. Setting up a birth control clinic in the school health office
    2. Attending health curriculum meetings to ensure that contraceptive information is included in a unit on sexuality
    3. Teaching a group of parents about the problems of adolescent pregnancy
    4. Referring a pregnant adolescent for prenatal care

74. The nurse who assists Marge to learn about safe infant care is applying theoretical concepts of:
   ① Primary prevention
   ② Psychosocial intervention
   ③ Tertiary prevention
   ④ Developmental intervention

75. At 1 minute of age, the nurse suctions the nares of a neonate and notes cyanosis and respiratory distress during the procedure. The neonate's symptoms are most likely related to:
   ① Laryngomalacia
   ② Tracheoesophageal fistula
   ③ Choanal atresia
   ④ Bronchopulmonary dysplasia

76. The nurse knows that which of the following is a clinical manifestation of otitis media with effusion?
   ① Acute onset of pain
   ② Fever
   ③ Diminished hearing
   ④ Purulent ear drainage

77. The nursing care plan for a child who has acute otitis media should include goals for:
   ① Teaching parents how to administer ear drops
   ② Promoting compliance with antibiotic therapy
   ③ Preparing the child for myringotomy and insertion of a tympanostomy tube
   ④ Assessing parents to identify and eliminate environmental allergens

---

Joan, 11 years old, is admitted to the hospital for the treatment of an acute asthma attack.

---

78. When assessing Joan's respiratory status, the nurse should expect to note which of the following data?
   ① Accessory muscles of respiration in use as a factor contributing to inspiratory stridor
   ② Mild inspiratory stridor with audible wheezing on inspiration
   ③ Intercostal retractions on inspiration and expiratory wheezing
   ④ Rapid, shallow respiration markedly increased in rate, and a hoarse cough

79. Joan's father expresses concern about his daughter's asthma. In counseling her father about the disease, which of the following statements by the nurse is most appropriate?
   ① "Joan's illness is chronic and requires

that she be limited to quiet play activity."
   ② "Joan will outgrow her asthma; therefore, you do not have to worry about her future."
   ③ "Joan is likely to develop chronic obstructive pulmonary disease as she gets older."
   ④ "Joan's asthma can be controlled and she can participate in usual childhood activities."

80. Which clinical manifestations would alert the nurse that Joan is about to have an asthma attack?
   ① Prolonged expiration with wheezing
   ② Nasal flaring
   ③ Paroxysmal night-time cough with wheezing
   ④ Pallor and restlessness

81. Joan is receiving intravenous aminophylline to relieve bronchospasms. The nurse must observe for which of the following manifestations indicating toxicity?
   ① Tachycardia, agitation, vomiting
   ② Bradycardia, fatigue, increased blood pressure
   ③ Tachypnea, drowsiness, increased pulse
   ④ Fluid retention, ataxia, decreased blood pressure

82. The nurse's plan of care to meet body-image/self-concept needs in the adolescent with cystic fibrosis should include strategies for:
   ① Attractive hair styling, hats, or wigs that mask areas of alopecia
   ② Clothing selections that compensate for the protuberant abdomen and emaciated extremities
   ③ Discreet use of facial make-up to brighten pallor and mask acne
   ④ Activity/exercise routine that incorporates aerobics and long-distance running

83. A complete blood count is ordered for a child with cyanotic heart disease. The results are elevated hemoglobin and hematocrit levels. Which of the following statements reflects the correct interpretation of this information?
   ① The child is not anemic, because the hemoglobin and hematocrit are elevated.
   ② The body is compensating for tissue hypoxia by increasing red blood cell production.
   ③ The child is severely dehydrated and the loss of vascular fluid has elevated the hematocrit.
   ④ The child is hyperoxic due to the increased oxygen-carrying capacity of the blood.

Jenny, 2 years old, is to undergo a cardiac catheterization tomorrow morning.

84. Which of the following objective assessment data noted in the immediate post-cardiac catheterization period are indicative of serious complications in Jenny?
    1. Transient temperature elevations, apnea
    2. Apnea, dyspnea, asymmetrical motion of extremities
    3. Tachycardia, transient temperature elevations
    4. Bleeding from the catheterization site, hypertension

85. Which of the following instructions should the nurse include when advising Jenny's parents about home care following her cardiac catheterization?
    1. Give a liquid diet every 3 to 4 hours for 24 hours at home
    2. Maintain a dry, clean dressing over the catheterization site for 1 to 2 days
    3. Report slight discoloration at the catheter site to the physician
    4. Give only sponge baths for the first 24 hours at home

86. Which of the following is an appropriate goal for Mr. Johnson, 66 years old, who suffers from dysarthria following a stroke?
    1. Client will be able to use a picture board to communicate
    2. Client will be able to feed self
    3. Client will not develop sensory deprivation secondary to aphasia
    4. Client will regain speech with the help of speech therapy

87. Which of the following home instructions for the parents of a child taking digoxin is most correct?
    1. Mix the medication with a small amount of formula or food to ease the acceptance by the child
    2. If vomiting occurs a short time after the medication has been given, repeat the dose immediately
    3. If a dose is forgotten for more than 6 hours, give an extra dose of the medication
    4. If the child experiences nausea, vomiting, listlessness, or anorexia, notify the physician

88. Which of the following clinical manifestations should the nurse expect to see in an infant with pyloric stenosis?
    1. Choking and coughing with feeding
    2. Abdominal distention
    3. Projectile vomiting after feeding
    4. Hematemesis

89. Mari, 2 years old, has hepatitis and is being cared for at home. Assuming she likes all the following foods, which would be the best breakfast for her?
    1. Sausage, egg, whole milk
    2. Sugared cereal, banana, orange juice
    3. Pancakes, syrup, grape juice
    4. Scrambled eggs, toast, low-fat milk

90. Adam Prince, 27 years old, is hospitalized with an acute illness. Although he is normally well adjusted, he now seems dependent and demanding. This is probably an example of:
    1. Denial
    2. Dissociation
    3. Compensation
    4. Regression

91. Which of the following is the most realistic goal for a client with an acute exacerbation of Crohn's disease?
    1. Client will have no more than one bowel movement per day
    2. Client will less than four diarrheal stools per day
    3. Client will have no diarrheal stools
    4. Client will not develop constipation

92. Which of the following clients would benefit most from group therapy?
    1. Ms. Jones, who has a schizophrenic psychosis
    2. Mr. King, with an antisocial personality
    3. Ms. Will, with bipolar mania
    4. Mr. Vane, with active hallucinations

93. Which of the following is a common but manageable side effect of the anxiolytics?
    1. Nonintentional tremors
    2. Increased pigmentation
    3. Nonobstructive jaundice
    4. Ptosis

PRACTICE TEST PRE-TEST Answers and Rationales

Including Test-Taking Strategies

Legend: 1 to 5: Steps of the Nursing Process
           I to IV: Areas of Human Functioning

1. **This question asks for the most appropriate response. This means that more than one answer may be correct, but you are being asked to make a judgment as to which is most appropriate.**

1. ③ Paresthesia is a distortion of sensory stimuli, so testing for touch and pain are the best way to detect changes in the client's status. Proprioception is position sense, and discrimination and extinction are part of touch. 1, II. Neurological Examination.

2. **Again, this question asks for the most appropriate answer. Always look for the most complete answer.**

2. ① Tests for cerebellar function will give the most data, including information on muscle function, coordination, and balance. The brain stem is not involved in this case, and the other tests are not as complete. 1, II. Neurological Examination.

3. **Risk factor identification is an important concept in the NCLEX format. You will often be asked questions about who is most likely to develop or who should you screen first. These are all based on the graduate's ability to identify those at highest risk for a given condition.**

3. ① Jewish women of European descent are at higher risk for breast cancer. The other options are all low risk for breast cancer. 2, I. Breast Cancer.

4. **This question asks the opposite of the above question: who is at the lowest risk. This question will contain three high-risk factors and one low-risk factor. You need to find the one low-risk factor to correctly identify the answer.**

4. ② A low-risk factor is young age at the time of her first child. The other options are all high-risk factors for breast cancer. 2, I. Breast Cancer.

5. ② A common symptom of breast cancer is elevation of the nipple, because the lump is usually fixed to adjacent tissues. The mobile, encapsulated lump is usually fibrocystic breast disease. Absence of nipple discharge is normal. 1, I. Breast Cancer.

6. **This is a straightforward question. It is simply asking you which of the following is recommended. The other answers would contain some incorrect information.**

6. ③ The American Cancer Society recommends a baseline mammogram between the ages of 35 and 40; for low-risk women, only as needed between 40 and 50, and yearly after the age 50. For high-risk women, it is yearly after age 40. 1, IV. Breast Cancer.

7. **This is another example of a question that may have more than one correct answer, but you are asked to identify the priority goal. Think about breast cancer. You should know that the psychological impact of this disease is great, so the priority answer in this case is the one that reflects her sense of loss. Sometimes a physiological answer might be the priority; you have to decide if the condition has more psychological implications or more physiological ones.**

7. ③ It is very important to allow the client to express her sense of loss and possibly anger. There is no reason for her to have a skin graft or to go through menopause. The arm exercises are important, but not as important as the expression of grief. 3, I. Breast Cancer.

8. **This question has one appropriate action and three inappropriate ones. Think of it as a true–false question with three true answers and one false answer. You need to identify the false answer.**

8. ③ It is important for the Hemovac tubing to be able to drain freely without obstruction. The tubing should not be irrigated and must be emptied regularly. Pinning the Hemovac to the back of her gown could interfere with expansion of the Hemovac. 4, I. Breast Cancer.

9. ① Lymphedema is more likely to occur when the limb is dependent. Keeping it above the level of the heart will help it not to form lymphedema and to drain if it is present. Keeping the arm fixed at the side will only decrease mobility, as will using only the unaffected arm. It is potentially dangerous to apply heat to the arm. 4, I. Breast Cancer.

---

10. To answer a question of this type, you need to understand the precautions postmastectomy. It is important that the woman not abduct the affected arm until the sutures come out. At the same time, she should use that arm. You have to look at the answers and see which one accomplishes this.

---

10. ④ Washing her face will allow movement from the elbow down without moving it at the axilla. The other options require movement of the axilla, exercises which require a doctor's order, and are not done until more healing has occurred. 1 & 4, I. Breast Cancer.

---

11. This question asks two questions. First, what is a realistic goal, and then what is realistic after only 3 days? Choice 4 will not occur for several months after the surgery, whereas choice 2 would be accomplished by the day of surgery. You must also realize that with early discharge, women must learn to care for their own Hemovacs.

---

11. ③ With early discharge, most women are going home by the second to third postoperative day. The client must learn to care for her own Hemovac, because it is usually in place for 5 to 7 days. It is too early for either choices 1 or 4, and choice 2 should have been accomplished by the day of surgery. 3, I. Breast Cancer.

---

12. This question asks you to identify the reason behind a behavior. Be sure you understand whether this is a normal behavior, and then answer the question based on that.

---

12. ② It is normal to experience a feeling of ambivalence after a mastectomy, a sense of loss and happiness. The grieving process usually takes months to resolve. She does not need to be alone, but needs to know that what she is going through is normal. 2, I. Breast Cancer.

13. ④ It is even more important that the client do breast self-examination after a mastectomy because there is about a 25% risk that she will develop a second primary cancer in the contralateral breast. The cancer does not spread to the opposite breast; it is a second primary. No woman should depend only on the physician for a breast self-examination. 2 & 4, I. Breast Cancer.

---

14. To answer this question, you need to know what normal blood gas levels are. You must then decide what you should do based on your knowledge of these levels.

---

14. ④ These are all normal blood gas values for a client with COPD, so no action is needed. Although the PaO_2 is slightly low, it is well within normal limits for a client with COPD. 2 & 4, I & II. COPD.

---

15. This is a simple factual question. Given a set of clinical manifestations, what is the problem that the client is exhibiting?

---

15. ② Hypercapnia or increased blood carbon dioxide will result from smoking or exercise in this client. The symptoms of hypercapnea are an increased respiratory rate, headache, confusion, lethargy, nausea, and vomiting. 1 & 2, II. COPD.

16. ① In obstructive pulmonary disorders, the vital capacity or amount of air that can be maximally exhaled following maximal inspiration is decreased. There is an increased residual volume. The expiratory time and forced volume are both decreased. 1, I. COPD.

17. This question requires you to understand both the purpose of steroids and their side effects. All options are important assessments, but only one relates to steroid therapy and its side effects.

17. ④ Steroids are immunosuppressants that control some of the symptoms of COPD. These drugs can predispose the client to the development of infections because of the suppression of the immune system. The other options are important assessments; however, they do not address the question. 1, II. COPD/Corticosteroids.

18. This question requires a knowledge of the pathophysiology of COPD and an understanding of ways to correct for this problem.

18. ③ Pursing the lips slows or retards the flow rate of exhaled air; this keeps airways open and prevents alveolar collapse. The other options will not improve ventilation. 4, I. COPD.

19. This situation requires that you know where the apical section of the lung is, plus an understanding of the purpose of postural drainage.

19. ① The sitting position will allow gravity to help drain the apical or upper segments of the lungs. This will aid in the mobilization of secretions from this area. The other positions are more appropriate for other segments of the lungs. 2 & 4, I. Postural Drainage.

20. This answer requires an understanding of the danger of 100% oxygen in clients with COPD, plus a knowledge of how to decrease the hypoxia caused by suctioning.

20. ③ Suctioning always depletes oxygen levels. Hyperventilating the lungs before, during, and after tracheal suctioning will decrease the possibility of hypoxia, anoxia, and arrhythmias. The other options will not prevent hypoxia from occurring or are dangerous for a client with COPD. 4, I. Tracheal Suctioning.

21. This question requires a knowledge of the normal changes in blood gases for clients with COPD. This client has a higher than normal CO_2. It is also important to understand the danger of a high O_2 in these clients.

21. ① A client with COPD runs an elevated CO_2 level as a normal. It is important that the O_2 level remain slightly low, because the respiratory drive in these clients is responsive to hypoxia, not hypercapnia. Choices 2 and 3 would be dangerous for the client. The bicarbonate level is also usually elevated to balance the elevated CO_2. 3, II. COPD.

22. ② Tracheobronchial hydration may be done by parenteral or oral methods, aerosolization, or direct instillation of liquefying agents. Choices 1 and 3 will not help the secretions. Choice 4 would be ineffective if the secretions are thick and tenacious. 2 & 4, I. Lung Cancer.

23. This question asks you first to know the meaning of a specific diagnostic test and then to identify a therapeutic response. Psychosocial answers should always encourage further response on the part of the client.

23. ③ The CEA level is a tumor marker, not a test for the presence or absence of cancer. It is important to assess his understanding of the test, because it cannot be used to rule out lung cancer. You also want to choose a response that encourages the client to discuss, not simply respond. 4 & 5, I. Lung Cancer.

24. In this example, you are given the nursing diagnosis and asked what an appropriate goal would be.

24. ④ Splinting the chest will make him more comfortable; therefore, he will be more likely to cough and deep breathe effectively, preventing an ineffective gas exchange. Choice 1 is actually one reason behind teaching the client to splint the incision. Choices 2 and 3 may be

unrealistic, because the tumor itself may eventually cause a complete obstruction. 3, I. Lung Cancer.

---

25. This is another two-part question. First, the question asks you the meaning of the manifestations given; then, based on that understanding, asks what is the appropriate nursing action. When answering this type of question, think carefully about the given manifestation. It is true that if you don't understand this portion, it will be difficult to answer the question.

---

25. ③ Oscillating movements of the fluid in the water-seal chamber, called tidaling, reflects the client's ventilatory movements when the system is patent and functioning properly. All that is required is continued monitoring. The other choices contain actions that are unnecessary, because this is a normal and expected manifestation. 2 & 4, I. Water-Seal Drainage.

---

26. This is just like item #25. You must know whether this manifestation is normal or not; then, based on that knowledge, give the appropriate action.

---

26. ② Intermittent bubbling in the water-seal bottle is normal as the lung re-expands and air is removed from the pleural cavity. No unusual actions are needed; simply continue having the client deep breathe to aid in lung re-expansion. Clamping the chest tube is done only in an emergency, and choices 3 and 4 are unnecessary. 2 & 4, I. Water-Seal Drainage.

---

27. To answer this question, you must understand the principles of water-seal drainage.

---

27. ① Suction is regulated by pulling atmospheric air through water in the suction-control chamber. It is possible to obtain up to 30 cm of suction. Choices 2 and 3 will not affect the suction, and choice 4 would decrease the amount of suction. 4, II. Water-Seal Drainage.

28. ② Removal of the chest tubes causes some pain, so it is always best to premedicate

the client before they are removed. This way, the client is more likely to cooperate with the removal. The client should hold his breath with the removal and be in an orthopneic position for removal. The collection chambers do not need to be emptied before removal. 4, I. Chest Tubes.

---

29. To answer this question, you need to know what the risk factors are for heart disease and then whether or not these can be modified.

---

29. ③ Lifestyle behaviors can be changed, which would reduce the risk of heart attack but not prevent it; therefore, choices 1, 2, and 4 would not be correct. Because sex, age, and family history are the major risk factors and they are not modifiable, the client should be told that he can lower his risk but not prevent a heart attack. 4, I. Cardiovascular Disease.

30. ① The most likely problem after a catheterization is the formation of a hematoma. If a hematoma occurs, it could seriously impair circulation. The other choices are not likely to occur. 1, I & II. Cardiac Catheterization.

---

31. To answer this question, you need to understand the clinical manifestations of CHF and those of its complications.

---

31. ② Symptoms of acute pulmonary edema are dramatic and terrifying. Capillary pressure within the lungs becomes so elevated that fluid pours from the circulating blood into the interstitium and alveolar spaces of the lung. The other choices would not cause these symptoms. 1, II. CHF.

---

32. This question requires that you understand the purpose of rotating tourniquets and what their use accomplishes.

---

32. ③ Temporary pooling of the blood in the extremities slows venous return and helps to relieve the symptoms of pulmonary edema until more permanent methods can work. 3, II. CHF, Rotating Tourniquets.

33. Knowing the purpose of rotating tourniquets, you must then know the possible problems associated with their use.

33. ④ Tourniquets are applied with enough force to obstruct venous blood flow but not enough force to impair arterial blood flow. Choices 1 and 2 would be inappropriate, because pressure above the tourniquet is unimportant. Choice 3 would indicate that too much force had been applied. 1, I. CHF. Rotating Tourniquets.

34. Be sure to read all the distractors carefully in a question such as this, because there may be some true information in each, although only one will be completely true. This is a straightforward question that simply asks you the manifestations of compensated congestive heart failure.

34. ① Compensatory mechanisms assist the failing heart to maintain an adequate cardiac output and blood flow to the tissues. These changes will increase the blood flow. The other options would not increase cardiac output. 1, II. CHF.

35. This question wants you to identify the complications associated with a pacemaker insertion versus the possibly normal outcomes.

35. ④ Occasionally, the endocardial lead perforates the ventricle and comes into contact with the diaphragm. Should this happen, the client will develop hiccoughs at the pacemaker's set rate. Choices 1, 2, and 3 are expected after the insertion, so no action is needed concerning them. 4 & 5, II. Pacemaker.

36. The question asks for risk-factor identification with the answer reflecting the highest risk factor.

36. ② As a group, males have a four times greater risk of developing coronary heart disease than do females. Caucasian males die more frequently from coronary heart disease than do African Americans, although African Americans have a higher incidence of hypertension. Age is also a risk factor, especially in association with

women after menopause. 1, II. Coronary Heart Disease.

37. In a question such as this, there are three responses that indicate the client understands the teaching done and one that indicates the client doesn't. Again, think of this as a true–false question with three true answers and one false answer.

37. ④ Anginal pain is temporary and the myocardium is not damaged by the pain. The other choices show that the client understands angina. 3 & 5, I. Angina.

38. When a question asks which of the following is inappropriate, you are looking for the one false answer. Three of the answers are true.

38. ④ Tolerance does not develop to NTG. If it seems less effective, it may be that the angina is progressing to a myocardial infarction. NTG should be taken whenever it is needed. The other options contain information that the client should understand. 3, I. Angina.

39. In diet questions, you must understand what diet prescription is most appropriate for a specific client with a specific disease. Then you must choose the foods that best meet that prescription. It is best to first identify the prescription and then think to yourself what foods best meets that, then look at the menus you are given. Be sure that any menu you choose does not contain any food that would not be in this diet. When you are studying for the NCLEX, you might want to put together several diets, such as a low-cholesterol breakfast or lunch.

39. ① This diet is the highest fiber diet. High fiber can prevent constipation, decrease the number and severity of anginal attacks, and may also lower serum cholesterol and triglyceride levels. Choice 2 contains eggs; choice 3, cream and caffeine; and choice 4 is high calorie. 3 & 5, I. Heart Disease.

40. In this case, the diet prescription is given to you. Decide whether a food is high or low in the areas covered by the prescription and then look at the menus offered. Again, be sure you don't pick a

menu that contains any item that would violate the prescription.

---

40. ④ Chinese food and soy sauce contain monosodium glutamate, which is high in sodium. The other options contain food that would fit into the prescribed diet. 3 & 5, I. Hypertension.

---

41. This question has three choices that are high in calcium and one that is not.

---

41. ③ An increase in dietary calcium may help protect against high blood pressure. Foods high in calcium include milk products, leafy green vegetables, fish, dried beans and peas, and citrus fruit. Yellow vegetables are not high in calcium. 3 & 5, I. Hypertension.

---

42. It is generally correct to choose responses that encourage the client to continue discussing a topic, rather than simply giving an answer that closes off discussion.

---

42. ③ Home blood pressure monitoring fosters compliance with the treatment of hypertension. The recording documents trends in the client's blood pressure that may represent the client's condition more accurately. It is not a difficult skill, and home monitoring units are easy to learn to use. This will foster independence on the client's part. Choice 3 also offers the client an opportunity to continue the discussion. 4, I & IV. Hypertension.

43. ② Clients undergoing amputations experience a sense of loss, not only for the limb but also for the loss of functional ability. Grieving is, therefore, normal and expected. Physical attractiveness and wholeness are issues the client faces that may precipitate grief. There are no data to suggest that she is angry or fearful. 1, III. Amputations.

---

44. You need to think about what the client's needs will be after the amputation and then decide what action would facilitate meeting these needs. In this case,

you should know that the client will need some sort of assistive device; therefore, upper body strengthening is important.

---

44. ③ Strengthening the upper extremities will help the client manipulate assistive devices postoperatively. Upper extremity strength is also needed to compensate for the changed center of gravity that occurs when a lower limb is lost. The other activities will not help or are potentially detrimental, such as choice 2. 4, II. Amputations.

45. ④ Wrapping the stump with an Ace bandage in a figure-eight style helps to control edema and maintain the stump in a tapered shape that can more easily be fitted for a prosthesis. The other choices are immaterial. 4, II. Amputations.

---

46. To answer this question, you need to be aware of the changes associated with an amputation; then, based on this knowledge, you must give the most appropriate nursing intervention.

---

46. ③ The center of gravity changes when a lower limb is amputated. A client of Mrs. Mason's age would be expected to have problems maintaining balance after surgery. The nurse is best able to prevent falls by assisting the client from the affected side, letting the client move her unaffected side. Choices 1 and 2 would limit her independence and choice 4 is unnecessary. 4, I. Amputations.

---

47. This is a true–false type question. There will be three choices that will limit the use of a prosthesis and one that will not; so there are three true, limiting factors and one false factor that does not limit the use of a prosthesis.

---

47. ① In a motivated client, age is not a barrier to the use of a prosthetic device. Diseases of a chronic nature often leave a client in a debilitated state that is a contraindication to a prosthesis. Choices 2 and 4 may also limit success. Her diabetes may also be a factor in successful prosthetic rehabilitation, but not her age. 1 & 3, I. Amputations.

48. This question is the same type as question 47.

48. ④ A client must be highly motivated and committed to be successful at intermittent catheterization. He or she must also be willing to learn a routine and follow it consistently. Sterile technique is not needed, and a significant other could perform the procedure. Only clients unwilling to follow a regular schedule would be unsuccessful. 1 & 3, IV. Urinary Tract Infections.

49. This is another diet question that requires you to know what makes up an acid–ash diet and what foods either increase or decrease the acidity of the urine. This is also a true–false question.

49. ① Carbonated beverages are not included in an acid–ash diet because they alkalinize the urine. The other options acidify the urine. 4, I. Urinary Tract Infections.

50. This question requires you to know what affects medication effectiveness and what orders the nurse should question.

50. ① Aminoglycosides have diminished action in acid urine and would, therefore, not be as effective. Choice 2 would acidify the urine, and choice 3 and sometimes choice 4 need acid urine to be effective. 2, I. Urinary Tract Infections.

51. This is a straightforward question that asks you to identify symptoms associated with a particular disease process. Because the answers contain multiple parts, be careful that every part is true before you choose it.

51. ③ As renal disease reaches end stage, all body systems will become involved and the kidneys typically decrease in size unless a condition such as polycystic kidneys is involved. The creatinine may be stable or begin to slowly increase. Anemia is common because of the decrease in erythropoietin. 1, II. Renal Failure.

52. This question asks you about the effects of dialysis on medications. You must know whether medications are affected by dialysis or if the medications themselves affect dialysis to answer this question correctly.

52. ④ Antihypertensive medications are often essential in maintaining an acceptable blood pressure level between treatments. When administered before a treatment, these medications augment the hypotensive effects of fluid removal during dialysis. 2, I & II. Hemodialysis.

53. To answer this question correctly, you must carefully look at the stem of the question. It states that the drowsiness occurs after meals. This means that something in the diet is causing the problem. If you understand cirrhosis, you would know that protein in the diet can lead to elevated serum ammonia, a CNS depressant. The question then asks you to identify other signs of an elevated ammonia level.

53. ② The protein in his diet may not be metabolized appropriately and he is demonstrating signs of hepatic encephalopathy. When the blood ammonia level is highly elevated, the client will exhibit liver flap or asterixis. Assess for these flapping tremors by asking him to dorsiflex his hand with the rest of the arm resting on the bed. Choice 3 is not specific enough, because it does not specify what blood work. Either stimulants or sedatives are dangerous for these clients. 1 & 4, II. Cirrhosis.

54. This question simply requires a knowledge of normal anatomy and physiology. If you know where the head of the pancreas lies, the manifestation should be obvious.

54. ① Tumors at the head of the pancreas usually block the flow of bile. Weight loss may occur before the jaundice is noted, but it is usually mild. Severe weight loss might occur with cancer of the pancreas, but it is usually a late sign. Choices 2 and 4 are not clinical manifestations of a pancreatic tumor. 1, II. Pancreatic Tumor.

55. ① Myxedema causes hypoglycemia and hypotension and does not alter liver function. It does increase blood cholesterol levels and therefore the client's risk of cardiac disease. 1, II. Hypothyroidism.

56. **This is a straightforward knowledge question that simply asks the effect of maternal nutrition on the fetus.**

56. ① Poor nutrition on the part of the mother during pregnancy, especially during the last trimester, is associated with low–birth-weight infants. Overeating is more harmful to the mother, and brain damage will not occur if the diet is not followed rigidly. Infant obesity is not linked to maternal diet. 5, IV. Maternal Nutrition.

57. **This is another knowledge question, asking why starch causes diarrhea in an infant under 4 months old. The age of the infant should be a clue to answer, because it probably refers to something a very young infant lacks.**

57. ④ Intestinal amylase is present in reduced amounts during the first 4 months of life; therefore, starch, a polysaccharide, cannot be digested in large quantities, leading to diarrhea. Choice 3 is a result of the diarrhea, and choices 1 and 2 are incorrect. 4, I. Infant Nutrition.

58. **This question requires you to remember the meaning of the growth norms for children.**

58. ④ Conditions that indicate the need for nutritional counseling are growth at the extremes of the norms, either too high or too low. The other choices are normal variations. 1, II. Childhood Nutrition.

59. **This question simply tests your knowledge of normal principles of nutrition, in this case as it applies to a child.**

59. ② It should be stressed to the mother that if sweets and ''junk food'' are curtailed and excessive milk intake is not permitted, a healthy child will eat when hungry without any coercion. The other choices would cause more nutritional problems. 3, IV. Childhood Nutrition.

60. **First you must determine how serious a fever is in a child of this age. Then you must decide the best course of action.**

60. ③ The nurse recognizes that a fever in any child under 6 months is likely to be caused by a potentially serious illness and that a febrile neonate should be seen promptly by a physician. Lowering the fever without identifying the problem could be dangerous, as could waiting another day. 4, I. Infant Fever.

61. ④ The nurse must recognize the possible deleterious effects of a muscle relaxant or narcotic on the child's respiratory function. 5, II. Pediatric Surgical Intervention.

62. **This question asks for a priority answer. Remember, this means that more than one answer may be correct, but only one will be the priority. Life, limb, function is the usual way to think about priority setting when the question is physiological.**

62. ③ The nurse recognizes priority and appropriate activities to perform when attending to the postoperative child. The nurse must first assess the child, then attend to other duties such as a report. Choices 2 or 4 could be dangerous, and choice 1 is not the priority. 4, I & II. Pediatric Surgical Intervention.

63. **This question requires a knowledge of the physiological differences between neonates and infants. Questions of this type usually are looking for a system or function that neonates do not possess at birth, but develop during the first year of life. You also need to understand the absorption of medications.**

63. ④ Gastric emptying time does not reach the adult level of 2 hours until 6 to 8 months of age. Prolonged exposure of certain drugs to gastric contents can increase destruction of the drug. Reduced gastric motility delays entry of orally administered drugs into the lower intestinal tract, where most absorption takes place. 1, I. Pediatric Medications.

64. This is a safety and priority setting question. This means that all the actions are probably appropriate, but one is the priority. Again, think of which answer provides the most safety.

64. ② The nurse recognizes that the first step to take to ensure safe administration of medication to children is to check the amount of drug to be administered. Children have a lower range of tolerance for medications than adults. The other options contain information that should also be checked, but choice 2 is first. 4, I & II. Pediatric Medications.

65. A question like this requires a knowledge of growth and development. If you understand the developmental level of the child, you will be able to know which action is best for the child.

65. ④ Preschoolers need assistance to achieve control and will feel better once a task has been successfully accomplished. Prolonged reasoning and arguing should be avoided. Children will quickly learn if medication is hidden in other foods, leading to distrust on the part of the child. 4, IV. Pediatric Growth and Development.

66. This question simply requires a knowledge of the correct way to administer ear drops to a child.

66. ① The nurse recognizes that this is the correct procedure for the instillation of ear drops given the child's age. Choice 2 will cause pain if the drops are too cold, and choices 3 and 4 are unnecessary. 4, II. Pediatric Medications.

67. This question asks you to set a realistic goal. You must first understand the implications of the disease, and then decide which goal is realistic for a child with this diagnosis.

67. ② Cerebral palsy originates during the prenatal period through the early years of life as a result of cerebral hypoxia. Brain damage is permanent, but not progressive. Intelligence may or may not be affected, depending on the extent of damage, but is

assessed at periodic intervals as the child grows. 3, I. Cerebral Palsy.

68. This question is the first one in a series following a situation. For all the following questions, remember that you are dealing with questions concerning a pregnant teenager. The girl's age will influence all your answers. The situation also tells you that she has had minimal prenatal care, which is typical of mothers in this age group. This first question is simply a knowledge question.

68. ② The nurse knows that according to research, some of the problems experienced by the offspring of adolescent mothers include academic difficulties, low intellectual functioning, and more behavioral problems in school. There is no evidence for choice 1, and these children have more physical problems and less interaction. 2, IV. Adolescent Pregnancy.

69. You need to understand the growth and development of adolescents and the facts about adolescent pregnancy to correctly answer this and several other questions.

69. ② The nurse knows that it is normal for the adolescent to display egocentrism, focus primarily on themselves, and this may be the cause of Marge's behavior. There are no data to support choices 1 or 3. 1, IV. Adolescent Pregnancy.

70. ② The nurse understands the concept of personal fable and can apply it to this situation of adolescent sexual behavior. Adolescents feel that if they believe something will or won't happen, it is true. 1, IV. Adolescent Pregnancy.

71. Remember, psychosocial questions are best answered with a response that promotes communication. Unless the request is for simple information, choose an answer that encourages discussion on the part of the client.

71. ③ The nurse understands that adolescents have difficulty in making independent decisions, and the nurse can be helpful by exploring possible solutions and consequences. Choice 3 best exemplifies this. Choices 2 and 4 imply value judgments, and choice 1 does not help her identify her feelings. 4, III. Adolescent Pregnancy.

This question and the next two require you to understand the levels of prevention. Primary prevention refers to preventing the problem; secondary to early diagnosis; and tertiary to prevention of complications.

---

72. ④ The nurse knows that primary prevention activities are directed toward decreasing the probability of encountering illness or stressors. Choice 4 is the only one directed at helping to prevent teenage pregnancy. The others reflect other levels of prevention. 4, IV. Adolescent Pregnancy.

73. ④ The nurse knows that secondary prevention efforts are directed toward promoting early case finding so that prompt intervention can be instituted. Secondary prevention is early detection of a disease or problem, and choice 4 is the only choice directed at this early detection. 4, IV. Adolescent Pregnancy.

74. ③ The nurse knows that tertiary prevention includes all those interventions to help clients live full and productive lives while managing the limitations imposed by their condition. It is the act of rehabilitation or preventing complications. 3, IV. Adolescent Pregnancy.

75. ③ Choanal atresia, congenital blockage of the passageway between the nose and the pharynx, should be suspected if, during suctioning of the nares, the nurse observes respiratory difficulty and cyanosis. 2 & 5, IV. Neonate, Respiratory Distress.

---

76. This is a simple knowledge question, asking the clinical manifestations of a specific disease.

---

76. ③ The nurse recognizes that otitis media with effusion describes a collection of fluid in the middle ear that is not infectious; therefore, signs and symptoms of acute infection are not present. Choices 1, 2, and 4 are symptoms of infection. 1, II. Otitis Media.

77. ② In order to promote resolution of middle ear infection, the nurse must emphasize to parents the importance of completing the full course of antibiotic therapy, even though the child seems completely well. 3, IV. Otitis Media.

---

78. This question requires you to know the usual manifestations of asthma.

---

78. ③ Clinical manifestations of asthma, acute narrowing of the lower airway, include prolonged expiration, wheezing on expiration, and intercostal retractions. The other options are not associated with an acute attack of asthma. 1, II. Asthma.

---

79. This question is one that simply asks for information. You need to look at the answers to see which one offers completely correct information for the father.

---

79. ④ Parents should be assisted in helping a child with asthma to achieve optimal growth and development while continuing to be aware of the chronicity of this disease, as well as measures to control exacerbations. Limitation of activities should not be needed and there is reason to assume either that she will outgrow it or that it will progress to COPD. 4, IV. Asthma.

80. ③ Early manifestations of an impending attack of asthma include increased sputum production accompanied by a paroxysmal cough. Progressive distress is characterized by signs of lower airway obstruction, such as in the other options. 1, II. Asthma.

---

81. Medication questions are sometimes hard to study for. To prepare for this type question, look at the drug tables and become familiar with the characteristics of drug classes, rather than trying to learn a lot of individual drugs.

---

81. ① Classic manifestations of aminophylline toxicity are irritability, marked restlessness, tachycardia, and vomiting. The other choices contain opposite responses or at least one incorrect answer. 1, II. Asthma.

82. This question asks about goal setting. To answer this one, you need to be sure you understand the disease process and then decide which is a realistic goal.

82. ② Children with cystic fibrosis are often malnourished as a result of poor digestion and absorption of fats and fat-soluble vitamins. They should be assisted in ways to enhance their body image. There is no alopecia or acne, and excessive exercise is contraindicated. 3, III & IV. Cystic Fibrosis.

83. This question requires you to know the rationale behind a compensatory mechanism for a disease. You need to know the pathophysiology of cyanotic heart disease.

83. ② The body compensates for tissue hypoxia by stimulating the bone marrow to produce increased red blood cells, elevating the hemoglobin and hematocrit. Choice 1 is not wrong, but does not really answer the question, and the other options are incorrect. 2, II. Cyanotic Heart Disease.

84. This requires you to know first what the most common complication of a cardiac catheterization is and then what the signs of this complication are. Many NCLEX questions require this type of two-step thinking process. Before you try to answer this question, think about the likely complication, and then the symptoms of it.

84. ② Postcardiac catheterization complications include arterial thrombus and spasms of the vessels, which can result in asymmetrical alteration of the extremity. Accurate assessment is necessary for early detection of these complications, which are potentially life-threatening. It is vital to have a baseline assessment of the extremities so that postcatheterization changes can be noted. The other options are incorrect. 1, II. Cardiac Catheterization.

85. This question again asks for knowledge of the potential problems after a catheterization and then what the family should do to prevent or detect these problems.

85. ④ The child's nutritional status is important to promote wound healing, but diet usually need not be altered once the child is home. The nurse recognizes that the catheterization site is a potential source of infection and must be kept clean, dry, and open to the air. Discoloration of the insertion site is normal and expected. 4, I. Cardiac Catheterization.

86. This question is again a two-part one. You must first decide what dysarthria is and then what an appropriate goal would be for a client with this.

86. ④ Dysarthria is a muscular problem that develops following a stroke. This problem is very amenable to speech therapy. The client does not have aphasia, so he will not develop problems associated with this. There are no data to suggest he has trouble with eating, although the dysarthria may lead to some difficulties with swallowing. 3, I. Strokes.

87. This is another medication question. The problems associated with digitalis toxicity are the same for both children and adults.

87. ④ The nurse recognizes that digoxin is a potent medication and must be administered with caution. Choices 2 and 3 are potentially dangerous practices. The best answer is choice 4. Signs of digitoxicity such as nausea, vomiting, listlessness, anorexia, bradycardia, or dysrhythmias warrant immediate medical attention. 4, I & II. Pediatric Cardiac Medications.

88. This question asks you to differentiate the clinical manifestations of one GI disease from the others. It is actually a simple knowledge question.

88. ③ In pyloric stenosis, the sphincter is hypertrophied, resulting in a narrowed opening that impedes the peristaltic movements and emptying of the stomach. Forceful stomach contractions against resistance are responsible for projectile vomiting. The other choices are associated with other GI conditions, such as tracheoesophageal fistula and lower GI obstructions. 1, II. Pyloric stenosis.

---

89. This is another diet question. Again, decide what the correct diet would be for a client with liver disease. Once you have decided on the correct diet prescription, then look at the menus given to see which one best fits your choice.

---

89. ④ In hepatitis, a low-fat, high-protein diet in small, frequent servings is best. Nausea, which usually occurs with hepatitis, is less intense in the morning and it is therefore the time when nutritious foods are better tolerated. Choice 4 is the highest in protein and lowest in fat. 2 & 5, II. Hepatitis.

---

90. This question requires a knowledge of the effects of anxiety and the fact that anxiety can lead to regression.

---

90. ④ It is not unusual for a client in a highly stressful situation to regress to a stage provoking less anxiety in an attempt to cope with his severe anxiety. Although denial may occur, it does not cause dependence. Choices 2 and 3 are not related to dependent behavior. 1, III. Defense mechanisms.

---

91. As with all goal questions, this question requires you to first understand the client's condition and then identify appropriate goals for this specific situation.

---

91. ② During an acute exacerbation of Crohn's disease, the client may have up to 10 or more diarrheal stools a day. Lowering the number to just four would be a significant improvement. Choices 1 and 3 are probably unrealistic until the acute phase of the disease is over. Choice 4 is highly unlikely, and would never occur while the disease is active. 3, I. Crohn's Disease.

92. ② Group therapy allows the sharing of problems with others who have similar problems, thoughts, and feelings. It can help the client learn new ways of coping. Choices 1, 3, and 4 cover clients who are unlikely to recognize the need for help, a requirement for successful treatment. 1, III. Group Therapy.

---

93. This question requires you to know the side effects of a major category of medications.

---

93. ① Nonintentional tremors are one of the extrapyramidal symptoms associated with major tranquilizers, and are common and easily managed. Choice 3 is not common, but if it occurs, liver function studies should be ordered. The others are not common side effects of anxiolytics. 5, III. Psychotropic Medications.

UNIT II

The Adult Client

3

Adult Growth
and Development

PRE-TEST Growth and Development

1. Physical changes associated with middle age include:
   ① Decrease in organ size and capability
   ② Decreased visual acuity beginning about age 40
   ③ Major decrease in deep sleep
   ④ Decrease in sex drive and libido

2. The major nutrient needed by women after menopause are foods rich in:
   ① Iron
   ② Potassium
   ③ Calcium
   ④ Vitamin C

3. Which of the following is a common problem of men in late middle age?
   ① Urinary dysfunction
   ② Decreased sex drive
   ③ Frequent impotence
   ④ Chronic constipation

4. Which of the following is NOT a developmental task of middle age?
   ① Coping with grown children
   ② Increasing leisure activity
   ③ Increasing emphasis on advancing career
   ④ Coping with role reversal with parents

5. Which of the following would NOT be a part of a middle-aged client's psychosocial development?
   ① Attitude toward aging
   ② Acceptance of retirement
   ③ Coping with new family relationships
   ④ Coping with changing body image

6. The "middle old" are described as those between 75 and 85 years old. Which of the following would be a physical change associated with this age group?
   ① Decreased response to physical stress
   ② Inability to carry out normal ADLs
   ③ Rapid progression of aging changes
   ④ Normal response time

7. The elderly have a decrease in total body fluids, causing:
   ① Increased thirst
   ② A decreased risk of dehydration
   ③ An increase in urine output
   ④ More side effects from water-soluble drugs

8. The elderly are more susceptible to overdoses from fat-soluble drugs because they have:
   ① A decreased percentage of body fat
   ② An increased percentage of body fat
   ③ A decrease in renal function
   ④ An increase in bowel transit time

9. Usual respiratory changes in the elderly include:
   ① Decrease in dead space
   ② Increased vital capacity
   ③ Decreased cough effectiveness
   ④ Increased respiratory rate

10. The elderly have changes in the integument. Which of the following is NOT an appropriate problem associated with these skin changes?
    ① Increased ability for scar formation
    ② Dry cracking skin from decreased turgor
    ③ Decreased sweating due to decreased sweat glands
    ④ Increased risk of hypothermia

PRE-TEST Answers and Rationales

1. ② Visual acuity begins to decrease by age 40, requiring the use of magnification. The other items do not occur in middle age as normal changes. If they do occur, they may indicate some pathology. 1, IV. Middle Age.

2. ③ Calcium requirements increase in women after menopause due to the drop in estrogen levels. If calcium is not taken in adequate amounts, osteoporosis may occur. Iron needs increase slightly; needs for the other nutrients remain unchanged. 4, II & IV. Middle Age.

3. ① Urinary dysfunction is a common symptom of benign prostatic hypertrophy, a common problem in late middle age. There is no reason for any of the other symptoms to occur unless severe problems exist. 2, II & IV. Middle Age.

4. ③ Developmental tasks of middle age include coping with grown children, increased amounts of leisure time, and coping with one's aging parents. Career advancement is not a major goal at this point, because most middle-aged people have reached their maximum potential by then. 1, IV. Middle Age.

5. ② Important psychosocial needs for middle-aged clients include their attitude toward aging, coping with new roles within the family, and coping with changes in body image. They may begin to prepare for retirement, but acceptance of retirement is a task for the elderly. 1, IV. Middle Age.

6. ① The major physical change experienced by the "middle old" is a decreased response to physical stress. They are still able to carry out normal ADLs, but they do have a slightly slowed response time. The aging changes are usually gradual. 1, IV. Elderly.

7. ④ Because the elderly have a decrease in body water, water-soluble drugs can become increasingly concentrated, leading to an increase in side effects. Their thirst is normally decreased and they have an increased risk of dehydration. Their urine output is usually decreased and concentrated. 2, II & IV. Elderly.

8. ② The elderly have an increase in the percentage of fat in the body, which leads to an increase in the amount of fat-soluble drugs that can be absorbed. This can result in possible overdose. Renal function should not affect these drugs, and an increase in bowel transit time would decrease their absorption, which leads to underdosing. 2, II & IV. Elderly.

9. ③ The elderly have an increase in dead space, a decrease in vital capacity, and little change in their respiratory rate. A decrease in the effectiveness of the cough is the most common and potentially serious change. 1, II & IV. Elderly.

10. ① There is a decreased ability to form granulation tissue in the elderly, which impairs healing and scar formation. The other items are normal problems associated with aging skin. 2, IV. Elderly.

GROWTH AND DEVELOPMENT in Middle Age (40 to 65 years)

Physical Growth and Development: General Considerations

  I. Organ size and capacity similar to those in young adult
 II. Maintenance of physical function; slight decrease in endurance
III. Able to perform daily tasks without difficulty or discomfort
 IV. Sensory: decreased visual acuity with need for magnification beginning around age 40
  V. Sleep pattern without major interruption
     A. Slight decrease in time spent in deep sleep
     B. Slight decrease in total hours of sleep
 VI. Sexual activity and interest continue at satisfactory level
VII. Reproductive function
     A. Males: slight decrease in testosterone and sperm production
     B. Females: ceases at menopause (see female reproductive disorders)
VIII. Nutritional status
     A. Caloric intake appropriate for adequate weight for height and age

B. Nutrient distribution per RDAs for age and sex (Table 3–1)

C. Calcium supplements needed by many females to prevent osteoporosis (postmenopause)

Nursing Process Applied to Physical Growth and Development

I. Assessment
A. Physical assessment similar to that in young adults
B. Lifestyle extremely important, due to relationship of lifestyle (smoking, alcohol use, exercise, stress management) to health maintenance
C. Vocation and work environment
D. Nutrition
E. Sexual function
F. Elimination: be alert for early signs of age-related dysfunction
1. Males: hesitancy and difficulty initiating urination suggest prostatic hyperplasia
2. Females: loss of small amounts of urine with coughing, laughing, sneezing suggests stress incontinence

II. Analysis
A. High risk for body image changes related to aging process
B. High risk for ineffective individual coping related to inability to reach life goals

III. Planning/goals, expected outcomes
A. Client will not experience body image changes, as evidenced by acceptance of aging process

B. Client will cope with life changes effectively, as evidenced by the establishment of realistic goals

IV. Implementation
A. Nursing process utilized in planning for client
B. Client assumes active role in own health care

V. Evaluation
A. Client maintains or returns to health status appropriate for age and sex
B. Client meets developmental tasks of middle age

Psychosocial Growth and Development: General Considerations

I. Occupational satisfaction
A. Work performance peak usually reached at this time
B. Women may return to work force when children are grown

II. Satisfying leisure-time activities
A. Less emphasis on advancing careers and raising children leads to more available free time
B. May need to find less strenuous leisure activities due to physical changes
C. Must develop interests outside of work environment in preparation for retirement

III. Family relationships
A. Children
1. Coping with adolescent children
2. Adjustment to increasing independence of children ("letting go")
3. Adjusting to role of grandparent

TABLE 3–1 Nutrient Distribution per RDAs for Age and Sex

Age (years)	Weight (kg)	Weight (lb)	Height (cm)	Height (in.)	(g) Protein	(RE) Vitamin A	(μg) Vitamin D	(mg) Vitamin E	(mg) Vitamin C	(mg) Thiamin	(mg) Riboflavin	(mg equiv.) Niacin	(mg) Vitamin B₆	(μg) Folacin	(μg) Vitamin B₁₂	(mg) Calcium	(mg) Phosphorus	(mg) Magnesium	(mg) Iron	(mg) Zinc	(μg) Iodine
Males																					
11–14	45	99	157	62	45	1,000	10	8	50	1.4	1.6	18	1.8	400	3.0	1,200	1,200	350	18	15	150
15–18	66	145	176	69	56	1,000	10	10	60	1.4	1.7	18	2.0	400	3.0	1,200	1,200	400	18	15	150
19–22	70	154	177	70	56	1,000	7.5	10	60	1.5	1.7	19	2.2	400	3.0	800	800	350	10	15	150
23–50	70	154	178	70	56	1,000	5	10	60	1.4	1.6	18	2.2	400	3.0	800	800	350	10	15	150
51+	70	154	178	70	56	1,000	5	10	60	1.2	1.4	16	2.2	400	3.0	800	800	350	10	15	150
Females																					
11–14	46	101	157	62	46	800	10	8	50	1.1	1.3	15	1.8	400	3.0	1,200	1,200	300	18	15	150
15–18	55	120	163	64	46	800	10	8	60	1.1	1.3	14	2.0	400	3.0	1,200	1,200	300	18	15	150
19–22	55	120	163	64	44	800	7.5	8	60	1.1	1.3	14	2.0	400	3.0	800	800	300	18	15	150
23–50	55	120	163	64	44	800	5	8	60	1.0	1.2	13	2.0	400	3.0	800	800	300	18	15	150
51+	55	120	163	64	44	800	5	8	60	1.0	1.2	13	2.0	400	3.0	800*	800	300	10	15	150

* Many experts now recommend 1200 mg calcium for women in this age group to prevent or decrease osteoporosis.

B. Aging parents
   1. May need to assume responsibility for frail aging parents
   2. Coping with role reversal in child–parent relationship
C. Spouse
   1. Changing relationship with spouse due to decreased focus on career and childrearing; family once again consists of only husband and wife
   2. May experience great satisfaction because time is now available for intimate relationship
   3. Prior dissatisfaction in marital relationship may increase due to lack of outside distractions
IV. Retirement planning
   A. Financial
   B. Fulfilling activities
   C. Housing
V. Coping with physical and physiological changes
   A. Climacteric
      1. Female: menopause (see section on menopause)
      2. Male (between ages 55 to 65): degree of physiological changes determines need for coping
   B. Changing body image
      1. Male: baldness, decrease in height, shift of muscle mass to adipose tissue with decreased exercise
      2. Female: wrinkling of skin, shift of adipose tissue
VI. Developmental theories (Table 3–2)
   A. Erikson
      1. Definition: choice between primary concern for own needs (stagnation) versus concentrating on needs of others and examining accomplishments (generativity)
      2. Developmental tasks
         a. Stagnation versus generativity
         b. Achievement depends upon successfully accomplishing tasks of prior levels; positive attitude toward own aging
   B. Peck's expansion of Erikson
      1. Definition: looks at biological as well as psychosocial; multiple factors
      2. Developmental tasks
         a. Valuing wisdom versus valuing physical powers
         b. Socializing versus sexualizing (companionship versus sexual activity and reproduction)
         c. Flexibility versus rigidity
   C. Havighurst
      1. Definition: developmental tasks culturally related; successful accomplishment leads

TABLE 3–2 Developmental Theories

Theorist	Middle Age	Old Age
Erikson	Stagnation vs. generativity	Integrity vs. despair
Peck	Wisdom vs. physical powers Socializing vs. sexualizing Flexibility vs. rigidity	Ego differentiation vs. work-role preoccupation Body transcendence vs. body preoccupation Ego transcendence vs. ego preoccupation
Havighurst	Helping children become responsible Civic and social responsibility Satisfaction in occupation Leisure activities Relating to spouse Coping with physical changes Adjusting to aging parents	Adjust to: Physical changes of aging Retirement, decreased income Death of spouse Age group New social roles Living arrangements for age
Freud	Ability to love Work in harmony	Ability to love Cope with pending death
Maslow	Maintain self-esteem Growth: self-actualization	Self-actualization Maintain self-esteem
Kohlberg	Social contract orientation: concern for human dignity	Universal ethics orientation: "elder statesperson"

to happiness and satisfaction versus unhappiness, difficulty with later life
      2. Developmental tasks
         a. Helping children become responsible adults
         b. Civic and social responsibility
         c. Satisfaction in one's occupation
         d. Developing leisure-time activities
         e. Relating to spouse as an individual
         f. Coping with physical changes of mid-life
         g. Adjusting to aging parents
   D. Freud
      1. Definition: difficulty with mid-life related to unresolved conflict in childhood
      2. Developmental tasks
         a. To love
         b. To work in harmony
   E. Maslow
      1. Definition: pyramidal hierarchy of needs; basic physiological needs, moving to safety and security, belonging, self-esteem, self-actualization
      2. Developmental tasks
         a. Growth toward self-actualization
         b. By mid-life, self-esteem should be established

c. All individuals do not reach self-actualization during lifetime
F. Kohlberg
  1. Definition: identifies six stages of moral development
    a. Obedience and punishment orientation
    b. Satisfying own needs; moral behavior to obtain rewards
    c. Approval seeking: moral behavior to win approval
    d. Law and order orientation: respect law and rules to avoid penalty of disobeying; faith in existing authority, fixed rules; maintenance of social order at all costs
    e. Social contract orientation: moral behavior concerned with human rights, equality; moral principles agreed upon by society as a whole
    f. Universal ethical principles: highest stage; morality equals decisions of conscience; rises above code agreed to by society
  2. Developmental tasks
    a. Social contract orientation appropriate at mid-life; achieved by only one third
    b. Law and order orientation prevalent
    c. Universal ethical principles orientation rarely achieved

Nursing Process Applied to Psychosocial Growth and Development

  I. Assessment
    A. Attitude toward aging
    B. Family relationships
    C. Leisure activities
    D. Occupation: satisfaction; retirement planning
    E. Developmental level; task accomplishment
 II. Analysis: high risk for altered growth and development related to inability to meet developmental tasks of middle age
III. Planning/goals, expected outcomes: client will not develop altered growth and development, as evidenced by having a positive attitude toward own aging; coping with changing family relationships; developing satisfying leisure activities; maintaining satisfaction with work; beginning retirement planning; and accomplishing developmental tasks appropriate to mid-life
IV. Implementation
    A. Nursing process will be utilized
    B. Client will assume active role
 V. Evaluation: client successfully copes with emotional demands of mid-life; maintains positive outlook on life; and successfully accomplishes tasks of middle age

GROWTH AND DEVELOPMENT IN THE ELDERLY (65+ YEARS)

Physical Growth and Development: General Considerations

  I. Definitions
    A. Young-old (65 to 75 years):
      1. Normally vital and active
      2. Some slowing of responses; however, function often similar to middle age
    B. Middle-old (75 to 85 years):
      1. Gradual progression of aging changes
      2. Decreased response to physical stress
      3. Able to carry out daily activities without undue fatigue in absence of debilitating chronic disease
    C. Old-old (85+ years):
      1. Increasing frailty, but many still are independent
      2. 50% decrease in renal function
      3. Medications must be tailored to renal function
      4. Further decreased response to physical stress
 II. General: although some generalizations can be made, rate at which one ages highly individualistic; dependent upon heredity, lifestyle, exposure, stress, presence or absence of chronic disease that may affect aging process; aging is normal stage of development and is decremental; leads to reduced function in each body system; becomes more difficult to maintain homeostasis under physical stress; however, sufficient reserve present under ordinary circumstances; little difficulty with basic daily activities
    A. Total body fluid decreases
      1. Increased risk of dehydration
      2. Higher concentration of water-soluble drugs
    B. Increased percentage of body fat
      1. Increased storage
      2. Possible prolongation of effect of fat-soluble drugs
    C. Renal function decreases by approximately 50%
      1. Decreased renal blood flow
      2. Decreased excretion of drugs
    D. Cardiac output decreased
    E. Pulmonary function decreased
      1. Increased "dead space"

2. Decreased vital capacity
3. Decreased cough effectiveness

F. Mobility
1. Loss of calcium from bone: greater for Caucasian women (osteoporosis)
2. Decreased position sense in feet but not in hand; cane may alleviate associated unsteadiness

G. Integument
1. Wrinkling of skin with loss of moisture
2. Decreased skin turgor
3. Decreased sweat gland secretion
4. Loss of subcutaneous fat; risk of hypothermia
5. Thinning of hair
    a. Hereditary baldness (males)
    b. Loss or thinning of hair on extremities and pubis

H. Sensory
1. Vision
    a. Decreased visual acuity with need for magnification
    b. Decreased depth perception
    c. Decreased accommodation to dark or bright light
2. Hearing
    a. Difficulty hearing high-pitched sounds
    b. Delayed processing: speak slowly

I. Sleep pattern
1. Marked changes compared with younger clients
2. Almost total absence of deep sleep
3. Stage I sleep (lightest level with no awareness of having slept) predominates
4. Frequent awakening (up to ten times per night)
5. Frequent complaints of insomnia due to changes in sleep pattern; often in spite of client's obtaining adequate sleep for maintenance of health
6. Sedative use and requests common due to dissatisfaction with sleep pattern

J. Sexual function
1. Interest undiminished
2. Longer time for male to achieve erection
3. Decreased vaginal secretions may lead to need for lubricant

K. Nutrition
1. Caloric needs decreased; 7.5% for each decade after 25 years old
2. Nutrient needs remain unchanged (see Table 3-1 for RDAs)
3. Nutrition often compromised by
    a. Continued nutrient needs in face of decreased caloric needs

    b. Difficulty chewing secondary to tooth loss
    c. Difficulty preparing meals or shopping for food
    d. Social isolation
    e. Decreased income

Nursing Process Applied to Physical Growth and Development

I. Assessment
A. Careful and thorough history; allow more time for responses
B. Drug history assumes great importance due to
1. Use of multiple drugs
2. High usage of over-the-counter drugs
3. Increased incidence of drug toxicity due to changes of aging
    a. Decreased total body fluid
    b. Increased percentage of body fat
    c. Decreased albumin for binding of protein-bound drugs leads to more unbound (active) drug
4. Symptoms often secondary to drug use, rather than indicating new problem
C. Findings considered abnormal in young may be normal in elderly
D. Sudden change in function indicates problem present, rather than normal aging
E. Assess cognitive function through use of mental status test when possibility of confusion or dementia exists
F. When confusion noted, assess for possible reversible causes such as drugs, infection, relocation trauma
G. Obtain client's perception of sleep pattern; if dissatisfied with sleep, but not tired next day, sleep most likely adequate and teaching will be needed regarding normal aging and sleep
H. Nutritional assessment critical for this age group; recent unintentional loss of weight or body weight less than 80% of ideal suggests nutritional problem and need for further assessment

II. Analysis: high risk for impaired home maintenance management related to decreased functional ability

III. Planning/goals, expected outcomes
A. Client will manage self-care at home as evidenced by ability to maintain functional ability as long as possible
B. Client focuses on maximizing or maintaining remaining function; because of frequency of chronic problems, goals do not focus on cure, as with younger clients

IV. Implementation
  A. Nurse recognizes need for increased support systems when physical function decreased
  B. Nurse considers community resources and caregivers when client no longer independent
  C. Nurse provides client teaching appropriate to cognitive level
V. Evaluation: client maintains or is restored to maximal functional ability

Psychosocial Growth and Development: General Considerations

I. Multiple losses (actual or potential)
  A. Income
  B. Friends, family members
    1. Relocation
    2. Death
  C. Spouse
  D. Home
  E. Physical function
  F. Cognitive ability
  G. Social status
II. Need for productive activity
  A. Volunteering
  B. Gainful employment
  C. Helping others
III. Must cope with changing body image
IV. Potential for loneliness; social isolation
V. Need for adaptation to change
VI. Realization that end of life is near
VII. Spirituality
  A. More personal relationship with God
  B. Assists in coping with life stresses and end of life
VIII. Psychosocial theories
  A. Disengagement (Cumming and Henry)
    1. Society and older individuals mutually withdraw from each other
    2. Disputed as being comforting to society, discomforting for elderly
    3. Does not consider differences among aged
  B. Activity
    1. Old age can be abolished by remaining active
    2. Does not consider diversity among elderly
  C. Continuity
    1. People tend to continue lifestyle already established
    2. Attempts to cope with diversity among older individuals
IX. Developmental tasks; theories (see Table 3–2)
  A. Erikson
    1. Definition: conflict between integrating, appreciating one's own life experiences (ego integrity) versus bitterness, resentment, feeling that life has been wasted, negative outlook (despair)
    2. Developmental task
      a. Integrity versus despair
      b. Successful outcome: acceptance of own life and self without regret; coming to terms with pending death
      c. Ideal outcome: maturity, independence, wisdom, positive attitude, positive outlook
  B. Peck's expansion of Erikson
    1. Definition: more specific than Erikson; expands on integrity versus despair
    2. Developmental tasks
      a. Ego differentiation versus work-role preoccupation: value placed on job and family; when integrity based on work, retirement threatens; when integrity based on family, independence of children threatens
      b. Body transcendence versus body preoccupation: enjoyment of life despite physical change or discomfort
      c. Ego transcendence versus ego preoccupation; able to devote self to future generations versus preoccupation with pending death
  C. Havighurst
    1. Definition: difference between tasks of mid-life and late life is disengagement from mid-life roles to take on new roles
    2. Developmental tasks; adjustments
      a. Physical changes of aging
      b. Retirement and decreased income
      c. Death of spouse
      d. One's age group, developing associations at time of disengagement
      e. New social roles
      f. Need for living arrangement to meet physical, emotional, social needs
  D. Freud
    1. Definition: similar to mid-life, difficulties relate to unresolved earlier conflicts
    2. Developmental tasks
      a. Focus remains on ability to love
      b. Emphasis on ability to cope with pending death rather than work
  E. Maslow
    1. Definition: hierarchy of needs
    2. Developmental tasks
      a. Growth toward or achievement of self-actualization
      b. Maintenance of self-esteem
  F. Kohlberg
    1. Definition: moral development
    2. Developmental tasks

a. Movement from law and order orientation to social contract orientation; concern for human rights and dignity
b. Universal ethics orientation highest level; only occasionally achieved; transcends social codes; "elder statesperson"

Nursing Process Applied to Psychosocial Growth and Development

I. Assessment
   A. Outlook
   B. Coping abilities
   C. Support systems
   D. Losses
   E. Adaptation to change
   F. Spirituality
II. Analysis
   A. High risk for altered growth and development related to inability to meet developmental tasks of old age
   B. High risk for spiritual distress related to aging and inevitable death
III. Planning/goals, expected outcomes
   A. Client will develop normally as evidenced by client's ability to meet developmental tasks of old age
   B. Client will not develop spiritual distress, as evidenced by client's statements of acceptance of own eventual death as a natural part of life
IV. Implementation
   A. Use reminiscence to assist client toward ego integrity, sense of self-worth
   B. Gear teaching to client's cognitive level
   C. Use regular routine, maintained to provide security, improve coping ability in presence of decreased cognitive function
   D. Maintain independence wherever possible to assist in maintenance of self-worth
V. Evaluation
   A. Client accepts physical changes of aging; adapts to new roles; adjusts to losses associated with aging; and maintains positive attitude, sense of self-worth
   B. Client copes successfully with death and dying and maintains spiritual satisfaction

POST-TEST Growth and Development

1. Middle-aged people should:
   ① Exercise less each decade after 50
   ② Increase their sleep after 50
   ③ Decrease their calories by 7.5% for each decade after 25
   ④ Decrease their fluid intake

2. The leading cause of death in middle-aged men is:
   ① Heart disease
   ② Colon cancer
   ③ Cirrhosis
   ④ Stroke

3. Which of the following physiological factors does NOT decrease in middle age?
   ① Peristalsis
   ② Metabolic rate
   ③ Rigidity of lung tissue
   ④ Visual accommodation

4. A normal visual change associated with aging is:
   ① Tunnel vision
   ② Decreased accommodation to light or dark
   ③ Loss of central vision
   ④ Decreased vision from clouding of the lens

5. The average number of calories a 65-year-old woman should consume daily to maintain her ideal body weight is about:
   ① 1000
   ② 1500
   ③ 2000
   ④ 2500

6. The elderly suffer from many nutritional problems. Which of the following is NOT a likely cause of their nutritional problems?
   ① Difficulty chewing due to lost teeth
   ② Difficulty shopping for food
   ③ Decreased caloric needs
   ④ Social isolation during meals

7. The elderly are more prone to drug overdose because:
   ① They have a lower body fat content
   ② Their body water content is high proportionally
   ③ They often forget to take their medication
   ④ Their serum albumin levels are lower

8. You are caring for an elderly person in the hospital. The client is exhibiting severe confusion. The family says that the client's mind has been perfectly clear and that the client has never been confused before. The most likely cause of the confusion is:
   ① Relocation trauma
   ② Alzheimer's disease
   ③ Organic brain syndrome
   ④ A side effect of medication

9. One of the most appropriate developmental tasks of the elderly is:
   ① Preparation for retirement
   ② Beginning parenting of adult children
   ③ Preparation for death
   ④ Reassessment of roles within the family

POST-TEST Answers and Rationales

1. ③ The middle-aged adult has a natural decrease in metabolism, requiring a 7.5% decrease in calories to maintain the same body weight. Exercise and fluid intake should remain the same or increase, while the need for sleep stays the same and then decreases. 4, II. Middle Age.

2. ① Heart disease is the leading cause of death in middle-aged men; therefore, the major health need in this group is centered on prevention of cardiovascular disease. 2, IV. Middle Age.

3. ③ The rigidity of lung tissue increases during middle age. The other options decrease. 5, IV. Middle Age.

4. ② Tunnel vision may be a sign of glaucoma; loss of central vision may be a sign of retinal detachment and cloudy vision may be characteristic of cataracts. Decreased accommodation is the only normal visual change associated with aging. The key word is *normal*. 2, IV. Elderly.

5. ② The rule is that caloric intake should decrease about 7.5% for each decade after age 25. The normal caloric intake would be about 1500 calories from age 65 on. 1, II & IV. Elderly.

6. ③ The elderly often need more calories than they receive and more nutritious foods. The other answers are common causes of poor nutrition in the elderly. 2, II & IV. Elderly.

7. ④ Many drugs that the elderly take, such as cardiac glycosides, are protein-bound drugs. The low serum albumin common in many elderly means that higher levels of the drugs are in circulation, which can lead to overdose. The elderly have a higher percentage of fat, a low level of body water. Forgetting their drugs would lead to underdosing, not overdosing. 2, II & IV. Elderly.

8. ① The most common cause of sudden acute confusion in this client is probably due to relocation trauma associated with the change in the environment. Alzheimer's disease and organic brain syndrome occur gradually and the family would have noticed some changes. There is no mention of medication administration and it *cannot* be assumed. 2, IV. Elderly.

9. ③ One of the most common developmental tasks of the elderly is acceptance of and preparation for death. The other options are tasks of the middle-aged person. 1, IV. Elderly.

PRE-TEST Female Reproductive Disorders

1. Before an appointment for a Pap smear, the client should be cautioned against:
   ① Coming if she is experiencing a vaginal discharge
   ② Douching immediately before the appointment
   ③ Having sexual intercourse the day before the appointment
   ④ Having a bath the morning of the appointment

2. Prior to the pelvic examination, the nurse should:
   ① Have the client void
   ② Administer an enema
   ③ Catheterize the client
   ④ Scrub the perineal area with antiseptic soap

3. The main rationale for the above action is to:
   ① Obtain a stool specimen
   ② Obtain a sterile urine specimen
   ③ Decrease discomfort during the pelvic exam
   ④ Remove flatus and feces from the rectum

4. Your client is encouraged to ambulate frequently after she has an abdominal hysterectomy. The nurse knows this intervention will prevent:
   ① Abdominal distention
   ② Wound infection
   ③ Diarrhea
   ④ Urinary retention

5. Your client is recovering from a total abdominal hysterectomy and a bilateral salpingo-oophorectomy that she had for severe bleeding caused by fibroid tumors. She asks if she will continue to have periods postoperatively. Your best answer would be that because of the surgery she will:
   ① Experience surgical menopause

② Not have the uncontrolled bleeding she
　 had preoperatively

③ Experience some changes associated with
　 menses, but she will not have a period

④ Return to a normal menstrual cycle

**Martha Reyes is a 50-year-old woman who visits a clinic
complaining of heat intolerance, irregular menses, and
heavy bleeding.**

---

6. The most likely cause of Mrs. Reyes' irregular
　 bleeding is:
　 ① Uterine cancer
　 ② Ovarian cancer
　 ③ Uterine fibroids
　 ④ Menopause

7. Psychological symptoms that Mrs. Reyes may
　 exhibit include:
　 ① Irritability and emotionalism
　 ② Lack of sexual urge
　 ③ Increased drowsiness
　 ④ Lethargy

8. Hormone replacement therapy is often
　 prescribed to control the symptoms of
　 menopause. Which of the following would
　 NOT be considered a common side effect of
　 hormone replacement therapy?
　 ① Abdominal distention
　 ② Fluid retention
　 ③ Osteoporosis
　 ④ Gallbladder disease

9. Nursing interventions to reduce the
　 complications of menopause include:
　 ① Increasing the client's caloric intake to
　 　 avoid weight loss
　 ② Reducing calcium in the diet to avoid
　 　 hypercalcemia
　 ③ Avoiding increased exercise to prevent
　 　 fatigue
　 ④ Recommending the use of water-soluble
　 　 lubricants to decrease vaginal dryness

**Ann Grant is a 50-year-old woman who is seen by a doctor
for the possibility of breast cancer.**

---

10. Which of the following is considered a high
　 risk factor for breast cancer?
　 ① Jewish women of European descent
　 ② Multiparity
　 ③ Japanese women in Japan
　 ④ Early artificial menopause

11. Which of the following would place Mrs.
　 Grant at lower risk for breast cancer?
　 ① Family history of breast cancer
　 ② First child before 25
　 ③ No children
　 ④ Early menarche, late menopause

12. Symptoms of breast cancer that Mrs. Grant
　 might have noticed include:
　 ① Mobile, encapsulated lump
　 ② Retraction or eversion of the nipple
　 ③ Painful regular lump
　 ④ Absence of nipple discharge

13. A mammogram is a screening test for breast
　 cancer. The American Cancer Society
　 recommends the following screening
　 schedule:
　 ① Every 5 years for women under 50
　 ② Yearly, starting at the age of 60
　 ③ A baseline study between 35 and 39
　 ④ Only as recommended by the physician

14. Mrs. Grant had a breast biopsy that was
　 positive for cancer. She is scheduled for a
　 modified radical mastectomy tomorrow
　 morning. Nursing interventions that should be
　 part of her preoperative preparation should
　 include:
　 ① Preparation for a skin graft
　 ② Teaching her side effects of hormone
　 　 replacement therapy
　 ③ Allowing her to express her sense of loss
　 ④ Teaching her the symptoms of
　 　 menopause

PRE-TEST Answers and Rationales

1. ② The purpose of a Pap smear is to check the cells that are sloughed off from the cervix and uterus. It is important that these cells not be washed out with a douche. If the client is experiencing discharge, she especially needs to see the doctor. Neither a bath nor sexual intercourse should interfere with the smear. 1, II & IV. Pap Smear's.

2. ① It is important that the client void before the examination, but there is no need to catheterize her or administer an enema. There is also no need for the procedure to be sterile. 4, II & IV. Pelvic Exam.

3. ③ The rationale for the client to void is to decrease discomfort during the pelvic examination. A full bladder can cause pressure and interfere with the examination. None of the other options are relevant. 2, II & IV. Pelvic Exam.

4. ① The most common problem after an abdominal hysterectomy is abdominal distention and ambulation helps to decrease this by stimulating peristalsis. Ambulation has no effect on wound infections or diarrhea and a minimal effect on urinary retention. 2, II & IV. TAH.

5. ① Removal of the ovaries causes surgical menopause. None of the other options are correct, because without her ovaries she will have no symptoms associated with her menses. 4, II & IV. TAH-BSO.

6. ④ Considering the limited history given, the most likely cause of the irregular bleeding is menopause. The heat intolerance is most likely hot flashes, a sign of menopause. 2, IV. Menopause.

7. ① Common psychological symptoms of menopause are irritability and emotionalism caused by unpredictable estrogen levels. Other symptoms are insomnia and jitteriness. Sexual urges should not be affected. 1, IV. Menopause.

8. ③ Hormone replacement therapy prevents osteoporosis. The other options are all side effects associated with hormone replacement therapy. 1, IV. Menopause.

9. ④ Vaginal dryness and atrophy are common problems following menopause. The use of a lubricant or estrogen cream is recommended. Weight gain and hypocalcemia are other common problems and exercise is recommended to help control the weight. 1, IV. Menopause.

10. ① Jewish women of European descent are at higher risk for breast cancer. The other options are all low risks for breast cancer. 1, II. Breast Cancer.

11. ② A low-risk factor is giving birth to her first child before age 25. The other options are all high-risk factors for breast cancer. 1, II. Breast Cancer.

12. ② A common symptom of breast cancer is eversion or retraction of the nipple, because the lump is usually fixed to adjacent tissues. The mobile, encapsulated lump is usually fibrocystic. Initially, pain is not associated with breast cancer. Absence of nipple discharge is normal. 1, II. Breast Cancer.

13. ③ The American Cancer Society recommends a baseline mammogram between the ages of 35 and 40, then for low-risk women every 1 to 2 years between 40 and 50 and yearly after the age of 50. For high-risk women, it is yearly after age 40. 4, II & IV. Breast Cancer.

14. ③ It is very important to allow the client to express her sense of loss and possibly anger. There is no reason for her to have a skin graft or to go through menopause. Hormone replacement therapy is contraindicated with a breast cancer client. 4, I & II. Breast Cancer.

NURSING PROCESS APPLIED TO FEMALE REPRODUCTIVE DISORDERS

Cervical Cancer

I. Assessment
   A. Definition/pathophysiology: usually squamous cell
   B. Incidence
      1. Occurrence of carcinoma *in situ* increasing dramatically, but 100% curable at this stage
      2. Occurrence of invasive cancer decreased by about 50%
   C. Predisposing/precipitating factors
      1. Low socioeconomic groups
      2. Early first marriage
      3. Early and frequent intercourse
      4. Multiple sex partners and sex partners with multiple sex partners
      5. High parity
      6. Poor medical care postpartum
      7. Poor hygiene
      8. Herpes, chronic cervical irritation, or human papillomavirus (HPV)
      9. Smoking started in early teenage years
      10. Nuns and Jewish women have lowest incidence
   D. Clinical manifestations
      1. Cytologic changes on Pap smears
      2. Lesion apparent on examination
      3. Vaginal bleeding postmenstrually and postcoitally
      4. Foul-smelling vaginal discharge
      5. Serosanguineous discharge
      6. Pelvic, lower back, leg, or groin pain
      7. Leakage of urine and feces from vagina
      8. Anorexia and weight loss
   E. Diagnostic tests
      1. Cytology—Pap smears
      2. Colposcopy—not screening, but diagnostic if lesions found or highly suspected
      3. Direct biopsy—endocervical curettage
      4. Conization if:
         a. Colposcopy done and abnormal cells are found in endocervical region
         b. Entire lesion not seen with colposcopy
         c. For better diagnosis
      5. Schiller test—Lugol's solution; abnormal tissue does not pick up stain; easier to biopsy
   F. Complications
      1. Liver metastasis
      2. Lung metastasis
      3. Bone metastasis
   G. Medical management

      1. Radiation therapy
         a. Often for invasive
         b. Internal implants or external radiation, often preoperatively
         c. Some potential for fistula formation
      2. Chemotherapy
         a. Minimal response at present; cisplatin most promising
   H. Surgical management
      1. Staging
         a. Premalignant lesion—cervical intraepithelial neoplasia (CIN)
            (1) CIN-I: mild dysplasia
            (2) CIN-II: moderate dysplasia (progressive changes)
            (3) CIN-III: severe dysplasia (carcinoma *in situ*)
         b. 0 (in situ)–IV (highly invasive)
      2. Work-up
         a. Complete blood count, liver function tests
         b. Chest x-ray, bone scan, and intravenous pyelogram (IVP)
         c. Cystoscopy for bladder involvement
         d. Sigmoidoscopy, barium enema
         e. Magnetic resonance imaging (MRI)
      3. Biopsy
      4. Prestaging laparotomy done sometimes
      5. Types of surgery
         a. Conization
         b. Hysterectomy—total abdominal hysterectomy with bilateral salpingo-oophorectomy (TAH-BSO)
         c. Radical lymph node dissection
         d. Pelvic exenteration with permanent ileostomy or colostomy and ileal conduit for persistent disease
II. Analysis
   A. Knowledge deficit related to gynecological examination and Pap smear requirements
   B. Knowledge deficit related to diagnostic testing associated with abnormal Pap smear results
   C. Knowledge deficit related to cervical cancer treatment, i.e., surgery or radiation therapy
   D. Body image disturbance related to loss of organs associated with sexual identity
   E. Knowledge deficit related to cervical cancer follow-up treatment
III. Planning/goals, expected outcomes
   A. Client will see physician for regular Pap smears
   B. Client will understand diagnostic tests
   C. Client will be prepared for surgical intervention or radiation therapy
   D. Client will adjust to changes in body image

E. Client will continue follow-up after treatment for cancer

F. Cancer will not recur

IV. Implementation

A. Explain to all female clients importance of scheduling yearly gynecological examinations and of following physician's recommendation on Pap smear schedules

B. Assist client in scheduling and understanding cervical cancer diagnostic test procedures

C. Nursing care of clients undergoing radiation therapy or surgery

  1. Radiation
    a. Internal
      (1) Implant usually in place for 48 to 72 hours
      (2) Client must move minimally to prevent overexposure of bladder or rectum to implant
        (a) Rectovaginal and vesicovaginal fistulas may occur
        (b) Enemas pre-insertion to empty rectum
        (c) Foley catheter to decompress bladder
        (d) Low-residue diet to prevent bowel movement during insertion
        (e) Raise head of bed no more than 10 degrees
      (3) Private room and limited visitors
      (4) Have lead-lined container and long-handled forceps available
      (5) Wear radiation badge to measure amount of exposure
    b. External, may be done preoperatively or postoperatively

  2. Surgery
    a. Preoperatively
      (1) Psychosocial support for tests and surgery
      (2) Preparation for surgically induced menopause
      (3) Routine preoperative preparation plus enemas and vaginal cleansing douche
    b. Postoperatively
      (1) Abdominal distention common after hysterectomy
        (a) Avoid codeine
        (b) Ambulate
      (2) Bladder function monitored carefully
      (3) Antiembolic hose to decrease lower extremity lymphedema
      (4) Monitor closely for phlebitis

  3. Recurrence
    a. Need for follow-up appointments
    b. Monitor for occurrence of fistulas

V. Evaluation

A. Client maintains regular gynecological examination and Pap smear appointments

B. Client completes diagnostic testing

C. Client recovers from surgery without complications

D. Client recovers from radiation therapy without complications

E. Client accepts altered body image

F. Client adjusts to surgical menopause without complications

G. Client continues follow-up visits

H. Client free from recurrence

Uterine Disorders

Prolapse With or Without Cystocele or Rectocele

I. Assessment

A. Definition/pathophysiology

  1. *Prolapse*—downward displacement of uterus through the vaginal canal
    a. First degree—uterus appears at vaginal opening
    b. Second degree—cervix protrudes through vaginal opening
    c. Third degree—entire uterus outside vagina
  2. *Cystocele*—downward displacement of bladder toward vaginal orifice
  3. *Rectocele*—upward displacement of rectum into posterior vaginal wall

B. Predisposing/precipitating factors
  1. Multiparity
  2. Lacerations of perineum postpartum
  3. Aging with weakening of vaginal muscles

C. Clinical manifestations
  1. Incontinence of urine or feces
  2. Urgency
  3. Constipation or retention
  4. Heaviness in perineal area
  5. Sacral back pain, especially at the end of the day

D. Diagnostic examination: physical examination and presence of weakness

E. Complications
  1. Incontinence
  2. Cervical erosion
  3. Urinary tract infections

F. Medical management: conservative therapy, use of pessary to keep pelvic organs in proper alignment

G. Surgical management
  1. Anterior colporrhaphy for cystocele
  2. Posterior colporrhaphy for rectocele
  3. Vaginal hysterectomy

II. Analysis
  A. Anxiety related to alteration in bowel or bladder elimination
  B. Knowledge deficit related to precipitating factors, treatment, and surgery (if indicated)
  C. Body image disturbance related to displacement of uterus

III. Planning/goals, expected outcomes
  A. Client will understand reasons for elimination changes and maintain adequate bowel and bladder elimination
  B. Client will understand precipitating factors, treatment, and surgery (if indicated) as evidenced by compliance with exercises, prosthesis use following treatment plan as indicated
  C. Client will accept condition as common and benign

IV. Implementation
  A. Assure client that condition is common and benign
  B. Help client learn to properly fit pessary and to wear it
  C. Teach perineal exercises if prolapse mild to prevent severe symptoms
  D. Preoperative care
    1. Cleansing douche and enemas
    2. Provide necessary sexual counseling
  E. Postoperative care
    1. Monitor bowel and bladder function carefully
      a. Prevent pressure on suture line
      b. Prevent infection from urinary catheter
    2. Maintain bedrest as ordered
    3. Apply heat lamp to dry incision as ordered
    4. Clean well after bowel movements or urination
    5. Teach perineal exercises to strengthen muscles and prevent recurrence
    6. Utilize mineral oil and stool softeners as ordered
    7. Use antiembolic hose and exercises to prevent thrombophlebitis

V. Evaluation
  A. Client maintains adequate bowel or bladder function without surgery
  B. Client uses pessary or perineal exercises as indicated
  C. Client recovers from surgery without complications
  D. Client returns to normal bowel and bladder elimination

E. Condition does not recur

Endometrial Cancer

I. Assessment
  A. Incidence
    1. Most common genital malignancy
    2. Incidence has increased over the past 20 years
    3. Postmenopausal disorder
  B. Predisposing/precipitating factors
    1. Obesity
    2. Nulliparity
    3. Late menopause
    4. Hypertension and diabetes
    5. History of breast or ovarian cancer
    6. Infertility
    7. Irregular menses
    8. Prolonged use of unopposed exogenous estrogen
  C. Clinical manifestations
    1. Postmenopausal bleeding
    2. Unusual heavy or irregular flow in a premenopausal woman
    3. Yellow or serosanguineous vaginal drainage
    4. Lumbosacral or pelvic pain
  D. Diagnostic examinations
    1. Pelvic examination
    2. Pap smear positive only about 50% of the time
    3. Endometrial biopsy
    4. Fractional dilation and curettage (D & C)
    5. Blood studies, chest x-ray, and IVP
    6. Cystoscopy and proctoscopy to check for spread
  E. Complications
    1. Lung metastasis
    2. Liver metastasis
    3. Peritoneal cavity metastasis
    4. Bone metastasis
  F. Medical management
    1. Hormonal manipulation
    2. Chemotherapy used to improve survival
  G. Surgical management: radical hysterectomy and lymph node dissection

II. Analysis
  A. Knowledge deficit related to risk factors, diagnostic testing, endometrial cancer treatment; i.e., radiation therapy or surgery
  B. Body image disturbance related to loss of organs associated with sexual identity and reproductive function

III. Planning/goals, expected outcomes
  A. Client will understand risk factors and seek treatment when appropriate; understand need for diagnostic testing and cancer treatment as

indicated by completion of tests and participation in treatment; and be prepared for surgery or radiation therapy, evidenced by recovery without complications
  B. Client will maintain a healthy body image, as evidenced by the continuation of normal sexual relations
IV. Implementation
  A. Explain risk factors
  B. Explain diagnostic test purpose and procedures
  C. Teach client about treatment options
  D. Preoperative and postoperative care (see cervical cancer section)
  E. Radiation therapy care (see cervical cancer section)
V. Evaluation
  A. Client recovers from surgery without complications
  B. Client complies with follow-up care
  C. Cancer does not recur
  D. Client and significant others cope with altered body image

Ovarian Cancer

I. Assessment
  A. Definition/pathophysiology: usually epithelial tumor
  B. Incidence
    1. Leading cause of death from gynecologic cancer
    2. Represents 25% of all gynecologic cancers in United States
  C. Predisposing/precipitating factors
    1. Risk increases with age
    2. Late menopause
    3. Nulliparity
    4. Caucasian race
    5. May be familial link in some families
    6. History of breast or colon cancer
    7. Living in an industrialized country
  D. Clinical manifestations
    1. Early disease often asymptomatic or presents with vague abdominal or pelvic discomfort/pressure
    2. Palpable ovary in postmenopausal woman
    3. Urinary frequency
    4. Increasing abdominal girth
  E. Diagnostic examinations
    1. Pelvic examination
    2. Vaginal ultrasound or computed tomography (CT) scan—determine pelvic mass or ovarian status
    3. Barium enema, proctoscopy—determine presence of gastrointestinal metastasis

    4. Tumor marker, CA 125 blood level
    5. Chest x-ray—determine presence of lung metastasis
  F. Prognosis
    1. Poor because tumor usually detected late in stage III or IV
    2. Good prognosis for stage I
  G. Complications
    1. Bowel obstruction
    2. Peritoneal cavity metastasis
    3. Liver metastasis
    4. Lung metastasis
  H. Medical management
    1. Adjuvant chemotherapy—cisplatin or carboplatin most active
    2. External beam pelvic irradiation
  I. Surgical management
    1. Total abdominal hysterectomy/bilateral salpingo-oophorectomy, omentectomy
    2. Surgical tumor debulking
II. Analysis
  A. Knowledge deficit related to disease process, diagnostic tests, and treatment; i.e., surgery, chemotherapy, or radiation therapy
  B. Anxiety related to ovarian cancer diagnosis
  C. Body image disturbance related to loss of organs associated with sexual/reproductive function
  D. Anticipatory grieving related to poor prognosis
III. Planning/goals, expected outcomes
  A. Client will understand disease process, diagnostic tests, and treatment as evidenced by client's ability to follow the diagnostic and treatment regimen
  B. Client will discuss feelings about alterations in life related to cancer diagnosis
  C. Client will maintain a healthy body image as evidenced by the continuation of a normal sexual relationship
  D. Client will cope with poor prognosis by discussing feelings with family and significant other
IV. Implementation
  A. Explain and help schedule diagnostic tests
  B. Surgery (see cervical cancer section)
  C. Chemotherapy (see Chapter 6, chemotherapy)
  D. Radiation therapy (see Chapter 6, radiation therapy)
  E. Discuss client's feelings related to sexual function
  F. Be available to client and family to discuss feelings of grief and loss concerning the disease and poor prognosis
V. Evaluation
  A. Client completes diagnostic work-up

B. Client recovers from surgery without complications

C. Client completes chemotherapy or radiation therapy with minimal side effects

D. Client and family accept the serious prognosis associated with ovarian cancer

Menopause

I. Assessment

A. Definition: menopause is physiological cessation of menses due to ending of ovarian function, end of biological reproductivity; climacteric is transition period during which reproductive function gradually diminishes and eventually ceases

B. Physiology

1. Occurs naturally, sometime between mid-forties and mid-fifties, plus or minus a few years

2. Ovarian function diminishes

a. Menstruation ceases

b. Reproductive organs and mammary glands atrophy

c. No further ova produced

d. Estrogen levels drop

3. Complex physiological and psychological process related to normal aging

C. Clinical manifestations

1. Decreased estrogen levels

a. Menses decreases, becomes irregular, finally stops

b. Vascular disturbances such as hot flashes occur

c. Atrophic changes

(1) Stress incontinence

(2) Senile vaginitis

(3) Dry skin

d. Weight gain

e. Osteoporosis

f. Increased risk for cardiovascular disease

2. Psychological effects

a. Normal sexual urges remain

b. May be seen as end of "womanhood"

c. May be welcome relief to burden of reproductivity and menstruation

d. Often vague symptoms such as dizziness, headaches, insomnia, nervousness

D. Medical management

1. Hormone replacement therapy (HRT), low-dose estrogen in conjunction with progesterone (Table 3–3)

2. Patient education

TABLE 3–3 Hormone Replacement Therapy

Sequential Method
Conjugated estrogen 0.625 mg days 1–25
Medroxyprogesterone acetate 5–10 mg days 15–25
Monthly withdrawal bleeding is experienced with the sequential method

Continuous Method
Conjugated estrogen 0.625 mg daily
Medroxyprogesterone acetate 2.5 mg daily
The 0.625-mg estrogen dosage appears to be the lowest dosage effective in preventing osteoporosis
Progestin is added to reduce the incidence of endometrial hyperplasia and endometrial carcinoma. Progestin is not required if the woman does not have a uterus

Side Effects of Hormone Replacement Therapy
Nausea
Abdominal bleeding
Monthly withdrawal bleeding
Fluid retention
Breast tenderness
Gallstones

II. Analysis

A. Knowledge deficit related to physiological and psychological changes and appropriate health measures required

B. Anxiety related to menopausal physiological and psychological changes

III. Planning/goals, expected outcomes

A. Client will understand physiological and psychological changes associated with menopause

B. Client will cope with changes produced by menopause

C. Client will practice health measures designed to reduce changes associated with menopause

IV. Implementation

A. Teach use and side effects of hormone replacement therapy (see Table 3–3)

B. Encourage client to express feelings associated with life changes

C. Teach client to follow nutritious low-fat diet to control possible weight gain and risk of cardiovascular disease

D. Encourage routine exercise to maintain vitality and decrease osteoporosis risk

E. Encourage client that sexual function remains normal

F. Encourage the use of oils or lotion for dry skin and lubricants for vaginal atrophy

G. Encourage yearly physical examinations

V. Evaluation

A. Client copes effectively with the climacteric period

B. Client verbalizes understanding of physiological and psychological changes of menopause

C. Client maintains healthy lifestyle

Breast Cancer

I. Assessment
   A. Incidence
      1. Increases with age
      2. Lowest in Japanese women in Japan
      3. Highest in Jewish women of European descent
   B. Predisposing/precipitating factors
      1. Lowest risk
         a. Women with multiple pregnancies or those whose first child born before age 30
         b. Early artificial menopause
      2. Highest risk
         a. Female gender
         b. Family history, first-degree relative: mother/sister
         c. Early menarche, late menopause
         d. Previous cancer of breast, endometrium, or ovary
         e. Nulliparity
         f. Obesity, diet high in fat (controversial)
         g. High-dose radiation exposure to the chest
   C. Clinical manifestations
      1. Usually found in upper outer quadrant or beneath nipple
      2. Fixed, irregular, nonencapsulated mass
      3. Painless mass except in very late stages
      4. Nipple retraction or elevation
      5. Bloody or clear nipple discharge
      6. Skin dimpling or retraction
      7. Skin edema or peau d'orange
      8. Ulceration
      9. Lymphadenopathy, usually axillary
      10. Lymphedema of affected arm
      11. Symptoms of bone or lung metastasis
   D. Diagnostic examinations
      1. Screening
         a. Breast examination part of annual physical examination
         b. Monthly self-examination of breast
      2. History and physical examination
      3. Mammography
         a. Baseline between ages of 35 and 40
         b. Every 1 to 2 years between ages 40 and 50, yearly for high-risk women
         c. Yearly after age 50
      4. Biopsy: aspiration, needle, incisional, or excisional
      5. Hormone receptor assay: estrogen and progesterone
      6. Staging
         a. Bone, lung, and liver scans
         b. Serum enzymes for bone and liver metastasis
         c. Carcinoembryonic antigen (CEA) and CA 15-3 as tumor markers
         d. Cellular kinetics
   E. Prognosis
      1. Unpredictable, because spread through both lymph and blood
      2. Stages 1 and 2 very treatable, but even later stages often amenable to hormonal manipulation
      3. Better for women with estrogen receptor–positive nodes
      4. Poorer with aneuploid tumors with high S-phase
   F. Complications
      1. Bone metastasis
      2. Spinal cord compression
      3. Brain metastasis and meningeal involvement
      4. Chronic lymphedema
   G. Medical management
      1. Chemotherapy (see Table 6–7)
      2. Radiation therapy
      3. Hormonal manipulation
         a. Estrogen in postmenopausal women
         b. Tamoxifen for estrogen receptor–positive tumors
         c. Oophorectomy for estrogen receptor–positive tumors, although now being replaced with tamoxifen therapy
         d. Ablative therapy
            (1) Adrenalectomy or chemical ablation with aminoglutethimide (Cytadren), which blocks the production of cortisol, androstenedione, and aldosterone
            (2) Hypophysectomy (seldom done)
   H. Surgical management
      1. Surgery (all with axillary node dissections)
         a. Excisional biopsy
         b. Lumpectomy
         c. Wedge resection
         d. Simple mastectomy
         e. Modified radical mastectomy
      2. Reconstructive surgery post-mastectomy
II. Analysis
   A. Knowledge deficit related to screening methods, diagnostic testing, treatment options, and breast reconstruction options
   B. Knowledge deficit related to treatment; i.e., surgery, radiation therapy, or chemotherapy
   C. Body image disturbance related to loss of organ associated with sexual identity
   D. Anxiety related to diagnosis of cancer
   E. Impaired physical mobility; arm, related to lymphedema
   F. Anticipatory grieving related to terminal prognosis

III. Planning/goals, expected outcomes
   A. Client will utilize recommended screening techniques for early detection
   B. Client will understand treatment options
   C. Client will recover from surgery without complications
   D. Client will accept body image changes
   E. Lymphedema will not develop
   F. Client will not suffer long-term impairment of arm function
   G. Client will understand and comply with chemotherapy, radiation therapy, or hormonal manipulation
   H. Client will obtain breast reconstruction if desired
   I. Client and significant other will cope with cancer diagnosis
   J. Client will cope with terminal prognosis
IV. Implementation
   A. Preoperative
      1. Help client explore available options
      2. Support beginning grieving process
   B. Postoperatively
      1. Hemovac care
      2. Position with affected arm above heart to promote drainage
      3. Exercises to decrease lymphedema or muscle weakness
         a. Immediately begin using affected hand and forearm
         b. With doctor's order, start stretching upper arm and shoulder

TABLE 3–4 Hand and Arm Care after Mastectomy with Axillary Node Dissection

DO'S

Protect affected hand and arm.
Wear gloves when gardening or cleaning.
Always use oven mitts when cooking.
Use a thimble when sewing.
Apply lanolin hand cream several times daily.
Use cream cuticle remover.
See doctor if any signs of inflammation occur in the affected arm.
Wear a Medic-Alert tag stating lymphedema arm.
Avoid strong sunlight.

DON'TS

Don't allow temperature extremes.
Don't let arm hang dependent.
Don't carry pocketbook or anything heavy.
Don't hold a cigarette in affected hand.
Don't allow any trauma, cuts, bruises, or burns.
No tourniquets or injections, no blood pressure readings or tests in the affected arm.
Don't pick nails or cuticles.
Don't wear any constrictive clothes or jewelry on affected side.

   c. Avoid overuse of arm first 2 months
   4. To prevent lymphedema, after axillary node dissection
      a. Short term
         (1) Keep affected arm elevated
         (2) Provide sign above bed: "No IVs, no IMs, no BPs; lymphedema arm"
      b. Discharge teaching (Table 3–4)
      c. Use of pressure sleeve if edema is severe
      d. Diuretics and low-salt diet for severe edema
   5. Encourage use of prosthesis
      a. Immediate, "Reach for Recovery"
      b. Permanent, after further treatment completed
         (1) Surgical, reconstruction
         (2) Nonsurgical
   6. Teach incision care with lanolin to soften skin and prevent wound contracture
   7. Encourage use of the "Reach for Recovery" volunteers
   8. Prepare client for delayed grieving 3 to 6 months postoperatively
   9. Encourage client to perform self-examination of the remaining breast
   10. Teach female family members about early detection
V. Evaluation
   A. Client practices breast screening
   B. Client's breast cancer detected early
   C. Client adequately prepared for surgery
   D. Client and significant others cope with altered body image
   E. Client recovers from surgery without complications
   F. Lymphedema does not develop or is controlled
   G. Client complies with follow-up therapy
   H. Client and significant others cope with cancer diagnosis
   I. Client and significant others cope with terminal prognosis

POST-TEST Female Reproductive Disorders

1. Prolapse of the uterus outside of the vaginal orifice is termed:
   ① Cystocele
   ② Rectocele
   ③ Third-degree prolapse
   ④ Vesico-vaginal fistula

2. Common risk factors for prolapse would include all of the following EXCEPT:
   ① Multiparity
   ② Postpartum lacerations
   ③ Chronic constipation
   ④ Aging

3. Which of the following is a curative procedure to treat prolapse?
   ① A vaginal hysterectomy and an anterior and posterior repair
   ② Insertion of a pessary
   ③ An anterior colporrhaphy
   ④ A posterior colporrhaphy

4. Which of the following is a risk factor for endometrial/uterine cancer?
   ① Malnutrition
   ② Multiparity
   ③ History of breast cancer
   ④ Early menopause

5. Which of the following is NOT a common symptom of uterine cancer?
   ① Postmenopausal bleeding
   ② Palpable ovary postmenopause
   ③ Irregular flow in premenopausal women
   ④ History of infertility

6. The major diagnostic test to confirm the presence of uterine cancer is:
   ① Pap smear
   ② Cystoscopy
   ③ Fractional D & C
   ④ Proctoscopy

7. Ovarian cancer is the leading cause of death from gynecological malignancy because:
   ① There is no known treatment
   ② There is a high mortality rate from surgery
   ③ There are few early symptoms
   ④ Ovarian cancer is the most common gynecological malignancy

---

Ann Grant is a 50-year-old woman who has a mastectomy because of breast cancer.

---

8. Mrs. Grant returns from surgery with a Hemovac in place. Nursing interventions for the client with a Hemovac include:
   ① Irrigating the tubing as needed
   ② Avoiding emptying the Hemovac
   ③ Preventing kinks in the tubing
   ④ Pinning the Hemovac to the back of the patient's gown

9. In order to decrease the postoperative lymphedema of the affected arm, the client should:
   ① Elevate her arm on pillows above heart level
   ② Keep the arm fixed at her side
   ③ Apply a warm pad over the affected arm
   ④ Use only the unaffected arm for all activities

10. On the first postoperative day, the nurse recommends that Mrs. Grant begin arm exercises. The best exercise at this time is:
    ① Abducting the affected arm and flexing the elbow
    ② "Wall walking" exercises every 4 hours
    ③ Using a rope pulley to extend her shoulder
    ④ Washing her face with the affected arm

11. Mrs. Grant seems depressed about her loss at times and happy about the positive outcome of her surgery at other times. The nurse realizes that:
    ① Mrs. Grant is neurotic and should see the social worker
    ② Clients often need time to adjust to this loss
    ③ Mrs. Grant is simply vain and needs to see a cosmetician
    ④ Clients often need some time alone after a loss like this

12. Mrs. Grant asks if she still has to do a monthly self-examination of her breast. Your best response would be:
    ① Yes, the cancer is likely to spread to the other breast
    ② No, there is no further risk of breast cancer
    ③ No, the doctor will do it every three months
    ④ Yes, there is an increased risk of a new cancer in the other breast

POST-TEST Answers and Rationales

1. ③ The correct term is third-degree prolapse. A cystocele occurs when the bladder prolapses through the anterior vaginal wall and a rectocele occurs when the rectum prolapses through the posterior vaginal wall. A fistula is an abnormal opening between two cavities. 1, IV. Uterine Prolapse.

2. ③ Having many children, especially with postpartum lacerations of the perineum, is a major risk factor for prolapse, as is aging with the accompanying muscle weakness. Chronic constipation does not directly cause prolapse. 1, IV. Uterine Prolapse.

3. ① The only way to cure a prolapse is with a hysterectomy, usually a vaginal approach. It is often necessary to do an anterior and posterior repair at the same time. A pessary is only a temporary palliative treatment for less severe prolapses. 4, IV. Uterine Prolapse.

4. ③ One of the major risk factors for endometrial uterine cancer is a previous history of breast cancer. Other risk factors are obesity, no children, and possibly exogenous estrogen. 1, IV. Uterine Cancer.

5. ② A palpable ovary postmenopause is a sign of ovarian cancer, not uterine cancer. The other options are all common symptoms of uterine cancer. 1, IV. Uterine Cancer.

6. ③ Uterine cancer can be diagnosed only by obtaining endometrial tissue. A fractional D & C provides this tissue. A Pap smear is positive only about 50% of the time in the presence of uterine cancer. A cystoscopy and proctoscopy are done to check for possible spread of the cancer. 2, II & IV. Uterine Cancer.

7. ③ Ovarian cancer has few early symptoms. The early symptoms are vague and nonspecific gastrointestinal complaints. Treatment involves surgery, chemotherapy, and radiation therapy. The surgery (TAH-BSO, omentectomy) carries a low mortality rate. Endometrial cancer is the most common gynecologic malignancy. 1, II. Ovarian Cancer.

8. ③ It is important for the Hemovac tubing to be able to drain freely without obstruction. The tubing should not be irrigated and must be emptied regularly. Pinning the Hemovac to the back of the patient's gown could interfere with expansion of the Hemovac. 4, II & IV. Breast Cancer.

9. ① Lymphedema is more likely to occur when the limb is dependent. Keeping the arm above the level of the heart will facilitate lymphatic drainage. Keeping the arm fixed at the side will only decrease mobility, as will using only the unaffected arm. It is potentially dangerous to apply heat to the arm. 4, II & IV. Breast Cancer.

10. ④ Washing her face will allow movement from the elbow down without disturbing the axilla. The other options require movement of the axilla, exercises that require a doctor's order, and are not done until more healing has occurred. 4, II & IV. Breast Cancer.

11. ② It is normal to experience a feeling of ambivalence after a mastectomy, a sense of loss and happiness. The grieving process usually takes months to resolve. She does not need to be alone, but needs to know that what she is going through is normal. 2, II & IV. Breast Cancer.

12. ④ It is even more important that the client do a self-examination of the breast after a mastectomy because there is about a 25% risk that she will develop a second primary in the contralateral breast. 4, II & IV. Breast Cancer.

PRE-TEST Male Reproductive Disorders

1. Testicular cancer is an age-limited cancer. It occurs between what ages?
   ① 10 to 30 years
   ② 20 to 40 years
   ③ 30 to 50 years
   ④ 40 to 60 years

2. Which of the following is NOT a risk factor for testicular cancer?
   ① Cryptorchidism
   ② Use of birth control pills after pregnancy begins
   ③ Use of diethylstilbestrol (DES) by pregnant mother to prevent miscarriage
   ④ Decreased testosterone levels after puberty

3. The major symptom of testicular cancer is:
   ① Painful scrotal enlargement
   ② Painless testicular swelling
   ③ Pain and swelling along epididymis
   ④ Enlarged groin lymph nodes

Mr. Anthony is admitted for a suprapubic prostatectomy.

---

4. Which of the following is a priority postoperative nursing implementation?
   ① Irrigating the Foley catheter
   ② Changing the dressings
   ③ Measuring the output
   ④ Administering pain medication
5. Which of the following is the most common long-term complication that could occur after a suprapubic prostatectomy?
   ① Bladder neck strictures
   ② Osteitis pubis
   ③ Continued bladder spasms
   ④ Urinary fistula
6. Four days postoperatively, Mr. Anthony goes to the bathroom and has a bowel movement. When he returns to bed, you notice the urine in the catheter tubing has become dark red. Which of the following is the most appropriate nursing intervention?
   ① Check him again in 15 minutes
   ② Call the doctor
   ③ Irrigate the catheter
   ④ Restart the constant bladder irrigation
7. Nitrofurantoin (Macrodantin) is commonly used to treat urinary tract infections. Which of the following best describes the action of this drug?
   ① Urinary antiseptic
   ② Urinary antibiotic
   ③ Urinary analgesic
   ④ Sulfonamide
8. Anticholinergics such as propantheline bromide (Pro-Banthine) are used to treat which urinary problem?
   ① Incontinence
   ② Retention
   ③ Infection
   ④ Spasms

Arnold Gold is a 67-year-old man admitted for prostatic cancer.

---

9. Which of the following diagnostic tests is a good example of effective secondary prevention for prostatic cancer?
   ① Serum acid phosphatase level
   ② Yearly cystoscopy
   ③ Yearly digital rectal exam
   ④ Serum alkaline phosphatase level
10. Mr. Gold undergoes a perineal prostatectomy. Postoperatively, which of the following interventions would be CONTRAINDICATED?
    ① Administering rectal suppository for constipation
    ② Leaving the Foley catheter in for 10 days
    ③ Providing a warm sitz bath after the sutures are out
    ④ Teaching him perineal exercises
11. Which of the following is NOT a likely follow-up treatment if his cancer has spread?
    ① Bilateral orchiectomy
    ② Radiation therapy
    ③ A radical lymph node dissection
    ④ Diethylstilbestrol (DES)
12. Which of the following outcomes is important and realistic for Mr. Gold after his surgery?
    ① Client regains normal urinary control
    ② Client copes with impotency
    ③ Client regains normal bowel function
    ④ Client adjusts to lower extremity lymphedema
13. The client asks you why he is having a vasectomy after his prostatectomy. The rationale for this is to prevent:
    ① Impotence
    ② Retrograde ejaculation
    ③ Epididymitis
    ④ Prostatitis

PRE-TEST Answers and Rationales

1. ② Testicular cancer is limited to young men between 20 and 40. It is very uncommon outside this age range. 1, IV. Testicular Cancer.

2. ④ Risk factors for testicular cancer include undescended testicles, the use of birth control pills after pregnancy begins, and DES during pregnancy. Testosterone levels do not pose a specific risk factor. 1, IV. Testicular Cancer.

3. ② Painless swelling of the testicles and a dragging sensation in the scrotum are the main symptoms of testicular cancer. The other options are not symptoms. 1, IV. Testicular Cancer.

4. ② A suprapubic prostatectomy requires a large incision into the bladder, resulting in large amounts of urinary drainage and frequent dressing changes. The other options are interventions that will be done, but none have the priority of the dressing changes because of the potential infection and need to measure urine output. 4, II & IV. Prostatectomy.

5. ④ Because there is an incision into the bladder with urinary drainage, there is a risk of fistula development if the wound does not heal properly. None of the other options are appropriate for this surgery. 5, I & IV. Prostatectomy.

6. ① It is normal for some bleeding to occur after the first bowel movement, because the rectum and prostatic capsule are in such close proximity. The best answer is to simply check him in 15 minutes to make sure no new bleeding has occurred. The nurse should also teach the client not to strain at a bowel movement. 4, I & IV. Prostatectomy.

7. ① Macrodantin is classified as a urinary antiseptic that reduces the bacteria in the urinary tract. It is good for chronic usage. 2, II. Urinary Tract Infections.

8. ④ The best treatment for bladder spasms is an anticholinergic such as propantheline bromide. It would increase retention and not affect continence or infection. 4, II. Urinary Tract Infections.

9. ③ Secondary prevention for prostatic cancer is a yearly digital rectal examination, which can detect both BPH and prostatic cancer. The cancer appears as a hard nodule in the posterior lobe of the prostate. The acid and alkaline phosphatase and cystoscopy are used to check for spread of the cancer. 4, IV. Prostatic Cancer.

10. ① Anything rectally can cause severe problems because of the proximity of the rectum and prostate. The Foley catheter is left in longer to help healing, and the sitz bath helps both healing and discomfort. The perineal exercises are important for the client to regain urinary control. 4, II & IV. Prostatic Cancer.

11. ③ A radical lymph node dissection is not done to treat prostate cancer, because the lymph nodes are not the common route of spread. The other options are treatments used to treat metastatic prostate cancer. 5, IV. Prostatic Cancer.

12. ② After a perineal prostatectomy, the client will be impotent and have some degree of incontinence. Altered bowel function and lymphedema are inappropriate for this surgery. 5, IV. Prostatic Cancer.

13. ③ Epididymitis is usually caused by a retrograde infection migrating from the urethra or prostate. A prostatectomy increases the risk of organisms being introduced and migrating to the epididymis. Impotence will not occur, and the client will experience sterility and retrograde ejaculation after the surgery. Prostatitis cannot occur after removal of the gland. 1, II. Epididymitis.

NURSING PROCESS APPLIED TO MALE REPRODUCTIVE DISORDERS

Testicular Cancer

I. Assessment
  A. Definition/pathophysiology
    1. Cancers arising from germinal epithelium
    2. Two major histological types
      a. Seminomas
        (1) About 40% of tumors
        (2) Spread slowly, through lymphatics
        (3) Responsive to radiation therapy
      b. Nonseminomas (embryonal, teratoma, interstitial cell, and gonadal stroma)
        (1) Invades spermatic cord and spreads to lungs
        (2) More sensitive to chemotherapy
  B. Etiology: exact cause not known
  C. Incidence: Most common solid tumor in men between 29 and 35
    1. Increasing incidence in white men
    2. Occurs between ages of 20 to 40
  D. Predisposing/precipitating factors
    1. Cryptorchidism—undescended testicles
    2. Exogenous estrogens
    3. Birth control pills after conception
    4. Diethylstilbestrol (DES) to prevent spontaneous abortions
  E. Clinical manifestations
    1. Early
      a. Painless testicular swelling
      b. Dragging sensation in the scrotum
      c. Gynecomastia
      d. Infertility
    2. Late
      a. Back or bone pain
      b. Respiratory symptoms
  F. Diagnostic examinations
    1. Transillumination of the testis
    2. Intravenous pyelogram (IVP)
    3. Abdominal and lung scans, MRI
    4. Blood studies
      a. Serum alpha-fetoprotein
      b. Serum beta human chorionic gonadotropin
    5. Lymphangiogram—injection of dye into small lymph vessels on tops of both feet (done less with the advent of MRI)
      a. Pre-test: warn client that test is long and painful
      b. Post-test
        (1) Monitor for swelling
        (2) Warn client that blue discoloration will remain
  G. Complications: lung, liver, bone, and adrenal metastases

  H. Medical management
    1. Radiation therapy for seminomas for cure
    2. Chemotherapy postoperatively for cure with cisplatin, vinblastine, bleomycin, etoposide, ifosfamide, and doxorubicin (see Table 6–6)
  I. Surgical management: high radical inguinal orchiectomy as biopsy and cure
    1. May have radical retroperitoneal lymph node dissection on affected side
    2. Resection of single metastatic lesion of lung, liver, or retroperitoneum
  J. Prognosis
    1. Improved survival over last 10 years
    2. Now considered curable in about 95% of all cases
    3. Recurrence usually occurs within first 2 years; recurrence responds to further treatment
II. Analysis
  A. Knowledge deficit related to lack of understanding for need for testicular self-examination (TSE)
  B. Knowledge deficit related to diagnosis and treatment for testicular cancer
  C. High risk for altered body image related to removal of testicle
  D. High risk for sexual dysfunction related to removal of testicle and possible impotence secondary to radical retroperitoneal lymph node dissection
III. Planning/goals, expected outcomes
  A. Client will practice routine testicular self-examination and find testicular tumors early
  B. Client will be physically and psychologically prepared for surgery, radiation therapy, or chemotherapy
  C. Client will cope with altered body image
  D. Client will adapt to altered sexuality and learn alternate methods of sexual gratification
IV. Implementation
  A. Teach young men how to examine testicles monthly
  B. Assist client in expressing fears associated with orchiectomy
  C. Care after radical retroperitoneal lymph node dissection same as after any major abdominal surgery
  D. Care for client receiving radiation therapy (see Chapter 6, Radiation Therapy)
  E. Care for client receiving chemotherapy (see Chapter 6, Chemotherapy)
    1. Maintain nutritional status
      a. Control nausea and vomiting from cisplatin (see Table 6–8)
  F. Provide sexual counseling as needed
    1. Treatment may affect fertility and ejacula-

tory capacity, but client should be able to achieve erection
  2. Encourage testicular implants if bilateral orchiectomy was done
V. Evaluation
  A. Client correctly practices testicular self-examination and discovers testicular cancer early
  B. Client recovers from surgery without complications
  C. Client complies with follow-up radiation therapy and chemotherapy
  D. Client and significant others cope with altered body image and sexuality

Benign Prostatic Hypertrophy (BPH)

I. Assessment
  A. Definition/pathophysiology: hypertrophy and hyperplasia of the normal prostatic tissue
  B. Etiology
    1. Exact cause of BPH not known
    2. Factors such as diet, effects of chronic inflammation, socioeconomic factors, heredity, and race have all been considered without definite conclusion
    3. Hormonal alteration probably responsible: testicular androgen seems most common hormone suspected
  C. Incidence
    1. Occurs in 50% of men over 50
    2. Increases to more than 75% in men over 80
    3. More common in Caucasian men
  D. Clinical manifestations
    1. Urinary symptoms
      a. Urgency
      b. Frequency
      c. Hesitancy
      d. Changes in the size and force of stream
      e. Infection
      f. Retention
      g. Dribbling
      h. Nocturia
    2. Enlarged prostate on digital rectal examination
  E. Diagnostic examinations
    1. Prostate easily palpated on rectal examination; smooth, diffuse enlargement
    2. Cystoscopy (see Chapter 8, Bladder Cancer)
    3. Blood studies
      a. Prostate-specific antigen to rule out cancer
      b. Acid phosphatase to rule out metastatic cancer

F. Complications
  1. From BPH
    a. Hydroureter
    b. Hydronephrosis
    c. Pyelonephritis
    d. Renal failure
  2. From surgery
    a. Bladder neck strictures after transurethral resection (TUR)
    b. Retrograde ejaculation
    c. Urinary incontinence, most commonly after TUR
    d. Epididymitis
G. Medical management
  1. Decompression bladder drainage for severe distention
  2. Insertion of suprapubic catheter
  3. Medication (Table 3–5)
    a. Androgen-deprivation agents to inhibit prostatic hypertrophy, such as estrogen, cyproterone acetate, or the nonsteroidal veterinary antiandrogen flutamide

TABLE 3–5 Medications Used to Treat Benign Prostatic Hypertrophy (BPH) or Prostatic Cancer

Selected Medications for BPH	Action
Testosterone-ablating agents Diethylstilbestrol (DES) Flutamide (Eulexin) Gonadotropin-releasing hormone (GnRH) analogs Nafarelin acetate (Synarel) Buserelin (Suprefact, investigational) Leuprolide (Lupron) Goserelin acetate (Zoladex) Cyproterone acetate (Androcur)	**Testosterone-ablating agents** decrease the amount of circulating testosterone levels, leading to suppression of prostatic tissue growth. **Estrogens** inhibit prostatic growth by suppressing release of luteinizing hormone–releasing agent, leading to a decrease in testosterone. **Flutamide** is an antiandrogen that competes with testosterone for androgen receptor sites. **GnRH** inhibits the release of pituitary gonadotropin, preventing testosterone biosynthesis. **Cyproterone** is a synthetic antiandrogen that acts as an androgen-receptor inhibitor.
Testosterone-sparing agents Finasteride (Proscar)	A 5-alpha reductase inhibitor that blocks dihydrotestosterone without suppressing circulating testosterone. Decreases prostatic tissue without affecting potency or libido.
Alpha-blocking agents Phenoxybenzamine (Dibenzyline) Terazosin (Hytrin) Prazosin (Minipress)	There is abundant autonomic innervation of the bladder neck and prostatic smooth muscle. Prostatic obstruction is due in part to the neurogenic tone of the bladder neck and prostatic smooth muscle. These agents block the alpha receptors, improving urination by decreasing outlet obstruction.

   b. Testosterone-sparing agents without side effects of estrogens or antitestosterones
   c. Alpha-adrenergic blocking agents used to decrease muscle tone and improve voiding
   H. Surgical management
   1. Prostatectomy (Table 3–6)
      a. TUR
      b. Retropubic prostatectomy
      c. Suprapubic prostatectomy
      d. Balloon dilation
   2. Vasectomy to prevent epididymitis
II. Analysis
   A. Altered patterns of urinary elimination: frequency, urgency, hesitancy, change in stream, incontinence, retention, or nocturia related to urethral obstruction
   B. High risk for disturbance in self-concept related to threats to sexuality from disease and treatment
   C. Pain related to surgery and bladder spasms
   D. Knowledge deficit related to postoperative exercises and return of urinary function
   E. High risk for sexual dysfunction related to removal of prostate, retrograde ejaculation, and sterility
III. Planning/goals, expected outcomes
   A. Client will not develop symptoms of BPH as evidenced by absence of frequency, urgency, hesitancy, change in stream, incontinence, retention, or nocturia
   B. Client will not develop a disturbance in self-concept as evidenced by client's willingness to discuss sexual issues
   C. Client will have pain relieved or controlled as evidenced by client's report
   D. Client will understand postoperative exercises and will have return of normal urinary function
   E. Client will not develop sexual dysfunction as evidenced by client's statements and client's ability to discuss fears and concerns with staff
IV. Implementation
   A. Administer medications to shrink size of prostate as ordered (see Table 3–5)
   B. Preoperatively
   1. Maintain bladder drainage
   2. Apply antiembolic hose
   3. Ensure that client understands implications of surgical approach
   C. Postoperatively
   1. Monitor constant bladder irrigation (CBI), used to decrease bleeding and prevent clots
      a. Use normal saline or physiological solution to prevent water intoxication
      b. Run at rate to keep urine light pink
   2. Monitor for bleeding or clot formation

TABLE 3–6 Comparison of Types of Prostatectomies

Surgical Approach	Clinical Problems	Nursing Implications
Transurethral resection	Lithotomy position; often under spinal anesthesia; low morbidity; no abdominal incision; done through cystoscope; not all gland removed; bleeding common; uses CBI; bladder spasms common; bladder neck strictures may occur; dribbling and incontinence postoperatively; may or may not be sterile	Monitor for hemorrhage; run CBI to keep urine pink; use antispasmodics for bladder spasms; teach perineal exercises for return of control; monitor for recurrence
Suprapubic	Large abdominal incision with bladder incision; severe hemorrhage possible; urinary drainage on abdomen copious; bladder spasms common; CBI to keep urine pink; urinary fistula possible; longer healing; sterility occurs	Change abdominal dressing frequently using sterile technique; monitor blood loss; use antispasmodics for spasms; maintain patency of Foley catheter; teach perineal exercises
Retropubic	Abdominal incision without opening bladder; bleeding more controlled; low mortality rate; osteitis pubis possible; few spasms; minimal abdominal drainage; may use CBI; may be used for cancer; sterility occurs	Monitor for bleeding; teach perineal exercises to regain control; maintain patency of Foley catheter
Perineal	Perineal incision in lithotomy; used for cancer only; little bleeding; causes sterility and impotency; urinary incontinence common; increased risk of infection	Avoid rectal tubes, thermometers, enemas; monitor for infection; provide sexual counseling; teach perineal exercises

CBI—Continuous bladder irrigation.

3. Maintain patency of Foley catheter
4. Use antispasmodics for bladder spasms
5. Teach client perineal exercises to improve bladder control
6. Maintain traction on Foley catheter to decrease bleeding
7. Provide stool softeners to prevent rectal straining and bleeding
8. Obtain serial urine samples after Foley catheter is removed to monitor bleeding
9. Increase fluid intake
10. Teach client to watch for bleeding about 2 weeks after TUR

V. Evaluation
  A. Client does not develop symptoms of BPH
  B. Client does not develop a disturbance in self-concept
  C. Client has pain relieved or controlled
  D. Client understands and practices postoperative exercises and normal urinary function returns
  E. Client does not develop sexual dysfunction

Cancer of the Prostate

I. Assessment
  A. Definition/pathophysiology
    1. Primarily adenocarcinoma
    2. More common in posterior lobe
    3. Spreads through blood stream and lymphatics
  B. Etiology: exact cause of prostate cancer not known
  C. Incidence
    1. More common in African-Americans than in Caucasians
    2. Most common cancer of the reproductive/urinary tract in men and the third leading cause of death among men in the United States
    3. Man's risk of prostatic cancer increases with each decade after age 50
    4. Young men seem to have more aggressive disease and more likely to have metastasis at time of diagnosis
    5. Japanese-Americans have the lowest incidence
  D. Predisposing/precipitating factors
    1. Exposure to cadmium
    2. Viral link
    3. May have hormonal basis; is testosterone dependent
  E. Clinical manifestations
    1. Asymptomatic in early stages: hard, pea-size nodule in posterior lobe of prostate palpated on rectal examination

2. Later symptoms
  a. Weight loss
  b. Back pain
3. Symptoms of BPH often at same time
4. Hematuria
F. Diagnostic examinations
  1. Digital rectal examination
  2. Transrectal ultrasound
  3. Needle biopsy or through TUR
  4. Blood studies
    a. Prostate-specific antigen (PSA)
    b. Acid phosphatase for spread
    c. Alkaline phosphatase for bone metastases
  5. IVP and cystoscopy
G. Complications: bone metastases
H. Medical management
  1. Radiation therapy to prostate and bony metastasis
    a. External
    b. Internal
  2. Castration
    a. Bilateral orchiectomy
    b. Diethylstilbestrol (DES) (see Table 3–5)
    c. Aminoglutethimide to destroy adrenal androgen function
  3. Hormonal manipulation (see Table 3–5)
    a. Estrogen therapy
    b. Antiandrogens
    c. Gonadotropin-releasing factors
  4. Chemotherapy in hormone-resistant tumors
I. Surgical management
  1. Radical perineal or retropubic prostatectomy for cure
  2. TUR for palliation
J. Prognosis
  1. In early stages, 85% 5-year survival
  2. Survival may approximate usual life expectancy in early stages
  3. Late stages, survival 1 to 3 years
II. Analysis
  A. Knowledge deficit related to diagnostic examinations and surgery
  B. Altered body image related to surgery and castration
  C. Knowledge deficit related to postoperative exercises and return of urinary function
  D. High risk for sexual dysfunction related to removal of prostate, retrograde ejaculation, and sterility
III. Planning/goals, expected outcomes
  A. Client will understand diagnostic examinations
  B. Client will be physically and psychologically prepared for surgery

C. Client will cope with altered body image and sexuality

D. Client will recover without complications

E. Client will regain urinary control after radical prostatectomy

IV. Implementation

   A. Preoperatively

     1. Help client discuss fears associated with altered body image and sexuality

     2. Administer laxatives, enemas, antibiotics, and low-residue diet to clean out bowel

     3. Maintain adequate urinary drainage

   B. Postoperatively

     1. See postoperative prostatectomy under BPH

     2. Change dressing as needed

     3. Avoid rectal tubes, suppositories, or rectal thermometers

     4. Maintain patency of catheter

     5. Use propantheline (Pro-Banthine) for bladder spasms

     6. Avoid constipation or rectal straining

     7. Teach perineal exercises; have client practice hourly

     8. Provide good wound care for perineal wound

     9. Counsel about altered sexuality

   C. Provide care for internal or external radiation (see Chapter 6, Radiation Therapy)

   D. Administer DES as ordered; teach about side effects (see Table 3–5)

   E. Prepare client for bilateral orchiectomy

V. Evaluation

   A. Client recovers from surgery without complications

   B. Client and significant others cope with altered body image and sexuality

   C. Client regains urinary control

   D. Client complies with follow-up treatments

Epididymitis

I. Assessment

   A. Definition/pathophysiology

     1. Infection of epididymis; may result from infection of prostate

     2. Usually retrograde infection with organism migrating from the prostate or urethra

   B. Predisposing/precipitating factors

     1. Often secondary to gonorrhea or other sexually transmitted disease

     2. May occur after prolonged use of a Foley catheter, after a prostatectomy without a vasectomy, or, rarely, following cystoscopy

   C. Clinical manifestations

     1. Pain along the inguinal canal and vas deferens

     2. Swelling in groin and scrotum

     3. Pyuria and bacteriuria with fever and chills may occur

     4. Abscess may form

   D. Diagnostic examinations

     1. History and presence of risk factor with associated clinical manifestations may be way to diagnose

     2. Ultrasound to differentiate swelling from possible tumor

   E. Complications: abscess requiring an orchiectomy

   F. Medical management

     1. Bedrest with scrotum elevated

     2. Antibiotics appropriate for organism

     3. Application of cold compresses or sitz baths for pain relief

II. Analysis

   A. Sexual dysfunction related to pain and scrotal swelling

   B. Pain related to scrotal swelling

III. Planning/goals, expected outcomes

   A. Client will not develop sexual dysfunction

   B. Client will have pain relieved

IV. Implementation

   A. Apply cold compresses or help client with sitz baths as ordered

   B. Apply scrotal support or Bellevue bridge

   C. Administer antibiotics as ordered

   D. Instruct client to avoid heavy lifting, straining, or sexual intercourse until the infection subsides

V. Evaluation

   A. Client does not develop sexual dysfunction

   B. Client pain is relieved

Prostatitis

I. Assessment

   A. Definition/pathophysiology

     1. Inflammation of the prostate gland

     2. May be bacterial or abacterial

   B. Predisposing/precipitating factors

     1. Abacterial

       a. May occur after a viral illness

       b. May result from sudden decrease in sexual activity, especially in young men

     2. Bacterial

       a. Bacteria may reach prostate through bloodstream or migrate in a retrograde manner from the urethra

       b. *Escherichia coli* common causative organism

   C. Clinical manifestations

1. Fever and chills
2. Dysuria
3. Boggy, tender prostate
4. Urethral discharge
5. Backache, perineal pain, mild dysuria, and hematuria may be present with chronic prostatitis
   D. Diagnostic examinations
   1. History and presence of symptoms
   2. Prostatic fluid analysis may show increased white blood cells
   E. Complications
   1. Epididymitis
   2. Cystitis
   3. Prostatic abscess
   F. Medical management
   1. Antibiotics
   2. Sitz baths
   3. Stool softeners
   4. Prostatic massage, masturbation, or sexual intercourse to drain prostatic fluid
II. Analysis
   A. Sexual dysfunction related to pain and scrotal swelling
   B. Pain related to scrotal swelling
III. Planning/goals, expected outcomes
   A. Client will not develop sexual dysfunction
   B. Client will have pain relieved
IV. Implementation
   A. Force fluids to decrease risk of urinary tract infections
   B. Instruct client in methods to drain prostate such as massage, intercourse, or masturbation
   C. Administer antibiotics and stool softeners as ordered
   D. Provide comfort measures such as sitz baths and analgesics as ordered
   E. Instruct client to take full course of antibiotics; may be up to 30 days
V. Evaluation
   A. Client does not develop sexual dysfunction
   B. Client pain is relieved

POST-TEST Male Reproductive Disorders

Your 28-year-old client is diagnosed with a testicular tumor.

1. He has a lymphangiogram preoperatively to determine possible spread. An important nursing assessment that should be made before the examination is his:
   ① Respiratory status
   ② Renal function
   ③ Knowledge of the disease
   ④ Lower extremity circulatory status

2. Your client asks why he is scheduled for a radical orchiectomy and radical lymph node dissection when the doctor has not even done a biopsy. Which of the following is the rationale for this surgery?
   ① The doctor is already sure it is malignant because of the laboratory tests
   ② It is very dangerous to do a biopsy because of potential spread and there is every indication that it is malignant
   ③ It is the doctor's prerogative to decide the surgical approach
   ④ There are no benign diseases that could cause the same symptoms, so the assumption is that it is malignant

3. An example of secondary prevention for testicular cancer is:
   ① Yearly physical examination
   ② Monthly testicular self-examination
   ③ Yearly rectal examination
   ④ Avoiding hormone usage

4. After the radical orchiectomy with a radical retroperitoneal lymph node dissection, which of the following sexual problems would be most likely to occur?
   ① Impotency
   ② Decreased ejaculatory capacity
   ③ Absence of sperm
   ④ Inability to maintain an erection

5. Which of the following is a risk factor for benign prostatic hypertrophy?
   ① Decreased testosterone level
   ② Aging
   ③ Homosexuality
   ④ High level of sexual activity

6. Which of the following is NOT a common symptom of benign prostatic hypertrophy?
   ① Gross hematuria
   ② Nocturia
   ③ Hesitancy
   ④ Dribbling

7. Which of the following is NOT a potential complication of benign prostatic hypertrophy?
   ① Hydroureter
   ② Pyelonephritis
   ③ Renal failure
   ④ Impotence

8. Secondary prevention for the client at risk for benign prostatic hypertrophy would include yearly:
   ① Physical examination
   ② Acid phosphatase levels
   ③ Digital rectal examination
   ④ Cystoscopy

9. One of the major goals preoperatively for the client with BPH would be that the client will:
   ① Regain urinary control with perineal exercises
   ② Have adequate urinary output
   ③ Accept the inevitable impotence caused by surgery
   ④ Return to a normal voiding pattern

10. Which of the following is important teaching for the nurse to accomplish preoperatively?
    ① Perineal exercises
    ② Coughing and deep breathing
    ③ Leg exercises
    ④ The importance of early ambulation

POST-TEST Answers and Rationales

1. ① It is important to monitor respiratory function, because that is how the dye from the lymphangiogram is excreted. None of the other options are relevant to this procedure. 1, I & IV. Testicular Cancer.

2. ② Testicular tumors are all malignant; if it is determined that there is a growth, a biopsy is never done because of the risk of spread. The other options are inappropriate for this situation. 2, I. Testicular Cancer.

3. ② A young man should perform a monthly testicular self-examination, just as a woman should do a breast examination. This is the best secondary prevention (early detection) against testicular cancer. The other options are inappropriate. The only hormone use would be that of the mother and that would be an example of primary prevention (preventing the disease). 2, I & IV. Testicular Cancer.

4. ② The radical lymph node dissection usually decreases ejaculatory capacity. There is a slight chance of impotence. Absence of sperm occurs only if both testicles are removed. 2, IV. Testicular Cancer.

5. ② The main risk factor for BPH is aging. The incidence goes up steadily with age.

Testosterone is not implicated nor is homosexuality or sexual activity. 2, IV. BPH.

6. ① Hematuria is not a symptom of BPH. All of the other options are common symptoms. 1, II. BPH.

7. ④ Impotence is not a risk with BPH. With obstruction of the ureter, all of the other options are real possibilities. 2, IV. BPH.

8. ③ The best secondary prevention for prostate is yearly digital rectal examination in men over 40. A physical examination is not specific and acid phosphatase is elevated only when there is prostate cancer that has spread. A cystoscopy is a much more invasive procedure. 2, IV. BPH.

9. ② The major goal preoperatively is to establish urine output, usually with a catheter or a suprapubic tube. Urine control and return to normal voiding pattern will not be possible until after surgery. Impotency is not an inevitable outcome after surgery. 3, IV. BPH.

10. ① Perineal exercises will help the client to regain urinary control postoperatively, so it is important that the client learn and practice them before surgery. The other options are simply routine teaching needs. 4, IV. BPH.

BIBLIOGRAPHY

GROWTH AND DEVELOPMENT
Albert, M. (1987). Health screening to promote health for the elderly. *Nurse Practitioner* 12: 42–56.

American Association of Retired Persons. (1988). *Using the experience of a lifetime* (publication #D13343). Washington, DC: American Association of Retired Persons.

American Association of Retired Persons. (1986). *Miles away and still caring: A guide for long distance caregivers* (publication #D12748). Washington, DC: American Association of Retired Persons.

American Association of Retired Persons, and Administration on Aging. (1988). *A profile of older Americans* (DHHS publication #D996). Washington, DC: Department of Health and Human Services.

Black, J., and Matassarin-Jacobs, E., eds. (1993). *Luckmann and Sorensen's medical/surgical nursing: A psychophysiologic approach.* 4th ed. Philadelphia: W. B. Saunders.

Erikson, E. H. (1968). *Childhood and society,* 2nd ed. New York: W. W. Norton.

Esberger, K. K., and Hughes, S. T., eds. (1989). *The aging person: A holistic perspective.* St. Louis: C. V. Mosby.

Havinghurst, R. (1972). *Developmental tasks and education.* New York: David McKay.

Matteson, M. A., and McConnell, E. S., eds. (1988). *Gerontological nursing.* Philadelphia: W. B. Saunders.

Yurick, A. G., Spier, B. E., Robb, S. S., Ebert, N. J., and Magnussen, M. H., eds. (1989). *The aged person and the nursing process.* Norwalk, CT: Appleton & Lange.

FEMALE REPRODUCTIVE DISORDERS
Baird, S. B., McCorkle, R., and Grant, M. (1991). *Cancer nursing: A comprehensive textbook.* Philadelphia: W. B. Saunders.

Beard, M., and Curtis, L. (1988). *Menopause and the years ahead.* Tucson: Fisher Books.

Black, J., and Matassarin-Jacobs, E., eds. (1993). *Luckmann and Sorensen's medical/surgical nursing: A psychophysiologic approach.* 4th ed. Philadelphia: W. B. Saunders.

Cohen, S., Kinner, C., and Hollingsworth, A. (1991). *Maternal, neonatal, and women's health nursing.* Springhouse, PA: Springhouse Corp.

Erikkson, J., and Walczak, J. (1990). Ovarian cancer. *Seminars in Oncology Nursing* 6(3): 214–227.

Hammond, C., Haseltine, F., and Schiff, I. (1989). *Menopause: Evaluation, treatment and health concerns.* New York: Alan R. Liss.

Holleb, A., Fink, D., and Murphy, G. (1991). *American Cancer Society textbook of clinical oncology.* Atlanta: American Cancer Society.

Hubbard, J., and Holcombe, J. (1990). Cancer of the endometrium. *Seminars in Oncology Nursing* 6(3): 206–213.

Love, S. (1990). *Dr. Susan Love's breast book.* Reading: Addison-Wesley.

Osteen, R. (1990). *Cancer manual,* 8th ed. Boston: Boston American Cancer Society, Massachusetts Division.

Otto, S. (1991). *Oncology nursing.* St. Louis: Mosby–Year Book.

Thompson, L. (1990). Cancer of the cervix. *Seminars in Oncology Nursing* 6(3): 190–197.

MALE REPRODUCTIVE DISORDERS

Benson, R. C., Beard, C. M., Kelalis, P. P., and Kurland, L. T. (1991). Malignant potential of cryptorchid testis. *Mayo Clinic Proceedings* 66: 372–378.

Black, J., and Matassarin-Jacobs, E., eds. (1993). *Luckmann and Sorensen's medical/surgical nursing: A psychophysiologic approach.* Philadelphia: W. B. Saunders.

Bostwick, D. G. (1989). The pathology of early prostate cancer. *CA: A Cancer Journal for Clinicians* 39(3): 376–393.

Brawer, M. K., and Lange, P. H. (1989). Prostate-specific antigen and premalignant change: Implications for early detection. *CA: A Cancer Journal for Clinicians* 39(3): 361–375.

Drago, J. R. (1989). The role of new modalities in the early detection and diagnosis of prostate cancer. *CA: A Cancer Journal for Clinicians* 39(3): 326–336.

Gaillard-Moguilewsky, M. (1991). Pharmacology of antiandrogens and value of combining androgen suppression with antiandrogen therapy. *Urology* (suppl) 37(2): 5–11.

Gershman, S. T., and Stolley, P. D. (1988). A case-controlled study of testicular cancer using Connecticut tumor registry data. *International Journal of Epidemiology* 17: 738–742.

Goodman, M. (1988). Concepts of hormonal manipulation in the treatment of cancer. *Oncology Nursing Forum* 15(5): 639–647.

Hayes, R. B., Brown, L. M., Pottern, L. M., Gomez, M., Kardaun, J. W. P. F., Hoover, R. N., O'Connell, K. J., Sutzman, R. E., and Javadpour, N. (1990). Occupation and risk for testicular cancer: A case-control study. *International Journal of Epidemiology* 19(4): 825–831.

Heinrich-Tynning, T. (1987). Prostatic cancer treatments and their effects on sexual functioning. *Oncology Nursing Forum* 14(6): 37–41.

Hill, D. J. (1990). The patient with testicular cancer: Nursing management of chemotherapy. *Oncology Nursing Forum* 17(2): 243–249.

Joseph, A. C., and Chang, M. K. (1989). A bladder behavior clinic for post prostatectomy patients. *Urologic Nursing* 9(3): 15–19.

Klein, L. (1990). Current approaches to balloon dilatation of the prostate. *Astra Urologue* May: 1–7.

Lee, F., Torp-Petersen, S. T., and Siders, D. B. (1989). The role of transrectal ultrasound in the early detection of prostate cancer. *CA: A Cancer Journal for Clinicians* 39(3): 337–360.

Lepor, H., ed. (1988). Pharmacologic intervention in benign prostatic hypertrophy. *Urology* (suppl 6) 32: 2–31.

Loughlin, K. R. (1991). Medical and nonmedical therapy for benign prostatic hypertrophy. *Geriatrics* 46(6): 26–31.

Mahon, S. M., Casperson, D., and Wozniak-Petrofsky, J. (1990). Prostate cancer: Screening through treatment and nursing implications. *Urologic Nursing* 2: 5–11.

Matzkin, H., and Braf, Z. (1991). Endocrine treatment of benign prostatic hypertrophy: Current concepts. *Urology* 37(1): 1–13.

Murphy, G. P. (1989). Progress against prostatic cancer. *CA: A Cancer Journal for Clinicians* 39(3): 325.

Reddy, E. K., Burke, M., Giri, S., Krishnan, L., Gemer, L., Evans, R., Mebust, W. K., and Weigel, J. (1990). Testicular neoplasms: Seminoma. *Journal of the American Medical Association* 82(9): 651–655.

Rudolf, V. M., and Quinn, L. M. (1988). The practice of TSE among college men: Effectiveness of an educational program. *Oncology Nursing Forum* 15(1): 45–48.

Sawyer, P. F. (1987). Prostatectomy: Nursing care radical prostatectomy for cancer of the prostate. Nursing diagnoses and interventions. *Journal of Urologic Nursing* 6(4): 266–276.

Silverberg, E., and Lubera, J. A. (1989). Cancer survival rates. *CA: A Journal for Clinicians* 39: 3–32.

Stepp, C. (1991). Balloon dilatation of the prostate: A historical review. *Urologic Nursing* 5: 21–24.

Walsh, P., Gittes, R., Perlmutter, A., and Stamey, T., eds. (1986). *Campbell's urology,* 5th ed. Philadelphia: W. B. Saunders.

4

Cardiopulmonary Disorders in the Adult Client

PRE-TEST Cardiovascular Disorders

Mr. Adams, aged 75, has a persistent blood pressure of 180/110 and a history of long-standing primary hypertension.

1. Which of the following statements is true concerning primary hypertension?
   1. It occurs only in the elderly population
   2. The exact cause is unknown
   3. It accounts for 10% of all hypertension
   4. It is a curable disease
2. Which of the following data concerning his diagnosis would Mr. Adams report?
   1. Elevated serum level
   2. Elevated heart rate
   3. Chest pain
   4. Peripheral edema
3. Mr. Adams is started on furosemide (Lasix) 20 mg, PO, BID and methyldopa (Aldomet) 250 mg, PO, TID. Which of the following is a true statement about Lasix?
   1. It is a thiazide diuretic
   2. It can decrease the blood urea nitrogen (BUN)
   3. It can cause hyperkalemia
   4. It can produce orthostatic hypotension
4. The nurse will hold the methyldopa and call the physician if Mr. Adams experiences:
   1. Sedation
   2. Oliguria
   3. Constipation
   4. Dry mouth
5. Mr. Adams needs a low-salt diet. What is the best approach for meal planning?
   1. Let the dietician select proper foods
   2. Allow Mr. Adams to select his own foods
   3. Assist Mr. Adams to select appropriate foods that he likes
   4. Ask Mrs. Adams to select foods because she does the cooking at home
6. Which food group is not a source of dietary potassium?
   1. Fruits
   2. Meats
   3. Carbohydrates
   4. Vegetables
7. A person with mild hypertension would be treated with:
   1. Antianxiety agents
   2. Vasodilators
   3. Adrenergic inhibitors
   4. Diuretics

8. Which risk factor is most modifiable in prevention of hypertension?
   1. Stress
   2. Smoking
   3. Cholesterol
   4. Family history

Mr. Jackson is a 45-year-old executive who is admitted to the coronary care unit with a diagnosis of acute myocardial infarction. Mr. Jackson has a history of smoking and he is overweight. His father died at age 40 from a heart attack.

9. Mr. Jackson is exhibiting typical symptoms of myocardial infarction. When assessing Mr. Jackson's chest pain, the nurse would most likely note which complaint?
   1. Pain easily relieved by nitroglycerin SL
   2. Severe, viselike substernal pain that radiates
   3. Mild pain relieved by rest
   4. Pain upon inspiration accompanied by a friction rub
10. Mr. Jackson appears anxious. Nursing care that would help decrease his anxiety would be:
    1. Telling him that there is nothing to be afraid of and not to worry
    2. Acting in a calm, reassuring manner and providing simple, brief explanations of procedures and routines
    3. Giving him a copy of hospital regulations
    4. Giving him printed materials on myocardial infarction
11. In the first 48 hours after myocardial infarction, the nurse will observe Mr. Jackson for which common complication?
    1. Sepsis
    2. Endocarditis
    3. Dysrhythmias
    4. Pulmonary embolism
12. An intravenous line is inserted. The primary reason for this is to:
    1. Provide a route for administration of drugs if complications occur
    2. Lessen the stress and energy used in having the patient take sufficient amounts of oral fluids
    3. Facilitate keeping accurate records of all fluids given to a patient
    4. Replace fluids, because most patients become somewhat dehydrated following myocardial infarction

13. To confirm the diagnosis of myocardial infarction, the nurse should prepare Mr. Jackson for which diagnostic tests?
    1. Amylase, SGPT
    2. CPK, LDH, SGOT/AST
    3. PT, PTT, sedimentation rate
    4. BUN, creatinine

14. The 12-lead ECG shows large Q-waves in the inferior leads. The nurse knows this is an indication of:
    1. Nonspecific myocardial changes
    2. Myocardial ischemia
    3. Electrolyte-induced hypokalemia
    4. Myocardial tissue necrosis

15. Morphine sulfate is ordered for Mr. Jackson. The rationale for administration of this drug is to:
    1. Lower his pulse rate
    2. Increase myocardial contractility
    3. Relieve pain and decrease venous return
    4. Suppress a rapid respiratory rate

16. The physician's order does not indicate the desired route of administration. The nurse should:
    1. Give the drug PO to avoid muscle damage with IM injections
    2. Give the drug SQ to promote rapid absorption
    3. Clarify the order with the physician
    4. Give the drug IM, because this is the method most frequently used

17. The cardiac monitor shows Mr. Jackson having frequent premature ventricular contractions (PVCs). The medication that should be administered for this is:
    1. Digoxin (Lanoxin)
    2. Furosemide (Lasix)
    3. Lidocaine (Xylocaine)
    4. Dopamine hydrochloride (Intropin)

18. Mr. Jackson is ordered to stop smoking. The primary reason for this is that nicotine:
    1. Dilates peripheral blood vessels and removes blood from the heart
    2. Acts as a stimulant and causes constriction of blood vessels
    3. Will alter clotting time
    4. Causes lung cancer

Mrs. White is diagnosed with left-sided congestive heart failure (CHF). She complains of dyspnea; her respirations are rapid and shallow and she has bilateral rales.

---

19. Mrs. White's dyspnea is primarily caused by:
    1. Jugular venous distention
    2. Anxiety associated with dyspnea
    3. Elevation of diaphragm due to ascites
    4. Fluid accumulation in alveoli

20. Mrs. White will breathe best if the nurse positions her in:
    1. Sims
    2. Trendelenburg
    3. High Fowler's
    4. Prone

21. An early sign that the nurse will observe that might indicate Mrs. White's decreasing tissue oxygenation would be:
    1. Restlessness
    2. Cyanosis
    3. Confusion
    4. Incoordination

22. The rate of oxygen flow Mrs. White will receive is based upon:
    1. Changing respiratory rate
    2. Lung sounds
    3. Arterial blood gases
    4. Degree of dyspnea

23. Mrs. White develops pulmonary edema. The first priority for the nurse is to:
    1. Obtain emergency crash cart
    2. Transfer client to the CCU
    3. Establish patent airway
    4. Maintain IV site for medications

Mrs. Brown has been admitted to the hospital with acute thrombophlebitis of the right lower extremity and is placed on bedrest.

---

24. Along with pain and redness, the affected extremity will probably show evidence of:
    1. Edema
    2. Negative Homans sign
    3. Absence of peripheral pulse
    4. Coolness

25. While Mrs. Brown is confined to bed, which action should the nurse encourage to prevent pulmonary emboli?
    1. Coughing and deep breathing
    2. Elevation of the knee gatch
    3. Limiting fluid intake
    4. Frequent movement of legs

26. Mrs. Brown is being treated with the anticoagulant heparin. Which is a true statement about heparin?
    1. It helps prevent formation of new clots
    2. Vitamin K is the antidote
    3. It may be given by mouth

④ The dose is determined by prothrombin time (PT)

27. Mrs. Brown has been told to stop smoking by her physician. The nurse finds a pack of cigarettes in her room. The first action the nurse should take is:
    ① Dispose of the cigarettes without telling Mrs. Brown
    ② Notify the physician immediately
    ③ Keep the cigarettes at the nurse's desk until Mrs. Brown's discharge
    ④ Inform Mrs. Brown of your finding

28. When teaching Mrs. Brown prevention of future recurrent thrombophlebitis, the nurse should focus on:
    ① Application of heat
    ② Management of diet, exercise, and drugs
    ③ Cleaning of feet with disinfectants
    ④ Massage of lower extremities with lotion

Mr. Horner is admitted with a diagnosis of abdominal aortic aneurysm. He has a history of hypertension and coronary artery disease (CAD). He will undergo surgery tomorrow.

29. The most significant complication that can occur with Mr. Horner at this stage is:
    ① Preoperative anxiety
    ② Dilation of the aorta
    ③ Mural thromboembolism
    ④ Aortic dissection

30. Which of the following would be crucial for the nurse to assess while doing Mr. Horner's admission assessment?
    ① Previous experience with surgery
    ② Pedal pulses
    ③ Chest x-ray
    ④ Family history of cardiac disease

PRE-TEST Answers and Rationales

1. ② Although the incidence of primary hypertension increases with age, due to arteriosclerosis, it does occur in other age groups and accounts for 90% of all hypertension. This is a chronic, incurable disease. Despite many risk factors and theories, the exact cause is unknown. 1, II. Hypertension.

2. ③ Although choices 1, 2, and 4 are associated with hypertension, they represent objective data and the physical examination. Reported chest pain is a subjective complaint obtained from a history. 1, II. Hypertension.

3. ④ Lasix is a potent loop diuretic, causing an elevated BUN, hypokalemia, and orthostatic hypotension related to the extracellular fluid shift secondary to a hyperosmolar state. 1, II. Hypertension.

4. ② Sedation, dry mouth, and constipation are common and expected side effects, especially during the initiation of therapy. Oliguria indicates decreased renal perfusion, which could lead to drug toxicity. 2, II. Hypertension.

5. ③ The dietician and the client's wife should be included in meal planning. However, the client should make informed decisions assisted by the professional nurse. 3, II. Hypertension.

6. ② Meats are not high in potassium; the other food groups are. 1, II. Hypertension.

7. ④ A person may be given an antianxiety drug as an adjunct to treatment but not in place of a diuretic, which eliminates fluids and relieves vessel pressure. 1, II. Hypertension.

8. ② Although cessation of smoking may be extremely difficult, it is still the most easily modified risk factor. A person cannot do much about family history or cholesterol, which is also genetically linked. Stress can be modified, but smoking is a greater risk factor. 1, IV. Hypertension.

9. ② The typical pain associated with myocardial infarction is severe and often radiates. The other distractors describe angina and a friction rub is associated with pericarditis or pleurisy. 1, II. Coronary Artery Disease (CAD).

10. ② Initially, anxiety is commonly severe in the presence of acute myocardial infarction. Simple explanations and reassurance help to correct misconceptions and decrease anxiety. Printed and detailed materials are not appropriate at this time. 4, III. CAD.

11. ③ Dysrhythmias are the most common complication associated with acute myocardial infarction. The others are not associated with an MI. 1, I. CAD.

12. ① Life-threatening complications may occur with acute myocardial infarction. An intravenous line is necessary for emergency administration of drugs if complications occur. The other options are inappropriate. 2, II. CAD.

13. ② CPK, LDH, and SGOT/AST are cardiac enzymes that aid in the diagnosis of myocardial infarction. Choice 1 is pancreatic and liver enzymes, choice 3 bleeding and inflammation indicators, and choice 4 kidney function indicators. 1, II. CAD.

14. ④ The 12-lead ECG is an important diagnostic tool for myocardial infarction. Q-waves are a definitive sign of myocardial cell death and infarction. 1, II. CAD.

15. ③ Morphine sulfate is the drug of choice to treat severe pain associated with myocardial infarction. Morphine also causes peripheral vasodilation. This results in decreased venous return and decreased myocardial oxygen demand. 2, II. CAD.

16. ③ For legal reasons, this is the action that must be taken. Every order must specify route. 3, II. CAD.

17. ③ Lidocaine is an antidysrhythmic agent and is the drug of choice for premature ventricular contractions associated with acute myocardial infarction. Choice 1 a cardiac glycoside, choice 2 a diuretic, and choice 4 a vasopressor. 3, II. CAD.

18. ② Nicotine causes vasoconstriction, increases blood pressure, and increases myocardial oxygen demand. 2, II. CAD.

19. ④ The heart's inability to pump blood effectively causes a back-up of fluid into the alveoli with resulting dyspnea. Anxiety is secondary and will aggravate the dyspnea. Abdominal ascites and JVD are signs of right-sided failure. 2, II. Congestive Heart Failure (CHF).

20. ③ The high Fowler's position allows for descent of the diaphragm and full lung expansion. The other positions would limit lung expansion. 4, II. CHF.

21. ① Restlessness, a vague but early sign of tissue hypoxia, gives the nurse an opportunity to intervene and perhaps prevent the late signs (choices 2, 3, and 4). 1, II. CHF.

22. ③ Although the other signs may reflect hypoxia, arterial blood gases (ABGs) are the only direct measure of oxygenated blood. 2, II. CHF.

23. ③ The airway must be patent to prevent cardiac arrest. The others are important, but not the highest priority. 1, II. CHF.

24. ① Choices 3 and 4 indicate arterial disease; Homans sign is likely to be positive. Edema is a common sign. 1, II. PVD.

25. ④ Movement of legs prevents venous stasis and clots; fluid should be increased to decrease blood viscosity; use of the knee gatch can compress the popliteal artery. 4, I. PVD.

26. ① Protamine sulfate is the antidote. Heparin is given IV or subcutaneously because it is destroyed by gastric enzymes; dose is titrated to the PTT blood level. Anticoagulants help prevent new clot formation. 2, II. PVD.

27. ④ The nurse should protect a client's human rights but should also inform the physician, because continued smoking may impede the treatment plan. 4, II. PVD.

28. ② Prevention is based on self-care; choices 1, 3, and 4 are inappropriate and potentially injurious. 4, IV. PVD.

29. ④ All of these would be a concern to the nurse. Anxiety is expected in any preoperative client. Dilation of the aorta is the cause of the aneurysm. Mural thromboemboli are possible, but aortic dissection would be the most significant problem at this time. 2, II. Aortic Aneurysm.

30. ② It is the physician's responsibility to examine the chest x-ray. The nurse needs to know the status of Mr. Horner's pedal pulses as baseline data to assess any complications that may occur (i.e., aortic dissection, thromboembolic). Previous surgical experience and family history are not crucial at this time. 1, I. Aortic Aneurysm.

NORMAL CARDIOVASCULAR–PERIPHERAL VASCULAR SYSTEM

I. Cardiac cycle: period of relaxation, diastole, followed by period of contraction, systole
II. Impulse formation and conduction
   A. Electrical behavior
      1. Series of cellular electrochemical changes known as the action potential
         a. Depolarization: electrochemical event associated with impulse formation that results in the mechanical event of myocardial contraction
         b. Repolarization: immediately follows depolarization; represents recovery or return to resting state and is associated with myocardial relaxation
      2. Electrical properties of cardiac tissue
         a. Automaticity: characteristic of cardiac tissue, especially specialized conductive tissue, for self-excitation
         b. Conductivity: ability to conduct an impulse or wave of depolarization along a specialized conductive pathway that results in myocardial contraction
   B. Conductive pathway
      1. Sinoatrial node, "pacemaker"
      2. Atrioventricular node
      3. Bundle of His
      4. Right and left bundle branches
      5. Purkinje fibers
III. Autonomic nervous system control of heart
   A. Sympathetic system: increases heart rate and force of contraction
   B. Parasympathetic system: decreases heart rate and force of contraction
IV. Regulation of cardiac function; cardiac output
   A. Definition of cardiac output: volume of blood pumped by the heart per minute (cardiac output equals heart rate times stroke volume)
   B. Factors affecting cardiac output
      1. Preload: left ventricular filling volume, left ventricular end-diastolic volume
      2. Afterload: resistance of impedance left ventricle must overcome to eject blood into aorta

3. Contractility: inotropic state
4. Heart rate

V. Coronary circulation (Figure 4–1)
   A. Coronary vasculature
      1. Left coronary artery
         a. Left anterior descending artery (LAD)
         b. Left circumflex
      2. Right coronary artery
      3. Posterior descending artery
      4. Collateral circulation: intercoronary channels that develop in response to tissue ischemia

B. Factors influencing coronary artery blood flow
   1. Aortic pressure, blood pressure
   2. Diastolic filling time, heart rate

VI. Blood pressure regulation
   A. Definition of blood pressure: blood pressure equals cardiac output times total peripheral resistance
   B. Factors that affect blood pressure (see section on Hypertension)

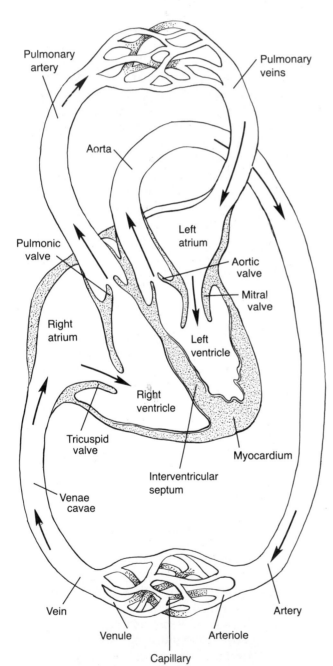

FIGURE 4–1. Cardiopulmonary circulation. Representation of blood flow through the cardiovascular system.

NURSING PROCESS APPLIED TO ADULTS WITH CARDIOVASCULAR DISORDERS

Hypertension

I. Assessment
   A. Normal function of blood pressure (BP) control maintained by balance between vasodilation and vasoconstriction of arterioles that allow for changing needs for oxygen by various bodily tissues; the following events occur when individual becomes hypotensive or vasodilated, or when the individual develops progressive and uncontrolled hypertension or is vasoconstricted
      1. Sensory baroreceptors located in carotid arteries and aortic arch respond by sending message to medulla in order to: increase heart rate, force of contraction, and cardiac output
      2. Sympathetic nervous system causes peripheral vessel constriction by releasing
         a. Norepinephrine
         b. Epinephrine
      3. Renin–angiotensin–aldosterone mechanism is activated
         a. Renin converted to angiotensin to constrict arterioles
         b. Secretion of aldosterone
         c. Release of antidiuretic hormone
   B. Pathophysiology
      1. Balance for normal BP control is lost and there is persistent increased peripheral resistance
      2. Arterioles abnormally resist blood flow, causing pathological changes of small and large vessels and eventual ischemia/infarction in vital organs such as brain (CVA); heart (MI, CHF); kidneys (failure); eyes (retinal hemorrhage/detachment); extremities (PVD)
   C. Classification
      1. Primary; essential; idiopathic: persistent

elevation of 140 mm Hg systolic; 90 mm Hg diastolic, or higher
   a. Benign: a form of primary that is slowly progressive
   b. Malignant: a form of primary with accelerated course; diastolic greater than 110 mm Hg
2. Secondary: occurs as a result of other conditions such as pheochromocytoma; hyperaldosteronism; renal disease; Cushing's disease; coarctation of the aorta; eclampsia associated with pregnancy

D. Incidence
   1. Primary; essential; idiopathic
      a. Benign
         (1) Occurs in all age groups, but increases with age
         (2) 90% of all hypertension (HTN)
         (3) Leading cause of death in United States
      b. Malignant
         (1) Highest in African-American males
         (2) Death in 1 to 2 years if untreated
   2. Secondary
      a. 10% of all hypertension
      b. May be cured if primary cause eliminated

E. Predisposing/precipitating factors
   1. Family history of hypertension and cardiovascular disease
   2. Client history of cardiovascular, cerebral, and renal disease; diabetes mellitus
   3. Obesity
   4. Elevated serum lipids
   5. Smoking
   6. Heavy alcohol consumption
   7. Dietary sodium
   8. Stress
   9. Drugs—for example, contraceptives, nonsteroidal anti-inflammatory

F. Clinical manifestations
   1. Early stage: may be asymptomatic
      a. Headache: occipital, early morning
      b. Vertigo
      c. Flushed face
      d. Epistaxis
      e. Nocturia
   2. Progressive stage
      a. Dyspnea/orthopnea
      b. Chest pain
      c. Leg edema
      d. Diminished or absent peripheral pulses
      e. Increased heart rate
      f. Dysrhythmias
      g. Nausea/vomiting
      h. Confusion
      i. Papilledema
      j. Distended neck veins
      k. Carotid bruit
      l. Oliguria

G. Diagnostic examinations
   1. Routine lab to determine severity of vascular disease and primary versus secondary cause
      a. CBC
      b. Electrolytes, including cholesterol and triglycerides
      c. Urinalysis
   2. Determine cardiac size and condition of pulmonary vasculature: chest x-ray
   3. Determine cardiac conduction: ECG
   4. Determine specific renal cause
      a. Urine for catecholamines: pheochromocytoma
      b. Urine for 17 ketosteroids; 24-hour collection and serum corticoids: Cushing's disease
   5. Nurse's role
      a. Explain all tests
      b. Know that drugs such as steroids can alter urine tests

II. Analysis
   A. Acute hypertensive crisis
      1. Altered tissue perfusion related to decreased cardiac output
      2. High risk for injury related to altered tissue perfusion and risk of emboli
      3. High risk for ineffective individual coping related to severity of diagnosis and risks of injury
   B. Chronic hypertension
      1. Knowledge deficit related to risk factors, medication, dietary modifications, and blood pressure control
      2. High risk for noncompliance with medication, dietary modifications, and blood pressure control related to denial and lack of observable symptoms

III. Planning/goals, expected outcomes
   A. Acute hypertensive crisis (malignant hypertension)
      1. Client will maintain adequate systemic perfusion
      2. Client will maintain adequate comfort and safety
      3. Client will maintain adequate coping skills
   B. Chronic hypertension
      1. Client will identify and modify risk factors
      2. Client will verbalize understanding of prescribed drugs

TABLE 4–1 Drugs Used in Hypertension (HTN)

Class	Example	Action	Use	Common Side Effects	Nursing Implications
Diuretics	*Thiazide and thiazide type:* chlorothiazide (Diuril), hydrochlorothiazide (HydroDiuril), chlorthalidone (Hygroton), metolazone (Zaroxolyn)	Promotes excretion of Na^+, Cl^-, H_2O	Mild HTN	Headache, dry mouth, vertigo, postural hypotension, GI upset, hypokalemia (thiazide/loop), hyperkalemia (potassium-sparing), hyponatremia, hypocalcemia, hyperglycemia	Teach potassium-rich diet (hypokalemia potentiates digoxin toxicity); monitor serum electrolytes and BUN and creatinine for renal function
	Loop: furosemide (Lasix), ethacrynic acid bumetanide (Bumex)	Inhibits reabsorption of Na^+ and Cl^- in ascending loop of Henle	Thiazide-resistant edema		
	Potassium-sparing: spironolactone (Aldactone), triamterene (Dyrenium)	Inhibits reabsorption of Na^+ and Cl^- while retaining K^+ in distal loop of Henle	Ascites, edema with high serum Na^+	Prone to hyperkalemia	
Adrenergic inhibitors	*Beta blocker:* propranolol (Inderal) *Alpha blocker:* prazosin (Minipress)	Blocks sympathetic activity at beta or alpha receptor sites	Mild to moderate HTN	Headache, dry mouth, bradycardia (Inderal), tachycardia (Minipress), fluid retention or loss, postural hypotension, GI upset, sexual impotence, sedation	Record baseline heart rate and BP sitting and lying; safety measures to prevent falls; assess need for information about sexual dysfunction
	Central blockers: methyldopa (Aldomet), clonidine (Catapres)	Decreases sympathetic outflow of norepinephrine from brain	Moderate to severe HTN		
	Peripheral blockers: reserpine (Serpasil), guanethidine (Ismelin)	Depletes storage sites of peripheral norepinephrine			
Vasodilators	Hydralazine (Apresoline)	Direct relaxation of smooth muscle of peripheral arterioles	Moderate to severe HTN	Dizziness, headache, bradycardia, tachycardia, fluid retention or loss, postural hypotension, GI upset; depression (Apresoline)	Record baseline heart rate and BP and take frequently; keep recumbent; always use infusion pump; protect Nipride from light; monitor drug levels and serum electrolytes
	Diazoxide (Hyperstat)	Same as hydralazine	Hypertensive crisis		
	Sodium nitroprusside (Nipride)	Direct relaxation of both arteriolar and venous smooth muscle	Same as diazoxide		
Calcium channel blockers	Diltiazem (Cardizem), nifedipine (Procardia, Adalat), verapamil (Calan, Isoptin)	Inhibits the influx of calcium across the cell membrane of peripheral arterioles	Used investigationally for HTN	Headache, dizziness, flushing, peripheral edema, bradycardia, tachycardia, hypotension	Record baseline heart rate and BP sitting and lying; verapamil decreases urinary excretion of digoxin and may lead to toxicity
Angiotensin-converting enzyme inhibitor	Captopril (Capoten) Enalapril (Vasotec)	Suppresses the renin-angiotensin aldosterone mechanism	HTN refractory to other agents very potent	Tachycardia, bradycardia, angina, flushing, neutropenia, agranulocytosis, proteinuria	Monitor WBCs, BUN, creatinine; teach client to report infections, bleeding, bruising

3. Client will verbalize understanding of dietary requirements and restrictions
4. Client will develop plan for life-long blood pressure control

IV. Implementation
 A. Acute hypertensive crisis
  1. Transfer to ICU
  2. Monitor for signs and symptoms of de-

creasing perfusion and report changes (see section I, Assessment)

3. Give sodium nitroprusside or diazoxide (Table 4–1)
4. Monitor electrolytes and drug levels
5. Provide rest
   a. Control environmental factors
   b. Give analgesics
6. Provide for relief of nausea and vomiting
   a. Give antiemetics
   b. Oral hygiene
   c. Smaller meals
7. Provide safety
   a. Monitor for progressive visual deficits
   b. Protect from injury
   c. Monitor for alteration in level of consciousness
8. Identify cause of hypertensive crisis for follow-up teaching when stable
9. Allay fears
   a. Reinforce coping skills
   b. Explain all treatments
   c. Include significant others for support

B. Chronic hypertension
   1. Identify readiness for learning
      a. Explain hypertension in basic terms
      b. Assist client in identifying ways to reduce modifiable risk factors
      c. Explain drug actions and side effects; assist in setting up administration schedule to fit lifestyle; i.e., diuretic timing
      d. Teach dietary restrictions
         (1) Explain that sodium increases intravascular fluid
         (2) Explain that potassium is needed for cardiac conduction (Table 4–2)
         (3) Explain need to limit foods high in fat, cholesterol, and calories (if client is overweight)

   e. Explain need for regular exercise to increase vasodilation and to relieve stress
   f. Provide information about community resources such as smoking clinics and stress management
   g. Teach client to report new symptoms
   2. Anticipate risk for noncompliance and communicate openly with client
      a. Sexual impotence related to drug therapy
      b. Cost
      c. Denial
   3. Reinforce life-long care because there is no cure and client can be asymptomatic despite pathology
   4. Reinforce need for follow-up and periodic re-evaluation of drug therapy

V. Evaluation
   A. Acute hypertensive crisis
      1. Adequate systemic perfusion maintained
      2. Blood pressure stabilized at a safe level
      3. Safety, comfort, and adequate coping skills maintained
   B. Chronic hypertension
      1. Client identifies and modifies risk factors
      2. Client verbalizes understanding of drug and diet therapy
      3. Client develops effective plan for life-long blood pressure control

Coronary Artery Disease

I. Assessment
   A. Pathophysiology
      1. Condition characterized by decreased coronary artery blood flow resulting in a disruption in the balance between myocardial oxygen supply and demand; usually caused by atherosclerosis
      2. Imbalance between oxygen supply and demand causes myocardial cellular and tissue ischemia, impairs ventricular function, alters cardiac rhythm, and decreases cardiac output
      3. Clinical manifestations
         a. Angina pectoris: transient myocardial ischemia, without cell death
         b. Myocardial infarction (MI): prolonged ischemia with irreversible cellular damage and muscle death
      4. Major complications
         a. Dysrhythmias: disorder in cardiac impulse formation (automaticity) or conduction affecting heart rate and rhythm

TABLE 4–2 Sources of Dietary Potassium

Fruits	Vegetables	Carbohydrates
Apples, apricots, bananas, cantaloupes, dates, figs, grapefruits, honeydews, nectarines, oranges, papayas, peaches, pears, pineapples, prunes, raisins, strawberries, tangerines, watermelons	Asparagus, broccoli, brussels sprouts, cabbage, carrots, cauliflower, celery, mushrooms, parsnips, beans, potatoes, pumpkins, peas, rhubarb, rutabagas, squash, tomatoes, yams	Bran cereal, wheat germ, whole-grain cereal

b. Heart failure—(see Congestive Heart Failure and Shock)

B. Incidence: leading cause of death in the United States

C. Predisposing/precipitating factors
1. Unmodifiable risk factors
   a. Age: middle age usual onset of clinical symptoms
   b. Sex: males are affected more than females until age 60
   c. Race: African Americans are affected more than whites
   d. Family history of heart disease
2. Modifiable risk factors
   a. Elevated serum lipids and diet
   b. Cigarette smoking
   c. Hypertension
   d. Diabetes
   e. Obesity
   f. Stressful lifestyle
   g. Sedentary lifestyle

D. Clinical manifestations
1. Chest pain (Table 4–3)
   a. Precipitating factors
   b. Location
   c. Description
   d. Duration
   e. Associated symptoms
2. Clinical manifestations of decreased cardiac output associated with complications of dysrhythmias and heart failure (Figure 4–2)
3. Anxiety, depression, and denial due to symptoms, lack of information regarding condition, procedures, equipment, perceived future impact of heart disease on lifestyle, and/or perceived effect of illness on others

E. Diagnostic examinations/laboratory values
1. Electrocardiogram; 12-lead ECG and continuous cardiac monitoring
   a. Angina pectoris: ST-segment depression
   b. Myocardial infarction: T-wave inversion, ST-segment elevation, pathological Q-wave (permanent change)
   c. Dysrhythmias: life-threatening ventricular dysrhythmias common with acute myocardial infarction (Table 4–4)
2. Cardiac enzymes and isoenzymes with myocardial infarction
   a. CPK; MB isoenzyme
   b. SGOT/AST
   c. LDH; LDH-1 higher than LDH-2 isoenzyme
3. Arterial blood gas levels; hypoxemia, acidosis
4. Other
   a. Coronary angiography (cardiac catheterization)
   b. Exercise stress test
   c. Myocardial imaging with radioactive isotopes
   d. 24-hour Holter monitor
   e. Echocardiogram

F. Complications
1. Myocardial infarction
2. Death

G. Medical management
1. Preventive medications such as vasodilators
2. Low fat, low cholesterol, low sodium diet
3. Thrombolytic therapy (see Table 4–6)

H. Surgical management
1. Bypass surgery
2. Angioplasty (see Table 4–7)

II. Analysis
A. Pain related to decreased myocardial perfusion
B. High risk for decreased cardiac output related to decreased cardiac function
C. High risk for ineffective individual coping related to fear of disability and death
D. Knowledge deficit related to diagnosis, therapy, and lifestyle changes

III. Planning/goals, expected outcomes
A. Client will be free from chest pain

TABLE 4–3 Assessment of Chest Pain Associated with Angina Pectoris and Myocardial Infarction

Angina Pectoris	Myocardial Infarction
Precipitating Factors	
Physical exertion, stress, temperature extremes	Often no precipitating factors; may occur at rest
Location	
Usually retrosternal, localized, but may radiate to neck, jaw, epigastrium, shoulders, and arms	Substernal, usually radiates
Description/Duration	
Less severe than pain associated with MI, shorter in duration, usually relieved with rest or nitroglycerin SL	Severe, longer in duration or continuous, often described as viselike, crushing, squeezing sensation, relieved with morphine sulfate IV
Associated Symptoms	
	Nausea, vomiting, diaphoresis, dizziness, palpitations, apprehension, severe anxiety

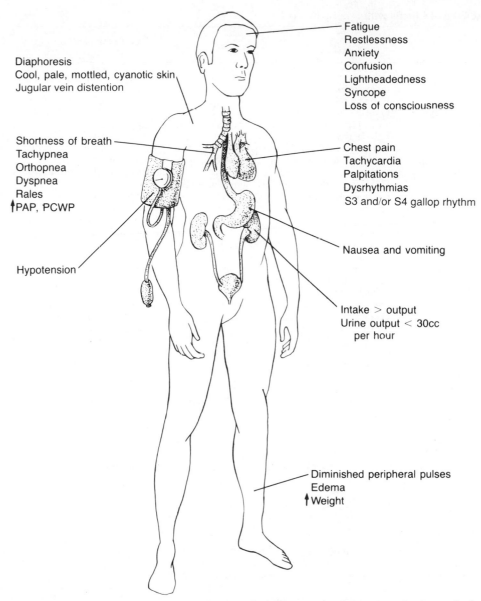

Fatigue
Restlessness
Anxiety
Confusion
Lightheadedness
Syncope
Loss of consciousness

Diaphoresis
Cool, pale, mottled, cyanotic skin
Jugular vein distention

Shortness of breath
Tachypnea
Orthopnea
Dyspnea
Rales
↑PAP, PCWP

Chest pain
Tachycardia
Palpitations
Dysrhythmias
S3 and/or S4 gallop rhythm

Nausea and vomiting

Hypotension

Intake > output
Urine output < 30cc
    per hour

Diminished peripheral pulses
Edema
↑Weight

FIGURE 4–2. Signs and symptoms of decreased cardiac output due to impaired ventricular function and alterations in cardiac rhythm.

B. Client will maintain adequate cardiac output
C. Client will demonstrate effective coping behavior
D. Client will participate in an exercise program of progressive activity
E. Client will demonstrate understanding of disease process and participate in therapeutic treatment regimen
IV. Implementations
  A. To prevent/control chest pain
    1. Respond immediately to complaints of chest pain due to potential life-threatening complications
    2. Obtain full description of pain; see signs and symptoms; differentiate between

chest pain associated with angina and MI and other sources
3. Initiate bedrest to decrease myocardial oxygen demand
4. Perform therapeutic measures to decrease anxiety and decrease oxygen demand
5. Administer diet restricted in cholesterol, saturated fats, and sodium; soft, bland diet during acute phase
6. Implement pharmacological interventions
  a. Oxygen therapy to increase oxygen supply to ischemic myocardium
  b. Patent intravenous infusion line for

TABLE 4–4 Nursing Care of Clients with Dysrhythmias

Dysrhythmia	Etiology	*Goal: Intervention
Bradycardia (HR < 60) Examples: 　Sinus bradycardia, heart block	Ischemia, MI Increased parasympathetic tone (Valsalva) Hypothermia Drug effects: digitalis toxicity 　　　　　　beta blockers	Drug therapy: cholinergic blockers (atropine), sympathomimetics (isoproterenol)* Pacemaker; temporary or permanent Measures to treat underlying cause (hold digoxin, stool softener to avoid Valsalva's maneuver)
Tachycardia (HR > 100) Examples: 　Sinus tachycardia, PAT, SVT	Ischemia, MI Normal physiological response to: anxiety, fear, fever, exertion, hypotension, decreased cardiac output Drug effects: digitalis toxicity; stimulants such as caffeine and nicotine	Drug therapy: beta blockers (propranolol),* cardiac glycosides (digoxin), calcium antagonists (verapamil) Vagal maneuvers (Valsalva, carotid sinus massage) Cardioversion Measures to treat underlying cause (relieve anxiety, hold digoxin, remove stimulants, treat the infection)
Ventricular dysrhythmias Examples: 　PVCs, ventricular tachycardia, ventricular fibrillation, ventricular standstill	Most common, life-threatening dysrhythmias associated with ischemia and acute MI Other: electrolyte imbalance (hypokalemia), hypoxia, acidosis Digitalis toxicity Mechanical irritation (pacemaker wire, Swan-Ganz catheter)	Drug therapy: lidocaine (Xylocaine), procainamide (Pronestyl), bretylium tosylate (Bretylol), quinidine, disopyramide phosphate (Norpace) Defibrillation Measures to treat underlying cause (e.g., electrolyte replacement, oxygen therapy, pulmonary care; hold digoxin) CPR
Atrial dysrhythmias Examples: 　Atrial fibrillation, atrial flutter	Congestive heart failure Valvular heart disease	Drug therapy: digoxin (Lanoxin), quinidine, procainamide (Pronestyl), anticoagulation therapy (heparin, Coumadin) Cardioversion Measures to treat CHF

Nursing Interventions

† Goal: Client will be electrophysiologically stable

Monitor for signs and symptoms associated with dysrhythmias; notify physician of presence; document
　Irregular apical pulse
　HR less than 60 or more than 100 beats per minute
　Apical-radial pulse deficit
　Palpitations
　Syncope, dizziness
　Other signs of reduced cardiac output
Initiate continuous cardiac monitoring; ensure that high- and low-rate alarms are set; obtain 12-lead ECG;
Interpret type of dysrhythmias; investigate underlying cause
Participate with physician; implement and monitor response to medical therapy and interventions
Administer IV antidysrhythmic drugs cautiously
　Administer slowly and at prescribed rate; hypotension common side effect
　Ensure IV remains patent
　Use infusion pump for continuous administration; check frequently to ensure adequate dosage being delivered
　Be alert to signs and symptoms of drug toxicity
Ensure that emergency equipment readily available

* Isoproterenol must be used with EXTREME caution in clients with suspected/confirmed MI because it severely increases MVO$_2$ and increases tachydysrhythmias.
† Use beta blockers with caution in CHF: further decreases CTX.

emergency administration of drugs if necessary
　c. Nitroglycerin SL for anginal pain
　d. Morphine sulfate IV for chest pain associated with MI
　e. Antianginal agents (Table 4–5)
　f. No IM injections, because cardiac serum enzyme levels may elevate from skeletal muscle damage
　7. Prepare patient for thrombolytic therapy if appropriate (Table 4–6)

　8. Prepare patient for PTCA if appropriate (Table 4–7)

B. To maintain an adequate cardiac output
　1. Utilize coronary care unit for continuous electrocardiographic and hemodynamic monitoring if required, and specialized nursing care
　2. Assess frequently for complications of acute myocardial infarction and decreased cardiac output; report immedi-

TABLE 4–5 Antianginal Agents

Class	Example	Action	Common Side Effects	Nursing Implications
Analgesic	Morphine sulfate	Narcotic CNS analgesic used to relieve severe pain and anxiety associated with acute myocardial infarction; also reduces venous return, thereby decreasing myocardial workload	Respiratory depression, hypotension, nausea and vomiting, constipation	When administering IV, monitor closely for hypotension and respiratory depression
Vasodilators	Nitrates/nitrites: nitroglycerin SL and nitroglycerin IV; long-acting: isosorbide dinitrate (Isordil, Sorbitrate, and other manufacturers), nitroglycerin topical (Nitro-Bid Transderm, and other manufacturers)	Relax smooth muscle of coronary and peripheral blood vessels causing an increase in their diameter, thereby improving blood flow and decreasing resistance primarily caused by venule dilation, thereby reducing preload; as peripheral resistance decreases, workload on heart is reduced and oxygen demand/supply ratio improves	Flushing, headache, dizziness, hypotension	Monitor blood-pressure closely

Postural hypotension may occur; caution clients to change position slowly, to sit or lie down, especially when taking nitroglycerin tablets SL

Give Tylenol for heart attack

When taking nitroglycerin tablets SL for anginal pain, instruct client to take additional tablets (up to 3) at 5-minute intervals if necessary. If pain is not relieved after 15 minutes, physician should be contacted immediately or client should report to hospital

Tablets are inactivated by light, heat, cold, air, and moisture; store at room temperature, in tight-fitting, amber glass container

A potent nitroglycerin tablet should produce a burning sensation under tongue when taken SL; check expiration |
| Beta-adrenergic blocking agents | Propranolol (Inderal), atenolol (Tenormin) | Block sympathetic stimulation of beta receptors; decrease myocardial workload and oxygen demand by decreasing contractility, HR, and BP | Hypotension, bradycardia, decreased myocardial contractility, congestive heart failure, (bronchospasm, and wheezing with Inderal). | Administer cautiously in clients with congestive heart failure and with respiratory conditions such as bronchitis and asthma; beta blockers may mask symptoms of hypoglycemia

Do not discontinue beta-adrenergic blocking therapy abruptly; results in exacerbation of symptoms |
| Calcium channel blockers | Diltiazem (Cardizem), nifedipine (Procardia) verapamil (Calan) | Reduce vascular smooth muscle tone by interfering with the ability of free calcium ions to initiate muscular contraction; act on coronary and peripheral arteries, causing vasodilation, increased myocardial oxygen supply, and decreased peripheral resistance | Dizziness, hypotension, bradycardia with diltiazem, verapamil | Monitor BP and HR |

TABLE 4–6 Thrombolytic Therapy

Goal	Lyse intracoronary clot to restore blood flow, salvage ischemic myocardium, limit infarct size, and save left ventricular function
Agents Used	Streptokinase, urokinase, recombinant tissue plasminogen activator (rt-PA), anistreplase
Selection Criteria	<65–70 years of age; significant ST elevation; <6° since onset of symptoms
Contraindications	History of CVA; recent surgery or trauma, hypertension, coagulopathy
Complications	Hemorrhagic stroke or bleeding from other sites
Effective if	Decrease in chest pain, ST elevation resolves, CPKs peak rapidly, reperfusion dysrhythmias (PVCs, ventricular tachycardia)

Client Goals	Implementations
Prevent harm from hemorrhage	Monitor PTT if on heparin Monitor neurological status frequently (LOC, complaints of headache) Monitor puncture sites for bleeding Monitor urine, stool for occult blood Avoid unnecessary punctures No IM injections Monitor hemoglobin and hematocrit Apply direct pressure to bleeding sites for 30 minutes or until bleeding stops
Maintain cardiac tissue perfusion	Monitor for chest pain, ST elevation, reperfusion dysrhythmias Notify physician if chest pain, hypotension, SOB, or ECG changes occur
Reduce client/family anxiety	Explain procedures and treatments Check on patient frequently Allow verbalization of fears Provide calm, reassuring environment

ately, carefully document, and follow hospital protocol for treatment
3. Place client in semi-Fowler's position to decrease venous return and enhance lung expansion
4. Maintain patent intravenous line for emergency drug administration
5. Ensure that emergency drugs and equipment are available and in good working order; ensure that cardiac alarm systems are activated
6. Be alert to altered electrolyte levels
7. Implement pharmacological interventions
   a. Antidysrhythmic agents (see Table 4–4)
   b. Drugs to treat heart failure (see Table 4–1)
8. Participate in emergency measures if cardiac output severely compromised
   a. Measures to treat dysrhythmias
      (1) Defibrillation/cardioversion
      (2) Pacemaker insertion
      (3) CPR (see CPR)
   b. Measures to treat congestive heart failure and shock (see CHF and Shock)
C. Ensure participation in program of progressive activity
   1. Restrict activity; bedrest for first 24 to 48 hours and if stable, supervised program of increased activity based on measure of energy expenditure (METs)
   2. Assess for complications secondary to reduced activity
      a. Thrombophlebitis; pain, redness, swelling
      b. Constipation; also from effects of opiates
   3. Provide measures to prevent complications secondary to reduced activity
      a. Anti-embolic hose
      b. Ankle flexion/extension exercises
      c. SQ heparin
      d. Stool softener; prevents Valsalva's maneuver, which may cause changes in BP and heart rate
   4. Nitroglycerin SL may be used prophylactically prior to exercise
D. Help client develop effective coping behavior
   1. Assess behavioral coping reactions
   2. Assess and utilize client's support systems
   3. Implement measures to decrease anxiety

TABLE 4–7 Percutaneous Transluminal Coronary Angioplasty (PTCA)

Purpose	Nonoperative procedure where a balloon is inserted into the coronary artery to increase its diameter and improve blood flow
Preparation	Explain the procedure to the client and answer questions Obtain baseline blood work, including type and crossmatch Have operating room on standby for emergency coronary artery bypass
Postprocedural Care	Patient will return with introducer sheaths in place (done to decrease chance of bleeding) Monitor closely for development of chest pain Be prepared to obtain STAT 12-lead ECG and give calcium channel blockers and nitrates If chest pain continues, prepare for another PTCA or surgery

Complications	Similar to cardiac catheterization
	  Dye reactions, blood loss from site, hypotension, bradycardia, hematoma formation; treat with diphenhydramine (Benadryl), fluids as appropriate
	
	Restenosis
	  Administer antiplatelet drugs (ASA, dipyridamole [Persantine])

a. Act with calmness and efficiency and minimize environmental activity and noise

b. Correct client's misconceptions; reassure, educate, explain environment, procedures, and routines

c. Bolster optimism, offer support and encouragement, and ensure early mobilization by participation in supervised progressive activity program

d. Mild sedation

4. Participate in management of client's coping mechanisms

E. Help client understand disease process and participate in therapeutic treatment regimen

1. Assess readiness to learn, time teaching appropriately

2. Instruct client on the following:

a. Purpose of coronary care unit and routines

b. Anatomy, physiology, pathophysiology of CAD and MI in language client can understand

c. Purpose and explanation of procedures, diagnostic tests, and therapeutic interventions including home management

(1) Cardiac catheterization (Table 4–8)

(2) Coronary artery bypass surgery (Table 4–9)

(3) Pacemaker (Table 4–10)

(4) Thrombolytic therapy (see Table 4–6)

(5) IABP (Table 4–11)

d. Risk factor reduction

e. Activity guidelines

(1) Pulse taking

(2) Return to work

(3) Return to sexual activity

f. Dietary guidelines

g. Medications

(1) Dose and schedule

(2) Action

(3) Side effects

h. Warning signs of MI

i. Follow-up care

V. Evaluation

A. Client will verbalize comfort

B. Client will be hemodynamically and electrophysiologically stable

C. Client will demonstrate decreased anxiety and integrate treatment plan into lifestyle

D. Client will maintain a prescribed activity level without complications

E. Client will verbalize understanding of the following:

1. Coronary artery disease process

2. Diet low in sodium, saturated fats, and cholesterol

3. Medication therapy including dose, schedule, rationale for, side effects of, and importance of taking as prescribed

4. Activity restrictions and activity progression

5. Signs and symptoms important to report to health care provider

6. Plan for follow-up care, including future appointments

F. Client will participate in modifiable cardiovascular risk factor reduction

G. Client will demonstrate pulse-taking

TABLE 4–8 Nursing Care for Individuals Undergoing Cardiac Catheterization

Precardiac Catheterization Nursing Care

- Provide thorough explanation of procedure and rationale
- Ensure that written consent is obtained
- Maintain NPO status 6 to 18 hours before procedure

Postcardiac Catheterization Nursing Care

Potential Complications	Nursing Interventions
Hemorrhage	• Closely observe insertion site for bleeding or hematoma formation • Assess BP and HR at frequent intervals according to physician order and hospital policy • Maintain pressure dressing over insertion site; sandbag may be utilized • Instruct client to avoid flexing femoral area if femoral site used

Postcardiac Catheterization Nursing Care

Potential Complications	Nursing Interventions
	• Instruct client to maintain bedrest for 12 to 24 hours according to physician order and hospital policy
Impaired peripheral circulation secondary to clot dislodgement	• Assess frequently presence and quality of peripheral pulses • Assess color, sensation, and temperature of extremity
Injury, renal impairment, due to nephrotoxic effects of cardiac catheterization contrast medium	• Encourage fluids • Monitor intake and output • Observe for signs of acute renal failure (increasing BUN and serum creatinine, decreased urine output, oliguria, anuria, edema, weight gain, lethargy, and confusion)

TABLE 4–9 Guidelines for Preoperative and Postoperative Care of Individuals Experiencing Open Heart Surgery

Problem: Patient/family anxiety related to impending surgery and associated risks

Goal: Patient/family will demonstrate decreased anxiety

Interventions:

- Collaborate with physician on teaching to be done

- Provide opportunity for patient/family to discuss surgery, encourage questions, verbalization of feelings and anxieties

- Explain operative procedure according to client's readiness to learn and need for information

- Preoperative teaching
    Chest physiotherapy (cough and deep breathing techniques, incentive spirometry, postural drainage)
    NPO status after midnight
    Medication for sleep if needed
    Preoperative body hair removal, morning shower
    Preoperative medications
    Operating room
    Anesthesia

- Postoperative teaching
    Recovery room/critical care unit environment, environmental noise, close proximity of nurse and other health care providers
    Monitoring devices; purpose and anticipated time of removal
        Endotracheal tube and mechanical ventilation
        IV, arterial line, hemodynamic monitoring devices
        Chest tubes
        ECG monitor
        NG tube
        Foley catheter
    Medication for pain
    Ways to communicate while breathing tube in place
    Activity; chest physiotherapy, and activity progression
    Anticipated time in the critical care unit
    Emotional response; depression, nightmares

Problem: Decreased cardiac output related to hypovolemia, impaired ventricular function, dysrhythmias

Goal: Client will maintain an adequate cardiac output

Interventions:

- Etiology: hypovolemia due to hemorrhage, inadequate blood/fluid replacement, and coagulopathy caused by cardiopulmonary bypass machine

- Monitor for signs of hypovolemia
    Hypotension, tachycardia
    Low CVP, PAP, PCWP
    Signs of peripheral hypoperfusion (skin temperature, color, peripheral pulses)
    Altered mental status
    Oliguria
- Observe for hemorrhage
    Excessive amounts of wound and chest tube drainage
    Falling HCT
- Observe for signs of coagulopathy
    Blood oozing from incisions and puncture sites
    Bloody secretions from endotracheal tube
    Petechiae, ecchymotic areas
    Hematuria
    Heme-positive NG aspirate and stool
    Altered coagulation profile (e.g., prothrombin time, partial thromboplastin time, platelet count, bleeding time)

- Notify physician of presence of abnormalities; document carefully

- Perform measures to prevent hypovolemia; implement and monitor response to medical therapy
    Replacement fluids (0.9 NaCl lactated Ringer's solution), blood and blood products (albumin plasma, platelets)
    Measures to prevent and control bleeding (e.g., prolonged pressure after giving injections, avoidance of activities that increase the potential for trauma such as stiff toothbrushes or straight-edge razors)
    Protamine sulfate to reverse heparin effects after cardiopulmonary bypass machine

- Etiology: impaired ventricular function due to pre-existing, intraoperative or perioperative myocardial ischemia and infarction, metabolic abnormalities, residual cardiac depressant effects of anesthesia, cardiac tamponade

- Monitor for signs and symptoms of heart failure

- Notify physician of presence of abnormalities; document carefully

- Implement measures to maintain an adequate cardiac output
    Semi- to high-Fowler's position to facilitate breathing and decrease venous return
    Promote rest to decrease myocardial oxygen demand
    Diet low in sodium to decrease fluid retention
    Maintain patent chest tube (strip or milk prn)

- If heart failure present, implement and monitor response to medical therapy and interventions
    Oxygen therapy
    Inotropic, vasopressor agents (digoxin, dopamine, dobutamine, amrinone)
    Vasodilator agents (sodium nitroprusside IV, nitroglycerin IV)
    Diuretics
    Intra-aortic balloon pumping (See Table 4–11)

- Etiology: dysrhythmias due to myocardial ischemia, acid–base imbalance, hypoxia, electrolyte imbalance (hypokalemia), surgical injury of conduction system, pre-existing enlarged heart chambers; edema around valve anulus can cause heart block J MVR/AVR—usually temporary—NOT considered a TRUE surgical injury.

- Maintain continuous ECG monitoring for dysrhythmias; high- and low-rate alarms set at all times

- Perform actions to prevent dysrhythmia development (e.g., monitor arterial blood gas levels and electrolytes; perform pulmonary care)

- If present, document carefully, notify physician

- Implement and monitor response to medical therapy as ordered; treat underlying cause of dysrhythmia
    Oxygen therapy
    Electrolyte replacement
    Antidysrhythmic agents and treatment measures (see Table 4–4)

Problem: Respiratory insufficiency related to hypoventilation, atelectasis, pneumothorax, hemothorax, thromboemboli

Goal: Client will demonstrate adequate ventilation and oxygenation

Intervention:

- Etiology: hypoventilation, atelectasis

- Perform frequent assessments of respiratory status
    Presence of spontaneous respirations
    Respiratory rate; tachypnea
    Quality of respirations; dyspnea, labored shallow respirations
    Breath sounds; rales, rhonchi, wheezing
    Confusion, restlessness
    Cyanosis

- Monitor arterial blood gas levels

- Verify and document ventilator settings

- Implement measures to prevent respiratory problems
    Endotracheal suction (hyperinflate ambu and hyperoxygenate)
    Cough and deep-breathing exercises
    Use of incentive spirometry
    If on bedrest, turn every 2 hours; early mobilization and activity progression

- Etiology: pneumothorax, hemothorax

- Perform frequent respiratory assessments as above

TABLE 4–9 Guidelines for Preoperative and Postoperative Care of Individuals Experiencing Open Heart Surgery *Continued*

- Maintain patent chest drainage system
- Etiology: thromboemboli
- Monitor for deep vein thrombosis
  Calf pain, redness, swelling
  Positive Homans' sign
- Encourage leg exercises q 10; discourage crossing of legs
- Monitor for evidence of pulmonary emboli; implement and monitor response to medical and nursing interventions

Problem: Infection; sternotomy, IV cutdown sites, cardiopulmonary bypass machine, hypoventilation, atelectasis, mechanical ventilation, urethral catheter

Goal: Client will be free of infection

Intervention:

- Monitor temperature
- Assess for wound, catheter site infections; redness, drainage, swelling
- Assess for pulmonary infections; change in color and character of sputum, diminished breath sounds
- Monitor for urinary tract infections; cloudy urine, dysuria, flank pain, hematuria, foul-smelling urine
- Maintain appropriate aseptic technique during procedures
- Be aware of length of time IV and hemodynamic monitoring lines have been in place; plan replacement as necessary; remove Foley catheter as soon as possible
- Observe for signs of sepsis, fever, chills, diaphoresis, hypotension, tachycardia, altered level of consciousness
- Monitor laboratory values: CBC, blood cultures, wound, urine and sputum cultures
- Medical therapy, antibiotics, antipyretics
- Provide appropriate wound care

Problem: Anxiety; pain; difficulty with communication while intubated; disorientation with environment and procedures; feelings of helplessness

Goal: Client will demonstrate decreased anxiety and participate in plan of care

Intervention:

- Orient to time, situation, location
- Assist with communication
- Anticipate needs
- Allow family support and participation
- Reassure client on daily progress
- Encourage verbalization of fears and feelings regarding operation, recovery, and discharge

Problem: Knowledge deficit; discharge care

Goal: Client will demonstrate understanding of surgical procedure and will participate in the discharge plan of care

Intervention:

Instruct on the following:

- Diet: avoid foods high in cholesterol, saturated fats, and sodium
- Discharge medications: purpose, dosage, side effects
- Activity allowances, limitations (include discussion of sexual activity as appropriate)
- Care of incision and symptoms of wound infection to report
- Risk factor modification
- Avoidance of stress, fatigue

Evaluation:

- Client/family will demonstrate decreased anxiety and integrate treatment plan into lifestyle
- Client will be hemodynamically and electrophysiologically stable
- Client will demonstrate no signs and symptoms of respiratory insufficiency
- Client will be free from infections
- Client/family will demonstrate sufficient information to comply with discharge regimen

Congestive Heart Failure (CHF)

I. Assessment
   A. Compensatory mechanisms for maintaining cardiac output
      1. Tachycardia
      2. Ventricular dilation: Starling's law
      3. Myocardial hypertrophy
      4. Vasoconstriction secondary to norepinephrine and epinephrine
      5. Sodium and water retention related to aldosterone and antidiuretic hormone
   B. Pathophysiology
      1. Heart fails as a pump to meet the body's need for oxygen and removal of waste after compensatory mechanisms are exhausted and decompensation occurs
      2. Left-sided CHF: blood backs up into pulmonary circulation
      3. Right-sided CHF: blood backs up into systemic circulation
   C. Incidence
      1. Affects 50 to 60% of those with organic heart disease
      2. Frequent complication of myocardial infarction (MI)
   D. Predisposing/precipitating factors
      1. Hypervolemia: IV fluids; HTN due to sodium and water retention and increased peripheral resistance (afterload)
      2. Hypovolemia: dehydration, valve damage
      3. Decreased contractility: MI, coronary atherosclerosis, dysrhythmias

TABLE 4–10 Pacemaker Insertion—Postoperative Nursing Care Plan

Problem: Decreased cardiac output related to pacemaker malfunction	**Problem:** Knowledge deficit
Goal: Client will maintain adequate cardiac output with normal pacemaker function	**Goal:** Client will demonstrate understanding of pacemaker function and its care

Intervention:

Intervention (left column):

- Note method of pacing (demand/fixed rate) and rate set by physician in surgery; use information to assess pacemaker function

- Monitor for signs and symptoms of pacemaker malfunction; immediately notify physician, document carefully
  Apical pulse rate less than preset pacemaker rate
  Ventricular dysrhythmias (PVCs) due to mechanical irritation of displaced pacemaker wire
  Signs of decreased cardiac output

- Obtain ECG and assess for malfunction

- Maintain an electrically safe environment; ensure that all electrical equipment is grounded

- Initiate measures to prevent pacemaker dislodgement
  Limit arm and shoulder movement on side of permanent pacemaker insertion for first 72 hours
  Assist with gentle full ROM and progress activity but limit vigorous movement or stress on operative side usually for first 6 weeks as ordered by physician

Intervention (right column):

Instruct client on the following:

- Rationale and function of pacemaker

- Pulse taking

- Safety precautions
  Avoid participation in contact sports
  Avoid close proximity with high voltage electrical equipment (older model microwaves, radar equipment)
  Wear Medic-Alert tag
  Have pulse generator monitored regularly at physician's office, pacemaker clinic, or telephone monitoring device

- Signs and symptoms to report to health care provider
  Fever and signs of inflammation or infection at operative site
  Pulse rate less than preset permanent pacemaker rate
  Fatigue
  Dizziness
  Chest pain
  Palpitations
  Shortness of breath
  Swelling of extremities
  Weight gain

4. Various heart diseases: rheumatic, pericarditis, cardiomyopathy
5. Increased and prolonged metabolic needs: hypoxia, fever, pregnancy

E. Clinical manifestations, in varying degrees, are dependent upon cause, years present, and existing damage to myocardium (Table 4–12)

TABLE 4–11 Care of the Patient with an Intra-aortic Balloon Pump

Purpose: To increase coronary artery perfusion, and decrease afterload, thus conserving myocardial work
Uses: Intractable angina, myocardial infarction, CHF

Analysis	Goal	Implementation
Decreased cardiac output related to left ventricular failure	Adequate cardiac output	Check for proper functioning of balloon Monitor PAP, PCWP, and cardiac outputs Maintain proper timing of balloon
Impaired tissue perfusion related to occlusion/embolus	Maintain perfusion to distal extremity/kidneys	Check pulses q 1-2°, especially distal to insertion site Monitor color, temperature of extremities May use prophylactic heparin drip Never turn balloon off for long periods of time Check urine output q1°; notify physician if urine flow stops abruptly (occlusion of renal arteries by balloon) Keep alarms on at all times
High risk for infection related to altered skin integrity	No evidence of infection	Inspect balloon insertion site q shift Site dressing changes per policy
High risk for injury related to anticoagulants	No evidence of hemorrhage	Monitor PTT if on heparin Monitor platelets qd (balloon destroys platelets) Instruct client to keep insertion site extremity straight
Anxiety related to apparatus/ICU	Reduce anxiety	Inform client/family of purpose for balloon; answer questions; allow verbalization of fears

TABLE 4–12 Congestive Heart Failure: Clinical Manifestations and Interventions

Manifestations of Left-sided CHF	Interventions
Dyspnea/orthopnea	Position in Fowler's or semi-Fowler's; humidified oxygen
Cheyne-Stokes respirations	Ensure airway patency; monitor ABGs; avoid sedatives
Cough/rales	Assess lung sounds; give Lasix
Oliguria	Strict I & O; monitor BUN, creatinine
Confusion	Orient to person, place, time; protect from harm

Manifestations of Right-Sided CHF	
Edema of lower extremities	Protect from thermal/ mechanical injury; elevate periodically
Sacral edema	Turn every 2 hours; prevent decubiti
Jugular vein distention (JVD)	Assess for other signs of fluid retention and need for Lasix, digoxin, and Na^+-restricted diet
Abdominal ascites	Measure girth, weight
Hepatomegaly	Know all drugs and effects on impaired liver function; serum digoxin level
Abdominal pain, anorexia, nausea and vomiting	Avoid gas-forming foods; serve small, frequent meals; frequent oral hygiene; antiemetics

General Manifestations	
Fatigue	Bedrest; assist with ADLs
Anxiety	Quiet, relaxed environment; anti-anxiety agents
Chest pain	Short- and long-acting nitrates; oxygen

1. Left-sided
   a. Dyspnea/orthopnea
   b. Cheyne-Stokes respirations
   c. Cough—frothy and possibly blood-tinged
   d. Rales
   e. Oliguria—related to impaired renal blood flow
   f. Confusion due to cerebral hypoxia
2. Right-sided
   a. Peripheral edema: lower extremities, sacrum, jugular venous distention
   b. Abdominal ascites
   c. Hepatomegaly
   d. Abdominal pain, anorexia, nausea/vomiting
3. General
   a. Fatigue

   b. Anxiety
   c. Chest pain
F. Diagnostic examinations
   1. Routine: CBC, electrolytes, ECG, chest x-ray
   2. Noninvasive: echocardiogram to assess position, size, and movement of valves/ chambers by ultrasound; arterial blood gas (ABG) to assess pO_2, pCO_2 and acid–base balance of blood
   3. Invasive: cardiac catheterization to assess valves/chambers and cardiac output using catheters, contrast dye, fluoroscopy, and x-rays (see Table 4–6)
G. Pulmonary complications
   1. Pulmonary edema: left ventricular pressure so high that fluid escapes from blood vessels into pulmonary vasculature
      a. Emergency treatment
         (1) IV digitalis to promote contractility and diuresis
         (2) IV furosemide (Lasix) to promote diuresis
         (3) IV aminophylline to relieve bronchospasm
         (4) IV morphine sulfate to relieve chest pain, provide sedation, and decrease venous return (i.e., preload)
         (5) IV arterial dilators (sodium nitroprusside) to decrease peripheral resistance (i.e., afterload)
         (6) IV venous dilators (isorbide) to decrease venous return (i.e., preload)
         (7) Oxygenation with possible intubation
H. Medical management
   1. Medications
      a. Digitalis (Table 4–13)
      b. Furosemide (Lasix) (see Table 4–1)
   2. Low sodium diet with fluid restriction
II. Analysis
   A. Decreased cardiac output related to decreased pumping ability of heart
   B. Altered tissue perfusion related to decreased cardiac output
   C. Impaired gas exchange related to pulmonary edema and decreased cardiac output
   D. Fluid volume excess related to decreased cardiac output and decreased renal perfusion
   E. Altered nutrition: less than body requirements related to dietary modifications, fluid restrictions, and fatigue
   F. Activity intolerance related to fatigue and decreased cardiac output
   G. High risk for injury related to hypoxia

III. Planning/goals, expected outcomes
  A. Client will maintain adequate cardiac output and systemic tissue perfusion
  B. Client will maintain adequate gas exchange and respiratory function
  C. Client will maintain adequate hydration and nutrition status
  D. Client will maintain adequate rest and activity
  E. Client will be free of physical and emotional harm
IV. Implementation
  A. To maintain adequate cardiac output and systemic perfusion
    1. Monitor for signs and symptoms of decreasing perfusion and report (see section I, Assessment)
    2. Give digitalis (see Table 4–13)
    3. Give furosemide (Lasix) (see Table 4–1)
    4. Prepare and care for patient undergoing IABP therapy (see Table 4–11)
  B. To maintain adequate gas exchange and respiratory function
    1. Monitor ABGs and report
    2. Position in high Fowler's to improve lung expansion
    3. Give humidified oxygen to decrease cardiorespiratory workload
    4. Assist to turn, cough, and deep breathe every 2 hours to increase gas exchange and remove secretions
    5. Give expectorants, mucolytics, and aminophylline when ordered
  C. To maintain adequate hydration and nutrition status
    1. Monitor for excess fluids such as weight gain, edema, rales, output less than intake
    2. Monitor for dehydration such as hypotension, elevated BUN, dry mucous membranes
    3. Restrict sodium, usually 2 to 3 grams per day (Table 4–14)
    4. Give smaller, frequent meals (prevent increased blood flow to GI tract), high protein (increases serum albumin and colloidal oncotic pressure), bland, low residue (prevent nausea and vomiting)
    5. Monitor for impaired renal function such as elevated BUN, creatinine, oliguria, hyperkalemia
  D. To maintain adequate rest and activity
    1. Promote complete bedrest during acute stage; minimize noise, ADLs to decrease oxygen consumption
    2. Space activities and assist client to gradually increase activity level
  E. To prevent physical and emotional harm
    1. Protect from injury, especially with cerebral hypoxia; use side rails, orient to environment, provide close supervision
    2. Give thorough skin care to prevent breakdown due to immobility, decreased perfusion, and malnutrition
    3. Give stool softener to prevent Valsalva's maneuver
    4. Monitor for thromboembolus
    5. Monitor for impaired liver function such as unusual bleeding, jaundice, decreased albumin
    6. Offer realistic reassurance to client and significant others

TABLE 4–13 Cardiac Glycosides

Class	Example	Action	Use	Common Side Effects	Nursing Implications
Cardiac glycosides	Digoxin (Lanoxin)	Increases stroke volume and contraction while decreasing heart rate and size (therefore increases cardiac output), improve systemic/pulmonary circulation; decrease venous pressure and promote diuresis	CHF Pulmonary edema, supraventricular tachycardias	Cardiovascular: bradycardia, tachycardia, and other dysrhythmias; hypotension Gastrointestinal: anorexia, nausea, vomiting, diarrhea CNS: headache, confusion, fatigue, visual disturbances	Not to be confused with digitoxin, a longer-acting form of digitalis, used in renal impairment; check apical pulse one full minute and hold if pulse is below 60 or above 120; report to physician; teach client to do same at home; monitor blood level for toxicity, especially in elderly; monitor for hypokalemia when on diuretics; potentiates toxicity

TABLE 4–14 Approximate Sodium Content in Common Food Items

Food Item	Amount	Sodium (mg)	Food Item	Amount	Sodium (mg)
Dairy			**Fats/Oils**		
Whole or low fat milk	1 cup	122	Butter or margarine	1 tbsp	125
Swiss cheese	1 oz	74	Corn, olive, safflower	1 tbsp	none
Swiss cheese, processed	1 oz	388			

General facts for healthful eating

- Processed and canned foods contain the most sodium; fresh and frozen the least

Food Item	Amount	Sodium (mg)
Breads/Cereals		
White bread	1 slice	127
White bread, low sodium brand	1 slice	7
Whole wheat, cooked	1 cup	519
Bran flakes	1 cup	207

- Fish and smoked and sausage-type foods contain more sodium than meat and poultry

- Read food labels and over-the-counter drug labels carefully for sodium content

Food Item	Amount	Sodium (mg)
Fruits/Vegetables		
Green beans, frozen	1 cup	5
Green beans, canned	1 cup	319
Orange juice	1 cup	3

- Avoid use of table salt in preparation and seasoning; all foods contain some natural sodium

- Investigate other nonsodium seasonings and low-sodium food brands

Food Item	Amount	Sodium (mg)
Fish/Shellfish		
Tuna	3 oz	680
Clams, canned	3 oz	850

- Avoid snack type foods; these are very high in sodium; fruits and vegetables are very low in sodium

Meanings of sodium labels for food

"Sodium free"	Less than 5 mg of Na^+ per serving
Very low sodium	35 mg or less of Na^+
Low sodium	140 mg or less of Na^+
Reduced sodium	Process to reduce usual level of Na^+ by 75%
Unsalted	Processed without salt

Food Item	Amount	Sodium (mg)
Meat/Poultry		
Egg, fried	1	155
Egg, boiled	1	61
Ground beef	3 oz	41
Ham	3 oz	559
Chicken, broiled	3 oz	60
Hot dog	1	607

7. Support grieving process related to loss of health/lifestyle and chronicity of CHF

V. Evaluation

A. Client returns from a state of acute CHF to a state of chronic compensated CHF

B. Adequate rest and activity maintained

C. Client free from physical and emotional harm

Peripheral Vascular Disease (PVD)

Arterial Disease

I. Assessment

A. Definition: structural changes of arteries, veins, and nerves related to blood flow obstruction

B. Etiology, incidence, predisposing/precipitating factors

1. Arteriosclerosis obliterans

a. Accumulation of fatty atherosclerotic plaques in the intimal lining of large arteries of lower extremities

b. Occurs in men ages 50 to 70, postmenopausal women, diabetics

c. High-fat diet, obesity, sedentary lifestyle, smoking, stress

2. Raynaud's disease

a. Intermittent arterial vasospasm producing pain and cyanosis of arteries in hands and feet

b. Most common in women ages 18 to 40; can also occur in males and children

c. Cold, stress, smoking

3. Buerger's disease (thromboangiitis obliterans)

a. Inflammatory disorder producing spasm and thrombosis of smaller arteries in hands and lower extremities

b. Occurs in men ages 16 to 40

c. Smoking

C. Clinical manifestations

1. Pain

a. Upper extremities: numbness or tingling in one or more digits

b. Lower extremities: intermittent claudication, severe and sharp, increased with activity and relieved by rest

2. Peripheral pulses decreased or absent

3. Edema, infrequent

4. Skin changes

a. Upper extremities: hands may be

cool/cold, pale/cyanotic; ulceration and gangrene of digits may occur with advanced tissue hypoxia
   b. Lower extremities: legs may be cool/cold, pale/cyanotic, texture smooth/shiny, hair loss, nails thickened; ulcers when present are severely painful with pale grey bases and defined edges found on toes, heels, dorsum of foot, and lateral malleolus
D. Diagnostic examinations
   1. Noninvasive
      a. Ultrasound
      b. Skin temperature studies: arterial damage exists when both hands (legs) placed in warm water and occluded extremity does not vasodilate
      c. Treadmill test for intermittent claudication: degree of ischemia measured by the amount of exercise needed to produce pain
   2. Invasive
      a. Angiography (arteriography): contrast dye injected into brachial or femoral artery and x-ray films expose obstruction (see Table 4–7)
E. Surgical intervention
   1. Aortic bifurcation graft; femoral popliteal bypass graft
      a. Preoperative nursing care

      (1) Reduce anxiety by assessing client's understanding, reinforcing surgeon's explanation, and explaining routine postoperative care
      (2) Monitor for existing infection and report; administer prophylactic broad spectrum antibiotic given 48 hours before surgery
      (3) See Chapter 6, ''Nursing Process Applied to Adults Undergoing Surgery,'' for general measures
   b. Postoperative nursing care
      (1) Monitor for graft occlusion, most common complication; indicated by absence of peripheral pulses, cool, pale/cyanotic extremity
      (2) Monitor for hemorrhage: bleeding at incision site; signs and symptoms of shock
      (3) Monitor for thrombus: warmth, redness, pain of extremities
      (4) Monitor for pulmonary embolus (Table 4–15)
      (5) Monitor for infection: purulent wound drainage; *Staphylococcus aureus* most common
   2. Amputation
      a. Preoperative nursing care

TABLE 4–15 Nursing Care Plan—Pulmonary Embolus

Assessment: Know clients at high risk; for example, history of previous PE, cardiac or pulmonary disease, postoperative, trauma (for example, hip fracture), pregnancy

Analysis: High risk for injury related to hypoxia

Goal: Client will not develop pulmonary emboli

Implementation: Perform a comprehensive nursing history asking specific close-ended questions to avoid missing important risk factors

Evaluation: Client or family answers yes or no to specific questions

---

Assessment: Know that signs/symptoms can be sudden or insidious; for example, chest pain, dyspnea, apprehension, cough, hemoptysis, rapid, weak pulse, tachypnea, hypotension, fever

Analysis: Impaired gas exchange related to altered tissue perfusion

Goal: Client's cardiopulmonary status remains within normal limits

Implementation:
   Cardiovascular; elevate head of bed; administer oxygen; monitor lung sounds, vital signs, Homans' sign, and ABGs; give morphine sulfate, dopamine, and anticoagulants (heparin in acute stages)

   Renal: monitor IV intake and urinary output; Foley catheter usually inserted, daily weights

   Cerebral: monitor level of consciousness; stay closely with client for reassurance; explain procedures used to diagnose PE: ABGs, chest x-ray, lung scan, ECG

Evaluation:
   Cardiovascular: vital signs stable: afebrile; HR 60 to 80 bpm; respirations 12 to 20 per minute; systolic BP greater than 100; client denies dyspnea and chest pain and does not appear short of breath; lung sounds audible in all lobes with absence of wheezing and rales; absence of cyanosis; ABG within normal limits; PTT PT within therapeutic range

   Renal: output greater than 30 mL per hour

   Cerebral: alert and oriented; absence of apprehension

---

        (1) Emotional support for loss of limb, body image

        (2) Strengthening exercises for arms and unaffected leg for using crutches and transfers

        (3) See Chapter 6, "Nursing Process Applied to Adults Undergoing Surgery," for general measures

    b. Postoperative nursing care

        (1) Monitor for pulmonary embolus, most common complication (see Table 4–14)

        (2) Monitor for hemorrhage/infection of stump site

        (3) Elevate stump for first 24 hours to reduce edema, then keep flat to prevent hip (knee) flexion contractures

        (4) Encourage client to look at stump and assist with stump care to promote acceptance of new body image

        (5) Wash stump with mild soap and water when incision healed; massage toward the suture line to increase circulation

        (6) Prepare stump for future prosthesis by showing client how to bear weight against footstool and wrapping with pressure bandage, figure-eight method, to shape stump

        (7) Prevent brachial plexus (arm paralysis) by assuring that crutches are correctly measured

        (8) Inform client that phantom limb sensation/pain is common and may persist for a time; visualization techniques and whirlpool helpful

        (9) Instruct in transfers to wheelchair

II. Analysis

  A. Altered tissue perfusion related to arterial changes

  B. Pain related to decreased tissue perfusion

  C. Knowledge deficit related to disease, treatment, and prevention of recurrence

III. Planning/goals, expected outcomes

  A. Client will maintain adequate arterial blood flow

  B. Client will be free of physical/emotional discomfort

  C. Client will develop plan to prevent future blood flow obstruction

IV. Implementation

  A. Monitor for signs and symptoms of decreasing arterial blood flow (see section on Assessment)

  B. Generally, affected extremity kept below heart level to prevent dislodging thrombus; enhance arterial flow to distal portion of extremity

  C. Push fluids, 2 to 3 liters per day, unless contraindicated by CHF or renal failure, to decrease blood viscosity

  D. Administer drugs as ordered

    1. Anticoagulants (Table 4–16)

    2. Fibrinolytics: streptokinase, urokinase; actively dissolve clots; high rate of anaphylaxis

    3. Dextran: plasma expander to decrease blood viscosity

    4. Peripheral vasodilators such as nylidrin (Arlidin), papaverine, isoxsuprine (Vasodilan) for direct relaxation of arteriolar and venous smooth muscle

    5. Antiplatelets: dipyridamole (Persantine) and aspirin to decrease platelet aggregation

  E. Monitor for pulmonary embolus and prepare client for embolectomy if necessary

  F. Give narcotic analgesics for severe pain, but know that drugs that increase arterial blood flow also help to decrease pain

  G. Ulcer care: keep area clean, dry, and pressure free; limit activity to reduce oxygen needs; apply topical corticosteroids and antibiotics to stimulate granulation of new tissue; oral antibiotics may also be used

  H. Anticipate and support the grieving process should bypass or amputation be required

  I. Teach avoidance of smoking, which causes vasoconstriction

  J. Teach reduction of calories if overweight; reduction of cholesterol

  K. Teach need for regular walking within limits of discomfort to increase collateral circulation

  L. Teach safety measures that prevent compromised circulation:

    1. Avoid restrictive clothing such as belts, girdles, garters

    2. No leg crossing at the knees; both legs on the floor

    3. Avoid too warm or too cold temperatures

    4. Never go barefoot; wear correct-fitting shoes

    5. Seek licensed podiatrist for trimming thickened toenails, removal of corns, and so on

    6. Teach need to inspect feet daily for signs of infection and report promptly

  M. Stress importance of follow-up appointments for life-long care of a chronic disease

V. Evaluation

  A. Client has adequate arterial blood flow

TABLE 4–16 Anticoagulants

Example	Action	Use	Common Side Effects	Nursing Implications
Heparin	Exert direct effect on blood coagulation, blocking the conversion of prothrombin to thrombin and fibrinogen to fibrin; does not dissolve existing clots but prevents their extension and the formation of new clots; IV	Prophylaxis and treatment of venous and arterial thrombosis, pulmonary embolus	Spontaneous bleeding, such as epistaxis, gums, hematuria, black, tarry stools; subcutaneous injections, pain, itching, ecchymoses, GI disturbances	Protamine sulfate antidote for heparin; vitamin K antidote for Coumadin; monitor prothrombin time (PT) for Coumadin and partial thromboplastin time (PTT) or APTT for heparin; never aspirate or rub site after subcutaneous injection; always use infusion pump with heparin IV; always check heparin dose with second nurse; monitor for guaiac stools and other signs of bleeding; teach client safety: no aspirin or ASA products; read labels carefully; report bleeding gums, etc.; electric razors only; follow-up for regular PT levels
Warfarin sodium (Coumadin)	Cumulative and more prolonged; interfere with the hepatic synthesis of the vitamin K–dependent clotting factors; oral route used for maintenance when heparin therapy is complete			

B. Client free of physical and emotional discomfort
C. Client verbalizes a plan to prevent future blood flow obstruction

Venous Disorders

I. Assessment
   A. Etiology, incidence, predisposing/precipitating factors
      1. Varicose veins
         a. Abnormally dilated veins and incompetent valves leading to venous pooling of superficial veins in lower extremities
         b. Men and women affected equally
         c. Occupations requiring prolonged standing; pregnancy; familial tendency
      2. Thrombophlebitis
         a. Vein inflammation and clot formation of deep small veins in lower (upper) extremities
         b. Men and women affected equally
         c. IV catheters, surgery, immobilization
      3. Chronic venous stasis
         a. Prolonged increased venous and capillary pressure
         b. Men and women affected equally
         c. Long-standing varicose veins, recurrent episodes of thrombophlebitis, and deep vein thrombosis (DVT)
   B. Clinical manifestations
      1. Pain—aching type relieved with elevation (varicose veins, thrombophlebitis); throbbing severe type (DVT)
      2. Peripheral pulses usually present unless edema severe
      3. Skin changes
         a. Warm temperature
         b. Thickened texture
         c. Color—pigmentation change; bluish (varicose veins); reddish/brownish (thrombophlebitis); pallor/cyanosis (DVT)
         d. Edema present
         e. Ulcers when present moderately painful; pink bases with irregular edges; found on medial aspect of ankle
         f. Positive Homans sign
   C. Diagnostic examinations
      1. Ultrasound
      2. Trendelenburg test—leg raised until vein empties and tourniquet applied above knee; client stands and tourniquet removed; varicose vein fills from above instead of from below
      3. Venography (phlebography)—invasive procedure whereby thrombi are identified with radiopaque dye and x-rays; the most useful diagnostic test; nurse asks about dye allergy and obtains informed consent
   D. Complications
      1. DVT
         a. Pulmonary embolus
         b. Death
      2. Varicose veins: thrombophlebitis

E. Medical management
  1. DVT
     a. Bedrest
     b. Elevate extremity
     c. Anticoagulants
  2. Varicose veins
     a. Support stockings
     b. Avoid prolonged standing or sitting
II. Analysis
  A. Altered tissue perfusion related to arterial changes
  B. Pain related to decreased tissue perfusion
  C. Knowledge deficit related to disease, treatment, and prevention of recurrence
III. Planning/goals, expected outcomes
  A. Client will maintain adequate venous blood flow
  B. Client will be free of physical/emotional discomfort
  C. Client will develop a plan to prevent future blood flow obstruction
IV. Implementation
  A. Monitor for signs of decreasing venous blood flow (see section on Assessment)
  B. Generally, affected extremity kept above heart level to decrease edema and pain
  C. Push fluids unless contraindicated
  D. Drugs same as for arterial disorders
  E. Teach ankle flexion/dorsiflexion if on bedrest to increase venous return
  F. Apply correctly measured elastic support hose to compress superficial veins, directing flow into deeper veins and back to heart
  G. Monitor for pulmonary embolus (see Table 4–12)
  H. Give narcotic analgesics for severe pain but know that drugs that increase venous blood flow also help decrease pain
  I. Ulcer care—warm, moist packs; wet to dry saline dressings; topical corticosteroids/antibiotics; monitor for cellulitis and need for debridement
  J. Support client's potential negative feelings related to cosmetic disfigurement from varicose veins and know that vein ligation may be an option; also, skin grafting for nonhealing ulcers
  K. Teach safety measures that prevent compromised circulation (same as section on Arterial PVD)
V. Evaluation
  A. Client has adequate venous blood flow
  B. Client is free of physical and emotional discomfort
  C. Client verbalizes a plan to prevent future blood flow obstruction

Aneurysms

I. Assessment
  A. Definition: A localized dilation of a blood vessel primarily due to atherosclerotic disease, described according to:
    1. Structure
       a. True: abnormal widening involving all three layers of the vessel wall
       b. False: disruption of inner and medial layers of vessel, usually from trauma
       c. Dissecting: blood enters a weakened area of intima and splits the aortic media
    2. Shape
       a. Saccular: weakened area on one side of vessel
       b. Fusiform: weakening involves entire circumference of the vessel (most common)
    3. Location: refers to the arteries involved, or portion of aorta involved
  B. Pathophysiology
    1. Arises from areas of dense atherosclerosis, which destroys medial layer, causing weakening and widening of the aorta
    2. Increased widening increases wall tension, which increases widening
    3. Hypertension contributes to this phenomenon
  C. Aortic aneurysms
    1. Clinical manifestations: symptoms suggestive of origin of aneurysm
       a. Chest or back pain of sudden onset ("tearing" quality)
       b. Feelings of distention in chest or abdomen
       c. Paraplegia related to spinal cord ischemia
       d. Symptoms suggestive of cardiac tamponade or aortic insufficiency
       e. Symptoms of hemothorax
       f. Limb ischemia (cool, pulseless)
       g. Renal ischemia (decreased urine output)
       h. Mesenteric ischemia (cramping abdominal pain)
    2. Diagnostic examinations
       a. Chest x-ray shows widening mediastinum (most definitive)
       b. ECG and cardiac enzymes to rule out MI
       c. Angiogram to determine exact location
    3. Medical management
       a. Consists of pain management and treatment of CHF (i.e., morphine, re-

duce the blood pressure, and blood transfusions for blood loss)
    b. Death occurs in 90% of patients within 3 months
  4. Surgical management
    a. Surgical intervention necessary if hemodynamically unstable
    b. Dissected segment removed and replaced with prosthetic graft
    c. May need to replace aortic valve in ascending aneurysm
    d. Surgical complications
      (1) Graft infection
      (2) False aneurysm develops at surgical site
      (3) Graft thrombosis and occlusion
    e. Survival rate good if treated immediately, decreases with time
  5. Complications
    a. Mural thrombi
      (1) Thrombi formation on the wall of vessel results from roughened intima
      (2) May embolize to other areas
    b. Organ pressure—increasing size of aneurysm may place pressure on surrounding organs and cause pain/malfunction
    c. Aortic dissection: the *major* complication.
      (1) Occurs most frequently in African-American males, 50 to 70 years of age, with a history of hypertension
      (2) Other factors include: Marfan's syndrome, chest trauma, cardiac enlargement, and iatrogenic causes (i.e., aortic tears from insertion of IABP)
D. Thoracic aneurysms
  1. Clinical manifestations
    a. Horner's syndrome (ischemia to the ipsilateral stellate ganglia): ptosis, anhidrosis (lack of sweating) on affected side related to spinal cord ischemia
    b. Tracheal deviation and tracheal tug (downward pull)
    c. Unequal blood pressure in arms related to interruption of blood flow through the subclavian arteries
    d. Edema of the head or neck
    e. Specific to type
      (1) Ascending—angina
      (2) Transverse aortic arch—dysphagia, hoarseness, pulsation in upper anterior chest wall, signs and symptoms of cerebral ischemia

      (3) Descending—constant shoulder or back pain
  2. Diagnostic examinations
    a. Chest x-ray
    b. CT scan
    c. MRI
    d. Ultrasound
    e. Aortography
  3. Medical and surgical management—see Aortic Aneurysms
  4. Complications
    a. Major preoperative complication
      (1) Aortic dissection
      (2) Operative mortality less than 10%
      (3) Same postoperative complications as with aortic dissection
E. Abdominal aortic aneurysms
  1. Clinical manifestations
    a. Usually asymptomatic, often found on routine physical examination
    b. May be tender to palpation with an audible bruit over lesion
    c. Pain—abdominal or back, often with urologic and gastrointestinal symptoms present
    d. With a leak or rupture, severe, tearing pain develops with signs of shock with general circulatory collapse
    e. May show evidence of embolization to lower extremities
  2. Diagnostic examinations
    a. Ultrasound
    b. MRI
    c. CT scan (most accurate)
    d. Simple x-ray may be misleading
  3. Medical management—rarely done except for aneurysms less than 6 cm
  4. Surgical management
    a. Open aneurysmal segment and sew graft in place; wall of original aneurysm wrapped around
    b. Decreases late complications (infection, development of false aneurysm, thrombus, embolus)
    c. Surgery necessary, unless refused, if aneurysm is tender, enlarged, or producing other symptoms
  5. Complications
    a. Rupture (see Aortic dissection)
    b. 5-year postoperative survival rate is 70%
II. Analysis
  A. Altered tissue perfusion related to decreased blood flow secondary to:
    1. Aortic dissection
    2. Thoracic aneurysm
    3. Abdominal aortic aneurysm
    4. Thrombi formation

5. Embolization to extremities
B. Decreased cardiac output related to aortic dissection
C. Fluid volume deficit related to hemorrhage
D. Pain related to ischemia or dissection
E. Anxiety related to fear of death
F. Knowledge deficit related to diagnostic measures; preoperative/postoperative routines
G. High risk for impaired gas exchange

III. Planning/goals, expected outcomes
A. Client will evidence adequate tissue perfusion as measured by:
　　1. Warm, dry extremities
　　2. Palpable pulses
　　3. Capillary refill of 3 seconds or less
　　4. Color of extremities pink
　　5. Normal neurologic function, if thoracic aneurysm
B. Client will evidence adequate cardiac output as measured by:
　　1. Blood pressure greater than 90 mm Hg systolic
　　2. Urine output 30 mL/hour or greater
　　3. No complaints of angina
C. Client will evidence adequate fluid volume as measured by:
　　1. CVP 5 to 10 cm H_2O
　　2. BP greater than 90 mm Hg
　　3. Urine output 30 mL/hour or greater
　　4. Hemoglobin and hematocrit stable
D. Client will evidence relief of pain as measured by:
　　1. Verbalization of relief
　　2. No grimacing or guarding
E. Client/family will evidence decreased anxiety/fear as measured by ability to:
　　1. Verbalize source of anxiety/fear
　　2. Concentrate on dialogue
　　3. Verbalize effective coping strategies
F. Client/family will evidence understanding of diagnostic, pre-/postoperative routines/procedures as measured by:
　　1. Verbalization of understanding of need for diagnostic studies
　　2. Demonstration of turning, coughing, and deep breathing postoperatively
　　3. Verbalization of necessary postprocedural/postoperative restrictions
G. Client will not experience impaired gas exchange as evidenced by:
　　1. Normal respiratory rate and excursion
　　2. Clear lung sounds in all fields
　　3. Arterial blood gases within normal limits

IV. Implementation—preoperative
A. To maintain adequate tissue perfusion
　　1. Assess vital signs and peripheral circulation (pulses and capillary refill) frequently
　　2. Monitor level of consciousness and urine output
　　3. Prevent any constriction (clothing, etc.) on peripheral extremities
　　4. Assess for blood transfusion reactions, if given
　　5. Supplemental oxygen as needed
　　6. Assess movement and sensation of lower extremities as soon as client is conscious
　　7. Monitor vital signs, CVP, PCWP as appropriate
　　8. Monitor peripheral pulses capillary refill frequently
　　9. Monitor extremity skin color and temperature
　　10. Discourage flexion at groin in early postoperative phase
B. To maintain adequate cardiac output
　　1. Assess BP, CVP, PCWP as appropriate
　　2. Use inotropic agents, venous/arterial dilators to improve cardiac output as needed
　　3. Institute bedrest
C. To maintain adequate fluid volume
　　1. Maintain adequate IV access
　　2. Monitor fluid intake and output frequently
　　3. Foley catheter usually needed
　　4. Monitor BUN, creatinine
　　5. Monitor urine output
　　6. Monitor specific gravity
　　7. Monitor BP, CVP, PCWP
D. To provide pain relief
　　1. Assess type and intensity of pain
　　　　a. Notify physician STAT for back pain or chest pain
　　　　b. Medicate for pain *after* the pain has been assessed by physician
　　2. Assess degree of pain relief
　　3. Position change as needed
　　4. Provide appropriate distraction
E. To decrease anxiety and fear
　　1. Allow client/family to verbalize fears or concerns
　　2. Give simple, short explanations
　　3. Check client/family frequently
　　4. Provide quiet, calm reassurance
F. To maintain adequate gas exchange
　　1. Monitor respiration, lung sounds, ABGs as needed
　　2. Provide supplemental, humidified oxygen
　　3. See Chapter 6, ''Nursing Process Applied to Adults Undergoing Surgery''

V. Evaluation
A. Adequate tissue perfusion is maintained
B. Adequate cardiac output is maintained

C. Adequate fluid volume is maintained
D. Adequate pain relief is achieved
E. Anxiety and fear are decreased

POST-TEST Cardiovascular Disorders

Mr. Boyd, a 34-year-old African-American man with a long smoking history, is diagnosed with malignant hypertension.

1. The most significant risk factor Mr. Boyd has is:
   ① Age
   ② Sex
   ③ Race
   ④ Smoking
2. Which of the following nursing interventions is the most important for preventing malignant hypertension?
   ① Administering antihypertensives
   ② Assessing for signs and symptoms of decreasing tissue perfusion
   ③ Educating persons at high risk
   ④ Providing safety and comfort measures
3. Mr. Boyd's chest x-ray reveals left ventricular enlargement. This is significant for increased:
   ① Capillary pressure
   ② Venous pressure
   ③ Arterial pressure
   ④ Pulmonary pressure
4. Mr. Boyd develops hypertensive crisis. The most effective medications to be used are:
   ① Adrenergic inhibitors
   ② Vasodilators
   ③ Angiotensin convertors
   ④ Calcium channel blockers
5. Of all the activities Mr. Boyd enjoys, his physician would probably restrict:
   ① Bicycling
   ② Hiking
   ③ Swimming
   ④ Ice skating
6. Which test will a client be least likely to have when being worked up for hypertension?
   ① CBC
   ② Urinalysis
   ③ Arteriogram
   ④ Electrocardiogram
7. When your client suddenly becomes hypotensive, which action will best increase tissue perfusion?
   ① Elevate legs
   ② Give vasodilators
   ③ Apply elastic support stockings
   ④ Increase intravenous infusion rate

8. When teaching a client about multiple medications for hypertension, it is important to first:
   ① Establish what the client wants to know
   ② Check with the physician first
   ③ Determine what the client needs to know
   ④ Stress drug interactions and side effects

Mr. B., aged 50, has angina pectoris. He takes nitroglycerin tablets and he knows that he should not overexercise.

9. Angina pectoris results from:
   ① Reduction in myocardial blood supply
   ② An increase in muscle metabolism
   ③ Hypertensive crisis
   ④ Increased viscosity of coronary artery blood flow
10. When Mr. B. develops chest pain, his first action should be:
    ① Cease activity immediately
    ② Prepare to go to the hospital immediately
    ③ Take nitroglycerin SL
    ④ Continue with what he is doing because he probably is not having a heart attack
11. Nitroglycerin taken sublingual (SL) is expected to:
    ① Block nervous stimulation of myocardial muscle
    ② Interfere with calcium ion influx
    ③ Produce coronary artery and peripheral vasodilation
    ④ Diminish heart rate
12. When taking nitroglycerin SL, Mr. B. knows to:
    ① Store the pills in a plastic envelope
    ② Take a nitroglycerin tablet at approximately 3-hour intervals throughout the day
    ③ Allow at least a 20- to 30-minute interval between doses of nitroglycerin
    ④ Take the pill while sitting or lying down
13. Mr. B. has been instructed that nitroglycerin may produce which possible side effect?
    ① Nausea
    ② Headache
    ③ Drowsiness
    ④ Tinnitus
14. The LEAST effective activity for Mr. B. to do in order to decrease his risk of CAD would be to:
    ① Reduce his weight
    ② Decrease dietary intake of saturated fats
    ③ Use isometric exercises
    ④ Modify his stressful lifestyle

15. Mr. B. has a prescription to take a daily dose of propranolol (Inderal). Before this medicine is prescribed, Mr. B. should be questioned if he has a history of asthma. The rationale for this is that:
   ① Bronchial constriction occurs as a side effect
   ② Propranolol decreases cardiac output and pulmonary congestion is likely
   ③ A rapid heart rate is necessary to maximize alveolar gas exchange
   ④ Asthmatic symptoms are masked with propranolol

16. Propranolol (Inderal) produces a negative inotropic effect. Inotropy refers to:
   ① Heart rate
   ② Strength of contraction
   ③ Ability to suppress dysrhythmias
   ④ Impulse conduction

Mr. Lewis is diagnosed with right-sided CHF and is complaining of anorexia and nausea; his liver is slightly enlarged.

17. The nurse will assess right-sided CHF by noting:
   ① Oliguria
   ② Cheyne-Stokes respirations
   ③ Peripheral edema
   ④ Rales

18. The nurse will provide which diet for Mr. Lewis?
   ① Acid ash
   ② Bland
   ③ High residue
   ④ High roughage

19. The best indicator of Mr. Lewis's nutritional status is his:
   ① Weight
   ② Serum glucose
   ③ Appetite
   ④ Serum albumin

20. Mr. Lewis is receiving digoxin and furosemide (Lasix). He is at risk for electrolyte imbalances caused by:
   ① Sodium restriction
   ② Inadequate hydration
   ③ Diuresis
   ④ Diaphoresis

21. A chest x-ray reveals that Mr. Lewis has an enlarged heart. This is due to:
   ① Increased cardiac workload
   ② End-stage CHF
   ③ Pulmonary edema
   ④ Cardiac inflammation

Mrs. King is an obese 65-year-old housewife who has been suffering from intermittent claudication. She has been admitted with the diagnosis of possible arterial occlusion.

22. Assessment data the nurse collects to support this diagnosis would include asking questions about:
   ① Age of menopause
   ② Daily activity
   ③ Dietary habits
   ④ Medications taken

23. An arteriogram confirms a severe occlusion of the left lower extremity. When Mrs. King is supine, the nurse observes the color of the affected extremity to be:
   ① Reddish
   ② Brownish
   ③ Pale
   ④ Unchanged

24. Mrs. King must undergo a femoral-popliteal bypass graft. The nurse's first priority postoperatively is to immediately:
   ① Relieve pain
   ② Assess circulation
   ③ Reinforce dressing
   ④ Administer antibiotics as ordered

25. After surgery, Mrs. King is at risk for developing a pulmonary embolus. The earliest indication of this will be:
   ① Dyspnea and shortness of breath
   ② Cyanosis
   ③ Tachypnea
   ④ Decreased breath sounds

26. Unfortunately, the bypass is unsuccessful and a below-the-knee amputation is required. Immediately after surgery, Mrs. King's stump should be kept:
   ① Elevated for 12 hours
   ② Elevated for 24 hours
   ③ Elevated for 48 hours
   ④ Flat to prevent hip and knee contractures

Mr. Horner undergoes repair of his aneurysm. He returns to you still unconscious from the anesthesia.

27. Which of the following data would give you the best information regarding Mr. Horner's graft patency?
   ① Urine output
   ② Level of consciousness
   ③ Pedal pulses
   ④ Blood pressure

28. As soon as Mr. Horner regains consciousness, the nurse would:
① Orient him to his surroundings
② Assess his pain
③ Ask him to move his legs
④ Ask him to cough

POST-TEST Answers and Rationales

1. ③ Although all are risk factors, race is the most significant empirical variable for malignant hypertension. 1, II. Hypertension.
2. ③ The key word is prevention; education is the most effective defense against the disease. 4, IV. Hypertension.
3. ③ Left ventricular enlargement is secondary to increased systolic arterial pressure. The others cause other problems. 2, II. Hypertension.
4. ② Diazoxide (Hyperstat) and nitroprusside (Nipride), vasodilators, are given intravenously for the treatment of hypertensive crisis. The other drugs are simply used to treat hypertension in general. 3, II. Hypertension.
5. ④ Ice skating is associated with cold weather, and constricting footwear causes vasoconstriction. The other exercises increase cardiac blood flow. 4, IV. Hypertension.
6. ③ An arteriogram is an invasive and risky diagnostic procedure and would not routinely be performed. The others are routine tests that might be done. 1, II. Hypertension.
7. ④ IV fluids would add volume and thus vessel pressure. Choices 1 and 3 are important also but slower. Vasoconstrictors, not vasodilators, would be given to raise blood pressure. 4, II. Hypertension.
8. ① Always take a client-centered approach; this includes choices 3 and 4. Client teaching is a nurse's responsibility and independent function. 4, II. Hypertension.
9. ① Angina pectoris is chest pain associated with myocardial ischemia. Ischemia occurs as a result of decreased myocardial perfusion and decreased coronary artery blood flow. 2, I. CAD.
10. ① Angina pectoris is commonly relieved by rest. Activity increases myocardial oxygen demand. Nitroglycerin is used if rest does not work. 3, II. CAD.
11. ③ Nitroglycerin is a vasodilator. It increases oxygen supply through coronary artery dilation and it decreases oxygen demand by reducing venous return. 5, II. CAD.
12. ④ Nitroglycerin and other vasodilators cause orthostatic hypotension and therefore should be taken when sitting or lying.

Nitroglycerin should be stored in an airtight, dark container. It should be taken at 5-minute intervals, three doses only. If pain is not relieved after three doses, the individual should contact his or her physician immediately or go to an emergency room. 3, II. CAD.

13. ② The common side effect associated with nitroglycerin is headache. 5, II. CAD.
14. ③ Isometric exercises have a high oxygen demand. All others are ways to reduce risk factors associated with coronary artery disease. 4, II. CAD.
15. ① Propranolol causes bronchial constriction. Constriction of the bronchi will worsen an asthmatic condition. 1, II. CAD.
16. ② Propranolol is an adrenergic blocking agent. It blocks sympathetic stimulation in the myocardium and decreases force of contraction. Inotropy refers to force of contraction. 2, II. CAD.
17. ③ Choices 1, 2, and 4 indicate left-sided heart failure. Peripheral edema is a sign of right-sided heart failure. 1, II. Congestive Heart Failure.
18. ② An acid ash diet is used to increase urinary acidity, while choices 3 and 4 may aggravate gastrointestinal symptoms. A bland diet is the best. 4, II. Congestive Heart Failure.
19. ④ Mr. Lewis's enlarged liver can cause albumin, normally formed there, to decrease. This would lead to alteration in protein metabolism and a nutritional deficit. It is therefore the best indicator. 2, II. Congestive Heart Failure.
20. ③ The combination of a diuretic and the increased pumping action of the heart, from digoxin, leads to diuresis which may cause loss of electrolytes. 2, II. Congestive Heart Failure.
21. ① The heart, like any muscle, will enlarge due to overwork. Choices 2 and 3 are more associated with left-sided failure. There is no reason to assume inflammation. 2, II. Congestive Heart Failure.
22. ② Although choices 1, 3, and 4 are relevant to the long-term development of ASHD, intermittent claudication is best identified by assessing whether activity causes pain and rest relieves the pain. 1 & 2, II. Peripheral Arterial Disease.
23. ③ Because of gravity, the extremity is maximally perfused when below heart

24. ② Graft occlusion is the most common complication of a bypass graft. Decreased circulation would indicate this. 4, I & II. Peripheral Arterial Disease.

25. ③ Tachypnea would occur prior to choices 1 and 4 and cyanosis is a late sign of hypoxia. 1, I. Peripheral Arterial Disease.

26. ② After 24 hours, elevation of the stump can lead to hip and knee flexion contractures. 4, II. Peripheral Arterial Disease, Amputations.

27. ① Urine output gives the best indicator of graft patency because of the location of

level and pale when at or above heart level. 1, II. Peripheral Arterial Disease.

the renal arteries on the aorta. Abrupt cessation of urine flow could indicate graft occlusion or rupture. Given that clients with aneurysms usually have atherosclerotic changes, pedal pulses are not always reliable; however, skin color and temperature are. Level of consciousness and blood pressure are unreliable indicators at this time. 1, II. Aneurysms.

28. ③ Because of possible ischemia to the lower extremities, it is essential to assess for function in this area immediately. The others are not of immediate priority. 1, I. Aneurysms.

PRE-TEST Shock States

1. Your client is suffering from hypovolemic shock. Signs and symptoms you would expect to assess include:
   ① Increased venous return
   ② Increased cardiac output
   ③ Decreased tissue perfusion
   ④ Decreased pulse rate

2. Cardiogenic shock is caused by:
   ① Decreased venous return
   ② Decreased pumping ability of heart
   ③ Increased blood pressure
   ④ Massive vasodilation

3. The major pathophysiological mechanism causing distributive shock is:
   ① Failure of the heart as a pump
   ② Massive blood loss
   ③ Increased cardiac output
   ④ Massive vasodilation

4. Which is NOT a cause of hypovolemic shock?
   ① Acute myocardial infarction
   ② Prolonged vomiting
   ③ Overuse of diuretics
   ④ Diabetes insipidus

5. Which of the following would NOT be a cause of neurogenic shock?
   ① Decompression of vasomotor center
   ② Spinal anesthesia
   ③ Blood transfusions
   ④ Medullary trauma

6. In early shock, urine output is decreased primarily due to:
   ① Renal hypoperfusion
   ② Decreased blood volume
   ③ Massive shunting
   ④ Aldosterone

PRE-TEST Answers and Rationales

1. ③ The ultimate problem associated with all forms of shock is a decrease in tissue perfusion. The cardiac output and venous return are decreased and the pulse increased. 1, II. Shock.

2. ② Cardiogenic shock is also known as pump failure. The heart fails to adequately pump the blood. Decreased venous return is a symptom of cardiogenic shock but not a cause. Choices 3 and 4 have no relevance. 1, II. Shock.

3. ④ The major pathophysiological mechanism in distributive shock is massive vasodilation from a variety of causes. Choices 1 and 2 are causes of other types of shock and 3 is not associated with shock. 1, II. Shock.

4. ① An acute MI causes cardiogenic shock, not hypovolemic shock. The other options are all causes of hypovolemic shock. 1 & 2, II. Shock.

5. ③ Neurogenic shock is caused by all options except blood transfusions. A transfusion reaction can cause anaphylactic shock. 1 & 2, II. Shock.

6. ④ Aldosterone is released in response to renal hypoperfusion, resulting in the retention of sodium and water, thus decreasing the urine volume. Massive shunting does not occur until later in shock. Decreased blood volume would lead to renal hypoperfusion. 1, II. Shock.

NURSING PROCESS APPLIED TO ADULTS IN SHOCK STATES

I. Assessment
 A. Definition: failure of circulatory system to provide tissue perfusion necessary for normal cellular function and failure to remove waste products of metabolism that accumulate due to inadequate venous return
 B. Etiology/pathophysiology
   1. Hypovolemic shock
     a. Cause: results from decreased intravascular volume of at least 15 to 25%, causing decreased venous return
     b. Pathophysiology: decreased volume leads to decreased venous return leads to decreased cardiac output leads to decreased blood pressure leads to decreased tissue perfusion
   2. Cardiogenic shock
     a. Cause: results from inability of heart to effectively pump blood
     b. Pathophysiology: decreased pumping ability leads to decreased cardiac output leading to decreased blood pressure leading to decreased tissue perfusion
   3. Distributive shock
     a. Cause: results from massive vasodilation of blood vessels due to effects of histamines or toxins or problems with central nervous system (neurogenic)
     b. Pathophysiology: vasodilation leads to decreased venous return leading to decreased cardiac output leading to decreased blood pressure leading to decreased tissue perfusion
 C. Predisposing/precipitating factors
   1. Hypovolemic shock
     a. Hemorrhage: loss of blood due to
       (1) Injury/trauma
       (2) Surgery
       (3) Gastrointestinal bleeding
       (4) Delivery of a baby
       (5) Bleeding disorders
         (a) Platelet deficiency/thrombocytopenia
         (b) Defects in coagulation
           (i) Hemophilia
           (ii) Disseminated intravascular coagulation (DIC)
           (iii) Vitamin K deficiency
           (iv) Liver disease
     b. Dehydration: loss of blood, fluid volume due to
       (1) Prolonged vomiting
       (2) Excessive diarrhea
       (3) Excessive gastrointestinal drainage
       (4) Overuse of diuretics
       (5) Endocrine disorders
         (a) Diabetes insipidus (decreased antidiuretic hormone [ADH])
         (b) Diabetes mellitus (ketoacidosis)
         (c) Addison's disease (decreased aldosterone)
     c. Third space fluid loss: movement of fluid into interstitial spaces or body cavity, thus unavailable for circulation
       (1) Burns

(2) Peritonitis
(3) Bowel obstruction
(4) Liver disease
(5) Major surgical procedures
2. Cardiogenic shock
a. Coronary: abnormal perfusion of coronary circulation causing inadequate supply of oxygen to myocardium
(1) Acute myocardial infarction (most common)
(2) Other causes
(a) Congestive heart failure
(b) Cardiac tamponade/constrictive pericarditis
(c) Pulmonary emboli
(d) Arrhythmia
(e) Cardiac surgery
(f) Severe valvular disease
(g) Rupture of any cardiac structure
b. Noncoronary: perfusion of coronary circulation normal but deficit in myocardial cell causes an impairment in contractility
(1) Cardiomyopathy
(2) Myocarditis
(3) Ventricular aneurysms
3. Distributive shock
a. Sepsis: bacteria liberate toxins that cause massive vasodilation (especially in elderly or immunocompromised client)
(1) Urinary tract
(a) *Escherichia coli*
(b) *Klebsiella*
(c) *Pseudomonas*
(2) Respiratory tract
(a) *Escherichia coli*
(b) *Pseudomonas*
(c) *Pneumococci*
(3) Gastrointestinal
(a) *Escherichia coli*
(b) *Klebsiella*
(c) *Salmonella*
(d) *Bacterioides*
b. Anaphylaxis—allergic reaction liberates histamine, causing widespread dilation of arterioles
(1) Drugs (antibiotics—penicillin, sulfa)
(2) Foods
(3) Insect and snake venom
(4) Blood transfusion reactions
(5) Contrast media dye (iodine)
c. Neurogenic—loss of sympathetic tone causes widespread vasodilation
(1) Injury/disease of spinal cord
(2) Spinal anesthesia

(3) Decompression of vasomotor center (drugs, pain, hypoglycemia)
(4) Direct medullary damage
D. Clinical manifestations
1. Vital signs
a. Blood pressure
(1) Normal or even elevated in early shock secondary to compensatory vasoconstriction
(2) Severely low (less than 90 mm Hg systolic) in progressive shock due to sustained vasoconstriction and decreased cardiac output
(3) Narrowing pulse pressure
b. Pulses
(1) Rapid, weak, thready
(2) Irregular/dysrhythmias
(3) Major vessels may be palpable
(4) Peripheral pulses easily obliterated
c. Respiration
(1) Rapid, shallow
(2) Dyspnea
(3) Rales, rhonchi, wheezes auscultated
(4) Use of accessory muscles in neck, shoulder, and abdomen as ventilatory failure ensues
d. Temperature
(1) May be elevated in sepsis
(2) Generally subnormal, due to decreased cellular metabolism secondary to poor tissue perfusion
2. Level of consciousness
a. Restlessness, agitation, and confusion in early shock due to decreased cerebral blood flow
b. Lethargy, stupor, and coma in progressive shock due to inadequate oxygen to brain cells, and accumulation of cellular toxic substances
3. Skin and mucous membranes
a. Flushed, warm, and moist in early sepsis
b. Dry with poor skin turgor in early hypovolemia
c. Flushed with macular or papular lesions in anaphylaxis
d. Cool, pale, moist in progressive shock due to poor tissue perfusion; presence of cyanosis and possible peripheral edema
4. Urine output
a. Decreased, less than 20 mL per hour
b. Decreased in early stages as a result of aldosterone mechanism
c. In progressive shock, specific gravity

decreased due to kidneys' inability to concentrate urine

    d. Anuria in end stages of shock

E. Diagnostic examinations

  1. Central venous pressure (CVP)

    a. Decreased CVP (usually below 5 cm H_2O) if hypovolemic shock due to loss of volume

    b. Increased CVP (usually above 15 cm H_2O) if cardiogenic shock due to poor cardiac output

  2. Arterial blood gases (ABG)

    a. Hypoxemia (low oxygen level in blood) due to problems with ventilation, diffusion, or perfusion, depending on etiology of shock (i.e., PaO_2 <80)

    b. In early shock, client has tendency to hyperventilate in order to provide more oxygen to tissues, resulting in respiratory alkalosis (i.e., ↑ pH, $PaCO_2$)

    c. In progressive shock, persistent hypoxemia causes hypoxia; body switches from aerobic (presence of oxygen) to anaerobic (absence of oxygen) metabolism, resulting in metabolic and respiratory acidosis

  3. Serum lactate levels: elevate from metabolic acidosis described above

  4. Chest x-ray (CXR): may reveal cardiomegaly and/or pulmonary congestion due to poor cardiac output, particularly in cardiogenic shock

  5. Electrocardiogram (ECG)

    a. Arrhythmias may be present due to hypoxia of myocardium

    b. Changes indicative of acute myocardial infarction may be present in cardiogenic shock

  6. CBC

    a. Hematocrit may be elevated in hypovolemic shock due to hemoconcentration; exception: hemorrhage, then lowered hematocrit

    b. Leukopenia (decreased WBC) may occur in early septic shock, later followed by leukocytosis (increased WBC)

  7. Electrolytes: changes particularly in serum potassium and calcium level may occur because of acid–base imbalance, altered renal function, and possible fluid shifts

  8. BUN/creatinine: may increase due to poor renal function from shock state

F. Complications of prolonged shock

  1. Adult respiratory distress syndrome (ARDS) may occur in all types of prolonged shock

  2. Acute tubular necrosis (ATN) may occur in all types of prolonged shock

  3. Disseminated intravascular coagulation (DIC), complication of septic shock

II. Analysis

A. Altered tissue perfusion related to decreased volume

B. Decreased cardiac output related to decreased volume

C. Altered gas exchange related to decreased volume

D. Fluid volume deficit related to blood loss

E. Anxiety: client/family related to severity of condition

III. Planning/goals, expected outcomes

A. Client will evidence adequate cardiac output

  1. Systolic blood pressure of 90 to 110 mm Hg

  2. Diastolic blood pressure of 60 to 90 mm Hg

  3. Absence of arrhythmias with normal heart rate

B. Client will evidence adequate tissue perfusion by

  1. Cardiopulmonary: absence of chest pain and respiratory distress

  2. Cerebral: alert and oriented to person, place, and time

  3. Renal: urine output of at least 20 to 30 mL per hour

  4. Peripheral: skin warm and dry with strong peripheral pulses, absence of cyanosis

C. Client will evidence adequate gas exchange by

  1. Respiratory rate of 16 to 20 breaths per minute

  2. Absence of dyspnea, cyanosis

  3. Blood gases at normal baseline

  4. Chest x-ray clear

D. Client will evidence adequate fluid volume by

  1. Normal CVP (5 to 15 cm H_2O)

  2. Blood pressure (systolic) greater than 90 mm Hg; pulse 110/min

  3. Urine output of 30 mL/hr or greater

  4. Clear breath sounds

E. Client and family will verbalize fears and concerns

  1. Visit calmly with each other

  2. Client able to rest comfortably

IV. Implementation

A. Maintain appropriate cardiac output

  1. Monitor vital signs frequently

  2. Monitor and control arrhythmias (Table 4–17)

  3. Administer medications to enhance cardiac contractility (inotropic agents) and de-

TABLE 4–17 Antiarrhythmic Therapy

Class	Examples	Action	Use	Common Side Effects
Antiarrhythmic	Lidocaine hydrochloride (Xylocaine), procainamide (Pronestyl), bretylium tosylate (Bretylol)	Decrease ventricular excitability and arrhythmias	For use in shock that precipitates arrhythmias and/or arrhythmias that precipitate a shock-like state; used most often in cardiogenic shock	May cause hypotension and depress myocardial contractility, may cause confusion in the elderly

crease vascular resistance (vasodilators) (Table 4–18)

B. Maintain appropriate tissue perfusion
  1. Positioning: horizontal supine position with pillow under head recommended; Trendelenburg position not advised because it will not facilitate venous blood flow from brain and causes increased pressure on diaphragm, thus decreasing ventilation
  2. Administer medications that enhance tissue perfusion (vasopressors) (see Table 4–12) and correct causative factors of shock (Table 4–19)
  3. Intra-aortic balloon pump: used in treatment of cardiogenic shock; balloon inflates during diastole to maintain coronary perfusion to myocardium and deflates during systole to decrease left ventricular workload
C. Maintain adequate gas exchange
  1. Monitor ABG for respiratory and metabolic acidosis

  2. Administer sodium bicarbonate (see Table 4–18) to treat acidosis
  3. Oxygen therapy and mechanical ventilation instituted to correct hypoxemia; client needs to be intubated and generally placed on volume-cycled ventilator; PEEP (positive end-expiratory pressure) may be added to ventilator and hyperinflates alveoli to improve gas exchange
D. Maintain adequate fluid volume
  1. Insert Foley catheter and monitor I & O every hour
  2. Assess for signs of fluid overload such as congestive heart failure with symptoms such as rales, peripheral edema, and jugular venous distention, particularly in cardiogenic shock
  3. Administer medications such as diuretics (see Table 4–1) in cases of fluid overload or cardiogenic shock
  4. Monitor CVP to assess appropriate fluid restriction/replacement needs
  5. Administer appropriate fluid therapy, par-

TABLE 4–18 Primary Medications in Shock Therapy

Class	Examples	Action	Use	Nursing Implications
Inotropic drugs	Dopamine (Intropin), dobutamine (Dobutrex), amrinone (Inocor)	Increase force of myocardial contractility	For use in shock states where there is a need to increase stroke volume, increase cardiac output, increase BP, and increase tissue perfusion	May increase myocardial oxygen need and therefore precipitate angina pectoris or myocardial infarction
Vasodilators	Sodium nitroprusside (Nipride), nitroglycerin (Tridil)	Act on smooth muscles to dilate both arteries and veins	For use in shock states where there is a need to decrease venous return and decrease peripheral resistance	May decrease cardiac output and therefore cause a decrease in coronary perfusion
Vasopressors	Norepinephrine bitartrate (Levophed), epinephrine hydrochloride (Adrenalin), phenylephrine hydrochloride (Neo-Synephrine), metaraminol bitartrate (Aramine)	Increase HR and force of contraction and/or arteriolar constriction, thereby increasing cardiac output and BP	For use in shock states where there is a need to increase cardiac output by increasing HR contractility	At high doses, alpha stimulation may cause severe vasoconstriction especially in renal, skin, and splanchnic circulation

TABLE 4–19 Other Medications in Shock Therapy

Class	Examples	Action	Use	Nursing Implications
Diuretics	Furosemide (Lasix), mannitol (Omsitrol)	Decrease fluid volume	For use in shock that causes edema and pulmonary congestion, as in cardiogenic shock	Monitor fluid and electrolyte balance, particularly hypokalemia
Steroids	Methylprednisolone (Medrol), dexamethasone (Decadron)	Reduce capillary permeability, stabilize lysosomal enzymes, and prevent endotoxin action	For use in shock states due to sepsis or anaphylaxis	Monitor water retention with increased BP, also hyperglycemia
Bronchodilators	Epinephrine (1:1000 solution) (Adrenalin)	Stimulate sympathetic nervous system for bronchodilation	For use in relief of bronchospasm and itching seen in anaphylactic shock	Monitor for increased BP and possible cardiac arrhythmias
Antihistamines	Diphenhydramine hydrochloride (Benadryl)	Block histamine receptors and reduce inflammation	For use in the relief of swelling, rash, and itching in anaphylactic shock	Monitor central nervous system depression
Parenteral electrolyte: sodium bicarbonate	Sodium bicarbonate	Buffer the hydrogen ion concentration in the blood	For metabolic acidosis seen in late stages of shock	Alkalosis and signs and symptoms of tetany should be monitored if administered too rapidly
Antibiotics	*Broad spectrum:* ampicillin (Omipen) *Gram negative:* ticarcillin disodium (Ticar) *Gram positive:* vancomycin (Vancocin) *Aminoglycosides:* gentamycin (Garamycin) *Cephalosporins:* cefotaxime (Claforan)	Depending on the type of antibiotic, action will differ; overall goal is to decrease the presence and action of the infecting organism	For use in shock due primarily to sepsis	Monitor signs and symptoms of allergic reaction

ticularly in hypovolemic shock (Table 4–20)

E. Encourage patient and family to express fears and concerns
  1. Have family verbalize their fear of acute life-threatening illness
  2. Have family speak with clergy and available support systems

V. Evaluation
  A. Client responds to therapy and demonstrates adequate cardiac output as evidenced by
    1. Stable baseline blood pressure and heart rate
    2. No cardiac arrhythmias
  B. Client responds to therapy and demonstrates adequate tissue perfusion by
    1. No damage to cardiopulmonary system as evidenced by no complaints of chest pain or shortness of breath
    2. No damage to brain as evidenced by appropriate levels of consciousness and motor movement
    3. No damage to renal system as evidenced by urine output greater than 30 mL per hour
    4. No damage to peripheral vascular system as evidenced by strong distal pulses and warm, dry lower extremities
  C. Client responds to therapy and demonstrates adequate gas exchange as evidenced by
    1. Normal respiratory rate
    2. Normal ABG
    3. Normal chest x-ray
  D. Client responds to therapy and demonstrates adequate fluid volume as evidenced by
    1. Normal CVP
    2. Intake relatively equivalent to output
    3. Urine output 30 mL/hr or greater
    4. No presence of rales on auscultation
    5. Baseline vital signs
  E. Client and family cope effectively with fears and concerns as evidenced by
    1. Verbalize fear of potential death
    2. Share feelings openly with each other

TABLE 4–20 Fluid Replacement Therapy

Class	Examples	Action	Use	Nursing Implications
Whole blood or blood products	Whole blood, packed red blood cells (PRBC), plasma	Replace volume in hypovolemic shock	If hematocrit less than 30, or if there is a need to limit fluid therapy (i.e., increased CVP), PRBCs given; if plasma volume decreased but not due to blood loss, plasma given; whole blood given in extreme emergencies only	Monitoring for signs and symptoms of an allergic reaction essential
Plasma expanders	Dextran (Rheomacrodex, Macrodex), (Hetastarch) (Hespan), 5% albumin	Increase osmolality of fluid in intravascular space so that fluid shifts from interstitial to vascular space	Used to expand plasma volume when hemorrhage rapid	Can cause formation of hyperosmolar urine and lead to renal tubular damage. Hespan may cause coagulopathies
Crystalloid solutions	Normal saline (.9NS), lactated Ringer's solution, Ringer's solution	Restores intravascular volume; lactate ion buffers acidosis	Used to replace volume when blood loss usually less than 1500 ML	Can cause interstitial and intracellular edema

POST-TEST Shock States

1. Which of the following clinical manifestations are a direct outcome of the altered tissue perfusion associated with shock?
   ① Elevated body temperature
   ② Tachypnea
   ③ Urine output greater than 30 mL per hour
   ④ Peripheral vasodilation
2. When a client is suffering from cardiogenic shock, the CVP reading will be:
   ① High, usually above 15 cm H_2O
   ② Low, usually below 5 cm H_2O
   ③ Between 5 and 10 cm H_2O
   ④ Extremely low, less than 1 cm H_2O
3. The acid–base imbalance that would probably be evident in early stages of shock would be:
   ① Respiratory acidosis
   ② Metabolic acidosis
   ③ Respiratory alkalosis
   ④ Metabolic alkalosis

4. Inotropic drugs such as dobutamine are often used to treat shock. One of the negative effects of this drug is:
   ① Increased myocardial oxygen need
   ② Increased cardiac output and tissue perfusion
   ③ Increased renal blood flow and output
   ④ Decreased coronary perfusion
5. Which of the following is the proper position for the client suffering from hypovolemic shock?
   ① Trendelenburg
   ② Reverse Trendelenburg
   ③ Supine with the feet elevated
   ④ Supine with the head on a pillow
6. Which of the following clinical manifestations reflects an improvement in the client's shock?
   ① Systolic pressure between 80 and 90
   ② Respiratory rate greater than 24
   ③ Urine output greater than 30 mL per hour
   ④ CVP greater than 10 cm H_2O

POST-TEST Answers and Rationales

1. ② The altered tissue perfusion results in hypoxia and the body attempts to compensate for the low oxygen by hyperventilating. The body temperature is usually low during shock and high fever would further increase hypoxia, as would vasodilation. Urine output would be low in shock. 5, I. Shock.

2. ① With cardiogenic shock, the venous pressure is often elevated because of the back-up of pressure into the venous system when the heart fails. 2, II. Shock.

3. ③ In early shock, the client is hyperventilating and blowing off CO_2. When this happens, the client will be in respiratory alkalosis. This usually corrects itself as the shock resolves. 2, II. Shock.

4. ① The inotropic drugs cause an increase in myocardial oxygen need, which can then result in angina because of the decreased tissue perfusion. Choice 3 is a positive effect of the drugs as is choice 2. The drugs do not cause decreased coronary perfusion. 2, II. Shock.

5. ④ Trendelenburg is not recommended for the client in shock since it shifts the organs upward against the diaphragm and decreases respirations. Raising the head slightly increases venous return from cerebral circulation. 4, II. Shock.

6. ③ When the urine output is above 30 mL per hour, it means that the kidneys are being adequately perfused, which means that the shock has resolved. Choices 1 and 2 are signs of continuing shock and choice 4 could indicate fluid overload or cardiogenic shock. 5, I & II. Shock.

PRE-TEST Cardiopulmonary Resuscitation

1. Which of the following would most influence the decision to terminate CPR?
   ① Twenty-five minutes have passed without successful resuscitation
   ② The client's pupils are fixed and dilated
   ③ The client has suffered some brain damage
   ④ The cardiovascular and pulmonary systems have failed to respond to maximum effort

2. If CPR is performed on a victim by two persons, which of the following ratios of cardiac compression to pulmonary ventilation would be used?
   ① 6 compressions to 2 ventilations
   ② 4 compressions to 4 ventilations
   ③ 5 compressions to 1 ventilation
   ④ 15 compressions to 2 ventilations

3. Which of the following is LEAST likely to precipitate a respiratory arrest?
   ① Drowning
   ② Stroke
   ③ Drug overdose
   ④ Myocardial infarction

4. Which of the following statements is correct in the priority of treating an unconscious victim?
   ① Determine unresponsiveness, call for help, begin chest compressions
   ② Determine unresponsiveness, call for help, position the victim on a flat firm surface
   ③ Begin cardiac compressions, call for help, open the airway
   ④ Determine unresponsiveness, begin cardiac massage, position the victim on a flat firm surface

5. If you suspect an unconscious victim of having sustained a cervical spine injury, which of the following methods would you use to open the victim's airway?
   ① Head-tilt/chin-lift maneuver
   ② Head-tilt/neck-lift maneuver
   ③ Jaw-thrust maneuver
   ④ None of the above

PRE-TEST Answers and Rationales

1. ④ A decision about ending CPR is best based on cardiovascular-pulmonary unresponsiveness. Time is not the most important factor, and brain damage cannot be assessed at this point. Other factors may cause pupil changes. 5, I. CPR.

2. ③ The compression/ventilation ratio for two rescuers is 5 compressions to 1 ventilation. 4, II. CPR.

3. ④ Drowning, stroke, and drug overdose all predispose respiratory arrest. A myocardial infarction predisposes cardiac arrest. 1, II. CPR.

4. ② First determine unresponsiveness, then call for help and position the victim on a firm flat surface, then assume rescuer position and open the airway. 2 & 4, II. CPR.

5. ③ If a cervical spine injury is suspected, the jaw-thrust method is recommended to open the airway with minimal disruption to the spine. 4, II. CPR.

CARDIOPULMONARY RESUSCITATION (CPR)

I. Definition: externally supporting artificial ventilation and circulation with rescue breathing and external cardiac compression

II. Pathophysiology: cessation of breathing and circulation; heart, circulation, and respirations suddenly cease

III. Etiology and indications, precipitating factors
   A. Primary respiratory arrest
      1. When there is primary respiratory arrest, heart can continue to pump blood for several minutes
      2. Existing stored oxygen in lungs and blood will continue to circulate to brain and other vital organs
      3. Causes of respiratory arrest: drowning, stroke, smoke inhalation, drug overdose, suffocation, electrical shock, airway obstruction, head and chest trauma
   B. Primary cardiac arrest
      1. When heart fails, ventilation ceases within seconds
      2. Oxygen not circulated, and oxygen stored in vital organs depleted in a few seconds
      3. Heart consumes more oxygen per minute than any other organ of body
      4. Brain cells are most sensitive to oxygen depletion
      5. Immediate action must be instituted within 4 minutes following arrest or biological death—death of brain cells—will occur with irreversible brain damage
      6. Causes of cardiac arrest: ventricular fibrillation, ventricular tachycardia, asystole, electromechanical dissociation, myocardial infarction, respiratory arrest

IV. Clinical manifestations
   A. Abrupt and complete unconsciousness
   B. Absence of breathing or gasping respirations
   C. Absence of pulses or heart beat
   D. Cyanosis of lips and nailbeds
   E. Dilation of the pupils (approximately 2 minutes after the heart stops beating)

V. Medical management (the ABCs of basic resuscitation)
   A. Airway (open and maintain *airway*)
      1. Determine unresponsiveness
         a. Ascertain the absence of spontaneous respirations and carotid pulse
         b. Tap or gently shake the victim and ask "Are you okay?"
      2. Call for help
      3. Position the victim; place victim on firm, flat surface in supine position, arms alongside the body
      4. Assume rescuer position: kneel at level of victim's shoulders in rescuer position
      5. Open airway with the head-tilt/chin-lift maneuver (if no spinal injury)
         a. Place one hand on victim's forehead and tilt head back
         b. Place fingers of other hand under chin and lift up
            (1) This lifts tongue away from back of throat
            (2) Prevents airway obstruction from tongue and relaxed muscles
      6. If cervical spine or neck injury suspected, use jaw-thrust method to open airway
         a. Pull forward victim's entire jaw
         b. Place fingers of both hands behind angles of jaw
         c. Lift forward while pressing chin down
      7. Avoid obstructing airway
      8. Open airway may initiate spontaneous respirations

9. If dentures are loose and cannot be managed in place, remove
10. If dentures are secure, leave in to form a tighter fitting seal

B. Determine breathlessness (provide ventilation through rescue *breathing*)
    1. Look, listen, and feel for breathing
    2. Assess and determine breathlessness
        a. Look for rise and fall of chest
        b. Listen for air exhalation
        c. Feel for exhaled air movement
        d. Assess for 3 to 5 seconds
    3. If victim is breathing
        a. Monitor breathing
        b. Maintain open airway. Place in recovery position if no spinal injury (victim rolls onto side)
        c. Call for help
    4. If breathing is absent
        a. Use mouth-to-mouth barrier device if available; position correctly
        b. Use your thumb and index finger on forehead and pinch victim's nostrils
        c. Take a deep breath and put your lips around victim's mouth to create an airtight seal, mouth to mouth
        d. Deliver two full breaths, each lasting 1½ to 2 seconds
        e. Pause to take a breath after each ventilation you deliver
        f. Adequate artificial ventilation established if you can
            (1) See chest rise 1 to 2 inches
            (2) Feel lungs inflate as they fill with air
            (3) Feel victim exhale between ventilations
        g. Mouth-to-nose technique if you cannot
            (1) Establish tight seal around the victim's mouth
            (2) Open victim's mouth
        h. Mouth-to-stoma
            (1) If victim has a tracheostomy
            (2) Not necessary to do head-tilt/chin-lift
        i. If resistance felt when forcing air into airway
            (1) Airway may be obstructed
            (2) Reposition airway and repeat
            (3) If artificial ventilation still difficult, remove the airway obstruction and repeat

C. Circulation (provide artificial *circulation* through use of external cardiac compressions)
    1. Determine pulselessness
        a. Check carotid pulse for 5 to 10 seconds
        b. Palpate carotid artery gently to avoid compressing artery
        c. If pulse is present, continue rescue breathing at 12 times per minute, then call for help
        d. If pulse is absent, call for help at once
        e. Note sternal landmarks by marking off two fingerbreadths above xyphoid process
    2. Perform external cardiac compressions
        a. Place heel of hand over lower half of body of sternum
        b. Interlock hands and compress chest 3.8 to 5 cm or 1½ to 2 inches for adult
        c. Keep arms straight, with elbows locked with fingers off chest wall to prevent rib fractures
        d. Perform 15 external chest compressions at a rate of 80 to 100 per minute
        e. Allow chest to return to normal position after each compression
        f. Do not remove hands from chest wall between compressions
    3. Maintain ventilation/compression ratio
        a. One rescuer:
            (1) Open the airway
            (2) 15 chest compressions at a rate of 80 to 100 per minute
            (3) Administer two rescue breaths
            (4) Repeat cycle of 15 compressions to two breaths
            (5) Deliver four complete cycles of ventilation/compression (15:2)
            (6) Reevaluate the victim and assess for carotid pulse
        b. Two rescuers:
            (1) Compression/ventilation ratio 5:1
            (2) Deliver the rescue breath during the 1- to 1½-second pause that follows compression 5
            (3) Reassess after 10 cycles
            (4) Palpate carotid pulse to determine effectiveness of compressions
    4. Continue CPR until
        a. Victim regains cardiac rhythm and spontaneous respirations
        b. Resuscitation efforts are assumed by another responsible person who continues basic life support and CPR
        c. Rescuer exhausted and unable to continue resuscitation
        d. Victim pronounced dead by physician

POST-TEST Cardiopulmonary Resuscitation

1. In a hospital, the decision to terminate CPR must be made by the
   1. Nurse
   2. Respiratory therapist
   3. Physician
   4. All of the above
2. If CPR were performed on a victim by a single rescuer, which of the following ratios of cardiac compressions to pulmonary ventilations should be used?
   1. 10 compressions to 2 ventilations
   2. 5 compressions to 1 ventilation
   3. 15 compressions to 2 ventilations
   4. 15 compressions to 3 ventilations
3. When assessing the unconscious victim for pulselessness, which of the following is the best artery to check?
   1. Radial
   2. Femoral
   3. Carotid
   4. Brachial
4. How long should the nurse assess for pulselessness?
   1. 1 full minute
   2. 30 seconds
   3. 15 to 25 seconds
   4. 5 to 10 seconds
5. Which of the following is LEAST likely to precipitate cardiac arrest?
   1. Ventricular tachycardia
   2. Myocardial infarction
   3. Electrical shock
   4. Stroke

POST-TEST Answers and Rationales

1. ③ The physician is the only one in the hospital who may legally decide to terminate CPR. 4, II. CPR.
2. ③ The compression/ventilation ratio for one rescuer is 15 compressions to 2 ventilations. 4, II. CPR.
3. ③ The carotid artery is the most accessible

and reliable, and the most easily learned and found. 4, II. CPR.

4. ④ When assessing the victim for pulselessness, check the carotid pulse for 5 to 10 seconds. 1, II. CPR.
5. ④ Ventricular tachycardia, myocardial infarction, and electrical shock all predispose cardiac arrest. Strokes precipitate respiratory arrest. 2, II. CPR.

PRE-TEST Respiratory Disorders

3/24/02

Mr. Cole is a 40-year-old unemployed factory worker. He has a history of alcoholism and is poorly nourished.

1. Mr. Cole's Mantoux test shows an induration of 12 mm after 48 hours. Which of the following statements accurately explains this result?
   ① The test is considered negative as long as there is no clinical evidence of tuberculosis (TB)
   ② The test shows that Mr. Cole has been infected with a tuberculosis organism
   ③ The test shows that Mr. Cole is positive for active tuberculosis
   ④ The test shows doubtful reaction and needs to be repeated
2. Which of the following statements is true regarding tuberculosis?
   ① Reactivation of tuberculosis will not occur after being dormant for 5 years
   ② A negative sputum examination alone rules out active or inactive tuberculosis infection
   ③ Tuberculosis is essentially not an airborne infection
   ④ Diagnosis of tuberculosis is confirmed by a positive tuberculin test, chest x-ray, and sputum culture
3. After diagnostic work-up, Mr. Cole is placed on INH, rifampin, and PAS (para-aminosalicylic acid). Which statement is correct about the side effects of the medications?
   ① PAS may impair Mr. Cole's ability to discriminate color

   ② Mr. Cole will have decreased hearing ability from prolonged use of INH
   ③ A red-orange discoloration of urine results from use of rifampin
   ④ Gout is a common side effect of these drugs
4. Mr. Peters is suspected of having lung carcinoma. Which of the following symptoms of lung cancer is usually noted initially?
   ① Dyspnea
   ② Dysphagia
   ③ Chest pain
   ④ Chronic cough
5. Which of the following is true regarding lung carcinoma?
   ① Lung cancer is often detectable by physical examination
   ② The risk of developing lung cancer increases in proportion to smoking
   ③ The most definitive diagnostic test for lung cancer is the chest x-ray
   ④ Lung cancer has better prognosis when cancer cells are found in pleural effusion
6. After a lobectomy, Mr. Peters had a chest tube draining to Pleur-Evac on low continuous suction. Which of the following initial assessments by the nurse is abnormal?
   ① 100 mL bloody drainage during the first 2 hours
   ② Constant bubbling in the suction chamber
   ③ Oscillation of fluid in the water-seal during respirations
   ④ Crepitations around chest tube site
7. The nurse notes later that bubbling in the suction chamber had stopped. Which of the following actions is appropriate?
   ① Apply high continuous suction
   ② Check suction equipment
   ③ Check for air leak and disconnection
   ④ Assess patient for respiratory distress

Mr. Brown, diagnosed with COPD, is admitted with increasing shortness of breath, productive cough with thick sputum, and wheezing.

8. The nurse encourages him to do pursed-lip breathing in order to:
   ① Increase oxygen supply to the lungs
   ② Prevent airway closure and air trapping
   ③ Mobilize bronchial secretions
   ④ Promote rapid exhalation of air

9. The nurse administers 2 L O_2 per nasal cannula to Mr. Brown. Higher flow O_2 would cause Mr. Brown to have:
   ① An elevated $PaCO_2$
   ② Improved PaO_2
   ③ Apnea
   ④ Dyspnea

10. Mr. Brown was given Robitussin to:
    ① Liquefy tenacious secretions
    ② Facilitate a productive cough
    ③ Relax bronchial smooth muscles
    ④ Suppress the cough reflex

PRE-TEST Answers and Rationales

1. ② An induration of 10 mm or more is considered positive. A positive reaction indicates that the individual has, at some time, been infected with the tubercle bacillus. It does not solely, however, provide definitive proof of either an active or inactive infection. 1, II. TB.

2. ④ Diagnosis of pulmonary tuberculosis is confirmed by a positive skin test, appearance of areas of infection on chest films, and identification of *Mycobacterium tuberculosis* from cultured specimens. Tuberculosis is essentially transferred from person to person via inhalation of infected droplet nuclei. It can also reactivate after being latent for years if the person's resistance is lowered. 1, II. TB.

3. ③ Rifampin causes a red-orange discoloration of all body secretions including tears, saliva, urine. PAS and INH cause GI symptoms and INH causes hepatotoxicity and peripheral neuropathy. 5, II. TB.

4. ④ Lung cancer is a "silent" disease with the client being asymptomatic until the cancer has progressed. Symptoms vary depending on the location and size of the tumor. However, cough is the most common symptom of bronchogenic carcinoma, which is 90% of lung cancer. 1, II. Lung Cancer.

5. ② Cigarette smoke contains chemical carcinogens and causes cellular changes that increase in degree as more cigarettes are smoked. 1, II. Lung Cancer.

6. ④ Crepitations, crackly sensations palpated around chest tube site, would indicate the presence of subcutaneous emphysema. This occurs when air escapes into the subcutaneous spaces from an existing pneumothorax. The other choices are normal assessments. 5, I & II. Lung Cancer.

7. ② Absence of bubbling in the suction control chamber means that the suction is not being maintained either because of mechanical failure of the suction equipment or because the suction is turned off. High continuous suction should never be applied, and an air leak would cause continuous bubbling. 1–5, II. Lung Cancer.

8. ② Pursed-lip breathing retards the flow rate of exhaled air creating a back pressure in the airway and preventing airway collapse. 1, IV. COPD.

9. ③ High flow of oxygen will eliminate the hypoxic drive in a COPD client with chronic respiratory acidosis. Because the client has adapted to a high carbon dioxide level, some degree of hypoxemia becomes the stimulus to breathe. 5, II. COPD.

10. ② Robitussin, an expectorant, facilitates removal of secretions by reducing the adhesiveness of secretions to the respiratory tract and promoting ciliary action. 1, II. COPD.

NORMAL RESPIRATORY SYSTEM

I. Upper airways (include nasal cavity, paranasal sinuses, pharynx, and larynx)
  A. Airway conduction
  B. Defense mechanisms
  C. Provides humidity

II. Lower respiratory tract
  A. Conducting airways (include trachea, right and left main stem bronchi, secondary bronchi, and bronchioles)
  B. Acinus (gas exchange units that include the respiratory bronchioles, alveolar ducts and sacs, and alveoli)

III. Thorax and lungs
  A. Thorax boundaries are sternum, 12 ribs, and 12 thoracic vertebrae
  B. Muscles of respiration include diaphragm and intercostals, and accessory muscles include the abdominal, sternocleidomastoid, and the pectoral muscles
  C. The right lung has three lobes, whereas the left lung has two lobes
  D. The lungs are lined by the visceral pleura, but the chest wall is lined by the parietal pleura; the negative pressure in the pleural space prevents the lungs from separating from the chest wall
    1. Lungs contain about 500 million alveoli
    2. Alveolar cells manufacture surfactant, which acts to lower the surface tension of the alveoli and prevent collapse of the alveoli (atelectasis)
    3. Gas exchange takes place across the al-

veolar–capillary membrane, which is thin and has an immense surface area, thereby promoting diffusion

IV. Respiration: defined as process of gas exchange (uptake of oxygen and the elimination of carbon dioxide) between living cells and the environment
   A. Ventilation: defined as flow of mixture of gases into and out of lungs
      1. Hyperventilation defined as a low $PaCO_2$ and hypoventilation defined as a high $PaCO_2$ level
      2. Pulmonary function testing identifies five volumes and four capacities that measure ventilation (Figure 4–3); generally, volumes and capacities increase with COPD and decrease with restrictive diseases
      3. Compliance: measure of distensibility or elasticity of lungs or chest wall. Compliance equal to the change in volume divided by change in pressure. Clients with restrictive lung diseases tend to have lungs with decreased compliance, whereas clients with obstructive diseases tend to have lungs with increased compliance
      4. Ventilation–perfusion inequalities occur when either ventilation or perfusion is decreased. A major cause of hypoxia. If an alveolus is perfused, but has no ventilation (for example, atelectasis), it is termed right-to-left shunting or intrapulmonary shunting
      5. Control of breathing: neural (medulla and pons); mechanical (stretch and irritant receptors); chemical control includes central chemoreceptors that respond to high $PaCO_2$ levels and peripheral chemoreceptors that respond to low PaO_2 levels
   B. Transport
      1. Oxygen: a small amount is dissolved in plasma, whereas most is bound to hemoglobin. The PaO_2 reflects the dissolved oxygen and relates to oxyhemoglobin saturation by the oxygen dissociation curve (see Figure 4–3). Room air 21% oxygen
      2. Carbon dioxide: produced in mitochondria of cells, and present in room air in only minimal amounts; carbon dioxide carried dissolved, as bicarbonate, and as carbamino (a carbon dioxide-amino acid)
      3. Gases diffuse by diffusion gradients
   C. Cell respiration: metabolites oxidized to obtain energy for life processes, whereas CO_2 released as waste product of metabolism

V. Normal respiratory assessment
   A. History
      1. General health

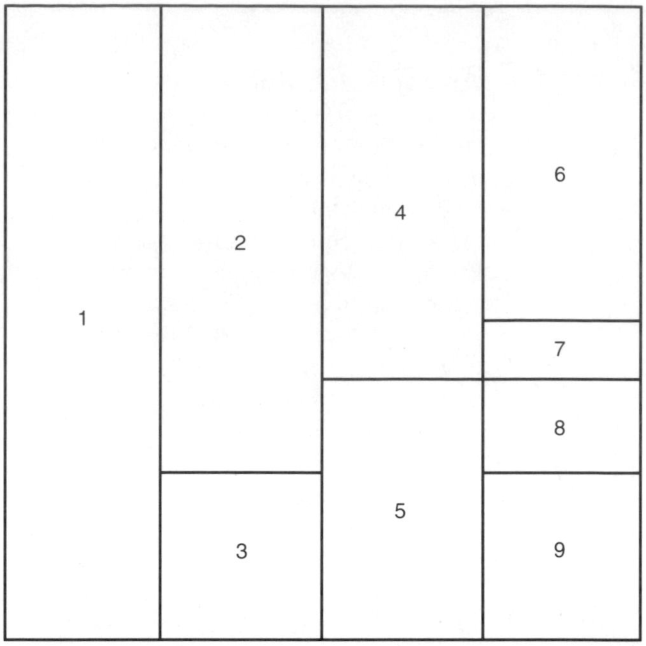

Name of Volume or Capacity	Abbreviation	Approximate Measurement
1. Total lung capacity	TLC	6000 mL
2. Vital capacity	VC	75% TLC= 4500 mL
3. Residual volume	RV	25% TLC= 1500 mL
4. Inspiratory capacity	IC	60% TLC= 3600 mL
5. Functional residual capacity	FRC	40% TLC= 2400 mL
6. Inspiratory reserve volume	IRV	50% TLC= 3000 mL
7. Tidal volume	TV	10% TLC= 600 mL
8. Expiratory reserve volume	ERV	15% TLC= 900 mL
9. Residual volume	RV	25% TLC= 1500 mL

FIGURE 4–3. Diagram of lung volumes and capacities. Approximate measurements are based on a total lung capacity (TLC) of 6000 mL. These are *not* absolutes. Texts vary as to normals; normals also vary with a person's size, sex, and age.

      2. Smoker (packs/day times number of years smoked)
      3. Occupation
      4. Complaints
         a. Cough
         b. Sputum/hemoptysis
         c. Dyspnea
         d. Chest pain

B. Inspection
   1. General
   2. Clubbing of nails (indicates chronic hypoxia)
   3. Truncal or central cyanosis (indicates late and unreliable sign of hypoxia because blood must be less than 80% saturated before it shows (Figure 4–4)
   4. Respiratory rate (normals are 30 to 60 for newborn; 20 to 40 for infant; 15 to 25 for young child; 12 to 20 for adolescent or adult)
   5. Respiratory pattern: normal; tachypnea (fast); bradypnea (slow); Cheyne-Stokes (progressively deeper respirations followed by shallower respirations and a period of apnea; hyperpnea (increased depth); apnea (cessation of air flow)
   6. Use of accessory muscles
   7. Chest symmetry: increased anterior-posterior (A-P) diameter or barrel chest seen with COPD
C. Palpation
   1. Expansion (decrease with restrictive diseases)
   2. Tactile fremitus: increased if consolidation preceded by an open airway; decreased if consolidation preceded by a closed airway, in COPD, obesity, pleural effusion
   3. Deviated trachea: deviates to side of least pressure

D. Percussion
   1. Resonance: normal
   2. Dullness: indicates consolidation
   3. Hyperresonance: heard with COPD
E. Auscultation
   1. Normal breath sounds (sometimes called vesicular)
   2. Abnormal breath sounds include decreased breath sounds (heard with consolidation or when sounds are blocked as with COPD, obesity, or pleural effusion); bronchovesicular or vesicular (heard with consolidation)
   3. Extra sounds
      a. Crackles (sometimes called rales): from air bubbling through fluid or sudden opening of closed airways (heard with pneumonia, pulmonary, and atelectasis)
      b. Rhonchi: due to narrowed airways (heard during excess mucus production, as with COPD)
      c. Wheeze: generated by vibrations of narrowed airways (heard in COPD, especially asthma)
      d. Pleural friction rub: due to roughened pleurae rubbing against each other (heard in pleurisy)
      e. Bronchophony and egophony: due to altered transmission of voice sounds (heard with consolidation and pneumonia)

NURSING PROCESS APPLIED TO ADULTS WITH RESPIRATORY DISORDERS

Oxygen Therapy

I. Assessment
   A. Definition and purpose
      1. Oxygen therapy is the administration of increased concentrations of oxygen (over 21%)
      2. Used to treat both acute and chronic hypoxia
   B. Indications
      1. PaO_2 less than 60 or saturation less than 90%
      2. Above normal, but significant signs of hypoxia present
      3. Myocardial infarction
      4. Carbon monoxide poisoning
      5. Anemia
      6. After anesthesia
      7. After cardiopulmonary arrest

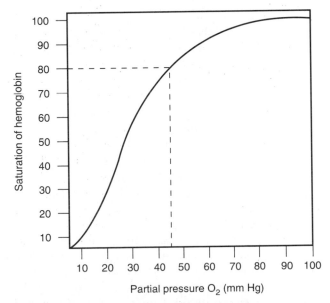

FIGURE 4–4. The oxyhemoglobin curve, which relates hemoglobin saturation to pO_2 levels. It can be seen that central cyanosis is a late sign of hypoxia, because cyanosis is seen at about 80% saturation.

8. During stressful procedures and situations (for example, suctioning or bronchoscopy)
C. Early signs of hypoxia subtle
D. Tachypnea and hyperpnea
E. Confusion
F. Tachycardia and hypertension
G. Cyanosis late sign (seen with saturation of less than 80%)
H. PaO_2 between 60 and 80 is relative hypoxemia; PaO_2 less than 50 defined as respiratory failure

II. Analysis
A. Impaired gas exchange related to decreased concentrations of oxygen
B. Altered breathing pattern related to tachypnea and hyperpnea
C. Impaired verbal communication related to confusion
D. Potential for injury related to oxygen being flammable

III. Planning/goals, expected outcome
A. Client will have increased PaO_2
B. Client will not have symptoms of hypoxia
C. Client will verbalize safety procedures with oxygen therapy

IV. Implementation
A. Nasal cannula
1. Most commonly used system
2. Check for proper position
3. Give good oral care
4. Not accurate for more than 4 L/min
B. Face mask
1. Client inhales from mask and exhales through the side
2. Mask inconvenient because it must be removed for eating, expectoration, and drinking
3. Chosen above the cannula when humidification needed
4. Never use with less than 5 L/min to avoid rebreathing of exhaled CO_2
5. More accurate when secure
C. Partial rebreathing mask
1. Similar to a mask with a reservoir bag added
2. Oxygen flow of 5 L/min required to limit rebreathing of CO_2
3. More accurate than nasal cannula and face mask and used for acutely ill patients requiring 40 to 60% oxygen
D. High-flow systems: non–rebreathing masks and the Venturi mask
1. These systems can accurately provide high oxygen percentages
2. Venturi mask most accurate

E. Monitor client for adverse effects of oxygen, including hypoventilation, absorption atelectasis, and oxygen toxicity
1. Signs of oxygen toxicity occur after administration of 100% oxygen for 24 hours
2. Oxygen toxicity causes pulmonary edema, reduced surfactant and atelectasis, hyaline membrane, and focal hemorrhage
3. Symptoms of oxygen toxicity include a dry cough, chest tightness, crackles, wheezes, and retrolental fibroplasia in infants
F. Teach client not to smoke around oxygen; it should be at least 10 feet away from any open flame, including pilot lights
G. Monitor client's blood gases or pulse oximetry for effectiveness of oxygen therapy

V. Evaluation
A. Client uses oxygen safely
B. Client's PaO_2 improves with therapy
C. Client is not confused and has normal vital signs

Mechanical Ventilation/Suctioning

I. Assessment
A. Definition and purpose
1. Mechanical ventilation uses a machine to provide ventilation when clients cannot oxygenate adequately themselves
a. Negative pressure ventilation uses iron lung concept
(1) Helps to increase the chest size and draw air into the lungs, as in natural ventilation
(2) Does not require intubation, but is painful
b. Positive pressure ventilation more commonly seen
(1) Requires intubation
(2) Forces air into the lungs and client passively expires
2. Suctioning is removal of secretions with a catheter
B. Indications
1. Two main indications for mechanical ventilation include inadequate ventilation and hypoxemia (PaO_2 of less than 50)
2. Clients need to be suctioned when they cannot remove the secretions themselves or when they are intubated
C. Decreased venous return can result from positive pressure ventilation, causing hypoten-

sion, decreased cardiac output, tachycardia, confusion, and oliguria

D. Barotrauma can result from high pressures, resulting in deterioration of blood gases and absent breath sounds, along with sudden agitation

E. Positive pressure ventilation associated with release of antidiuretic hormone (ADH) so clients often retain fluid; crackles, decreased compliance, and decreased vital capacity also seen

F. Gastric distention and gastrointestinal bleeding often associated with positive pressure ventilation; abdominal distention and bloody nasogastric drainage can result

G. Malnutrition can result due to previous health status, extent of this hospitalization, weight and percentage of ideal weight, serum albumin and transferrin levels, and muscle atrophy

H. Complications
1. Infection
2. Pneumomediastinum (barotrauma)
3. Oxygen toxicity
4. Difficulty weaning
5. Gastrointestinal bleeding

II. Analysis

A. Impaired communication related to intubation

B. Decreased cardiac output related to decreased venous return

C. High risk for infection related to endotracheal tube and suctioning

D. High risk for injury related to barotrauma, malfunctioning of equipment, gastrointestinal bleed; oxygen toxicity

E. High risk for fluid volume excess related to excessive ADH secretion

F. High risk for dysfunctional weaning response related to injury

III. Planning/goals, expected outcome

A. Client will be able to communicate to nurse in some way

B. Client's vital signs will be normal

C. Client will not develop pneumonia as evidenced by chest x-ray

D. Client will be able to be weaned safely from the ventilator with no complications

IV. Implementation

A. Monitor blood gases and pulse oximeter

B. Suction when coarse crackles are heard; suction with sterile technique; hyperinflate the patient with 100% oxygen before and after suctioning to avoid complications

C. Measure abdominal girth and bowel sounds; guaiac stools and nasogastric drainage

D. Provide enteral or parenteral feedings; if high levels of carbohydrate, watch for high CO_2 levels and difficulty in weaning; better to provide calories with fat emulsions

E. Watch for signs of fluid overload (crackles, positive fluid balance)

F. Closely watch cardiac monitor for arrhythmias

G. Monitoring ventilator alarms

H. Evaluate for readiness to wean
1. Tidal volume, negative inspiratory force, and other pulmonary function parameters
2. Oxygenation criteria
3. Vital signs and evaluation of right-to-left shunt

V. Evaluation

A. Client successfully weaned from the ventilator with no complications

B. Client relaxed and able to communicate

C. Client has normal vital signs and PaO_2

Chronic Obstructive Pulmonary Disease

I. Assessment

A. Definition: a diagnostic category for respiratory conditions that involve a persistent obstruction/limitation of airflow; collectively referring to chronic bronchitis, emphysema, and asthma

B. Pathophysiology/clinical manifestations: clinically difficult to distinguish among these three disorders, as all cause diffuse limitation in airflow and have common manifestations; often coexisting in same individual; however, pathogenesis of airflow obstruction differs among these three disorders
1. Chronic bronchitis: defined by the American Thoracic Society as excessive sputum production with cough for a minimum of 3 months per year and for 2 consecutive years
   a. Hypertrophy and hyperplasia of submucosal bronchial glands
   b. Excessive mucus production
   c. Impaired ciliary function
   d. Recurring infections of the lower respiratory tract
   e. Inflammatory process causes narrowing of airways and mucus plugs
   f. Bronchioles become damaged and fibrotic
   g. Decreased V/Q ratio
   h. Clinical manifestations
      (1) Chronic productive cough
      (2) Shortness of breath

(3) Often marked hypoxemia and respiratory acidosis

(4) Frequent episodes of associated right ventricular failure (cor pulmonale)

(5) May have crackles and wheezes due to secretions

(6) Frequent respiratory infections

(7) Called "blue bloater" because of cyanotic, bloated appearance

2. Emphysema

a. Destructive changes in the alveolar walls, ducts, and respiratory bronchioles, slowly progressing over many years; this loss of tissue distinguishes emphysema from chronic bronchitis and asthma

b. Enlargement of air spaces as alveoli fuse together

c. Alveoli lose inherent elastic recoil

d. Collapse of small, poorly supported, distal airways

e. Decreased expiratory flow rates causing air trapping

f. The impaired diffusion is balanced by the destruction of the capillary bed, so V/Q imbalance is slight

g. Some types are associated with alpha-1-antitrypsin deficiency

h. Clinical manifestations (for emphysema)

(1) Cough with minimal sputum

(2) Shortness of breath

(3) Downhill course

(4) Often near-normal PaO_2 and $PaCO_2$

(5) Anorexia and weight loss

(6) Cor pulmonale a late sign

(7) Barrel chest, hyperresonance, distant breath sounds, prolonged expiration

(8) Fatigue

(9) Called "pink puffer" because of shortness of breath and skin appearance

3. Bronchial asthma

a. Intermittent airway obstruction is present during asthmatic attack

b. May be immunological (allergic) or nonimmunological (nonallergic) type

c. Bronchial hyperreactivity to stimuli

d. Contraction of smooth muscles of airways (bronchospasm)

e. Edema of membranes that line the airways

f. Excessive amount and viscosity of mucous secretions

g. May become chronic and develop into emphysema, chronic bronchitis, or both

h. Decreased V/Q ratio

i. Clinical manifestations for asthma

(1) Wheezing

(2) Increased eosinophils in sputum and blood

(3) Often precipitated by exposure to allergens or irritants

(4) Shortness of breath, prolonged expiration, cough, use of accessory muscles

(5) Sudden onset of symptoms, and symptoms can be reversed with medication

C. Incidence

1. Approximately 10 to 25% of adult United States population is diagnosed with chronic bronchitis

2. Approximately 3 to 5% of adult United States population is diagnosed with asthma

3. Incidence of emphysema cannot be accurate because it often coexists with chronic bronchitis

4. Chronic bronchitis and emphysema have higher incidence rates among smokers and older men; asthma commonly seen in childhood

D. Predisposing/precipitating factors

1. Smoking

2. Air pollution and occupational hazards— for example, smoke, coal, asbestos, chemicals, dust, gases

3. Chronic respiratory infections

4. Allergic factors

5. Familial and genetic factors

6. Aging

F. Diagnostic examinations

1. Chest x-ray: may show presence of bullae and hyperinflation of lung in emphysema; vascular shadow prominence; pulmonary infiltrates and so on

2. Pulmonary function tests (PFTs): functional residual capacity, residual volume, and total lung capacity may be increased in the three disorders (but more markedly in emphysema) and may disappear in asthma when in complete remission; these abnormal pulmonary functions indicate airway obstruction and decrease in vital capacity

3. Arterial blood gases: hypoxemia with an

accompanying hypercapnia common during exacerbation and as disease progresses; with bicarbonate level rising due to compensation by kidneys

II. Analysis
- A. Impaired gas exchange related to excessive secretions or loss of tissue
- B. Ineffective airway clearance related to secretions
- C. High risk for infection related to increased secretions and altered breathing pattern
- D. Fatigue related to increased work of breathing
- E. Altered nutrition: less than required related to anorexia
- F. Knowledge deficit related to knowledge needs with daily living and medications

III. Planning/goals, expected outcomes
- A. Client's hypoxemia and hypercapnia will be minimized
- B. Client will maintain a clear and patent airway
- C. Client will tolerate gradually increased activities
- D. Client will evidence resolution/absence of infection
- E. Client will maintain optimum nutritional status
- F. Client will verbalize understanding of disease process, treatment, and health maintenance

IV. Implementation
- A. Assess character of breathing patterns, breath sounds, and extra sounds, percuss for resonance, and observe sputum
- B. Promote mobilization of secretions through mucolytic agents, increased humidification, fluid intake of 1½ to 2 L per day (unless contraindicated), suctioning, and chest physiotherapy
- C. Position client upright to allow maximum breathing
- D. Teach client to use pursed-lip and abdominal breathing
- E. Administer low flow O_2 because with COPD clients with high $PaCO_2$ levels, use hypoxia as the stimulus to breathe
- F. Monitor therapeutic and side effects of medications and treatment
- G. Provide adequate rest periods and pace activities
- H. Encourage range of motion exercises
- I. Assist with activities of daily living as needed and assess response
- J. Involve client and family in planning care including goal setting
- K. Assess client for signs of infection: fever, chills, increase in cough and sputum, WBC, and abnormal breath sounds (crackles, wheezes, rhonchi)
- L. Teach client to avoid contact with infected people
- M. Provide proper caloric requirements, small feedings high in protein; if on enteral or parenteral feedings, avoid high levels of carbohydrate, as this increases CO_2 levels
- N. Assess nutritional status: body weight, percentage of ideal weight, caloric intake, muscle tone, and size
- O. Discuss health maintenance and treatment regimen
  1. Avoidance of smoking, irritants, and infection
  2. Avoidance of extremes of temperature
  3. Use measures to conserve energy
  4. Proper nutrition and hydration
  5. Rest and activity program
  6. Disease process including signs of infection and complications
  7. Medications and treatment including O_2 therapy
  8. Monitor use of tranquilizers and drugs that depress respiration (opiates)

V. Evaluation
- A. Client demonstrates improvement of dyspnea with PaO_2 and $PaCO_2$ within expected ranges for COPD
- B. Overall improvement in activity tolerance and nutritional intake are evident
- C. Client shows adequate knowledge of disease, medications, treatments, and signs and symptoms to report to physician
- D. No evidence of complications such as respiratory failure, pneumonia, atelectasis

Pneumonia

I. Assessment
- A. Definition: acute infection causing inflammation of lung tissue and alveoli filled with exudate
- B. Pathophysiology
  1. Infectious viral, fungal, or bacterial agents may be introduced by inhalation, aspiration, or spread from primary infection through circulation
  2. Extent of inflammatory process varies and may involve different areas of lung parenchyma and pleura depending on type of pneumonia and host condition
  3. Some pathological changes include
     a. Hypertrophy and hypersecretion of mucous membranes lining the lungs

b. Congestion as alveoli become fluid-filled
c. Massive dilation of capillaries
d. Infiltration of affected lung area with RBCs, leukocytes, and fibrins with subsequent consolidation
e. Inflammation of pleurae
f. Atelectasis and impaired gas exchange
g. Bacteremia
h. Right-to-left shunting and hypoxemia

C. Etiology
1. Gram-negative bacteria: *Streptococcus pneumoniae, Staphylococcus aureus, Streptococcus pyogenes*
2. Gram-positive bacteria: *Klebsiella pneumoniae, Pseudomonas aeruginosa, Haemophilus influenzae, Legionella pneumophila*
3. Anaerobic bacteria: anaerobic streptococci, *Bacteroides* species
4. *Mycoplasma pneumoniae*
5. Viruses
6. Fungal: *Histoplasma capsulatum, Coccidioides immitis, Aspergillus*
7. *Pneumocystis carinii* (has been considered a protozoan, but is probably closer to a fungus)

D. Incidence
1. Leading infectious cause of death; accounts for 10% of hospital admissions; fifth leading cause of death in the United States; estimated that there are 1 million cases of bacterial pneumonia per year in the United States
2. Can occur at any season, but most common during winter and early spring
3. More common among infants and elderly

E. Predisposing/precipitating factors
1. Chronic obstructive pulmonary disease
2. Respiratory tract infection—for example, influenza
3. Smoking and air pollution
4. Tracheal intubation
5. Conditions in which there is risk for aspiration: for example, post-anesthesia, drug overdose
6. Impaired immune response: for example, leukemia; use of immunosuppressive drugs
7. Prolonged bedrest and immobility
8. Malnutrition

F. Clinical manifestations
1. Typical manifestations
a. Fever and chills
b. Productive cough with greenish or rusty spots

c. Tachypnea, nasal flaring, and intercostal retraction, dyspnea
d. Pleuritic chest pain
e. Crackles, dullness over area of consolidation, bronchophony, and egophony

2. Atypical manifestations
a. Malaise and fatigue
b. Headache
c. Sore throat, pharyngitis
d. Gastrointestinal manifestations: nausea, vomiting, abdominal pain, diarrhea

3. Manifestations of pneumocystis pneumonia
a. Seen in immunocompromised patients and in AIDS patients
b. Severe dyspnea
c. Fever
d. Prominent hypoxia and right-to-left shunting
e. Rapidly progresses to respiratory failure and death when untreated

G. Diagnostic examinations
1. Chest x-ray: lobar, interstitial, or necrotizing pneumonia; empyema may also be present
2. Sputum: Gram's stain, sputum and blood culture, and sensitivity
a. Sputum: Gram's stain allows for classifying causative organism into gram-negative or -positive so that appropriate therapy can be initiated while awaiting culture results
b. Cultures done to identify the bacterial agents and properly select an effective antibiotic or to evaluate effectiveness of the therapy
c. Sputum culture collected for 3 consecutive days when client awakens in the morning; use sputum trap if client being suctioned
d. Tracheal suctioning may be done if client unable to voluntarily cough
e. Fiberoptic bronchoscopy for diagnosing pneumocystis
3. Complete blood count shows elevated leukocytes
4. Arterial blood gases reveal hypoxemia

H. Complications
1. Pleural effusion: collection of fluid in the pleural cavity compresses lung tissue and interferes with normal ventilation
2. Atelectasis: alveolar collapse causes abnormally uneven distribution of ventilation within the lung with right-to-left shunting

3. Pleurisy: inflammation of pleura
4. Empyema: accumulation of purulent exudate in the pleural cavity
5. Lung abscess: commonly caused by aspiration of material into the lung resulting into a pus-containing lesion and cavitation
6. Pericarditis: spread of infection to the pericardium via the bloodstream

I. Medical management
1. Expectorants (Table 4–21)
2. Antibiotics (Table 4–22)
3. Bronchodilators (Table 4–23)

II. Analysis
A. Ineffective airway clearance related to secretions
B. Impaired gas exchange related to alveolar exudate
C. Altered pattern of breathing related to pleuritic pain and dyspnea
D. Infection related to offending organism
E. Knowledge deficit related to disease process, therapy, and preventive measures

III. Planning/goals, expected outcomes
A. Client will maintain a patent airway and clearance of secretions

TABLE 4–21 Drugs Used to Treat Respiratory Disorders

Class	Example	Action	Use	Common Side Effects	Nursing Implications
Bronchodilators: Xanthine derivatives	Theophylline (Theo-Dur)	Relax bronchial smooth muscle and inhibit release of histamine and slow release substance A (SRS-A) from mast cells; they are mild diuretics and cardiac stimulants	Symptomatic relief of asthma and bronchial spasms	GI upset, nausea, nervousness, frequency, diarrhea, insomnia, tachycardia, palpitations, esophageal reflux	Use with caution in clients with hypertension, tachycardia, hypoxemia, glaucoma, hyperthyroidism, BPH, diabetes; monitor for CNS symptoms; give with food or antacids; avoid smoking; check theophylline levels
Antihistamines	Diphenhydramine hydrochloride (Benadryl)	Block action of histamine at H1 receptor sites, smooth muscles of the blood vessels, bronchioles, and GI tract	Relieve symptoms of allergies; in adjunct in treatment of anaphylaxis; prevent and treat motion sickness, relieve insomnia; prevent and treat nausea due to surgery and anesthesia	Sedation, epigastric distress, hypotension, palpitations, tachycardia, thickening of bronchial secretions, vertigo, urinary frequency	Warn about sedation; use carefully in patients with convulsions, hyperthyroidism, cardiovascular and renal disease, HTN, diabetes; avoid use with alcohol; monitor for dry mucous membranes; give with meals or antacids
Cough preparations: expectorants	Guaifenesin (Robitussin)	Facilitate removal of thick mucus from lungs and act as soothing demulcent by stimulating secretion of a lubricant	Facilitates productive cough	Nausea and vomiting, GI irritation, drowsiness	Instruct client not to use more than 1 week without seeing physician; use high fluid intake and humidity to loosen secretions; do not follow with water, except potassium iodide
Antitussives	Narcotics: any product with codeine; non-narcotics: dextromethorphan	Suppress cough reflex; act centrally on the cough center or peripherally within the tracheobronchial tree	To treat dry nonproductive coughs that interfere with sleep or other activities	Dizziness, sedation, sweating, nausea, dry mouth, constipation, urinary retention, palpitations	Caution client about possible sedation; administer with caution to clients with asthma, COPD, cardiac disease, convulsions, renal or hepatic disease, CNS depression, BPH, alcoholism, or hypothyroidism

TABLE 4–22 Antibiotic Therapy for Pneumonia

Class	Examples	Use	Common Side Effects	Nursing Implications
Penicillins	Penicillin G Na/K; procaine penicillin G (Wycillin); potassium penicillin V (Pen-Vee-K); nafcillin (Unipen); ampicillin; amoxicillin; carbenicillin; ticarcillin; cloxacillin (Tegopen); methicillin (Staphcillin)	Bactericidal against a wide variety of gram-positive and some gram-negative organisms; most effective in the treatment of bacterial pneumonia	Allergic reactions (skin rashes, anaphylaxis); GI disturbances (nausea and vomiting, epigastric distress); CNS toxicity manifested by hallucinations, hyperreflexia, seizures when administered in very high doses to patients with neurological reactions (thrombocytopenia, agranulocytosis, anemia); impaired renal function	Check for history of penicillin allergy prior to administration of drug; observe for allergic manifestations and other side effects; evaluate effects of drug especially when given concurrently with drugs that may increase or decrease its action—for example, gentamicin is synergistic to penicillin; probenecid decreases its renal excretion; tetracycline and erythromycin both inhibit bactericidal activity of penicillin; monitor for development of resistant organisms; susceptibility testing should be done before and during the course of therapy
Cephalosporins	Cephalexin (Keflex), cefamandole (Mandol), cefazolin (Ancef, Kefzol, cephalothin, Keflin), cefoxitin (Mefoxin), cephapirin (Cefadyl), ceftazidime (Fortaz)	Effective against numerous infections but used primarily for *Klebsiella pneumoniae* along with aminoglycoside	GI disturbances, nephrotoxicity (decreased urine output and creatinine clearance, hematuria, proteinuria), phlebitis with IV administration	Assess for allergic reactions to cephalosporins and penicillins; it is controversial whether cephalosporins can be given without causing allergic reactions when there is a known hypersensitivity to penicillin; monitor for toxic side effects; check BUN and creatinine; assess effectiveness when administered with bacteriostatic antibiotics—for example, tetracyclines and erythromycins, which may decrease or destroy its effects
Aminoglycosides	Kanamycin (Kantrex), neomycin, amikacin sulfate, gentamicin (Garamycin), tobramycin, streptomycin	Bactericidal against a wide range of gram-positive and gram-negative bacteria and mycobacteria; however, they differ in clinical uses Streptomycin: used in the treatment of tuberculosis in combination with other tuberculostatic drugs Neomycin: used for reducing intestinal flora and thereby decreasing blood ammonia levels Gentamicin: used to treat bacteremia caused by proteus, pseudomonas, *E. coli,* and klebsiella Amikacin and tobramycin: used to treat gentamicin-resistant infection	Ototoxicity, nephrotoxicity, neuromuscular blockade, peripheral neuritis, resistant infection	Assess client for beginning auditory and vestibular damage—for example, vertigo, ataxia, roaring in the ears, hearing loss; monitor renal function, especially when administered to elderly persons or to those with renal insufficiency; monitor peak and trough levels and drug dosages; assess neuromuscular effects, especially when administered with muscle relaxants and sedatives
Tetracyclines	Chlortetracycline HCL (Aureomycin), demeclocycline HCL	Bacteriostatic for many gram-negative and gram-positive organisms,	GI disturbances, allergic reactions, hepatotoxicity, enamel hypoplasia, and	Avoid use in children, during pregnancy, and when there is impaired

TABLE 4–22 Antibiotic Therapy for Pneumonia *Continued*

Class	Examples	Use	Common Side Effects	Nursing Implications
	(Declomycin), doxycycline hyclate (Vibramycin)	including mycobacteria, rickettsiae, mycoplasma, and agents of psittacosis	permanent staining of teeth when used during tooth development	hepatic or renal function; do not administer with food, milk, milk products, antacids since they inhibit tetracycline absorption; monitor client for a developing superinfection; monitor liver function in long-term therapy; instruct client to avoid direct sunlight because sunburn reaction or erythema is likely to occur
Antifungal	Amphotercin-B	Histoplasmosis, coccidioidomycosis, aspergillus	Nephrotoxic convulsions, thromobcytopenia, leukopenia, fever, chills, pain at injection site, nausea, vomiting	Check for extravasation, protect from light, symptomatic relief of adverse reactions, check BUN and creatinine and I & O
Miscellaneous anti-infectives	Trimethoprim-sulfamethoxazole (TMP-SMZ); pentamidine (Pentam)	Pneumocystis pneumonia	TMP-SMZ: rash, fever, leukopenia, failure to respond to Pentam: severe hypoglycemia	Clients with AIDS have a peculiar predisposition to allergic reactions to sulfonamides, making the switch to Pentam imperative sometimes; careful monitoring of drug effectiveness

B. Client will show improved respirations
C. Client will verbalize decrease in discomforts from pleuritic chest pains and coughing
D. Client will progressively assume activities of daily living without shortness of breath, tachycardia, and fever
E. Client and family will verbalize understanding of disease process, therapy, and preventive measures
IV. Implementation
   A. Administer expectorants and cough suppressants (see Table 4–21), antibiotics (see Table 4–22), bronchodilators (see Table 4–23)
   B. Teach client how to cough effectively by splinting chest and how to prevent spread of infection
   C. Evaluate effects of treatments (IPPB, incentive spirometry and postural drainage)
   D. Position client in semi-Fowler's to promote adequate ventilation
   E. Suction client as needed
   F. Administer oxygen as indicated

TABLE 4–23 Bronchodilators

Class	Example	Use	Common Side Effects	Nursing Implications
Bronchodilators; beta-adrenergic	Metaproterenol (Alupent); albuterol (Ventolin)	COPD	Tremor, palpitations, headache, hypertension, nervousness, dizziness, nausea, worse V/Q ratio and decreased PO_2	With all inhalants: after shaking, exhale; hold inhaler four fingers in front of mouth; activate MDI and breathe in slowly for 5–6 seconds; hold breath for 10 seconds; wait 1–5 minutes for repeat puff; rinse out mouth, if bad taste. Watch blood gases and vital signs
Bronchodilators; anticholinergic	Ipratropium (Atrovent)	COPD	Anxiety, dizziness, headache, cough, dry mouth	As above with inhalants; observe effectiveness
Steroids	Beclomethasone (Beclovent); triamcinolone (Azmacort)	Asthma	Throat irritation, hoarseness, dry mouth, cough	As above with inhalers; evaluate effectiveness of drug, listen for wheezes, crackles

G. Monitor respirations, breath sounds, blood gases
H. Increase fluid intake to 2 to 3 L per day unless contraindicated
I. Assess for signs of dehydration: poor skin turgor, dry mucous membranes, hypotension, tachycardia
J. Assess character of pain and effect on respiration
K. Provide comfort measures: analgesics as ordered, comfortable position, cool bath, and skin care
L. Good handwashing to prevent spread of infections; sometimes on respiratory isolation
M. Increase activities as tolerated with adequate rest periods
N. Provide balanced diet, liquid initially, and advance to solids high in protein, calories, vitamins, and minerals
O. Instruct client regarding maintenance of good nutrition, fluid intake, rest, and avoidance of infection and predisposing factors such as smoking
P. Encourage client to adhere to post-discharge care, including completion of antibiotics and vaccinations for influenza and pneumococcal pneumonia
V. Evaluation
A. Client's respiratory infection will be resolved as evidenced by absence of respiratory distress and a decrease in sputum production
B. Client's pain controlled and normal breathing pattern reestablished
C. Client complies with post-discharge care with sufficient understanding of disease and treatment regimen

Tuberculosis

I. Assessment
A. Definition: bacterial infection caused by *Mycobacterium tuberculosis;* usually involves lungs but may also cause extrapulmonary infections in bones, lymph nodes, kidneys, and meninges and may spread throughout bloodstream (miliary tuberculosis)
B. Pathophysiology
1. Inhaled bacilli implanted in bronchioles and alveoli
2. Inflammation occurs to counteract infection
3. Granulomatous lesion called tubercle formed and surrounded by lymphocytes
4. Lesion undergoes necrosis characterized by cheesy consistency in center, which may become liquefied and cause cavitation

5. When lesion heals, tubercle bacilli remain in lung in walled-off, dormant state and may be reactivated if organisms rapidly multiply and body defenses lowered
C. Etiology: organisms spread by inhalation of minute tubercle-laden droplets when an infected person speaks, coughs, or sneezes
D. Predisposing/precipitating factors
1. Overcrowded, poorly ventilated dwellings
2. Poor nutritional status
3. Prolonged exposure to individuals infected with tuberculosis
4. Alcoholism
5. Inadequate treatment of previous tuberculosis (TB) infection
6. Presence of medical conditions that lower the resistance to infection
E. Incidence
1. Older persons, especially males age 65 and over, and children under 5
2. High incidence among African Americans, Native Americans, homeless, low socioeconomic groups, and persons with HIV
3. Incidence increasing rapidly over last 5 years
F. Clinical manifestations
1. Systemic, nonspecific manifestations: fatigue, malaise, anorexia, weight loss, low-grade fever, night sweats
2. Pulmonary manifestations: cough with productive mucopurulent sputum, pleuritic chest pain, dyspnea, hemoptysis (advanced cases)
G. Diagnostic examinations
1. Tuberculin test: positive reaction indicates evidence of tuberculous exposure; most accurate tuberculin test is Mantoux test or intracutaneous injection of either PPD (purified protein derivative) or OT (old tuberculin prepared from dead tubercle bacilli); significant reaction is 10 mm or more in diameter
2. Chest x-ray: shows evidence of active infection—i.e., pulmonary infiltration, nodules, cavitations
3. Sputum exam: three or more specimens may be needed to confirm diagnosis; usually acid-fast bacilli identified with sputum smears is the first bacteriological evidence; however, the most accurate means of identifying the mycobacterium is culture technique that can detect small quantities of the bacteria
H. Medical management: antitubercular medications (Table 4–24)

TABLE 4–24 Antituberculosis Medications

Class	Use	Common Side Effects	Nursing Implications
First-line drugs: isoniazid (INH), rifampin, ethambutol, streptomycin Second-line drugs: viomycin, capreomycin, kanamycin, pyrazinamide, para-aminosalicylic acid (PAS)	Either bacteriostatic or bactericidal against *Mycobacterium tuberculosis:* usually prescribed as combination therapy to be more effective and to lessen development of resistant organisms; standard therapy usually includes a 9-month regimen of INH and rifampin, supplemented by ethambutol, streptomycin, or a second-line drug; course of treatment ranges from 9 to 24 months beyond time client converts to a negative sputum and symptoms are ameliorated; INH, the most potent tuberculostatic drug, may be used as a single prophylactic agent for those who convert to positive PPD	INH: peripheral neuropathy, GI distress, hepatic toxicity, agranulocytosis, thrombocytopenia, hemolytic anemia Ethambutol: loss of visual acuity, disturbances of color discrimination, dermatitis, GI symptoms, elevated liver function tests, precipitation of gout Rifampin: red-orange urine and secretions, GI distress, liver dysfunction, hematologic reaction Streptomycin, viomycin, kanamycin, and capreomycin: all cause auditory and vestibular damage and impairment of renal function PAS: GI intolerance, allergic reaction	Emphasize importance of completing and not interrupting medication regime to achieve sufficient treatment and to decrease susceptibility of family members to infection; instruct client on side effects of medications and report adverse side effects; monitor drug dosage, liver and renal function as indicated; administer pyridoxine with INH to control peripheral neuritis; administer INH on an empty stomach or 1 hour prior to intake of antacids for maximum absorption; evaluate visual acuity and color vision for those receiving ethambutol and hearing function and balance for those receiving streptomycin and similar drugs

II. Analysis

   A. Knowledge deficit related to need for health teaching and compliance with regimen

   B. Impaired gas exchange related to infected alveoli

   C. Altered pattern of breathing related to dyspnea

   D. Fatigue related to generalized malaise

   E. Altered nutrition: less than required related to anorexia and possible pre-existing malnutrition

III. Planning/goals, expected outcomes

   A. Client will explain drug actions, dosage, side effects, and the importance of continuing medications uninterruptedly

   B. Client's breathing pattern and gas exchange will return to pre-illness level

   C. Client will practice measures to prevent infection

   D. Client will return to pre-illness activity level

   E. Client will maintain a nutritionally adequate diet

IV. Implementation

   A. Assist with diagnostic testing to detect tuberculosis

   B. Administer antituberculosis drugs and observe for toxic effects (see Table 4–24)

   C. Instruct client on preventing spread of infection (careful handwashing, covering nose and mouth when coughing and sneezing, proper handling and disposal of sputum)

   D. Teach client and family about multiple drug therapy and completion of treatment (at least nine months or longer as necessary)

   E. Provide nutritious diet and evaluate general nutritional status

   F. Explain nature of the disease and signs and symptoms of recurrence of tuberculosis

V. Evaluation

   A. Client maintains measures to control spread and transmission of tuberculosis

   B. Client complies with medications, diet, rest, and activity

   C. Tuberculosis goes into remission

Lung Cancer

I. Assessment

   A. Definition: group of malignant processes that may arise from within and involve the bronchial epithelium (bronchogenic), lung parenchyma (bronchoalveolar), or visceral pleurae (mesothelioma)

   B. Pathophysiology

     1. May be either metastatic (extends from a malignancy anywhere in the body) or primary tumor (bronchopulmonary origin)

     2. Approximately 90% of lung cancer bronchogenic carcinoma; tumor grows slowly over several years until it is large enough to be detected on roentgenogram; i.e., 0.5 to 1.0 cm in diameter

3. Pathological features include nonspecific, inflammatory changes, hypersecretion of mucus, desquamation and hyperplasia of cells
4. Four different cell types of primary lung cancer
   a. Squamous cell (most common)
   b. Adenocarcinoma, alveolar cell
   c. Large cell
   d. Small cell
5. Primary lung cancers metastasize by direct extension and via the blood and lymph systems

C. Incidence
1. Leading cause of cancer deaths in men and women
2. There are over 150,000 new cases diagnosed yearly in the United States with more than 140,000 deaths annually
3. Occurs most frequently in individuals ages 40 to 75 with long history of smoking

D. Predisposing/precipitating factors
1. Cigarette smoking and passive exposure to smoking
2. Exposure to occupational carcinogens: for example, asbestos, radiation, arsenic, coal products, iron oxide
3. Pre-existing pulmonary diseases: for example, COPD, tuberculosis, bronchiectasis

E. Clinical manifestations
1. When lung cancer presents with symptoms, usually advanced and unresectable
2. Initial symptoms usually persistent cough and expectoration
3. If bronchial obstruction, wheezing and dyspnea noted
4. Nonspecific symptoms that may be due to regional spread of tumor include dysphagia, hoarseness, anorexia, fatigue, nausea and vomiting, and weight loss
5. Extrathoracic metastases: neurological deficits, bone pain, liver and biliary dysfunctions

F. Diagnostic examinations
1. Chest x-ray: indicated for anyone who has had cough for two or three weeks; may show presence of tumor when large enough to be detected by x-ray
2. Sputum cytologic examination—for identifying malignant cells
3. Computed tomography (CT): to identify location and extent of masses in the chest
4. Fiberoptic bronchoscopy
   a. For direct visualization and biopsy of tumor; biopsy is the only true diagnosis for cancer
   b. Keep NPO after test until gag reflex returns
   c. Some blood-tinged sputum normal post-test
5. Bone scan for metastasis
6. MRI to see if it is a primary tumor

G. Medical management
1. Radiation therapy
2. Chemotherapy

H. Surgical management
1. Pneumonectomy
2. Lobectomy
3. Wedge resection

II. Analysis
A. Altered airway clearance related to secretion
B. High risk for ineffective individual coping related to poor prognosis
C. Alteration in nutrition: less than required related to anorexia due to disease and treatment
D. Knowledge deficit related to type and course of treatment, side effects, and potential complications
E. High risk for infection related to lowered resistance and retained secretions

III. Planning/goals, expected outcomes
A. Client and family will be able to deal with diagnosis of cancer
B. Client will verbalize palliative relief of symptoms of pain and dyspnea
C. Client will show improvement in nutrition—increase in caloric and protein intake, minimal weight loss, less nausea and anorexia
D. Client and family will verbalize understanding of type and course of treatment; i.e., surgery, chemotherapy, and radiation and potential side effects and complications
E. Client will not develop infection

IV. Implementation
A. Provide explanations and psychological support during diagnostic testing and treatment
B. Provide measures to relieve pain including drugs and relaxation technique
C. Maintain an open airway and oxygen support
D. Provide a high calorie, high protein, palatable diet
E. Assess degree of malnutrition and requirements for nutritional support
F. Monitor client's response to therapy and onset of complications
G. Teach client and family regarding treatment, side effects, and signs of complications

V. Evaluation

A. Client able to cope with own fears
B. Client copes with distressing symptoms associated with radiation and chemotherapy

Pulmonary Edema

I. Assessment
   A. Definition: Abnormal accumulation of extravascular fluid in lungs; edema can be due to left ventricular failure (cardiogenic pulmonary edema) or noncardiogenic edema due to pulmonary hypertension and breakdown of alveolar-capillary membrane
   B. Pathophysiology
      1. Cardiogenic pulmonary edema: left ventricular failure; pulmonary vascular congestion; increased capillary hydrostatic pressure; movement of edema to alveoli; alveolar flooding occur
      2. Noncardiogenic pulmonary edema: hydrostatic pressures normal, but alveolar-capillary membrane damaged; with resultant flooding of alveoli
      3. Either type: fluid-filled alveoli decrease diffusion; disruption of surfactant predisposes the alveoli to collapse; "foam" created as air and fluid mix; lung compliance decreases; both right-to-left shunting and decreased V/Q ratios can limit oxygenation
   C. Incidence
      1. Noncardiogenic pulmonary edema
         a. Occurs as a complication in adult respiratory distress syndrome (ARDS)
         b. About 150,000 cases of ARDS annually in the United States
      2. Cardiogenic pulmonary edema
         a. More common
         b. Occurs as a complication of left ventricular failure, myocardial infarction, mitral stenosis, or fluid overload
   D. Predisposing/precipitating factors
      1. ARDS (life-threatening condition that leads to respiratory failure with about a 50% mortality rate; is a complication from a variety of disorders, including sepsis, trauma, and pneumonia)
      2. Left ventricular failure
      3. Fluid overload
      4. Myocardial infarction
      5. Mitral stenosis
   E. Clinical manifestations
      1. Cardiogenic
         a. Dyspnea
         b. Orthopnea
         c. Paroxysmal nocturnal dyspnea
         d. Pink, frothy sputum
         e. Crackles
         f. S_3 or S_4 present
         g. Hypotension
         h. Hypoxia
      2. Noncardiogenic
         a. Tachypnea
         b. Hypoxia to the point of cyanosis
         c. Crackles
         d. Acute respiratory distress and rapid deterioration
   F. Medical management
      1. Medications
         a. Ionotropic (see Table 4–1)
         b. Diuretics (see Table 4–1)
      2. O_2
II. Analysis
   A. Impaired gas exchange related to right-to-left shunting and decreased V/Q ratios
   B. Altered pattern of breathing related to severe dyspnea
   C. Fluid volume excess related to left ventricular failure in cardiogenic pulmonary edema
   D. Decreased cardiac output related to left ventricular failure in cardiogenic pulmonary edema
III. Planning/goals, expected outcome
   A. Client's oxygenation will improve; blood gases will show normal PaO_2
   B. Client's breathing will ease; rate will decrease
   C. Client's left cardiac function will improve; no S_3 or S_4 will be heard
IV. Implementation
   A. Monitor blood gases
   B. If on ventilator, suction frequently
   C. Maintain oxygenation with ventilator or nasal cannula; if on ventilator, use of PEEP (positive end-expiratory pressure)
   D. Restrict fluids and sodium
   E. Administer inotropic drugs, diuretics in cardiogenic pulmonary edema (see Table 4–1)
   F. Prevent pulmonary infection with strict asepsis in suctioning and handwashing
   G. Maintain nutrition with parenteral or enteral feedings in noncardiogenic pulmonary edema
V. Evaluation
   A. Client's oxygenation improves with normal PaO_2 values and absence of crackles
   B. Work of breathing decreases and client's respiratory rate decreases
   C. Client no longer needs the ventilator
   D. Client's dyspnea and use of accessory muscles decreases
   E. Client's heart no longer fails, no S_3 or S_4, increased blood pressure, and no crackles

Pulmonary Embolism

I. Assessment
  A. Definition: obstruction to blood flow in a pulmonary artery or capillary caused by a thrombus
  B. Pathophysiology
    1. Layers of platelets and fibrin collect (often near a venous valve) to produce a clot; often fibrinolysis occurs to dissolve the clot; however, an embolism occurs when clot dislodges and travels to the lung
    2. Once thrombus lodges, it decreases the size of the pulmonary vasculature resulting in hypoxia from V/Q mismatching
    3. Surfactant is lost in the region of the emboli so that atelectasis occurs, resulting in right-to-left shunting
    4. Loss of surfactant also results in increased permeability of the alveolar-capillary membrane, with resultant pulmonary edema and decreased diffusion
    5. The mechanical stimulus of the embolism causes an intense pulmonary vasoconstriction, promoting pulmonary hypertension and pulmonary edema
  C. Etiology
    1. Blood clot
    2. Fat
    3. Amniotic fluid
    4. Air
    5. Tumor fragments
    6. Foreign material, such as sutures or bullets
    7. Sepsis
    8. Parasites
  D. Incidence
    1. At least 500,000 cases of pulmonary embolism in United States annually
    2. At least 50,000 deaths are attributed to pulmonary embolism yearly in the United States
  E. Predisposing/precipitating factors
    1. Venous stasis
    2. Increased blood coagulability
    3. Damage to the vascular wall
    4. Postoperative clients, especially elderly clients with hip surgery or pelvic surgery
    5. Obesity
    6. Pregnancy
    7. Immobility
    8. Multiple fractures
    9. Congestive heart failure
    10. COPD
    11. Cancer
  F. Clinical manifestations
    1. Dyspnea
    2. Chest pain
    3. Acute anxiety
    4. Cough
    5. Hemoptysis
    6. Tachycardia
    7. Decreased PaO_2
    8. Unfortunately, symptoms variable, so it is frequently misdiagnosed
  G. Diagnostic examinations
    1. First test is V/Q scan
    2. When V/Q scan is not diagnostic (does not show embolus), pulmonary angiogram performed
    3. ECG and blood gases also done
  H. Complications: pulmonary infarction occurs in less than 10% of the cases; an area of the lung is destroyed
  I. Medical management: anticoagulant therapy (see Table 4–16)
II. Analysis
  A. Impaired gas exchange related to right-to-left shunting, V/Q mismatching, and decreased diffusion
  B. Altered pattern of breathing related to dyspnea
  C. Pain related to pleural irritation
  D. Anxiety related to hypoxia
  E. High risk for injury related to anticoagulant therapy
III. Planning/goals, expected outcomes
  A. Client's dyspnea will decrease and PaO_2 improve
  B. Client's pain will cease or will be controlled
  C. Client's anxiety will decrease
  D. Client will not suffer further injury such as respiratory arrest
IV. Implementation
  A. *Prevent formation:* measures to prevent formation of emboli include early ambulation, using thromboembolic stockings and mechanical leg compression devices, and stabilizing injured limbs
  B. Once emboli have developed, treat with anticoagulants, vena caval filters, embolectomy, and sometimes thrombolytic therapy (urokinase or streptokinase)
  C. Begin oxygen or mechanical ventilation as ordered
  D. Administer steroids and diuretics (fat emboli only) as ordered
V. Evaluation
  A. Blood gases show an increased PaO_2 level
  B. No complaints of dyspnea
  C. Client no longer complains of pain
  D. Anxiety decreases

E. Respiratory arrest does not occur, client suffers no further injury

Chest Injuries

I. Assessment
   A. Definition: blunt or penetrating injuries to chest wall, parenchyma, or heart and surrounding structures
   B. Pathophysiology
      1. Ribs can fracture in blunt or penetrating trauma; limiting expansion and oxygenation
      2. Flail chest (Figure 4–5) is a fracture of two or more ribs producing an unstable rib cage, such that inspiration produces sucking in of the chest wall and expiration produces a ballooning out of the same section of the chest wall, preventing full expansion and promoting hypoxia
      3. Pneumothorax is a perforation of the lung, collection of air in the pleural space, with a collapsed lung, causing severe hypoxia
      4. Cardiac contusion with tamponade is contusion of the heart with life-threatening accumulation of blood in the pericardial sac, causing dysrhythmias and decreased cardiac output
      5. Pulmonary contusion results from compression or decompression injury that ruptures lung tissue, small airways, and alveoli, with resultant alveolar edema, right-to-left shunting, and V/Q mismatching, leading to hypoxia and decreased pulmonary compliance
   C. Predisposing/precipitating factors
      1. Automobile or motorcycle accidents
      2. Homicide attempts with guns or knives
      3. Bleats or explosions
      4. Falls
   D. Clinical manifestations
      1. Flail chest on assessment (see Figure 4–5)
      2. Severe hypoxia
      3. Shock
      4. Decreased or absent breath sounds with pneumothorax; if hemothorax, dullness over the area with blood collection
      5. Dyspnea
      6. Cardiac contusion: ECG with results similar to ischemia
      7. Cardiac tamponade: muffled heart sounds, midthoracic pain, elevated central venous pressure, distended neck veins and decreased cardiac output
      8. Tachypnea, tachycardia, hypotension
      9. Crackles with pulmonary contusion
      10. Decreased or asymmetrical chest expansion
      11. Chest pain
   G. Diagnostic examinations
      1. Chest x-ray
      2. ECG
      3. CT scan
   H. Complications
      1. Shock and hemorrhage
      2. ARDS
      3. Sepsis
   I. Surgical management
      1. Chest tubes or other aspiration (pericardial tap)

Inspiration

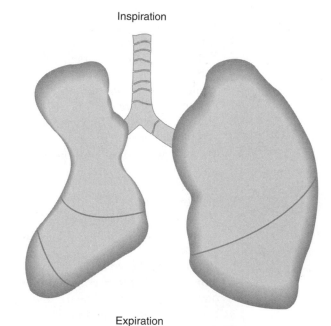

Expiration

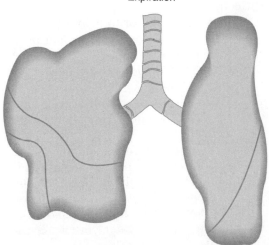

FIGURE 4–5. Flail chest.

2. Surgical fixation of fractures

II. Analysis
A. Ineffective breathing pattern related to specific trauma disorder
B. Decreased cardiac output related to hypotension, hemorrhage, cardiac trauma
C. Pain related to specific injury
D. Anxiety related to dyspnea
E. Impaired gas exchange related to atelectasis and specific injury

III. Planning/goals, expected outcomes
A. Client's PaO_2 will return to normal level
B. Client will experience relief of anxiety and dyspnea
C. Client will verbalize decreased pain
D. Client will have normal blood pressure, pulse, and respirations
E. Client will have a normal cardiac rhythm

IV. Interventions
A. Maintain patent airway, oxygenation, and possible mechanical ventilation
B. Provide adequate analgesia as ordered
C. Closely monitor vital signs
D. Monitor chest tube for pneumothorax or hemothorax
E. Provide cardiac monitoring
F. Prepare client for possible surgery
G. Suction frequently if on mechanical ventilation

V. Evaluation
A. Client's blood gases are in normal range
B. Vital signs are within normal limits
C. Cardiac monitor in normal sinus rhythm
D. Client does not complain of pain or shortness of breath

Closed Chest Water-Seal Drainage

I. Assessment
A. Definition and purpose
1. Treatment involving insertion of a chest tube with a water-seal drainage for the purpose of draining air and fluid from the pleural space in order to restore negative intrapleural pressure and thereby re-expand collapsed lung
2. May consist of one-, two-, or three-bottle system or a disposable Pleur-Evac unit, essentially the same as the three-bottle system (Figures 4–6 and 4–7). Currently, disposable systems are more common

B. Indications
1. Pneumothorax
2. Hemothorax
3. Empyema
4. Chest surgery: for example, resection of the lung except pneumonectomy where there is no lung to re-expand; any surgery where the chest is entered, such as open heart surgery

C. Monitor for impairment of respiration, dyspnea, rapid, shallow respirations, decreased breath sounds, asymmetry of chest expansion, restlessness, anxiety, chest pain, deviated trachea, subcutaneous emphysema (crepitus)

D. Functioning of drainage system
1. Water-seal
a. Prevents atmospheric air from entering chest tube and pleural space by having glass rod in collection bottle below surface of water; water heavier than air so when client inspires, water rises up the tube
b. Fluctuation of fluid normally observed in water-seal during inspiration and expiration; fluctuation ceases when lung re-expanded; however, absent fluctuation can also mean obstructed tube
c. Continuous bubbling after lung re-expansion indicates air leak either from insertion site or break in tubing or connection
d. Be sure water-seal section of disposable system adequately filled with water (at least 5 mL)

2. Collection bottle
a. In both one- and two-bottle system, water-seal bottle also serves as collection bottle
b. In three-bottle and Pleur-Evac systems, one chamber collects drainage, one provides water-seal, and third chamber controls suction

3. Suction
a. Applied in two- or three-bottle system when large amounts of air and blood to be removed
b. Amount of suction needed between 10 and 20 cm H_2O either through an Emerson pump or wall suction unit; amount of suction depends on water depth
c. With an uncontrolled suction source, amount of suction determined by formula $H - h$ with H being amount of tubing under water in suction control bottle, and h being amount of tubing under water in water-seal bottle
d. In Pleur-Evac unit, suction chamber

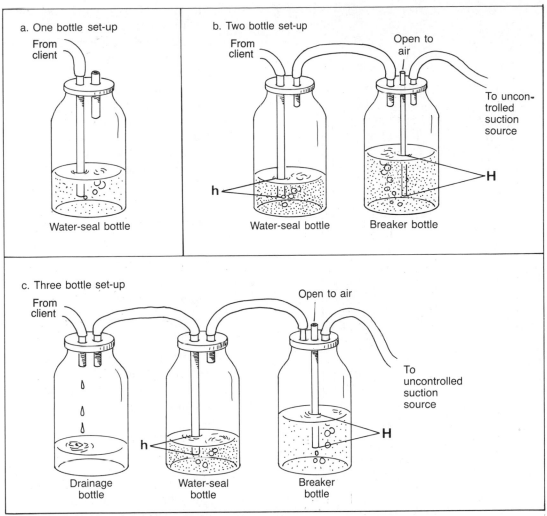

a. One bottle set-up
From client
Water-seal bottle

b. Two bottle set-up
From client
Open to air
To uncontrolled suction source
h
H
Water-seal bottle
Breaker bottle

c. Three bottle set-up
From client
Open to air
To uncontrolled suction source
h
H
Drainage bottle
Water-seal bottle
Breaker bottle

FIGURE 4–6. Water-seal drainage: *a,* **One-bottle set-up;** *b,* **two-bottle set-up, suction control added;** *c,* **three-bottle set-up, suction control and drainage bottle added.**

filled with sterile water up to 20-cm level

E. Complications
1. Tension pneumothorax
2. Mediastinal shift
3. Infection
4. Subcutaneous emphysema

II. Analysis
A. High risk for injury
B. Altered pattern of breathing related to insertion of tube

III. Planning/goals, expected outcomes
A. Client will demonstrate adequate respirations
B. Client will achieve full lung re-expansion
C. Client will remain infection-free

IV. Implementation
A. Promote adequate respirations
1. Assess rate and quality of respirations, chest movement, breath sounds, sub-

cutaneous emphysema, and for signs of increasing respiratory distress
2. Position client in semi-Fowler's to facilitate breathing
3. Administer supplementary O_2 as indicated
4. Encourage deep breathing and incentive spirometry, especially postoperatively
5. Encourage ambulation as tolerated
6. Assist with diagnostic procedures and treatment: for example, arterial blood gases, daily chest x-ray, chest physiotherapy
7. Provide comfort measures and pain medication as ordered

B. Maintain proper functioning of system
1. Keep drainage bottles below chest level
2. Insure that connections intact
3. Monitor for fluctuations or bubbling in

* watch for tube obstructions

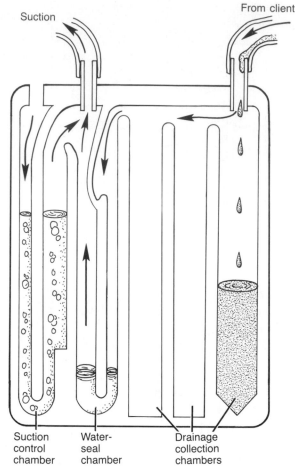

FIGURE 4–7. Pleur-Evac-type drain.

Suction control chamber

Water-seal chamber

Drainage collection chambers

1. Monitor vital signs, especially temperature, CBC, chest x-ray
2. Send cultures of drainage, sputum, blood when infection suspected
3. Maintain aseptic technique when changing dressing
4. Administer prophylactic antibiotics as ordered (see Table 4–22)

V. Evaluation
   A. Client's lung fully re-expanded and respirations adequate

POST-TEST Respiratory Disorders

Mr. Brown is a 75-year-old man admitted with fever and congestion over the last 3 days.

1. Mr. Brown's chest x-ray shows consolidation in his left lower lung. Which of the following would NOT be noted over the area of consolidation on physical examination?
   ① Resonance
   ② Bronchophony
   ③ Egophony
   ④ Dull percussion sound

2. Prior to collection of sputum for culture, the nurse should instruct Mr. Brown to:
   ① Brush his teeth to obtain uncontaminated sputum
   ② Completely fill sputum container
   ③ Keep container's opening and interior sterile
   ④ Collect at least a teaspoonful of sputum in the evening

3. Mr. Brown was placed on ticarcillin IV piggyback. Which side effect is important to assess?
   ① Blurring of vision
   ② Allergic reaction
   ③ Nausea and vomiting
   ④ Constipation

water-seal; locate air-leak source if continuous bubbling noted
4. Maintain patency of tubes by avoiding dependent loop and kinking; milking not routinely done as it increases negative pressure exerted on pleural space
5. Never clamp off tube except when bottle accidentally broken or bottles must be raised above chest
6. Monitor amount of suction applied
7. Assess character and amount of drainage
8. Evaluate readiness for chest tube removal
   a. Absence of respiratory distress
   b. Equal and normal breath sounds
   c. Fully expanded lungs on x-ray
   d. Absence of fluctuations in water-seal bottle
   e. Instruct client to perform Valsalva maneuver on removal so that air does not leak into pleural space
C. Prevent infection

Mr. Allen is a 45-year-old unemployed African-American man admitted with the diagnosis of tuberculosis.

4. Mr. Allen is receiving INH to treat his tuberculosis. Because he is receiving the INH he will also be on:

① Aspirin
② Neomycin
③ Lorazepam (Ativan)
④ Pyridoxine

5. Mr. Allen should be taught what activity to decrease the risk of spread of his tuberculosis?
① Coughing and deep-breathing exercises
② To avoid using the same bathroom as his family
③ Covering his nose and mouth when sneezing or coughing
④ Disinfecting his dishes after he eats

Mark Weaver is a 24-year-old man admitted with a spontaneous pneumothorax. He has had a chest tube inserted to remove the air.

---

6. Mark has had his chest tube in for 24 hours. How can the nurse evaluate if his lung has re-expanded?
① Absence of bubbling in the breaker bottle
② Absence of bubbling in the water-seal bottle
③ Fluctuation in the breaker bottle
④ Bubbling in the water-seal bottle

7. In order to further assess Mark's lung re-expansion, the physician orders that the chest tube be clamped. Clinical manifestations the nurse would observe indicating that the lung has not re-expanded would include:
① Slow, deep respirations at rest
② Dyspnea after exertion
③ Shortness of breath at rest
④ Coughing on activity

8. Mark is to have his chest tube removed. While this is being done, the nurse should ask Mark to:
① Breathe in, hold breath, and bear down
② Breathe out, hold breath, and bear down
③ Breathe out and then rapidly breathe in
④ Either breathe out or in then hold breath

9. The doctor comes in to remove the chest tube. Immediately after the removal, the site should be:
① Sutured closed by pulling the purse string suture closed
② Covered with a Vaseline gauze dressing
③ Covered with a moist saline dressing
④ Covered with dry 4-by-4 dressings

POST-TEST Answers and Rationales

1. ① Resonance is a loud, low-pitched sound elicited over normal lungs on percussion. Bronchophony (increased intensity and clarity of voice sound), egophony, and dullness all indicate consolidation. 1, II. Pneumonia.

2. ③ If a culture is to be done on a sputum, the container's opening and interior must be kept sterile to accurately identify bacterial growth and any organisms in the respiratory tract. 4, I. Pneumonia.

3. ② Ticarcillin is a penicillin derivative and hypersensitivity is a common side effect. It is important to assess a history of allergies prior to administration as it can produce serious allergic reactions. Although nausea may occur, it is not as serious as an allergic reaction. 5, II. Pneumonia.

4. ④ One toxic effect of INH is peripheral neuropathy, which is thought to be due to a vitamin B_6 deficiency since it can be controlled by daily administration of pyridoxine (vitamin B_6). It plays an important role in the metabolism of amino acids and fatty acids and is said to participate in energy transformation in the brain and nerve tissue. 4, II. TB.

5. ③ Tuberculosis is an airborne infection. Hence, covering the nose and mouth when sneezing or coughing prevents the spread of droplet infection. This should be a priority of client teaching. The other interventions are unnecessary. 4, I. TB.

6. ② Absence of bubbling in the water-seal bottle with no respiratory distress indicates that the lung has fully expanded after a pneumothorax. The nurse can verify this finding by auscultating for breath sounds over the area of collapse. 4, I & II. Chest Tubes.

7. ③ If the client becomes short of breath after clamping the chest tube, this indicates that there is still air that needs to be drained out. The clamp must be released to prevent air from accumulating further in the pleural space, which could cause a tension pneumothorax. 4, I & II. Chest Tubes.

8. ① Removal of a chest tube is done at the end of a full inspiration because the increased intrathoracic pressure pushes air out of the pleural space. Holding the breath and bearing down prevents air from being drawn back in. 1, I & II. Chest Tubes.

9. ② Vaseline gauze is used to seal the opening in the chest from the insertion of the chest tube so that air will not gain entrance into the intrapleural space. 4, I & II. Chest Tubes.

PRE-TEST Diseases of the Blood

Mary Brown, a 34-year-old mother, has just been diagnosed with Hodgkin's disease.

1. She is scheduled for a lymphangiogram. A lymphangiogram is an
   ① Injection of radiopaque dye into the brachial artery
   ② Computerized tool used to identify metastasis
   ③ Radiographic examination of the lymphatic system
   ④ Ultrasound examination of the lymphatic system

2. Several hours after Mrs. Brown had returned to your unit from having a lymphangiogram, she put on her call light screaming, "My urine is blue!" Your best response would be:
   ① "That's okay. Everything will be all right."
   ② "I'll call the doctor and he or she can explain the cause of the discolored urine."
   ③ "This is a predictable response after the examination. This indicates you are excreting the dye given during the test."
   ④ "This is an expected side effect of the test. It will go away by itself in a few hours."

3. Which of the following signs and symptoms are NOT characteristic of Hodgkin's disease?
   ① Fatigue
   ② Night sweats
   ③ Lymph node enlargement
   ④ Hemoptysis

4. Hodgkin's disease is a malignant disorder that primarily involves the
   1. Lymphoid system
   2. Biliary system
   3. Bone marrow
   4. Hematopoietic system
5. A definitive diagnostic test used to confirm the diagnosis of Hodgkin's disease is
   1. Complete blood count (CBC)
   2. Lymph node biopsy
   3. Chest x-ray
   4. Abdominal CT scan

Mary Smith, aged 22, is admitted to the hospital with a diagnosis of possible acute leukemia.

---

6. Mary is scheduled for a bone marrow biopsy. Which of the following is important in preparing Mary for her biopsy?
   1. An explanation of the procedure
   2. Assessing her coagulation studies
   3. Administering sedation and assessing for anesthetic allergies prior to the procedure
   4. All of the above
7. Which of the following interventions would be INAPPROPRIATE after Mary's bone marrow biopsy?
   1. Applying firm pressure to the site for 5 minutes post-procedure
   2. Assessing the biopsy site for bleeding
   3. Charting the date, time, location, and tolerance of the procedure
   4. Encouraging Mary to ambulate as much as possible to prevent muscle stiffness
8. Acute leukemia is characterized by
   1. Slow, insidious onset
   2. Normal, mature white blood cells
   3. Prolonged disease course if untreated
   4. Rapidly fatal disease progression if untreated
9. The leading cause of death in adult clients with leukemia is
   1. Hemorrhage
   2. Anemia
   3. Infection
   4. Lymphatic obstruction
10. Mary's CBC results show a WBC of 1000 mm^3, a hemoglobin of 8.0 g, a hematocrit of 22%, and a platelet count of 40,000. Which of the following interventions is INAPPROPRIATE considering these laboratory results?
    1. Preventing contact with visitors or personnel with colds
    2. Administering aspirin to Mary for her complaints of headache
    3. Monitoring Mary's temperature every 4 hours
    4. Checking of Mary's stools, urine, and emesis for occult blood
11. Mary's temperature is 39°C. Which of the following interventions is LEAST appropriate?
    1. Administer acetaminophen by rectal suppository to control the fever
    2. Continue to monitor temperature every 2 to 4 hours
    3. Obtain cultures of sputum, urine, and blood
    4. Promptly administer antibiotic therapy
12. The highest incidence of chronic leukemia is in which of the following populations?
    1. Children
    2. Young adults
    3. Infants
    4. Elderly individuals

PRE-TEST Answers and Rationales

1. ③ A lymphangiogram is a radiographic examination of the lymphatic system. 1, II. Lymphoma.
2. ③ After a lymphangiogram, veins of the lower extremities, dorsal skin of the feet, and urine may have blue-green discoloration from dye extraction for 2 to 5 days. 1, I and II. Lymphoma.
3. ④ Hemoptysis is a characteristic sign of advanced lung cancer. The rest are potential symptoms of Hodgkin's disease. 1, II. Lymphoma.
4. ① Hodgkin's disease is a malignant disorder of the lymphoid tissues. 1, II. Lymphoma.
5. ② A lymph node biopsy is a definitive means of establishing the diagnosis of Hodgkin's disease. The presence of the Reed-Sternberg cell is ascertained through this biopsy. 2, II. Lymphoma.
6. ④ Explaining this procedure, assessing coagulation studies, assessing for anesthetic allergies, and administering sedation are all essential in preparing a client for this procedure. 1, I and II. Leukemia.
7. ④ Because bleeding is a potential complication after a bone marrow biopsy, pressure on the biopsy site and limited activity are indicated. 4, I. Leukemia.
8. ④ Acute leukemia is characterized by a rapid onset and disease progression, with death resulting in days to months if untreated. The others are more characteristic of chronic leukemia. All leukemias involve abnormal white blood cells. 1, II. Leukemia.
9. ③ Although hemorrhage, anemia, and lymphatic obstruction are also severe complications, most clients die from overwhelming infection due to immunosuppression. 1, II. Leukemia.
10. ② Laboratory results indicate an increased risk for infection and bleeding due to decreased white cell, red cell, and platelet counts. Aspirin potentiates bleeding risk and may also mask the onset of infection by suppressing fever. The other interventions are appropriate. 4, I. Leukemia.
11. ① Acetaminophen may mask further fever elevations. Rectal suppositories should be avoided because they may introduce colonic bacteria into the blood stream. Promptly obtaining cultures, administering antibiotics, and monitoring fever are more appropriate interventions. 4, I. Leukemia.
12. ④ Chronic leukemia is more common in the elderly. 2, IV. Leukemia.

NURSING PROCESS APPLIED TO ADULTS WITH DISEASES OF THE BLOOD

Leukemia

I. Assessment
   A. Definition: leukemia is a malignant blood disorder affecting the bone marrow, spleen, and lymph tissue; characterized by an abnormal proliferation and accumulation of hematopoietic cells; in most cases, these are immature white blood cells (leukocytes) and their precursors that infiltrate the bone marrow and peripheral blood as well as other body tissues and organs
   B. Pathophysiology
      1. Control factors regulating orderly differentiation and maturation of white blood cells absent, resulting in the arrest of the maturation process of a specific cell line
      2. Abnormal or immature white blood cells do not function properly; as a result of the massive proliferation of these abnormal or immature cells, fewer normal white blood cells produced; abnormal white blood cells continue to multiply and infiltrate, and may damage
         a. Bone marrow
         b. Spleen
         c. Lymph nodes
         d. Liver
         e. Kidneys
         f. Lungs
         g. Gonads
         h. Skin
         i. Central nervous system
      3. Normal bone marrow becomes diffusely replaced with abnormal or immature

white blood cells, interfering with bone marrow's ability to produce other types of cells such as erythrocytes and thrombocytes; bone marrow becomes functionally incompetent with resulting bone marrow suppression

4. With incompetent bone marrow, client predisposed to
   a. Anemia from decreased erythrocyte production
   b. Infection from inadequate numbers of mature, functioning white blood cells to defend the body against pathogens
   c. Hemorrhage from thrombocytopenia

C. Classification and incidence
   1. Categorized by course and duration of disease
      a. Acute involves more immature, usually blast cells; has a rapid onset and disease progression
      b. Chronic involves more mature (differentiated) cells; more insidious onset and prolonged disease course
   2. Categorized by type of hematopoietic cell affected
      a. Lymphocytic involves abnormal maturation and proliferation of the lymphocyte cell series
      b. Myelocytic involves the myeloid series; also referred to as nonlymphocytic
   3. Acute lymphocytic (lymphoblastic) leukemia (ALL)
      a. Immature lymphocytes proliferate in the bone marrow
      b. Abnormal leukemic cell resembles an immature lymphocyte or lymphoblast
      c. Although uncommon in adults, ALL comprises 85% of childhood leukemias
      d. Although peak incidence between ages 2 and 10, second rise occurs in middle and older adults
   4. Acute myelogenous (myelocytic, myeloblastic) leukemia (AML); also referred to as acute nonlymphocytic leukemia (ANLL)
      a. Immature myeloid cells proliferate and accumulate in the bone marrow
      b. More common in adults than ALL; majority 35 to 65 years old
   5. Chronic lymphocytic leukemia (CLL)
      a. Abnormal and incompetent lymphocytes proliferate, accumulate, and spread to other lymphatic tissue
      b. Occurs most frequently ages 50 to 70
      c. More common in men

   6. Chronic myelogenous leukemia (CML)
      a. Stem cell abnormality leads to uncontrolled proliferation of the granulocytic (myeloid) cells; this results in a marked increase in number of circulating granulocytes
      b. In most cases (95%), a characteristic chromosomal abnormality, referred to as the Philadelphia chromosome, is present
      c. Eventually evolves into acute form (blast crisis), evidenced by increased leukocyte/blast count
      d. Peak age of onset between 40 and 50
      e. Incidence slightly higher in men
   7. Chronic leukemias more common among the elderly

D. Predisposing/precipitating factors
   1. Exposure to large amounts of radiation
   2. Exposure to benzene, arsenic, and other chemicals
   3. Genetic factors and disorders such as Down's syndrome
   4. Chemotherapeutic agents—secondary to therapy for other types of cancer; especially alkylating agents (see Table 6–6)
   5. Possible viral etiology (HTLV-I, HTLV-II)

E. Clinical manifestations
   1. Will vary based on the type of leukemia, the extent of involvement of other organs, and the degree of bone marrow depression (BMD)
   2. Acute leukemias have rapid onset, progress rapidly, with short clinical course; left untreated, death will result in days to months; symptoms related to BMD, infiltration of leukemic cells into other organ systems, and hypermetabolism of leukemia cells
   3. Chronic leukemias have more insidious onset with more prolonged clinical course; asymptomatic early in disease; life expectancy may be more than 5 years; symptoms related to hypermetabolism of leukemic cells infiltrating other organ systems; cells more mature and function more effectively
   4. Central nervous system manifestations related to abnormal WBCs infiltrating central nervous system
   5. Clinical manifestations include shortness of breath, fatigue, malaise, dyspnea, weakness, weight loss, decreased activity tolerance, chills, bone or joint pain, headaches, visual disturbances, anorexia, fever, anemia, thrombocytopenia, petechiae or other ecchymoses, gingival

bleeding, epistaxis, pallor, generalized lymphadenopathy, hyperuricemia, spleno-megaly, hepatomegaly, increased WBCs, history of recurrent infections, skin and soft tissue infiltrates

F. Diagnostic examinations
1. Complete blood count with differential
   a. Hemoglobin, platelets, and RBCs may be decreased; WBC may be low, normal, or elevated; differential will include many immature cells or blasts, and one type of WBC may predominate
   b. CBC norms
      (1) WBC: 4.5 to 11.0 × 10³
      (2) RBC
          (a) Male: 4.6 to 6.2 × 10⁶
          (b) Female: 4.2 to 5.4 × 10⁶
      (3) Hemoglobin
          (a) Male: 13.5 to 18.0 g
          (b) Female: 12.0 to 16.0 g
      (4) Hematocrit
          (a) Male: 40 to 54%
          (b) Female: 38 to 47%
      (5) White cell differential
          (a) Segmented neutrophils, 56%
          (b) Bands, 3%
          (c) Eosinophils, 2.7%
          (d) Basophils, 0.3%
          (e) Lymphocytes, 34%
          (f) Monocytes, 4%
      (6) Platelets: 150,000 to 400,000/mm³
2. Uric acid will be increased secondary to destruction of large number of leukocytes
3. Lactic dehydrogenase (LDH) elevated
4. Bone marrow aspiration and biopsy reveal increased numbers of immature WBCs or blast cells; confirms diagnosis; establishes type of cells involved
   a. Nursing implications
      (1) Pre-test
          (a) Reinforce physician's explanation of procedure to ease anxiety and ensure cooperation
          (b) Assess coagulation studies (PT, PTT, platelet count) before procedure
          (c) Procedure performed at the bedside
          (d) Remind client of importance of remaining immobile
          (e) Site will be anesthetized with a local anesthetic; assess allergies
          (f) Sedation often ordered
          (g) Signed consent before sedation
          (h) Support client and family
      (2) Preferred sites
          (a) Posterior iliac crest, sternum
          (b) Client may experience pressure or discomfort over the specimen site with marrow aspiration
          (c) May need more than one marrow specimen; e.g., bilateral iliac crests
      (3) Post-test
          (a) Apply firm pressure to site for 5 minutes to prevent hemorrhage
          (b) Apply sterile pressure dressing; position client or apply sandbag or pillow to provide additional pressure to biopsy site
          (c) Limited activity or bedrest as directed by physician
          (d) Assess dressing site for bleeding and inflammation
          (e) Assess vital signs as clinically indicated
          (f) Administer analgesics as required
5. Lumbar puncture (spinal tap)
   a. Performed to rule out CNS involvement or when CNS involvement suspected
   b. Refer to Table 5–1: Diagnostic Tests—Neurological Dysfunction

G. Complications: vary with the type of leukemia and severity of disease
1. Three most common
   a. Anemia
   b. Hemorrhage
      (1) Potential for bleeding occurs with platelet count of less than 50,000 cells/mm³
      (2) Spontaneous bleeding may occur with platelet count of less than 20,000 cells/mm³
   c. Infections: leading cause of death; most arise from client's own bacterial flora
2. Leukostasis: syndrome caused by exceptionally high numbers of circulating leukemic blasts that aggregate and invade capillary walls, causing rupture and bleeding
   a. Treatment includes chemotherapy to decrease WBC count and leukaphere-

sis (WBC removal accomplished by plasmapheresis technology)

3. Tumor lysis syndrome
   a. Occurs when large numbers of rapidly proliferating cells are lysed (as a result of cytotoxic chemotherapy), releasing intracellular components and uric acid into the blood
   b. Hyperkalemia, hyperphosphatemia, hyperuricemia, and hypocalcemia result; electrolyte levels must be monitored closely
   c. Treatment and prevention include allopurinol administration, aggressive hydration with alkaline solutions, and correction of electrolyte abnormalities

H. Medical management: varies with type of leukemia
   1. Goal for acute leukemia is the eradication of all leukemic cells, achievement of a normal bone marrow blast count, and reconstitution of bone marrow with normal elements
   2. Treatment of chronic leukemias generally palliative and directed at control of WBCs and platelet count
   3. Response to treatment, therapy, and prognosis differ according to type
   4. Chemotherapy (see Table 6–6)
      a. Acute leukemias are treated with combination drug therapies over a period of time often referred to as phases:
         (1) Induction: intensive chemotherapeutic course to destroy as many leukemic cells as possible and induce a remission
         (2) Consolidation: additional chemotherapy to eliminate any undetected remaining leukemic cells
         (3) Maintenance: an extended program of low-dose therapy given to maintain a remission
      b. May use intrathecal chemotherapy (Ara-C or methotrexate) to destroy leukemic cells invading CNS
   5. Blood transfusions to restore deficient blood components, especially packed red blood cells and platelets
   6. Radiation therapy to sites of organ infiltration including the spleen, lymph nodes, and CNS
   7. Biotherapy being investigated
   8. Antibiotic, antiviral, and antifungal therapy for infections
   9. Bone marrow transplantation
      a. Donor marrow replaces deficient hematopoietic elements
      b. Technological advances and increased knowledge of supportive care have decreased morbidity and mortality
      c. No longer considered "a last resort"
      d. Sources of donor marrow include:
         (1) Autologous: collected from the patient
         (2) Syngeneic: identical twin donor
         (3) Allogeneic: histocompatibly matched, usually a sibling

II. Analysis
   A. Knowledge deficit related to disease process; treatment; potential complications; and community resources
   B. High risk for infection related to disease process and bone marrow depression from chemotherapy
   C. High risk for injury related to thrombocytopenia from disease process and bone marrow depression from chemotherapy
   D. Activity intolerance related to fatigue, anemia, and generalized weakness
   E. Altered nutrition: less than body requirements related to anorexia, nausea, vomiting, stomatitis from chemotherapy
   F. Anxiety related to diagnosis, uncertain outcome of therapy, loss of control, stress, and potential alterations in interpersonal relationships

III. Planning/goals, expected outcomes
   A. Client will verbalize knowledge of disease process, treatment, potential side effects, and community resources
   B. Client will be without evidence of infection
   C. Client will not exhibit signs of bleeding
   D. Client will increase or adjust activities within tolerance level
   E. Client will maintain adequate nutritional and fluid intake
   F. Client will demonstrate decreased anxiety

IV. Implementation
   A. Provide information on disease process, treatment, potential complications, and community resources
      1. Assess baseline knowledge; reinforce previous information given; clarify misconceptions
      2. Explain pathophysiology of leukemia in lay terms
      3. Individualize information for specific type of leukemia and extent of disease
      4. Explain symptoms of potential complications
      5. Explain principles of chemotherapy, names of specific agents, treatment schedule, management of possible side effects

6. Provide written materials to reinforce teaching
7. Encourage questions, verbalization of fears and concerns
8. Initiate referrals to other health care members as needed
9. Provide information about national and local community resources

B. Exercise infection precautions
1. Use meticulous handwashing
2. Perform all procedures with strict asepsis
3. Monitor CBC and differential; markedly decreased WBC count increases risk of infection
4. Place client in protective isolation if necessary; this may include low-bacteria diet as well
5. Screen visitors and staff members for colds or infections; restrict contact with client
6. Teach infection control measures to client and family
7. Provide frequent oral hygiene
8. Avoid rectal temperatures, suppositories, enemas

C. Monitor closely for the development of infection and promptly intervene when infection develops
1. Monitor client's temperature at frequent intervals (usual signs and symptoms of infection may be absent; fever is often the first and only sign)
2. Monitor chest x-ray interpretations for evidence of infiltrates, pneumonia
3. Insure prompt medical evaluation of temperatures; in neutropenic individuals, life-threatening septic shock can develop in a matter of hours
4. Obtain blood, urine, sputum, and other cultures as necessary
5. Remember that certain medications (steroids, acetaminophen) may mask signs of fever
6. Administer antibacterial, antiviral, and antifungal therapy as ordered; maintain a regular schedule; delays in antibiotic administration can further predispose to the development of septic shock
7. Observe for altered skin integrity, especially the oral mucosa
8. Assess IV access sites frequently, especially central venous access devices, for signs of inflammation
9. Teach signs and symptoms of infection; emphasize prompt reporting of these to health care provider
10. Assess client's ability to take a temperature prior to discharge

D. Prevent bleeding
1. Avoid IM or SQ punctures; if necessary, maintain gentle pressure on site; use smallest gauge needle possible
2. Avoid invasive or traumatic procedures
3. Avoid the use of ASA or aspirin-containing products
4. Monitor CBC and platelet counts; notify physician of critical values
5. Administer transfusions as necessary (RBCs and platelets) and monitor for transfusion reaction
6. Avoid the use of toothbrushes, dental floss and razors; encourage foam toothettes or electric razors
7. Assess the client frequently for signs of bleeding: skin, mouth, nose, urine, feces, emesis, sputum
8. Guaiac all stool, urine, and emesis
9. Protect client from falls and other injuries
10. Teach client signs and symptoms of bleeding; instruct to report immediately
11. Avoid repeated venipunctures; central venous access device indicated
12. Monitor for signs of hypotension, tachycardia, and changes in level of consciousness
13. Observe for fatigue and weakness
14. Administer stool softeners as ordered
15. Instruct client to avoid straining at stool, blowing nose

E. Prevent fatigue related to anemia
1. Monitor CBC
2. Administer packed RBCs and monitor for transfusion reaction
3. Assess and document client's level of tolerance to all activities
4. Assist with ADLs as necessary
5. Encourage and adjust activities within client's tolerance level as condition permits
6. Plan activities/procedures so client receives periods of undisturbed rest
7. Observe for symptoms of anemia: pallor of skin, nailbeds, fatigue, weakness, palpitations, dizziness, shortness of breath

F. Maintain nutrition and hydration
1. Monitor serum albumin levels (an indicator of protein stores)
2. Monitor electrolytes
3. Monitor I & O
4. Weigh daily
5. Assist client with meals as necessary
6. Provide pleasant surroundings during meals

7. Assess client's food preferences
8. Confer with dietician
9. Document calorie count
10. Provide soft, bland, cold foods as necessary
11. Administer antiemetics or oral anesthetic as necessary
12. Allow family to bring foods from home if possible
13. Offer small, frequent meals with nourishing snacks
14. Encourage fluids
15. Encourage high-protein, high-calorie diet
16. Assess skin turgor and mucous membranes
17. Assess urine specific gravity
18. Administer total parenteral nutrition (TPN) and intravenous fluids as required

G. Assist client to verbalize anxiety and maintain control
1. Identify client's support system, resources, prior coping strategies, and communication patterns
2. Explore concerns related to uncertainty of the future, physical symptoms, changes in self-concept, and effect of illness on daily life and interpersonal relationships
3. Assist client to recognize stressors and assist with problem solving
4. Reassure with information about care and disease process as needed
5. Refer to appropriate counselor as needed: social service, chaplain
6. Provide client/family with information about local support groups
7. Provide continuity of care if possible
8. Encourage diversional activities
9. Involve client in decision making about care and flexibility in scheduling activities

V. Evaluation
A. Client describes disease process, treatment plan, potential side effects, and available community resources
B. Client is without evidence of infection
C. Client does not exhibit signs of bleeding
D. Client maintains ADLs within tolerance level
E. Client maintains weight and adequate hydration
F. Client verbalizes anxiety and identifies ways to decrease/control it

Lymphoma

I. Assessment
A. Definition: a group of malignant neoplasms that affect the lymphoid tissues

1. Two major subgroups
a. Hodgkin's disease (HD): characterized by the presence of Reed-Sternberg cells
b. Non-Hodgkin's lymphoma (NHL): broad and heterogeneous group of lymphoid cancers characterized by a natural history ranging from indolent to aggressive
2. Clinical course, prognosis, and treatment are different

B. Pathophysiology: uncontrolled proliferation of abnormal lymphocytes infiltrate and compromise the function of other organs, including the bone marrow, spleen, liver, lungs, and skin
1. Immune deficiency results
2. Death usually results from infection or bleeding due to compromise of bone marrow function
3. HD spreads from one lymph node group to an immediately adjacent lymph node group; referred to as contiguous spread; NHL tends to skip to noncontiguous groups
4. NHL rarely presents as stage I (limited disease); frequently disseminated at the time of diagnosis; early involvement of the oropharyngeal lymphoid tissue, skin, gastrointestinal tract, and bone marrow common

C. Classification
1. By staging (Ann Arbor classification) to detect the extent and involvement of the malignancy and determine treatment protocol
a. Stage I: limited to single lymph node or single extralymphatic organ
b. Stage II: involvement of two or more lymph node areas on the same side of the diaphragm or local involvement of an extra lymphatic organ
c. Stage III: involvement of lymph node regions on both sides of the diaphragm, with involvement of an extralymphatic region or the spleen
d. Stage IV: diffuse involvement of one or more extralymphatic regions or tissues
2. By the absence (A) or presence (B) of systemic symptoms: weight loss, fever, night sweats
3. By histologic cell type: an important prognostic indicator
4. NHL also categorized as indolent versus aggressive; low grade, intermediate grade, or high grade; clinical course and prognosis varies with each

D. Etiology
   1. Unknown; infectious/viral etiology implicated; immune system aberrations; genetic
E. Incidence
   1. HD: peaks in two age groups, the late 20s and steadily increases with age after age 45 with a second peak occurring in the sixth decade
   2. NHL: incidence rises steadily starting in the fourth and fifth decades
   3. More common in men than women
F. Predisposing/precipitating factors
   1. Increased frequency of NHL in individuals with congenital or acquired immunodeficiencies, including AIDS, those with autoimmune diseases, and the immunosuppressed following organ transplantation
G. Clinical manifestations
   1. Onset insidious
   2. Usually occur from pressure exerted by large nodes on surrounding tissues
   3. Typical presentation for HD: painless lymphadenopathy which may be accompanied by constitutional symptoms of malaise, fever, night sweats, and weight loss; adenopathy most commonly found in neck and supraclavicular areas
   4. Massive mediastinal adenopathy may result in cough, wheezing, dyspnea, or superior vena cava obstruction
   5. NHL: commonly asymptomatic with history of "waxing and waning" adenopathy over several months; usually more widely disseminated at time of diagnosis
   6. Intermittent fever may occur
   7. Progressive anemia
   8. Hepatomegaly; splenomegaly
   9. CNS involvement more common in the aggressive types of NHL
H. Diagnostic examinations
   1. Lymph node biopsy
      a. Surgical excision of an active lymph node to obtain a specimen for histological examination; definitive means of establishing diagnosis; distinguishes between benign and malignant tumors
      b. Nursing implications
         (1) Pre-test
            (a) Explain procedure to client
            (b) Excisional biopsy: NPO after midnight or clear liquids on morning of test
            (c) Consent necessary
            (d) Approximate time, 15 minutes
            (e) Check for hypersensitivity to local anesthetics
            (f) Record baseline vital signs
         (2) Post-test
            (a) Monitor dressing for bleeding, tenderness and signs of inflammation at the biopsy site
            (b) Monitor vital signs
   2. Laboratory work-up including CBC, differential, erythrocyte sedimentation rate (ESR), liver, and renal function studies
   3. Radiological studies
      a. Chest x-ray or CT to assess mediastinal or hilar lymphadenopathy
      b. Abdominal CT to detect abdominal lymph node enlargement
      c. Lymphangiogram to assess lower aortic, iliac, and retroperitoneal lymph nodes
         (1) Radiologic procedure: oil-based dye infused into the lymph vessels via small needles in the dorsum of the foot
         (2) Nursing implications
            (a) Pre-test
               (i) Explain procedure
               (ii) Lasts approximately 4 hours
               (iii) Remind of the importance of remaining immobile
               (iv) Consent required
               (v) Assess for iodine allergy
               (vi) Sedation may be ordered
            (b) During test, be alert for dye reactions: fever, headache, burning, unusual taste sensations
            (c) Post-test
               (i) Observe the dorsum of the feet for signs and symptoms of bleeding, infection, inflammation
               (ii) Resume normal activities but keep feet dry until sutures are removed
               (iii) Instruct client that malaise, headache, fever may occur during the first 12 to 24 hours after the test
               (iv) Advise that urine, veins of lower extremities, and dorsal skin of feet may have blue-green discoloration from dye excretion for 2 to 5 days
               (v) Monitor for signs of complications: oil-based embolus; cough; dyspnea; pleuritic pain; hemoptysis
   4. Staging laparotomy with possible liver bi-

opsy and splenectomy performed only when the extent of disease cannot be determined by other diagnostic tests and confirmation of abdominal disease would alter the choice of therapy

  a. Abdomen is surgically opened to visualize the abdominal organs for diagnosis and biopsy

  b. Pre-test: plan for surgical procedure; consent required

  c. Post-test: routine postoperative care for abdominal surgery

5. Bone marrow aspiration and biopsy to assess for bone marrow involvement: see diagnostic examinations for leukemia

6. Lumbar puncture if suspicious of CNS involvement: refer to Table 5–1: Diagnostic Tests—Neurological Dysfunction

I. Complications

1. Bone marrow depression related to disease and therapy increases risk of infection, bleeding, and anemia

2. Systemic side effects from chemotherapy

3. Radiation induced pneumonitis, pericarditis, and hypothyroidism

4. Increased risk of developing second malignancies (especially acute nonlymphocytic leukemia) as a result of chemotherapy (alkylating agents) or radiation therapy

5. Spinal cord compression, renal failure, bowel obstruction, superior vena cava obstruction caused by pressure from surrounding enlarged lymph nodes

J. Medical management

1. Irradiation in patients with limited disease

2. Combination chemotherapy with or without radiation therapy for more advanced disease states; chemotherapeutic agents include (see Table 6–6)

  a. Alkylating agents: nitrogen mustard, chlorambucil, cyclophosphamide, carmustine, lomustine

  b. Vinca alkaloids: vincristine, vinblastine

  c. Antibiotics: doxorubicin, bleomycin

  d. Other: prednisone, procarbazine, methotrexate, DTIC

3. High-dose chemotherapy with autologous or allogeneic bone marrow transplant for refractory disease

4. Biological response modifier therapies under investigation

K. Surgical management

1. Primary roles of surgery are to obtain diagnostic tissue and perform laparotomy when indicated

2. Splenectomy in selected cases only

II. Analysis

A. Knowledge deficit related to disease process, treatment, potential complications, and community resources

B. High risk for infection related to disease process and bone marrow depression from therapy

C. High risk for injury related to systemic complications of chemotherapy or radiation therapy

D. Nutrition, altered: less than body requirements related to anorexia, nausea, vomiting, stomatitis from chemotherapy

E. Anxiety related to diagnosis, uncertain outcome of therapy, loss of control, stress, and potential alterations in interpersonal relationships

III. Planning/goals, expected outcomes

A. Client will verbalize knowledge of disease process, treatment, potential side effects, and community resources

B. Client will be without evidence of infection

C. Chemotherapy- or radiation-induced complications will be minimized

D. Client will maintain adequate nutritional and fluid intake

E. Client will demonstrate decreased anxiety

IV. Implementation

A. Provide information on disease process, treatment, potential complications, and community resources (same as for leukemia)

B. Exercise infection precautions (same as for leukemia)

C. Monitor closely for the development of infection and promptly intervene when infection develops (same as for leukemia)

D. Prevent and control therapy-induced complications through continuous assessment, prompt intervention, and teaching (refer to Chapter 6, Chemotherapy and Radiation Therapy, Implementations)

E. Maintain nutrition and hydration (same as for leukemia)

F. Assist client to verbalize anxiety and maintain control (same as for leukemia)

V. Evaluation

A. Client describes disease process, treatment plan, potential side effects, and available community resources

B. Client is without evidence of infection

C. Client exhibits minimal to no chemotherapy- or radiation-induced complications

D. Client maintains weight and adequate hydration

E. Client verbalizes anxiety and identifies ways to decrease/control it

POST-TEST Diseases of the Blood

Martha Jones is a 21-year-old secretary with acute lymphocytic leukemia. Her WBC is 1000 mm³; hemoglobin, 7.0 g; hematocrit, 20%; and platelet count, 20,000.

---

1. Which of the following procedures is diagnostic for leukemia?
   1. Serum uric acid level
   2. Bone marrow aspiration and biopsy
   3. Lumbar puncture
   4. Complete blood count
2. The nurse should observe Martha for signs of infection because there is a disturbance of function in the
   1. Bone marrow
   2. Musculoskeletal system
   3. Central nervous system
   4. Endocrine system
3. Which of the following nursing actions would be indicated in view of Martha's platelet count?
   1. Call the physician and anticipate an order for stat vitamin K administration
   2. Promptly notify the physician of the laboratory result
   3. Call the laboratory to redraw the specimen
   4. No action is necessary, as this is not a dangerous platelet count
4. Nursing intervention(s) for Martha would include which of the following:
   1. Monitor platelet count, erythrocytes, hemoglobin and hematocrit levels
   2. Monitor urine, stool, and emesis for bleeding
   3. Teach Martha to use a soft toothbrush
   4. All of the above
5. Therapy for Martha is aimed chiefly at
   1. Increasing lymphocytes
   2. Increasing serum iron levels
   3. Preventing infection
   4. Preventing electrolyte imbalance
6. One of the nursing goals in the care of the client with leukemia is to maintain adequate nutrition. Which of the following laboratory tests would be most useful in assessing nutritional status?
   1. Serum electrolytes
   2. Urinalysis
   3. Serum albumin
   4. Sedimentation rate
7. A common metabolic abnormality in leukemia that results from the destruction of leukocytes is

1. Hypokalemia
2. Hyperuricemia
3. Hypercalcemia
4. Hyperglycemia

John Brown is a 19-year-old construction worker admitted to your unit for a diagnostic work-up. Leukemia is highly suspected, and tomorrow he is scheduled for a bone marrow aspiration and biopsy.

---

8. When preparing John for his bone marrow aspiration and biopsy, you should explain that the biopsy site is usually the
   1. Anterior tibia
   2. Distal humerus
   3. Posterior iliac crest
   4. Posterior fossa
9. One of the important daily nursing assessments in your care of John would be to monitor his
   1. Urinalysis results
   2. Serum glucose level
   3. Complete blood count
   4. Serum cholesterol level
10. John asks you if he will be "out" for the bone marrow biopsy. Your best answer to him would be:
    1. "Yes, you will be totally unaware of the procedure."
    2. "No, but you will receive both a sedative to relax you and a local anesthetic to numb the biopsy site."
    3. "No, but you will receive something for pain after the procedure if you request it."
    4. "Yes, you will receive general anesthesia."

Mr. James, a 40-year-old businessman, is admitted to your unit to rule out Hodgkin's disease.

---

11. Which of the following tests would routinely be included in the diagnostic work-up of Mr. James?
    1. Lymph node biopsy
    2. Open lung biopsy
    3. Needle liver biopsy
    4. Intravenous pyelogram (IVP)

12. Once the diagnosis of Hodgkin's disease is confirmed, which of the following would NOT be a consideration when planning nursing care for this client?
    ① Implementing fluid restrictions
    ② Assisting Mr. James to verbalize his anxiety
    ③ Monitoring Mr. James for the development of infections
    ④ Controlling radiation- or chemotherapy-induced side effects

13. Mr. James confides in you that he is worried about keeping his job. Your best response would be:
    ① "You have every right to be concerned. Therapy for Hodgkin's disease is really tough."
    ② "Your wife seems very understanding. Why don't you talk to her about it?"
    ③ "Your feelings are very normal. What are some of your concerns?"
    ④ "I'll call our social worker to talk with you."

POST-TEST Answers and Rationales

1. ② Although serum uric acid level may be increased, the CBC abnormal, and lumbar puncture may show evidence of leukemic cells, the only definitive test for leukemia is bone marrow aspiration and biopsy. 1, II. Leukemia.

2. ① In leukemia, the normal bone marrow becomes diffusely replaced with the abnormal or immature white blood cells, interfering with the bone marrow's ability to produce other types of cells. 1, II. Leukemia.

3. ② The physician should be notified of this low platelet count, because spontaneous hemorrhaging may occur. Administration of platelets are indicated to prevent bleeding, not vitamin K. 4, I. Leukemia.

4. ④ Monitoring the CBC, assessing body fluids for bleeding, and preventing further trauma such as that caused by a hard toothbrush are all important because of the increased risk of bleeding with thrombocytopenia. 4, I. Leukemia.

5. ③ Prevention of infection is most important because Martha's WBC is 1000 mm³ and infection is the leading cause of death in leukemia patients. 4, I. Leukemia.

6. ③ The serum albumin level provides an indication of protein reserve. 1, II. Leukemia.

7. ② Hyperuricemia occurs in leukemia and is caused by hypermetabolism of leukemia cells. 1, II. Leukemia.

8. ③ The posterior iliac crest is the site of choice for bone marrow aspiration and biopsy. 4, II. Leukemia.

9. ③ Monitoring the complete blood count allows the nurse to check for anemia, thrombocytopenia, leukopenia, and the presence of blast cells in peripheral blood. 1 & 4, II. Leukemia.

10. ② A sedative and local anesthetic are both administered. The procedure is done at the bedside, not in the operating room. 1 & 4, II. Leukemia.

11. ① A lymph node biopsy is routinely done to examine tissue for the presence of Reed-Sternberg cells. 2, II. Lymphoma.

12. ① All are appropriate interventions except fluid restrictions. 4, I. Lymphoma.

13. ③ Encouraging the client to talk about his specific concerns allows the nurse to explore the client's perceptions of the effect of illness on his daily life and interpersonal relationships. 4, III. Lymphoma.

PRE-TEST Fluid/Electrolyte Disorders

52-year-old Martha Gates was seen in the clinic for complaints of muscle spasms, cramps, and tingling sensations. She was diagnosed as having hypocalcemia.

1. The nurse performed a nutritional assessment to determine Martha's daily dietary intake of calcium-rich foods. Which of the following are high in calcium?
   ① Milk
   ② Beets
   ③ Almonds
   ④ Cocoa

2. In addition to a dietary deficiency of calcium, which of the following could cause hypocalcemia?
   ① Hyperparathyroidism
   ② Vitamin D deficiency
   ③ Acidosis
   ④ Hypophosphatemia

3. On the second day of hospitalization, Martha had a convulsion and was given calcium gluconate IV. Which of the following is an appropriate nursing intervention for a client receiving IV calcium infusions?
   ① Encourage the client to ambulate during the infusion
   ② Increase the infusion rate if the client complains of a sensation of heat
   ③ Monitor the ECG and blood pressure
   ④ If the client is receiving digitalis, ask the physician to increase the dose

4. Which of the following mechanisms explains the client's muscle cramps and spasms?

① When serum calcium is decreased, more sodium becomes bound to protein; therefore, less sodium is available for nerve and muscle excitability

② When serum calcium is decreased, less calcium is available for muscle contraction

③ When serum calcium is decreased, more potassium enters nerve and muscle cells, bringing these cells farther away from threshold of excitation

④ When serum calcium is decreased, nerve and muscle cell membrane permeability to sodium is increased, leading to increased neuromuscular excitability

---

John Green has hypertension and cardiac insufficiency. He is receiving digitalis and a thiazide diuretic. He recently developed hypokalemia.

---

5. Which of the following foods should the nurse avoid giving Mr. Green because they are NOT high in potassium?
   ① Bananas
   ② Citrus fruits
   ③ Raisins
   ④ Pickles

6. Mr. Green is to receive potassium replacement in the form of IV KCl. Which of the following guidelines should the nurse observe in regard to IV potassium chloride (KCl) therapy?
   ① KCl should not be administered unless urine output is at least 200 mL per hour
   ② A priming dose of KCl should be given IV push
   ③ The fastest that KCl should ever be given is 20 mEq per hour
   ④ KCl should be diluted in a small volume of fluid and given IV piggyback

7. What effect, if any, will hypokalemia have on his digitalis therapy?
   ① No effect
   ② As long as he has hypokalemia, the need for digitalis therapy will be eliminated
   ③ He is at higher risk for digitalis toxicity
   ④ Hypokalemia causes the liver to increase its rate of clearance of the digitalis

8. Mr. Green is being discharged and will be maintained on KCl supplements in the form of an effervescent tablet three times a day. The nurse should instruct Mr. Green to:
   ① Dissolve the KCl in water, never in juice
   ② Take the KCl at mealtimes

③ Dissolve the tablets at least 1 hour prior to taking them
④ Chew the tablets if he does not like taking them in dissolved form.

A client was admitted to the emergency room after having a convulsion. The following arterial blood values were obtained:

pH	7.55
PaCO$_2$	45 mm Hg
PaO$_2$	90 mm Hg
SO$_2$	94%
HCO$_3^-$	36 mEq/L
H$_2$CO$_3$	1.35 mEq/L

---

9. The arterial blood values listed are indicative of:
   ① Metabolic acidosis
   ② Metabolic alkalosis
   ③ Respiratory acidosis
   ④ Respiratory alkalosis

Janet Smith is a 21-year-old woman brought into the emergency room after an automobile accident in which she lost a large amount of blood. The admission laboratory report indicates that she has metabolic acidosis.

---

10. A sign or symptom that would NOT substantiate the diagnosis of metabolic acidosis is:
    ① Weakness
    ② Confusion
    ③ Nausea or vomiting
    ④ Muscle tetany

11. A sign that the body is attempting to compensate for the metabolic acidosis is:
    ① Decreased serum potassium
    ② Kussmaul's respirations
    ③ Alkaline urine
    ④ Decreased ammonia in urine

12. Ms. Smith is to receive sodium bicarbonate IV to correct the acidosis. Which of the following guidelines is correct in regard to sodium bicarbonate administration?
    ① It should be added to IV solutions that contain calcium
    ② It should never be given IV push
    ③ Calcium gluconate should be made available in case muscle tetany occurs
    ④ Therapy is judged to be effective if rebound alkalosis develops

PRE-TEST Answers and Rationales

1. ① Milk and milk products are high in calcium. Beets, almonds, and cocoa are rich in oxalate which inhibits calcium absorption. 4, II. Fluid & Electrolytes.

2. ② Vitamin D is required for calcium absorption in the GI tract. Hyperparathyroidism, acidosis, and hypophosphatemia can cause hypercalcemia. 1, II. Fluid & Electrolytes.

3. ③ Calcium gluconate can cause hypotension and cardiac dysrhythmias. Increasing digitalis would increase the risk of cardiac problems. 4, I. Fluid & Electrolytes.

4. ④ When Na^+ enters nerve and muscle cells, they become less negative and therefore closer to the threshold for excitation—that is, they become more excitable. 1, I & II. Fluid & Electrolytes.

5. ④ Bananas, citrus fruits, and raisins are rich in K^+ and should be increased in the client's diet to replace K^+ lost from thiazide diuretics. Pickles are high in Na^+ and therefore not recommended. 4, II. Fluid & Electrolytes.

6. ③ K^+ affects the electrical stability of heart cells and should not be given IV push or at IV infusion rates faster than 20 mEq per hour, which is the fastest rate used in emergency situations. 4, I & II. Fluid & Electrolytes.

7. ③ Digitalis and K^+ bind to the same site on the Na^+–K^+ pump on heart cell membranes. When serum K^+ is low, more digitalis binds to the heart cells and therefore its potency is enhanced. 1, I. Fluid & Electrolytes.

8. ② Taking KCl at mealtimes will decrease GI irritation. Effervescent tablets can be dissolved in juice to disguise the taste. KCl tablets should not be chewed because they can lead to mouth ulcers. 4, II. Fluid & Electrolytes.

9. ② A pH of 7.55 indicates alkalosis. The $PaCO_2$ is normal, thus eliminating a respiratory origin. The elevated HCO_3^- indicates a metabolic origin to the alkalosis. 2, II. Acid/Base.

10. ④ H^+ competes with Ca^{++} and therefore interferes with muscle contraction; therefore tetany would not occur. 1, II. Acid/Base.

11. ② The deep, rapid breaths of Kussmaul's respirations result in increased elimination of CO_2, which is a source of acid. 2, II. Acid/Base.

12. ③ If acidosis is over-corrected with sodium bicarbonate, resulting in alkalosis, tetany may occur because in alkalosis more Ca^{++} is on the nerve and muscle cell membranes blocking the entry of Na^+. 4, II. Acid/Base.

Fluid Balance

I. Regulation of fluid shifts between intravascular and interstitial spaces
   A. Physical principles governing fluid and solute exchange between fluid compartments
      1. Simple diffusion: movement of solute from area where it is in higher concentration to area where it is in lower concentration
      2. Osmosis: movement of water from area where it is in higher concentration to area of lower concentration; osmotic pressure is attractive force for movement of water and it depends on number of solute molecules in solution; for example, solution with higher concentration of sodium draws water to it; proteins exert a type of osmotic pressure referred to as colloid osmotic pressure; since proteins are large molecules and normally do not move out of vascular compartment, they are important in maintaining blood volume
      3. Filtration: movement of water and solutes through membrane from an area of higher pressure to an area of lower pressure; force behind filtration is hydrostatic pressure
   B. Fluid and solute exchange at the capillaries
      1. Capillary structure: fluid and solute exchange between blood and tissue spaces occurs at capillaries; capillaries composed of layer of endothelial cells, which is per-

meable to solutes, water, and gases, but impermeable to larger molecules such as proteins; substances move through small gaps between adjacent endothelial cells and some substances such as O_2 and CO_2 move through cells themselves

2. Starling forces: regulate fluid and solute movement at capillaries
   a. The hydrostatic pressure exerted by blood at arterial end of capillary forces O_2, nutrients, and some fluid out into interstitial spaces surrounding cells; this outward fluid movement limited by plasma colloid osmotic pressure (COP) and interstitial pressure
   b. At venous end of capillaries, forces (lower blood pressure and higher plasma COP resulting from fluid loss at arterial end) favor movement of fluid back into vascular compartment
   c. Some of fluid and solutes that leak into tissue spaces are returned to circulation by lymphatic system

Basic Concepts of Water Metabolism

I. Body water: functions and compartments
   A. Body water constitutes approximately 60% of body weight in a normal-weight adult
   B. Water crucial for survival because it is medium in which metabolic processes occur and in which CO_2 and waste products removed
   C. Approximately two thirds of body water is located intracellular and one third located in extracellular compartment, composed of interstitial fluid and plasma
II. Mechanisms that regulate body water to prevent dehydration
   A. Physiological systems that regulate intake and urinary excretion of water respond to alterations in serum osmolarity that occur when there is water deficit or excess
      1. Antidiuretic hormone (ADH) is released from posterior pituitary gland in response to increase in serum osmolarity or decrease in blood volume; ADH causes solute free reabsorption of water in collecting ducts of kidney
      2. Thirst activated in response to increase in serum osmolarity
      3. Renin-angiotensin-aldosterone system activated in response to decreased blood volume or decreased NaCl concentration reaching kidneys; aldosterone causes sodium and water reabsorption in distal tubules and collecting ducts of kidney

NURSING PROCESS APPLIED TO ADULTS WITH FLUID/ELECTROLYTE DISORDERS

Edema

I. Assessment
   A. Definition: excess fluid in interstitial space, which may be localized or generalized
      1. Not a disease itself, but rather a manifestation of a disease process
      2. Focus of this section on subcutaneous edema; however, it should be kept in mind that edema may also form in potential spaces such as pleural, pericardial, and peritoneal cavities and in internal organs such as brain
   B. Predisposing/precipitating factors
      1. Increased capillary hydrostatic pressure
         a. Conditions causing venous obstruction: venous clots, right heart failure, varicosities, pressure on veins from casts or tight bandages
         b. Conditions causing arteriolar dilation: local or systemic allergic reactions, inflammation
         c. Increased extracellular fluid volume: endocrine disorders or compensatory mechanisms resulting in increased aldosterone (for example, Cushing's disease, liver disease, renal ischemia); renal failure; excessive fluid administration
      2. Increased capillary permeability
         a. Inflammation
         b. Allergic reactions
         c. Burns
         d. Mechanical injury
      3. Decreased plasma colloid osmotic pressure
         a. Conditions causing loss of albumin: burns, hemorrhage, diarrhea, nephrosis
         b. Conditions causing decreased albumin production: liver disease, dietary protein deficiencies
      4. Lymphatic obstruction
         a. Malignant invasion of lymph nodes
         b. Surgical removal of lymph nodes for cancer
         c. Infection and inflammation—beta hemolytic streptococcus or filariasis
   C. Clinical manifestations
      1. Weight gain: 1 L of fluid weighs approximately 1 kg; several liters of fluid may be retained before edema becomes visually evident

2. Elevated BP if edema associated with increased blood volume
3. Skin alterations: stretched, pale, and shiny from increased tension and fluid covering blood vessels
4. Alterations in body contours
   a. Pitting edema: indentation (pit) that forms over edematous area under pressure from examiner's finger; pit caused by fluid translocated away from area under the pressure point; roughly evaluated on four-point scale
      (1) 1+—edema barely detectable with slight pitting; 2+—deeper pit but fairly normal contours; 3+—deep pit and puffy appearance
      (2) 4+—excessive fluid accumulation with deep pit and frankly swollen appearance, note, when edema becomes so severe that there is no place for fluid to be displaced, tissues become hard and unable to be indented
   b. Dependent edema: gravitational flow of edema fluid to most dependent portion of body; for example, in ambulatory clients edema will most likely occur in feet and lower legs; in clients on bedrest, edema will most likely occur over sacrum and back
   c. Weeping edema: in very severe forms of edema, fluid leaks out of skin pores when pressure exerted over area
   d. Brawny edema: caused by trapping of fluid by coagulated proteins in tissue spaces; skin becomes thick and hardened with an orange-peel appearance due to severe stretching
D. Complications
   1. Plasma fluid volume deficit
   2. Plasma protein deficit
   3. Decubitus ulcers from breakdown of edematous tissues
   4. Ischemic tissue damage because as edema fluid accumulates, it pushes cells farther away from surrounding capillaries
   5. Decreased movement in edematous areas
II. Analysis
A. Fluid volume excess
B. High risk for injury related to altered tissue integrity from distention
C. High risk for injury related to altered perfusion
III. Planning/goals, expected outcomes
A. Cause of client's edema will be corrected or controlled

B. Client's edematous tissues will be protected from injury
C. Client will not develop complications from therapy for edema
IV. Implementation
A. Specific implementations depend on cause of edema
   1. Heart failure: digitalis, diuretics, sodium and fluid restriction (see CHF)
   2. Renal failure: dialysis, sodium and fluid restriction, renal transplant (see Renal Failure, Chapter 8)
   3. Malnutrition: increase dietary protein
   4. Trauma: apply cold to injured area (up to 24 hours) to decrease amount of plasma accumulating in area
B. General implementations for management of edema
   1. Monitor I & O
   2. Administer prescribed drugs such as diuretics or albumin
   3. Restrict fluid and sodium intake
   4. Instruct client to read food labels for sodium content
   5. Elevate body parts prone to edema without causing pressure or sharp bends
   6. Use elastic support stockings and sleeves to increase resistance to outward flow of fluid
C. Keep skin over edematous tissue clean and lubricated; change client's position frequently
D. Monitor electrolytes for signs of hypokalemia or hyponatremia and administer prescribed electrolyte supplements if needed
E. Pharmacology and nutrition
   1. Diuretics (Table 4–25)
   2. Refer to section on nutrition and hypernatremia for Na^+ content of foods (see Table 4–14)
V. Evaluation
A. Underlying cause of edema has been corrected or controlled
B. I & O balanced; no further weight gain or decrease; no further increase in circumference of the edematous extremity
C. Skin integrity maintained over edematous tissue
D. Serum electrolytes normal; no signs or symptoms of electrolyte imbalance

Dehydration

I. Assessment
A. Definition: dehydration is deficit of body water relative to solutes; extracellular fluid becomes hypertonic causing water to move out

TABLE 4–25 Diuretics

Class	Examples	Action and Use
Thiazide diuretics	Bendroflumethiazide, benzthiazide, chlorothiazide, chlorthalidone, chlorothiazide, hydrochlorothiazide, hydroflumethiazide, indapamide, polythiazide, quinethazone, trichlormethiazide	Produce diuresis by inhibiting Na^+ and Cl^- reabsorption in the thick ascending limb of the loop of Henle thus increasing their excretion; also increase K^+ excretion and uric acid retention; used for edematous states and hypertension
Loop diuretics	Bumetanide, ethacrynic acid, ethacrynate, furosemide	Block Cl^- reabsorption and therefore block passive Na^+ reabsorption along the thick portion of the ascending limb of the loop of Henle; also increase K^+ and H^+ excretion; used for chronic renal failure and edematous conditions
Potassium-sparing diuretics	Amiloride, spironolactone, triamterene	Spironolactone is an inhibitor of aldosterone, which interferes with Na^+–K^+ and Na^+–H^+ exchange in the collecting ducts, resulting in Na^+ retention; used in Na^+-retaining states in which aldosterone is elevated—for example, for CHF or cirrhosis of the liver; amiloride and triamterene are used for their K^+-sparing effect usually in combination with other diuretics

Common Side Effects

Hyponatremia, hypochloremic alkalosis, hypokalemia (except K^+-sparing diuretics), magnesium depletion, hyperkalemia (K^+-sparing diuretics in the presence of oliguria), hypovolemia, hyperuricemia, allergic reactions, photosensitivity (especially thiazides), potentiation of digitalis toxicity (in presence of hypokalemia), drowsiness, lethargy, headache, GI upset (nausea and vomiting, constipation or diarrhea), glucose intolerance (thiazides), hematuria (ethacrynic acid), reversible deafness (loop diuretics), orthostatic hypotension

Nursing Implications

Administer drugs so that diuresis occurs during the daytime and does not interrupt sleep; administer with meals to decrease GI irritation; monitor therapeutic response (weight loss, increased urine output, decreased blood pressure); monitor serum K^+ and instruct client to recognize and report signs of K^+ imbalance; monitor serum Na^+ and instruct client to recognize and report signs of low sodium syndrome; monitor need for adjustment of insulin dosage in diabetics; caution client, especially elderly, about possible orthostatic hypotension and measures to prevent falling (change to standing position slowly, lie down if lightheaded or dizzy, avoid hot baths and environmental temperatures); administer prescribed potassium supplements or K^+ rich foods when K^+-losing diuretics are used; determine client's sensitivity to sulfonamides prior to administration of thiazides or loop diuretics

of cells into extracellular fluid resulting in cell shrinkage and altered function
B. Precipitating/predisposing factors
 1. Decreased water intake
   a. Unavailability of fluids
   b. Impaired thirst mechanism (for example, from head injury)
   c. Impaired swallowing
   d. Inability to communicate needs (for example, aphasia, confusion, coma)
   e. Debilitating disorders in which clients cannot attend to their thirst
 2. Increased water loss
   a. Diabetes insipidus (deficiency of ADH)
   b. Severe burns
   c. Osmotic diuresis (diabetic ketoacidosis)
   d. Increased respiratory rate
 3. Excess solute intake
   a. High protein diet or tube feedings without adequate fluid intake
   b. Excessive IV infusion of hypertonic solutions
C. Clinical manifestations
 1. Thirst
 2. Acute decrease in body weight over few days (1 L of water weighs approximately 1 kg)
 3. Decreased urine output; increased urine osmolarity and specific gravity
 4. Elevated body temperature (lack of fluid for perspiration)
 5. Dry or cracked mucous membranes and tongue; decreased skin turgor
 6. Increased serum sodium and osmolarity
 7. Central nervous system (CNS) alterations (from shrinkage of brain cells)—agitation, confusion, lethargy, coma
 8. Manifestations of decreased circulating blood volume that occur in severe dehydration—postural hypotension, rapid, thready pulse, decreased vein prominence, and increased vein refill time

D. Complications
  1. Fever
  2. Dilutional hypernatremia
  3. Renal failure
  4. Shock
  5. Coma
II. Analysis
  A. Fluid volume deficit related to fluid loss
  B. High risk for injury related to altered sensorium
  C. High risk for altered skin integrity related to loss of turgor
  D. High risk for injury related to complications of treatment
III. Planning/goals, expected outcomes
  A. Clients at risk will not become dehydrated
  B. Dehydrated client's body water will be replaced
  C. Client will be protected from injury if an altered level of sensorium or weakness develop
  D. Client's skin and mucous membrane integrity will be preserved
  E. Client will not develop complications from therapy for dehydration
IV. Implementations
  A. Monitor I & O in clients at risk; place debilitated or confused clients on regular schedule of water administration
  B. With mild to moderate water deficit (less than 10% body weight), oral fluid replacement may be sufficient; more severe water deficits (greater than 10% body weight), administer prescribed IV fluids (usually 2.5% or 5% dextrose)
  C. Assist client while ambulating; use support strap when sitting; bed side rails kept up
  D. Apply skin lotion; change position frequently; keep lips and mucous membranes moist
  E. Replace body water gradually over 24 to 36 hours to prevent circulatory overload, pulmonary edema, and sudden compartmental shifts in water; monitor for signs of water intoxication (decreased serum sodium and osmolarity, polyuria, CNS alterations such as disorientation, muscle twitching, and coma, caused by cerebral edema); monitor for glucose overload if dextrose solutions are used, especially in diabetics
V. Evaluation
  A. Body water balance maintained in clients at risk for dehydration
  B. I & O balanced; body weight restored; serum sodium and osmolarity normal; skin turgor normal; body temperature normal; no alteration in sensorium

C. Client has not sustained injury
D. Client's skin and mucous membrane integrity maintained
E. No signs or symptoms of circulatory overload, glucose overload, or water intoxication

Electrolyte Imbalances

Basic Concepts of Electrolyte Balance
I. Functions and regulation of electrolytes
  A. Sodium (Na^+), potassium (K^+), calcium (Ca^{++}), and magnesium (Mg^{++}) are the principal cations
  B. Maintenance of normal concentration and distribution of these electrolytes in body fluid compartments essential to life; specific functions of each electrolyte discussed in following sections
  C. Adequate intake of electrolytes usually met by normal diet; electrolytes absorbed through gastrointestinal tract
  D. Excretion of electrolytes occurs primarily in urine and to lesser extent in feces or perspiration
  E. Various hormones or vitamins are necessary for absorption or excretion of certain electrolytes; this aspect of regulation discussed in sections on specific electrolytes
II. General concepts of electrolyte imbalances
  A. Deficit of an electrolyte may result from decreased intake or increased excretion or dilution of electrolyte by increased body water
  B. Excess of electrolyte may result from increased intake or decreased excretion or concentration of electrolyte by decreased body water
  C. Clinically, electrolytes are measured in serum; serum levels do not necessarily change in same direction as total body content or intracellular level of electrolyte; serum level is a measure of concentration of electrolyte in relation to volume of water in vascular compartment
  D. Usually, concentration of electrolyte in serum is related to presence or absence of associated signs and symptoms

NOTE: Electrolyte imbalances in following sections will be discussed in terms of serum level of electrolyte

Sodium Imbalances
Basic Concepts
I. Distribution in body
  A. Na^+ found in all fluid compartments of body with highest concentration occurring in extracellular fluid of which Na^+ is major cation

B. Normal serum Na^+ concentration in adult is 135 to 145 mEq/L
C. Na^+ usually found in combination with Cl^- or another anion
II. Sodium intake and excretion
   A. Minimum daily intake requirement for Na^+ in adult is 2 g, usually met in excess by normal diet which contains Na^+ found naturally in foods and that added during food preparation
   B. Na^+ excreted primarily in urine and to a lesser extent in feces and perspiration
   C. Na^+ excretion regulated by aldosterone, which promotes Na^+ reabsorption in distal tubules and collecting ducts of kidneys; water follows movement of Na^+
III. Functions of sodium
   A. Na^+ regulates osmotic pressure and therefore volume of extracellular fluid (interstitial and intravascular spaces)
   B. Conduction of neural impulses
   C. Muscular contraction

Hyponatremia
I. Assessment
   A. Definition: decreased serum Na^+ level below 135 mEq/L
   B. Predisposing/precipitating factors
      1. Increased Na^+ loss (usually accompanied by some water loss also)
         a. Renal losses (diuretics, osmotic diuresis, adrenal insufficiency, salt-washing nephritis)
         b. Gastrointestinal losses (vomiting, diarrhea, GI suction, bile drainage, small bowel fistula)
         c. Endocrine imbalances (hypopituitarism, hypoadrenalism)
         d. Skin losses (excessive perspiration, burns)
      2. Dilutional hyponatremia (excess extracellular water dilutes serum Na^+)
         a. Excessive ingestion of water (psychogenic polydipsia, rapid infusion of Na^+-free IV solutions, ingestion of tap water to replace both Na^+ and water loss)
         b. Water retention (drugs that increase ADH, such as morphine or barbiturates, heart failure, cirrhosis)
      3. Decreased sodium intake: overzealous dietary restriction of Na^+ intake for therapeutic reasons
   C. Clinical manifestations
      1. Manifestations of hypovolemia if Na^+ deficit occurs along with water deficit (decreased BP, weak, thready pulse, oliguria, postural hypotension)
      2. Manifestations of hypervolemia if Na^+ deficit occurs secondary to dilution by excess water (weight gain, increased blood pressure, pulmonary edema)
      3. Manifestations of cellular swelling when decrease in Na^+ in extracellular fluid is in excess of water loss because fluid moves into cells where osmolarity higher
         a. Manifestations of swelling of brain cells (altered level of sensorium—for example, anxiety, confusion, coma)
         b. Manifestations of swelling of neuromuscular cells (weakness, cramps, muscle twitching, convulsions)
         c. Manifestations of swelling of GI cells (anorexia, diarrhea, abdominal cramps)
   D. Diagnostic examinations
      1. History and physical to determine the underlying cause
      2. Serum Na^+ concentration
      3. Serum osmolarity
   E. Complications
      1. Shock
      2. Coma
      3. Coexisting electrolyte deficiencies
II. Analysis
   A. High risk for injury related to hyponatremia
   B. High risk for injury related to therapy
   C. Knowledge deficit related to causes and treatment
III. Planning/goals, expected outcomes
   A. Hyponatremia will be prevented in clients at risk
   B. Underlying cause of client's hyponatremia will be identified
   C. Client's sodium balance will be restored
   D. Client will not experience complications from therapy for hyponatremia
   E. Client safety will be maintained in event that weakness or confusion develop
IV. Implementation
   A. Prevention depends on situation
      1. Advise clients working in hot environments to drink sodium-containing fluids or add salt to diet or ingest salt tablets
      2. Monitor clients on diuretics for sodium depletion
      3. Irrigate NG tubes with normal saline
      4. Teach outpatients to recognize and report signs and symptoms of hyponatremia
   B. Nursing history and assessment
   C. Specific implementations depend on underly-

ing cause; listed below are common causes of hyponatremia and related implementations

1. Absolute Na^+ deficit: administer prescribed NaCl solutions; isotonic solutions used except in severe deficits, which may require more rapid reversal with a hypertonic solution such as 3% NaCl
2. Water retention (for example, CHF): restrict water intake, administer prescribed diuretics
3. To relieve CNS alterations from cellular swelling: administer prescribed mannitol, hypertonic glucose, or urea to induce osmotic diuresis

D. Replace Na^+ slowly so that it can be distributed among body compartments; monitor electrolytes to prevent overshoot hypernatremia; assess for manifestations of fluid overload, especially in elderly clients and those with cardiac disorders

E. Assist client while ambulating, support while sitting; keep side rails up; observe client frequently

V. Evaluation
  A. Hyponatremia prevented in clients at risk
  B. Underlying cause of hyponatremia identified
  C. Serum Na^+ within normal limits; no signs or symptoms of hyponatremia
  D. No signs or symptoms of overshoot hypernatremia or fluid overload
  E. Client has not sustained injury

Hypernatremia

I. Assessment
  A. Definition: increased serum Na^+ level above 145 mEq/L
  B. Precipitating/predisposing factors
    1. Primary hypernatremia (actual Na^+ gain)
      a. Infusion of saline solutions
      b. Salt water drowning
      c. Renal disease
      d. Hyperaldosteronism
      e. Cushing's syndrome/disease
      f. Excessive Na^+ intake in client with renal failure
    2. Decreased extracellular water resulting in increased concentration of serum Na^+
      a. Excessive water loss (diuretics, diabetes insipidus, watery diarrhea, heavy perspiration that results in more water than Na^+ loss)
      b. Decreased water intake (inability to attend to thirst, difficulty swallowing, withholding water for therapeutic reasons)

C. Clinical manifestations
    1. Manifestations associated with cell shrinkage (excess extracellular Na^+ draws water out of cells causing cellular dehydration and altered function)
      a. Thirst
      b. CNS alterations
      c. Dry, flushed skin
      d. Dry, fissured mucous membranes
    2. Manifestations associated with hypovolemia if it is cause of hypernatremia (weight loss, decreased blood pressure, weak, thready pulse, increased temperature)
    3. Edema, if there is both Na^+ and water excess

D. Diagnostic examinations
    1. History and physical to determine underlying cause
    2. Serum Na^+ concentration
    3. Serum osmolarity
    4. Lab tests to detect concentration of other blood components (protein, urea, hematocrit), if there is a coexisting water deficit
    5. Urine specific gravity to determine if kidneys are retaining water in face of a water deficit

E. Complications
    1. Manic excitement
    2. Hypovolemia
    3. Coma

II. Analysis
  A. High risk for injury related to hypernatremia
  B. High risk for injury related to therapy
  C. Knowledge deficit related to causes and treatment

III. Planning/goals, expected outcomes
  A. Hypernatremia will be prevented in clients at risk
  B. Underlying cause of client's hypernatremia will be identified
  C. Client's sodium balance will be restored
  D. Client will not develop complications from therapy for hypernatremia
  E. Client safety will be maintained in event that weakness or confusion develop

IV. Implementations
  A. Prevention depends on situation
    1. Those with decreased ability to excrete Na^+ (renal failure, CHF) should have Na^+ intake restricted
    2. Those at risk for water deficit, such as elderly, confused, or debilitated, should be placed on regular schedule of water administration

3. Check for adequacy of renal function prior to administration of IV electrolytes
B. Take careful nursing history
C. Specific implementations depend on the underlying cause; listed below are common causes of hyponatremia and related implementations
   1. Primary hypernatremia: diuretics to remove Na^+; discontinue Na^+-containing IV fluids, renal dialysis for severe hypernatremia unresponsive to other forms of therapy
   2. Decreased extracellular water-liberal administration of water after assessment of renal and cardiac function
D. Monitor electrolytes to prevent overshoot hyponatremia; assess for manifestations of fluid overload in cases of water-replacement therapy
E. Assist client while ambulating; support while sitting; keep side rails up; observe client frequently
F. Maintain adequate nutrition
   1. Table 4–4 lists Na^+ content of foods
   2. Table 4–4 describes the meaning of Na^+ labels for food
V. Evaluation
A. Hypernatremia prevented in clients at risk
B. Underlying cause of hypernatremia identified
C. Serum Na^+ within normal limits; no signs or symptoms of hypernatremia or associated hypovolemia
D. No signs or symptoms of overshoot hyponatremia or fluid overload
E. Client has not sustained injury

Potassium Imbalances
Basic Concepts
I. Distribution in body
A. K^+ found in all fluid compartments of body with highest concentration occurring in intracellular fluid of which K^+ is the major cation
B. Only 2% of total body K^+ found in extracellular fluid compartment
C. Normal serum K^+ 3.5 to 5.0 mEq/L
II. Potassium intake and excretion
A. Daily requirement for K^+ intake 0.5 to 1.5 g, which is supplied in slight excess by normal diet
B. Urinary excretion primary route of K^+ loss, with smaller amounts of K^+ excreted in feces and perspiration
C. Kidneys can increase K^+ excretion, via effects of aldosterone, when K^+ intake increases; however, kidneys cannot conserve K^+ when intake is low

D. Acid–base balance affects K^+ excretion; in acidosis, increased amounts of H^+ excreted in urine and more K^+ retained; opposite occurs in alkalosis; H^+ and K^+ compete for secretory sites in renal tubules
E. Acid–base imbalances cause intercompartmental shifts in K^+; in acidosis, H^+ moves into cells to be buffered by intracellular proteins and K^+ moves out; opposite effect occurs in alkalosis
F. Maintenance of normal intracellular concentration of K^+ depends to large extent on Na^+-K^+ pump, which pumps K^+ into cell and Na^+ out; ATP supplies energy to run this pump
III. Functions of potassium
A. Regulates intracellular osmotic pressure and fluid volume
B. Participates in acid–base balance
C. Cofactor in metabolic reactions
D. Critical in neuromuscular excitability of skeletal, cardiac, and smooth muscle

Hypokalemia
I. Assessment
A. Definition: decreased serum K^+ below 3.5 mEq/L
B. Predisposing/precipitating factors
   1. Inadequate K^+ intake
      a. Diet or IV solutions deficient in K^+
      b. Inability to eat
   2. Increased K^+ loss from body
      a. Renal losses (osmotic diuresis, renal tubular necrosis, K^+-losing diuretics, increased aldosterone levels)
      b. GI losses (vomiting, diarrhea, gastric suction, intestinal fistulas)
      c. Skin losses (excessive diaphoresis, burns—late stage when K^+ initially lost from injured cells has been excreted in the urine)
   3. K^+ shift into cells
      a. Alkalosis or alkalinizing drugs
      b. Insulin and glucose therapy
C. Clinical manifestations
   1. Manifestations of altered cell polarization, which affects neuromuscular activity (intracellular K^+ moves out to replenish extracellular K^+ level)
      a. CNS (confusion, irritability, lethargy, coma)
      b. Altered neuromuscular activity (weakness, cramps, paresthesia, paralysis)
      c. Cardiovascular system (ECG alterations—arrhythmias, prominent U-wave, prolonged interval widening

QRS complexes; postural hypotension)

  d. Respiratory system (shallow breathing, respiratory muscle paralysis)

  e. GI system (decreased bowel mobility, paralytic ileus, anorexia, nausea and vomiting)

  2. Metabolic alkalosis (as intracellular K^+ moves out to replenish extracellular K^+, H^+ moves into cells which increases extracellular pH)

  D. Diagnostic examinations

  1. History and physical to determine underlying cause

  2. Serum K^+ concentration

  3. Serum pH (alkalosis causes K^+ to move into cells)

  E. Complications

  1. Ventricular fibrillation

  2. Respiratory arrest from respiratory muscle paralysis

  3. Potentiation of digitalis toxicity

II. Analysis

  A. High risk for injury related to hypokalemia

  B. High risk for injury related to therapy

  C. Knowledge deficit related to causes and treatment

III. Planning/goals, expected outcomes

  A. Hypokalemia will be prevented in clients at risk

  B. Underlying cause of client's hypokalemia will be identified

  C. Client's potassium balance will be restored

  D. Client will not experience complications from therapy for hypokalemia

  E. Client safety will be maintained in the event that weakness or confusion develop

IV. Implementations

  A. Prevention depends on the situation; for example, instruct clients on K^+-losing diuretics to ingest foods high in K^+; monitor clients on insulin therapy for hypokalemia

  B. Take accurate nursing history

  C. Replenish K^+, preferably by oral route by providing foods high in K^+ or administering prescribed K^+ supplements; in more severe cases, administer prescribed intravenous K^+

  D. Monitor client for signs and symptoms of potassium toxicity (refer to Hyperkalemia), assess adequacy of renal function prior to K^+ administration, monitor ECG, pulse, muscle strength

  E. Assist client while ambulating, support while sitting; keep side rails up; observe client frequently

  F. Administer medications and nutrition as ordered

  1. Table 4–26 lists K^+ supplements

  2. Table 4–27 lists foods high in K^+

TABLE 4–26 Potassium Supplements

Examples	Action and Use	Common Side Effects	Nursing Implications
Liquid: Cena-K, Kaochlor Kay, Ciel, Klor-Con, Rum-K, SK-potassium chloride *Powder:* K-Lor, Kay Ciel, Klor-Con, Klorvess *Effervescent tablets:* Kaochlor-Eff, K-lyte, K-lyte/Cl *Plain tablets:* Klotrix, K tab, Slow K, Kaon, Kaon-Cl, Kao Nor *Intravenous:* potassium chloride, potassium gluconate *Liquid:* Kaon, Kaylixir, K-G Elixir	Treat or prevent K^+ deficit	GI upset (nausea and vomiting, abdominal distention, diarrhea, esophageal or gastric ulceration); hyperkalemia (refer to section on signs and symptoms and complications of hyperkalemia)	Assess adequacy of renal function prior to administration; administer with meals to decrease GI irritation; dilute with at least 4 oz of fluids to prevent GI irritation and rapid absorption; administer in milk or fruit juice to disguise unpleasant taste; dissolve effervescent tablets immediately prior to administration; position client upright when swallowing large tablets (do not crush, chew, or suck on tablets); teach client and/or family importance of drug compliance; instruct client not to use salt substitutes or OTC drugs containing K^+ without first consulting the physician; do not administer KCl IV push; mix well in IV bag; do not administer IV KCl faster than 20 mEq/hour; carefully monitor IV flow rate; stop infusion if oliguria develops; monitor ECG of client on IV K^+ supplementation

TABLE 4–27 Foods High in Potassium

Meats: Beef, ham, turkey, chicken, veal

Fish

Milk products

Fruits: Bananas, dates, prunes, dried fruits, citrus fruits and juices, raisins, avocados

Vegetables: Spinach, brussels sprouts, beans, yams, potatoes

V. Evaluation
   A. Hypokalemia prevented in clients at risk
   B. Underlying cause of hypokalemia identified
   C. Serum K^+ within normal limits; no signs or symptoms of hypokalemia
   D. No clinical manifestations of overshoot hyperkalemia
   E. Client has not sustained injury

Hyperkalemia
   I. Assessment
      A. Definition: increased serum K^+ above 5.5 mEq/L
      B. Predisposing/precipitating factors
         1. Excessive K^+ intake
            a. Rapid infusion of K^+-containing IV solutions
         2. Decreased K^+ excretion
            a. Decreased renal excretion (renal failure, adrenocortical insufficiency)
            b. Decreased fecal excretion (intestinal obstruction)
         3. K^+ shift out of cells
            a. Cell injury (burns, trauma, crushing injuries)
            b. Acidosis or acidifying drugs
      C. Clinical manifestations
         1. Manifestations of altered cell polarization, which affects neuromuscular activity
            a. Neural and skeletal muscle alterations (weakness, cramps, dizziness, paresthesia)
            b. Cardiac alterations (arrhythmias, ECG-peaked T-waves and wide QRS complex, cardiac fibrillation, and arrest)
            c. Smooth muscle alterations (nausea, diarrhea, vomiting, intestinal cramps)
         2. Metabolic acidosis (high extracellular K^+ causes more K^+ to move into cells with subsequent H^+ exit from cells into extracellular fluid)
      D. Diagnostic examinations
         1. History and physical to determine the underlying cause
         2. Serum K^+ concentration
         3. Serum pH (acidosis causes K^+ to move out of cells)
      E. Complications
         1. Ventricular fibrillation and arrest
         2. Respiratory arrest
   II. Analysis
      A. High risk for injury related to hyperkalemia
      B. High risk for injury related to therapy
      C. Knowledge deficit related to causes and treatment
   III. Planning/goals, expected outcomes
      A. Hyperkalemia will be prevented in clients at risk
      B. Underlying cause of client's hyperkalemia will be identified
      C. Client's K^+ balance will be restored
      D. Client will not experience complications from therapy for hyperkalemia
      E. Client safety will be maintained in event of weakness or dizziness
   IV. Implementations
      A. Prevention depends on situation
         1. Monitor serum K^+ in clients receiving K^+-containing medications and in clients in acidosis
         2. Avoid transfusion with old, stored blood because of cell lysis and release of K^+
         3. Do not infuse IV solutions containing K^+ until urine output assessed to be adequate
      B. Take accurate nursing history
      C. Instruct client to decrease intake of foods high in K^+ and to avoid salt substitutes containing K^+
      D. Increase K^+ excretion with prescribed dialysis or ion exchange resins
      E. Increase cellular uptake of K^+ by administering prescribed insulin and glucose
      F. Decrease K^+ release from cells by preventing injury and infection
      G. Monitor client for signs and symptoms of hypokalemia (refer to section on hypokalemia)
      H. Monitor ECG
      I. Institute safety precautions
      J. Administer K^+-reducing medication described in Table 4–28
   V. Evaluation
      A. Hyperkalemia prevented in clients at risk
      B. Underlying cause of hyperkalemia identified
      C. Serum K^+ within normal limits; no signs or symptoms of hyperkalemia
      D. No signs or symptoms of overshoot hypokalemia
      E. Client has not sustained injury

TABLE 4–28 Potassium-Reducing Medication

Example	Action and Use	Common Side Effects	Nursing Implications
Sodium polystyrene sulfonate (Kayexalate)	Cation exchange resin that removes K^+ from the body by exchanging it with Na^+ (and to a lesser extent, other cations); the K^+-containing resin is then excreted in the feces; used to decrease K^+ in cases of hyperkalemia	GI upset, hypokalemia, hypocalcemia, hypernatremia	Administer with prescribed laxative to ensure rapid movement of resin in GI tract; monitor serum Na^+ and instruct client on prescribed Na^+ restrictions; monitor serum K^+ and acid-base balance and signs and symptoms of hypokalemia; if resin used as retention enema, encourage client to retain it for one to several hours

Magnesium Imbalances

Basic Concepts

I. Distribution in body
  A. Magnesium (Mg^{++}) found in all fluid compartments of body with highest concentration occurring in intracellular fluid
  B. Normal serum Mg^{++} concentration 1.5 to 2.5 mEq/L
  C. Approximately 50% of total body Mg^{++} located in bone

II. Magnesium intake and excretion
  A. Minimum daily requirement for Mg^{++} in non-pregnant adult is 250 mg, which is met by normal diet
  B. Absorption of Mg^{++} in GI tract is increased by parathyroid hormone and decreased by high calcium levels, excess fat, and phosphorus and in alkalosis
  C. Excretion of Mg^{++} by normal kidneys regulated by plasma concentration of Mg^{++}

III. Functions of magnesium
  A. Regulation of synaptic transmission at neuromuscular junction and in CNS
  B. Cofactor in variety of enzymatic reactions in metabolic pathways

Hypomagnesemia

I. Assessment
  A. Definition: decreased serum Mg^{++} level below 1.5 mEq/L
  B. Predisposing/precipitating factors
    1. Inadequate intake
      a. Malnutrition or starvation
      b. High dietary intake of Ca^{++} without increasing Mg^{++} intake
      c. Prolonged IV infusion of Mg^{++}-free IV solutions without oral Mg^{++} intake
    2. Decreased absorption of Mg^{++}
      a. Diarrhea
      b. Genetic Mg^{++} absorption defect
      c. Malabsorption syndromes
      d. Presence of high Ca^{++}, fat, or phosphorus in GI tract
    3. Excessive excretion or fluid loss
      a. Diuretics
      b. Diabetic ketoacidosis
      c. Prolonged GI suction
      d. Hyperaldosteronism
  C. Clinical manifestations
    1. Manifestations of increased CNS and neuromuscular excitability resulting from increased acetylcholine release
      a. CNS alterations (agitation, confusion, convulsions, insomnia)
      b. Neuromuscular alterations (hyperactive reflexes, positive Chvostek's sign and Trousseau's sign, cramps, nystagmus, muscle tremors, and twitching)
    2. Cardiovascular alterations
      a. Arrhythmias
      b. Hypertension
      c. Tachycardia
  D. Diagnostic examinations
    1. History and physical to determine underlying cause
    2. Serum Mg^{++} level
  E. Complications
    1. Convulsions
    2. Cardiac arrhythmias

II. Analysis
  A. High risk for injury related to hypomagnesemia
  B. High risk for injury related to therapy
  C. Knowledge deficit related to causes and treatment

III. Planning/goals, expected outcomes
  A. Hypomagnesemia will be prevented in clients at risk
  B. Underlying cause of client's hypomagnesemia will be identified

C. Client's magnesium balance will be restored

D. Client will not experience complications from therapy for hypomagnesemia

E. Client safety will be maintained in event that confusion or convulsions occur

IV. Implementations

  A. Prevention depends on situation

    1. Encourage malnourished client to ingest foods high in Mg^{++} (green vegetables, nuts, seafood, whole grains, dried beans, cocoa)

    2. Decrease Ca^{++} intake in client on high dietary Ca^{++}

    3. Administer prescribed magnesium supplements to clients at risk

  B. Take accurate nursing history

  C. Increase dietary intake of Mg^{++}; administer prescribed Mg^{++} supplements

  D. Monitor client for manifestations of Mg^{++} excess (refer to section on clinical manifestations of hypermagnesemia)

  E. Have calcium gluconate available because it antagonizes the sedative effects of Mg^{++}

  F. Maintain safety and institute seizure precautions

  G. Administer Mg^{++} supplements (Table 4–29)

V. Evaluation

  A. Hypomagnesemia prevented in clients at risk

  B. Underlying cause of hypomagnesemia identified

  C. Serum Mg^{++} within normal; no signs or symptoms of hypomagnesemia

  D. No signs or symptoms of overshoot hypermagnesemia

  E. Client has not sustained injury

Hypermagnesemia

I. Assessment

  A. Definition: increased serum Mg^{++} greater than 2.5 mEq/L; associated signs and symptoms usually do not occur until Mg^{++} exceeds 4 mEq/L

  B. Predisposing/precipitating factors

    1. Decreased renal excretion

      a. Renal insufficiency

      b. Severe dehydration causing oliguria

      c. Adrenal insufficiency

    2. Increased intake or absorption

      a. Excessive IV Mg^{++} administration

      b. Salt water drowning

      c. Overuse of Mg^{++}-containing antacids or cathartics

NOTE: Increased Mg^{++} intake usually results in hypermagnesemia only if there is coexisting decreased renal output

  C. Clinical manifestations

    1. Manifestations of neuromuscular depression

      a. CNS (lethargy, sedation, confusion)

      b. Skeletal muscles (flaccid paralysis, weak or absent reflexes, respiratory depression)

      c. Cardiovascular system (vasodilation causing a sensation of warmth and hypotension, cardiac arrhythmias)

  D. Diagnostic examinations

    1. History and physical to determine underlying cause

    2. Serum Mg^{++} level

  E. Complications

    1. Oversedation

    2. Respiratory depression

    3. Cardiac arrhythmias and arrest

    4. Coma (if Mg^{++} greater than 15 to 20 mEq/L)

II. Analysis

  A. High risk for injury related to hypermagnesemia

TABLE 4–29 Magnesium Supplement

Example	Action and Use	Common Side Effects	Nursing Implications
Magnesium sulfate	Used to treat severe hypomagnesemia; used IV to control convulsions	Diarrhea (oral form), hypermagnesemia (respiratory and cardiac depression, muscle weakness, sedation, hypotension, diaphoresis, confusion)	Assess renal function prior to administration; keep calcium gluconate available in case of cardiotoxicity; for IM injection, give deep IM and massage to enhance absorption, frequent observation of client receiving IV magnesium (test deep tendon reflexes, monitor cardiac and renal function, stop IV if client becomes hypotensive, excessively diaphoretic, or reflexes become weak or absent)

B. High risk for injury related to therapy
C. Knowledge deficit related to causes and treatment
III. Planning/goals, expected outcomes
 A. Hypermagnesemia will be prevented in clients at risk
 B. Underlying cause of the client's hypermagnesemia will be identified
 C. Client's magnesium balance will be restored
 D. Client will not experience complications from therapy for hypermagnesemia
 E. Client safety will be maintained in event that sedation or confusion occur
IV. Implementations
 A. Prevention depends on situation
  1. Do not administer Mg^{++}-containing medication if renal function inadequate
  2. Provide adequate fluids to dehydrated client to ensure adequate urine excretion
  3. Teach client proper use of antacids and cathartics containing Mg^{++}
 B. Take accurate nursing history
 C. Decrease intake of foods high in Mg^{++}
 D. Withhold Mg^{++}-containing medications
 E. Provide adequate fluid intake
 F. Conduct prescribed dialysis procedures
 G. Administer prescribed Ca^{++} gluconate to antagonize cardiotoxic and sedative effects of Mg^{++}
 H. Monitor client for manifestations of Mg^{++} deficit or calcium toxicity (if treated with calcium gluconate)
 I. Institute safety precautions
V. Evaluation
 A. Hypermagnesemia prevented in clients at risk
 B. Underlying cause of hypermagnesemia identified
 C. Serum Mg^{++} within normal; no signs or symptoms of Mg^{++} excess
 D. No signs or symptoms of overshoot hypomagnesemia or hypercalcemia
 E. Client has not sustained injury

Calcium and Phosphorus Imbalances
Basic Concepts
I. Relationship between calcium and phosphorus
 A. Ca^{++} and phosphorus (PO_4) discussed together in this section because there are some common elements in their regulation and because there is an inverse relationship in their serum levels
 B. Increase or decrease in Ca^{++} accompanied by opposite change in PO_4
 C. Inverse relationship between alterations in serum levels of Ca^{++} and PO_4 helps prevent

formation of Ca^{++}-PO_4 precipitates, which would alter cellular function
II. Distribution in body
 A. Approximately 99% of body Ca^{++} and PO_4 is in bone and teeth
 B. Normal serum Ca^{++} level 9 to 11 mg/dL or 4.5 to 5.8 mEq/L
 C. Normal serum PO_4 level 3 to 4.5 mg/dL or 1.7 to 2.6 mEq/L
 D. Ca^{++} in blood either bound to protein (inactive Ca^{++}) or in free, ionized form (active Ca^{++})
 E. When plasma protein levels decrease, more calcium is in free, ionized form
III. Ca^{++} and PO_4 is equal to intake and excretion
 A. Approximately 75% of Ca^{++} and PO_4 intake derived from milk and milk products, the rest from vegetables and fruit
 B. Recommended daily allowance for Ca^{++} in non-pregnant adult 800 mg
 C. Approximately 30% of ingested Ca^{++} absorbed in intestines and remainder excreted in feces
 D. Approximately 70% of PO_4 ingested is absorbed; PO_4 excreted mainly in urine
 E. Vitamin D increases absorption of Ca^{++} and renal excretion of PO_4
 F. When blood Ca^{++} low, parathyroid hormone secreted and it increases Ca^{++} absorption from GI tract and CA^{++} resorption from bone
 G. When blood Ca^{++} increased, calcitonin secreted, causing bone to take up Ca^{++}, thereby decreasing its serum level
 H. Increase in serum PO_4 stimulates bone uptake of Ca^{++}
IV. Functions of Ca^{++} and PO_4
 A. Ca^{++} and PO_4 essential components of bone and teeth
 B. PO_4 involved in metabolic reactions and cellular energy production
 C. PO_4 functions in acid–base balance by assisting in renal excretion of H^+
 D. Ca^{++} regulates membrane permeability and nerve transmission
 E. Ca^{++} triggers muscle contraction
 F. Ca^{++} involved in blood coagulation
 G. Ca^{++} essential for hormone secretion

NOTE: Alterations in Ca^{++} and PO_4 are discussed with focus on primary alteration in Ca^{++}, which then causes a secondary and inverse alteration in PO_4

Hypocalcemia
I. Assessment
 A. Definition: decreased serum calcium below 9 mg/dL or 4.5 mEq/L

B. Predisposing/precipitating factors
1. Decreased dietary Ca^{++}
2. Decreased Ca^{++} absorption
   a. Vitamin D deficiency
   b. Overuse of antacids
3. Increased calcium losses
   a. GI losses (diarrhea, intestinal fistulas, pancreatitis)
   b. Loss in exudates (burns, infection, peritonitis)
4. Decreased availability of physiologically active free Ca^{++}
   a. Alkalosis (more Ca^{++} bound to protein)
   b. Massive transfusions with citrated blood (citrate binds Ca^{++})
5. Hypoparathyroidism
C. Clinical manifestations
1. Manifestations of increased neuromuscular excitability (when serum Ca^{++} decreases, nerve and muscle cell membrane permeability to Na^+ increases leading to cell depolarization)
   a. Numbness and tingling
   b. Muscle spasms, tetany, cramps, convulsions
   c. Positive Trousseau's sign and Chvostek's sign
   d. Laryngospasm
2. Manifestations of depressed cardiac contractility (lack of Ca^{++} to sustain strong cardiac contractions)
   a. Weak cardiac contractions
   b. Cardiac arrhythmias
D. Diagnostic examinations
1. History and physical to determine underlying cause
2. Serum Ca^{++} concentration
E. Complications
1. Convulsions
2. Respiratory arrest from laryngospasm
3. CHF
4. Cardiac arrest
5. Pathological fractures

II. Analysis
A. High risk for injury related to hypocalcemia
B. High risk for injury related to therapy
C. Knowledge deficit related to causes and treatment

III. Planning/goals, expected outcomes
A. Hypocalcemia will be prevented in clients at risk
B. Underlying cause of client's hypocalcemia will be identified
C. Client's calcium balance will be restored
D. Client will not experience complications from therapy for hypocalcemia

E. Client safety will be maintained in event that muscle spasms or convulsions develop
F. Fractures will be prevented

IV. Implementations
A. Prevention depends on the situation
1. Instruct clients with poor nutritional habits regarding importance of adequate Ca^{++} and vitamin D intake
2. Monitor clients who have potential Ca^{++} loss in exudates for hypocalcemia
3. Monitor alkalotic clients for hypocalcemia
4. Keep calcium gluconate available for emergency use for clients after thyroid surgery (possibility of injury to parathyroid glands)
B. Take accurate nursing history
C. Replenish Ca^{++} preferably by oral route by increasing client's dietary intake of Ca^{++} and vitamin D; if oral route not appropriate, administer prescribed IM or IV Ca^{++} supplements
D. Monitor client for signs and symptoms of hypercalcemia (refer to section on Hypercalcemia); assess adequacy of renal function prior to administering IV Ca^{++}
E. Assist client while ambulating; keep side rails up; support while sitting; seizure precautions
F. Administer medications and nutrition
1. Table 4–30 lists Ca^{++} supplements
2. Dietary sources of calcium are milk and milk products, green leafy vegetables, and sardines, clams, and oysters

V. Evaluation
A. Hypocalcemia prevented in clients at risk
B. Underlying cause of hypocalcemia identified
C. Serum Ca^{++} within normal limits; no signs or symptoms of hypocalcemia
D. No signs or symptoms of overshoot hypercalcemia
E. Client has not sustained injury

Hypercalcemia

I. Assessment
A. Definition: an increased serum calcium above 11 mg/dL or 5.8 mEq/L
B. Predisposing/precipitating factors
1. Excess Ca^{++} or vitamin D intake
2. Hyperparathyroidism
3. Increased Ca^{++} mobilization from bone
   a. Multiple fractures
   b. Prolonged immobilization
   c. Bone tumors
   d. Tumors (for example, breast, lung, kidney) secreting bone demineralizing hormones

TABLE 4–30 Calcium Supplements

Examples	Action and Use	Common Side Effects	Nursing Implications
Calcium chloride (IV), calcium gluceptate (IV or IM), calcium gluconate (oral or IV), calcium lactate (oral)	Used to prevent hypocalcemia or to replenish Ca^{++}	Tingling sensation, metallic taste, local tissue irritation and burning; after IV infusions—sensation of heat, vasodilation, hypotension, dysrhythmia, cardiac arrest	Monitor ECG and blood pressure; advise client to remain in bed during IV infusion; observe digitalized client for signs and symptoms of digitalis toxicity; observe infusion site closely to avoid extravasation, which causes cellulitis and necrosis; avoid oxalate rich foods (spinach, beets, almonds, cashews, cocoa) in client on oral Ca^{++} supplements since these foods interfere with calcium absorption

4. Increased availability of physiologically active free Ca^{++}

C. Clinical manifestations
1. Manifestations of decreased neuromuscular excitability (elevated Ca^{++} decreases cell membrane permeability in Na$^+$)
   a. CNS: depression, altered level of sensorium
   b. Muscular system: decreased deep tendon reflexes, muscle weakness
   c. GI system: decreased motility, nausea and vomiting, constipation
   d. Cardiac arrhythmias

D. Diagnostic examinations
1. History and physical to determine underlying cause
2. Serum Ca^{++} concentration

E. Complications
1. Renal failure
2. Cardiac arrest
3. Pathological fractures
4. Potentiation of digitalis toxicity

II. Analysis
A. High risk for injury related to hypercalcemia
B. High risk for injury related to therapy
C. Knowledge deficit related to causes and treatment

III. Planning/goals, expected outcomes
A. Hypercalcemia will be prevented in clients at risk
B. Underlying cause of client's hypercalcemia will be identified
C. Client's calcium balance will be restored
D. Client will not experience complications from therapy for hypercalcemia
E. Client safety will be maintained

IV. Implementations
A. Prevention depends on situation
1. Instruct clients to avoid excessive Ca^{++} or vitamin D supplementation
2. Promote early ambulation for clients on bedrest; use tilt table to achieve weight-bearing position in immobilized clients; encourage use of trapeze bar
3. Monitor acidotic clients for hypercalcemia

B. Take accurate nursing history
C. Restrict dietary intake of Ca^{++}
D. Hydrate client to promote renal excretion of Ca^{++}
E. Administer prescribed mithramycin to decrease serum Ca^{++} in clients with cancer
F. Maintain an acid urine to increase Ca^{++} solubility by encouraging intake of acid ash fruit juices, cranberry and prune juice
G. Prevent urinary tract infections that cause an alkaline urine and Ca^{++} precipitates
H. Monitor client for signs and symptoms of rebound hypocalcemia
I. Institute safety precautions

V. Evaluation
A. Hypercalcemia prevented in clients at risk
B. Underlying cause of hypercalcemia identified
C. Serum Ca^{++} within normal limits; no signs or symptoms of hypercalcemia
D. No signs or symptoms of overshoot hypocalcemia
E. Client has not sustained injury

Chloride Imbalances
Basic Concepts
I. Distribution in body
A. Chloride (Cl$^-$) found in all fluid compartments of body, with highest concentration in extracellular fluid of which it is major anion
B. Normal serum Cl$^-$ concentration 96 to 106 mEq/L

II. Chloride intake and excretion

A. Cl^- usually ingested with Na^+ in form of NaCl

B. Cl^- absorbed in intestines with only small amount lost in feces

C. Because Cl^- combines with Na^+, its excretion in urine indirectly regulated by aldosterone

D. Cl^- usually varies in relation to Na^+ and water balance

III. Functions of chloride

A. Helps maintain osmotic pressure and fluid volume of extracellular compartment

B. Essential for production of HCl by gastric parietal cells

C. Participates in regulation of acid–base balance

1. Cl^- competes with HCO_3^- for Na^+—for example, in acidosis, more HCO_3^- reabsorbed from urine and more Cl^- excreted with Na^+

2. Cl^- shifts into or out of cells in exchange for HCO_3^-

Hypochloremia

I. Assessment

A. Definition: decreased serum Cl^- level below 96 mEq/L

B. Predisposing/precipitating factors

1. Cl^- loss most commonly parallels Na^+ loss or dilution by excess water (refer to section on Hyponatremia)

2. Cl^- loss occurring independent of Na^+ loss—for example, vomiting gastric fluid

3. Decreased Cl^- intake most commonly occurs from NaCl restricted diet

C. Clinical manifestations

1. Signs and symptoms are those of hypochloremic metabolic alkalosis (when Cl^- is decreased, HCO_3^- is retained to maintain electrical neutrality of body fluids); (refer to section on Acid–base imbalances)

2. Signs and symptoms of hypervolemia if Cl^- deficit caused by dilution by excess water

3. Signs and symptoms of hyponatremia, if associated with Na^+ deficit

D. Diagnostic examinations

1. History and physical to determine underlying cause

2. Serum Cl^- concentration

E. Complications (refer to Hyponatremia and Metabolic alkalosis)

II. Analysis

A. High risk for injury related to hypochloremia

B. High risk for injury related to therapy

C. Knowledge deficit related to causes and treatment

III. Planning/goals, expected outcomes

A. Hypochloremia will be prevented in clients at risk

B. Underlying cause of client's hypochloremia will be identified

C. Client's chloride balance will be restored

D. Client will not experience complications from therapy for hypochloremia

E. Client safety will be maintained

IV. Implementations

A. Refer to preventive measures discussed under hyponatremia

B. Take accurate nursing history

C. Specific implementations depend on underlying cause

1. Refer to implementations discussed under Hyponatremia

2. Refer to implementations discussed under Metabolic alkalosis

3. Administer prescribed saline solutions, KCl or ammonium chloride

D. Monitor electrolytes to prevent overshoot hyperchloremia

E. Institute safety and seizure precautions

V. Evaluation

A. Hypochloremia prevented in clients at risk

B. Underlying cause of hypochloremia identified

C. Serum Cl^- within normal limits; no signs or symptoms of hypochloremia

D. No signs or symptoms of overshoot hyperchloremia

E. Client has not sustained injury

Hyperchloremia

I. Assessment

A. Definition: increased serum Cl^- above 106 mEq/L

B. Predisposing/precipitating factors

1. Primary hyperchloremia

a. Excessive ingestion or infusion of Cl^--containing compounds such as KCl, NaCl, ammonium chloride

b. Refer to factors listed under primary hypernatremia

2. Decreased extracellular water resulting in increased concentration of serum Cl^-

a. Refer to Hypernatremia

C. Clinical manifestations

1. Signs and symptoms are those of metabolic acidosis (when Cl^- is in excess, more HCO_3^- excreted by kidneys); refer to section on manifestations of metabolic acidosis

2. Manifestations of hypovolemia if Cl^- excess caused by water deficit
3. Manifestations of hypernatremia if associated with Na^+ excess

D. Diagnostic examinations
1. History and physical to determine underlying cause
2. Serum Cl^- concentration

E. Complications (refer to Hypernatremia and Metabolic acidosis)

II. Analysis
A. High risk for injury related to hyperchloremia
B. High risk for injury related to therapy
C. Knowledge deficit related to causes and treatment

III. Planning/goals, expected outcomes
A. Hyperchloremia will be prevented in clients at risk
B. Underlying cause of client's hyperchloremia will be identified
C. Client's chloride balance will be restored
D. Client will not experience complications from therapy for hyperchloremia
E. Client safety will be maintained

IV. Implementations
A. Refer to preventive measures discussed under hypernatremia
B. Take accurate nursing history
C. Refer to implementations discussed under Hypernatremia and Metabolic acidosis
D. Monitor electrolytes to prevent overshoot hypochloremia
E. Institute safety and seizure precautions

V. Evaluation
A. Hyperchloremia prevented in clients at risk
B. Underlying cause of the hyperchloremia identified
C. Serum Cl^- within normal limits; no signs or symptoms of hyperchloremia
D. No signs or symptoms of overshoot hypochloremia
E. Client has not sustained injury

Acid–Base Imbalances

Basic Concepts of Acid–Base Balance
I. Acid: a substance that dissociates into ions and in so doing donates protons (H^+ ions) to solution; strength of an acid determined by degree to which it dissociates; for example, a stronger acid dissociates to greater extent and donates larger amount of H^+ ions
II. Base: a proton (H^+ ion) acceptor; stronger base has greater affinity for H^+
III. pH: a measure of the acidity of solution and equal to negative logarithm of H^+ ion concentration (pH = $-$ log H^+); for example, if H^+ concentration is equal to 10^{-7} g/L, pH is equal to 7; as pH decreases, H^+ ion concentration increases and the more acidic the solution becomes; as pH increases, the H^+ ion concentration decreases and the more basic the solution becomes

IV. Buffer: a mixture of a weak acid and its base, which minimizes changes in pH when either acid or base added to solution; base in buffer mixture functions as H^+ ion acceptor when acid added to solution; acid in buffer mixture functions as H^+ ion donor when base added to solution

V. Types of acids produced in body
A. Volatile acids
1. Can be eliminated by lungs in gaseous form as CO_2
2. Source is aerobic metabolism, for example: glucose + $O_2 \rightarrow CO_2 + H_2O \rightleftharpoons H_2CO_3 \rightleftharpoons H^+ + HCO_3^-$

B. Fixed (nonvolatile) acids
1. Nongaseous acids
2. Eliminated by kidneys
3. Source is various metabolic pathways; for example, anaerobic metabolism of glucose $\rightarrow$ lactic acid aerobic metabolism of amino acids $\rightarrow H^+ + SO_4^-$ incomplete oxidation of fats $\rightarrow$ ketoacids

VI. Physiological buffer systems: arterial blood pH normally regulated between 7.35 and 7.45 despite daily endogenous production and ingestion of acids and bases; this regulation is accomplished through actions of chemical buffers and respiratory and renal systems (Table 4–31)

VII. Acid–base imbalances
A. A decreased arterial pH indicates a state of acidosis that may be of either metabolic or respiratory origin; in metabolic acidosis, the serum bicarbonate level is below normal; in respiratory acidosis, the $PaCO_2$ is elevated
B. An increased arterial pH indicates a state of alkalosis that may be of either metabolic or respiratory origin; in metabolic alkalosis, the serum bicarbonate level is above normal; in respiratory alkalosis, the $PaCO_2$ is decreased

Metabolic Acidosis
I. Assessment
A. Definition: condition in which arterial blood pH below 7.35 caused by either accumulation of fixed (nonvolatile) acids or base deficit
B. Predisposing/precipitating factors
1. Increase in metabolic acids

TABLE 4–31 Physiological Buffer Systems

Buffer System	Components	Examples of Buffering Actions	Comments
Chemical Buffer Systems			
Bicarbonate buffer system	$CO_2 + H_2O \rightleftharpoons H_2CO_3 \rightleftharpoons H^+ + HCO_3^-$ Carbonic acid — Controlled by the lungs Bicarbonate — Controlled by the kidneys	$NaHCO_3 + HCl \rightarrow H_2CO_3 + NaCl$ Strong acid — Weak acid $H_2CO_3 + NaOH \rightarrow NaHCO_3 + H_2O$ Strong base — Weak base	Chemical buffers react immediately to an acid–base imbalance; however, once they are used up, they are not immediately replaced
Phosphate buffer system	Na_2HPO_4 and NaH_2PO_4 Disodium hydrogen phosphate — Sodium dihydrogen phosphate	$Na_2HPO_4 + HCl \rightarrow NaH_2PO_4 + NaCl$ Strong acid — Weak acid $NaH_2PO_4 + NaOH \rightarrow Na_2HPO_4 + H_2O$ Strong base — Weak base	Normally, the HCO_3^-/H_2CO_3 ratio is 20/1
Protein buffer system	Plasma proteins Intracellular proteins Hemoglobin		As H^+ ions enter the cell to be buffered by intracellular proteins, K^+ ions leave the cell in order to maintain electrical neutrality; therefore, in acidosis the serum K^+ tends to rise; opposite reaction occurs in alkalosis
Respiratory Buffer Mechanisms	Alterations in rate and depth of respiration to excrete or retain CO_2	An increase in H^+ concentration or P_{CO_2} stimulates the respiratory center, resulting in hyperpnea and increased CO_2 excretion A decrease in H^+ concentration or P_{CO_2} depresses the respiratory center, resulting in hypoventilation and CO_2 retention	Respiratory system responds within minutes to an acid–base imbalance; however, it can only regulate volatile acids; pulmonary compensation is not complete because as P_{CO_2} returns to normal, stimulus affecting respiratory center is removed; hypoventilatory response to metabolic alkalosis is limited by resulting hypoxemia; pulmonary compensation may be inadequate in clients with pulmonary disease
Renal Buffer Mechanisms	Variable reabsorption of HCO_3^- Addition of new HCO_3^- to the blood Excretion of H^+ in combination with HPO_4 or NH_3^+	In acidosis, renal excretion of H^+ increases and reabsorption and production of HCO_3^- increases In alkalosis, renal excretion of H^+ and reabsorption of HCO_3^- decrease	It takes several hours to several days for renal system to effectively compensate for an acid–base imbalance; renal system will be able to compensate only if it is not the cause of imbalance and if renal function is adequate

a. Excess production of metabolic acids
  (1) Fasting/starvation
  (2) Ketotic diet
  (3) Diabetic ketoacidosis
  (4) Lactic acidosis
  (5) Salicylate poisoning
 b. Retention of metabolic acids: renal failure
2. Increase in bicarbonate loss
  a. Diarrhea

b. GI suctioning

c. GI fistulas

d. Increased chloride levels

C. Clinical manifestations

1. Nausea/vomiting

2. Weakness

3. Lethargy

4. Coma

5. Warm, flushed skin

6. Compensatory signs

a. Kussmaul's respirations

b. Acidic urine

c. Increased serum potassium

7. Clinical manifestations

a. Clinical manifestations of primary disorder causing metabolic acidosis

b. Clinical manifestations caused by altered cellular functions resulting from acidosis

(1) Depressed muscular function resulting from competition between H^+ and Ca^{++} for binding sites on muscle contractile proteins

(2) Depressed neuromuscular function resulting from increased level of free (ionized) Ca^{++} caused by increased H^+ ions displacing Ca^{++} from protein; increased free Ca^{++} then binds to nerve and muscle cell membranes, blocking entry of Na^+ and therefore decreasing electrical excitation

c. Clinical manifestations resulting from compensatory mechanisms

D. Diagnostic examinations

1. History and physical to determine underlying cause of acidosis

2. Blood gas, pH, and electrolyte levels

E. Complications

1. Fluid and electrolyte loss from vomiting and diarrhea

2. Cardiac dysrhythmias from elevated serum K^+

3. Hypotension

4. Congestive heart failure

5. Shock

II. Analysis

A. High risk for injury related to metabolic acidosis

B. High risk for injury related to therapy

C. Knowledge deficit related to causes and treatment

III. Planning/goals, expected outcomes

A. Underlying cause of client's metabolic acidosis will be identified

B. Client's acid–base balance will be restored

C. Client will not develop complications from metabolic acidosis

D. Client safety will be maintained in event of weakness or altered level of sensorium

E. Client will not develop complications from therapy for metabolic acidosis

F. Client will be comfortable

IV. Implementations

A. Take accurate nursing history

B. Specific implementations depend on the underlying cause; listed below are some common causes of metabolic acidosis and implementations

1. Diabetic ketoacidosis: administer prescribed insulin, fluids, and K^+; instruct client on insulin and diet therapy

2. Renal tubular disease: replace bicarbonate kidneys unable to reabsorb

3. Lactic acidosis: improve tissue perfusion via cardiovascular support

4. Renal failure: dialysis

5. Drug overdose: instruct client regarding use of salicylates, ethanol, etc.

6. If therapy of underlying cause will not reverse acidosis rapidly enough, administer prescribed drugs, such as sodium bicarbonate or sodium lactate to neutralize the acid.

C. Monitor I & O; replace fluid and electrolytes lost from vomiting, diarrhea, or osmotic diuresis

D. Assist client when mobile; use supporting straps when sitting; keep side rails up; position on side to prevent aspiration

E. Monitor client for manifestations of overshoot metabolic alkalosis; monitor for manifestations of hypokalemia, because as acidosis is corrected, K^+ reenters cells; administer prescribed K^+ supplements after determining adequacy of renal function; encourage foods high in K^+

F. Provide alkaline mouthwash to neutralize mouth acids; provide lemon and glycerine swabs to lubricate lips dried out from compensatory hyperpnea

G. Administer alkalinizing drugs (Table 4–32)

V. Evaluation

A. Underlying cause of metabolic acidosis identified

B. Blood pH and HCO_3^-/H_2CO_3 and urine pH normal; no signs or symptoms of metabolic acidosis

C. No evidence of fluid or electrolyte imbalance

D. Client has not sustained injuries

E. Serum K^+ maintained within normal limits; no evidence of overshoot metabolic alkalosis

TABLE 4–32 Pharmacology of Alkalinizing Drugs

Example	Action and Use	Common Side Effects	Nursing Implications
Sodium bicarbonate	Dissociates into Na^+ and HCO_3^- thereby increasing the plasma alkaline reserve; used to treat acidosis; effect is immediate if given IV	Metabolic alkalosis, hypocalcemia, hypokalemia, gastric distention, fluid retention	Administer with caution, monitoring acid–base status, to avoid rebound alkalosis; have calcium gluconate and ammonium chloride available for therapy of tetany and alkalosis if they occur; avoid addition to IV solutions with calcium, which may result in formation of precipitates
Sodium lactate	Metabolized to bicarbonate in the liver and thereby increases the plasma alkaline reserve; used to treat acidosis; effect takes 1 to 2 hours	Metabolic alkalosis, hypocalcemia, hypokalemia	Administer with caution to avoid rebound alkalosis; avoid use in clients with liver disease or lactic acidosis

Respiratory Acidosis

I. Assessment
  A. Definition: condition in which arterial blood pH below 7.35 caused by the retention of CO_2, which combines with H_2O to form carbonic acid (H_2CO_3)
  B. Predisposing/precipitating factors
    1. Increased CO_2
    2. Decreased ventilation
      a. Central nervous system depression
      b. Asthma
      c. COPD
      d. Pulmonary edema
    3. Chest trauma
    4. Respiratory paralysis
  C. Clinical manifestations
    1. Headache
    2. Confusion/disorientation
    3. Tremors
    4. Warm, flushed skin
    5. Compensatory sign: acid excretion in urine
    6. Bases of clinical manifestations
      a. Clinical manifestations of hypoventilation or impaired gas exchange, which is underlying cause of acidosis
      b. Clinical manifestations caused by altered cellular functions resulting from acidosis
        (1) Depressed neuromuscular function (see mechanisms listed under Metabolic acidosis)
        (2) Vasodilatory effect of CO_2 on cerebral blood vessels
      c. Clinical manifestations resulting from compensatory mechanisms
  D. Diagnostic examinations
    1. History and physical to determine the underlying cause of the respiratory impairment
    2. Blood gas, pH, and electrolyte levels
  E. Complications
    1. Respiratory depression from blunting of respiratory drive caused by H^+ deficiency
    2. Tetany, convulsions
    3. Hypokalemia
    4. Decreased oxygen release at tissue level secondary to shift in oxyhemoglobin association curve to left
II. Analysis
  A. Altered gas exchange related to hypoventilation
  B. High risk for injury related to respiratory acidosis
  C. High risk for injury related to therapy
  D. Knowledge deficit related to causes and treatment
III. Planning/goals, expected outcomes
  A. Client will have adequate ventilation
  B. Client will not develop complications from respiratory acidosis
  C. Client will not develop complications from oxygen therapy
  D. Client safety will be maintained in the event of weakness or altered level of sensorium
IV. Implementations
  A. Specific implementations depend on the cause of the ventilatory impairment; the following are general measures to increase ventilation
    1. Establish a patent airway
    2. Administer mechanical ventilatory aids as prescribed
    3. Facilitate removal of tracheobronchial secretions by teaching and encouraging client to cough and deep breathe
    4. Take in adequate fluids
    5. Perform postural drainage and clapping and manual chest vibration
    6. Prevent respiratory infections

7. Teach client about risks associated with smoking and provide information to assist in smoking cessation
8. Support medical therapy for specific respiratory disorders—for example, administer antibiotics or bronchodilators

B. Observe client's blood gases and signs and symptoms of worsening hypoventilation and acidosis

C. Administer prescribed drugs, such as sodium bicarbonate, if necessary to neutralize excess acid

D. Cautiously administer oxygen, especially to clients with chronic hypercapnia, in order to increase tissue oxygenation without causing respiratory depression
   1. Monitor for signs of CO_2 narcosis, such as respiratory depression, decreasing level of sensorium, cardiac dysrhythmias
   2. Monitor for signs of oxygen toxicity, such as pulmonary edema, presence of blood in tracheobronchial secretions
   3. Monitor use of mechanical ventilators to prevent rebound respiratory alkalosis

E. Assist client when mobile; use supporting straps when sitting; keep side rails up; position on side to prevent aspiration

F. Pharmacology
   1. Most effective therapy for respiratory acidosis is improvement of alveolar ventilation
   2. Drug therapy with alkalinizing agents may be contraindicated since increasing pH removes stimulatory effect of H^+ on respiration and may therefore further reduce ventilation and increase the hypercapnia

V. Evaluation
   A. Client effectively coughs and deep breathes; client performs postural drainage with production of sputum; client stops smoking; blood gases are normal; no signs of respiratory distress
   B. Blood pH, gases, and electrolytes are normal
   C. No evidence of CO_2 narcosis or O_2 toxicity or rebound respiratory alkalosis
   D. Client has not sustained injuries

Metabolic Alkalosis
I. Assessment
   A. Definition: condition in which arterial blood pH greater than 7.45; caused by either loss of H^+ or gain of bicarbonate
   B. Predisposing/precipitating factors
      1. Excessive bicarbonate
         a. Bicarbonate antacids
         b. Loss of body fluids

2. Hydrogen ion gain
   a. Vomiting
   b. Gastric suctioning
   c. Potassium loss
      (1) Diuretics
      (2) Steroid therapy
      (3) Potassium loss or decreased intake

C. Clinical manifestations
   1. Nausea/vomiting
   2. Confusion
   3. Tetany
   4. Convulsions
   5. Compensatory signs
      a. Hypoventilation
      b. Increased urinary pH
   6. Bases of clinical manifestations
      a. Manifestations of primary disorder causing metabolic alkalosis
      b. Increased neuromuscular excitability resulting from decreased level of free calcium (with a decrease in H^+, more Ca^{++} is bound to protein and thus inactive), which allows more Na^+ to enter nerve and muscle cells
      c. Manifestations resulting from compensatory mechanisms

II. Analysis
   A. High risk for injury related to metabolic alkalosis
   B. High risk for injury related to therapy
   C. Knowledge deficit related to causes and treatment

III. Planning/goals, expected outcomes
   A. Underlying cause of client's metabolic alkalosis will be identified
   B. Client's acid–base balance will be restored
   C. Client will be protected from injury in event of convulsions
   D. Client will be free from complications from therapy of metabolic alkalosis

IV. Implementations
   A. Take accurate nursing history
   B. Specific implementations depend on underlying cause; listed below are some common causes of metabolic acidosis and implementations
      1. Excessive ingestion of sodium bicarbonate: instruct client regarding appropriate use of sodium bicarbonate-containing drugs
      2. Chloride loss: administer prescribed chloride replacements
      3. Potassium deficit: administer prescribed potassium supplements; encourage foods high in potassium
      4. If therapy of underlying cause will not reverse alkalosis rapidly enough, administer

prescribed acidifying drugs such as ammonium chloride or acetazolamide (Diamox) (Table 4–33)
C. Institute seizure precautions
D. Monitor blood gases and electrolytes during therapy to detect overshoot metabolic acidosis
V. Evaluation
   A. Underlying cause of metabolic alkalosis identified
   B. Blood pH, HCO_3^-/H_2CO_3 normal; no signs or symptoms of alkalosis
   C. Client has not sustained injuries
   D. No evidence of overshoot metabolic acidosis; serum K^+ within normal

Respiratory Alkalosis

I. Assessment
   A. Definition: condition in which arterial blood pH greater than 7.45 caused by decrease in P_{CO_2} secondary to increased alveolar ventilation
   B. Predisposing/precipitating factors
      1. Hyperventilation
         a. Salicylate poisoning (early)
         b. Anxiety
         c. Hypoxia
         d. Increased blood ammonia
   C. Clinical manifestations
      1. Numbness, tingling fingers and toes
      2. Lightheadedness
      3. Tetany/convulsions
      4. Positive Chvostek's sign and Trousseau's sign
      5. Bases of clinical manifestations
         a. Clinical manifestations of primary disorder causing respiratory alkalosis
         b. Increased neuromuscular excitability (refer to Metabolic alkalosis)
         c. Signs and symptoms resulting from compensatory mechanisms

D. Diagnostic examinations
   1. History and physical to determine underlying cause of alkalosis
   2. Blood gas, pH, and electrolyte levels
E. Complications
   1. Tetany, convulsions
   2. Hypokalemia
   3. Decreased oxygen release at tissue level secondary to shift in oxyhemoglobin association curve to left
   4. Dizziness and fainting
II. Analysis
   A. Altered breathing pattern related to hyperventilation
   B. High risk for injury related to respiratory alkalosis
   C. High risk for injury related to therapy
   D. Knowledge deficit related to causes and treatment
III. Planning/goals, expected outcomes
   A. Underlying cause of respiratory alkalosis will be identified and eliminated
   B. Client's acid–base balance will be restored
   C. Client will be protected from injury in event of convulsions
   D. Client will be free from complications resulting from therapy of respiratory alkalosis
IV. Implementations
   A. Take accurate nursing history to identify underlying cause of respiratory alkalosis, which will serve as basis for therapy. For example:
      1. Salicylate abuse: instruct client regarding appropriate use of drugs
      2. Anxiety reaction: assist client to recognize and cope with situations that provoke anxiety; teach client to take slow deep breaths or temporarily hold breath in situations that precipitate hyperventilation or use of rebreathing mask
      3. Mechanical ventilation: monitor ventila-

TABLE 4–33 Pharmacology of Acidifying Drugs

Example	Action and Use	Common Side Effects	Nursing Implications
ammonium chloride	Ammonium (NH_4^+) is converted to urea in liver, resulting in release of H^+ and Cl^-, which decreases pH; used to correct alkalosis	GI irritation, metabolic acidosis, hypokalemia	Minimize GI irritation by administering with or immediately after meals; monitor blood gases and electrolytes to avoid overshoot acidosis; avoid use in clients with liver or renal failure
acetazolamide (Diamox)	A carbonic anhydrase inhibitor that enhances renal bicarbonate excretion; used to correct alkalosis	Nausea and vomiting, polyuria, paresthesias, metabolic acidosis, hypokalemia, volume depletion	Minimize GI irritation by administering with or immediately after meals; monitor for overshoot acidosis; monitor I & O; instruct client to report paresthesias and drowsiness

tory settings and client's blood gases and electrolytes
B. Administer rebreathing mask or prescribed sedatives or 5% CO_2 for inhalation
C. Institute seizure precautions
D. Monitor blood gases and electrolytes during therapy to detect overshoot metabolic acidosis
E. Pharmacology: therapy directed at underlying cause; in severe, acute cases, sedatives may be prescribed
V. Evaluation
A. Underlying cause of client's respiratory alkalosis identified and corrected
B. Blood pH, HCO_3^-/H_2CO_3, and electrolytes normal; no signs or symptoms of alkalosis
C. Client has not sustained injuries
D. No evidence of overshoot metabolic acidosis

Mixed Acid–Base Imbalances
I. Assessment
A. Definition: mixed acid–base imbalance consists of more than one type of acid–base imbalance occurring in client at same time
B. Predisposing/precipitating factors
1. Mixed acid–base imbalance may be caused by disorders resulting in similar directional change in pH—for example, metabolic acidosis and respiratory acidosis that occur during cardiac arrest
2. Mixed acid–base imbalance may be caused by disorders resulting in opposite directional changes in pH—for example, metabolic acidosis and respiratory alkalosis that occur with salicylate poisoning; in this type of mixed acid–base imbalance, pH tends to be within normal range; however, HCO_3^- and $PaCO_2$ move in direction affected by primary disorder
C. Clinical manifestations (see individual acid–base imbalances)
D. Diagnostic examinations
1. History and physical to determine underlying causes of the imbalances
2. Blood gas, pH, and electrolyte levels to determine whether alterations in HCO_3^- and $PaCO_2$ are as expected or indicative of mixed acid–base imbalance; if alteration greater or less than that expected as compensatory change, mixed acid–base imbalance may exist
II. Analysis (refer to individual acid–base imbalances)
III. Planning/goals, expected outcomes (refer to individual acid–base imbalances)
IV. Implementations (refer to individual acid–base imbalances)
V. Evaluation (refer to individual acid–base imbalances)

Stepwise Approach to Assessment of Acid–Base Imbalances
I. Suspect presence of acid–base imbalance based on clinical presentation, laboratory data, and history
II. Determine arterial pH, blood gases, and HCO_3^-
III. If pH acidic, determine cause
A. $PaCO_2$ above 45 mm Hg indicates respiratory acidosis
B. HCO_3^- below 22 mEq/L indicates metabolic acidosis
IV. If pH alkalotic, determine cause
A. $PaCO_2$ below 35 mm Hg indicates respiratory alkalosis
B. HCO_3^- above 26 mEq/L indicates metabolic alkalosis
V. If pH within normal range, check at which end it is at; if it is close to acidic or basic side, it may be indicative of compensated acidosis or alkalosis:
A. If pH toward acidic side
1. It may indicate respiratory compensation for metabolic acidosis if $PaCO_2$ low
2. It may indicate renal compensation for respiratory acidosis if HCO_3^- high
B. If pH toward basic side
1. It may indicate respiratory compensation for metabolic alkalosis if $PaCO_2$ high
2. It may indicate renal compensation for respiratory alkalosis if HCO_3^- low
VI. Determine if acid–base imbalance simple or mixed by applying rules for expected compensation

POST-TEST Fluid/Electrolyte Disorders

A 30-year-old construction worker has been working outdoors in extremely hot weather for the past week. He was admitted to the hospital today with a diagnosis of hypernatremia. His renal function is assessed and found to be normal.

---

1. The hypernatremia in this situation most likely indicates that the client needs which of the following?
   ① A sodium-restricted diet
   ② Both sodium and water restrictions
   ③ Less fluid intake
   ④ More fluid intake

2. Which of the following manifestations would NOT occur in this client?
   1. Dry, fissured mucous membranes
   2. Central nervous system alterations
   3. Hypotension
   4. Lack of thirst

Carol Washington is a 50-year-old diabetic who is currently hospitalized with renal failure. Her serum electrolytes taken shortly after admission were Na$^+$: 155 mEq/L, Mg^{++}: 3.4 mEq/L, Ca^{++}: 12 mg/dL.

---

3. Which of the following electrolyte imbalances does this client have?
   1. Hypernatremia and hypercalcemia
   2. Hypernatremia, hypermagnesemia, and hypocalcemia
   3. Hypernatremia, hypermagnesemia, and hypercalcemia
   4. Hypermagnesemia and hypercalcemia
4. A subsequent laboratory report indicates that Mrs. Washington has hyperkalemia. Which of the following is an INAPPROPRIATE nursing intervention for a client with hyperkalemia?
   1. Monitor client's ECG
   2. Monitor client's pH
   3. Encourage intake of bananas, orange juice, and dried fruit
   4. Assess client for neuromuscular alterations
5. Mrs. Washington has a 2+ pitting edema of the lower extremities. Which of the following should be assessed to help evaluate the effectiveness of therapy for edema?
   1. Daily weight
   2. Plasma pH
   3. Arterial blood gases
   4. Plasma glucose

Twenty-four-year-old Tamara Hemingway was brought to the emergency room for treatment of a fracture she sustained in a skiing accident. She is in pain, extremely anxious, and hyperventilating.

---

6. Her admission laboratory report shows an arterial blood pH of 7.54. The most likely diagnosis of her pH imbalance is:
   1. Metabolic acidosis from tissue hypoxia caused by blood loss
   2. Respiratory alkalosis caused by hyperventilation
   3. Respiratory acidosis caused by hyperventilation
   4. Metabolic alkalosis caused by overexertion
7. Which of the following is the most appropriate nursing intervention to correct this client's acid–base imbalance?
   1. Administer sodium bicarbonate IV push as ordered
   2. Administer ammonium chloride IV push as ordered
   3. Provide emotional support and assist client with a rebreathing mask
   4. Call respiratory therapy to set up mechanical ventilation

POST-TEST Answers and Rationales

1. ④ Situations in which there is more water loss than sodium loss, as occurs with heavy perspiration in a hot environment, results in concentration of the serum sodium—that is, dilutional hypernatremia. If dietary intake of sodium is too high, excess sodium will be excreted if renal function is normal. 1, II. Fluid & Electrolytes.

2. ④ In hypernatremia, excess extracellular sodium draws water out of the cells causing cellular dehydration and altered function. When a water deficit is the cause of hypernatremia, there will also be manifestations of hypovolemia. 1, II. Fluid & Electrolytes.

3. ③ The upper limit of normal serum sodium is 145 mEq/L; for magnesium it is 2.5 mEq/L; and for calcium it is 11 mg/dL. Therefore all three are elevated in this client. 1, II. Fluid & Electrolytes.

4. ③ Foods listed are high in K^+ and therefore inappropriate in this condition. ECG, neuromuscular alterations, and metabolic acidosis should be assessed for, because they are likely to develop in clients with hyperkalemia. 1, II. Fluid & Electrolytes.

5. ① Edema is caused by Na^+ and water retention. If therapy for edema is effective, weight loss should occur as excess body water is lost. 5, II. Fluid & Electrolytes.

6. ② An arterial pH 7.54 is indicative of alkalosis. Based on the client's history, the alkalosis was most likely caused by hyperventilation, which causes too much CO_2 to be excreted. CO_2 combines with water to form carbonic acid and when CO_2 is lost in excess, an acid deficit develops. 2, I & II. Fluid & Electrolytes.

7. ③ A rebreathing mask forces the client to inhale CO_2 that was exhaled, thus replacing a source of body acid. This is usually effective and thus eliminates the need for drug therapy. 4, II. Fluid & Electrolytes.

BIBLIOGRAPHY

CARDIOVASCULAR

Black, J., and Matassarin-Jacobs, E., eds. (1993). *Luckmann and Sorensen's medical/surgical nursing: A psychophysiologic approach.* Philadelphia: W. B. Saunders.

Burrell, L. O. (1992). *Adult nursing in hospital and community settings.* Norwalk, CT: Appleton & Lange.

Cohen, J., Pantaleo, N., and Shell, W. (1982). What isoenzymes tell you about your cardiac patient. *Nursing 82* (April): 47–49.

Cromwell, V., Huey, R., Korn, R., Weiss, J., and Woodley, R. (1980). Understanding the needs of your coronary artery bypass patients. *Nursing 80* (March) 10: 34–40.

Johanson, B. C., Dungca, C. U., Hoffmeister, D., and Wells, S. J. (1985). *Standards for critical care,* 2nd ed. St. Louis: C. V. Mosby.

Kern, L. and Gawlinski, A. (1983). Stage-managing coronary artery disease. *Nursing 83* 4 (13): 34–40.

Kinney, M. R., Packa, D. R., Andreoli, K. G., and Zipes, D. P. (1991). *Comprehensive cardiac care,* 7th ed. St. Louis: Mosby-Year Book.

Kinney, M. R., Packa, D. R., and Dunbar, S. B. (1988). *AACN's clinical reference for critical care nursing,* 2nd ed. St. Louis: Mosby-Year Book.

Lewis, S. M., and Collier, I. C. (1987). *Medical-surgical nursing: Assessment and management of clinical problems,* 2nd ed. New York: McGraw-Hill.

Malseed, R. T. (1982). *Pharmacology: Drug therapy and nursing considerations.* Philadelphia: J. B. Lippincott.

Norton, L., and Conforti, C. (1985). The effects of body position on oxygenation. *Heart and Lung* 14 (1): 45–51.

Penckofer, S., and Holm, K. (1984). Early appraisal of coronary revascularization on quality of life. *Nursing Research* 33 (2): 60–63.

Phipps, W., Long, B., and Woods, N. (1987). *Medical surgical nursing: Concepts and clinical practice,* 3rd ed. St. Louis: C. V. Mosby.

Spenser, R. T., Nichols, L. W., Waterhouse, H. P., West, F. M., and Bankert, E. G. (1983). *Clinical pharmacology and nursing management.* Philadelphia: J. B. Lippincott.

Ulrich, S. P., Canale, S. W., and Wendell, S. A. (1986). *Nursing care planning guides: A nursing diagnosis approach.* Philadelphia: W. B. Saunders.

HEMORRHAGIC DISORDERS: SHOCK

Barrett, J., and Nyhus, L. (1986). *Treatment of shock,* 2nd ed. Philadelphia: Lea and Febiger.

Barrows, J. (1982). Shock demands drugs. *Nursing 82* 12 (2): 34–41.

Beckwith, N., and Carriere, S. (1985). Fluid resuscitation in trauma. *Journal of Emergency Nursing* 11 (6): 293–299.

Guzzetta, C., and Dossey, B. (1984). *Cardiovascular nursing: Bodymind tapestry.* St. Louis: C. V. Mosby.

Johnson, B., Dungca, C., Hoffmeister, D., and Wells, S. (1985). *Standards for critical care,* 2nd ed. St. Louis: C. V. Mosby.

Klein, D. (1984). Shock: Physiology, signs and symptoms. *Nursing 84,* 44–46.

Kneisl, C., and Ames, S. (1986). *Adult health nursing: A biopsychosocial approach.* Menlo Park, CA: Addison-Wesley.

Luckmann, J., and Sorensen, K. (1987). *Medical-surgical nursing: A psychophysiologic approach.* 3rd ed. Philadelphia: W. B. Saunders.

Moorhouse, M., Geissler, A., and Doenges, M. (1987). *Critical care plans: Guidelines for patient care.* Philadelphia: F. A. Davis.

Phipps, W., Long, B., and Woods, N. (1987). *Medical-surgical nursing: Concepts and clinical practice,* 3rd ed. St. Louis: C. V. Mosby.

Rice, V. (1984). Shock management. Part I: Fluid volume replacement. *Critical Care Nurse* 4 (6): 69–82.

Rice, V. (1985). Shock management. Part II: Pharmacologic intervention. *Critical Care Nurse* 5 (1): 42–57.

Scherer, J. (1985). *Lippincott's nurses' drug manual.* Philadelphia: J. B. Lippincott.

CARDIOPULMONARY RESUSCITATION

National Conference on Cardiopulmonary Resuscitation and Emergency Cardiac Care. (1992). New recommendations for CPR and ECC. *Journal of the American Medical Association* 268 (16): 2172–2183.

PULMONARY

Rau, J. L. (1989). *Respiratory care pharmacology.* Chicago: Yearbook Medical.

Dettenmeier, P. A. (1992). *Pulmonary nursing care.* St. Louis: Mosby-Year Book.

Keraten, L. D. (1989). *Comprehensive respiratory nursing: A decision making approach.* Philadelphia: W. B. Saunders.

Mitchell, R. S., Petty, T. L., and Schwarz, M. I. (1989). *Synopsis of clinical pulmonary disease.* St. Louis: C. V. Mosby.

Weinberger, S. E. (1992). *Principles of pulmonary medicine.* Philadelphia: W. B. Saunders.

Traver, G. A., Mitchell, J. T., and Flodquist-Priestly, G. (1991). *Respiratory care: A clinical approach.* Baltimore: Aspen.

Wilkins, R. L., Sheldon, R. L., and Krider, S. J. (1990). *Clinical assessment in respiratory care.* St. Louis: C. V. Mosby.

DISEASES OF THE BLOOD

Anderson, M. G. (1991). The lymphomas and multiple myeloma. In S. B. Baird, ed., *A cancer source book for nurses* (6th ed.) (pp. 286–295). Atlanta: American Cancer Society.

DeVita, V. T., Jaffe, E. S., Mauch, P., and Longo, D. L. (1989). Lymphocytic lymphomas. In V. T. DeVita, S. Hellmann, and S. A. Rosenberg, eds., *Cancer: Principles and practice of oncology,* 3rd ed. (pp. 1741–1798). Philadelphia: J. B. Lippincott.

Eyre, H. J., and Farver, M. L. (1991). Hodgkin's disease and non-Hodgkin's lymphomas. In A. I. Holleb, D. J. Fink, and G. P. Murphy, eds., *American Cancer Society textbook of clinical oncology* (pp. 377–398). Atlanta: American Cancer Society.

Fialkow, P. J., and Singer, J. W. (1989). Chronic leukemias. In V. T. DeVita, S. Hellman, and S. A. Rosenberg, eds., *Cancer: Principles and practice of oncology,* 3rd ed. (pp. 1836–1852). Philadelphia: J. B. Lippincott.

Grodecki, J. (1991). Malignant lymphoma. In S. E. Otto, ed., *Oncology nursing* (pp. 200–214). Chicago: C. V. Mosby.

Hellman, S., Jaffe, E. S., and DeVita, V. T. (1989). Hodgkin's disease. In V. T. DeVita, S. Hellman, and S. A. Rosenberg, eds., *Cancer: Principles and practice of oncology,* 3rd ed. (pp. 1696–1740). Philadelphia: J. B. Lippincott.

Jedlow, C. R. (1991). Leukemia. In S. B. Baird, ed., *A cancer source book for nurses,* 6th ed. (pp. 276–285). Atlanta: American Cancer Society.

Meili, L. (1991). Leukemia. In S. E. Otto, ed., *Oncology nursing* (pp. 215–244). Chicago: C. V. Mosby.

Mitus, A. J., and Rosenthal, D. S. (1991). Adult leukemias. In A. I. Holleb, D. J. Fink, and G. P. Murphy, eds., *American Cancer Society textbook of clinical oncology* (pp. 410–432). Atlanta: American Cancer Society.

Schilter, L., and Rossman, E. (1991). Bone marrow transplantation. In S. B. Baird, ed., *A cancer source book for nurses,* 6th ed. (pp. 91–98). Atlanta: American Cancer Society.

Wiernik, P. H. (1989). Acute leukemias. In V. T. DeVita, S. Hellman, and S. A. Rosenberg, eds., *Cancer: Principles and practice of oncology,* 3rd ed. (pp. 1809–1835). Philadelphia: J. B. Lippincott.

Wujcik, D. (1990). Leukemia. In S. L. Groenwald, M. H. Frogge, M. Goodman, and C. H. Yarbro, eds., *Cancer nursing: Principles and practice,* 2nd ed. (pp. 930–950). Boston: Jones & Bartlett.

Yarbro, C. H., ed. (1990). Adult leukemia. *Seminars in Oncology Nursing,* 6 (1).

Yarbro, C. H. (1990). Lymphomas. In S. L. Groenwald, M. H. Frogge, M. Goodman, and C. H. Yarbro, eds., *Cancer nursing: Principles and practice,* 2nd ed. (pp. 974–989). Boston: Jones & Bartlett.

FLUID AND ELECTROLYTES

Barta, M. (1987). Correcting electrolyte imbalances. *RN* 50 (2): 30–34.

Benner, B., Coe, F. L., and Rector, F. C. Jr. (1987). *Renal physiology in health and disease.* Philadelphia: W. B. Saunders.

Black, J., and Matassarin-Jacobs, E., eds. (1993). *Luckmann and Sorensen's medical/surgical nursing: A psychophysiologic approach,* 4th ed. Philadelphia: W. B. Saunders.

Cardin, S. (1980). Acid–base balance in the patient with respiratory disease. *Nursing Clinics of North America* 15 (3): 593–600.

Chenevey, B. (1987). Overview of fluids and electrolytes. *Nursing Clinics of North America,* 22: 749–850.

DuBose, T. (1983). Clinical approach to patients with acid–base disorders. *Medical Clinics of North America* 67 (4): 799–813.

Felver, L. (1980). Understanding the electrolyte maze. *American Journal of Nursing* 80 (9): 1591–1595.

Govani, L., and Hayes, J. (1985). *Drugs and nursing implications.* Norwalk, CT: Appleton-Century-Crofts.

Guyton, A. C. (1991). *Textbook of medical physiology,* 8th ed. Philadelphia: W. B. Saunders.

Halpern, M. L., and Goldstein, M. B. (1988). *Fluid, electrolyte, and acid–base emergencies.* Philadelphia: W. B. Saunders.

Herlihy, B., and Herlihy, J. (1987). Physiologic role and regulation of potassium. *Critical Care Nurse,* 7 (5): 10–14.

Menzel, L. (1980). Clinical problems of electrolyte balance. *Nursing Clinics of North America* 15 (3): 559–575.

Metheny, N., and Snively, W. (1983). *Nurses' handbook of fluid balance.* New York: J. B. Lippincott.

Rice, V. (1982). The role of potassium in health and disease. *Critical Care Nurse* (May/June): 54–74.

Romanski, S. (1986). Interpreting ABG's in four easy steps. *Nursing 86* 16 (9): 58–64.

Stroot, V., Lee, C., and Barrett, C. (1986). *Fluids and electrolytes: A practical approach.* Philadelphia: F. A. Davis.

5

Sensory/Perceptual Functions in the Adult Client

PRE-TEST Neurological Disorders

1. Your client is scheduled for a cerebral arteriogram to rule out carotid stenosis. Which of the following is NOT an important assessment post-test?
   1. Circulation and sensation distal to insertion site
   2. Symptoms of a cerebral embolus
   3. Presence of a headache
   4. Hematoma formation at the insertion site

2. In preparing a client for an EEG, before the test the nurse should:
   1. Sedate the client
   2. Wash the client's hair
   3. Administer phenytoin (Dilantin) as ordered
   4. Keep the client awake for 48 hours

3. Your client is suspected of having increased intracranial pressure. Which of the following is a common clinical manifestation of this condition?
   1. Decreased pulse pressure
   2. Tachycardia
   3. Hypothermia
   4. Projectile vomiting

4. Which of the following is CONTRAINDICATED in the client with increased intracranial pressure?
   1. Elevating the head of the bed 15 to 30 degrees
   2. Avoiding Valsalva maneuver
   3. Providing a footboard to prevent footdrop
   4. Avoiding neck flexion

5. In administering a tube feeding to an unconscious client, the nurse should:
   1. Lower the head of the bed
   2. Test for tube placement by immersing the end of the tube in water
   3. Administer tube feedings at room temperature
   4. Administer at least 3 L of feeding per day

6. Which of the following is a correct nursing intervention for a client who has had a supratentorial craniotomy?
   1. Elevate the head of the bed 30 degrees
   2. Take only oral temperatures
   3. Administer analgesics as ordered
   4. Position client on operative side

7. Which of the following is appropriate nursing care for a client who has had an infratentorial craniotomy?
   1. Elevate the head of the bed 45 degrees
   2. Position on sides first 24 hours, not back

3. Suction nasally as needed
4. Apply heat for periocular edema

8. Which of the following is NOT a risk factor for cerebrovascular accidents?
   1. Hypertension
   2. Diabetes mellitus
   3. Peripheral vascular disease
   4. Chronic bronchitis

9. Your client is suffering from a cerebrovascular accident (CVA) as a result of a thrombus. Which of the following is appropriate care for this client?
   1. Cough and deep breathe hourly
   2. Use a footboard for isometric exercises
   3. Administer warfarin (Coumadin) as ordered
   4. Position the client flat in bed

10. Which of the following is NOT a vital assessment to make on the client with a spinal cord injury?
    1. Loss of perspiration below level of injury
    2. Ability to speak
    3. Presence of spontaneous respirations
    4. Level of loss of sensation

11. Your client has had a spinal cord injury and is suffering from autonomic dysreflexia. Which of the following would NOT be a symptom of dysreflexia?
    1. Severe headache
    2. Rapidly increasing blood pressure
    3. Profuse sweating
    4. Tachycardia

12. Which of the following is NOT an effective preventive measure to prevent the occurrence of autonomic dysreflexia?
    1. Maintain the client in a prone position
    2. Prevent bladder distention
    3. Maintain a bowel regime
    4. Prevent pressure sores

13. Which of the following would NOT be a treatment for autonomic dysreflexia?
    1. Relieving bladder distention
    2. Keeping the client flat in bed
    3. Administering ganglionic blocking agents as ordered
    4. Removing pressure from lower extremities

14. Your client is suffering from Parkinson's disease. Which of the following is a common clinical manifestation of this disease?
    1. Increased perspiration and salivation
    2. Diarrhea and nausea
    3. Tremors at rest
    4. Muscle weakness

15. Your client is started on carbidopa (Sinemet) to control the symptoms of Parkinson's. Which of the following would NOT be considered a side effect of this drug?
    1. Nausea and vomiting
    2. Ataxia
    3. Orthostatic hypotension
    4. Urinary frequency
16. Your client is suffering from multiple sclerosis. Which of the following is NOT considered a clinical manifestation of this disease?
    1. Nonintentional tremors
    2. Diplopia
    3. Nystagmus
    4. Scanning speech
17. Martin is an 18-year-old admitted with a diagnosis of epilepsy. Martin exhibits brief lapses of consciousness and vacant stares. The nurse knows that he is exhibiting what type of seizures?
    1. Grand mal
    2. Petit mal (absence)
    3. Jacksonian
    4. Psychomotor
18. If Martin has a severe seizure in his bed, which of the following is a priority for the nurse to do for this client?
    1. Observe the characteristics of the seizure
    2. Monitor the client's vital signs
    3. Protect the client's head
    4. Note the duration of the seizure
19. Martin is started on phenytoin (Dilantin). Which of the following is a common side effect of Dilantin?
    1. Constipation
    2. Hyperalertness
    3. Loss of color vision
    4. Gum hyperplasia

PRE-TEST Answers and Rationales

1. ③ A headache is neither a common finding nor a sign of serious problems. The other options contain important findings post–cerebral angiogram. There is a risk of a stroke after this test, and also bleeding at the insertion site. 1, I & II. Cerebral Arteriogram.

2. ② An EEG requires a clean, oil-free surface for recording electrical activity of the brain. The nurse must wash the client's hair so it is clean and oil free. The client should not be sedated and phenytoin (Dilantin) is often withheld so maximal seizure activity can be recorded. Sometimes the client is kept awake for 24 hours, but not 48 hours. 4, II. EEG.

3. ④ Increased intracranial pressure is characterized by increased pulse pressure, bradycardia, and hyperthermia plus projectile vomiting. 1 & 2, II. Increased Intracranial Pressure.

4. ③ When a client is experiencing increased intracranial pressure, it is important to avoid activities that would increase that pressure. A footboard would increase the likelihood that the client would perform isometric exercises, which would increase intracranial pressure. All other options help to prevent an increase in pressure, and choice 1 also helps to increase venous drainage, which can help lower the pressure. 4, II. Increased Intracranial Pressure.

5. ③ Tube feedings should always be administered at room temperature because if the feeding is hot or cold it can cause cramping or regurgitation. The head of the bed should be elevated to prevent regurgitation and aspiration. Tube placement should never be assessed by immersion in water, and only 2 L of feeding are given daily. 4, II. Unconscious Client/Tube Feedings.

6. ① With a supratentorial craniotomy, the head of the bed should be elevated 30 degrees to allow for venous drainage. The client should be positioned on the unaffected side to prevent shifting. Oral temperatures should never be taken and analgesics would not be given because they may mask changes in level of consciousness. 4, II. Intracranial Surgery.

7. ② With an infratentorial craniotomy, the client must be positioned flat in bed on either side, not on the back, for the first 24 hours. Neck flexion must be avoided. Use ice only for periorbital edema and never suction nasally. 4, II. Intracranial Surgery.

8. ④ Chronic bronchitis is not a risk factor for cerebrovascular accident (CVA). The other options are all risk factors for strokes. 1 & 2, II. CVA.

9. ③ When a CVA results from a thrombus, anticoagulants such as warfarin (Coumadin) are used to help prevent additional clots. Coughing and deep breathing, isometrics, and positioning flat in bed all increase intracranial pressure and so should be avoided. 4, II. CVA.

10. ② When a client suffers a spinal cord injury, it is important to determine the level of injury so that probable complications can be anticipated. Loss of speech is more likely to occur with head injury than spinal injury. The others are vital assessments to be made by the nurse. 1, II. Spinal Cord Injuries.

11. ④ Bradycardia, not tachycardia, is a symptom of autonomic dysreflexia. The other options contain common symptoms of autonomic dysreflexia. 1 & 2, II. Spinal Cord Injuries.

12. ① If the client is prone, there is likely to be pressure on the penis or catheter, which leads to dysreflexia. The other options are appropriate ways to prevent autonomic dysreflexia from occurring. 4, I & II. Spinal Cord Injuries.

13. ② Treatment for autonomic dysreflexia includes removing the cause, administering ganglionic blocking agents, and elevating the head of the bed to decrease the hypertension. 4, I & II. Spinal Cord Injuries.

14. ③ The tremors associated with Parkinson's disease are nonintentional or rest tumors. Clients may also exhibit constipation, decreased perspiration and salivation, and muscle rigidity. 1 & 2, II. Parkinson's Disease.

15. ④ Urinary retention is not a side effect of carbidopa (Sinemet). All of the other options are typical side effects of Sinemet. 1, II. Parkinson's Disease.

16. ① The tremors associated with multiple sclerosis are intentional, not

nonintentional, tremors that increase with movement. Diplopia, nystagmus, and scanning speech are typical symptoms of MS. 1 & 2, II. Multiple Sclerosis.

17. ② A petit mal (absence) seizure is a momentary loss of consciousness often seen as a lapse of attention. The other options are other types of seizures. 1 & 2, II. Epilepsy.

18. ③ The most important action is to protect the client's head and maintain a patent airway. The other options are important for the nurse to do, but they are not the priority actions. 4, I & II. Epilepsy.

19. ④ A side effect of phenytoin (Dilantin) is gum hyperplasia. This is a very distressing side effect for most clients, requiring ongoing oral care. The other options are not side effects of Dilantin. 1 & 2, II. Epilepsy.

NORMAL NERVOUS SYSTEM

I. Central nervous system
  A. Brain
  B. Spinal cord
II. Peripheral nervous system
  A. Somatic (voluntary)
  B. Visceral (involuntary)
    1. Afferent
    2. Efferent (autonomic nervous system)
      a. Parasympathetic nervous system
      b. Sympathetic nervous system
III. The functions of the nervous system are to receive stimuli, interpret them at various levels, and transmit them for action; nervous system responsible for an individual's perception of his or her environment

NURSING PROCESS APPLIED TO ADULTS WITH NEUROLOGICAL DISORDERS

Trauma

Head Injury
I. Assessment
  A. Definition: mild to extensive damage transmitted to brain tissue as result of mechanical force resulting in various degrees of injuries
  B. Types of injuries
    1. Open head: interruption in
      a. Scalp
      b. Skull (fractures)
      c. Dura
    2. Closed head: nonpenetrating
      a. Concussion: mild
      b. Contusion
      c. Hematoma
        (1) Epidural (arterial bleed)
        (2) Subdural (venous bleed)
  C. Incidence
    1. 90% of nervous system trauma
    2. Majority less than 35 years old
    3. Males outnumber females
  D. Predisposing/precipitating factors
    1. Accidents: motor vehicle, industrial
    2. Falls, abuse
    3. Blows: sports injuries, crime-related injuries
    4. Construction: occupational hazards
  E. Clinical manifestations: dependent upon injury; usually result of increased intracranial pressure (IICP)
    1. Level of consciousness: varying degrees
      a. Alert: oriented
      b. Confused: disoriented
      c. Lethargic: obtunded
      d. Comatose: various levels
    2. Pupillary response: affected side
      a. Unilateral dilation
      b. Sluggish reaction to light
      c. Nonreactive
      d. Fixed
    3. Papilledema
    4. Visual disturbance
      a. Blurred
      b. Diplopia
    5. Extraocular movements (EOM)
    6. Vital signs
      a. Blood pressure: increased
      b. Pulse pressure: widening
      c. Pulse: decreased
      d. Respirations: decreased, irregular
      e. Temperature: elevated
    7. Motor function
      a. Extraocular movements not intact
      b. Weakness—flaccid, paresis
      c. Paralysis of limbs; extremities
        (1) Monoplegia
        (2) Hemiplegia

d. Posture
    (1) Decorticate
    (2) Decerebrate
8. Sensory function
    a. Decreased sensation: paresthesia
    b. Absence of feeling
9. Reflex activity
    a. Corneal: decreased, absent
    b. Gag: decreased, absent
    c. Babinski: positive, present
    d. Deep tendon (DTR): hyper, hypoactive
10. Headache
11. Nausea and vomiting
12. Seizure activity
    a. Focal
    b. Generalized
F. Diagnostic examinations (Table 5–1)

G. Complications
    1. Cerebral bleeding
    2. Hematomas
    3. Uncontrolled IICP
    4. Infections
    5. Seizures
II. Analysis
    A. Altered tissue perfusion: cerebral related to decreased cerebral arterial blood flow
    B. Altered sensory perceptions related to cerebral trauma
    C. Impaired physical mobility related to trauma
III. Planning/goals, expected outcomes
    A. Client will have tissue perfusion to the brain
    B. Client will breathe unassisted
    C. Client will be oriented to person, place, and time
    D. Client will have pre-injury cognitive function

TABLE 5–1 Diagnostic Tests—Neurological Dysfunctions

Test	Diagnostic Purpose	Specific Preparation	Nursing Care Post-Test
Skull x-ray	Fractures, space-occupying lesions	Explain procedure; no specific preparation	No specific care
Scans (CT) 20–45 minutes	Space-occupying lesions, brain contusions, brain atrophy, hydrocephalus, infections	Explain procedure; lying still and flat on table; hold breath when requested; IV injection of dye when used (ask if allergic to iodine or shellfish); written consent when using dye	Observe allergic response; push fluids to eliminate dye if used
NMR—MRI (noninvasive) 30 minutes	Neoplasms, vascular abnormalities, hemorrhage	Explain procedure; no specific preparation	No specific care
Angiography (invasive) 30–45 minutes	Vascular abnormalities; displacement of vessels caused by hematoma, abscesses, tumors	Explain procedure; obtain written consent; lying still; local veins shelter area surrounding artery to be injected; ask if allergic to iodine or shellfish; hydrate 2 days before test; NPO for 6 to 12 hours; established baseline neuro assessments; premedication	Neuro assessment every 15 to 30 minutes until VS stable; elevate head of bed 15 to 30 degrees only; bedrest 24 hours; assess pulses (distal): subclavian, brachial, carotid; bed flat when femoral artery is used; immobilize puncture site for 6 to 8 hours; apply ice to the site; observe for signs, symptoms of complications; push fluids
Lumbar puncture (invasive) (15 minutes)	Measure CSF pressure; infections, hemorrhage, neoplasms; contraindicated for IICP and brainstem herniation	Explain procedure; obtain written consent; L3 L4 or L4 L5 site of puncture; lateral recumbent position	Neuro assessment; push fluids for 48 hours; monitor I & O
Myelography (invasive) 1 hour	Detect abnormalities of cord or vertebrae; locate obstruction of CSF flow (herniated disc, neoplasm, abscess)	Explain procedure; obtain written consent; NPO 4–6 hours; pre-test; ask if allergic to iodine; premedication to sedate; post-test; same as LP (#5)	Neuro assessment every 2 hours for 24 hours; position: pantopaque (oil base) *flat* 6 to 24 hours; metrizamide (water base) elevate head of bed 15 to 30 degrees for 8 hours; analgesics for headache; push fluids; monitor I & O; assess for distended bladder; complications
EEG (noninvasive) 45–60 minutes	Epilepsy, tumors, hematomas, abscesses, drug overdose, determine brain death	Explain procedure and that it is painless; clean hair; stimulants and alcohol withheld 24 hours prior; may have breakfast; premedication to sedate	Wash hair; provide restful environment; side rails up if sedated

E. Client will not develop complications of IICP
F. Client will have increased self-esteem
IV. Implementation
  A. Establish baseline neurological assessment
  B. Establish and maintain an open airway
    1. Insert oral airway if necessary
    2. Prevent neck flexion
    3. Monitor vital signs
    4. Turn client every 2 hours
    5. Suction as needed only if necessary
  C. Control bleeding, if any
  D. Monitor, assess, evaluate neurological status in terms of baseline
    1. Level of consciousness
      a. Reorient to person, place, and time
      b. Call by familiar name
    2. Vital signs
    3. Pupillary signs, EOM
    4. Motor and sensory response
    5. Cranial nerve function
    6. Reflexes
  E. Control intracranial pressure (ICP)
    1. ICP monitoring, if done
    2. Elevate head of bed 30 degrees
    3. Prevent flexion of neck and hips
    4. Avoid Valsalva maneuver
    5. Avoid straining activities—coughing, sneezing, bending
    6. Limit unnecessary talking about condition of client
    7. Provide periods of rest
    8. Offer reassurance and use therapeutic touch
    9. Administer appropriate medications
      a. Osmotic diuretics—mannitol (Osmitrol) (Table 5–2)
      b. Corticosteroids—dexamethasone (Decadron) (Table 5–3)
      c. Anticonvulsants—phenytoin (Dilantin) (Table 5–4)
      d. Ranitidine (Zantac) (Table 5–5)
  F. Limit fluid intake
  G. Maintain accurate I & O
  H. Maintain quiet environment
  I. Provide passive exercises, provide range of motion (ROM)
  J. Administer daily hygiene
  K. Insert foley catheter if necessary
V. Evaluation
  A. Client has patent airway
  B. Client does not have symptoms of IICP
  C. Client's neurological status stable
    1. States name, time, and location
    2. Vital signs stable
  D. Client asks for family, significant other
  E. Client's skin clean, dry, and without breakdown
  F. Client does range of motion

Spinal Cord Injury
I. Assessment
  A. Definition: fracture or displacement of one or more vertebrae with or without concurrent trauma to the spinal cord itself: if cord involved, there are alterations in sensory and motor function below this level
  B. Types of injuries
    1. Flexion
    2. Rotational
    3. Lateral
    4. Compression
    5. Hyperextension
  C. Incidence
    1. About 10,000 to 20,000 annually
    2. Younger age groups
  D. Predisposing/precipitating factors
    1. Trauma—automobile and motorcycle accidents, falls, diving injuries, sports injuries
    2. Infectious diseases

TABLE 5–2 Osmotic Diuretics

Example	Action	Use	Common Side Effects	Nursing Implications
Mannitol (Osmitrol)	Increase osmotic pressure of glomerular filtrate; inhibit reabsorption of water; increase excretion of water, sodium, potassium, calcium, chloride, phosphorus, magnesium, urea, and uric acid	To treat renal failure, increased intracranial or intraocular pressure, and to promote excretion of certain toxic substances	Transient volume expansion, hyponatremia or hypernatremia, hypokalemia, tachycardia, thirst, nausea and vomiting, phlebitis	Monitor vital signs, urine output, CVP, and pulmonary artery pressure prior to and hourly after administration; assess for signs and symptoms of dehydration; monitor neurological status; monitor serum electrolytes; assess client for nausea and vomiting, muscle weakness, numbness, confusion, thirst; infuse dose over 30 to 60 minutes with increased intracranial pressure

TABLE 5–3 Anti-Inflammatories

Class	Example	Action	Use	Common Side Effects	Nursing Implications
Steroids	Cortisone acetate (Cortistan), dexamethasone (Decadron)	Block inflammatory, allergic, and immune responses, as do glucocorticoids	To treat a wide variety of inflammatory, autoimmune/allergic disorders, to replace natural glucocorticoids	Na^+ and water retention; GI ulceration, hypertension, CHF, delayed wound healing, protein breakdown, osteoporosis, cataracts, leukopenia, diabetes, hypokalemia	Warn patient to avoid infections; increased need during stress and illness; monitor for Addison's disease; give with antacids; use low salt, high potassium diet; teach patient not to stop taking drug without doctor's approval
Nonsteroidal	Ibuprofen (Motrin)	Act by inhibiting prostaglandin synthesis	To reduce inflammation of arthritis and other disorders	Prolonged bleeding time, edema, tinnitus, GI distress, rash	Avoid in patients with ulcers or asthma; teach that it takes weeks to reach full effect; give with food or milk; watch for side effects

3. Malignancy
4. Aging and osteoporosis
5. Herniated nucleus pulposa
6. Congenital defects—spina bifida

E. Clinical manifestations (Figure 5–1)
   1. Loss of sensation below level of injury
   2. Respiratory distress if high fracture
   3. Cardiac abnormalities
   4. Loss of sweating below level of injury with loss of thermal control
   5. Unpredictable autonomic responses
   6. Loss of vasomotor tone below level of injury with marked reduction of blood pressure
   7. Pain
   8. Loss of bowel and bladder control
   9. Loss of reflexes below level of injury

F. Diagnostic examinations
   1. Complete neurological examination
   2. Spinal x-rays
   3. CT scan of spine
   4. Search for other injuries

G. Complications
   1. Death

TABLE 5–4 Anticonvulsants

Example	Action	Use	Common Side Effects	Nursing Implications
Hydantoins: phenytoin (Dilantin)	Decrease nerve cell excitability in various ways	To treat epilepsy and other seizure disorders	GI irritation, dizziness, apathy, nervousness, ataxia, gingival hyperplasia, blurred vision, nystagmus, insomnia, irritability, diarrhea, depression, liver damage	Teach client to comply with consistent medication regime; avoid use of alcohol; warn client about drowsiness or decreased alertness; give with meals to decrease GI distress; monitor for rash or other signs of allergy; consider risk to pregnant women and fetus and use vitamin K prophylactically to increase clotting before delivery; warn client urine may be pink or reddish brown; use with caution in elderly or with clients with impaired renal or liver function, hypotension, MI, or CHF; do not let client switch brands of phenytoin; wear Medic Alert tag

TABLE 5–5 Histamine H$_2$ Receptor Antagonist

Example	Action	Use	Common Side Effects	Nursing Implications
Cimetidine (Tagamet), ranitidine (Zantac), nizatidine (Axid), famotidine (Pepcid)	Decrease gastric acid secretion, total acidity, and pepsin activity	To prevent and treat duodenal ulcers; reduce gastric acid secretion and concentration; prevent stress ulcers; prevent ulcer recurrence	Diarrhea, dizziness, rash, gynecomastia, alopecia, neutropenia, impotence, bradycardia, headache; not safe for long-term use in pregnancy or lactation	Do not give within 1 hour of antacids; decrease dosage in patients with renal failure; relapse following therapy may occur; monitor for relief of symptoms; does not cause rebound acidity when discontinued; may potentiate oral anticoagulants; may increase the half-life of diazepam

2. Respiratory failure
3. Permanent paralysis
4. Autonomic dysreflexia
5. Spinal shock
6. Further damage to cord

II. Analysis
   A. Altered sensory perception related to trauma to spinal cord
   B. Impaired physical mobility related to neurological impairment

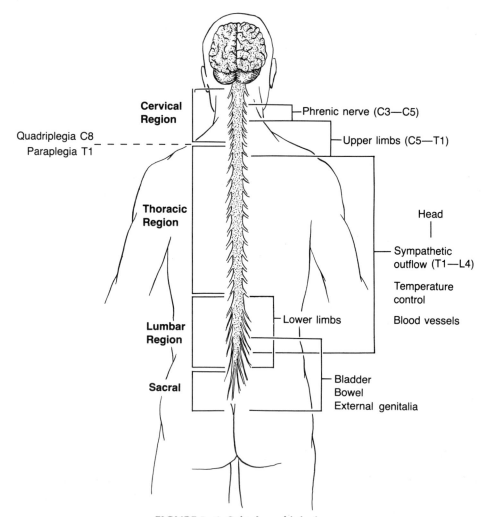

FIGURE 5–1. Spinal cord injuries.

C. Powerlessness related to immobility and difficulty in performing self-care

D. Fear related to effects of loss of body part or function

III. Planning/goals, expected outcomes

A. Client will not suffer further injury to spinal cord

B. Client will not develop respiratory distress

C. Client will not suffer from undetected spinal shock

D. Client will not develop autonomic dysreflexia

E. Client will not develop complications of immobility

F. Client will adapt to loss

IV. Implementation

A. Maintain spine in stable position from time of injury on

B. Log-roll client

C. Use special turning beds—Stryker frame, Roto bed

D. Apply traction as needed—Crutchfield, Gardner tongs, halo traction

E. Prepare for decompression laminectomy

F. Administer dexamethasone (Decadron) or mannitol as ordered (see Tables 5–2, 5–3)

G. Monitor respiratory status
   1. Suction as needed
   2. Prepare for intubation and ventilation as needed

H. Assess for and treat spinal shock
   1. Occurs within first hour and lasts days or months
   2. Major manifestations: hypotension, respiratory difficulty, flaccid paralysis, bladder and bowel atony, absence of perspiration
   3. Administer vasopressors, plasma expanders, and analgesics as ordered

I. Monitor fluid and electrolyte balance

J. Prevent autonomic dysreflexia
   1. Prevent bowel and bladder distention
   2. Monitor urinary drainage for obstruction
   3. Prevent pressure sores
   4. Avoid pain or unnecessary pressure below level of injury, especially to penis or testes while male clients prone

K. Assess for autonomic dysreflexia, occurs after several months
   1. Malignant hypertension
   2. Bradycardia
   3. Severe throbbing headache
   4. Flushing and profuse perspiration
   5. Goose flesh

L. Treat autonomic dysreflexia
   1. Identify and remove cause
   2. Elevate head of bed
   3. Administer ganglionic blocking agents, reserpine

M. Administer tube feedings as ordered

N. Prevent complications of immobility (see Chapter 7)

O. Provide emotional support as needed

P. Arrange for counseling or group support as needed

V. Evaluations

A. Client suffers no further injury to spinal cord

B. Client does not develop respiratory distress

C. Client has spinal shock successfully treated

D. Client does not develop autonomic dysreflexia

E. Client does not develop complications of immobility

F. Client adapts to loss

Meningitis

I. Assessment

A. Definition: infection of meninges (pia, arachnoid, and subarachnoid space) caused by a bacterial, viral, or fungal organism

B. Incidence
   1. Bacterial
      a. Pneumococcus, meningococcus, hemophilus
      b. Children: 3 months to 3 years, teenagers
      c. Over age 40: pneumococcus
      d. Serious
   2. Viral
      a. Virus
      b. Children: 2 months to 6 years (90%)
      c. All age groups
      d. Not fatal
   3. Fungal: cryptococcal

C. Predisposing/precipitating factors
   1. Immunoglobulin deficiency
   2. Radiation therapy
   3. Immunosuppression
   4. Debilitation
   5. Malnutrition
   6. Infections in other parts of body
   7. Malignancy of reticuloendothelial system
   8. Crowded conditions, poor hygiene

D. Clinical manifestations: dependent on type of meningitis (*indicates most common)
   *1. Headache
   *2. Fever with chills, temperature elevated 104°F to 105°F (40°C to 40.5°C)
   *3. Nausea and vomiting
   *4. Decreased level of consciousness
      a. Confusion
      b. Irritability
   *5. Signs of meningeal irritation
      a. Positive Kernig's sign
      b. Positive Brudzinski's sign
      c. Stiff neck, nuchal rigidity

d. Opisthotonos position
6. Photophobia
7. Seizure activity
8. Petechial rash
9. Cranial nerve dysfunction
10. Signs of IICP
E. Diagnostic examinations (see Table 5–1)
1. History and physical
2. Skull x-ray
3. Cerebrospinal fluid examination
a. Color—turbid
b. Protein elevated
c. Pressure increased
F. Complications
1. Headache
2. Seizure activity
3. Deafness
4. Paresis
5. Paralysis
II. Analysis
A. High risk for infection related to invading organisms
B. Altered sensory perception related to overwhelming infection decreasing level of consciousness
C. Altered body temperature related to infectious process
III. Planning/goals, expected outcomes
A. Client will have decreased signs of infection
B. Client will not develop respiratory distress
C. Client will show signs of increasing level of consciousness
D. Client will have no signs of complications
E. Client will not develop seizure activity
F. Client/family will comprehend preventive and therapeutic measures
IV. Implementations
A. Establish baseline neurological assessments
B. Maintain patent airway
1. Bedrest
2. Position, turn every 2 hours
3. Suction as needed
4. Oxygen as needed
C. Observe, monitor vital signs
D. Monitor and control temperature
1. Administer antipyretics orally or rectally
2. Cool sponge bath
3. Cool room temperature
4. Hypothermia blanket
5. Antimicrobial drugs as ordered
6. Isolate, if necessary
E. Give daily hygiene
F. Maintain quiet environment
1. Bedrest
2. Offer reassurance, therapeutic touch
3. Avoid stimulation
4. Control environmental noise

G. Relieve pain
1. Administer analgesics (salicylates, acetaminophen)
2. Quiet environment
3. Elevate head of bed 30 degrees
H. Seizure precautions
1. Airway at bedside
2. Pad siderails, up position
3. Suction, if necessary
I. Diet
1. As tolerated
2. IV fluids, if necessary
3. Strict I & O
4. Oral fluids
a. Increase as tolerated
b. Increase calories, carbohydrates
J. Include family in care
1. Explain all procedures to family/client
2. Communicate client's status
3. Prophylactic antimicrobials for family if necessary
4. Include prevention in discharge plan
V. Evaluation
A. Signs of infection decrease
B. Client's airway patent
C. Client alert and oriented
D. Client has no headache
E. No signs of seizure activity
F. Client taking fluids orally
G. Client expresses interest in learning about prevention and treatment
H. Family involved in care
I. Family/client comprehends prevention, therapeutic, and supportive measures

Brain Tumors

I. Assessment
A. Definition: new growth of tissue (benign or malignant) within brain, space-occupying lesion
B. Incidence: dependent upon type of tumor
1. Cause unknown
2. 2% of yearly cancer deaths
3. Persons affected
a. All ages
b. Peaks
(1) Second half of first decade: 5 to 10 years
(2) 40 to 50 years
4. 12,000 primary brain tumors every year
5. Men more than women
6. Classification—varies
a. Primary (90% originating within cranium)
b. Metastatic (10% originating outside brain)

    c. Histological—degree of malignancy
      (1) Benign
      (2) Malignant (stages I to IV)
- C. Predisposing/precipitating factors
  1. Heredity
  2. Congenital
  3. Immunological deficits
  4. Viruses
  5. Chemical
  6. Radiation
  7. Secondary to cerebral trauma
  8. Toxin
  9. Metastases
- D. Clinical Manifestations: dependent on location and rate of growth (*most common)
  *1. Headache especially early morning
  *2. Nausea and vomiting
  *3. Papilledema
  *4. Signs of IICP
  *5. Dizziness
  *6. Personality changes
  *7. Localized clinical manifestations
    a. Seizure activity
    b. Motor deficits
    c. Sensory deficits
    d. Speech deficits
- E. Diagnostic examinations (see Table 5–1)
  1. History and physical
  2. Visual and fundoscopic examination
  3. Skull x-ray
  4. Electroencephalogram (EEG)
  5. Angiogram
  6. Nuclear magnetic resonance imager (NMRI)
  7. CT scan
- F. Complications
  1. Shock
    a. Hemorrhagic
    b. Hypovolemic
  2. Uncontrolled IICP
  3. Seizures
  4. Infection—meningitis
  5. Residual paralysis, paresthesia
  6. Diabetes insipidus
  7. Complications of immobility
- G. Medical management—alone or in combination
  1. Radiation
  2. Chemotherapy
- H. Surgical management: craniotomy
II. Analysis
- A. Altered thought processes and confusion related to effects of disease process
- B. Impaired physical mobility related to weakness, motor deficits
- C. Chronic pain related to effects of disease process
- D. Self-care deficit: all ADLs related to progressive physical debilitation
- E. Body-image disturbance related to treatment regimen
III. Planning/goals, expected outcomes for craniotomy
- A. Client will maintain patent airway
- B. Client will have stable vital and neurological signs
- C. Client will have no signs of IICP
- D. Client will have minimal drainage from incisional area
- E. Client's pain will be controlled
- F. Client will have no complications of immobility
IV. Implementations
- A. Establish and maintain open airway
  1. Assess vital signs
  2. Prevent neck flexion
  3. Turn every 2 hours
  4. Maintain alignment
  5. Lie on unaffected side
  6. Body position: dependent on type of craniotomy
    a. Supratentorial: elevate head of bed 30 degrees
    b. Infratentorial: position from side to side, not on back
  7. Deep breathe without coughing
- B. Establish baseline neurological assessment
- C. Check dressings for drainage: wet, blood, or cerebrospinal fluid
- D. Monitor, assess, evaluate neurological status in terms of baseline data
  1. Level of consciousness
  2. Vital signs
  3. Pupillary signs plus EOMs, periorbital edema
  4. Motor and sensory response—bilateral
  5. Cranial nerve function
- E. Monitor and control IICP
  1. Monitor ICP lines (4 to 15 mm HG if client has one)
  2. Position properly with head of bed elevated 30 degrees, unaffected side
  3. Prevent flexion and hyperextension of neck
  4. Avoid coughing, straining, Valsalva maneuver, isometric exercises
  5. Monitor fluid and electrolyte balance
  6. Fluid intake limited (1500 to 1800 mL in 24 hours)
  7. Foley catheter
    a. Measure output hourly
    b. Specific gravity hourly
  8. Monitor arterial blood gases for hypoxia and/or hypercapnia

9. Administer appropriate medications as ordered
    a. Dexamethasone (Decadron) IV (see Table 5–3)
    b. Osmotic diuretics, IV mannitol (see Table 5–2)
    c. Phenytoin (Dilantin) to prevent seizures (see Table 5–4)
    d. Ranitidine (Zantac) (see Table 5–5)
10. Control environment
    a. Quiet atmosphere
    b. Reassuring touch

F. Assess for pain and administer analgesic
  1. Codeine as needed
  2. Acetaminophen (Tylenol) as needed
  3. Narcotic analgesics (morphine and meperidine [Demerol]) CONTRAINDICATED; mask symptoms of IICP

G. Administer daily hygiene
  1. Skin care
  2. Mouth care
  3. Log-rolling (if necessary)
  4. Eye care: patches to prevent corneal ulcerations if no blink reflex
  5. ROM, passive exercises

H. Include family in care of client
  1. Keep family informed of condition
  2. Let client/family participate in care, activities, ADLs
  3. Teach client/family ADLs, diet, activity, medication, safety measures
  4. Prepare for discharge
  5. Include social worker, other members of health team
  6. Discuss follow-up care

V. Evaluation
A. Client has patent airway and is off respirator
B. Client afebrile
C. Client's neurological status stable
D. Client's incision clean, dry, approximated, and not inflamed
E. Client states pain relieved
F. Client dangles on side of bed and progresses to chair at bedside
G. Client develops no complications
H. Client/family verbalize fears and concerns
I. Client has positive body image
J. Client/family aware of ADLs and limitations

Strokes (Acute and Chronic)

I. Assessment
A. Definition: syndrome in which cerebral circulation interrupted, causing an onset of various neurological deficits
B. Incidence
  1. 10% of deaths in United States each year
  2. Third leading cause of death (200,000 per year)
  3. 2 million Americans affected each year
  4. Second most common cause of disability
  5. Familial tendencies
  6. More men than women
  7. More African Americans than whites
  8. Age 65 to 85: highest incidence of thrombosis
  9. Younger clients, cerebral hemorrhage

C. Etiology/classification
  1. Thrombus (50%): most common interference in blood supply
    a. Transient ischemic attack (TIA)
    b. Stroke-in-evolution
    c. Completed stroke
  2. Embolus: result of heart disease
  3. Hemorrhage: rupture of vessel
    a. Intracerebral
    b. Aneurysm

D. Predisposing/precipitating factors—multicombination
  1. Hypertension
  2. Smoking
  3. Oral contraceptives
  4. High-risk factors
    a. Stress
    b. Elevated cholesterol, lipoprotein, triglycerides
    c. Obesity
    d. Sedentary work with little exercise
  5. Pre-existing conditions
    a. Heart disease
    b. Atherosclerosis
    c. Arteriovenous malformations
    d. Vasospasm
    e. Aneurysm
    f. Diabetes
    g. Polycythemia vera

E. Clinical manifestations: dependent upon involved area of brain (Figure 5–2)
  1. Headache
  2. Nausea and vomiting
  3. Dizziness, vertigo
  4. Signs of IICP
  5. Seizures
  6. Visual changes
    a. Homonymous or bitemporal hemianopsia (loss of vision in one half of visual field on same side or both temporal sides)
    b. Nystagmus
    c. Diplopia
    d. Blindness
    e. Papilledema
  7. Motor changes

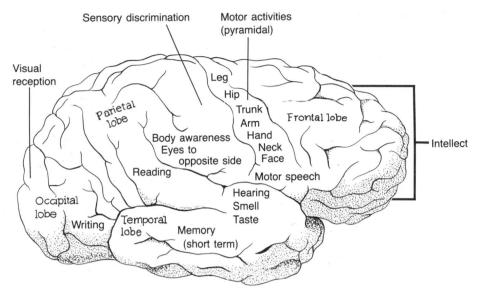

FIGURE 5–2. Brain areas and functions.

a. Paralysis, hemiplegia (side of body opposite cerebral accident)
b. Hemiparesis, (side of body opposite cerebral accident)
c. Ataxia
d. Dysarthria
e. Dysphagia

8. Sensory changes
   a. Decreased sensation (pressure, heat, cold)
   b. Pain
   c. Perceptual deficits (usually left-sided hemiplegia) identifying client or environment
      (1) Apraxia (unable to use objects correctly)
      (2) Right/left orientation

9. Speech changes (usually right-sided hemiplegia)
   a. Aphasia—inability to speak
      (1) Expressive: difficulty expressing self in understandable speech
      (2) Receptive: does not comprehend spoken word or written word
      (3) Global: combination of expressive and receptive aphasia

10. Emotional changes
    a. Labile
    b. Cries easily
    c. Inappropriate laughter
    d. Fear, anger
    e. Withdrawal
    f. Depression

11. Bowel and bladder changes
    a. Urgency
    b. Incontinence
    c. Constipation and fecal impactions
    d. Loose stool

F. Diagnostic examinations (see Table 5–1)
   1. History and physical
   2. Neurological examination
   3. CT scan
   4. NMRI
   5. Cerebral blood flow studies
   6. Angiogram
   7. Lumbar puncture

G. Complications: dependent upon extent of damage and upon management and care given
   1. Alterations in mobility
      a. Contractures, hip flexion
      b. Footdrop
      c. Decubitus ulcers
      d. Respiratory complications
      e. Thrombophlebitis
   2. Residual paralysis, paresthesia
   3. Residual communication problems
   4. Paralytic ileus

II. Analysis
   A. Ineffective breathing pattern related to decreased mobility
   B. High risk for aspiration related to retained secretions, impaired swallowing
   C. Impaired verbal communication related to dysphasia, dysarthria
   D. Impaired physical mobility related to left-, rightsided weakness
   E. Impaired skin integrity related to prolonged immobility

III. Planning/goals, expected outcomes
   A. Acute phase

1. Client will maintain patent airway
2. Client's vital signs and neurological signs will be stable
3. Client will have no signs of IICP
4. Client will have adequate tissue perfusion to brain
5. Client will have minimal pain

B. Chronic phase
   1. Client will be free of skin breakdown
   2. Client will not develop complications of immobility, motor and/or sensory changes
   3. Client will not develop bladder or bowel problems
   4. Client/family will communicate fears and anxieties
   5. Client will function as independently as possible
   6. Client/family will become comfortable and knowledgeable enough to care for client at home
   7. Client/family will become knowledgeable about community resources

IV. Implementations
   A. Acute phase
      1. Establish and maintain open airway
         a. Assess vital signs
         b. Suction as needed, not more than 15 seconds to prevent IICP, never nasally
         c. Administer oxygen per nasal cannula
         d. Position client on side to prevent aspiration
         e. Elevate head of bed 15 to 30 degrees
         f. Turn every two hours
         g. Cough, deep breathe every hour/or chest PT
      2. Establish baseline assessments
      3. Monitor, assess, evaluate neurological status in terms of baseline
         a. Level of consciousness
         b. Pupillary signs, EOMs
         c. Motor and sensory response
         d. Cranial nerve function
         e. Reflexes
      4. Insert Foley catheter if necessary
         a. Monitor
         b. Measure, record output
      5. Administer IVs as ordered
      6. Monitor electrolyte balance
      7. Administer medications as ordered—heparin IV (see Table 4–16)
   B. Post-acute phase—continue above
      1. Give daily hygiene
         a. Skin care
         b. Mouth care
         c. Eye care
         d. ROM, passive exercises

2. Apply support hose
3. Initiate bladder, bowel program
   a. Stool softeners
   b. If Foley catheter out, offer bedpan or assist to commode every 2 hours
4. If conscious, offer fluids
   a. Check gag reflex intact
   b. Sip slowly
   c. Involve family with care
5. Explain procedures

C. Chronic phase
   1. Continue hygienic care
   2. Evaluate vision deficits; provide eye care as needed
   3. Increase mobility as tolerated
      a. Transfer to chair
      b. Wheelchair
      c. Walker
      d. Physical therapy, cane, braces, splints
   4. Teach transfer technique: chair/bed, bed/chair
   5. Encourage independence in ADLs with client
      a. Hygiene
      b. Dressing: affected side first
      c. Toileting: bowel, bladder program, stool softeners
      d. Eating: encourage independence, high-fiber diet, push fluids
      e. Gait training
   6. Encourage client/family to express feelings
   7. Provide emotional and psychological support to client/family
      a. Reassurance
      b. Control environment
      c. Reality orientation
      d. Support in relearning skills
      e. Use therapeutic communication techniques
      f. Establish form of communication system
   8. Refer client/family to appropriate rehabilitation and community resources
      a. Dietician
      b. Physical therapy
      c. Occupational therapy
      d. Speech therapy
      e. Social worker
      f. Home health, Visiting Nurse Association (VNA)

V. Evaluation
   A. Acute phase
      1. Client's airway patent
      2. Client's neurological status stable
      3. Client oriented
   B. Post-acute phase

1. Client aware of environment
2. Client transfers to chair two times each day
3. Client swallows sips of water without difficulty
4. Client transfers to chair alone

C. Chronic phase
   1. Client's skin free of breakdown
   2. Client expresses interest in self-care
   3. Client/family ask for information about referral services
   4. Client discharged to rehabilitation or home

Degenerative Diseases

Parkinson's Disease

I. Assessment
   A. Definition: chronic, degenerative process of neurons of basal ganglia, thalamus, and substantia nigra of brain, which are responsible for control and regulation of movement
   B. Etiology/pathophysiology
      1. Cause unknown
      2. Decrease in dopamine in cells of substantia nigra
      3. Arteriosclerosis: decrease in blood supply to basal ganglia
      4. Inherited genetic deficit
   C. Incidence
      1. Onset insidious and progressive
      2. Affects elderly, age 60 and older
      3. Males more than females
      4. 1 to 1.5 million cases in United States
      5. Course of disease: 15 to 20 years
   D. Predisposing/precipitating factors: none clearly documented
   E. Clinical manifestations (Figure 5–3)
      1. Tremors: moves
         a. Head to and fro
         b. Tremulous voice
         c. Feet
         d. Tongue
         e. Lips
         f. Jaw
      2. Muscular rigidity
         a. Jerky interrupted movements
         b. Lack of free-flowing movements-bradykinesia
         c. Shuffling gait with stooped position
         d. Loss of normal arm swing
      3. Mask-like face
         a. Expressionless
         b. Less blinking
      4. Restlessness, pacing
      5. Weakness, fatigue
      6. Mental depression
      7. Autonomic nervous system dysfunctions
         a. Drooling
         b. Dysphagia
         c. Seborrhea

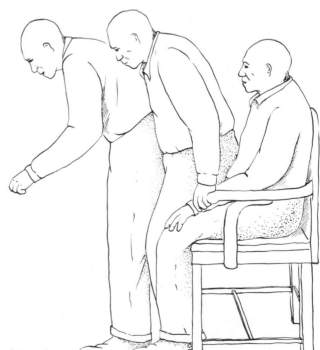

Constipation
- increase fluid intake and dietary fiber
- use stool softeners and mild laxatives
- establish a bowel routine

Impaired physical mobility
- physical therapy
- ROM exercises in all joints to prevent deformities
- gait training to prevent shuffling

Self-care deficiency
- allow extra time for dressing, bathing, and meals
- may need supplementary feedings to maintain weight
- mechanical devices to help in eating, toileting

Impaired verbal communication
- voice may be weak
- do exercises using facial muscles
- read aloud to help maintain intonation and articulation

Ineffective individual coping
- depression common, refer for professional help

High-risk for injury, due to gain, weakness, tremors
- check home for safety hazards
- may need a walking aid
- install safety devices in home, i.e., safety rails, raised toilet seat

FIGURE 5–3. Parkinson's disease: nursing diagnoses and interventions.

d. Oculogyric crisis (eyeballs jump up and down)

8. May have cognitive deficits

F. Diagnostic examinations
1. History and physical examination
2. Neurological examination
3. Clinical signs
4. Handwriting analysis for signs of small tremors
5. Electromyogram (EMG)

G. Complications
1. Falls
2. Self-care deficits
3. Depression
4. Debilitation
5. Failure of body systems

H. Medical management
1. Anticholinergics (Table 5–6)
2. Antiparkinsonian medications (Table 5–7)

II. Analysis
A. Impaired physical mobility related to neuromuscular impairment
B. Activity intolerance related to impaired motor function
C. Self-care deficit related to effects of chronic illness
D. Powerlessness related to debilitating condition
E. High risk for injury related to weakness and tremors
F. Constipation related to decreased muscle tone

III. Planning/goals, expected outcomes
A. Client will have reduced tremors
B. Client will manage self-care deficits
C. Client will have increased self-esteem
D. Client will perform ADLs
E. Client will adhere to drug therapy

IV. Implementations
A. Establish baseline neurological assessments
1. Assess posture, gait, rigidity
2. Assess ability to swallow, chew
3. Assess ability to speak
B. Administer appropriate medications at correct intervals to control symptoms
1. Anticholinergics (see Table 5–6): control tremor and rigidity

a. Trihexy phenidyl (Artane)
b. Benztropine (Cogentin)
2. Amantadine (Symmetrel) used in combination with other drugs (see Table 5–7)
3. Levodopa, dopamine precursor
4. Carbidopa (Sinemet), combination drug

C. Assess side effects of drugs
D. Encourage ambulation with safety measures
E. Teach client/family about side effects and interactions of drugs
F. Give supportive care to client
1. Give reassurance to build self-esteem
2. Encourage participation in previous activities
3. Encourage communication of feelings
G. Encourage independence
H. Encourage proper diet
1. High calorie
2. High protein
3. Soft diet
4. Small, frequent feeding
5. Fluids, 2000 mL per day
I. Encourage general hygienic care
J. Encourage family to modify home environment for safety factors
K. Refer family/client to community resources

V. Evaluation
A. Client functions as independently as possible
B. Client complies with medication regimen
C. Client/family states side effects and interactions of drugs
D. Client acknowledges progression of disease

Multiple Sclerosis

I. Assessment
A. Definition: chronic, degenerative disease that causes demyelination of the CNS white matter
B. Etiology/pathophysiology
1. Cause unknown
2. Viral infection (measles)
3. Autoimmune response
4. Destruction of myelin sheath of neuron with collection of scar tissue
5. Periods of remission and exacerbation
C. Incidence
1. Prevalent in Northern temperate zones

TABLE 5–6 Anticholinergics

Example	Action	Use	Common Side Effects	Nursing Implications
Atropine sulfate, Artane, Cogentin	Inhibit the effect of acetylcholine as transmitter for impulses in parasympathetic nervous system at synapses	To treat Parkinson's, to decrease saliva and respiratory secretions preoperatively	Dry mouth, blurred vision, acute glaucoma, constipation, dilated pupils, urinary retention, tachycardia	Avoid use in patients with glaucoma, BPH, myesthenia gravis, CHF, and hypertension; monitor vital signs; check for side effects; monitor I & O

TABLE 5–7 Antiparkinsonians

Example	Action	Use	Common Side Effects	Nursing Implications
Dopamine precursor: levodopa (Dopar, Larodopa); dopamine-releasing agents: carbidopa/levodopa (Sinemet), amantadine (Symmetrel)	Increase level of dopamine in CNS; often given in conjunction with anticholinergics, since cholinergic activity is increased when a deficit of dopamine exists; drug forms include dopamine precursors (levodopa) or dopamine-releasing agents (amantadine)	Control of symptoms of Parkinson's disease	Nausea and vomiting, anorexia, orthostatic hypotension, dry mouth, dysphagia, ataxia, headache, insomnia, anxiety, hypertension, urinary retention, skin rash, CHF, visual disturbances, tremors, and salivation	Use cautiously in clients with cardiovascular, respiratory, endocrine, or hepatic disease, peptic ulcers, wide-angle glaucoma, diabetes, and psychoses; not for use during pregnancy or lactation; watch BP; do not administer close to bedtime to decrease insomnia; do not discontinue drug abruptly; give with food to decrease GI irritation; observe for tremors; be alert for sudden worsening of symptoms with high doses; avoid vitamins containing vitamin B_6; monitor diabetics closely; warn that levodopa may darken urine and perspiration; advise patients that improvement is often gradual

2. Ages 20 to 40 years, young adult
3. Only 20% in 40 to 50 age range
4. 500,000 cases in United States yearly
5. Females more than males
6. Familial tendency with family member with MS 15 times greater than general population

D. Predisposing/precipitating factors
  1. Stress
  2. Infection
  3. Trauma
  4. Pregnancy
  5. Cold weather
  6. Fatigue

E. Clinical manifestations: vary with location and extent of disease (*most common early symptoms)
  1. Motor dysfunctions
    a. Weakness
    *b. Fatigue
    *c. Intention tremors
    d. Ataxia
    e. Spasticity of lower extremities
    f. Scanning speech
    g. Dysphagia
  2. Sensory dysfunction
    *a. Paresthesias (numbness, tingling)
    b. Decreased perception to pain, touch, temperature
  3. Visual and auditory disturbances
    *a. Optic neuritis
    *b. Blurred vision
    *c. Diplopia
    *d. Nystagmus (70% of clients)
    e. Vertigo
  4. Emotional changes
    a. Apathy
    b. Euphoria
    c. Irritability
    d. Labile emotions
    e. Depression
    f. Confusion
    g. Memory changes
  5. Bladder and bowel disturbances
    a. Urgency
    b. Frequency
    c. Retention
    d. Incontinence
  6. Abnormal reflexes: significant diagnostic value
    a. Hyperreflexia
    b. Absent reflexes
    c. Positive Babinski's reflex

F. Diagnostic examinations (see Table 5–1)
  1. History and physical
  2. Exacerbation and remission cycle
  3. CSF
    a. Increased gamma globulin
    b. Decreased protein
  4. Visual evoked response: slowing of conduction
  5. Abnormal reflexes (see signs and symptoms)

G. Complications—dependent upon course of disease; many potential problems of chronic nature

H. Medical management
   1. Anti-inflammatories/immunosuppress-
      ants (see Table 5–3)
   2. Muscle relaxants (Table 5–8)

II. Analysis
  A. Impaired physical mobility related to debilitat-
     ing condition
  B. Altered sensory perception and motor func-
     tion related to chronic illness; decreased
     vision
  C. Self-care deficit related to debilitating con-
     dition
  D. Powerlessness related to difficulty in perform-
     ing self-care
  E. Hopelessness related to effects of deterio-
     rating physical status

III. Planning/goals, expected outcomes
  A. Client/family will have realistic assessment of
     disease
  B. Client will understand activity limitations
  C. Client will be aware of neurological deficits
  D. Client will be free of complications of immo-
     bility
  E. Client will have adequate elimination patterns
  F. Client will remain as independent as possible
  G. Client will have increased self-esteem
  H. Client will understand therapeutic modalities
  I. Client/family will seek appropriate resources
  J. Client/family will ask appropriate questions
     about therapeutic modalities

IV. Implementations—supportive according to symp-
  toms, based on assessment of individual needs
  A. Establish baseline neurological assessments
     and changes
     1. Motor functions
     2. Sensory functions
     3. Visual and auditory perception
     4. Reflexes
  B. Monitor, assess, evaluate neurological status
     in terms of baseline
  C. Protect from injury by ensuring safety mea-
     sures while in chair or bed or when mobile
  D. Encourage independence in all ADLs
  E. Assist when necessary in all ADLs
  F. Administer medications dependent upon se-
     verity of symptoms
     1. ACTH
     2. Prednisone (see Table 5–3)
     3. Dexamethasone (Decadron) (see Table
       5–3)
     4. Muscle relaxants (see Table 5–8)
  G. Encourage proper diet
     1. Increase K^+ foods (see Table 4–2)
     2. Increase fluids
     3. Increase bulk in diet
     4. Low fat diet
     5. Increase fiber
  H. Encourage client/family to verbalize fears,
     concerns
  I. Give support and reassurance as appropriate
  J. Encourage physiotherapy as required
  K. Implement client/family teaching plan with ul-
     timate goal to keep client as independent as
     possible for as long as possible
     1. Assess client/family readiness for
       learning
     2. Assess client/family knowledge
     3. Alternate periods of rest and exercise
     4. Avoid extremes in temperature
     5. Encourage independence in ADLs
     6. Teach proper safety measures
     7. Suggest alternate sexual methods/suggest
       sexual counselor
     8. Assess knowledge deficits in therapeutic
       modalities
     9. Teach about medications
       a. Administration, dosage, time
       b. Side effects, adverse effects, interac-
         tions
     10. Teach about diet: importance of fluids,
       bulk, increased K^+
     11. Introduce to National Multiple Sclerosis
       Society

V. Evaluation
  A. Client/family verbalizes understanding of
     multiple sclerosis
  B. Client/family verbalizes fears and concerns
  C. Client demonstrates safety measures
  D. Client verbalizes correct diet, medications,
     activities
  E. Client maintains maximum level of function
  F. Client maintains continence

TABLE 5–8 Muscle Relaxants

Example	Action	Use	Common Side Effects	Nursing Implications
Methocarbamol (Robaxin)	Reduces transmission of impulses from spinal cord to skeletal muscles	To treat painful skeletal muscle spasms or other disorders	Drowsiness, lightheadedness, headache, hypotension, GI distress, rash	Watch for sensitivity; warn patient about impaired mental functioning; avoid alcohol or other depressants; give with food or milk; watch for hypotension

G. Client/family compliant with therapeutic modalities

H. Client/family uses appropriate referrals and resources

I. Client/family recognizes important changes in condition

POST-TEST Neurological Disorders

Mr. Baker is admitted for a neurological work-up. The first test to be performed is a lumbar puncture.

1. Mr. Baker tells you that he does not understand the procedure and does not really know what to expect. Your best response to him would be to:
   1. Tell him that you will call the physician to come explain the procedure to him
   2. Explain the proper position for the procedure, tell him to relax and breathe normally, and that local anesthetic will be used to prevent pain
   3. Explain that the doctor will be inserting a large needle into his back and that some fluid will be withdrawn from around his spinal cord and brain to test for an infection
   4. Tell him that someone will explain the procedure when it is time and that there is no need to worry about being hurt or paralyzed by the test

2. The most effective way to help Mr. Baker relieve his anxiety over the test is to:
   1. Give him a brief explanation of the exact procedure
   2. Reassure him that his physician is experienced in this procedure
   3. Ask him exactly what he is anxious about and listen to him
   4. Ask him to write down his questions to give to the physician before the test

3. After the lumbar puncture is completed, Mr. Baker should be:
   1. Encouraged to ambulate
   2. Placed in Trendelenburg for 2 hours
   3. Encouraged to force fluids
   4. Placed on strict bedrest for at least 48 hours

4. Mr. Baker is also scheduled for an electroencephalogram (EEG). The main reason for an EEG is to:
   1. Identify the location of a brain tumor
   2. Diagnose epilepsy
   3. Administer small shocks and record brain response
   4. Record the normal electrical activity of brain cells

5. In preparing him for the EEG, the nurse should:
   1. Sedate him with phenobarbital
   2. Withhold all medications
   3. Keep him awake for 48 hours before the test
   4. Shampoo his hair

6. In trying to document a client's level of consciousness, the best description is:
   1. Alert and able to state name and time
   2. Seems to be comatose
   3. Remains unable to respond
   4. Somewhat stuporous and does not know location

7. Which of the following charting gives the most objective information concerning neuromuscular status?
   1. Paralysis of lower extremities
   2. Unable to grip nurse's hand with left hand, but strong grip with right
   3. Weak and lethargic most of the time, confused frequent intervals
   4. Poor response to painful stimuli

8. When checking a client's pupillary response, the nurse knows this is best done:
   1. In a well-lighted room with a flashlight
   2. In a darkened room with a penlight
   3. After the client has received a mydriatic
   4. After the client has received a miotic

9. When caring for a client who suffers from dysarthria, it is important for the nurse to:
   1. Administer tube feedings accurately
   2. Maintain adequate fluid intake
   3. Face the client when speaking
   4. Speak slowly and clearly and allow time for response

10. Meningitis can be caused by:
    1. Any bacterial infection
    2. Many different viruses
    3. Meningococcus
    4. All of the above

11. A client who has meningitis often exhibits photosensitivity and extreme irritability, making it important that the nurse:
    1. Provide a quiet, dimly lit environment for the client
    2. Ventilate the room properly and provide sufficient sunlight
    3. Eliminate strong odors and unpleasant sights to prevent vomiting
    4. Allow frequent visits from family to prevent depression from isolation

12. A high fever often accompanies meningitis. A nursing intervention most helpful in relieving febrile delirium would be to:
    1. Restrain the client to prevent self-injury
    2. Apply a warm water bottle to the posterior neck
    3. Increase fluid intake to prevent dehydration
    4. Apply cool compresses or an ice bag to the forehead

13. When a client is admitted with a head injury, one of the most important goals of nursing care would be to prevent or detect:
    1. Self-injury
    2. Convulsions
    3. Increased intracranial pressure
    4. Paralysis

14. Clients with head injuries are NOT given sedatives because these drugs may:
    1. Produce coma
    2. Mask the client's symptoms
    3. Depress the client's respirations
    4. Lead to cerebral hemorrhage

15. Cerebrospinal fluid leakage should be expected in head-injured clients with:
    1. Bleeding from the nose or mouth
    2. Purulent, thick drainage from the nose or ears
    3. Clear yellow or pink-tinged fluid from the nose or ears
    4. Watering of the eyes and drainage of mucus from the nose

16. In order to confirm the presence of cerebrospinal fluid drainage, the nurse should:
    1. Test the fluid for the presence of glucose
    2. Send a specimen to the laboratory for diagnosis
    3. Test the fluid for the presence of albumin
    4. Send for a culture and sensitivity

17. If leakage of cerebrospinal fluid is confirmed, the client should be:
    1. Cautioned against blowing or picking the nose
    2. Positioned with the head lower than the rest of the body
    3. Cautioned against moving the head at all
    4. Encouraged to blow the nose to remove secretions

18. Which of the following would NOT cause a stroke?
    1. Cerebral thrombosis
    2. Cerebral hemorrhage
    3. Encephalitis
    4. Atherosclerosis

19. A client who has had a stroke should have range of motion exercises done regularly. The importance of this nursing intervention is that:
    1. Muscles have been damaged by the interruption of blood flow
    2. Bone and joints have been affected and contractures may occur
    3. Part of the brain controlling muscles has been destroyed and will never function normally
    4. Use of muscles may return if complications involving the musculoskeletal system have been prevented

20. When a stroke has been caused by a hemorrhage, the nurse should:
    1. Position the client flat in bed
    2. Cough and deep breathe the client hourly
    3. Position the client in semi-Fowler's
    4. Administer warfarin (Coumadin) as ordered

21. If you come upon a client having a seizure, you should:
    1. Protect his or her head from injury and turn him or her to the side if possible
    2. Restrain the client to prevent injury
    3. Place an object between the teeth and move the client to an upright position
    4. Move the client to the floor and hold the client down

22. When log-rolling a client to the side, it is important for the nurse to:
    1. Elevate the head of the bed slightly to avoid pressure on the back
    2. Raise the knee gatch slightly to avoid pressure on the hips
    3. Support the back with pillows and place a pillow between the legs to avoid straining the back
    4. Remove the pillow from under the client's head and place it under the shoulders

POST-TEST Answers and Rationales

1. ② The nurse should explain the procedure in broad terms without interjecting information that will needlessly frighten the client. The information in choice 2 is clear and honest. There is no need to call the physician to explain the examination. 4, I & II. Lumbar Puncture.

2. ③ The best way to reassure a client is to first find out exactly what the client is anxious about. The other options assume that the nurse already knows the problem without consulting the client. 5, II & III. Lumbar Puncture.

3. ③ The loss of cerebrospinal fluid causes the headache; therefore, the best way to decrease the potential problem is to force fluids. 4, II. Lumbar Puncture.

4. ④ An EEG simply records the electrical activity of the brain. It can help to do both choices 1 and 2, but the main reason is to measure the electrical activity of the brain. 3, II. EEG.

5. ④ The electrodes need to make good contact with oil-free skin. Shampooing the hair decreases the amount of oil. The other options might be done to some degree but only if specifically ordered. For example, a sleep-deprived EEG is done with the client awake for 24 hours. 4, II. EEG.

6. ① When collecting and recording data, the most objective description should always be used. The rest of the options are vague and open to misinterpretation, such as unable to respond, verbally or to pain? 1 & 5, II & IV. Neurological Status.

7. ② The statements charted should be as objective and descriptive as possible. The other options are open to misinterpretation. 1 & 5, II & IV. Neurological Status.

8. ② To see a change in the pupils, the room should be dimly lit and a focused light source used for the test. A mydriatic or miotic would cause the pupil to dilate or constrict respectively. 1 & 5, II & IV. Neurological Status.

9. ④ Dysarthria means that the client has difficulty speaking because of muscle weakness, not damage to the speech center, so the nurse should speak slowly and clearly to the client and allow plenty of time for the response. Tube feedings are usually not required, and fluid intake is irrelevant. There is no need to face the client. 4, IV. Neurological Status.

10. ④ All of the organisms listed can cause meningitis if they are introduced into the spinal column and infect the meninges. 5, II. Meningitis.

11. ① With the photosensitivity and irritability exhibited in meningitis, the environment should be as calm and controlled as possible. Choice 3 is not wrong, but choice 1 is a more complete answer. 4, II. Meningitis.

12. ④ Cool compresses or ice bags to the forehead help relieve the febrile delirium. Restraints often cause injury to the client. Warmth may increase the fever and fluid intake will not relieve the fever even though it might help prevent dehydration. Choice 3 does not address the question. 4, II. Meningitis.

13. ③ Clients with head injuries may develop increased intracranial pressure and a widening pulse pressure (the difference between the systolic and diastolic blood pressure) is an early sign of this. The increased pressure itself might cause all the other options listed so it is the most complete answer. 3, I. Head Injuries.

14. ② Decrease in the level of consciousness is an important diagnostic sign in clients with head injuries and sedatives will themselves alter the level of consciousness since they are CNS depressants. They do not produce coma and usually they do not significantly depress the respirations. 5, I. Head Injuries.

15. ③ Cerebrospinal fluid is clear, yellowish fluid and often leaks from the nose or ears with severe head injuries. It is important to detect it because it indicates that the integrity of the CNS has been disrupted and infection is a real possibility. 5, I. Head Injuries.

16. ① Cerebrospinal fluid contains glucose whereas normal nasal drainage does not. Choice 2 would work but would take an unnecessarily long time. 4, II. Head Injuries.

17. ① If the integrity of the skull is disrupted in the nasal region, bacteria from the nose can easily migrate into the cerebrospinal fluid, causing a severe infection. Blowing the nose may actually force bacteria back into the brain. 4, II. Head Injuries.

18. ③ Encephalitis does not cause a stroke. The other options cause strokes. 1 & 2, II. CVA.

19. ④ A stroke may only cause temporary loss of function so it is important to prevent contractures so that the client has the opportunity to regain maximal function. 4, II. CVA.

20. ③ Positioning the client in a semi-Fowler's allows increased venous return. Also, intracranial pressure is lessened. Being in a flat position increases intracranial pressure and could increase hemorrhage. The same is true for coughing and Coumadin. 4, II. CVA.

21. ① Protecting the head from trauma and decreasing the risk of aspiration are the priorities for client safety. Restraints and holding the client down may increase the injury that occurs. Forcing something into the mouth after the seizure has begun is also likely to cause injury. 3 & 4, I & II. Seizures.

22. ③ Supporting the back and body as an immovable whole is the principle of log-rolling. If the spine has been injured or surgery been performed, it is important to move the client as a single unit. 4, II. Spinal Injury.

PRE-TEST Sensory Disorders, Visual

1. One of the causes of cataracts is aging. Another cause of cataracts can be:
① Antihypertensives
② Head injuries
③ Coronary artery disease
④ Steroids

2. The major symptom of cataracts is:
① Gradual loss of vision
② Painful loss of vision
③ Positive red reflex
④ Tunnel vision

3. Your client had a cataract removed this morning. He is now complaining of severe eye pain. Your best action would be to:
① Call the physician
② Turn the client to the unaffected side
③ Turn the client to the affected side
④ Administer pain medication as ordered

4. Which of the following would be INAPPROPRIATE in the care of the client post-cataract removal?
① Administer antiemetics as ordered
② Teach the client that he or she can bend at the waist and lift over 20 pounds of weight
③ Teach client to properly insert eyedrops
④ Teach the client to apply the eyeshield at bedtime

5. A common clinical manifestation of glaucoma would be:
① Loss of central vision
② Painless rapid loss of vision
③ Whitish haze over the eyes
④ Seeing halos around lights

6. Miotics directly:
① Cause the pupils to dilate
② Cause the pupils to constrict
③ Decrease intraocular pressure
④ Increase intraocular pressure

7. Side effects of pilocarpine eyedrops include:
① Photosensitivity
② Nausea and vomiting
③ Bronchospasms in asthmatics
④ Prolonged dilation of pupil

8. Epinephrine eyedrops are used to:
① Decrease the production of aqueous humor
② Decrease the outflow of aqueous humor
③ Dilate the pupil
④ Constrict the pupil

9. Which of the following drugs is CONTRAINDICATED in clients with acute glaucoma?
① Pilocarpine
② Atropine
③ Acetazolamide (Diamox)
④ Epinephrine

PRE-TEST Answers and Rationales

1. ④ Cataracts can be caused by steroid therapy, trauma to the eye, and diabetes. The other options do not cause cataracts. 2, IV. Cataracts.

2. ① When cataracts occur, there is a gradual clouding of the lens with a gradual painless loss of vision. A positive red reflex means that the lens is clear of opacity. Tunnel vision is characteristic of glaucoma. 1, IV. Cataracts.

3. ① Severe eye pain post-cataract extraction is a sign of increased intraocular pressure either from hemorrhage or acute glaucoma. There is no nursing intervention that can relieve this, only a surgical iridectomy. Thus, the only correct option is to call the physician. None of the other options are correct actions. 4, I. Cataracts.

4. ② Antiemetics are very important to administer, because vomiting can cause an elevation in intraocular pressure (IOP). Inserting eyedrops and applying an eyeshield at night are necessary for preventing infection and injury. *Never* teach the client to sneeze or bend at the waist or lift any object weighing over 20 pounds, because the IOP will increase lethally. 4, IV. Cataracts.

5. ④ Glaucoma is characterized by seeing halos around lights, loss of peripheral vision, and gradual, painless loss of vision with chronic glaucoma or sudden, painful loss of vision with acute glaucoma. The whitish haze is characteristic of cataracts. 2, II. Glaucoma.

6. ② Miotics cause the pupil to constrict, thereby opening the canal of Schlemm. This indirectly leads to decreased intraocular pressure because it increases the outflow of aqueous humor. 2, I & II. Glaucoma.

7. ③ Pilocarpine can cause bronchospasms in asthmatics so it must be used cautiously with these clients. It constricts the pupil and does not cause either photosensitivity or nausea and vomiting. 2, I & II. Glaucoma.

8. ① Epinephrine eyedrops actually decrease the production of aqueous humor, thereby lowering the intraocular pressure. The other options describe the effects of other eyedrops. 2, I & II. Glaucoma.

9. ② Atropine causes the pupil to dilate, thereby decreasing the opening at the canal of Schlemm, decreasing the outflow of aqueous humor, and increasing the intraocular pressure. For these reasons, atropine is contraindicated in glaucoma. The other options are drugs used to treat glaucoma. 2, I & II. Glaucoma.

NURSING PROCESS APPLIED TO ADULTS WITH SENSORY DISORDERS

Visual Disorders

Cataracts

I. Assessment
  A. Definition/pathophysiology: an opacity of crystalline lens or capsule leading to painless, gradual blurring and eventual loss of vision (see Figure 5–4 for normal eye)
  B. Etiology, predisposing/precipitating factors
    1. Senile: result of aging
    2. Traumatic: result of trauma or injury
    3. Congenital: occurring at birth
    4. Heredity
    5. Malignancy
    6. Secondary: resulting from other diseases or medications such as glaucoma, diabetes, steroids, or radiation exposure
  C. Clinical manifestations
    1. Gradual loss of vision
    2. Distorted, blurred, or hazy vision
    3. No pain
    4. Cloudlike opacity over lens or capsule
    5. Photophobia to glaring light
    6. Monocular diplopia in one eye
    7. Absence of red reflex
  D. Diagnostic examinations
    1. Ophthalmoscopic eye examination with ocular power tests
    2. Loupe (convex magnifying lens)
  E. Complications
    1. Blindness
    2. Hyphema (bleeding into the anterior chamber)
    3. Vitreous prolapse
    4. Intraocular infection
    5. Uveitis

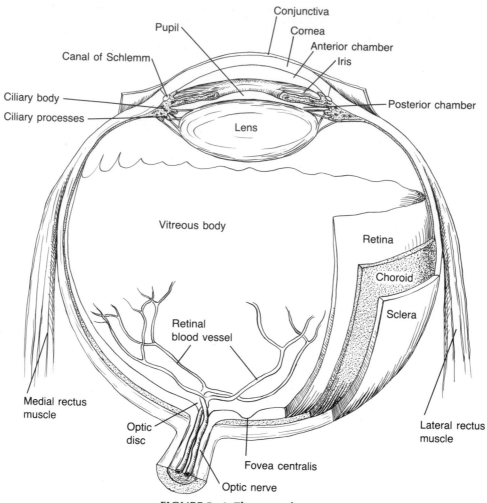

FIGURE 5–4. The normal eye.

6. Posterior capsule thickening after extra-capsular cataract extraction (ECCE)
7. Increased intraocular pressure (IOP)

F. Medical management
   1. No known medical treatment to cure or prevent cataract formation

G. Surgical management
   1. ECCE
      a. Manual
      b. Phacoemulsification (ultrasonic vibrations to fragment lens)
   2. Intracapsular cataract extraction (ICCE)
      a. Manual
      b. Cryoextraction (freezing)
   3. Peripheral iridectomy with ECCE or ICCE
   4. Intraocular lens implantation with ECCE
   5. Postoperative replacements
      a. Cataract glasses: magnifying glasses, central vision only
      b. Contact lenses: sharp visual acuity, need dexterity to insert
      c. Intraocular lenses: plastic, implanted during surgery

II. Analysis
   A. Sensory-perceptual visual alteration related to decreased visual acuity secondary to cataracts
   B. Impaired tissue integrity (visual) related to surgical procedure for removal of cataracts
   C. Impaired health maintenance related to visual changes
   D. High risk for injury related to decreased visual acuity

III. Planning/goals, expected outcomes
   A. Client will be adequately prepared physically and psychologically for surgery
   B. Client will recover from surgery without complications
   C. Client will regain vision to maximal level
   D. Client will remain safe in the hospital and home environment free of injury.

IV. Implementations
   A. Preoperatively

1. May be done as outpatient
2. Administer mydriatics and cycloplegics as ordered (Table 5–9)
3. Administer sedatives or tranquilizers as ordered
   B. Postoperatively
      1. Elevate head of bed 30 to 45 degrees for comfort
      2. Turn to back or unoperative side
      3. Orient eye-patched client to environment
      4. Position room and belongings to unoperative side
      5. Keep side rails up for safety
      6. Avoid straining, sneezing, coughing, bending, vomiting, lifting objects over 20 pounds
      7. Reapply eyeshield at bedtime
      8. Teach client to insert eyedrops on schedule and to use eyeshield after discharge
         a. Avoid eyestrain by listening to tapes,

TABLE 5–9 Medications to Treat Eye Diseases

Route	Class	Example	Action	Use	Common Side Effects	Nursing Implications
PO	Carbonic anhydrase inhibitors	acetazolamide (Diamox)	To treat glaucoma	Reduces production of aqueous humor	Paresthesias, drowsiness, headache, hypokalemia, hyponatremia, alkaline urine, diarrhea, anorexia	Use cautiously in clients with diabetes or on digoxin; monitor electrolyte levels; teach high potassium diet; administer in AM because of diuretic effect; watch for symptoms of blood dyscrasias or hypersensitivity; monitor for visual changes
Topical	Miotics (parasympatho-mimetics)	pilocarpine	Activate cholinergic receptors causing contraction of ciliary muscle and body	To treat open-angle glaucoma, narrow-angle glaucoma preoperatively; to reverse effects of cycloplegics and mydriatics	Ciliary spasms, headache, blurred vision, conjunctivitis, allergic reactions	Use carefully in clients with bronchial asthma; may cause bronchospasms; report symptoms of systemic cholinergics—salivation, sweating, cramping, and nausea; protect solution from light
	Mydriatics	epinephrine (Epitrate)	Direct stimulation of alpha and beta adrenergic receptors; decrease production and increase outflow of aqueous humor; produce mydriasis	Treatment of simple, open-angle glaucoma, dilation of the pupil for eye exams	Headache, stinging, blurred vision, lacrimation, rebound hyperemia, conjunctival irritation, scotomas	Warn client about blurred vision, increased sensitivity to light; monitor intraocular pressure frequently and adjust dosage as needed
	Cycloplegics	scopolamine	Competitive inhibition of acetylcholine at postsynaptic cholinergic receptor sites	To aid ophthalmic exams and surgery by producing mydriasis and cycloplegia	Blurred vision, photophobia, increased intraocular pressure, suppression of lacrimation	Tell client that effects last 4 to 6 hours; use neostigmine as antidote; warn about blurred vision and photophobia
	Beta-adrenergic blockers	timolol (Timoptic)	Nonspecific beta-adrenergic blocker that reduces formation of aqueous humor without producing miosis or hyperemia	To treat chronic, open-angle glaucoma and ocular hypertension	Ocular irritation, occasional hypersensitivity reaction	Warn client that use more than twice a day is ineffective; may need another antiglaucomic added for effectiveness; measure intraocular pressure at intervals

talking on phone, using dark protective lenses, etc.

  b. Advise against rubbing or placing pressure on eyes

  c. Advise to wipe excess drainage or tearing with a sterile, wet cottonball from inner to outer canthus

  d. Advise to contact physician immediately with any decrease in vision, severe eye pain, or increases in eye discharge

V. Evaluation

  A. Client recovers from surgery without complications

  B. Client able to care for self after discharge

  C. Client regains as much sight as possible

  D. Client remains free of injury

Glaucoma

I. Assessment

  A. Definition/pathophysiology: characterized by an increase in IOP resulting in optic nerve atrophy and blindness (Figure 5–5)

    1. Chronic, simple, open angle: thickening or obstruction in trabecular network, IOP greater than 30 to 50 mm Hg

    2. Acute, narrow angle, closed angle: impaired outflow from narrowing or closing of angle between iris and cornea, IOP greater than 50 to 70 mm Hg

    3. Congenital: abnormal development of filtration angle

    4. Secondary: results from inflammation, trauma, hemorrhage, tumors, iritis

  B. Incidence: increased risk with age

    1. Sixth leading cause of blindness in the world

    2. Over 40 years old, incidence is reported as 2% to 4%

    3. Glaucoma increases with aging

    4. Chronic open-angle glaucoma accounts for 90% of the cases of primary glaucoma

  C. Predisposing/precipitating factors

    1. Heredity

    2. Diabetes

  D. Clinical manifestations

    1. Progressive loss of peripheral vision

    2. Chronic open-angle

      a. Elevated IOP greater than 30 to 50 mm Hg

      b. Visual field irreversible loss

      c. Cupping of the optic disc

    3. Acute closed-angle

      a. Worse in the evening

      b. Blurred vision

      c. Halos around white lights

      d. Frontal headache

      e. Excruciating eye pain

      f. Photophobia

      g. Lacrimation

    4. Central vision loss (tunnel vision)

  E. Diagnostic examinations

    1. Tonometry to measure intraocular pressure, normal 10 to 20 mm Hg

    2. Physical examination revealing hardening of the eyeball

    3. Test of visual fields

    4. Ophthalmoscopic examination for cupping of optic disc

  F. Complication: blindness

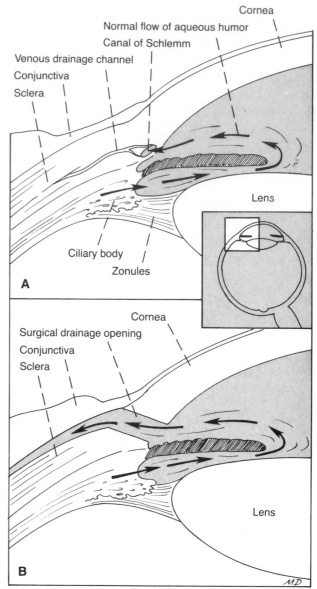

FIGURE 5–5. *A,* Normal flow of aqueous humor. *B,* Surgical procedure to create a new channel for aqueous humor for a person with glaucoma. (From Luckmann, J., Sorensen, K. C. Medical–Surgical Nursing: A Psychophysiologic Approach. 3rd ed. Philadelphia: W. B. Saunders, 1987.)

G. Medical management: for chronic, open-angle glaucoma (see Table 5–9)
   1. Miotics, pilocarpine—to constrict pupils
   2. Carbonic anhydrase inhibitors, acetazolamide (Diamox) (see Table 5–9), to decrease production of aqueous humor
   3. Anticholinesterase demecarium (Humorsol) to facilitate outflow of aqueous humor
   4. Epinephrine drops (see Table 5–9) to decrease production of aqueous humor and promote outflow
   5. Beta-blockers, timolol (Table 5–9) to decrease the production of aqueous humor and decrease IOP pressure without changing the pupil
   6. Honan IOP reducer (balloon)
H. Surgical management
   1. Peripheral iridectomy
   2. Trabeculoplasty
   3. Trabeculectomy
   4. Laser trabeculectomy
   5. Iridectomy or laser iridotomy

II. Analysis
A. Pain related to increased IOP
B. Anxiety related to decreased vision and loss of independence
C. High risk for injury related to loss of vision
D. Fear of blindness related to surgical intervention
E. Knowledge deficit related to lack of information about measures to reduce IOP

III. Planning/goals, expected outcomes
A. Acute pain will be relieved with medications or surgery
B. Client will have glaucoma diagnosed before vision is lost
C. Client will be safe from all injuries
D. Client will recover from surgery without complications
E. Client will understand and comply with lifelong use of medication

IV. Implementations
A. Postoperatively
   1. Keep client flat and quiet for 24 hours
   2. Turn to back or unoperative side
   3. Avoid activities that increase IOP
   4. Administer eyedrops as ordered
   5. Maintain eye patch for safety
B. Teach client
   1. Lifelong and proper medication use
   2. To carry identification—Medic Alert tag
   3. To avoid anticholinergics such as atropine
   4. Signs and symptoms of acute glaucoma
C. Administer medications as ordered

V. Evaluations

A. Client's glaucoma controlled without loss of vision
B. Client understands and correctly uses medications for life
C. Client recovers from surgery without complication
D. Client is restored to a state of independence

Retinal Detachment
I. Assessment
A. Definition/pathophysiology: when two layers of retina—outer pigmented epithelium and inner sensory layer—separate as result of fluid accumulation between layers as result of trauma or degeneration
B. Incidence: increased after 40 years old and peaks between 50 and 60 years old
C. Predisposing/precipitating factors
   1. Primary detachment: most common type
      a. Blunt or penetrating trauma
      b. High myopia (very near-sighted people)
      c. Retinal degeneration
      d. Aphakia (absence of crystalline lens)
   2. Secondary detachment
      a. Pressure from intraocular tumors or hemorrhage
      b. Scar formation after a vitrectomy
      c. Severe hypertension
      d. Diabetic retinopathy
      e. Toxemia in pregnancy
      f. Retrolental fibroplasia
D. Clinical manifestations
   1. Flashes of light or sparks
   2. Floaters and increases in blurred vision
   3. Sense of curtain being drawn
   4. Absence of pain
E. Diagnostic examination
   1. Ophthalmoscopic examination
   2. Visual field examination
   3. Refraction
   4. Color vision
F. Complication: irreversible blindness if untreated
G. Medical management
   1. Eye patch bilaterally
   2. Complete bedrest with detachment in dependent position
   3. Sedate as needed
H. Surgical management
   1. Photocoagulation: use of strong beam of light, laser beam, to burn retina to form inflammatory exudate
   2. Cryosurgery: supercooled probe applied to sclera over detachment, causing adherence due to scarring
   3. Electrodiathermy: use of electrode nee-

dle through sclera, allowing fluid to escape; exudate forms and retina adheres to choroid, which adheres to sclera

    4. Sclera buckle: splint to hold retina and choroid together until scar can form to hold them together permanently (Figure 5–6)

II. Analysis

  A. Ineffective individual coping related to fear of vision loss

  B. Knowledge deficit related to the treatment

  C. High risk for injury related to surgical procedure

  D. Fear related to vision loss

III. Planning/goals, expected outcomes

  A. Client will have retinal detachment diagnosed before permanent visual loss occurs

  B. Client will maintain complete bedrest to prevent further damage

  C. Client will be physically and psychologically prepared for surgery

  D. Client will recover from surgery without complications

IV. Implementation

  A. Preoperative

    1. Keep client eye-patched

    2. Keep client calm and correctly positioned

  B. Postoperative

    1. Keep client bilaterally eye-patched

    2. Maintain bedrest as ordered

    3. Assist with ADLs

    4. Administer eyedrops as ordered, mydriatics, cycloplegics, steroids, and antibiotics (see Table 5–9)

    5. Avoid sudden movements of head or anything that increases intraocular pressure

    6. Limit reading for 3 to 5 weeks

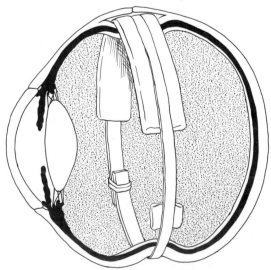

FIGURE 5–6. Sclera buckle for retinal detachment.

    7. Encourage follow-up ophthalmic care because of danger of recurrence or occurrence in other eye

V. Evaluation

  A. Client recovers from surgery without complication

  B. Client has near-normal vision restored

  C. Client complies with follow-up therapy

  D. Client interacts socially with family, friends, etc.

PRE-TEST Sensory Disorders, Auditory

1. The hearing loss that results when there is damage to the outer and/or middle ear is known as:
  ① Conductive loss
  ② Sensorineural loss
  ③ Mixed loss
  ④ Nerve deafness

2. Which of the following is a predisposing factor for a sensorineural hearing loss?
  ① Serous otitis media
  ② Otosclerosis
  ③ Perforation of the eardrum
  ④ Ototoxic drugs

3. Which of the following is useful in correcting a sensorineural hearing loss?
  ① Stapedectomy
  ② Myringotomy
  ③ Ossicular reconstruction
  ④ Nothing: it is irreversible

4. Nursing interventions appropriate after a tympanoplasty include:
  ① Inserting ear drops as ordered
  ② Avoiding the use of cotton in the ears
  ③ Teaching the client to avoid heavy physical activity for at least 3 weeks
  ④ Using hydrogen peroxide rinses in the ear three times a day as ordered

5. In order for Meniere's syndrome to be diagnosed, three symptoms must be present. These are paroxysmal vertigo, tinnitus, and:
  ① Vomiting
  ② Sensorineural hearing loss
  ③ Conductive hearing loss
  ④ Bilateral symptoms

6. Diagnostic tests used to diagnose Meniere's syndrome include all the following EXCEPT a(n):
  ① Caloric test
  ② Electronystagmogram
  ③ Electroencephalogram
  ④ Audiogram

7. Before the caloric test is done, the nurse knows it is important to withhold which drugs?
   1. Antihistamines
   2. Antihypertensives
   3. Steroids
   4. Anticonvulsants
8. Nonsurgical treatment for Meniere's syndrome includes:
   1. Administering vasodilators
   2. Avoiding tranquilizers such as diazepam
   3. Maintaining a salt-free diet
   4. Taking alcohol in small amounts

9. An outcome of the total labyrinthectomy would be:
   1. Periodic ear infections
   2. Unilateral hearing loss
   3. Nystagmus with motion
   4. Decreased tinnitus
10. The diagnostic tests in assessing hearing loss include all of the following EXCEPT:
   1. Electronystagmography
   2. Audiometry
   3. CT scan
   4. Myelogram

PRE-TEST Answers and Rationales

1. ① Conductive hearing loss occurs when there is damage to the outer and/or middle ear. If there is damage to the auditory nerve, it is sensorineural. Mixed loss contains elements of both. 2, II. Hearing Loss.

2. ④ A cause of auditory nerve damage is ototoxic drugs. This damage can lead to a sensorineural hearing loss. The other options are causes of conductive hearing loss. 1, II. Hearing Loss.

3. ④ Sensorineural hearing loss is irreversible and is not helped significantly by a hearing aid. The other options are treatments for conductive hearing loss. 4, II. Hearing Loss.

4. ③ The ear must be kept dry with cotton in it for about 6 weeks after a tympanoplasty. The client must avoid anything that would increase pressure within the ear such as sneezing, straining, or heavy lifting. 4, I & II. Tympanoplasty.

5. ② The three symptoms that must be present for the diagnosis of Meniere's syndrome are vertigo, tinnitus, and sensorineural hearing loss. Vomiting is a symptom, but not one of the cardinal ones. The symptoms may be unilateral. 2, II. Meniere's Syndrome.

6. ③ An electroencephalogram is not used to diagnose Meniere's syndrome. All of the other options are tests used to diagnose it. 2, II. Meniere's Syndrome.

7. ① Antihistamines may alter the results of the caloric test, decreasing the nystagmus, and so they are held before the test. None of the other drugs affect the results of this test. 4, II. Meniere's Syndrome.

8. ③ The excessive fluid in the inner ear and the labyrinth are a type of edema that salt may aggravate. Vasoconstrictors are used, as is diazepam. Alcohol and smoking are absolutely contraindicated. 4, II. Meniere's Syndrome.

9. ② A labyrinthectomy is done only after there is sensorineural hearing loss, because total unilateral loss is a result of the surgery. Tinnitus and nystagmus should disappear with the surgery. Ear infections are no more likely than normal. 5, I & II. Meniere's Syndrome.

10. ④ A myelogram is a neurological examination for herniated discs, spinal tumors, or spinal congenital defects. All the remaining tests are used to determine hearing loss. 1, II. Invasive Therapy, Hearing Loss.

Auditory Disorders

Hearing Loss

I. Assessment
   A. Definition/pathophysiology (Figure 5–7)
      1. Conductive hearing loss: inability to conduct sounds through the external and middle ear
      2. Sensorineural loss: loss of sensitivity to and discrimination of sounds due to damage of cochlea and auditory nerve (inner ear)
      3. Mixed loss: combination of both conductive and sensorineural loss; can include central hearing loss (CVA) or psychogenic hearing loss
   B. Etiology
      1. Acquired
      2. Congenital
   C. Incidence
      1. Most common disability in the United States
      2. 20 million Americans suffer some degree of hearing loss
      3. 10 million are over 65 years of age
   D. Predisposing/precipitating factors
      1. Conductive
         a. Earwax (cerumen)
         b. Infection (otitis media)
         c. Foreign body in the ear (bugs, beans, etc.)
         d. Trauma (external or internal)
         e. Perforation of the tympanic membrane
         f. Sclerosis of bone
         g. Tumor
         h. Fluid in the middle ear
      2. Sensorineural
         a. Ototoxic drugs
         b. Noise pollution

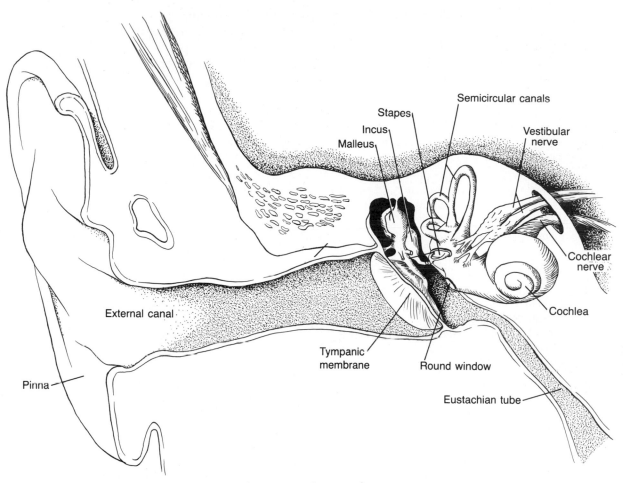

FIGURE 5–7. The normal ear.

c. Complications of infections (measles, mumps, meningitis)
d. Trauma
e. Neuromas
f. Aging process (presbycusis)

E. Clinical manifestations
1. Hearing loss
2. Pain (otalgia)
3. Discharge (otorrhea)
4. Tinnitus (sensation of noise—ringing, buzzing, or hissing)
5. Vertigo (spinning sensation)
6. Disequilibrium (i.e., unsteadiness, queasiness, faintness, etc.)

F. Diagnostic examination
1. Otoscopic examination
2. Tuning fork tests
   a. Weber
   b. Rinne
3. Culture and sensitivity of otorrhea
4. Audiometry
   a. Pure tone audiometry
   b. Speech audiometry
   c. Impedance audiometry
      (1) Tympanometry
      (2) Static impedance
      (3) Acoustic reflex tests
5. Vestibular tests
   a. Electronystagmography (ENG)
   b. Caloric test
6. Radiologic examination: CT scan of temporal bone

G. Complication: deafness

H. Medical/surgical management
1. Removal of foreign body
2. Myringotomy with tympanocentesis
3. Tympanoplasty
4. Ossicular/cochlear reconstruction
5. Stapedectomy
6. Removal of acoustic neuroma
7. Systemic antibiotics for otitis media
8. Hearing aid

II. Analysis
A. High risk for injury related to hearing deficit
B. Anxiety related to diagnostic tests and surgery
C. Knowledge deficit related to surgery and postoperative care

D. Sensory alterations: auditory related to hearing loss

E. Impaired social interactions related to withdrawal secondary to hearing loss

III. Planning/goals, expected outcomes
   A. Client will be safe in hospital environment
   B. Client will understand diagnostic tests
   C. Client will be physically and psychologically prepared for surgery by teaching preoperative and postoperative care
   D. Client will regain maximal amount of hearing
   E. Client will correctly use hearing aid or establish another method of communication

IV. Implementation
   A. Observe client's behavior to assess hearing loss
   B. Prepare client for diagnostic tests
   C. Prepare for surgery
   D. Postoperatively
      1. Avoid blowing nose
      2. Avoid heavy physical activity for at least 3 weeks
      3. Change sterile cotton ball in ear as prescribed
      4. Keep ear dry at least 6 weeks
      5. Avoid pressure changes such as airplane flights for 3 months
      6. Avoid loud noises from music, power tools, etc.
      7. Report any excessive bleeding or drainage immediately
      8. Monitor for dizziness or changes in balance

V. Evaluation
   A. Client recovers from surgery without complications
   B. Client regains hearing
   C. Client complies with wearing hearing aid
   D. Client will have an alternate way of communication

Meniere's Syndrome

I. Assessment
   A. Definition/pathophysiology: a labyrinthine disorder of inner ear
   B. Etiology: cause unknown
   C. Incidence
      1. Women between 40 and 60 years old
      2. Rare in children
      3. Five of every 100 people are affected in varying degrees by this disorder
   D. Predisposing/precipitating factors
      1. Defect in the function of the endolymphatic sac
      2. Sodium retention
      3. Viral infections
      4. Paroxysmal vasomotor changes

      5. Mental stress
      6. Endocrine disorders
      7. Allergies
      8. Impairment of microvasculature of inner ear related to abnormal metabolites such as sugar, insulin, triglycerides, or cholesterol
   E. Clinical manifestations (*symptoms must be present for diagnosis to be made)
      *1. Severe vertigo with nausea and vomiting
      2. Tinnitus
      *3. Sensorineural hearing loss on the involved side
      4. Nystagmus
      5. Uncomfortable full feeling in the involved ear
      6. Other
         a. Vertigo persists for 1 to 12 hours
         b. Followed by a period of unsteadiness
         c. Hearing loss fluctuation
         d. Tinnitus
         e. Personality changes
            (1) Anxious
            (2) Irritable
            (3) Depressed
         f. Uncoordinated and changes in gait
      7. Two to three acute attacks per year
   F. Diagnostic examinations
      1. Audiometric studies
      2. CT scan
      3. Allergic evaluation
      4. Blood tests such as glucose tolerance, insulin levels, cholesterol, and triglycerides
      5. Caloric test
         a. Iced or warm water introduced in ear canal
         b. Induces nystagmus
         c. Not done during acute attack
         d. Avoid antihistamines or tranquilizers before test
      6. Electronystagmography
      7. Electrocochleography
      8. Neurological examination
   G. Complication: Some degree of hearing loss after complete remission
   H. Medical management
      1. Atropine stops an attack in 20 to 30 minutes
      2. Diazepam (Valium) also used in an acute attack
      3. Antivertigo medications
         a. Meclizine hydrochloride (Antivert, Bonine)
         b. Dimenhydrinate (Dramamine)
         c. Diphenhydramine (Benadryl)
      4. Diuretics (ammonium chloride)
      5. Vasodilators

a. Nicotinic acid
b. Histamine
6. Salt-free diet
7. Alcohol and smoking eliminated
I. Surgical management
   1. Conservative procedures
      a. Ultrasound—depresses vestibular activity
      b. Endolymphatic subarachnoid shunt
      c. Sectioning of the vestibular portion of cranial nerve VII
   2. Destructive procedures
      a. Total labyrinthectomy
      b. Sectioning of cochlear nerve

II. Analysis
  A. Pain related to severe vertigo and dizziness
  B. High risk for injury related to dizziness and vertigo
  C. Fear of total hearing loss
  D. Knowledge of deficit related to course, medications, and treatment of symptoms

III. Planning/goals, expected outcomes
  A. Client will have nausea, vomiting, and headaches relieved
  B. Client will have vertigo and tinnitus controlled
  C. Client will maintain maximal amount of hearing
  D. Client will comply with therapeutic regimen

IV. Implementation
  A. Administer medications as ordered
    1. Teach the client about medications
  B. Teach the client to avoid jerking movements
    1. During an acute attack, encourage the client to stay in bed

    2. Instruct client to call for assistance with ambulating
  C. Teach the client to:
    1. Restrict fluid
    2. Maintain a salt-free diet
    3. Prevent loud noises
    4. Restrict smoking and alcohol
    5. Express concerns about the loss of hearing and changes in lifestyle

PRE-TEST Sensory Disorders, Laryngeal

1. Which of the following is NOT a common predisposing factor for laryngeal cancer?
  ① Smoking
  ② Alcohol abuse
  ③ Voice abuse
  ④ Smokeless tobacco

2. The earliest symptom of laryngeal cancer is:
  ① Hoarseness
  ② Throat pain
  ③ Dysphagia
  ④ Lymphadenopathy in throat

3. Which of the following is NOT a realistic goal for the client who is receiving curative therapy for laryngeal cancer?
  ① Client will cope with the altered body image.
  ② Client will regain speech after therapy completed.
  ③ Client will understand the side effects of radiation therapy.
  ④ Client will maintain adequate nutritional status.

PRE-TEST Answers and Rationales

1. ④ Smokeless tobacco predisposes oral cancer more than laryngeal cancer. The other options are all predisposing factors for laryngeal cancer. 1, II. Laryngeal Cancer.
2. ① Hoarseness is the only early symptom of laryngeal cancer. The other options are all late symptoms of the disease. 1, II. Laryngeal Cancer.
3. ② The client who is being treated for laryngeal cancer will have a radical laryngectomy as the core treatment. Because of this, all normal speech will be lost and the client will have to learn another form of communication. The other options are reasonable goals for this client. 3, I. Laryngeal Cancer.

Laryngeal Cancer

I. Assessment
   A. Definition/pathophysiology
      1. Usually squamous cell carcinoma
      2. Common malignancy of head and neck; may affect glottis, supraglottic, transglottic, false cords, pyriform sinuses, or true cords
      3. Grows slowly due to limited lymphatic distribution in this area
   B. Incidence
      1. Men affected eight times more than women
      2. Highest in smokers and drinkers
      3. Occurs between 55 and 70 years of age
      4. 2% to 3% occur in larynx
   C. Predisposing/precipitating factors
      1. Rare in nonsmokers
      2. Prolonged use of tobacco and alcohol
      3. Air pollution
      4. Occupational exposure to radiation
      5. Chronic pharyngeal infection
      6. Chronic laryngitis
      7. Voice abuse
      8. Often associated with bronchiogenic cancer
      9. Family predisposition to cancer
   D. Clinical manifestations
      1. Early
         a. Hoarseness longer than 2 weeks
         b. Voice changes
         c. Feeling of lump in throat
      2. Late
         a. Dysphagia
         b. Increasing dyspnea
         c. Cough
         d. Hemoptysis
         e. Weight loss
         f. Pain around adam's apple that radiates to ear on affected side
         g. Enlarged cervical lymph nodes
         h. Feeling of lump in throat
   E. Diagnostic examination
      1. X-rays of the head, neck, and chest
      2. Laryngeal tomography
      3. Direct examination with laryngoscopy and biopsy
      4. CT scan of neck
      5. Laryngograms
      6. Needle biopsy of enlarged cervical lymph nodes
   F. Complications: metastasis to head and neck
   G. Medical management
      1. Dependent on stage of cancer
      2. Radiation therapy; preoperatively, postoperatively, or instead of surgery in high risk or elderly clients
   H. Surgical management
      1. Partial laryngectomy
      2. Hemilaryngectomy
      3. Total laryngectomy and tracheostomy with or without radical neck dissection
      4. Laryngoplasty post-resection
II. Analysis
   A. Knowledge deficit related to diagnostic examinations and surgery
   B. Ineffective breathing pattern related to new airway, pain
   C. Fear related to inability to speak, isolation, mutilating surgery, diagnosis of cancer, drooling
   D. High risk for impaired skin integrity related to surgical incision, tracheostomy, wound drainage, radiation therapy to neck
   E. Altered nutrition: less than body requirements related to dysphagia, edema, decreased oral intake
   F. Pain related to operative incision
   G. Self-esteem disturbance related to disfiguring surgery

III. Planning/goals, expected outcomes
  A. Client will understand diagnostic tests and implications; will be physically and psychologically prepared for surgery; and will recover from surgery without complications
  B. Client will learn acceptable alternate form of communication
  C. Client will understand and tolerate tracheostomy radiation therapy without complications
  D. Client will cope with altered body image
  E. Client will maintain adequate nutritional status
  F. Client will be free from pain
  G. Client and significant others will cope with disfiguring surgery
IV. Implementation
  A. Preoperatively
    1. Allow verbalization of fears
    2. Establish alternate form of communication
    3. Provide meticulous mouth care
    4. Provide adequate nutritional intake (see Table 8–11)
      a. Liquids
      b. Enteral nutrition
      c. Hyperalimentation
    5. Prepare client for preoperative radiation therapy
      a. Provide skin care as needed
      b. Provide artificial saliva for decreased salivation

  6. Prepare client for tracheostomy, site of surgical incision, and nasogastric feeding tube
  B. Postoperative
    1. Assess respiratory rate every 1 to 2 hours
    2. Turn, cough, and deep breathe every 2 to 4 hours
    3. Auscultate lung sounds every 2 hours
    4. Provide constant humidity
    5. Medicate for pain frequently (Table 5–10)
    6. Suction as needed through mouth or tracheostomy
    7. Monitor for hemorrhage
    8. Remove nasal crusts
    9. Position in semi-Fowler's for maximal chest expansion: change position every 2 to 4 hours
    10. Ambulate early and encourage deep breathing to prevent pneumonia
    11. Maintain tube feedings or hyperalimentation as ordered
    12. Monitor closely for tracheal–esophageal fistula formation
    13. Monitor wound drainage carefully
    14. Offer support and encourage client to express grief
  C. Stoma care
    1. Suction as needed
    2. Clean inner cannula as needed
    3. Keep extra tracheostomy tube and obturator at bedside

TABLE 5–10 Analgesics

Class	Example	Action	Use	Common Side Effects	Nursing Implications
Non-narcotic	Salicylates: acetylsalicylic acid (aspirin); para-aminophenols: acetaminophen (Tylenol)	Decrease pain, often through anti-inflammatory actions without side effects of narcotics; major drugs are either salicylates (aspirin) or para-aminophenols (acetaminophen)	To relieve mild to moderate pain	Salicylates: salicylism (headache, nausea, vomiting, palpitations, hyperventilation), hypersensitivity, GI distress and bleeding, anticoagulant effect, liver damage; Acetaminophen: hypersensitivity, CNS stimulation, liver and renal damage, palpitations	Avoid use of salicylates in patients with GI disorders, anti-inflammatory or anticoagulant therapy, or history of aspirin sensitivity; avoid overuse; keep supply away from children; monitor liver and renal function; warn patient to avoid over-the-counter medicines that contain "hidden" aspirin
Narcotic	morphine sulfate, meperidine (Demerol)	Decrease pain by inhibiting the transmission of pain impulses, reducing cortical responses to pain stimuli, or altering activity in the pain-perception center of the brain	Treatment of moderate or severe pain	Drowsiness, dizziness, or lightheadedness, euphoria, respiratory depression, constipation, urinary retention, hypersensitivity, hypotension	Monitor effectiveness of analgesia; watch for hypotension and respiratory depression; monitor I & O, bowel movements; watch for possible tolerance and dependence

4. Always use two people to change ties
5. Teach client to care for own tracheostomy
6. Teach client to cover stoma when coughing
7. Suggest use of light porous covering over healed stoma
8. Teach safety precautions
   a. Protective cover over trachea when taking a shower
   b. Wear Medic Alert tag stating "neck breather"
D. Encourage client to stop smoking and drinking
E. Encourage client to work on alternate speech method
F. Encourage client to comply with postoperative radiation therapy or follow-up therapy as needed
V. Evaluations
A. Client recovers from surgery without complications
B. Client learns alternate form of communication
C. Client recovers from radiation therapy without complications
D. Client copes with altered body image
E. Client's nutritional status adequate
F. Client remains free of pain
G. Client and significant others cope with altered body image and lifestyle changes

POST-TEST Sensory Disorders, Visual, Auditory, Laryngeal

1. Timolol (Timoptic) eyedrops function by:
   ① Reducing the formation of aqueous humor
   ② Increasing the outflow of aqueous humor
   ③ Constriction of the pupil
   ④ Dilation of the pupil
2. Which of the following statements would indicate that your client with glaucoma needed more teaching?
   ① "I will not take any over-the-counter drugs without checking for the presence of anticholinergics."
   ② "I will wear a Medic Alert tag that states I have glaucoma."
   ③ "I will call the doctor if I develop severe eye pain."
   ④ "I'll use the medication for a full 2 weeks."
3. The expected outcome of successful cataract extraction with an intraocular lens implant would be:

① Total return of 20/20 vision
② Enlarged central vision with cataract glasses
③ Return to precataract vision with some improvement
④ Return to normal vision with the use of special contact lenses
4. Factors that would predispose the development of a retinal detachment include:
   ① Drugs such as steroids
   ② Sudden exertion after severe debilitation
   ③ Overuse of eyedrops
   ④ Prolapse of the iris after cataract surgery
5. Clinical manifestations that would indicate a retinal detachment include:
   ① Tunnel vision
   ② Loss of central vision
   ③ Gradual painless loss of vision
   ④ Blurred vision with floating spots
6. The proper position for a client with a retinal detachment would be lying:
   ① On the unaffected side
   ② With the detachment dependent
   ③ Supine
   ④ Prone
7. After a repair of a retinal detachment, the eyedrops used postoperatively should be:
   ① Mydriatics
   ② Miotics
   ③ Epinephrine
   ④ Timolol
8. Preoperatively, it is important for the client with laryngeal cancer to:
   ① Learn esophageal speech
   ② Avoid oral care
   ③ Increase intake of proteins
   ④ Avoid having dental work done
9. In caring for a client postoperatively after a radical neck dissection, the nurse will have to teach the client to care for the tracheostomy. Which of the following should the client be taught?
   ① Remove the tracheostomy tube if obstruction occurs
   ② Never put any covering over the tracheostomy
   ③ Leave the tracheostomy ties in place until the physician changes them
   ④ Remove and clean the inner cannula daily
10. Which of the following is NOT a symptom of laryngeal cancer?
    ① Hoarseness
    ② Hemoptysis
    ③ Dysphagia
    ④ Lymphadenopathy

11. The client who has Meniere's disease understands that he or she should avoid all of the following EXCEPT:
    ① Smoking
    ② Excess sodium intake
    ③ Alcohol
    ④ Antivertigo medication

12. A client who has suddenly developed hearing loss would be analyzed with which nursing diagnosis?

① High risk for infection related to left-sided hearing loss
② Pain related to hearing loss
③ Self-care deficit related to right-sided hearing loss
④ Impaired social interaction related to withdrawal due to hearing loss

POST-TEST Answers and Rationales

1. ① Timolol actually reduces the formation of aqueous humor, thereby lowering the intraocular pressure. It does not affect the pupil or the outflow of the humor. 2, I & II. Glaucoma.

2. ④ The medication to treat glaucoma must be taken for the rest of the client's life. This statement means that there is a need for more teaching. The other options reflect an understanding of glaucoma by the client. 5, I & II. Glaucoma.

3. ③ The client can expect a return to their former vision with some actual improvement, often requiring a new prescription about 6 weeks after the surgery. There is no need for special lenses or glasses. There will be only 20/20 vision, if that is what the client had preoperatively. 3, I. Cataracts.

4. ② Sudden exertion after a client has been severely debilitated can precipitate a retinal detachment. The other options are not related to this problem. 1, I & II. Retinal Detachment.

5. ④ Blurred vision with floating spots indicates the area where the retina has detached. The other options are symptoms of glaucoma or cataracts. 1, II. Retinal Detachment.

6. ② The client should lie with the detached portion of the retina dependent so that it can fall back into place and possibly reattach. The other positions would only cause it to pull away more. 4, II. Retinal Detachment.

7. ① Mydriatics are used to dilate the pupil after a retinal detachment. The other drugs are inappropriate in treating a retinal detachment. 4, I & II. Retinal Detachment.

8. ③ The client is often malnourished and there will be extensive healing postoperatively, so it is very important for the client to increase the intake of proteins either orally or through hyperalimentation. It is probably not practical to have the client learn esophageal speech preoperatively, and oral hygiene and dental care are absolute priorities. 4, II. Laryngeal Cancer.

9. ④ The client must learn to care for the tracheostomy, including the cleaning of the inner cannula. The stoma can be covered with a porous cloth to prevent aspiration of particles. If the airway is obstructed, the tube provides a way to suction the client and relieve the obstruction. The ties should be changed with assistance whenever the ties are soiled. 4, II. Laryngeal Cancer.

10. ② Hemoptysis is a sign of lung cancer, not laryngeal cancer. The other options are all signs of laryngeal cancer. 1, II. Laryngeal Cancer.

11. ④ Smoking, alcohol intake, and sodium retention are all precipitating factors that can aggravate an attack of Meniere's disease. Ingesting antivertigo drugs, i.e., Bonine, Antivent, assists in relieving the severe vertigo that is one of the classic signs of this disease. 4, II. Ear Disease.

12. ④ The only answer applicable to hearing loss is impaired social isolation. The remainder of the nursing diagnoses *assume* that there is a specific *cause* of hearing loss. 2, III. Ear Disease.

BIBLIOGRAPHY

NEUROLOGIC DISORDERS

Bauman, C. K., and Zumwalt, C. B. (1989). Intracranial neoplasms: An overview. *AORN Journal* 50: 240–256.

Black, J., and Matassarin-Jacobs, E., eds. (1993). *Luckmann and Sorensen's medical-surgical nursing: A psychophysiologic approach,* 4th ed. Philadelphia: W. B. Saunders.

Burns, E. M., and Buckwalter, K. C. (1988). Pathophysiology and etiology of Alzheimer's disease. *Nursing Clinics of North America* 23: 11–27.

Corderre, C. B. (1989). Meningitis: Dangers when the diagnosis is viral. *RN* 52 (8): 50–54.

Delgado, J., and Billo, J. M. (1988). Care of the patient with Parkinson's disease: Surgical and nursing interventions. *Journal of Neuroscience Nursing* 20: 141–150.

Doolittle, N. D. (1988). Stroke recovery: Review of the literature and suggestions for future research. *Journal of Neuroscience Nursing* 20:169–173.

Ferguson, J. M. (1987). Helping an MS patient live a better life. *RN* 50 (12): 22–27.

Harper, J. (1988). Use of steroids in cerebral edema: Therapeutic implications. *Heart and Lung* 17: 70–73.

Hartshorn, J. (1986). Nursing interventions for anticonvulsant drug interactions. *Journal of Neuroscience Nursing* 18: 250–256.

Hickey, J. V. (1986). *The clinical practice of neurologic and neurosurgical nursing,* 2nd ed. Philadelphia: J. B. Lippincott.

Hummel, S. K. (1989). Cerebral vasospasm: Current concepts of pathogenesis and treatment. *Journal of Neuroscience Nursing* 21: 216–224.

Kelly, B. (1988). Nursing care of the patient with multiple sclerosis. *Rehabilitation Nursing* 13: 238–243.

Lundgren, J. (1986). *Acute neuroscience nursing concepts and care.* Boston: Jones & Bartlett.

Santilli, N., and Sierzant, T. L. (1987). Advances in the treatment of epilepsy. *Journal of Neuroscience Nursing* 19: 141–155.

Zumwalt, C. B., and Bauman, C. K. (1989). Malignant glioma: A case study. *AORN Journal* 50: 256–260.

HEARING/VISION

Ames, S. W., and Kneisl, C. R. (1988). *Essentials of adult health nursing.* Menlo Park, CA: Addison-Wesley.

Beare, P. G., and Myers, J. L., eds. (1990). *Principles and practice of adult health nursing.* St. Louis: C. V. Mosby.

Bowers, A. C., and Thompson, J. (1991). *Clinical manual of health assessment,* 4th ed. St. Louis: C. V. Mosby.

Clayton, L. T., ed. (1990). *Taber's cyclopedic medical dictionary,* 15th ed. Philadelphia: F. A. Davis.

Doenges, M. E., and Moorhouse, M. F. (1991). *Nurse's pocket guide: Nursing diagnoses with interventions,* 3rd ed. Philadelphia: F. A. Davis.

Drance, S. M., and Heufeld, A. H., eds. (1984). *Glaucoma: Applied pharmacology in medical treatment.* New York: Grune & Stratton.

Engelstein, J. M., ed. (1984). *Cataract surgery: Current options and problems.* New York: Grune & Stratton.

Lewis, S. M., and Collier, I. C. (1987). *Medical-surgical nursing: Assessment and management of clinical problems,* 2nd ed. New York: McGraw-Hill.

Phipps, W. J., Long, B., and Woods, N. F. (1991). *Medical-surgical nursing: Concepts for clinical practice,* 4th ed. St. Louis: C. V. Mosby.

Swearingen, P. L., ed. (1990). *Manual of nursing therapeutics,* 2nd ed. St. Louis: C. V. Mosby.

6

Protective Functions in the Adult Client

PRE-TEST Communicable Diseases

1. Which of the following sexually transmitted diseases (STDs) are diagnosed with blood tests?
   1. Gonorrhea and HIV infection
   2. Genital herpes and syphilis
   3. HIV infection and syphilis
   4. Chlamydial infections
2. During a latency period in an STD, the infected person is usually:
   1. Noninfectious
   2. Capable of transmitting the disease
   3. Permitted to have unprotected sexual contact
   4. Very sick
3. Co-infections (having more than one STD simultaneously) are an important consideration in:
   1. Chlamydial infections and gonorrhea
   2. Genital herpes and syphilis
   3. Genital herpes and gonorrhea
   4. Genital warts and gonorrhea
4. Which of the following STDs are caused by bacteria?
   1. Herpes, gonorrhea, and HIV infection
   2. Genital warts (condyloma), syphilis, and chlamydial infections
   3. Syphilis, gonorrhea, and chlamydial infections
   4. Gonorrhea, syphilis, and herpes
5. The primary stage of syphilis is characterized by:
   1. No symptoms
   2. Chancre formation
   3. Fever, malaise, and rhinitis
   4. Diminished neurological function

6. High-risk behaviors that put a person at risk for HIV infection include:
   1. Using public swimming pools
   2. Sharing needles with HIV-infected injectable drug users
   3. Working as a volunteer in an AIDS assistance program
   4. Getting bitten by a mosquito

During a pre-employment physical, Anne Hill is told that she has a genital herpes infection.

---

7. Genital herpes is most accurately diagnosed by:
   1. A blood test
   2. History and physical
   3. Urinalysis
   4. Isolating the virus in tissue culture
8. HSV-1 or HSV-2 causes genital herpes. The clinic nurse tells Anne that characteristics of these viruses include the following:
   1. HSV is airborne
   2. HSV survives on inanimate objects for 1 hour
   3. HSV is found in the blood
   4. HSV enters the body via a break in the skin or mucous membrane
9. Anne is told by the nurse that:
   1. Herpes lesions seldom recur
   2. Asymptomatic genital herpes is more common in men
   3. She should abstain from intercourse until the lesions are healed
   4. There is NO risk of transmission when asymptomatic

PRE-TEST Answers and Rationales

1. ③ Only HIV infection and syphilis can be diagnosed with a blood test; the other STDs are usually diagnosed by taking specimens from the genital tract. 1, II. STD.
2. ② During latency in an STD, the infected person can often transmit the disease to a sexual contact or to a fetus. 1, II. STD.
3. ① Frequently chlamydial infections and gonorrhea are present simultaneously. This must be considered when a person is being diagnosed and treated. 1, II & IV. STD.
4. ③ Syphilis, gonorrhea, and chlamydia are all caused by bacteria. Herpes, condyloma and HIV infection are caused by viruses. 1, II. STD.

5. ② Chancre formation is the only symptom of primary syphilis. 1, II. STD.
6. ② Sharing needles and syringes contaminated with HIV-infected blood should be avoided. 1, IV. STD.
7. ④ Isolating HSV in a tissue culture is the best way of diagnosing genital herpes. 1, II. STD.
8. ④ Genital herpes is spread through direct contact with the lesion via a break in the skin or mucous membrane. 1, II. STD.
9. ③ One of the reasons why genital herpes is such a problem is because it often recurs, it can be asymptomatic, and it demands abstinence until lesions are healed for the most effective protection. 1, II & IV. STD.

NURSING PROCESS APPLIED TO ADULTS WITH COMMUNICABLE DISEASES

Sexually Transmitted Diseases: Overview

I. Sexually transmitted diseases (STDs) are one of 15 health priorities addressed in Surgeon General's report on health promotion and disease prevention; they represent a major health problem, with acquired immune deficiency syndrome (AIDS) now identified as the number one health problem in the United States
II. Venereal diseases, as STDs were previously called, are most common communicable diseases worldwide; they also cause enormous suffering and cost the nation billions of dollars annually
III. Significant changes in sexual behavior, including sexual activity at a younger age, multiple sex partners, and remaining single longer, have all contributed to the rising incidence of STDs
IV. STDs are transmitted by skin-to-skin contact or mucous membrane to mucous membrane; a person who develops an STD is at increased risk of contracting another STD
V. Six most common STDs, presented in order of incidence (Table 6–1)
   A. Chlamydial infections (3 to 5 million annually)
   B. Genital warts (1 million annually)
   C. Gonorrhea (700,000 annually)
   D. Genital herpes (500,000 annually)
   E. Syphilis (100,000 annually)
   F. AIDS (43,000 in 1991)

Chlamydial Infections

I. Assessment
   A. Definition: includes a spectrum of genital infections caused by the bacterium *Chlamydia trachomatis*
      1. Men—nongonococcal urethritis (NGU)
      2. Women—mucopurulent cervicitis (MPC)
   B. Incidence
      1. Most common STD in the United States, with an estimated 3 to 5 million cases per year
      2. Frequently co-infection of gonorrhea
      3. Highest infection rates occur in young men and women under age 20
   C. Transmission
      1. Sexual intercourse
      2. Two thirds of neonates of infected mothers, infected during passage through birth canal
   D. Clinical manifestations
      1. Women
         a. Asymptomatic 70% of time
         b. Dysuria
         c. Vaginal discharge
      2. Men
         a. Asymptomatic 25% of time
         b. Dysuria
         c. Penile discharge
         d. Swelling of testicles

TABLE 6–1 Six Most Common Sexually Transmitted Diseases

Disease	Cause/Incubation Period	Diagnosis	Signs and Symptoms	Complications	Treatment
Chlamydial infections	*Chlamydia trachomatis;* 5 to 10 days or longer	Cell cultures best; antigen detection from genital tract specimens	Women: 50 per cent asymptomatic, dysuria, vaginal discharge Men: dysuria, watery, mucoid penile discharge	Women: mucopurulent cervicitis, salpingitis, endometritis Men: epididymitis, prostatitis, proctitis Newborns: conjunctivitis, pneumonia	Tetracycline or doxycycline
Genital warts (Condyloma)	Human papillomavirus (HPV); 3 weeks to 9 months	Colposcopy; biopsy for definitive diagnosis	May carry HPV but remain asymptomatic; warts on penis, vagina, anus, occasionally mouth	Some types of HPV are associated with genital dysplasia and carcinoma; warts may enlarge and destroy tissue; may enlarge during pregnancy and bleed. Newborn rarely becomes infected with HPV at time of birth	Wart removal accomplished with cryotherapy with liquid nitrogen; applying podophyllin; there is no permanent cure for eliminating the human papillomavirus
Gonorrhea	*Neisseria gonorrhoeae;* 3 to 6 days	Culture from cervix, rectum, urethra, or pharynx	Women: dysuria, mucopurulent discharge Men: burning on urination, purulent, profuse discharge from urethra	Women: pelvic inflammatory disease (PID) progressing to sterility Men: prostatitis, epididymitis, proctitis Neonates: eye infections	Ceftriaxone followed by doxycycline
Genital herpes	Herpes simplex virus type 1 (HSV-1) or type 2 (HSV-2); 3 to 7 days	Isolation of virus in tissue culture; Papanicolaou or Tzanck smears	Vesicular lesions on cervix or penis; systemic including headache, malaise, low-grade fever	Biggest risk to neonate; may be localized or disseminated, seriously compromising infant's chances for survival	Treat symptomatically; acyclovir PO helps, but does not cure
Syphilis	*Treponema pallidum;* 10 to 90 days Primary stage: 2 to 12 weeks Secondary stage: 8 to 30 weeks Latency stage: approximately 10 weeks Tertiary stage: approximately 5 years	Blood tests: FTA-ABS; VDRL	Primary: chancre on genitals, mouth, or rectum Secondary: skin rash, malaise, fever, sore throat, generalized lymphadenopathy Latency: no symptoms Tertiary: cardiovascular, neurological, and skin changes	Blindness, deafness, brain damage, paralysis, heart disease Newborn: death in utero or after delivery if not treated	Penicillin, tetracycline, doxycycline
HIV infection/ AIDS	Human immunodeficiency virus (HIV); 7 to 10 years	Blood tests: ELISA; Western Blot; history and clinical evaluation; presence of clinical condition as defined by CDC	Fatigue, low-grade fever, weight loss, night sweats, thrush, lymphadenopathy, cough, shortness of breath (S.O.B.)	Depression of immune system puts client at risk for opportunistic infections;	Treat secondary infections; antivirus include zidovudine (AZT), ddI, ddC

TABLE 6–1 Six Most Common Sexually Transmitted Diseases *Continued.*

Disease	Cause/Incubation Period	Diagnosis	Signs and Symptoms	Complications	Treatment
				Pneumocystis carinii pneumonia and Kaposi's sarcoma are most common	

Universal Concepts of STDs

Transmission: All STDs are spread via sexual contact. The greater the number of sexual partners, the greater the likelihood of developing an STD.

Latency: Many STDs have a latency period when there are no symptoms—for example, for syphilis, AIDS, and genital herpes—but disease can still be transmitted during intercourse.

Effect on newborn: The presence of an STD during pregnancy will impact on the health of the fetus.

Co-infections: It is common to have more than one STD simultaneously—for example, AIDS and genital herpes, gonorrhea and chlamydia.

E. Diagnostic Examinations
  1. Cell cultures most reliable but expensive
  2. Antigen detection from genital tract specimens
F. Medical management
  1. Doxycycline 100 mg PO bid for 7 days
  2. Tetracycline 500 mg PO qid for 7 days
II. Analysis
  A. Knowledge deficit related to transmission, treatment, and complications
  B. Altered patterns of sexuality related to possibility of infecting partner and painful intercourse
  C. Altered patterns of urinary elimination related to infection involving urethra
III. Planning/goals, expected outcomes
  A. Client will understand mode of transmission, likelihood of serious complications, and importance of adhering to prescribed treatment regimen as evidenced by avoiding sexual intercourse until course of antibiotics is completed
  B. Client will advise sexual contacts of their need for treatment
  C. Client will experience freedom from dysuria and penile or vaginal discharge
IV. Implementation
  A. Clarify how Chlamydia is transmitted, possible complications, and why medical care is necessary
  B. Emphasize necessity of taking tetracycline 500 mg four times a day for 7 days or doxycylcline 100 mg two times a day for 7 days exactly as directed
  C. Encourage referral of sexual partner(s) for examination and treatment
  D. Advise avoiding sex until client and partner(s) are cured, using condoms and spermicide to prevent future infections
  E. Describe cause of dysuria and discharge and effect on urination
V. Evaluation
  A. Chlamydial infection resolves and does not recur
  B. Women do not develop pelvic inflammatory disease (PID) with subsequent infertility
  C. Men do not develop epididymitis, prostatitis, or urethral strictures
  D. Appropriate information empowers client to seek health care promptly
  E. Client experiences normal genitourinary function

Genital Warts

I. Assessment
  A. Definition: single or multiple painless growths around the anus, vulvovaginal area, penis, urethra, or perineum caused by human papillomaviruses (HPV); also known as condyloma, venereal warts, and HPV
  B. Incidence
    1. One million new infections annually, with 40 million Americans carrying HPV
    2. Often co-exist with other STDs
    3. Person carrying HPV may have it for life
  C. Transmission
    1. Genital warts remain in one place in body, spread by skin-to-skin contact
    2. HPV most often spread during vaginal, anal, and oral sex
    3. Following contact, warts may appear in 3

weeks to 9 months or may never appear at all

    4. Infected mothers rarely pass HPV to their babies during birth

D. Clinical manifestations

    1. Often asymptomatic; i.e., infected with HPV, but no lesions present

    2. Warts may be flat or raised; appear singly or in clusters; tendency to enlarge and bleed during pregnancy

    3. Warts may recur weeks, months, or years following treatment

E. Diagnostic examinations

    1. Based on clinical presentation

    2. Colposcopy may help diagnose cervical lesions

    3. Pap smear may indicate cell changes characteristic of HPV infection

    4. Some types of HPV are associated with anogenital dysplasia and epithelial carcinomas

    5. Definitive diagnosis requires biopsy, which is necessary for pigmented, persistent, or atypical warts

F. Medical management

    1. Goal is to remove warts; virus cannot be eradicated

    2. Cryotherapy with liquid nitrogen

    3. Applications of 10 to 25% solution of podophyllum or 80 to 90% trichloroacetic acid; podophyllum contraindicated in pregnancy because it may cause birth defects

II. Analysis

A. Impaired skin integrity related to presence of lesions

B. Altered health maintenance related to failure to seek appropriate health care services

C. Altered patterns of sexuality related to transmission of an STD

III. Planning/goals, expected outcomes

A. Client will experience resolution of warts, return of skin integrity following prescribed treatment

B. Client will adhere to treatment regimen until lesions are resolved; women will have annual Pap smears

C. Client will advise partners to be checked for presence of genital warts; abstain from sex or use condoms during course of treatment

IV. Implementation

A. Emphasize importance of adhering to prescribed treatment to achieve resolution of warts and decrease possibility of transmitting to sexual partners

B. Teach about mode of transmission, need to return for treatment should warts recur, importance of annual Pap smear for women

C. Advise that incidence of warts is increased in immunosuppressed patients and presence of genital warts is associated with higher rates of HIV infection

D. Encourage referral of sexual partners for examination and possible treatment, instruct about correct use of condoms

V. Evaluation

A. Client recognizes presence of warts and need to seek prompt treatment

B. Client abstains from sexual contact or uses condoms correctly to prevent transmission

C. Sexual partners are examined and receive treatment, if needed

D. Adequate information results in a decreased incidence of genital warts

Gonorrhea

I. Assessment

A. Definition: a sexually transmitted disease, caused by the bacterium *Neisseria gonorrhoeae,* which differs in men and women in terms of course, severity, and ease of diagnosis. Also known as Clap, Strain, Gleet, Dose, or GC

B. Incidence

    1. Estimated 700,000 cases annually

    2. Distribution is 60% men and 40% women

    3. Highest infection rates for ages 20 to 24, followed by ages 15 to 19

    4. Co-infection with *Chlamydia trachomatis* or syphilis

    5. Most commonly reported communicable disease in the United States, although number of reported cases has decreased by 22% since 1985

C. Transmission

    1. Contact with exudates of infected mucous membranes via oral, anal, or vaginal intercourse

    2. Neonate infected, usually eyes, during passage through birth canal

D. Clinical Manifestations

    1. Frequently asymptomatic; symptoms may appear 1 to 2 weeks after contact

    2. Women

        a. Dysuria

        b. Mucopurulent discharge

        c. PID with ensuing sterility a possible complication

    3. Men

        a. Burning on urination

        b. Purulent, profuse discharge from urethra

        c. Complications include prostatitis and epididymitis

E. Diagnostic examinations

1. Presumptive diagnosis based on history, symptoms, clinical evidence
2. Bacteriological cultures
   a. Cervix
   b. Urethra, rectum, and pharynx of both sexes
   F. Medical Management
      1. Ceftriaxone (Rocephin) 250 mg IM given one time
      2. Follow with doxycycline (Vibramycin) 100 mg PO bid for 1 week
II. Analysis
   A. Impaired tissue integrity related to presence of mucopurulent discharge
   B. Knowledge deficit related to transmission, treatment, and complications
   C. Altered patterns of sexuality related to presence of a sexually transmitted disease
III. Planning/goals, expected outcomes
   A. Client will experience cessation of mucopurulent discharge
   B. Client will understand treatment, transmission, and complications of gonorrhea as evidenced by client's statements and client's ability to follow the treatment plan
   C. Client will initiate appropriate behaviors to control spread of infection as evidenced by notification of sexual contacts, avoidance of sexual intercourse until cured, and use of condoms
IV. Implementation
   A. Reinforce need for treatment of sex partners; recurrent gonococcal salpingitis is primarily caused by failure to treat
   B. Reassure client that tracing and contacting sexual contacts can be done without jeopardizing client's confidentiality
   C. Instruct regarding correct use of prescribed oral medications
   D. Reinforce appropriate infection control methods, including
      1. Handwashing after toileting
      2. Avoid sexual intercourse until client and partner(s) are cured
      3. Correct use of condoms to prevent reinfection
   E. Instruct to return for evaluation if symptoms persist or recur following treatment
V. Evaluation
   A. Infection will resolve and not recur
   B. Complications will not develop
   C. Common co-infections like syphilis and chlamydia identified and treated
   D. Appropriate public health protocols of reporting and tracing sexual contacts observed
   E. Confidentiality of client and sexual contacts respected

Genital Herpes

I. Assessment
   A. Definition: a chronic sexually transmitted disease caused by herpes simplex virus type 1 or 2
      1. Oral herpes caused by herpes simplex virus 1 (HSV-1)
      2. Genital herpes caused by herpes simplex virus 2 (HSV-2), but HSV-1 can also cause genital involvement
   B. Incidence
      1. Estimated 500,000 cases annually
      2. Estimated 15 to 20% of Americans have genital herpes
   C. Transmission
      1. Skin-to-skin contact with an infected area; virus can infect any area of the body surface
      2. HSV enters through break in skin or mucous membrane
      3. HSV lives in nerve cell; not found in the blood
      4. Many carry HSV, but are asymptomatic and can still transmit HSV to their sexual partners
      5. May pose serious risk to newborns of infected mothers, at risk of infection during passage through birth canal
   D. Clinical Manifestations
      1. Vesicular lesions (cold sores) most frequently appearing on cervix or penis, often very painful
      2. Systemic symptoms
         a. Headache
         b. Malaise
         c. Low-grade fever
      3. Recurrence of lesions in 75% of cases
      4. Asymptomatic infection (cervical lesions) more common in women
      5. Cause of reactivation of genital herpes is unknown
   E. Diagnostic examinations
      1. History and clinical evaluation
      2. Isolation of virus in tissue culture is most accurate
      3. Scrapings from lesion; e.g., Papanicolaou (Pap) smear or Tzanck smear
   F. Medical management: acyclovir (Zovirax) PO 200 mg five times/day for 7 to 10 days
II. Analysis
   A. Impaired tissue integrity related to presence of lesions
   B. Pain related to presence of lesions
   C. Knowledge deficit related to mode of transmission and treatment
   D. Altered patterns of sexuality related to possibility of infecting partner and painful intercourse

E. High risk for neonatal infection related to presence of herpetic lesions in the birth canal

III. Planning/goals, expected outcomes
  A. Client will experience healing of lesions in 3 to 4 weeks
  B. Client will be pain-free as evidenced by client's statement of pain relief
  C. Client will understand transmission and treatment as evidenced by abstaining from sex while symptomatic and ability to follow prescribed treatment regimen
  D. Client will advise sexual contacts of presence of herpes infection
  E. Pregnant women should advise health providers of history of herpes

IV. Implementation
  A. Instruct concerning symptoms management, including
    1. Lesions kept clean and dry
    2. Sitz baths for pain relief, speed healing
    3. Acyclovir used orally does not cure, but alleviates symptoms and reduces shedding of virus; for first clinical episode, acyclovir 200 mg five times/day for 7 to 10 days; for recurrence, acyclovir 400 mg five times/day for 10 days or until clinical resolution occurs
    4. Aspirin, ibuprofen for pain; narcotics for severe pain
  B. Instruct client that abstinence is most effective way to avoid transmission when symptoms are present
  C. Reinforce refraining from intercourse when
    1. Lesions are present
    2. Last 4 to 6 weeks of pregnancy if woman's partner has HSV
  D. Reinforce importance of viral cultures during last 8 weeks of pregnancy to safeguard outcome of pregnancy

V. Evaluation
  A. Infection will be treated appropriately both initially and when it recurs
  B. Appropriate client teaching will afford protection for both client and sexual partners
  C. Newborn will not become infected with HSV
  D. When symptomatic, develop understanding of avoiding sex, but continue to enjoy acts of intimacy including cuddling, touching, and hugging

Syphilis

I. Assessment
  A. Definition: a systemic infection caused by the bacterium *Treponema pallidum;* characterized by three stages and a latency period; also known as lues
    1. Primary stage has incubation of 2 to 12 weeks, usually 3 weeks, and is characterized by a chancre (painless lesion) appearing at site of exposure, usually on genitals, mouth, or rectum; it disappears in 4 to 6 weeks with or without treatment
    2. Secondary stage appears 8 to 30 weeks after first stage; manifested by systemic symptoms of skin rash, malaise, fever, sore throat, lymphadenopathy, weight loss
    3. Latency appears 10 weeks later and may last indefinitely; there are no symptoms
    4. Tertiary stage includes neurological and cardiovascular damage; during latency and tertiary syphilis, it is thought that only the fetus is susceptible to transmission
  B. Incidence
    1. Primarily involves young people, ages 20 to 35
    2. Increasing rate of syphilis in the United States since 1986
    3. Syphilis increases risk of HIV infection
  C. Transmission
    1. Acquired: direct contact with open lesions of skin or mucous membranes, body fluids and secretions of infected person during sexual activity
    2. Congenital: passed on to fetus via placental transfer, delivery
    3. Via blood transfusion, if donor in early stages of disease
    4. Health professionals have developed primary lesions on hands following examination of infectious lesions
  D. Clinical manifestations
    1. Primary stage
      a. Chancre on genitals, mouth, or rectum
      b. Chancre often in vagina or on cervix in women
      c. May exhibit enlarged inguinal lymph nodes
    2. Secondary stage
      a. Systemic symptoms of skin rash, malaise, fever, sore throat, weight loss
      b. Lymphadenopathy usually present
    3. Tertiary stage
      a. Neurological damage
      b. Cardiovascular symptoms such as aortitis and aneurysms
  E. Diagnostic examinations
    1. Blood tests, especially accurate is the fluorescent treponemal antibody absorption test (FTS-ABS); rapid plasma reagin (RPR), Venereal Disease Research Laboratory (VDRL) tests also used
    2. History and clinical evaluation

F. Medical management
  1. Benzathine penicillin G 2.4 million units IM in one dose
  2. Doxycycline 100 mg tid PO for 10 days
  3. Tetracycline 500 mg qid PO for 10 to 15 days

II. Analysis
  A. Knowledge deficit related to transmission, course of disease, and treatment
  B. Altered patterns of sexuality related to possibility of infecting partner
  C. Potential for infection of fetus related to congenital transmission

III. Planning/goals, expected outcomes
  A. Client and sexual contacts will seek evaluation and treatment
  B. Client will take prescribed medication correctly
  C. Client will return for follow-up treatment and testing
  D. Client and partner will avoid sexual activity until cured
  E. Pregnant client will seek testing early in pregnancy

IV. Implementations
  A. Instruct concerning importance of sexual contacts being screened, examined, and treated
  B. Promote adherence to appropriate medication routine
    1. For primary, secondary, and early syphilis of less than 1 year in duration, benzathine penicillin 2.4 million units IM in one dose
    2. For syphilis of more than 1 year of duration, benzathine penicillin 2.4 million units IM weekly for 3 consecutive weeks
  C. Ensure cooperation with follow-up testing and treatment; blood tests at 3, 6, and 12 months after treatment; if HIV infected, require follow-up at 1, 2, 3, 6, 9, and 12 months
  D. Instruct in use of condoms to prevent future infections
  E. Instruct concerning risks of syphilis in pregnancy

V. Evaluation
  A. Syphilis will be cured as demonstrated by a nonreactive FTA-ABS or low VDRL titer
  B. Client and contacts receive adequate medications and follow-up testing
  C. Syphilis is prevented because safe sexual practices are used
  D. Penicillin-sensitive pregnant women should have allergy confirmed, be desensitized, and then given appropriate penicillin therapy
  E. Infected neonate receives IM penicillin for 10 days and follow-up VDRL titers

Acquired Immune Deficiency Syndrome (AIDS)

I. Assessment
  A. Definition: a severe, life-threatening clinical condition caused by the human immune deficiency virus (HIV) that suppresses the immune system and damages other organ systems, especially the CNS; AIDS is the clinical endpoint of HIV infection
  B. Incidence
    1. One million HIV infected in the United States
    2. At the end of 1992, more than 240,000 cases had been diagnosed since 1981, with a 67% case fatality rate
    3. Ages 20 to 49 most likely to be affected
    4. In 1992, disease escalating fastest among women and teens
  C. Transmission
    1. Unprotected oral, anal, or vaginal intercourse with an infected partner
    2. Injectable drug use with contaminated equipment
    3. 30% of infants born to HIV-infected mothers are infected before, during, or shortly after birth
    4. Infected blood or blood products
    5. Health care workers exposed to HIV-infected blood through injury with needles or other sharp instruments; current risk estimated to be 0.5%
  D. Clinical manifestations
    1. Progression of symptoms
      a. Initial acute HIV infection, which may manifest flu-like symptoms and last 1 to 2 weeks
      b. Asymptomatic HIV infection with no clinical signs or symptoms, lasting months to years
      c. Symptomatic HIV infection (AIDS-related complex [ARC])
        (1) Persistent generalized lymphadenopathy (PGL)
        (2) Chronic diarrhea
        (3) Fever of 38°C (100.5°F) or higher for 2 months or more
        (4) Drenching night sweats
        (5) Fatigue
        (6) Unexplained weight loss
      d. AIDS, final clinical stage of HIV infection; current case definition includes opportunistic infections, several cancers, extrapulmonary tuberculosis, wasting syndrome, and HIV dementia or sensory neuropathy

2. Clinical categories
   a. Category A: One or more of the following in adult/adolescent with documented HIV infection. No conditions in Category B or C present
     (1) Asymptomatic HIV infection
     (2) PGL
     (3) Acute HIV infection or history of acute HIV infection
   b. Category B: Symptomatic conditions in HIV-infected adult/adolescent that are not included in clinical category C and that meet at least one of the following criteria:
     (1) Conditions attributed to HIV and/or indicative of defect in cell-mediated immunity
     (2) Conditions considered to have clinical course or management complicated by HIV infection
   c. Category C: Any condition from 1987 case definition for AIDS in an adult/adolescent HIV-infected client classified on basis of both:
     (1) Lowest accurate CD4+ determination
     (2) Most severe clinical condition diagnosed regardless of client's current clinical condition

E. Diagnostic examinations
   1. Positive serologic test (ELISA or EIA and Western blot)
   2. History and clinical evaluation
   3. Presence of clinical condition as defined by CDC case definition for AIDS
   4. CD4+ levels categories
     a. Category 1: Greater than or equal to 500 CD4+ cells
     b. Category 2: 200 to 499 CD4+ cells
     c. Category 3: Fewer than 200 CD4+ cells

F. Medical management
   1. Antivirals
     a. Zidovudine (AZT)
     b. ddl (experimental)
     c. ddC (experimental)
   2. Prophylaxis for *Pneumocystis carinii* pneumonia
     a. Sulfamethoxazole (Bactrim)
     b. Pentamidine (Pentam)

II. Analysis
  A. Anxiety related to change in health status, loss of control, and threat of death
  B. Body-image disturbance realted to wasting, disfiguring skin conditions, loss of function
  C. High risk for altered body temperature related to infection, dehydration
  D. High risk for infection related to decreased immune function
  E. Knowledge deficit related to transmission, treatment, and course of disease
  F. Altered nutrition: less than body requirements related to stomatitis, impaired absorption, loss of appetite, and fatigue
  G. Social isolation related to effects of HIV infection and inadequate support system
  H. Altered patterns of sexuality related to possibility of infecting partner

III. Planning/goals, expected outcomes
  A. Client will experience decreased anxiety
  B. Client will develop strategies for coping with changes in appearance and function
  C. Client will experience body temperature within normal limits
  D. Client will protect self from people with infectious conditions to minimize likelihood of secondary infections and will seek prompt treatment at the first sign of illness
  E. Client will prevent spread of HIV infection, adhere to prescribed treatment regimen, and understand the course of the disease
  F. Client will maintain adequate nutrition as evidenced by good management of conditions that interfere with adequate intake of nutrients
  G. Client will use community resources to decrease loneliness and improve social support system
  H. Client will understand how to prevent infecting others with HIV as evidenced by avoiding sexual intercourse or employing safer sex techniques

IV. Implementation
  A. Assist in facilitating communication that will allay or relieve fears, anxieties, and concerns
  B. Suggest ways of coping with appearance changes; encourage independence and control whenever feasible
  C. Teach client to take and record temperature, identify signs and symptoms of incipient infections and dehydration, and seek care promptly
  D. Assist in identifying risks to client of exposure to infectious agents, including people, pets, molds, etc., and explain need for prompt intervention
  E. Identify client's need for information concerning transmission of HIV and living successfully with this diagnosis
  F. Explain the need for universal blood and body fluid precautions, which prevent parenteral, mucous membrane, and nonintact skin exposures of caregivers to blood-borne pathogens; identify the protective barriers that may be used including gowns, gloves, masks, and

protective eyewear; stress the importance of handwashing as the first line of defense for both client and caregiver

G. Evaluate diet for meeting nutritional needs, discuss strategies for control of symptoms that interfere with eating, and refer to nutritionist if necessary

H. Identify and refer to appropriate community resources

I. Review guidelines to prevent spread of HIV, including sexual abstinence, correct use of condoms and spermicides, avoiding the use of contaminated needles and syringes, and the need for HIV testing prior to becoming pregnant

V. Evaluation

A. Fears, anxieties, and concerns identified and controlled

B. Changes in appearance and level of functioning are managed effectively

C. Measures to maintain comfort and control fever succeed

D. Infections are avoided or identified promptly for treatment

E. Appropriate infection control measures are employed that protect client, caregivers, and sexual contacts

F. Adequate nutritional status achieved and maintained

G. Effectively used community resources decrease feelings of social isolation, improve quality of life

H. Spread of HIV is curtailed by safer sex practices, injectable drug users not sharing equipment, and identification of HIV seropositivity *prior* to becoming pregnant

POST-TEST Communicable Diseases

Jane Smith, school nurse at Center High School, has been assigned to teach the content on STDs for the sophomores' required health course.

1. In introducing the material to other faculty, she will explain that STDs are an important part of the health curriculum. The rising incidence of STDs is explained by which of the following?
   ① Lack of effective treatment
   ② Inadequate diagnostic testing
   ③ Sexual activity at a younger age
   ④ Poor personal hygiene practices
2. Understanding 15-year-olds, Nurse Smith knows teenagers:
   ① Are less likely to be at risk for gonorrhea and chlamydia
   ② Who are injecting drugs are at greatest risk for HIV infection
   ③ Need to know that unprotected vaginal, anal, and oral sex all pose risks
   ④ Will use condoms consistently if they know how to use them correctly
3. Prioritizing content according to numbers infected with specific STDs, Nurse Smith remembers that the STD affecting the largest population is:
   ① AIDS
   ② Chlamydial infections
   ③ Genital herpes
   ④ Syphilis

Sally Gray, a senior in high school, has been experiencing a vaginal discharge and episodic dysuria. She decides to seek help from an STD clinic run by the local health department.

---

4. To accurately diagnose Sally Gray's condition, the clinic nurse will explain that:
   ① A specimen from the vaginal tract secretions must be obtained
   ② A history and clinical examination will establish the diagnosis
   ③ Vaginal discharge and dysuria are often insignificant
   ④ Initiating the use of condoms and spermicide will cure the infection
5. When Sally returns to the clinic, she learns that she has a chlamydial infection. This type of STD responds well to:
   ① Injectable penicillin
   ② Doxycycline
   ③ Oral penicillin
   ④ Acyclovir
6. Because Sally has been sexually active with her boyfriend, he must:
   ① Also receive treatment
   ② Be notified that Sally is contagious for six months
   ③ Be quarantined for 1 week
   ④ Take medication prophylactically for 2 months

Brian Williams, a college senior, learns he is positive for HIV antibodies when he donates blood. He is advised to seek counsel at the university's student health service.

7. During counseling Brian is told:
   ① It is likely he will remain asymptomatic for a number of years
   ② That taking acyclovir will prevent progression of his HIV infection
   ③ He should use condoms and spermicide to protect his partner when he has symptoms (e.g., lymphadenopathy, fatigue, anorexia)
   ④ He should avoid public bathrooms to protect himself and others from infection

8. Brians' roommate, Joe, is concerned that he will get AIDS from sharing a room and a bathroom with Brian. Joe is advised that:
   ① HIV is not known to spread by casual contact
   ② He should not borrow Brian's sweatshirt
   ③ Using the same bathroom as Brian is very risky
   ④ HIV lives at least 24 hours outside blood or semen

9. Brian is advised that the meaning of HIV seropositivity is that:
   ① He is capable of transmitting the virus to sexual partners
   ② With appropriate medication, he will no longer be infectious after 2 months
   ③ He is not infectious
   ④ He can donate blood again in 5 years

10. In describing risky sexual practices, the nurse would be WRONG to tell Brian that:
   ① Anal intercourse is the primary way of spreading HIV
   ② Oral sex is considered risky
   ③ HIV can be transmitted during sexual intercourse from an infected man to a woman or from an infected woman to a man
   ④ Using birth control pills and foam will protect his girlfriend from HIV infection

POST-TEST Answers and Rationales

1. ③ Many feel that one of the reasons STDs continue to increase is because teenagers become sexually active sooner. Other reasons cited include staying single longer with greater likelihood of multiple sexual partners. 1 & 5, IV. STD.

2. ③ Teens need to know in clear-cut terms what types of sexual activity pose the greatest risks, including unprotected oral, anal, and vaginal sex. 4, IV. STD.

3. ② Chlamydia is often referred to as the silent epidemic. An estimated 3 to 5 million people are infected each year. 1, II. STD.

4. ① While history and examination are helpful, diagnosis can only be confirmed with a lab specimen. 1, II. STD.

5. ② Doxycycline is the treatment of choice for chlamydia. 4, I & II. STD.

6. ① Sexual contacts of those diagnosed with chlamydia are routinely treated for chlamydia to prevent reinfection of the patient and development of complications in the partner. 1, IV. STD.

7. ① Brian will probably remain asymptomatic for a number of years. Statistically, 50% of those with AIDS are so diagnosed 10 years after the initial HIV infection. 1, II. STD.

8. ① It is well documented that HIV is not spread by casual contact. The primary mode of transmission is anal intercourse. 1, IV. STD.

9. ① Positive results when tested for HIV antibodies mean that a person is capable of transmitting the virus and should either abstain or use condoms and spermicides. 1, IV. STD.

10. ④ Birth control pills and foam obviously are inadequate protection against sexual transmission of HIV. 4, IV. STD.

PRE-TEST Burns

1. Increased capillary permeability after a burn injury leads to:
① Edema
② Gastric ulcers
③ Hyperthermia
④ Paralytic ileus

2. Painful, blistered reddened skin are signs of a:
① Superficial partial-thickness (first-degree) burn
② Partial-thickness (second-degree) burn
③ Full-thickness (third-degree) burn
④ Deep full-thickness (fourth-degree) burn

3. Full-thickness burns heal:
① On their own in about 1 week
② Following heterografting
③ Following autografting
④ Quickly after escharotomy

4. Using the rule of nines to estimate percentage of body surface area burned, a burn of the entire chest and both arms in an adult would be:
① 18%
② 27%
③ 36%
④ 54%

5. After a major burn, which route is preferred for administration of narcotic analgesics?
① Oral
② Subcutaneous
③ Intramuscular
④ Intravenous

6. The usual source of burn wound contamination is:
① Contamination from the client's own flora
② Cross-contamination from other clients
③ Cross-contamination from the staff
④ Cross-contamination from visitors

7. Weight loss following a major burn is:
① Due to a metabolic reset of the appetite centers in the brain
② Preventable if the client is fed during the emergent phase
③ Inevitable due to the hypermetabolic state after injury
④ Treated by using several sources of nutrients

8. Psychological problems following burn injury are:
① Rare in adult burn clients
② Due to the prolonged intense pain
③ Common and adressed beginning in the emergent period
④ Seen most often in clients with maladaptive coping strategies

PRE-TEST Answers and Rationales

1. ① Increased capillary permeability after a burn injury allows plasma to escape from the blood vessels into interstitial space, leading to massive edema of burned and unburned skin. 1, I. Burns.

2. ② Partial-thickness burn is hallmarked by blisters and pain. The skin is open and sometimes wet from broken blisters. 1, I. Burns.

3. ③ Full-thickness burn, also called third degree, is the loss of the entire dermis and epidermis. The dermis cannot regenerate and the epidermis regenerates from outgrowths of epidermal cells that line the hair follicles in the dermis. Therefore, a full-thickness burn cannot heal on its own. It must be grafted from the client's own skin (autograft) for permanent healing to occur. Heterografts are temporary wound covers. Very small third-degree burns (size of a quarter) can heal by scarring and contracture. 1, I. Burns.

4. ③ The arms are each 9% and the chest is 18%, yielding a total of 36%. 2, I. Burns.

5. ④ Narcotics are given intravenously due to unpredicatable circulation to the periphery and ileus. If narcotics were given intramuscularly, they could pool in the extremity, not provide pain relief, and eventually flood the circulation when perfusion was restored. 4, I. Burns.

6. ① Autocontamination is the usual souce of burn wound contamination. 2, I. Burns.

7. ④ Weight loss is due to the hypermetabolism that follows burn injury and is best treated, once ileus resolves, through oral routes. It is common though to use parenteral and nasogastric feedings along with oral feedings to obtain the needed calories. 2, I. Burns.

8. ③ Psychological problems are common in all burn clients. They are due to several factors, such as pre-existent coping strategies, disfigurement, and pain. The management of these problems begins in the emergent period. 2, III. Burns.

NURSING PROCESS APPLIED TO CLIENTS WITH BURNS

I. Assessment
  A. Definition: burns are cutaneous injury from direct contact with or exposure to a thermal, chemical, electrical, or radiation source; extent of injury is related to the length of exposure and the intensity of the heat source
  B. Pathophysiology: complex and multisystem
    1. Cardiovascular release of vasoactive substances increases capillary permeability. Direct injury to the cells causes release of intracellular potassium and myoglobin (in the muscle cell). Fluid shift leads to edema in burned and unburned tissues and hypovolemia. Capillary membrane is restored in 36 to 48 hours and fluids return to usual spaces
    2. Renal and GI: initial shunting of blood from these organs leads to oliguria and ileus; gastric stress ulcerations may develop later (called Curling's ulcers)
    3. Respiratory: smoke inhalation may lead to carbon monoxide poisoning and inhalation injury when burns occur in enclosed space; burns may occur in upper and lower airways and lead to respiratory distress
    4. Immune: depressed function increases risk of infection
    5. Metabolic: hypermetabolic state develops that persists until wound closure
    6. Skin: loss of
      a. Thermoregulation
      b. Water via evaporation
      c. Protective barrier to microorganisms
  C. Etiology
    1. Thermal burns
      a. Fire
      b. Hot liquids
      c. Steam
      d. Semisolids (tar)
      e. Hot objects
    2. Chemical burns
      a. Strong acids
      b. Alkali
      c. Organic compounds
    3. Electrical burns
      a. Electricity

b. Lightning
4. Radiation burns
    a. Industrial radiation
    b. Therapeutic radiation
D. Incidence
    1. 70,000 people hospitalized yearly
    2. Third leading cause of death (as a form of accidents) for all ages
    3. Males most commonly injured under age 70
E. Predisposing/precipitating factors
    1. Age
        a. Scalds common in young children
        b. Flame and grease burns common in older children
        c. Clothing ignition common in the elderly
    2. Lifestyle
        a. Smoking in bed
        b. Hot water heater set too high
        c. Drug use impairing cognition
        d. No smoke detector
F. Clinical manifestations
    1. Depth of injury
        a. Superficial (first degree)
            (1) Epidermis only
            (2) Skin is pink or red
            (3) Painful
            (4) Heal in 3 to 7 days without scar
        b. Partial thickness (second degree)
            (1) Epidermis and into, not through, dermis
            (2) Skin is red, blistered (may be wet and shiny if blisters broken)
            (3) Very painful
            (4) Can heal on their own but may be grafted to speed healing and reduce risk of infection
        c. Full thickness (third degree)
            (1) Epidermis, dermis, and subcutaneous tissue and muscle
            (2) Skin dry, leathery (called eschar), black, brown, red, white, or yellow
            (3) Painless, but sensation of pressure retained
            (4) Does not heal without grafting, unless very small
    2. Extent of injury
        a. Calculated by rule of nines (Figure 6–1) or Lund and Browder charts (more accurate for children)
    3. Inhalation injury
        a. Facial burns
        b. Erythema or edema of the oropharynx or nasopharynx
        c. Singed nasal hairs

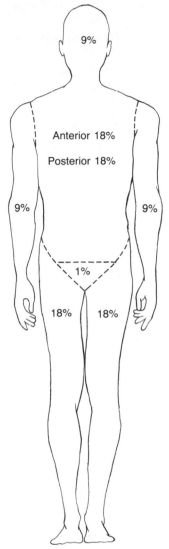

FIGURE 6–1. Rule of "nines" for burns.

    d. Agitation or anxiety
    e. Tachypnea
    f. Flaring nostrils
    g. Stridor
    h. Wheezing
    i. Dyspnea
    j. Voice change/raspy voice
    k. Carbonaceous sputum
    l. Cough
    m. Abnormal arterial blood gases: initial respiratory alkalosis due to tachypnea
4. Severity of injury (several factors)
    a. Burn depth
    b. Burn size
    c. Burn location: increased complications
        (1) Inhalation injury with head, neck, and chest burns
        (2) Eye injury with facial burns

(3) Loss of occupation with hand burns

(4) Infection with perineal burns

(5) Impaired circulation with extremity burns

(6) Impaired ventilation with chest burns

d. Age: mortality higher in

(1) Children

(2) Elderly over 65

e. Mechanism of injury: injury more severe with

(1) Electrical burns

(2) Chemical burns

(3) Inhalation injury

f. General health: previous history of

(1) Cardiac disorders

(2) Pulmonary disorders

(3) Diabetes

(4) Renal disorders

(5) Drug/alcohol dependence

G. Diagnostic examinations

1. Complete blood count

2. Serum electrolytes

3. Urinalysis

4. Chest x-ray

5. Xenon-133 lung scan/fiberoptic bronchoscopy if inhalation injury suspected

6. Carboxyhemoglobin levels

7. Arterial blood gases: maintain direct pressure on puncture site for 5 minutes

H. Complications: can involve any body system

1. Early

a. Hypovolemic shock

b. Pulmonary edema

c. Hyperkalemia

d. Cardiac dysrhythmias

e. Renal failure

f. Respiratory distress

g. Ileus

2. Mid

a. Weight loss/catabolism

b. Infection/sepsis

c. Gastric ulcerations

d. Pneumonia

e. Endocarditis

3. Late

a. Contractures

b. Keloid/hypertrophic scar

c. Depression, isolation

I. Medical management

1. Emergent: begins at time of injury and ends with restoration of fluid balance (diuresis begins)

a. Pre-hospital care

(1) Stop the burning process

(a) Flame

(i) Remove victim from flames

(ii) Smother clothing

(iii) Drop and roll on ground

(b) Chemical

(i) Brush off dry chemical

(ii) Copiously irrigate liquid chemicals

(iii) Remove chemical-laden clothes

(c) Electrical

(i) Shut off power source

(ii) Establish airway, breathing, circulation (ABCs)

(iii) Assess for other injuries

a) Cardiopulmonary arrest

b) Fractures

c) Lacerations

(d) Radiation

(i) Remove from power source

(ii) Decontaminate

b. Emergency department management

(1) Initiate or complete pre-hospital burn care (see previous section)

(2) Re-evaluate ABCs and other injuries

(3) Begin fluid resuscitation

(a) Large-bore peripheral IV placed

(i) In nonburned skin

(ii) Proximal to extremity burns

(iii) Common to use a central line

(b) fluid formulas used as a guideline

(i) 1 mL/kg/% burn

(ii) 70-kg man with a 70% burn needs 4900 mL first 24 hours

(c) calculation begins from time of injury

(d) noncolloid fluids given for 24 to 48 hours

(e) monitor response (urine output greater than 30 mL/hr in adults)

(4) Insertion of indwelling catheter

(5) Insertion of nasogastric tube

(6) Monitor vital signs

(7) Obtain baseline laboratory studies

(8) Initiate wound care

(a) Cover burn to prevent heat loss

(b) Elevate head and arms to reduce edema

(c) Apply topical antimicrobials to small wounds

(d) Debride large wounds if needed

(9) Pharmacological management

(a) Treat pain with intravenous narcotics: reliable absorption

(b) Provide tetanus prophylaxis

(c) Topical antimicrobial: silver sulfadiazine (Silvadene) usual agent

(10) Dietary management

(a) Major burns NPO until ileus resolves

2. Acute: begins at completed fluid resuscitation and ends when wounds have been covered or healed

a. Infection control

(1) Autocontamination usual source

(2) Infection control practices vary between hospitals

(3) Topical antimicrobials

(4) Systemic antibiotics not common, because they do not reach the wound (which is avascular)

b. Wound care

(1) Hydrotherapy

(2) Debridement

(a) Mechanical—scissors, water

(b) Enzymatic

(c) Surgical

c. Wound coverage

(1) Open method: cream alone applied to face, perineum

(2) Closed method: cream covered with dressings

(3) Temporary wound coverage:

(a) Biological

(i) Heterografts (pig skin)

(ii) Homografts (placenta, cadaver skin)

(b) Man-made: dressings

(4) Permanent wound coverage: autografting (from client)

d. Pharmacological management

(1) Narcotics/non-narcotics for pain

(2) Inhalation of nitrous oxide

e. Dietary management

(1) Aggressive due to increased need from hypermetabolism

(2) Various formulas to calculate need: 70-kg man with a 70% burn needs 4550 kcal/day

(3) Oral, IV, NG routes used

(4) Weight, wound healing, laboratory studies used to evaluate

(5) High protein, high calorie

f. Pain management

(1) Narcotics/non-narcotics

(2) Hypnosis, guided imagery, art and play therapy, biofeedback, music therapy

g. Physical therapy

(1) Therapeutic positioning: to avoid contracture

(2) Exercise: active range of motion (ROM)

(3) Splinting

3. Reconstructive

a. Promote complete wound healing

b. Minimize deformities

c. Increase strength and function

d. Provide psychosocial integration into society

e. Provide education/vocational rehabilitation

J. Surgical management

1. Escharotomy

a. Incisions made into the eschar to release pressure from edema beneath

b. For improving circulation/ventilation when burns are circumferential

2. Skin grafting: split-thickness skin grafts (STSG)

a. Sheet or meshed

b. Taken from a donor site

(1) Donor site painful

(2) Donor site encouraged to heal, can be used again as donor site

(a) Covered with synthetic film or fine-meshed gauze

(b) Covered initially, then left open to air

(c) May itch as it heals

c. Applied to a recipient site

(1) Clean or debrided burn wound

(2) Recipient site is immobilized

(3) Graft assessed for "take" (turns pale pink)

(4) Assessed for wound infection

d. May be harvested, stored, and applied to the wound at a later date without anesthesia

3. Scar revision

a. To lengthen contractures

b. Many required over years following injury

II. Analysis

A. Ineffective airway clearance related to tracheal edema, burn injury of the upper airway, and depressed ciliary action from inhalation injury

B. Fluid volume deficit related to increased capillary permeability and fluid shifts from intra-vascular space to interstitial space

C. Pain related to severe tissue injury

D. Hypothermia related to loss of thermoregulation provided by skin

E. High risk for altered peripheral tissue perfusion related to peripheral edema

F. Altered nutrition: less than body requirements related to hypermetabolic state

G. High risk for infection related to loss of primary defenses of intact skin

H. High risk for impaired physical mobility: contractures related to tendency of wounds to heal by contracture

I. Self-esteem disturbance related to disfiguring injury or threatened loss of self-concept

III. Planning/goals, expected outcomes

A. Client will have clear breath sounds, eupnea, clear sputum, effective cough

B. Client will have a urine output of greater than 30 mL/hr, stable vital signs, clear sensorium

C. Client will have controllable pain, be able to rest, and express desire to control factors that increase pain

D. Client will have normothermia with core temperature between 37.5°C and 38.3°C (99.6°F and 101.0°F)

E. Client will have palpable peripheral pulses, intact motor function and sensation in extremities, capillary refill less than 2 seconds, and no tingling or numbness

F. Client will have maintained 85 to 90% of pre-burn weight, healed wounds, and consume the needed calories every 24 hours

G. Client will have no burn wound infection, maintain stable body temperature, have no purulent drainage from puncture sites, and have negative sputum, urine, blood, and wound cultures

H. Client will maintain adequate ROM in all joints, be able to perform self-care and ambulate

I. Client will verbalize stressors and concerns and make use of support systems

IV. Implementation

A. Emergent phase
1. Assess for signs of respiratory distress
2. Monitor arterial blood gases and oxygen saturation levels
3. Administer oxygen
4. Turn, cough, and deep breathe
5. Incentive spirometer
6. Elevate head of bed
7. Monitor quality of sputum
8. Monitor lung sounds
9. Hourly I & O
10. Monitor laboratory studies: hematocrit (Hct), potassium
11. Infuse fluids per order to maintain urine output greater than 30 mL/hr
12. Assess vital signs
13. Administer narcotics routinely
14. Use IV route only until hemodynamically stable
15. Monitor core temperature
16. Use external heat shields
17. Keep room at 35°C (95°F)
18. Assess peripheral pulses
19. Assess capillary refill
20. Assess for numbness or tingling
21. Elevate affected extremities
22. Active ROM
23. Obtain pre-burn weight; weigh daily
24. Assess bowel sounds, NG tube patency
25. Maintain strict isolation
26. Apply topical antimicrobials
27. Clean and debride wounds
28. Maintain position of physiological function (splints, no pillows)
29. Reorient PRN
30. Assist client with coping skills (anxiety, fear)

B. Acute phase
1. Continue with above interventions
2. Explore alternative pain therapies
3. Use anxiolytic agents to supplement narcotics
4. Minimize exposure of open wounds
5. Record caloric intake
6. Frequent meals
7. Use feeding tube or total parenteral nutrition (TPN) as needed
8. Assess for signs of infection
9. Prepare for skin grafting
10. Immobilize after grafting
11. Provide donor site care
12. Wrap grafted legs before ambulating
13. Passive ROM to all joints
14. Teach about pressure garments for scar control
15. Determine pre-burn coping skills
16. Allow client to express feelings
17. Allow client to progress at own rate through grieving
18. Set limits on maladaptive behaviors
19. Promote self-confidence

C. Rehabilitation phase
1. Encourage ROM to reduce contractures
2. Use occupational therapy as needed
3. Teach client skin care to reduce itching: skin lubricants
4. Teach client/family wound care

5. Teach client to use pressure garments for 1 year
6. Encourage client to return to previous role(s) in society
7. Encourage ongoing use of psychological therapy

V. Evaluation
   A. Client's respiratory function remains within normal limits
   B. Client's fluid volume restored
   C. Client's pain controlled
   D. Client's temperature within normal limits
   E. Client maintains peripheral tissue perfusion
   F. Client maintains 85 to 90% of preburn weight
   G. Client heals burn wounds without infection
   H. Client did not develop contractures
   I. Client uses adaptive coping strategies while adapting to altered body image

POST-TEST Burns

David, a 37-year-old man, was burned in a house fire. When brought to the emergency department, the paramedics said that he was smoking in bed. David sustained burns of the face, chest, upper left arm, complete right arm, and neck. His burn wounds are blistered, red and yellow, and wet. He is screaming in pain.

1. Which of the following assessments should be given the highest priority in David's initial care?
   ① Degree of pain
   ② Airway patency
   ③ Hypovolemia
   ④ Signs of infection

2. Which of the following conclusions can be made about the extent and depth of the burn? The burn wound is about:
   ① 32% and superficial
   ② 45% and partial thickness
   ③ 36% and partial thickness
   ④ 32% and full thickness

3. A large-bore intravenous line is placed and David is given resuscitation fluids. What evaluation criteria should be used to determine the effectiveness of the fluid resuscitation?
   ① Hematocrit
   ② Urine output
   ③ Blood pressure
   ④ Extremity circumference

4. David is given intravenous morphine for pain control. What is the rationale for intravenous (IV) administration? IV morphine:
   ① Has the shortest half-life
   ② Is used because of ileus
   ③ Has a more rapid onset
   ④ Has a more predictable absorption

5. What position should David be placed in?
   ① Head and feet elevated
   ② Head of bed flat, hands elevated, no pillow
   ③ Head elevated on two pillows, hands dependent
   ④ Head of bed elevated, arms elevated, no pillow

6. David's family sees him for the first time. They are shocked at his appearance and ask the nurse why his face is so swollen. What facts should the nurse consider before addressing their concern? His facial edema is:
   ① Temporary and may resolve with diuretic therapy
   ② Permanent and a result of improper positioning
   ③ Temporary and a result of fluid shifts from tissue injury
   ④ Permanent but may be less noticeable once his face is skin grafted

David has daily wound care, during which time his burns are debrided and new topical antimicrobials are applied.

7. When the nurse is performing wound care on David's face, what technique should be used? The nurse should use a(n):
   ① Enzymatic debriding agent
   ② Temporary wound cover such as pig skin
   ③ Open method and just apply the ointment
   ④ Closed method and use dressings to cover the ointment

8. What complication is most likely to occur during hydrotherapy?
   ① Hypothermia
   ② Uncontrollable pain
   ③ Wound infection
   ④ Contracture

David's pre-burn weight was 176 pounds. He now weighs 155 pounds. David is begun on nasogastric feedings to meet his caloric needs.

9. David is assigned a student nurse who is administering his tube feeding. She places David in a left lateral position while infusing the feeding. Evaluate her technique. Her technique is:
   ① Correct
   ② Correct, as long as she checked placement of the tube before starting the infusion
   ③ Incorrect; semi-Fowler's is the preferred position
   ④ Incorrect; supine is the preferred position

10. When setting goal/expected outcome criteria for the nursing diagnosis "altered nutrition: less than body requirements," what goal/expected outcome criteria should be used for David? Client will:
    ① Maintain a body weight of 158.5 pounds
    ② Maintain a body weight of 139.5 pounds
    ③ Consume 4000 calories a day
    ④ Consume 2000 calories a day

11. David walks to the hospital gift shop. When he returns he is sullen. The nurse enters the room and asks him "How did your walk go?" David replies, "It was awful, everyone stared at me!" How should the nurse respond?
    ① "That's the way it will be for a while until you get used to the stares."
    ② "Why don't you think about how you are feeling and we will talk about this later."
    ③ "You probably went too far too fast, and you were just tired. I think you will be OK."
    ④ "You sound like you are upset at the stares. Can you talk about it now?"

12. David is to be discharged from the hospital. Which of the following ongoing treatments is necessary?
    ① High-calorie, high-protein diet to heal the wounds
    ② Range-of-motion exercises to reduce contractures
    ③ Pressure garments to reduce itching
    ④ Isolation to prevent infection

POST-TEST Answers and Rationale

1. ② Because David was burned in an enclosed space, that of a house fire, he is at increased risk of airway burn. Therefore, airway patency is the priority assessment. 1, I. Burns.

2. ③ A burn of the face is 4.5%, chest and neck is 18%, entire left arm is 9%, and upper right arm is 4%, which equals 36%. Blistered, wet, and red burns are superficial burns. 2, I. Burns.

3. ② Urine output of more than 30 mL/hr in the adult client is usually considered to be the criterion of adequate fluid resuscitation. Blood pressure is also used, but is not as sensitive of an evaluation measure. Following a burn, blood pressure may be elevated because of pain and may not fall as quickly when fluid resuscitation is inadequate. Hematocrit will drop to normal levels once the client is hydrated, but is an additional parameter of assessment, not a primary one. Extremities may develop increased edema, but the diameter of the extremities would not be an accurate measure of fluid resuscitation. 5, II. Burns.

4. ④ Intravenous morphine is the route of choice for pain because it has a known absorption. When narcotics are given orally or intramuscularly, they will not be absorbed due to ileus or limited perfusion of muscle. Theoretically, the drug could ''pool'' in areas of limited perfusion and be released in mass once perfusion is restored. The pharmacodynamics of the narcotic used are not the rationale for IV route. 2, II. Burns.

5. ④ David should be placed with his head and arms elevated to reduce the impact of edema and improve venous return. Due to his neck burns, he should not have a pillow to reduce the risk of contracture. 2 & 4, I. Burns.

6. ③ Edema following a burn is temporary due to interstitial fluid shifts. Edema is not treated with diuretics; in fact, the client is given fluids to restore intravascular fluid losses. Edema occurs in burned and unburned tissue; therefore, positioning helps reduce edema, but improper positioning seldom causes facial edema. 1 & 5, I. Burns.

7. ③ Facial burns are treated with an open method, which is just the application of the antimicrobial ointment. The closed method, which wraps the body part, can lead to disorientation and lack of ability to communicate. 4, I. Burns.

8. ① Hydrotherapy is most likely to lead to hypothermia, because the client's open wounds are exposed to the environment. Wound debridement in the tub can lead to pain, but it is controllable with narcotics given before tubbings. Wound infection can occur if the tank is not properly cleaned or with autologous contamination in the complete submersion style tank, but it is not common. Contractures are a late complication. 2, II. Burns.

9. ③ The student's technique is incorrect. The safest position for the client during tube feeding is semi-Fowler's to reduce the risk of aspiration. 2, I. Burns.

10. ① The goal is that the client maintain 85% of his pre-burn weight or 158.5 pounds for David. Weight is the best indicator of nutritional balance, not caloric intake. 3, I. Burns.

11. ④ In this situation, the nurse's best response is to reflect the client's feelings and allow him to converse about his feelings if he is able to. 4, III. Burns.

12. ② David will need to continue with range-of-motion exercises and elastic garments to reduce contractures. These garments can lead to itching, not prevent it. A high-protein, high-calorie diet and isolation are not needed once the wound is healed. 4, I. Burns.

PRE-TEST Adults Undergoing Surgery

1. Which of the following surgical clients is most likely to develop dehydration postoperatively?
   1. Adolescents
   2. Clients with history of melanoma
   3. Clients with history of hypothyroidism
   4. Elderly clients

2. Preoperative medications ordered for your client are meperidine (Demerol) 75 mg and atropine 0.3 mg. Dosages available are Demerol 50 mg/mL and atropine 0.4 mg/mL. You should prepare:
   1. Demerol 0.75 mL; atropine 1.2 mL
   2. Demerol 1.5 mL; atropine 0.5 mL
   3. Demerol 2 mL; atropine 1 mL
   4. Demerol 1.5 mL; atropine 0.75 mL

3. The purpose of giving atropine preoperatively is to:
   1. Provide general muscle relaxation
   2. Cause a decrease in pulse and respiration
   3. Produce a decrease in oral and respiratory secretions
   4. Enhance the effectiveness of meperidine (Demerol)

4. Which of the following statements is true regarding the nursing care of the recovery room client who had spinal anesthesia?
   1. The nurse should be alert to the possibility of hypotension.
   2. The semi-Fowler's position is optimal for these clients.
   3. The spinal anesthesia client is never given medication if unable to move his or her legs.
   4. High Fowler's position is best for these clients.

Mrs. Draper is scheduled for a colon resection. You have just given her preoperative medication of Demerol 50 mg IM and atropine 0.4 mg IM.

---

5. As you come to give her other preoperative medications, you find her sitting up in bed wringing her hands, perspiring, and unable to concentrate when you question her as to how she feels. Which of the following would be the most appropriate nursing action for Mrs. Draper?
   1. Ask her family to leave, lower the bed, put her in a supine position, and administer her medications
   2. Ask her family to leave, sit down, hold her hand, and ask her if she would like to talk to you about how she is feeling
   3. Call the family into the hall and ask if this is the way the client usually responds to stress
   4. Hold off giving the preoperative medications, call the OR, and describe the client's symptoms to the anesthesiologist or the surgeon

6. In the post-anesthesia recovery (PAR), which would be the best position for Mrs. Draper?
   1. Prone
   2. Trendelenburg
   3. Lithotomy
   4. Side-lying

7. Anticipating Mrs. Draper's return from the recovery room, which of the following equipment is LEAST necessary to have at the bedside?
   1. Gastric suction
   2. IV equipment
   3. An oral airway
   4. Tracheostomy set

8. Since returning from the recovery room, Mrs. Draper's blood pressure has dropped steadily, her dressing is soaked with blood, her urine output is low, and her skin is cold and clammy. Which of the following is the best nursing intervention for this client?
   1. Draw arterial blood gases
   2. Irrigate the nasogastric suction
   3. Increase the rate of the IV fluids
   4. Medicate with analgesics

9. What position would be best for Mrs. Draper, considering the above situation?
   1. Trendelenburg
   2. Supine, with feet elevated
   3. Side-lying
   4. Lithotomy

10. A possible early manifestation of a transfusion reaction is:
    1. Hypertension
    2. Flank pain
    3. Cyanosis
    4. Bradycardia

11. The postoperative client should always be assessed for the presence of a pulmonary embolus. Early clinical manifestations of a pulmonary embolus are:
    1. Restlessness and tachycardia
    2. Dull chest pain and tachycardia
    3. Low-grade fever and hypotension
    4. Localized, stabbing chest pain, and bradycardia

12. On her fifth postoperative day, Mrs. Draper complains of incisional pain. You assess her wound as red around edges, swollen with a

moderate amount of yellow drainage. The most appropriate nursing action would be to:

① Take vital signs and obtain a wound culture

② Apply sterile 4 × 4

③ Increase the dosage of antibiotic

④ Irrigate the wound with sterile normal saline and paint with Betadine

13. Which of the following would be considered normal for the first day postoperatively after upper abdominal surgery?

① Dyspnea

② Pain over the incision site when coughing

③ Yellow-green drainage from incision

④ Frequency and burning after urination

14. Which of the following is LEAST important in discharge teaching of Mrs. Draper?

① Instructions on wound care

② Instructions on the hospital telephone number to report any unusual signs and symptoms

③ Instructions on when to resume physical activities

④ Instructions on follow-up visit to surgeon

PRE-TEST Answers and Rationales

1. ④ The elderly are often dehydrated preoperatively and are very prone to fluid and electrolyte losses during surgery and postoperatively. None of the other clients are at particular risk. 2, II. Surgical Intervention.

2. ④ Demerol 50 mg/1 mL = 75 mg/X mL, 50X = 75, X = 1.5. Atropine 0.4 mg/1 mL = 0.3 mg/X mL, 0.4X = 0.3, X = 0.75. 4, I. Surgical Intervention.

3. ③ Atropine acts to reduce tracheobronchial secretions and dries the mucous membranes. It increases the pulse, is not a muscle relaxant, and does not affect Demerol. 4, II. Surgical Intervention.

4. ① Hypotension is the major complication of spinal anesthesia, because it causes peripheral vasodilation. None of the other answers are correct. 1, II. Surgical Intervention.

5. ④ The client is displaying extreme anxiety that would interfere with the course of the surgery. You should talk to her, but first you must notify the OR and staff of the delay. 1 & 5, III. Surgical Intervention.

6. ④ The side-lying position promotes maximum respiratory expansion and prevents aspiration. 4, II. Surgical Intervention.

7. ④ A client would not have a reason to have a tracheostomy after a colon resection. The other options would be necessary equipment postoperatively. 4, II. Surgical Intervention.

8. ③ The client who is experiencing hypovolemia and shock needs fluid volume replacement immediately. The most appropriate response is to increase the rate of the IV. 2 & 4, II. Surgical Intervention.

9. ② The client who is experiencing shock should be placed flat in bed with the legs elevated to an angle of 45 degrees. Trendelenburg puts unnecessary pressure on the diaphragm and decreases breathing. 4, II. Surgical Intervention.

10. ② An early clinical manifestation of a transfusion reaction is flank pain and low back pain because of the renal involvement. 2, II. Surgical Intervention.

11. ① Restlessness and tachycardia are caused by cerebral ischemia. These are physiological responses to the emboli. 4, II. Surgical Intervention and Respiratory.

12. ① The symptoms described indicate a wound infection. It is therefore important to assess if the client is febrile and to obtain a wound culture. 2 & 4, II. Surgical Intervention.

13. ② Incisional pain when coughing is normal after upper abdominal surgery because of the proximity of the wound to the diaphragm. 5, I. Surgical Intervention.

14. ② The client needs discharge information regarding physical activity, wound care, and follow-up care. It is not necessary to include the unit phone number. 3, IV. Surgical Intervention.

NURSING PROCESS APPLIED TO ADULTS UNDERGOING SURGERY

Preoperative Phase

Anxiety

I. Assessment
  A. Predisposing/precipitating factors
    1. Fear of unknown
    2. Fear of pain
    3. Fear of death
    4. Fear of anesthesia
    5. Fear of disfigurement
    6. Loss of control
    7. Financial difficulties
  B. Signs and symptoms
    1. Inability to concentrate, follow conversation
    2. Inability to verbalize fears
    3. Pacing, inability to rest, insomnia
    4. Anger, depression, confusion, or no emotional response
    5. Increase in pulse and respiratory rates
II. Analysis
  A. Fear of pain and discomfort
  B. Knowledge deficit related to surgical experience
  C. Ineffective individual coping related to impending surgery
III. Planning/goals, expected outcomes
  A. Client will verbalize fears/anxieties

B. Client will demonstrate decreased signs of anxiety

C. Client will demonstrate a knowledge of the surgical experience

IV. Implementations
 A. Allow for verbalization of fears, concerns
 B. Patient teaching
  1. Explain preoperative tests
  2. Explain preoperative routines
  3. Discuss what to expect postoperatively
   a. Recovery room
   b. Use of analgesia
   c. Use of special equipment
  4. Postoperative activities
   a. Turning, coughing, deep breathing
   b. Incisional splinting
   c. Leg exercises
 C. Include family/significant other in preoperative care and teaching
 D. Assess need for spiritual advisor prior to surgery
 E. Call surgeon if patient demonstrates unrelieved, elevated anxiety

V. Evaluation
 A. Client verbalizes fears about surgery
 B. Client and family/significant other demonstrate understanding of preoperative teaching (i.e., client demonstrates deep-breathing exercises)

Informed Consent

I. Assessment
 A. Definition: statement indicating the client understands the nature of the surgery as well as the risks and benefits involved.
 B. Assessment of client understanding and competence

II. Analysis: knowledge deficit related to surgical experience

III. Planning/goals, expected outcomes
 A. Client will be able to verbalize understanding of surgery
 B. Client will sign consent

IV. Implementations
 A. Assess client's level of understanding about surgery
 B. Act as client advocate in witnessing consent; answer and clarify client questions
 C. Contact surgeon if client has major questions or misunderstanding about surgery
 D. Assess language used, level of consciousness, use of drugs that may alter sensorium prior to patient signing consent

V. Evaluation
 A. Client verbalizes understanding of surgery
 B. Client signs informed operative consent

Older Adult

I. Assessment
 A. Etiology/incidence: elderly at higher risk to undergo surgery, as well as development of postoperative complications
 B. Predisposing/precipitating factors
  1. Presence of chronic diseases
  2. Frequently dehydrated
  3. Poor nutritional status
  4. Stress response diminished
  5. More sensitive to effects of analgesics, narcotics, and sedatives

II. Analysis
 A. High risk for fluid volume deficit related to decreased homeostatic mechanism
 B. High risk for decreased cardiac output related to decreased homeostatic mechanism
 C. High risk for ineffective airway clearance related to decreased cough reflex
 D. High risk for impaired physical mobility related to age and chronic illness

III. Planning/goals, expected outcomes
 A. Elderly clients will have risk factors identified
 B. Elderly clients will experience minimal postoperative complications

IV. Implementations
 A. Carefully evaluate intake and output postoperatively
 B. Reduce pain medications postoperatively; assess effectiveness
 C. Provide diet high in protein and vitamin C
 D. Assess and initiate preventive measures for the following frequently seen postoperative complications
  1. Shock
   a. Assess vital signs, level of consciousness (LOC)
   b. Assess urine output
  2. Atelectasis, pneumonia
   a. Assess respiratory status
   b. Good pulmonary hygiene
  3. Thrombophlebitis
   a. Early ambulation
   b. Support hose/sequential pressure boots
   c. Assess Homans sign
  4. Poor wound healing
   a. Assess wound for redness, swelling, tenderness
   b. Increase protein, vitamin C in diet

V. Evaluation
 A. Risk factors minimized during elderly client's postoperative course
 B. Elderly client free of complications postoperatively

Nutrition
I. Assessment
  A. Definition: nutritional problems of obesity and malnutrition can increase surgical risk
  B. Incidence
    1. Obesity
      a. Increases workload on heart
      b. More prone to wound infection, wound dehiscence, harder to heal
      c. More prone to pulmonary complications postoperatively
      d. Prolongs surgery
    2. Nutritional deficiency
      a. Protein and vitamins B, C, and K are essential for wound healing
      b. Prolonged postoperative recovery
II. Analysis
  A. Altered nutrition: less than body requirements related to malnutrition
  B. Altered nutrition: more than body requirements related to obesity
III. Planning/goals, expected outcomes
  A. Client will increase/decrease nutritional intake
  B. Client will not develop postoperative complications related to nutritional alteration
IV. Implementations
  A. Assess client preoperatively for nutritional status
    1. Weight
    2. Skin turgor, mucous membranes
    3. Serum protein, albumin levels
  B. Encourage weight reduction or diet high in protein, vitamins B, C, and K, if possible preoperatively
  C. Postoperatively assess for wound healing and pulmonary complications
V. Evaluation
  A. Client's nutritional intake improved
  B. Client has not developed wound or respiratory complications postoperatively

Past/Present Medical Diseases
I. Assessment
  A. Incidence: patient should be interviewed for history
    1. Pulmonary diseases (COPD)
    2. Cardiovascular diseases (MI, HTN, CHF)
    3. Liver disease
    4. Renal disease
    5. Endocrine disease (diabetes, hyperthyroidism, hypothyroidism)
    6. Infection
    7. Allergies
  B. Complications
    1. Pulmonary problems predispose clients to inadequate gas exchange and respiratory infection
    2. Clients with cardiovascular problems prone to shock and fluid imbalances postoperatively
    3. Clients with liver or renal disease may have problems metabolizing and excreting anesthetic and analgesic agents
    4. Clients with endocrine problems may have postoperative wound complications
    5. Clients with an infection present may have problems with postoperative healing
    6. Clients with allergies may have untoward effects to the anesthetic agents or postoperative medications
II. Analysis: high risk for injury related to pre-existing condition (COPD, MI, HTN, CHF, liver disease, renal disease, endocrine disease, infection, allergies)
III. Planning/goals, expected outcomes: client will not develop any operative or postoperative complications from past or present medical diseases
IV. Implementations
  A. Assess history of current diseases or previous health status that may interfere with the postoperative course
  B. Plan interventions that will treat/correct any existing health problems
  C. Monitor vital signs carefully postoperatively
  D. Monitor I & O
  E. Assess client's response to analgesics, anesthetic agents
  F. Assess wound healing
  G. Assess CBC, serum electrolytes, fasting blood sugar, ECG, CXR
V. Evaluation: client recovers from surgery without complications

Drug History
I. Assessment
  A. Incidence: client should be interviewed for use of medications prior to surgery
    1. Antibiotics
    2. Anticoagulants
    3. Antihypertensives
    4. Aspirin
    5. Diuretics
    6. Steroids
    7. Hypoglycemics
    8. Tranquilizers
    9. Recreational drugs
  B. Complications: medications that can adversely affect anesthesia or surgery (Table 6–2)
II. Analysis: high risk for injury related to medication use/history

TABLE 6–2 Drugs that Adversely Affect Surgery

Drug	Possible Effect
Corticosteroids	Delays wound healing; masks infection
	Increases risk of hemorrhage. Increases serum glucose
Thiazide diuretics	Interact with anesthesia, leading to excessive respiratory depression and decreased K^+
Antihypertensives	Interact with anesthesia to produce excessive hypotension
Antibiotics	Produces mild respiratory depression
	May mask infection
Anticoagulants and aspirin	Excessive bleeding or clotting if stopped suddenly
Antiparkinsonians	Interact with anesthesia to produce severe hypertension
Narcotics	Increased tolerance to sedation and anesthesia
Antiarrhythmics Propranolol (Inderal)	Affects patient's tolerance of anesthesia
Quinidine (gluconate)	Depresses cardiac function
Procainamide hydrochloride	Potentiates anesthetics that are neuromuscular blockers
Glaucoma medications	May cause respiratory or cardiovascular collapse during surgery
Hypoglycemic medications Chlorpropamide	Insulin needs decrease when client NPO
Glipizide Glyburide	Insulin needs increase in response to physiological stress and healing
Insulin	Insulin needs fluctuate in the postoperative course

III. Planning/goals, expected outcomes: client will not develop intraoperative or postoperative complications from previous drug therapy
IV. Implementations
 A. Assess and evaluate client's response to anesthetic agents and analgesics postoperatively
 B. Plan care based on individual need for medication (i.e., digoxin, insulin)
 C. Resume necessary drugs postoperatively
V. Evaluation
 A. Client recovers from surgery without complications

Diagnostic Examinations
 I. Assessment
 A. Definition: certain baseline diagnostic tests

performed to evaluate client's overall physical status
 B. Routine examinations (Table 6–3)
II. Analysis: high risk for injury related to present/potential problems that may interfere with the operative course
III. Planning/goals, expected outcomes: client will verbalize an understanding of diagnostic test, preparation for procedure, and care after procedure
IV. Implementations
 A. Assess learning needs
 B. Include client and family in teaching and learning plan
V. Evaluation: client successfully completes preoperative diagnostic work-up

Blood Transfusions
 I. Assessment
 A. Definition: administration of whole blood or blood components
 B. Complication: possible transfusion reaction
II. Analysis: high risk for injury related to blood transfusion
III. Planning/goals, expected outcomes
 A. Client will not experience complications as a result of blood transfusion
 B. Clients who are at high risk for blood loss (elderly, history of ASA intake, history of anemias or clotting disorders, clients having major surgery) will be identified
IV. Implementations
 A. Blood/blood components must be labeled and name and identification numbers checked prior to infusion
 B. Baseline vital signs obtained
 C. Blood must be hung with normal saline solution; tubing should be flushed with saline before and after administration of blood
 D. Assess for signs of transfusion reaction—low back pain, facial flushing, elevated temperature, headache, rapid, labored respirations, shock
 E. If transfusion reaction occurs, discontinue blood, and run normal saline
 F. If transfusion reaction occurs, obtain urine samples
 G. Save blood bag and tubing and send to blood bank for examination if transfusion reaction occurs
V. Evaluation: client has therapeutic response to the transfusion

Preoperative Medication
 I. Assessment
 A. Definition: medication given to client prior to surgery to facilitate induction of anesthesia

TABLE 6–3 Preoperative Diagnostic Tests

Test	Normal Ranges (may vary with different labs)	Purpose
Serum potassium	3.5–5.0 mEq/L	To identify hyperkalemia or hypokalemia
Serum sodium	136–145 mEq/L	To identify hypernatremia, hyponatremia, dehydration, or overhydration
Serum chloride	96–106 mEq/L	To identify hyperchloremia, hypochloremia, or metabolic alkalosis
Glucose	60–100 mg/dL	To identify hypoglycemia or hyperglycemia
Creatinine	0.7–1.4 mg/dL	To identify acute or chronic renal disease
Blood urea nitrogen (BUN)	10–20 mg/dL	To identify impaired liver or kidney function or excessive protein or tissue catabolism
Hemoglobin (Hgb)	Female: 12.0–15.0 g/dL Male: 13.0–17.0 g/dL	To identify the presence and extent of anemia
Hematocrit (Hct)	Female: 36–45% Male: 39–51%	To identify the presence and extent of anemia
Prothrombin time (PT)	11–18 seconds	To identify dysfunction of blood clotting (prothrombin level)
Partial thromboplastin time (PTT)	35–45 seconds	To identify deficiencies of coagulation factors
Chest x-ray	No abnormal heart or lung lesions	To determine size and contour of heart, lungs, and major vessels
Electrocardiogram (ECG)	Normal rate and rhythm	To determine the electrical activity of the heart

and reduce anxiety; usually central nervous system depressant and anticholinergic given

   B. Etiology/incidence (Table 6–4)

II. Planning/goals, expected outcomes

TABLE 6–4 Usual Preoperative Medications

Class	Example	Use and Common Effect
Sedatives: short-acting barbiturates	Sodium pentobarbital (Nembutal) Sodium secobarbital (Seconal) Midazolam hydrochloride (Versed)	Cause drowsiness and relaxation; facilitate and decrease amount of anesthesia
Tranquilizers: antianxiety agents (minor tranquilizers)	Diazepam (Valium), Hydroxyzine (Vistaril)	Reduce anxiety, fear; facilitate anesthesia induction; antiemetic; potentiate narcotics and sedatives
Narcotics	Morphine sulfate, meperidine (Demerol)	Facilitate anesthesia induction; produce drowsiness, euphoria
Anticholinergics	Atropine sulfate, glycopyrrolate (Robinul)	Decrease secretions; keep respiratory passages clear and dry; ease inhalation of anesthesia; decrease risk of atelectasis; prevent vagal bradycardia

   A. Client will have decreased level of anxiety

   B. Client will have easy induction of anesthesia

III. Analysis

   A. Anxiety related to impending surgery

   B. High risk for injury related to anesthesia induction

IV. Implementations

   A. Explain purpose of medication to client and family

   B. Reduce all environmental noises and stresses

   C. Client must stay in bed after receiving preoperative medication; must not smoke

   D. Assess response to preoperative medication

V. Evaluation

   A. Client has reduced anxiety prior to surgery

   B. Anesthetic induction occurs without difficulty

Preoperative Preparation

  I. Assessment: preparation to promote safety during surgery

 II. Analysis: high risk for injury related to inadequate preoperative preparation

III. Planning/goals, expected outcomes: client will be physically prepared for surgery

IV. Implementation
  A. Assess baseline vital signs and record
  B. Instruct and maintain NPO status
  C. Verify and implement any special orders such as enemas, inserting an IV line, skin prep
  D. Check the identification band
  E. Ensure that jewelry, nail polish, dentures, prosthetic devices have been removed
  F. Complete OR checklist: verify all information
V. Evaluation: client is physically prepared for surgery

Intraoperative Phase

Asepsis

I. Assessment
  A. Definition: absence of any infectious agents
  B. Etiology/incidence
    1. Asepsis practiced in operating room to prevent entrance of microorganisms into surgical wound
    2. Asepsis practiced to maintain client safety and decrease postoperative infections
II. Analysis: high risk for infection related to break in sterile technique
III. Planning/goals, expected outcomes: client will not be exposed to infection during surgery
IV. Implementations: principles of sterile technique must be followed to ensure a sterile environment for client (Table 6–5)
V. Evaluation
  A. Asepsis maintained
  B. No infection occurs

TABLE 6–5 Principles of Aseptic Technique in the Operating Room

- All materials that enter the sterile field must be sterile.
- Sterilization is the only means by which an item can be considered sterile. If anything comes in contact with an unsterile item, it becomes contaminated.
- Contaminated items should be removed immediately from the sterile field.
- Sterile team members must wear only sterile gowns. Once dressed for the procedure, they must recognize that all parts of the gown are considered unsterile except the front from chest to table level and the sleeves to 2 inches above the elbow.
- A wide margin of safety must be maintained between the sterile and unsterile field.
- Team members should move from sterile to sterile or from unsterile to unsterile.
- Tables are considered sterile only at table-top level, and items extending beneath this level are considered contaminated.
- The edges of a sterile package are considered contaminated once the package has been opened.
- Bacteria travel on airborne particles and will enter the sterile field with excessive air movements and currents.
- Bacteria travel with moisture and liquids by capillary action from surface to surface.
- Bacteria harbor on hair, skin, and respiratory tract of client, as well as those of surgical team members.

Positioning

I. Assessment
  A. Definition: correct positioning done for several purposes during surgery
    1. Provide functional alignment
    2. Prevent pressure on bony prominences
    3. Provide adequate respiratory expansion
    4. Avoid compression of nerve tissue, veins, and arteries
II. Analysis
  A. Impaired skin integrity related to improper positioning
  B. Altered peripheral tissue perfusion related to improper positioning
  C. Injury related to improper positioning
III. Planning/goals, expected outcomes: client will be properly positioned during surgical procedure
IV. Implementations
  A. Transfer cart is securely locked while moving client
  B. All bony prominences, muscles, and nerves padded
  C. Assess that straps do not constrict circulation
  D. Return from operative to supine position slowly to avoid hypotension
  E. Move both legs simultaneously
V. Evaluation: Client sustains no injuries as a result of positioning during surgery

Anesthesia

I. Assessment
  A. Types
    1. General: causes total loss of sensation, loss of consciousness, and loss of certain reflexes (i.e., blink, gag)
    2. Regional: reduces all painful sensation to one area of body without loss of consciousness
  B. Complications
    1. General
      a. Respiratory and cardiac depression
      b. Explosive hazards
    2. Regional
      a. Cannot be used for lengthy surgeries
      b. Hypotension secondary to peripheral vasodilation
II. Analysis
  A. Ineffective airway clearance related to anesthesia
  B. Altered tissue perfusion related to anesthesia
III. Planning/goals, expected outcomes: client will experience minimal complications from anesthesia
IV. Implementations
  A. Monitor vital signs closely; assess response to anesthetic agents
  B. Assess respiratory status

C. Assess for hypotension in clients receiving spinal anesthesia
D. Instruct clients who receive spinal anesthesia to remain flat for 24 hours and to take in 2000 mL fluid in 24 hours to reduce occurrence of spinal headache
V. Evaluation: client recovers from surgery without complications from anesthetic agents

Postoperative Phase

Respiratory Function

I. Assessment
   A. Definition: respiratory complications may develop postoperatively as a result of airway obstruction, laryngospasm, bronchospasm, and hypoventilation
   B. Incidence
      1. Respiratory complications are the most common postoperative problem
      2. High-risk factors for developing respiratory complications are smoking, history of COPD, and obesity
   C. Clinical Manifestations
      1. Restlessness
      2. Fast, thready pulse
      3. Rapid, shallow respirations
      4. Flaring of nostrils
      5. Decreased breath sounds
      6. Asymmetrical chest wall expansion
      7. Use of accessory muscles
      8. Decreased SaO_2
      9. Snoring
      10. Cyanosis
II. Analysis: ineffective airway clearance related to postoperative respiratory complications
III. Planning/goals, expected outcomes: client will not develop any respiratory complications postoperatively
IV. Implementations
   A. Position client on side with chin extended to prevent occlusion of airway, or in semiprone position
   B. Suction as needed
   C. Insert nasal airway
   D. Leave airway in until removed by client
   E. Deep breathing and coughing exercises
   F. Oxygen therapy, usually 60%, 6 L per minute
   G. Assess breath sounds, depth and rate of respirations, chest symmetry, use of accessory muscles
V. Evaluation: clear breath sounds postoperatively

Shock and Hemorrhage

I. Assessment
   A. Shock can develop postoperatively as a result of hemorrhage, effects of anesthesia, sepsis, cardiac arrest, and pulmonary emboli
   B. Clinical manifestations
      1. Restlessness, irritability, apprehension
      2. Lowered blood pressure
      3. Tachycardia
      4. Rapid, difficult respirations
      5. Dusky, pale, cold skin; pale lips and nailbeds
      6. Urine output decreased
II. Analysis
   A. Decreased cardiac output related to hypovolemia
   B. Altered peripheral tissue perfusion related to decreased cardiac output
III. Planning/goals, expected outcomes: client maintains adequate tissue perfusion postoperatively
IV. Implementation
   A. Assess vital signs frequently postoperatively
   B. Assess skin color and temperature
   C. Assess capillary filling
   D. Assess urine output
   E. Assess blood loss from incision and drains
   F. Position client in shock position—supine, legs elevated to 45 degrees
   G. Anticipate need for IV fluids
V. Evaluation: client does not develop manifestations of inadequate tissue perfusion postoperatively

Wound Infection

I. Assessment
   A. Etiology/incidence: most frequently causing invading organisms Staphylococcus and Streptococcus
   B. Predisposing/precipitating factors
      1. Poor nutrition prior to surgery
      2. Age (elderly)
      3. Obesity
      4. Use of steroids, radiation, or chemotherapeutic drugs
      5. Presence of other diseases (i.e., diabetes, cancer, peripheral vascular disease)
      6. Break in sterile technique in surgery or postoperatively
   C. Clinical manifestations
      1. Wound dehiscence: separation of wound edges
      2. Wound evisceration: protrusion of loops of bowel through incision
II. Analysis: high risk for infection related to surgical incision, poor nutrition and hydration, and immobility
III. Planning/goals, expected outcomes: client will not develop wound infection postoperatively
IV. Implementation

A. Assess for redness, swelling, increased drainage, or tenderness around wound
B. Assess for elevated temperature
C. Use aseptic technique with dressing changes
D. Change dressings with drainage immediately
E. Improve nutritional status of patient if necessary
F. Provide for good pulmonary hygiene, ambulation, splinting of incision for clients at high risk for developing wound dehiscence/evisceration
G. If dehiscence occurs, return client to bed (semi-Fowler's with knees gatched) and call physician
H. If evisceration occurs
   1. Return client to bed (semi-Fowler's with knees gatched)
   2. Cover intestines with wet dressing
   3. Call physician
   4. Prepare client for return to surgery
V. Evaluation
   A. Client's incision heals normally
   B. No infection occurs

Fluid and Electrolyte Balance
I. Assessment
   A. Etiology/incidence
      1. Fluid imbalances can develop postoperatively from blood loss, insensible fluid losses, physiological response of body to surgery, and improper intravenous fluid replacement
      2. Electrolyte imbalances can occur postoperatively from body fluids lost during surgery or gastrointestinal secretions lost through vomiting, nasogastric tubes, or diarrhea
   B. Predisposing/precipitating factors: elderly at high risk to develop fluid and electrolyte imbalances; and clients with pre-existing medical conditions
   C. Complications
      1. Pulmonary edema
      2. Water intoxication
      3. Hypovolemia
      4. Cardiac arrhythmias
      5. Hyponatremia
      6. Hypokalemia
      7. Acidosis/alkalosis
II. Analysis: high risk for fluid volume deficit/excess related to postoperative course
III. Planning/goals, expected outcomes: client will have normal fluid and electrolyte balance in postoperative period
IV. Implementations
   A. Assess I & O
   B. Assess serum electrolytes

C. Administer intravenous fluids properly
D. Irrigate nasogastric tubes with normal saline
E. Administer antiemetic if client experiencing unrelieved vomiting
F. Assess for signs of pulmonary edema
G. Encourage high-protein foods when client able to eat
V. Evaluation: client has normal fluid balance and electrolyte function postoperatively

Bowel Function
I. Assessment
   A. Predisposing/precipitating factors: decreased peristalsis may occur postoperatively because of anesthetics, narcotics, hypokalemia, decreased oral intake, or immobility
   B. Complications: paralytic ileus
II. Analysis: high risk for injury related to paralytic ileus
III. Planning/goals, expected outcomes: client will have normal bowel function postoperatively
IV. Implementations
   A. Auscultate bowel sounds every shift
   B. Assess stools
   C. Push fluids (2000 to 3000 mL daily, especially warm liquids)
   D. Maintain NPO until peristalsis returns
   E. Promote ambulation
   F. Stool softener or cleansing enema as ordered
   G. Assess for paralytic ileus—absence of bowel sounds, abdominal distension, nausea/vomiting
V. Evaluation: client has normal bowel movement after surgery

Ambulation
I. Assessment
   A. Etiology/incidence: early postoperative ambulation has been proven to hasten client's recovery and decrease postoperative complications
   B. Complications
      1. Atelectasis
      2. Pneumonia
      3. Thrombophlebitis
      4. Urinary retention
      5. Renal calculi
      6. Skin breakdown
      7. Muscle weakness/stiff joints
II. Analysis: high risk for impaired physical mobility related to postoperative pain and weakness
III. Planning/goals, expected outcomes: client will successfully ambulate in early postoperative period
IV. Implementations
   A. Encourage client to cough and deep breathe

and perform leg exercises in immediate post-operative period

  B. Assess client's ability to safely ambulate (i.e., check vital signs, LOC, color of skin)

  C. Encourage client to ambulate as soon as possible postoperatively; begin with dangling, assist to stand/walk, increase distance of ambulation daily

V. Evaluation: client ambulates postoperatively without difficulty or complications

Pain

I. Assessment

  A. Etiology/incidence: postoperative pain normal experience that may be caused by several factors

    1. Incision

    2. Organ manipulation

    3. Edema

    4. Muscle spasms

    5. Infection

    6. Distension

    7. Anxiety

II. Analysis: pain related to surgical incision, edema, infection, anxiety

III. Planning/goals, expected outcomes: client's postoperative pain will be reduced

IV. Implementations

  A. Assess client's complaint of pain and possible causes (i.e., urinary retention, anxiety, abdominal distension)

  B. Utilize nursing comfort measures for pain control (i.e., backrub, allowing client time to verbalize)

  C. Medicate with analgesics before pain becomes severe

  D. Assess respirations and pulse prior to administration of analgesic

  E. Assess pain for character, location, and effectiveness of pain relief measures

V. Evaluation: client comfortable postoperatively

Discharge Teaching

I. Assessment

  A. Etiology/incidence: discharge teaching should begin in preoperative period; specific teaching and preparation done postoperatively

II. Analysis: knowledge deficit related to postoperative care

III. Planning/goals, expected outcomes: client will be knowledgeable about discharge care

IV. Implementations

  A. Assess learning needs and level of understanding of client and family

  B. Client and family should be taught

    1. Incision care or dressing changes; clinical manifestations of infection

    2. Medications—how to take and possible side effects

    3. Activities allowed and restricted

    4. Symptoms to be reported

    5. Treatments to be performed

    6. Nutritional needs

    7. Follow-up care

V. Evaluation: client successfully cares for self at home

POST-TEST Adults Undergoing Surgery

Mr. LaGrille is a 55-year-old construction worker scheduled for a lumbar laminectomy.

---

1. Mr. LaGrille is very anxious about the pain he will experience postoperatively. Which of the following interventions would be most effective in initially helping this client deal with his fears?

  ① Describe in detail the type of pain he will most likely experience after surgery

  ② Avoid talking about the pain that he will experience

  ③ Explain the availability of pain medications after surgery

  ④ Teach him relaxation techniques

2. Mr. LaGrille is NPO after midnight. You explain to him that the rationale for this is to prevent:

  ① Fluid overload postoperatively

  ② Urinary incontinence during surgery

  ③ Vomiting and aspiration during surgery

  ④ Pneumonia postoperatively

3. One of the preoperative medications ordered for Mr. LaGrille is meperidine (Demerol). The purpose of administering this medication preoperatively is to:

  ① Facilitate anesthesia induction

  ② Provide an antiemetic effect

  ③ Reduce salivary and bronchial secretions

  ④ Reduce the hazards of atelectasis

4. Which of the following laboratory data would be necessary to report to the surgeon prior to Mr. LaGrille's surgery?

  ① Serum potassium 2.5 mEq/L

  ② Hematocrit 42 mL/100 mL

  ③ Platelet count 300,000 mm^3

  ④ Total serum protein 8 g/100 mL

5. IV fluids have been ordered to be started on Mr. LaGrille immediately prior to surgery. The order reads 1000 mL D_5/Water to infuse

over 8 hours. The drip factor is 15 drops (gtt)/mL. The correct rate of infusion is:
① 22 gtt/min
② 51 gtt/min
③ 42 gtt/min
④ 31 gtt/min

6. As soon as Mr. LaGrille enters the recovery room, the nurse should first:
① Remove the oropharyngeal airway
② Increase the IV fluid rate
③ Assess the level of consciousness and vital signs
④ Assess the wound and any drainage

7. Which of the following statements indicate that Mr. LaGrille has been adequately prepared for discharge?
① "I am planning on returning to work as soon as possible."
② "I will not do any heavy lifting or strenuous activity for 6 weeks."
③ "I am going to start a strict reducing diet tomorrow."
④ "Can I have a prescription for pain pills?"

8. Which of the following nursing actions are INAPPROPRIATE for a client recovering from general anesthesia?
① Encourage coughing and deep breathing
② Suction to remove excessive respiratory secretions
③ Position the client supine
④ Auscultate the client's lung fields

9. Which of the following assessments indicate probable respiratory problems postoperatively?
① Lungs clear bilaterally
② Afebrile
③ Nonproductive cough
④ Restlessness

10. After a nurse has assessed that a client is experiencing a transfusion reaction, the immediate nursing action will be to:
① Call the doctor
② Monitor the vital signs every 15 minutes
③ Discontinue the blood, infuse normal saline
④ Slow down the blood transfusion and notify the blood bank of the possible transfusion reaction

11. Midazolam (Versed) is ordered for your client as a preoperative medication. What is the primary purpose of this medication?
① Decrease emesis
② Produce drowsiness, relaxation
③ Decrease secretions
④ Prevent vagal bradycardia

12. Which of the following would NOT be a complication of prolonged bedrest postoperatively?
① Renal calculi
② Pneumonia
③ Muscle atrophy
④ Overhydration

Mrs. Alexis Conover, a 42-year-old white woman, had a cholecystectomy. On her third postoperative day, she calls you into her room. She states she feels nauseous. Your assessment findings are: T, 100; P, 100; R, 24; BP, 110/70; lung sounds clear; absent bowel sounds; negative Homan's sign; incision clear/no drainage.

---

13. Based on your assessments, what is your priority nursing diagnosis?
① High risk for decrease in cardiac output
② High risk for injury: paralytic ileus
③ High risk for wound infection
④ High risk for impaired gas exchange

14. On her seventh hospital day, Mrs. Conover is being discharged. Which of the following are INAPPROPRIATE discharge instructions to give this client?
① How to perform wound culture
② How to assess wound infection
③ Activity restrictions
④ When to schedule doctor visit

POST-TEST Answers and Rationales

1. ③ The client is experiencing anxiety because of fears related to the postoperative pain. The best intervention is to teach him that pain medication will be available to him as necessary to relieve his pain. 4, III. Surgical Intervention.

2. ③ Keeping the client NPO prevents aspiration of gastric contents during or after the surgery. 1, II. Surgical Intervention.

3. ① Demerol acts to facilitate the induction of anesthesia, promotes relaxation, and decreases anxiety preoperatively. Postoperatively it relieves pain. 3, II. Surgical Intervention

4. ① The normal serum potassium is 3.5 to 5.0 meq/L. A low level can lead to cardiac abnormalities and death. The other values are within normal limits. 4, II. Surgical Intervention.

5. ④ $1000/480 \times 15 =$ gtt/min, $100/48 \times 15 = 1500/48 = 31$ gtt/min. 1, I. Surgical Intervention.

6. ③ In the immediate postoperative period, the priority is to assess for respiratory distress. Always compare your assessments with the client's preoperative normals. 1, II. Surgical Intervention.

7. ② The client should not engage in any heavy lifting or strenuous activity for at least 6 weeks. He cannot return to work for about 6 weeks, and a severe diet would not be indicated. The request for pain pills should not be necessary unless the surgery is unsuccessful. 5, IV. Surgical Intervention.

8. ③ The best position for a client recovering from the effects of anesthesia is to position the head to the side and the chin extended forward to prevent airway obstruction. 4, II. Surgical Intervention.

9. ④ Restlessness is the earliest sign of cerebral anoxia. 1, II. Surgical Intervention.

10. ③ The transfusion should be stopped as the severity of the transfusion is directly related to the amount of blood transfused. Normal saline is administered to prevent agglutination of the blood. 4, II. Surgical Intervention, Hematology.

11. ② Midazolam (Versed) is a sedative that is used to induce sleep and reduce anxiety. 2, II. Surgical Intervention.

12. ④ Complications of immobility include renal calculi, pneumonia, muscle weakness and atrophy, thrombophlebitis, urinary retention, and skin breakdown. Overhydration is not a complication of immobility. 2, I. Surgical Intervention.

13. ② Based on the assessment data given— the nausea, absent bowel sounds—you would suspect possible paralytic ileus. Other assessment data given are normal. 2, II. Surgical Intervention.

14. ① It is not necessary to teach this client how to culture a wound. Essential discharge instructions include assessment of wound infection, activity restrictions, follow-up physician visit. 4, IV. Surgical Intervention.

PRE-TEST Immune Disorders

Mary Jones, a 39-year-old mother of two small children, has just been diagnosed with breast cancer. She will have a surgical excision of the tumor with postoperative external beam radiation therapy to the operative site.

1. Mrs. Jones is crying when you enter the room and tells you she is very frightened. Your most appropriate response would be:

① "Don't worry Mrs. Jones. Everything will be all right."
② "Look at some books and magazines to get your mind off the treatment."
③ "I can see that you're very upset. Let's talk about some of your concerns."
④ "I'll call our chaplain for you. He's comforted many patients with cancer."

2. In teaching Mrs. Jones about external radiation therapy, your instructions would include:
① Actual treatment takes only 2 to 5 minutes

② Bodily secretions will be radioactive

③ Treatment will be administered only once a week

④ Radioactive seeds will be implanted into the operative site

3. As part of your teaching regarding skin care, you would tell Mrs. Jones to:

① Wash the area daily with soap and water

② Apply lotion to the skin to keep it moist

③ Avoid wearing a tight-fitting bra to protect the area from irritation

④ Apply powder to keep the skin dry

John Carpenter is a 22-year-old college student admitted for chemotherapy treatment of acute lymphoblastic leukemia (ALL).

---

4. In addition to combination chemotherapy with intravenous drugs, John will also receive intrathecal methotrexate. This drug will be given into the:

① Bone marrow

② Cranium

③ Spinal fluid

④ Vertebra

5. John is engaged and was planning on being married when he graduated college. He and his fiance ask you about the reproductive consequences of chemotherapy. Which of the following is the most appropriate statement concerning the reproductive effects of chemotherapy?

① Contraception is no longer necessary

② John should consider sperm banking prior to beginning therapy

③ John will be permanently sterile as a result of therapy

④ John will be impotent as a result of therapy

6. John's white blood cell and platelet counts are critically low. He is febrile and complaining of a headache and constipation. Which is the most appropriate nursing intervention for this client?

① Administer aspirin every 4 hours to control the fever

② Monitor temperature and neurological status at least every 4 hours

③ Administer meperidine (Demerol) IM every 4 hours for headache

④ Administer a glycerin suppository

7. As a result of the intensive chemotherapy, John has extensive stomatitis. In order to alleviate the stomatitis pain, you would:

① Instruct John to use full-strength commercial mouthwash as an oral cleansing agent

② Provide John with hot soup and tea to soothe the irritated mucosa

③ Encourage orange juice with breakfast to increase vitamin C consumption and enhance wound healing

④ Administer acetaminophen elixir and oral topical anesthetic every 4 hours

8. The purpose of giving gamma-globulin injection to individuals exposed to hepatitis A is to:

① Actively immunize them against hepatitis A

② Induce life-long immunity to hepatitis A

③ Prevent the individual from transmitting the virus to another

④ Provide temporary passive immunity to hepatitis A

9. The body's inborn defense mechanism against bacteria, viruses, and fungi is called:

① Antigen memory system

② Immunity

③ Cell-mediated immunity

④ Humoral immunity

10. A mother's immunity is transferred to the fetus through the:

① Lymph system

② Venous circulation

③ Active and passive transport

④ Placenta

11. Which of the following is NOT a lymphoid organ?

① Thymus

② Spleen

③ Parathyroid gland

④ Bone marrow

12. The immune cells primarily responsible for organ transplant graft rejection are:

① T lymphocytes

② B lymphocytes

③ Natural killer cells

④ Granulocytes

13. The focus of teaching regarding cancer risk factors is:

① Prevention and detection

② Treatment protocols

③ Follow-up care

④ Rehabilitation

PRE-TEST Answers and Rationales

1. ③ Encouraging the venting of fears and concerns assists the client to verbalize anxiety. This also provides the nurse with baseline information upon which to plan further interventions. Cliches are not helpful. Diversional activities at this point in time just ignore the client's concerns. Initial assessment of concerns should be done prior to referral to the chaplain. 1, III. Cancer.

2. ① External beam therapy is administered daily over a period of weeks. Actual treatment lasts only a few minutes. Choices 2 and 4 are applicable to internal radiation therapy. 4, II. Radiation Therapy.

3. ③ Tight-fitting clothing should be avoided to protect the fragile skin from further irritation. Lotions, soap, and powder should not be applied to the treatment area without physician approval. 4, II. Radiation Therapy.

4. ③ Intrathecal drug administration refers to drugs given directly into the spinal fluid to treat leukemic infiltration of the brain. 1, II. Chemotherapy.

5. ② Sperm banking is an option for future procreation. Contraception is still necessary; sterility is a potential, but is not guaranteed. Impotence refers to impaired erectile function, not sperm production. 4, IV. Chemotherapy.

6. ② Temperature and neurological status need to be closely monitored in leukemic clients, who are at particular risk for infection and intracranial bleeding. Aspirin exacerbates bleeding and will mask further temperature elevations. Traumatic procedures (IM injections and rectal suppositories) are contraindicated in clients at risk for infection and bleeding. 4, I. Chemotherapy.

7. ④ Topical and systemic analgesics are indicated. Full-strength commercial mouthwash, hot beverages, and acidic foods will further irritate the inflamed oral mucosa. 4, II. Chemotherapy.

8. ④ Gamma-globulin injections confer temporary passive immunity. They are not a form of active immunization, nor do they confer life-long immunity. They do not prevent viral transmission. 1, II. Immunity.

9. ② Immunity is the correct terminology. The other options are subsumed under immunity. 1, II. Immunity.

10. ④ Immune transfer from the mother to fetus is through the placenta and colostrum. 1, II & IV. Immunity.

11. ③ The parathyroid gland is not a lymphoid gland. The thymus, spleen, and bone marrow are all portions of the lymphatic system. 1, II. Immunity.

12. ① T lymphocytes, specifically the cytotoxic T cells, are responsible for tissue rejection. 1, II. Immunity.

13. ① Teaching clients regarding risk factors should include prevention and early detection. The other options are more appropriate for the individual who has already been diagnosed with cancer. 4, IV. Cancer.

IMMUNITY: GENERAL CONCEPTS

I. Immune system: a complex network of specialized cells and organs that has evolved to defend the body against attacks by foreign invaders

II. Distinguishes between "self" and "nonself"
   A. Antigen: any "foreign" substance capable of triggering an imune response; e.g., virus, bacterium, fungus, parasite, foreign tissues or cells

III. Characterized by both diversity and specificity of response

IV. Memory capabilities

V. Components of the immune system
   A. Lymphoid system: where lymphocytes develop and congregate; includes the bone marrow, thymus, lymph nodes, spleen, tonsils and adenoids, appendix, lymphatic vessels and fluid, and other clusters of lymphoid tissue found throughout the body
   B. Cells of the immune system travel throughout the body by way of lymphatic and blood vessels
   C. Lymphocytes: white blood cells; major role in immune defense
      1. T lymphocytes: cellular immunity; reg-

ulate/orchestrate immune response as well as directly attack their targets; responsible for immunosurveillance and graft rejection

  a. Helper T cells: turn on antibody production, activate cytotoxic T cells, and initiate other immune responses

  b. Suppressor T cells: turn off antibody production and other immune responses; keep the immune system from overreacting

  c. Cytotoxic T cells: kill body cells infected by viruses or transformed by cancer; reject tissue and organ grafts

2. B lymphocytes: humoral immunity; differentiate into plasma cells; work chiefly by secreting antibodies (soluble proteins produced in response to specific antigens); antibodies also known as immunoglobulins

3. Natural killer (NK) cells: kill on contact; bind to target and deliver a burst of potent chemicals that lyse the target cell's membrane

D. Cytokines: substances released from activated immune system cells; affect behavior of other cells; help direct and regulate immune response

1. Interferons
2. Interleukins
3. Tumor necrosis factor
4. Colony-stimulating factors

E. Phagocytes: large white cells that engulf and digest foreign invaders

1. Monocytes and macrophages
2. Granulocytes: neutrophils, basophils, and eosinophils

F. Complement system: a complex series of blood proteins; actions "complement" the work of antibodies; complement destroys bacteria, produces inflammation, and regulates immune reactions; actions include

1. Cytolysis: destruction of cell membranes
2. Chemotaxis: chemical attraction of phagocytic cell to antigen
3. Adherence: adhesion of antigen–antibody complexes to surface of cell(s) or body tissues
4. Opsonization: antibody coats surface of antigen, making it more easy to digest by phagocytes
5. Neutralization: antibody neutralizes toxins released by bacteria
6. Anaphylactic reaction: activates release of mast cells and histamine

VI. Types of immunity
  A. Naturally acquired

1. Active: antigen-specific (bacteria, virus, fungus); develops slowly; long-term or lifelong effect (e.g., chickenpox)
2. Passive: antibodies transferred from mother to fetus through placenta and colostrum; develops immediately; effect temporary, but may last a few weeks

B. Artificially induced

1. Active: antigen-specific, produced slowly by immunization (live or killed vaccine or toxoid); effective for several years with extensions by booster doses (e.g., tetanus toxoid)
2. Passive: injection of antibodies via immune sera (human or animal); develops immediately; temporary effect, but may last several weeks (e.g., gamma globulin)

VII. Disorders of the immune system
  A. Autoimmune diseases: immune system wrongly identifies self as nonself

1. Hemolytic anemia
2. Rheumatic fever
3. Type I diabetes mellitus
4. Ulcerative colitis
5. Systemic lupus erythematosus (SLE)
6. Myasthenia gravis
7. Rheumatoid arthritis
8. Hashimoto's thyroiditis
9. Primary myxedema
10. Thyrotoxicosis
11. Primary biliary cirrhosis
12. Active chronic hepatitis
13. Scleroderma
14. Idiopathic thrombocytopenia purpura

B. Hypersensitivity reactions: overactive immune response

1. Atopic reactions (inherited)
2. Anaphylaxis
3. Allergic asthma
4. Rhinitis
5. Angioedema
6. Urticaria
7. Dermatitis

C. Allergies: apparently harmless substances provoke the immune system to set off inappropriate and harmful responses; antigens also known as allergens

D. Immunodeficiency: inability or incompetence of immune system to defend body because of primary (genetic) or secondary causes

1. Genetic defect in antibody (immunoglobulin) production
  a. Agammaglobulinemia
  b. Hypogammaglobulinemia
  c. Severe combined immunodeficiency disease (SCID): genetic; lack all major immune defenses

2. Acquired immune deficiency syndrome (AIDS)
3. Cancer: immune deficiencies may result from the disease process or from extensive therapy
4. Other causes of immune suppression
   a. Stress
   b. Malnutrition
   c. Age
   d. Radiation
   e. Burns
   f. Surgery
   g. Infections
   h. Blood transfusions

NURSING PROCESS APPLIED TO ADULTS WITH IMMUNE DISORDERS

Cancer

I. Assessment
   A. Definition/pathophysiology
      1. Cancer: a group of over 200 diseases characterized by uncontrolled growth and spread of abnormal cells
      2. Characteristics of malignant tumors
         a. Nonencapsulated
         b. Invasive
         c. Poorly differentiated
         d. Mitoses relatively common
         e. Rapid, uncontrolled growth
         f. Anaplastic (cells bear little similarity to tissue of origin) to varying degrees
         g. Metastases
      3. Named according to site of primary tumor and type of tissue involved
      4. Carcinogenesis: multistep process by which normal cells undergo malignant transformation
      5. Immune surveillance concept: because cancer cells are similar to foreign proteins, immune response is produced
         a. Many cancer cells believed to have tumor-associated antigens on surface that activate antibodies
         b. If surface antigen not detected or cells multiply rapidly, malignancy develops and continues beyond immune protection
      6. As tumor continues to grow, it destroys adjacent tissues through permeation, extension, and metastases through blood and lymph
      7. When cancer cells seed on vessels and organs, structural and functional site-dependent changes occur
         a. Break in integrity of vessel causes bleeding and entrapment of accumulated blood or lymph
         b. Inflammatory changes occur with fluid shifts between intracellular, intravascular, and interstitial spaces
         c. Pressure on organs causes pain with or without loss of function
            (1) Local effects: dysphagia, respiratory distress, impaired circulation, increased intracranial pressure, pain, bleeding, loss of function, spinal cord compression
            (2) Systemic effects, advanced carcinogenesis, and oncologic emergencies: anemia, thrombocytopenia, leukopenia, anorexia, nausea, vomiting, fatigue, electrolyte abnormalities such as hypercalcemia and hyperuricemia, infection, paraneoplastic syndromes (see Complications)
   B. Etiology: no specific single cause; multicausal theories and risk factors
      1. Genetics: somatic hereditary mutation (melanoma, glioblastoma, retinoblastoma)
      2. Physical agents: sunlight (skin cancer), radiation (leukemia, lymphoma), chronic trauma (colon, cervical cancer)
      3. Chemical agents: aniline dyes, asbestos, plastics, cobalt, aromatic amines, metals, hydrocarbons (lung, bladder, leukemia)
      4. Enzymes and hormones: increased enzyme activity and hormonal imbalance stimulate or inhibit development of cancer in hormone-dependent tissue; abnormal secretion of hormones or enzymes by cancer cells or tumors (prostate, breast, adrenal, lung cancer)
      5. Viruses (certain leukemias, lymphomas, cervical)
      6. Diet, health habits, lifestyle: low-fiber diet (colon cancer), smoking (lung cancer), alcohol (head and neck cancer), early sexual relations with different partners (cervical cancer)
      7. Immunological factors: depressed immune system (leukemia, Kaposi's sarcoma, lymphoma)
   C. Incidence
      1. About 30% of Americans will eventually develop cancer
      2. Increased incidence in the elderly
      3. Increased morbidity and mortality in African Americans
      4. Greatest incidence by site and sex

a. Women: lung, breast, colorectal

b. Men: lung, colorectal, prostate

5. Second leading cause of death in United States

   a. About 40% of newly diagnosed will be alive 5 years after diagnosis

   b. Survival depends on type, stage, and response to treatment

   c. Lung cancer leading cause of death in both sexes

D. Clinical manifestations: related to tissue histology (tumor type), stage (extent) of disease, and organs involved

E. Diagnostic examinations (Table 6–6)

  1. Goals of diagnostic evaluation: to determine

   a. Tissue type of the malignancy

   b. Primary site

   c. Extent of disease

  2. Tissue samples for histologic examination or cells for cytologic analysis crucial; determine type of therapy used

   a. Biopsy: tissue sample obtained via

     (1) Excision—entire mass removed

     (2) Incision—portion of tumor removed

     (3) Needle—core of tissue removed

   b. Cytology: cells obtained from tissue scrapings, fluids, secretions, or washings; e.g., Pap smears

  3. Endoscopies: direct visualization via endoscope in body cavity or opening

  4. Radiological examinations may include

   a. CT scans

   b. Radioisotope (nuclear medicine) examinations

   c. Ultrasound

   d. MRI scans

   e. Mammography

  5. Tumor markers: used to monitor course of a particular tumor and its response to therapy

   a. Alpha-fetoprotein (AFP): testicular, malignant trophoblastic

   b. Beta human chorionic gonadotropin (βHCG): testicular, malignant trophoblastic

   c. Carcinoembryonic antigen (CEA): colorectal, stomach, pancreas, breast, lung

   d. Prostatic-specific antigen (PSA): prostate

   e. CA-125: ovarian

F. Complications

  1. Related to extent of disease, specific tissues and organs involved, and treatment

  2. Oncologic emergencies

   a. Cardiac tamponade

   b. Superior vena cava (SVC) syndrome

   c. Spinal cord compression

   d. Syndrome of inappropriate antidiuretic hormone (SIADH)

   e. Hypercalcemia

   f. Septic shock

   g. Renal failure

   h. Respiratory distress: adult respiratory distress syndrome (ARDS), pleural effusion

   i. Disseminated intravascular coagulation (DIC)

   j. Tumor lysis syndrome

G. Medical and surgical management

  1. Single mode or combination of modes of treatment may be needed

   a. Goals of therapy include

     (1) Cure: complete eradication of disease with normal life span

     (2) Disease control: control spread and disease progression, prolongation of life

     (3) Palliation: relieve or reduce symptoms

   b. Choice of therapy depends on tumor histology and extent of disease

   c. Surgery: local treatment for prevention (colon polyps), tissue diagnosis, definitive treatment (early breast), rehabilitation (breast reconstruction), palliation (bowel obstruction)

   d. Chemotherapy (Table 6–7): systemic treatment; cure (testicular), control (colon), palliation (lung)

   e. Radiation therapy: local treatment; cure (early stage Hodgkin's disease), control (lung); prophylaxis (whole brain radiation therapy for lung cancer); palliation (pain from bone metastases)

   f. Biotherapy: use of agents or approaches that modify the relationship between tumor and host by modifying the host's biological response to tumor cells; under intense investigation in clinical trials; for example:

     (1) Interferons

       (a) Natural proteins/lymphokines produced by epithelial cells, macrophages, fibroblasts, and T lymphocytes

       (b) Alpha-, beta-, gamma-interferons

       (c) Alpha-interferons most commonly used in treating leukemias, lymphomas, mye-

TABLE 6–6 Selected Diagnostic Tests Used in Oncologic Evaluations

Test	Purpose	Pre-Care	Post-Care
Bronchoscopy	Assess trachea, bronchi, and lung parenchyma; obtain biopsy or washings for analysis	NPO past midnight; administer sedation, anticholinergic; local anesthetic applied to back of throat to prevent gag reflex; fiberoptic bronchoscope inserted through nares	Monitor vital signs and respiratory status; maintain NPO status until return of gag reflex
Computed tomography (CT)	Noninvasive procedure; produces cross-sectional pictures of internal structures; computer-generated three-dimensional image obtained; can visualize organs with greater detail than ordinary x-rays	May require NPO status depending on organ scanned; may be done with or without contrast; assess for contrast allergies; IV contrast dye may cause burning sensation as injected; client may report feelings of nausea, vomiting, flushing, itching, bitter taste	None
Colonoscopy/sigmoidoscopy	Examine left, transverse, and right colon and sigmoid; obtain specimen for biopsy	Clear liquid diet prior to examination; cathartics, enemas prior; NPO past midnight; sedation prior; scope inserted through anus; can be painful	Observe for unexpected bleeding or abdominal pain
Cystoscopy	Direct examination of the urethra and bladder for stricture or bleeding; obtain biopsy specimen of prostate, bladder, and urethra	May require sedation or anesthesia before procedure; may require NPO; cystoscope inserted into the urethra and advanced into the bladder	Monitor for urinary retention and bleeding; monitor vital signs
Esophagoscopy–gastroscopy	Direct visualization of esophagus and stomach; obtain biopsy specimens, brushings, or washings	NPO, sedation prior; local anesthetic applied to throat to prevent gag reflex; fiberoptic scope inserted through mouth	Monitor vital signs; maintain NPO status until return of gag reflex
Liver biopsy	Assess liver for malfunction or disease	Check coagulation studies and CBC; NPO, sedation prior; local anesthetic; biopsy needle inserted through right upper quadrant of abdomen to obtain specimen	Apply pressure to biopsy site; place client on right side; restrict activity (bedrest for several hours); observe for bleeding; monitor vital signs and CBC
Magnetic resonance imaging (MRI)	Noninvasive method; employs use of magnetic field rather than radiation; creates sectional images of the body, similar to CT scan; staging of malignant disease in the central nervous system, spine, head and neck, and musculoskeletal system	May require NPO; contraindicated for patients with aneurysm clips or pacemakers because of magnetic field; must remove all jewelry and metal objects for same reason; must lie still in confined area; pediatric or claustrophobic patients may require sedation; knocking or beating sound in machine is normal; contrast agent may be injected	None
Mammography	Determine presence of benign or malignant breast disease and cysts; to guide needle biopsy	Breast is compressed between the camera and film; may be momentarily uncomfortable	None
Nuclear medicine scans	Detect lesions and abnormalities in the bones, brain, liver, spleen, lung, kidney, and thyroid; assess myocardial function (MUGA, thallium scan)	Assess for previous reaction to contrast media; requires IV line for injection of dye; serial radiographs are taken; NPO may be required for selected tests	Encourage fluid intake to aid in urinary excretion of dye; monitor for allergic reaction
Paracentesis	Confirm presence of ascites; obtain specimens for analysis; provide symptomatic relief through removal of ascitic fluid	Local anesthetic to catheter insertion site; instruct client to void pre-procedure; insertion of trocar, then catheter for drainage; may be accompanied by albumin administration	Monitor vital signs (especially for hypotension); monitor characteristics of peritoneal drainage; observe and record fluid loss

TABLE 6–6 Selected Diagnostic Tests Used in Oncologic Evaluations *Continued.*

Test	Purpose	Pre-Care	Post-Care
Thoracentesis	Obtain pleural fluid for analysis; provide symptomatic relief of pleural effusion	Local anesthetic and sedation prior to trocar insertion; chest tube(s) may be placed for prolonged drainage; needle insertion for biopsy may be guided by fluoroscopy	Monitor vital signs and respiratory status (for evidence of pneumothorax); chest x-ray routinely done post-procedure; observe chest tube for proper function, note drainage characteristics and amount; observe for drainage and bleeding at insertion site; administer analgesics

lomas, renal carcinoma, Kaposi's sarcoma

II. Analysis
  A. Knowledge deficit related to cancer risk factors, prevention and detection
  B. Anxiety related to diagnosis; uncertain therapy outcome; potential for recurrence; concerns of pain, death, and disability; social stigma; loss of control; financial concerns; alterations in interpersonal relationships
  C. Knowledge deficit related to disease process, treatment, potential complications, and community resources

III. Planning/goals, expected outcomes
  A. Client identifies cancer risk factors, warning signals, prevention and detection practices
  B. Client demonstrates decreased anxiety
  C. Client verbalizes knowledge of disease process, treatment, potential side effects, and community resources

IV. Implementation
  A. Provide information on risk factors, recommended prevention and detection practices
    1. Seven warning signs of cancer (CAUTION)
      a. Change in bowel or bladder habits
      b. A sore that does not heal
      c. Unusual bleeding or discharge
      d. Thickening or lumps in a breast or elsewhere
      e. Indigestion or difficulty swallowing
      f. Obvious change in wart or mole
      g. Nagging cough or hoarseness
    2. Teach importance of physical examination and health screening; refer to American Cancer Society's recommendations for early detection of cancer in asymptomatic individuals
    3. Reinforce positive health habits and prevention practices (e.g., avoid smoking, excessive alcohol consumption, high-fat diet)

  B. Assist client to verbalize anxiety and maintain control
    1. Encourage ventilation of fears and concerns
    2. Avoid clichés such as "don't worry," "relax," or "everything will be all right"
    3. Explore concerns related to uncertainty of future, physical symptoms, changes in self-concept, and effect of illness on daily life and interpersonal relationships
    4. Identify client's support system, resources, prior coping strategies, and communication patterns
    5. Assist client to identify stressors and assist with problem solving
    6. Refer to appropriate counselor as needed: social service, chaplain
    7. Provide client/family with information about local support groups
    8. Provide continuity of care when possible
    9. Encourage diversional activities
    10. Involve client in decision making about care
    11. Provide flexibility in scheduling activities
  C. Provide information on disease process, treatment, potential complications, and community resources
    1. Determine baseline knowledge; reinforce previous information given; clarify misconceptions
    2. Explain disease process in terms appropriate for client's education level
    3. Identify type of therapy to be used (chemotherapy, radiation, surgery, biotherapy)
    4. Explain symptoms of potential complications
    5. Provide written materials to reinforce teaching
    6. Encourage questions, verbalization of fears and concerns

TABLE 6–7 Antineoplastics

Class	Example	Action	Use	Common Side Effects	Nursing Implications
Alkylating agents	Cyclophosphamide (Cytoxan)	Wide variety of drugs that act to destroy rapidly dividing cells; classified as cell-cycle specific (those that attack cells at a specific point in the process of cell division) or cell-cycle nonspecific (those that act at any time during cell division)	To treat a wide variety of cancers including leukemia, lymphoma, multiple myeloma, breast, lung, ovarian	Bone marrow depression in 7 to 14 days, nausea and vomiting, anorexia, alopecia, hemorrhagic cystitis, amenorrhea, sterility	Monitor blood counts closely; teach client safety precautions about low blood counts; use antiemetics preventively; increase fluid intake; administer IV slowly
	Cisplatin (Platinol)		To treat testicular, lung, ovarian, head and neck cancer	Severe nausea and vomiting, anorexia, nephrotoxicity, peripheral neuropathy, ototoxicity, moderate bone marrow depression at 14–21 days with high-dose therapy, potassium and magnesium wasting, hypersensitivity	Hydrate well with IV fluids and mannitol before therapy; monitor hearing; assess motor and sensory function; check weight daily; use antiemetics preventively; monitor for allergic reactions; monitor renal function, potassium, magnesium, and CBC
Antimetabolites	Methotrexate (Mexate)		To treat leukemia, lymphoma, ovarian, breast	GI ulceration, severe stomatitis, bone marrow depression in 10 to 14 days, nephrotoxicity, diarrhea, hepatotoxicity, pulmonary toxicity, neurological symptoms with intrathecal use, photosensitivity	With high-dose therapy, give leucovorin to prevent toxicity, hydrate well, and maintain alkaline urine; monitor CBC and renal function closely; oral hygiene and comfort measures; avoid sun exposure, use sunblock
Antibiotics	Doxorubicin (Adriamycin)		To treat breast, lung, head and neck, pancreas, soft-tissue sarcoma, ovarian	Bone marrow depression 10 to 14 days, severe tissue necrosis with extravasation, nausea and vomiting, anorexia, cardiotoxicity, alopecia, stomatitis, diarrhea, red discoloration of urine	Avoid extravasation; monitor cardiovascular function; warn about red urine; provide antiemetic therapy; warn about alopecia; monitor CBC; treat stomatitis
Plant alkaloids	Vincristine (Oncovin)		To treat testicular, neuroblastoma, leukemia, lymphoma, breast, lung, multiple myeloma	Neurotoxicity, constipation, peripheral neuropathies, abdominal pain, rare and mild bone marrow depression, alopecia, tissue necrosis with extravasation	Monitor for sensory or motor changes; administer stool softeners; avoid extravasation; observe for neurotoxicity; administer IV slowly
Hormones: Androgens	Testosterone, propionate	Growth of certain tumors (breast, thyroid, prostate,	Replacement therapy for males; to treat dysmenorrhea and	Males: impotence, gynecomastia, epididymitis, bladder	Warn about possible changes in sexual characteristics; use

TABLE 6–7 Antineoplastics *Continued.*

Class	Example	Action	Use	Common Side Effects	Nursing Implications
		uterine) depends on specific hormonal environment; altering this environment impairs/arrests tumor growth	menopause in women; to treat inoperable breast cancer in women	irritation; females: hirsutism, amenorrhea, masculinization; both: nausea and vomiting, fluid retention, hypercalcemia with bone metastases	with caution in patients on oral anticoagulants; monitor I & O; check for edema; monitor calcium levels
Anti-androgens	Flutamide (Eulexin)	Antagonizes androgen effects at cellular level; decreases growth in androgen-sensitive tumor	To treat metastatic prostate cancer; used with leuprolide	Diarrhea, nausea, vomitting, loss of libido, impotence, gynecomastia, hot flashes, edema, hypertension	Monitor for GI side effects, warn about side effects concerning sexuality; encourage compliance
Estrogens	Diethylstilbestrol (DES)		Postmenopausal syndrome, amenorrhea due to ovarian failure, suppression of lactation; prostatic cancer; breast cancer	Nausea and vomiting, anorexia, abdominal distension and bloating, spotting, menstrual changes, fluid retention, depression, hypercalcemia, migraines, breast tenderness and enlargement, reduced glucose tolerance, possible uterine cancer, thromboemboli, increased incidence of cardiovascular-associated deaths; males: similar but also development of female secondary sexual characteristics (impotence, loss of libido)	Contraindicated in pregnancy, some breast cancers, thrombophlebitis, thyroid and liver disease; use cautiously in patients with hypertension, migraines, diabetes, and asthma; monitor for edema and congestive heart failure; watch for depression; monitor serum calcium; counsel about sexual dysfunction
Anti-estrogens	Tamoxifen (Nolvadex)		To treat estrogen receptor positive breast cancer	Rare transient bone marrow depression, nausea, menstrual irregularity, hot flashes, "flare" reaction (bone and tumor pain), hypercalcemia in women with bone metastases, induces ovulation in premenopausal women	Monitor menstrual function; advise premenopausal women to use birth control; monitor serum calcium level; reassure that flare reaction will subside—not an indication of disease progression; rather, drug effectiveness
Synthetic luteinizing hormone	Leuprolide (Lupron)	Lowers testosterone level with continuous use	To treat advanced prostate cancer; used with flutamide; used in clients who cannot tolerate an orchiectomy or estrogen therapy	Dizziness, headache, decreased libido, impotence, anorexia, increased bone pain, hot flashes, paresthesias	Monitor for increase in bone pain; with vertebral metastasis, watch for loss of function; monitor acid phosphatase for response to therapy; teach client about side effects

7. Initiate referrals to other health care members as needed
8. Provide information about national and local cancer-related community resources

V. Evaluation
   A. Client identifies own risks and consults with health care member about warning signs of cancer
   B. Client practices positive health habits and lifestyle
   C. Client verbalizes anxiety and identifies ways to decrease/control it
   D. Client describes disease process, treatment plan, potential side effects, and available community resources

Chemotherapy and Radiation Therapy

I. Assessment
   A. Stage of disease and cell sensitivity to chemotherapy drugs or radiation determines choice of therapy
   B. Age of client, functional ability, and pre-existing health status impact on treatment toxicities
   C. Smaller tumor, less "tumor burden," more treatable; hence, early diagnosis important
   D. Rapidly dividing cells more sensitive to effects; hence, normal cells of bone marrow, gastrointestinal mucosa, hair, gonads experience most side effects
   E. Chemotherapy: chemical agents (drugs) used to destroy cancer cells
      1. Selection and use of chemotherapy: types of drugs (see Table 6–7) and indication(s) based on
         a. Cell (tumor) type
         b. Location of tumor
      2. Drug dose based on body surface area (mg/M^2) or weight (mg/kg)
      3. Combination treatment: more than one agent used to achieve maximum tumor effect with minimal toxicity
      4. Given intermittently, in repeated sequences referred to as cycles
      5. Given by a variety of routes: oral, IV, IM, subcutaneous, intra-arterial, intraperitoneal, intrathecal (into spinal fluid), topical
      6. Side effects/toxicities depend on specific drug(s) administered
         a. Bone marrow suppression: anemia, thrombocytopenia, neutropenia
         b. Gastrointestinal: stomatitis, diarrhea, anorexia, nausea, vomiting, constipation
         c. Alopecia (usually temporary)

d. Organ-specific: cardiac, hepatic, renal, pulmonary, neurological toxicities
e. Reproductive: potential sterility
f. Allergic reactions

F. Radiation therapy: high-energy ionizing radiation used to kill cancer cells; type and mode also based on location, size, and type of tumor; modes of administration include
   1. External
      a. Teletherapy: radiation delivered via external treatment machine
      b. Administered daily (in fractions) for a specified period of time, usually 2 to 6 weeks
      c. Actual treatment takes only 2 to 5 minutes
      d. Side effects depend on area treated, volume of tissue irradiated, fractionation, total dose, type of radiation, and individual differences
         (1) Integumentary: erythema, dry and moist desquamation, hyperpigmentation, alopecia (usually temporary)
         (2) Hematopoietic: bone marrow suppression
         (3) Gastrointestinal: mucositis, xerostomia (diminished salivary production), esophagitis, diarrhea
         (4) Respiratory: pneumonitis, fibrosis
         (5) Reproductive: sterility, hormonal changes
         (6) Urinary: cystitis, urethritis
         (7) Cardiovascular: pericarditis
         (8) Skeletal: osteoradionecrosis (children susceptible to bone deformities)
         (9) Neurological: inflammation and edema
         (10) Systemic: nausea, anorexia, malaise
      e. Client not radioactive
   2. Internal
      a. Sealed source: radiation delivered via internal implanted radioactive sealed source; for example, interstitially implanted radium needles; may be temporary or permanent
      b. Unsealed radioactive substances: radioactive iodine ingested orally (thyroid), radioactive phosphate injected intravenously, isotopes instilled into intrapleural or peritoneal spaces (ovarian)
      c. Radiation precautions necessary

II. Analysis
  A. High risk for injury related to side effects of therapy
  B. High risk for injury related to exposure to chemotherapy and radioactive sources
III. Planning/goals, expected outcomes
  A. Chemotherapy- and/or radiation-induced complications are minimized
  B. Client's significant others/family and health care providers will experience minimal exposure to and contamination from chemotherapy and radiation
IV. Implementations
  A. Prevent, minimize, relieve therapy-induced complications through continuous assessment, prompt intervention, and client/family education
    1. Monitor laboratory values to assess for organ toxicities
    2. Provide skin care for site of external radiation therapy
      a. No soap, oils, lotions, deodorants, powders except with doctor's approval
      b. Protect treatment area from sun, wind, and extreme heat or cold
      c. Do not wash off markings
      d. Avoid irritation (rubbing, scratching)
      e. Avoid tight-fitting clothing over treatment area
    3. Monitor for side effects of bone marrow depression
      a. Monitor CBC; report critical values promptly
      b. Exercise infection precautions
        (1) Meticulous handwashing
        (2) Isolate as indicated
        (3) Strict asepsis with procedures
        (4) Avoid invasive procedures, especially rectal temperatures, suppositories
        (5) Monitor temperature; report elevations
        (6) Monitor for signs of infection
        (7) Obtain cultures
        (8) Administer antibiotics
        (9) Acetaminophen may mask fever
        (10) Assess IV sites, especially central venous
      c. Exercise bleeding precautions
        (1) Avoid invasive procedures and trauma
        (2) Avoid aspirin
        (3) Monitor for bleeding: skin, mouth, nose, urine, feces, emesis, sputum; guaiac specimens
        (4) Observe for fatigue, weakness, hypotension, change in level of consciousness, tachycardia
        (5) Instruct to avoid straining at stool; administer stool softeners
        (6) Avoid razors, dental floss, tooth brushing with low platelet count
        (7) Administer blood transfusions as needed; monitor for reaction
      d. Prevent fatigue related to anemia
        (1) Assess activity tolerance
        (2) Assist with ADLs as needed
        (3) Encourage and adjust activities within client's tolerance level
        (4) Plan rest periods
        (5) Observe for symptoms: pallor, fatigue, weakness, palpitations, dizziness, shortness of breath
    4. Maintain nutrition and hydration
      a. Monitor weight
      b. Monitor electrolytes
      c. Assess I & O, skin turgor, mucous membranes
      d. Monitor serum albumin levels (indicator of protein stores)
      e. Confer with dietician
      f. Assess food preferences
      g. Document calorie count
      h. Provide soft, bland, cold foods
      i. Administer antiemetics (Table 6–8); prophylactic use preferred
      j. Offer crackers, toast for nausea
      k. Encourage small, frequent meals with nourishing snacks
      l. Encourage fluids
      m. Encourage high-protein, high-caloric diet
      n. Administer total parenteral nutrition (TPN) and IV fluids as needed
    5. Implement comfort measures for stomatitis
      a. Instruct to avoid irritants (e.g., alcohol, tobacco, spices, acidic foods, commercial mouthwashes, extreme temperatures in food and beverages)
      b. Instruct in oral hygiene measures
      c. Administer topical oral/systemic analgesics for pain
    6. Control diarrhea
      a. Provide clear liquid diet; advance to low residue: rice, bananas, applesauce, dry toast, mashed potatoes; avoid milk and milk products
      b. Encourage increased fluid intake
      c. Monitor number and consistency of bowel movements
      d. Monitor fluid and electrolyte status
      e. Administer antidiarrheal agents

TABLE 6–8 Antiemetics

Example	Action	Use	Common Side Effects	Nursing Implications
Phenothiazines Prochlorperazine (Compazine)	Vomiting center in the brain receives input from: —intestinal tract via vagus nerve —cerebral cortex and limbic system —vestibular apparatus in inner ear —sympathetic visceral afferents —chemoreceptor trigger zone (CTZ) Antiemetics act at one or more sites; rationale for combination therapy	Prevention and treatment of nausea and vomiting Chemotherapy drugs differ in their potential to induce nausea and vomiting	Drowsiness, dry mouth, flushing, hypotension, restlessness, fatigue, extrapyramidal effects (EPS) (parkinsonism, akathesia, tardive dyskinesia, dystonia)	Monitor I & O; monitor BP; when patient on long-term therapy, monitor for liver disease and EPS; warn about drowsiness; monitor effectiveness; use preventively; administer with Benadryl for EPS
Substituted benzamines Metaclopramide (Reglan)	Dopamine antagonist— blocks CTZ; —accelerates gastric emptying and small bowel transit		Sedation, restlessness, EPS, diarrhea	Administer with Benadryl to control EPS; monitor diarrhea
Benzodiazepines Lorazepam (Ativan)	CNS depressant; causes short-term amnesia; decreases anxiety		Arousable sedation, short-term amnesia (may be desirable to forget chemotherapy experience), hypotension, perceptual disturbances	Someone must accompany patient to drive if given with outpatient therapy; mix immediately prior to administration; slow IV push; reduce dose in elderly, hepatic or renal dysfunction
Serotonin antagonist Ondansetron (Zofran)	Serotonin receptor (5-HT$_3$) antagonist		Mild headache; no sedation—ideal for elderly, pediatric use; no EPS	Drug is very costly; current use limited to acute phase of nausea and vomiting; ideal for outpatient therapy

7. Prepare for alopecia
   a. Suggest scarves, hats, turbans, wigs
   b. Avoid trauma to remaining hair: frequent shampooing, hair dryers, perms, rollers, hair dye
   c. Stress temporary nature of loss
   d. Regrown hair may be slightly different color or texture
8. Advise of potential reproductive dysfunction
   a. Suggest sperm banking for males
   b. Discuss continued need for contraception
   c. Discourage pregnancy during therapy
   d. Advise of potential sterility
   e. Differentiate between impotence (erectile dysfunction) and sterility
B. Implement radiation precautions when internal radiation therapy sources used
   1. Instruct patient and family on procedure and visitation restrictions; follow institution specific policies and procedures
   2. Private room required; patient activity restricted to room or bedrest
   3. Pregnant visitors and caretakers restricted; no one under 18 allowed
   4. Maintain flat position and minimal movement in bed with cervical implants; prevent rectal and bladder distension
   5. Observe principles of time, distance, and shielding for visitors and caregivers
   6. Check linens, clothing, and bedpans for signs of dislodged implant; if dislodged, do not touch; notify appropriate personnel immediately
   7. Exercise precautions with secretions from clients receiving unsealed radioactive sources (orally, intravenously)
   8. Plan care and consolidate activities to decrease time at bedside
   9. Use appropriate radiation-monitoring devices (i.e., badges)
C. Implement precautions when handling che-

motherapy and patient excreta within 48 hours after therapy

  1. Routes of exposure: inhalation, absorption, and ingestion during drug preparation, administration, and disposal of contaminated materials

  2. Treat all contaminated equipment as hazardous waste

  3. Wear protective equipment when administering or handling drug(s) and body fluids from clients who have received drugs within previous 48 hours: disposable gloves; gowns per institutional policy; goggles if danger of eye splatter

  4. Accidental exposure: wash contaminated skin, rinse eyes if exposed, obtain medical evaluation

  5. Clean up spills immediately according to institutional policy

V. Evaluation

  A. Client exhibits minimal to no chemotherapy- and/or radiation-induced complications

  B. Client, family, healthcare providers are not exposed to radiation or chemotherapy contamination

POST-TEST Immune Disorders

Ms. Smith is undergoing an extensive work-up for a lung mass. She is scheduled for a bronchoscopy with washings and biopsy.

---

1. Ms. Smith asks you, "Is this procedure really necessary? I must have lung cancer after all of these years of smoking. Why doesn't the doctor just start treatment?" Your best response would be:
   1. "Your doctor wouldn't have ordered this unless it was absolutely necessary."
   2. "Because there are different kinds of lung cancer, your doctor needs to find out which one you have because it will determine the type of therapy."
   3. "Your doctor can't tell for certain that you even have lung cancer unless a tissue specimen is examined for the presence of cancer cells."
   4. "It is standard medical practice to evaluate all lung masses with a bronchoscopy."
2. Ms. Smith is diagnosed with small-cell lung

carcinoma. Her physician has chosen an intensive combination chemotherapy regimen with which to treat her. In preparation for chemotherapy, you would tell her:
   1. Chemotherapy is only given intravenously because the drugs are very irritating
   2. Chemotherapy is given intermittently, in repeated sequences referred to as cycles
   3. Chemotherapy has minimal side effects
   4. She will permanently lose all of her hair

3. One of the drugs Ms. Smith will receive is cisplatin. Which of the following is NOT a nursing implication associated with this particular drug?
   1. IV hydration and mannitol diuretic therapy
   2. Prophylactic antiemetic therapy
   3. Monitoring of renal function
   4. Administration of leucovorin

4. You are taking care of Ms. Smith the day that she receives her first chemotherapy treatment. Which of the following interventions is NOT indicated?
   1. Observe precautions when handling her excreta for the next 48 hours
   2. Isolate her from other patients to prevent cross contamination
   3. Wear protective apparel when handling drug(s)
   4. Treat all contaminated equipment as hazardous waste

5. Immunization with tetanus toxoid is an example of:
   1. Naturally acquired active immunity
   2. Naturally acquired passive immunity
   3. Artificially induced active immunity
   4. Artificially induced passive immunity

6. Allergies are an example of a(an):
   1. Immunodeficiency
   2. Autoimmune disease
   3. Genetic defect in antibody production
   4. Inappropriate immune response

7. Which of the following would NOT predispose a person to immunosuppression?
   1. Stress
   2. Malnutrition
   3. Chemotherapy
   4. Maladaptive behavior

8. Which of the following is NOT considered an autoimmune disorder?
   1. Cancer
   2. Ulcerative colitis
   3. Systemic lupus erythematosus (SLE)
   4. Rheumatoid arthritis

9. An example of active naturally acquired immunity is:
   1. Gamma-globulin injection
   2. Measles vaccination
   3. Chickenpox
   4. Placental transfer of maternal antibodies

10. Which of the following components of the immune system is directly responsible for antibody production?
    1. T lymphocytes
    2. B lymphocytes
    3. Cytokines
    4. Phagocytes

11. Another term for antibodies is:
    1. Complement
    2. Natural killer cells
    3. Macrophages
    4. Immunoglobulins

12. Which of the following interventions is NOT appropriate for clients receiving radiation via cervical implants?
    1. Restricting visitors and staff contact
    2. Encouraging frequent ambulation in the halls
    3. Exercising precautions with bodily secretions
    4. Isolating client in a private room

13. Which of the following is NOT a characteristic of malignant tumors?
    1. Controlled growth
    2. Ability to metastasize
    3. Poorly differentiated
    4. Invasiveness

POST-TEST Answers and Rationales

1. ③ Tissue and/or cell samples are crucial for cancer diagnosis. The first response offers no rationale for the procedure. Although true, the second response assumes that the client has cancer. The last response is incorrect. 1, II. Cancer.

2. ② Chemotherapy is administered intermittently over a specified period of time, in repeated sequences referred to as cycles. Chemotherapy can be given by a variety of routes. There are multiple potential side effects. Hair loss is usually only temporary, occurring during active therapy. 1 & 2, II. Chemotherapy.

3. ④ Leucovorin is given to prevent toxicity from methotrexate, not cisplatin. Because of the nephrotoxic and emetogenic effects of cisplatin therapy, the first three interventions are indicated. 4, I. Chemotherapy.

4. ② Isolation is not necessary. Precautions (including gowns and gloves) when handling drugs and excreta are necessary. All contaminated equipment should be considered hazardous waste. 4, I. Chemotherapy.

5. ③ Immunizations are examples of artificially induced active immunity. 1, II. Immunity.

6. ④ Allergies are inappropriate and harmful immune responses to harmless substances. Etiologies do not include genetic defects, autoimmunity, or immunodeficiency. 1, II. Immunity.

7. ④ Immunosuppression may be linked to or induced by stress, malnutrition, and chemotherapy, but not by maladaptive behaviors in and of themselves. 1, II. Immunity.

8. ① Cancer is not considered an autoimmune disorder, but rather a disease that may result from or further induce immunosuppression. Ulcerative colitis, SLE, and rheumatoid arthritis are considered autoimmune disorders. 1, II. Immunity.

9. ③ Chickenpox is an example of a naturally acquired active immunity. Placental transfer of maternal antibodies and gamma-globulin injections are examples of passive immunity. Measles vaccination is an example of artificially induced active immunity. 1, II. Immunity.

10. ② Although T lymphocytes help to turn on antibody production, it is the B lymphocytes that differentiate into plasma cells that secrete antibodies. Cytokines are released from activated immune cells and further regulate the immune response. Phagocytes engulf and digest foreign invaders. 1, II. Immunity.

11. ④ Antibodies are also referred to as immunoglobulins. Complement is involved in assisting antibodies. Natural killer cells are a type of lymphocyte that kills on contact. Macrophages are large white blood cells that act through phagocytosis. 1, II. Immunity.

12. ② A flat position in bed with minimal movement is important to prevent dislodgement of cervical implants. Isolation and radiation precautions are necessary. 4, I. Radiation Therapy.

13. ① Rapid, uncontrolled growth, as opposed to controlled growth, is characteristic of malignant tumors. The others are all characteristic of malignant tumors. 1, II. Cancer.

PRE-TEST Autoimmune Disorders

1. Systemic lupus erythematosus (SLE) is best defined as a(n):
   ① Inflammatory disease of the connective tissue
   ② Autoimmune disease of the joints
   ③ Infectious renal disorder
   ④ Vascular disorder

2. Which of the following can cause a lupus-like syndrome?
   ① Pregnancy
   ② Procainamide (Pronestyl)
   ③ Steroids
   ④ Prochlorperazine (Compazine)

3. Which of the following would NOT be considered a common clinical manifestation of lupus?
   ① Arthritic-like joint pain
   ② Fever
   ③ Fatigue and generalized weakness
   ④ Hypotension

4. Which of the following would NOT be considered a complication of lupus?
   ① Cirrhosis
   ② Renal failure
   ③ Congestive heart failure
   ④ Peripheral vascular disease

PRE-TEST Answers and Rationales

1. ① Lupus is an systemic autoimmune inflammatory disease of the connective tissue. Although the joints, kidneys, and vascular system are affected, it is caused by the inflammatory reaction. 1, II. Lupus.

2. ② Pronestyl causes a lupus-like syndrome. The other options do not cause a lupus-like syndrome. 1, II. Lupus.

3. ④ Hypertension, along with arthritic joint pain, fever, and fatigue are symptoms of lupus. Hypertension, not hypotension, is likely to occur. 5, I. Lupus.

4. ① Renal failure, CHF, PVD are all complications of lupus. The liver is not directly affected by lupus. 5, II. Lupus.

NURSING PROCESS APPLIED TO ADULTS WITH AUTOIMMUNE DISORDERS

Systemic Lupus Erythematosus

I. Assessment

A. Definition/pathophysiology (Figure 6–2): chronic, systemic, inflammatory disease involving connective tissue and multiple body systems; probably autoimmune in nature; characterized by remissions and exacerbations; with variable course of disease

B. Incidence
  1. African Americans 1 : 250
  2. Women during childbearing years

C. Predisposing/precipitating factors
  1. Drug-induced syndrome: hydralazine (Apresoline) and procainamide (Pronestyl)
  2. Stress
  3. Genetic predisposition
  4. Sunlight, any other form of ultraviolet light, and pregnancy exacerbate disease

D. Clinical manifestations
  1. Joint inflammation, arthritis-like
  2. Insidious onset
  3. Extreme fatigue, generalized weakness, and anorexia
  4. Weight loss
  5. Fever
  6. "Butterfly rash": raised rash across cheeks and bridge of nose
  7. Generalized rash
  8. Polymyositis
  9. Vasculitis: often direct cause of death

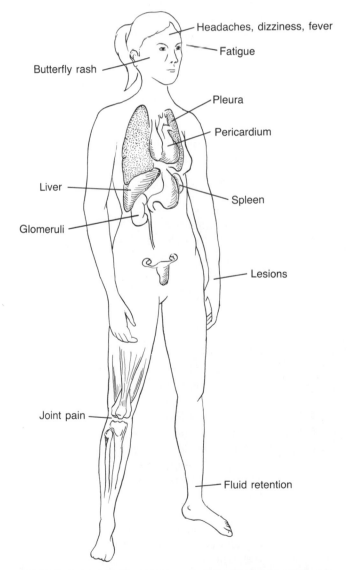

FIGURE 6–2. Manifestations of systemic lupus erythematosus.

a. Renal
b. Central nervous system
c. Cardiac, pericarditis, tachycardia, gallop rhythm
10. Hypertension
11. Peripheral vascular disease
12. Gastrointestinal problems
   a. Pain
   b. Cramping
   c. Nausea and vomiting
13. Pneumonitis, pleural effusion, basilar pneumonia
14. Raynaud's phenomenon
15. Generalized lymphadenopathy
16. Hepatosplenomegaly
17. Delirium, convulsions, psychosis, coma
E. Diagnostic examinations
   1. CBC showing mild to moderate, normochromic anemia and a mild leukopenia often present
   2. ESR is usually elevated
   3. Serum globulins may be increased
   4. LE prep
   5. Decreased complement levels, presence of immune complexes in the serum, presence of immune antibodies to DNA and antinuclear antibodies
   6. Assessments of affected organ systems
      a. Abnormalities in the kidneys will show up on an intravenous pyelogram (IVP)
      b. Barium enema would reveal colonic ulceration
      c. MRI might reveal CNS involvement
      d. ECG or echocardiogram might show cardiac changes
F. Complications
   1. Peripheral vascular disease and loss of limbs
   2. Hypertension
   3. Stroke
   4. Renal failure
   5. Congestive heart failure (CHF)
   6. Chronic obstructive pulmonary disease
G. Medical management
   1. Anti-inflammatories
      a. Steroids (see Table 5–3)
      b. Nonsteroidals (see Table 5–3) such as aspirin, ibuprofen
   2. Hydroxychloroquine (Plaquenil), antimalarial for skin lesions
   3. Topical steroids
   4. Cytotoxic agents, alkylating agents (cyclophosphamide), and antifolates (methotrexate)
   5. Plasmapheresis is used to remove circulating autoantibodies and immune complexes from the blood before organ and tissue damage occurs
   6. Symptomatic treatment to each affected body system; i.e., antihypertensives
II. Analysis
   A. Altered skin integrity related to rash
   B. Pain related to arthritic symptoms
   C. High risk for altered body image related to rash and amputations
   D. Activity intolerance related to symptoms of disease and complications
   E. Knowledge deficit related to medical treatment regimen
III. Planning/goals, expected outcomes
   A. Client's skin integrity will be maintained
   B. Client's pain and discomfort will be decreased
   C. Client will cope with altered body image
   D. Client will not suffer from excessive complications
   E. Client will maintain maximal level of independence
   F. Client will understand and comply with medical regimen
IV. Implementations
   A. Maintain skin integrity
      1. Use cool baths
      2. Avoid soaps and powders
      3. Apply topical steroids as ordered
      4. Administer Plaquenil as ordered
         a. Side effects
            (1) Nausea and vomiting
            (2) Rash
            (3) Retinal damage
      5. Administer steroids as ordered
   B. Avoid anything that exacerbates disease
      1. Sunlight
      2. Stress
      3. Pregnancy
   C. Provide frequent rest periods
   D. Encourage maximal independence
   E. Encourage client to express concerns over altered body image and chronic illness
   F. Assess affected body systems
   G. Provide high-protein (unless renal involvement), high-vitamin, and high-iron diet
   H. Monitor for easy bruising and injury
   I. Allow grieving over potential terminal nature of disease
V. Evaluations
   A. Client's skin remains intact
   B. Client states relief or control of pain and discomfort
   C. Client copes with altered body image
   D. Client understands and complies with medical regimen
   E. Client maintains maximal independence

POST-TEST Autoimmune Disorders

1. The major medication used to treat lupus is:
   1. Erythromycin
   2. Diazide
   3. Cortisone
   4. Gold
2. An important goal for the client with lupus would be that the client will:
   1. Exercise several hours per day
   2. Maintain normal skin integrity
   3. Be pain free
   4. Not develop wrist deformities
3. Which of the following nursing interventions is appropriate for the client with lupus?

   1. Administer Plaquenil as ordered
   2. Encourage the client to get plenty of sunlight
   3. Provide for frequent baths
   4. Provide a low-protein, high-carbohydrate diet
4. The most likely outcome from lupus is:
   1. Development of severe arthritis
   2. Disappearance of the disease after treatment
   3. Death from an infection or renal failure
   4. Appearance of a rash across the face

POST-TEST Answers and Rationales

1. ③ The major treatment for lupus is steroid therapy. Antibiotics would be used to treat infections secondary to infection and antihypertensives to treat the hypertension. Gold is used to treat rheumatoid arthritis. 4, I. Lupus.

2. ② The connective tissue is affected by lupus. Rash is a common symptom. A major goal is to maintain skin integrity. Deformities are not common from the arthritis, and some degree of discomfort is inevitable. It is important for the client with lupus to rest rather than exercise to prevent exacerbation of the disease. 3, I. Lupus.

3. ① Plaquenil is used for the skin symptoms of lupus. Sunlight increases the rashes; baths dry the skin further; and a low-carbohydrate, high-protein diet (with normal renal function) is recommended for the lupus client. 4, II. Lupus.

4. ③ Lupus is a fatal disease. Death is usually related to renal failure or infection. The other options are inappropriate. 5, IV. Lupus.

BIBLIOGRAPHY

SEXUALLY TRANSMITTED DISEASES

Bennett, J. (1986). AIDS: What precautions do you take in the hospital? *American Journal of Nursing* 8: 952–953.

Bennett, J. (1986). What we know about AIDS. *American Journal of Nursing* 9: 1016–1028.

Benenson, A. S., ed. (1990). *Control of communicable diseases in man,* 15th ed. Washington, DC: American Public Health Association.

Centers for Disease Control. (1989). *1989 Sexually transmitted diseases treatment guidelines.* Washington, DC: U.S. Department of Health and Human Services.

Centers for Disease Control. (1990). Progress toward achieving the 1990 objectives for the nation for sexually transmitted diseases. *Morbidity and Mortality Weekly Report* 39 (4): 1–3.

Chase, A. (1983). *The truth about STDs.* New York: Quill.

Corey, L. (1982). The diagnosis and treatment of genital herpes. *Journal of the American Medical Association* 9: 1041–1049.

Guinan, M. D., Wolinsky, S. M., and Reichman, R. C. (1985). Epidemiology of genital herpes simplex virus infection. *Epidemiologic Reviews* 7: 127–146.

Institute of Medicine, National Academy of Sciences. (1986). *Confronting AIDS.* Washington, DC: National Academy Press.

Loucks, A. (1987). Chlamydia: An unheralded epidemic. *American Journal of Nursing* 7: 920–922.

McCormack, W. M., ed. *Chlamydia.* Abbott Park, IL: Abbott Diagnostics Educational Services.

McFarlane, J. M. (1986). *The clinical handbook of family nursing.* New York: John Wiley & Sons.

Phipps, W. J., Long, B. C., Woods, N. F., and Cassmeyer, V. L., eds. (1991). *Medical-surgical nursing,* 4th ed. St. Louis: Mosby Year Book.

Public health service plan for the prevention and control of acquired immune deficiency syndrome (AIDS). (1985). *Public Health Reports* 5: 453–455.

Raab, B., and Lorincz, A. L. (1981). Genital herpes simplex—Concepts and treatment. *Journal of the American Academy of Dermatology* 3: 249–263.

Scherman, S. L. (1985). *Community health nursing care plans.* New York: John Wiley & Sons.

Sanders, L. L., Harrison, H. R., and Washington, A. E. (1986). Treatment of sexually transmitted chlamydial infections. *Journal of the American Medical Association* 13: 1750–1756.

Skidmore-Roth, L. (1992). *Mosby's 1992 nursing drug reference.* St. Louis: Mosby Year Book.

Taptich, B. J., Iyer, P. W., and Bernocchi-Losey, D. (1990). *Nursing diagnosis and care planning.* Philadelphia: W. B. Saunders.

BURNS

Baxter, C., and Waeckerle, J. (1988). Emergency treatment of burn injury. *Annals of Emergency Medicine* 17: 1305–1314.

Bernstein, N. R., and Robson, M. C. (1983). *Comprehensive approaches to the burned person.* Garden City, NY: Medical Examination Books.

Black, J., and Matassarin-Jacobs, E., eds. (1993). *Luckmann & Sorensen's medical-surgical nursing: A psychophysiologic approach,* 4th ed. Philadelphia: W. B. Saunders.

Demling, R. (1987). Fluid replacement in burned patients. *Surgical Clinics of North America* 67: 15–30.

Helvig, E., and Herndon, D. (1989). Airway and pulmonary management of burn patients. *Trauma Quarterly* 5 (4): 19–32.

Hurt, R. A. (1985). More than skin deep: Guidelines for caring for the burn patient. *Nursing 85* 15: 52–57.

Mancusi-Ungaro, S. (1989). Psychosocial issues in burn care. *Trauma Quarterly* 5 (4): 67–70.

Marvin, J. (1987). Pain management in the burn patient. *Journal of Burn Care and Rehabilitation* 8: 307–318.

Robertson, K. E., Cross, P. J., and Terry, J. C. (1985). Burn care: The first crucial days. *American Journal of Nursing* 7: 30–47.

SURGICAL INTERVENTION

Alverson, E. (1987). The preoperative interview: Its effect on perioperative nursing empathy. *AORN Journal* 45:1150–1159, 1162–1164.

American Society of Postanesthesia Nurses. (1986). *Standards of nursing practice.* Richmond, VA: American Society of Postanesthesia Nurses.

Andrews, D. R., and Taylor, C. (1985). Documenting postanesthesia recovery. *American Journal of Nursing* 85: 290–291.

Applegeet, C. J. (1987). Nursing aspects of outpatient surgery. *Urologic Clinics of North America* 14 (1): 21.

Ashby, D. M. (1987). Balancing fluids and electrolytes in the PACU. *Journal of Post Anesthesia Nursing* 2: 114–116.

Association of Operating Room Nurses (1988). *Standards of nursing practice.* Denver: Association of Operating Room Nurses.

Bailes, B. K. (1989). Perioperative nursing research, part IV: Intraoperative phase. *AORN Journal* 49: 1397–1409.

Barrett, J. E. (1985). Helping your postoperative patient breathe easier with incentive spirometry. *Nursing '85* 15 (10): 64.

Black, J., and Matassarin-Jacobs, E., eds. (1993). *Luckmann & Sorensen's medical-surgical nursing: A psychophysiologic approach.* Philadelphia: W. B. Saunders.

Blackwood, S. (1986). Back to basics: The preop exam. *American Journal of Nursing* 86: 39–44.

Boucher, B. A. (1986). The postoperative adverse effects of inhalation anesthetics. *Heart and Lung* 15: 590–608.

Bray, C. A. (1986). Postop pain: Altering the patient's experience through education. *AORN Journal* 43: 672, 674–675, 677.

Brent, N. (1987). How informed are you about consents? *Nursing Life* 6: 37–39.

Burge, S. (1986). How painful are postop incisions? *American Journal of Nursing* 86: 1263A, 1266D, 1266H.

Chitwood, L. B. (1987). Unveiling the mysteries of anesthesia. *Nursing '87* 17 (2): 52–55.

Cuzzell, J. Z. (1988). The new RYB color code. *American Journal of Nursing* 88: 1342–1346.

Drain, C. B., and Christoph, S. S. (1987). *The recovery room: A critical care approach to post anesthesia nursing,* 2nd ed. Philadelphia: W. B. Saunders.

Dripps, R. D., Eckenhoff, J. E., and Vandam, L. D. (1988). *Introduction to anesthesia,* 7th ed. Philadelphia: W. B. Saunders.

Erbostoesser, M. (1989). Care of the patient with malignant hyperthermia. *Journal of Post Anesthesia Nursing* 3: 71–74.

Faherty, B. S., and Grier, M. R. (1982). Analgesic medication for elderly people post surgery. *Nursing Research* 33: 369–372.

Fay, M. F. (1987). Drainage systems: Their role in wound healing. *AORN Journal* 46: 442–455.

Fraulini, K. E., and Borchardt, A. C. (1988). Guide to solving postanesthesia problems. *Nursing '88* 18 (5): 66–86.

Fraulini, K. E., and Gorski, D. N. (1983). Don't let perioperative medications put you in a spin. *Nursing '83* 13: 26–30.

Frost, E. A. M. (1985). *Recovery room practice.* Boston: Blackwell Scientific.

Goulart, D. (1987). Preoperative teaching for surgical patients. *Perioperative Nursing Quarterly* 3 (2): 8–13.

Groah, L. K. (1983). *Operating room nursing: The perioperative role.* Reston, VA: Reston Publishing.

Gruendenemann, B. J., and Meeker, M. H. (1987). *Alexander's care of the patient in surgery.* St. Louis: C. V. Mosby.

Hardy, E. B., Cirillo, B. C., and Gutzeit, N. M. (1988). Rewarming patients in the PACU: Can we make a difference? *Journal of Post Anesthesia Nursing* 3: 313–316.

Hardy, J. D. (1988). *Hardy's textbook of surgery,* 2nd ed. Philadelphia: J. B. Lippincott.

Hill, G. J. (1988). *Outpatient surgery,* 3rd ed. Philadelphia: W. B. Saunders.

Isreal, S. J., and De Kornfeld, T. J. (1987). *Recovery room care,* 2nd ed. Chicago: Year Book Medical.

Kneedler, J. A., and Dodge, G. H. (1987). *Perioperative patient care,* 2nd ed. Boston: Blackwell Scientific.

Latz, P. A., and Wyble, S. J. (1987). Elderly patients: Perioperative nursing implications. *AORN Journal* 46: 238–253.

Litwak, K., and Parnass, S. (1988). Practical points in the management of postoperative nausea and vomiting. *Journal of Post Anesthesia Nursing* 3: 275–277.

McCaffery, M. (1985). Narcotic analgesia for the elderly. *American Journal of Nursing* 85: 296–298.

McConnell, E. A. (1987). *Clinical considerations of in perioperative nursing.* Philadelphia: J. B. Lippincott.

Montanari, J. (1986). Action STAT! Wound dehiscence. *Nursing '86* 16 (2): 33.

Neuberger, G. B. (1987). Wound care: What's clear, what's not. *Nursing '87* 17 (2): 34–37.

Norheim, C. (1986). Spinal anesthesia: As bad as it sounds? *Nursing '86* 16 (4): 42–44.

Nyamathi, A., and Kashiwabara, A. (1988). Preoperative anxiety: Its effects on cognitive thinking. *AORN Journal* 47: 164–170.

Pierce, S. F., and Campbell, M. (1988). Return of bladder function: A research study. *AORN Journal* 47: 702–703, 706–712.

IMMUNITY, CANCER, CHEMOTHERAPY, RADIATION THERAPY

Alkire, K., and Groenwald, S. L. (1990). Relation of the immune system to cancer. In S. L. Groenwald, M. H. Frogge, M. Goodman, and C. H. Yarbro, eds. *Cancer nursing: Principles and practice,* 2nd ed. (pp. 72–88). Boston: Jones & Bartlett.

Baird, S. B., ed. (1991). *A cancer source book for nurses.* Atlanta: American Cancer Society.

Boring, C. C., Squires, T. S., and Heath, C. W. (1992). Cancer statistics for African Americans. *CA—A Cancer Journal for Clinicians* 42 (1): 7–17.

Boring, C. C., Squires, T. S., and Tong, T. (1992). Cancer statistics, 1992. *CA—A Cancer Journal for Clinicians* 42 (1): 19–38.

Brostoff, J., Scadding, G. K., Male, D., and Roitt, I. M. (1991). *Clinical immunology.* New York: Gower Medical.

Brown, J. K., and Hogan, C. M. (1990). Chemotherapy. In S. L. Groenwald, M. H. Frogge, M. Goodman, and C. H. Yarbro, eds. *Cancer nursing: Principles and practice,* 2nd ed. (pp. 230–283). Boston: Jones & Bartlett.

Burke, M. B., Wilkes, G. M., Berg, D., Bean, C. K., and Ingwersen, K. (1991). *Cancer chemotherapy: A nursing process approach.* Boston: Jones & Bartlett.

Cohen, R. F., and Frank-Stromberg, M. (1990). Cancer risk and assessment. In S. L. Groenwald, M. H. Frogge, M. Goodman, and C. H. Yarbro, eds. *Cancer nursing: Principles and practice,* 2nd ed. (pp. 103–118). Boston: Jones & Bartlett.

DeVita, V. T., Hellman, S., and Rosenberg, S. A., eds. (1989). *Cancer: Principles and practice of oncology,* 3rd ed. Philadelphia: J. B. Lippincott.

Fink, D. J. (1991). *Guidelines for the cancer-related checkup* (ACS Publication No. 3347-PE). Atlanta: American Cancer Society.

Frogge, M. H., and Goodman, M. (1990). Surgical therapy. In S. L. Groenwald, M. H. Frogge, M. Goodman, and C. H. Yarbro, eds. *Cancer nursing: Principles and practice,* 2nd ed. (pp. 189–198). Boston: Jones & Bartlett.

Hilderley, L. J. (1990). Radiotherapy. In S. L. Groenwald, M. H. Frogge, M. Goodman, and C. H. Yarbro, eds. *Cancer nursing: Principles and practice,* 2nd ed. (pp. 199–229). Boston: Jones & Bartlett.

Holeb, A. I., Fink, D. J., and Murphy, G. P. (1991). *American Cancer Society textbook of clinical oncology.* Atlanta: American Cancer Society.

National Cancer Institute. (1990). *Chemotherapy and you: A guide to self-help during treatment* (NIH Publication No. 91–1136). Bethesda, MD: National Cancer Institute.

National Cancer Institute. (1990). *Radiation therapy and you: A guide to self-help during treatment* (NIH Publication No. 91–2227). Bethesda, MD: National Cancer Institute.

National Cancer Institute. (1992). *Eating hints: Recipes and tips for better nutrition during cancer treatment* (NIH Publication No. 92–2079). Bethesda, MD: National Cancer Institute.

Odleske, D., and Groenwald, S. L. (1990). Epidemiology of cancer. In S. L. Groenwald, M. H. Frogge, M. Goodman, and C. H. Yarbro, eds. *Cancer nursing: Principles and practice,* 2nd ed. (pp. 3–30). Boston: Jones & Bartlett.

Oncology Nursing Society. (1988). *Cancer chemotherapy guidelines: Modules I–IV.* Pittsburgh, PA: Oncology Nursing Society.

Otto, S. E. (1991). *Oncology nursing.* Chicago: C. V. Mosby.

Schindler, L. W. (1988). *Understanding the immune system* (NIH Publication No. 88–529). Bethesda, MD: National Cancer Institute.

Yarbro, J. W. (1990). Carcinogenesis. In S. L. Groenwald, M. H. Frogge, M. Goodman, and C. H. Yarbro, eds. *Cancer nursing: Principles and practice,* 2nd ed. (pp. 31–42). Boston: Jones & Bartlett.

SYSTEMIC LUPUS ERYTHEMATOSUS

Balow, J. E. (1988). Lupus as a renal disease. *Hospital Practice* 23: 129–135, 139–140, 142–144.

Burlinghame, M. B., and Delafuente, J. C. (1988). Treatment of systemic lupus erythematosus. *Drug Intelligence and Clinical Pharmacology* 22: 283–288.

Fessel, W. J. (1988). Epidemiology of systemic lupus erythematosus. *Rheumatic Disease Clinics of North America* 14: 15–23.

Klipple, J. H. (1990). Systemic lupus erythematosus, treatment related complications, superimposed on chronic disease. *Journal of the American Medical Association* 263 (13): 1812–1815.

Pfeiffer, C. A., and Wetstone, S. L. (1988). Health locus of control and well-being in systemic lupus erythematosus. *Arthritis Care Research* 1 (3): 131–138.

Rothfield, N. F. (1989). The diagnostic pictures of systemic lupus erythematosus. *Hospital Practice* 24: 37–46.

Steinberg, A. D., and Klinman, D. M. (1988). Pathogenesis of systemic lupus erythematosus. *Rheumatic Disease Clinics of North America* 14: 25–41.

Townes, A. S. (1987). The "mask" of lupus. *Hospital Practice* 22: 93–97, 101–103, 107–108.

7

Mobility in the Adult Client

PRE-TEST Musculoskeletal Disorders

Ruth Fair is a 55-year-old woman who is admitted with a fractured femur. She will be in skeletal traction for at least 6 weeks.

1. Effects of immobility on Mrs. Fair's cardiovascular system include:
   1. Increased cardiac output
   2. Hypertension
   3. Vascular stasis
   4. Decreased cardiac workload

2. An important nursing intervention to reduce the stress on her cardiovascular system is:
   1. Keeping the head of the bed either flat or upright
   2. Encouraging the client to lie still as much as possible
   3. Warning the client not to use isometric exercises
   4. Teaching the client to move without Valsalva's maneuver

3. Which of the following would NOT be considered a common respiratory problem for Mrs. Fair, considering her immobility?
   1. Decreased cough reflex
   2. Decreased depth of respirations
   3. Productive cough
   4. Adventitious breath sounds

4. Mrs. Fair is bothered by a productive cough. Which of the following medications would be CONTRAINDICATED for her?
   1. Penicillin
   2. Theophylline
   3. Benylin expectorant
   4. Codeine cough syrup

5. Constipation is a common problem for the immobilized client. Which of the following would NOT contribute to Mrs. Fair's constipation?
   1. Inability to use bedpan
   2. High fiber diet
   3. Decreased fluid intake
   4. Decreased peristalsis

6. The nurse can help to decrease Mrs. Fair's constipation by:
   1. Encouraging her to use a bedside commode
   2. Turning her side to side every 2 hours
   3. Administering a Fleet enema every other day as ordered
   4. Administering Colace daily as ordered

7. Mrs. Fair is prone to musculoskeletal problems while she is in traction. Which of the following nursing interventions is INAPPROPRIATE to prevent these problems?
   1. Provide for active and passive range of motion of unaffected extremities
   2. Increase calcium and liquids in the diet
   3. Order a footboard to prevent footdrop
   4. Encourage her to perform isometric exercises

8. Mrs. Fair has complained of pain and burning on urination. Nursing implementations to help alleviate this include:
   1. Decreasing the fluid intake to decrease urination
   2. Providing orange juice to acidify the urine
   3. Catheterizing her to decrease the burning
   4. Increasing the amount of fish and cereal in her diet

9. Your client has an area of skin that is abraded, red, and warm. How would this type of injury be classified?
   1. Stage I
   2. Stage II
   3. Stage III
   4. Stage IV

10. Which of the following nursing interventions would be INAPPROPRIATE for the client with a stage III skin injury?
    1. Reposition the client hourly except on the affected side
    2. Place an Eggcrate on the bed
    3. Apply a dressing to contain the secretions
    4. Massage the area every 2 hours with lotion

11. Your client had a long leg cast applied for a fractured tibia. Which of the following is a priority assessment for the nurse to make?
    1. Numbness and tingling in the toes
    2. Uniform heat along the drying cast
    3. Decreased circulation proximal to the cast
    4. Cool areas along a dried cast

12. In caring for a wet cast, the nurse should:
    1. Use a hairdryer set on low to dry it
    2. Cover the cast to prevent client chilling
    3. Use a fan in the room to help dry the cast
    4. Move the cast using the fingertips only to lift it

13. Which of the following statements by the client concerning care of the cast at home would indicate a need for more client teaching?
    1. "I'll be careful not to get the cast wet when I bathe."
    2. "I'll pour a small amount of lotion inside the cast to help the itching."
    3. "I'll keep my cast elevated when I'm sitting to decrease swelling."
    4. "I won't put any weight on my casted leg until the doctor says I can."

PRE-TEST Answers and Rationales

1. ③ Immobility causes venous stasis, decreased cardiac output, hypotension especially orthostatic, and an increased cardiac workload. 2, II. Immobility.

2. ④ Valsalva's maneuver increases intrathoracic pressure and puts a great deal of stress on the heart. Having the client move without using it decreases the stress. Keeping the client still increases stress. Isometric exercises would help decrease it. 4, II. Immobility.

3. ① There is no reason for the cough reflex to be decreased in an immobilized client. The other options are common respiratory complications. 1, II. Immobility.

4. ④ Codeine suppresses the cough reflex and would increase the risk of atelectasis and pneumonia. Penicillin is an antibiotic; theophylline and Benylin should help the client to cough. 5, II. Immobility.

5. ② A high fiber diet is recommended to treat constipation. The other options are causes of constipation. 5, II. Immobility.

6. ④ Colace or other stool softeners help the client defecate more easily. Enemas should be avoided if at all possible. Mobility is limited by the traction, so the other options are impossible. 4, II. Immobility.

7. ③ A footboard would disrupt the traction and is therefore inappropriate for this situation. The other options are all appropriate actions to decrease musculoskeletal problems. 4, II. Immobility.

8. ④ Increasing the amount of fish, cereal, meats, and cranberry juice—all acid-ash foods—will decrease the pH of her urine, making it acid. Decreasing fluid increases the risk of infection, as does catheterizing her. Orange juice is alkaline-ash and will alkalinize the urine. 4, II. Immobility.

9. ② Stage II is as described. Stage I is redness; stage III is when there is an open, draining wound, and stage IV, a crater. 1, II. Immobility.

10. ④ With a stage III lesion, there is open skin and possible infection, so lotion is inappropriate. The other options are all appropriate treatments for a stage III lesion. 4, II. Immobility

11. ① The priority assessment is circulation and sensation. Uniform heat is a normal reaction to drying as it is coolness along the dry cast. Decreased circulation proximal to the injury is highly unlikely. 1, I & II. Fractures/Casts.

12. ③ Applying even low heat could burn the client. Covering the cast slows the drying process. Moving it with fingertips can create pressure areas. Using a fan to stir the air or opening a window are the only safe ways to help dry the cast. 4, I. Casts.

13. ② This statement would indicate misunderstanding. Nothing should ever be put into the cast. The other statements indicate proper understanding of discharge instructions. 5, I & IV. Casts.

NURSING PROCESS APPLIED TO ADULTS WITH MUSCULOSKELETAL DISORDERS

Hazards of Immobility

General Considerations
I. Adults need mobility to survive
II. Many and varied problems arise if client is immobilized even for 24 hours; problems increase with length of immobilization
III. Most problems can be avoided with proper nursing care
IV. Immobility affects all body systems

Cardiovascular System
I. Assessment
  A. Blood vessels
    1. Muscular activity aids in movement of blood
    2. With no activity, blood flow sluggish, inadequate nourishment to all cells
    3. Decreased flow predisposes stasis and clot formation
  B. Workload of heart
    1. Heart works harder when body at rest and supine
    2. More frequent use of Valsalva's maneuver every time client moves up in bed

C. Blood pressure
1. Orthostatic changes occur within hours
2. Client at risk for fainting or falling

II. Implementations
A. Exercises to maintain adequate circulation, within limits of client's condition
1. Passive range of motion
2. Active range of motion
3. Isometric exercises
4. Use of footboard and overhead trapeze, unless contraindicated
B. Positioning
1. Teach client to change position without using Valsalva's maneuver
2. Change position at least slightly every hour and completely every 2 hours
3. Elevate head of bed at intervals throughout day
4. Encourage client to move extremities as much as possible

Respiratory System

I. Assessment
A. Pulmonary stasis and accumulation of secretions
1. Wheezing
2. Productive cough
3. Altered respiratory depth and rate
4. Adventitious breath sounds
B. Inadequate aeration of lungs
1. Shortness of breath
2. Pain
3. Feeling of tightness in chest

II. Implementations
A. Have client cough and deep breathe
B. Have client turn frequently
C. Maintain adequate hydration
D. Change position to include semi-Fowler's to Fowler's
E. Medicate as needed to encourage coughing
F. Avoid codeine and other cough suppressants
G. Provide rest periods
H. Give frequent mouth care

Gastrointestinal System

I. Assessment
A. Ingestion
1. Decreased appetite
2. Emotions often low, so less willing to eat
3. Usually low protein intake
B. Elimination
1. Constipation caused by various factors
a. Decreased peristalsis
b. Physical inactivity

c. Inability to use bedpan
d. Decreased muscle tone
e. Embarrassment over using bedpan and asking for help
f. Amount and type of food eaten
g. Fluid intake
h. Pain medications
2. Impaction
a. Absence of stools for 3 days
b. May have diarrhea as liquid seeps around impaction

II. Implementations
A. Check client's dietary intake
1. Provide adequate liquids
2. Increase bulk and roughage in diet
B. Provide privacy for defecation
C. Use bedside commode if possible
D. Position sitting on bedpan if must remain in bed
E. Use fracture pan for comfort
F. Encourage client to follow normal bowel habits
G. Administer stool softeners (Colace) or bulk laxatives (Metamucil) as ordered (see Table 8–14).
H. Institute bowel training program
I. Avoid cathartics or enemas unless absolutely necessary

Musculoskeletal System

I. Assessment
A. Range of motion
1. Muscle activity maintains range of motion
2. Without joint motion, muscles lose elasticity and shorten
3. Fibrous tissue develops
4. Contractures may occur and cause permanent damage
B. Osteoporosis
1. New bone formed because of stress and strain placed on bones by walking and standing
2. Inactivity causes depletion of calcium, phosphorus, and nitrogen in bone
3. Demineralization causes increased bone porosity and increased risk of fractures

II. Implementation
A. Prevent footdrop with footboard, unless contraindicated
B. Use supportive devices to prevent contractures and deformities
C. Active and passive range-of-motion exercises
D. Stand and allow weightbearing if possible
E. Increase calcium in diet through foods such as yogurt, sardines, greens, milk, or cheese

Integumentary System

I. Assessment

A. Decubitus ulcers: lesions produced by sloughing of inflamed and necrotic tissue
1. Caused by pressure, especially over bony prominence
2. Caused by shearing force

B. Erythema begins within 1 to 2 hours of pressure and congestion because of impaired blood flow

C. Breakdown most likely to occur if individual malnourished, obese, aged, or with circulatory impairment

D. Other risk factors include skin that is moist, warm, and subjected to irritating substances such as urine, feces, sweat, or other discharges

E. Classification
1. Stage I (partial thickness)
   a. Skin deep pink, red, or mottled
   b. Skin warm and firm or tightly stretched
   c. Reversible, no permanent skin damage
2. Stage II (partial thickness)
   a. Skin blistered, cracked, or abraded
   b. Skin integrity disrupted
   c. Skin around area red and warm
3. Stage III (full thickness)
   a. Skin ulcerated with crater-like sore
   b. Underlying tissues involved
   c. Usually infected
   d. Infection causes continued erosion and copious secretions
4. Stage IV (full thickness)
   a. Deep ulceration and necrosis involving deep underlying muscle and maybe bone
   b. Extensively infected
   c. Ulcer either dry and covered with thick necrotic tissue, or wet and oozing purulent exudate

II. Implementations

A. Prevention of ulcers much easier than treatment
1. Frequent position changes
2. Pad all bony prominences
3. Support extremities
4. Turn at least every 2 hours, or more frequently
5. Use special devices such as Eggcrate, flotation pads, sheepskins, and mechanical flotation beds to distribute pressure and prevent breakdown
6. Keep client and all linens clean and dry
7. Use lotion to moisturize skin
8. Massage all potential breakdown areas
9. Maintain adequate nutrition and hydration
10. Reposition to avoid shearing force from sliding client against sheet

B. Treatment of pressure sores varies by institution
1. Keep ulcer clean and dry
2. Care required constantly to prevent further damage

Urinary System

I. Assessment

A. Stasis common when client not in upright position

B. When client supine, urine flows sluggish and pooling occurs

C. Calculi and infections common with stasis

D. Loss of bladder tone from distention

E. Lose control of urinary sphincters because of excessive pressure

F. Retention with overflow and incontinence common

II. Implementations

A. Encourage adequate fluid intake, at least 2 to 3 L per day

B. Have client empty bladder regularly

C. Restrict calcium intake

D. Encourage acid-ash foods such as cranberry juice, cereals, fish, meats, and vitamin C to acidify urine; avoid citrus fruits, which alkalinize urine

E. Have women sit and men stand to void to better empty bladder

F. Use catheter only as last resort

Psychological Aspects

I. Assessment

A. Loss of independence

B. Sense of hopelessness common

C. Feelings of isolation and depression

D. Worry over family and financial matters

II. Implementations

A. Allow maximum independence and decision making on part of client

B. Help client set realistic goals

C. Help client see own worth and maintain dignity

D. Arrange consultations with social services as needed

Traumatic Musculoskeletal Disorders

Casts

I. Assessment

A. Types of casts
1. Long or short leg casts
2. Walking casts with extra support for weightbearing
3. Spica casts cover trunk and one or two

extremities, either legs or shoulder and arm
4. Short arm cast
5. Body cast
B. Observe closely for pressure on nerves or blood vessels
C. Observe for numbness, tingling, or increased pain
D. Observe distal tissues for impaired circulation by checking color and for warmth by checking blanching
E. Monitor for elevated temperature, presence of foul odor
F. Check for warmth or "hot spots" under cast, which can signal inflammation
II. Implementation
A. Allow cast to dry completely before moving
B. Support cast on pillows
C. Leave cast exposed to air until dry
D. Do not use hairdryer or heat source on cast
E. Cast takes at least 24 hours to dry; longer in higher humidity
F. Keep cast clean, dry, and free from bodily secretions
G. Tape edges of cast to prevent irritation
H. Continually monitor circulation and sensation under cast
I. Monitor for complications
J. Teach client home cast care, especially not to stick objects down cast
K. Elevate casted extremities to decrease normal swelling
L. Use pillows to support leg cast when sleeping or sitting
M. Apply sling to support arm cast when up

Traction
I. Assessment
A. Types of traction (Figures 7–1, 7–2, 7–3)
1. Skeletal: traction applied directly to bone
2. Skin: traction applied to skin
a. Buck's traction—lower extremity, usually to treat factured hip
b. Russell's traction—for fractured hip or knee

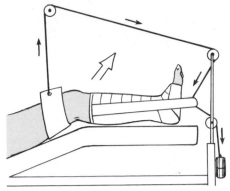

FIGURE 7–2. Russell's traction.

c. Cervical or pelvic—for cervical or lumbar strain
B. Traction: application of mechanical pull to body part to
1. Reduce and set fracture (skeletal)
2. Immobilize part
3. Relieve pain and muscle spasms
C. Be sure weights hanging free
D. Observe all skin for possible pressure sores
E. Monitor pin sites for possible infection
F. Assess for impaired circulation or undue pressure on nerves
II. Implementation
A. Maintain proper alignment for traction and countertraction
B. Turn and position client as allowed by type of traction
C. Clean pin sites daily and dress per institutional policy
D. Provide diversional activities
E. Use fracture bedpan

Fractures
I. Assessment
A. Definitions/types of fractures (Figure 7–4)
1. Complete: bone broken into two parts with complete separation of parts

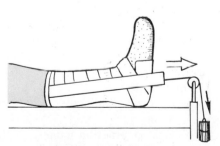

FIGURE 7–1. Buck's traction.

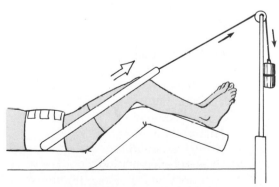

FIGURE 7–3. Pelvic traction.

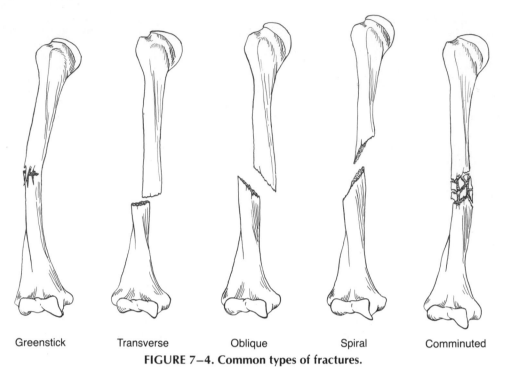

| Greenstick | Transverse | Oblique | Spiral | Comminuted |

FIGURE 7–4. Common types of fractures.

2. Incomplete: bone broken into two parts that do not separate
3. Comminuted: bone shattered into more than two fragments
4. Closed or simple: skin not broken
5. Open or compound: break in skin with protrusion of bone fragments
6. Greenstick: common in children, when bone partially bent and partially broken
7. Other types include pathological, longitudinal, spiral, transverse, oblique

B. Predisposing/precipitating factors
　1. Old age
　2. Osteoporosis, greatest in postmenopausal women
　3. Trauma
　4. Cancer

C. Clinical manifestations
　1. Pain
　2. Swelling
　3. Deformities
　4. Of fractured hip
　　a. Shortened
　　b. Abducted
　　c. Externally rotated

D. Diagnostic examinations
　1. History of injury
　2. X-ray examination
　3. Physical examination
　4. Arteriogram for certain fractures

E. Medical management

1. Goal to reunite bone fragments in as close to normal alignment as possible so bone can heal normally; healing occurs in five stages (Figure 7–5)
　a. Hematoma stage: blood from trauma clots and forms hematoma between broken ends of bone
　b. Cellular proliferation stage: granulation tissue forms, which becomes firm and becomes link between pieces of broken bone
　c. Callus formation stage: new bone tissue enters area, forming woven bone; ends begin to knit
　d. Callus ossification stage: immature cells replaced by mature cells, callus formed, tissue resembles normal bone
　e. Consolidation and remodeling stage: callus remodeled by osteoblastic and osteoclastic activity; excess bone absorbed from callus
2. Closed reduction
　a. Bones realigned without surgery
　b. Once bones in alignment, cast usually applied to hold bones in alignment

F. Surgical management
　1. Open reduction
　　a. Surgical realignment of bone fragments
　　b. Cast or traction usually applied postoperatively

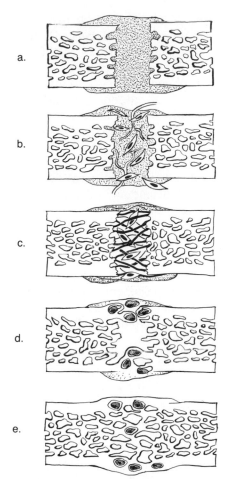

FIGURE 7–5. The five stages of bone healing. *A,* Hematoma stage; *B,* cellular proliferation stage; *C,* callus formation stage; *D,* callus ossification stage; *E,* consolidating and remodeling stage.

2. Internal fixation
   a. Follows open reduction
   b. Application of screws, plates, pins, nails, and so on to hold fragments in alignment
   c. May also involve removal of damaged bone and replacement with prosthesis
   d. Good for elderly, because it provides immediate bone strength
   e. Increased risk of infection
3. External fixation
   a. Sturdy external frame with multiple pins through bone
   b. Used with extensive open fractures with soft tissue damage
   c. Used if infected fractures do not heal properly
   d. Used with multiple traumas
   e. More freedom of movement than traction
   f. Greater risk of infection with multiple open pin sites

II. Analysis
   A. High risk for injury related to fracture and immobility
   B. Impaired physical mobility related to fracture
   C. Knowledge deficit related to treatment and home care
III. Planning/goals, expected outcomes
   A. Client will have fracture treated and it will heal without complications
   B. Client will not develop problems of immobility
   C. Client will understand and comply with home care instructions
IV. Implementation
   A. Monitor circulation and sensation distal to fracture
   B. Usual postoperative care
   C. Meticulous care of pin site and incision to prevent infection
   D. Monitor for pulmonary embolus or fat embolus
   E. Prevent complications of immobility
   F. Teach client and family home care for discharge
   G. For fractured femoral shaft—maintain skeletal traction for about 6 weeks, then prepare client for long leg cast
   H. For hip fracture
      1. Preoperative
         a. Maintain Buck's traction to decrease pain and immobilize leg
         b. Turn client every 2 hours from back to unaffected side and reapply traction
         c. Establish baseline vital signs
         d. Maintain maximal respiratory and cardiovascular systems
      2. Postoperative, hip pinning
         a. Turn client from back to unaffected side
         b. Up, non-weightbearing 1 to 2 days after surgery
         c. Non-weightbearing affected hip for 3 to 6 months
         d. Keep leg abducted, prevent internal or external rotation
      3. Postoperative, hip prosthesis
         a. Keep leg abducted with two to four pillows
         b. Turn to back or unoperative side
         c. Non-weightbearing for 3 months
         d. Up, non-weightbearing 2 to 4 days after surgery
         e. Prevent external rotation, use trochanter roll
         f. Administer antibiotics prophylactically to prevent infection
V. Evaluation
   A. Fracture heals without complications

B. No complications of immobility occur
C. Client and family understand and follow discharge instructions

Chronic Musculoskeletal Disorders

Rheumatoid Arthritis and Osteoarthritis

I. Assessment
   A. Definition/pathophysiology
      1. Rheumatoid arthritis
         a. Systemic, inflammatory, collagen disease causing pathological changes within joint and leading to permanent deformity
         b. Pathology—chronic inflammation of synovial membranes and formation of pannus
      2. Osteoarthritis
         a. Also called degenerative joint disease
         b. Nonsystemic, progressive, degenerative joint disease
         c. Degeneration of cartilage with wear and tear; formation of bony buildup, Heberden's nodes
   B. Incidence
      1. Rheumatoid arthritis
         a. Women 3:1
         b. Between 25 and 35 years old
         c. Exacerbations increased by physical or emotional stress
      2. Osteoarthritis
         a. Increases with age; most over 55 years old
         b. Women greater incidence
   C. Predisposing/precipitating factors
      1. Rheumatoid arthritis: unknown, probably autoimmune in nature
      2. Osteoarthritis
         a. Joints of wear and tear
         b. Highly stressed joints
         c. Obesity
         d. Onset rare before 40
   D. Clinical manifestations
      1. Rheumatoid arthritis
         a. Redness and swelling of joints
         b. Deformity and displacement of proximal joints
         c. Pain on motion
         d. Underweight
         e. Anemia
         f. Chronic low-grade fever, slight leukocytosis
         g. Presence of rheumatoid factors
         h. Muscle atrophy
         i. Morning stiffness
      2. Osteoarthritis
         a. Pain and stiffness on movement
         b. Distal joint enlargement
         c. Presence of Heberden's nodes
         d. Symptoms aggravated by humidity and temperature changes
         e. Weightbearing joint involvement
         f. Localized, nonsystemic symptoms
         g. Morning pain and stiffness
         h. Grating sound on movement (crepitus)
   E. Diagnostic examinations
      1. CBC
      2. Rheumatoid factor (RA factor)
      3. Antinuclear antibody (ANA)
      4. Complements
      5. Erythrocyte sedimentation rate (ESR or sed rate)
      6. X-rays
      7. Bone scan
   F. Medical management (rheumatoid arthritis)
      1. Anti-inflammatories
         a. Nonsteroidals (Table 7–1)
         b. Steroids
         c. Cyclophosphamide (Cytoxan) or azathioprine (Imuran)—side effects: bone marrow depression, rashes, alopecia, hemorrhagic cystitis, immune suppression
      2. Remissive agents
         a. Gold—side effects: dermatitis, blood dyscrasias, nephropathy
         b. D-penicillamine—side effects: loss of taste, GI distress, pruritus, proteinuria
         c. Hydroxychloroquine (Plaquenil)—side effects: headaches, dizziness, GI distress, ocular toxicity, retinopathy
      3. Orthopedic splints during acute inflammation to prevent deformity
      4. Heat therapy
      5. Balanced rest and activity
   G. Medical management (osteoarthritis)
      1. Weight loss
      2. Decreased stress on affected joints
      3. Balance rest and activity
      4. Use of nonsteroidal anti-inflammatories for pain relief only
   H. Surgical management (both): total joint replacement
II. Analysis
   A. High risk for self-care deficits related to arthritic joint changes
   B. High risk for ineffective individual coping related to deformities and impaired mobility
   C. Knowledge deficit related to disease and treatments
   D. High risk for injury related to surgical procedure
III. Planning/goals, expected outcomes

TABLE 7–1 Drugs Used to Treat Musculoskeletal Disorders

Class	Example	Action	Use	Common Side Effects	Nursing Implications
Nonsteroidal anti-inflammatories	Ibuprofen (Motrin), indomethacin (Indocin)	Large group of drugs with anti-inflammatory, and often analgesic, properties; act to reduce symptoms of inflammation, such as redness, swelling, fever, and pain	To treat mild to moderate pain due to inflammatory conditions; symptomatic relief of arthritic conditions	GI irritation, ulcers, bleeding, dyspepsia, bone marrow depression, headache, dizziness, bowel changes, allergy	Take with food or antacid to decrease GI distress; monitor blood counts; watch for GI bleeding; monitor for aspirin allergy; do not administer aspirin or other anti-inflammatory
Skeletal muscle relaxants	Methocarbamol (Robaxin), baclofen (Lioresal)	Interfere with nerve impulses in muscle tissues; CNS depressants with sedative properties; act on spinal and supraspinal sites to decrease frequency and amplitude of muscle spasms	To treat acute painful muscle spasms, muscle tension, and pains associated with anxiety; to treat spastic disorders such as multiple sclerosis	Headache, lethargy, dizziness, nausea and vomiting, hypotension, blurred vision, hypersensitivity, hypotonia	Give with meals; avoid orthostatic changes; warn about drowsiness; warn urine may change color; avoid alcohol or other CNS depressants; use cautiously with elderly and patients with seizure disorders; withdraw drugs slowly

A. Client will maintain functional abilities as long as possible

B. Client will cope with diagnosis of chronic disease

C. Client will understand and comply with therapy

D. Client will recover from surgery without complications

IV. Implementations

   A. Balance rest and activity

   B. Exercise only to point of pain

   C. Apply heat and cold to control pain

   D. Administer medications as ordered, monitor for side effects

   E. Assist with discharge planning including need for home assistance

   F. Encourage well-balanced diet

   G. After total hip replacement

      1. Monitor immediately for shock and hemorrhage

      2. Keep leg widely abducted (four pillows) and prevent flexion or external or internal rotation

      3. Prevent infection, give prophylactic antibiotics

      4. Maintain bedrest 2 to 7 days as ordered

      5. Apply support hose, monitor for phlebitis

      6. Turn from back to unoperative side, maintaining four-pillow abduction

      7. Avoid wheelchairs or low chairs when out of bed

      8. Assess circulation, motion, and sensation of affected foot frequently

      9. Teach client home care

         a. Do not lie on operative side

         b. Do not adduct legs, including crossing legs, for 1 year

         c. Do not bend or flex hip more than 90 degrees for 1 year

         d. Use special riser on toilet seat

         e. Use aids for dressing to avoid bending

         f. Do not sit for long periods of time

         g. Exercise only as ordered

         h. Partial weightbearing for 3 months

   H. Total knee replacement

      1. Care similar to total hip replacement

      2. Use of continuous passive motion (CPM) device to exercise knee

         a. Begun 24 to 48 hours after surgery

         b. Administer analgesics before application to decrease pain

V. Evaluation

   A. Client remains functional

   B. Client copes with diagnosis of chronic disease

   C. Client understands and follows therapeutic regimen

   D. Client recovers from total joint surgery without complications

Gouty Arthritis

  I. Assessment

   A. Definition/pathophysiology: primary disorder

of purine metabolism leading to abnormal amounts of uric acid in body

B. Incidence
1. More common in men
2. Probably hereditary
C. Predisposing/precipitating factors
1. Intake of foods high in purine—organ meats, wines, aged cheeses
2. Low urine output of uric acid
D. Clinical manifestations
1. Arthritis in terminal joints of foot; i.e., big toe
2. Periodic episodes of acute joint pain, swelling, inflammation
3. Systemic symptoms of fever, headache, tachycardia, anorexia
4. May exhibit symptoms of renal stones if urine output low
E. Medical management
1. Antigout medications such as colchicine and allopurinol (Zyloprim) (Table 7–2)
2. Low purine diet
3. High fluid intake
4. Probenecid to increase excretion of uric acid
II. Analysis
A. Pain related to inflammation

B. Knowledge deficit related to diet and medications
III. Planning/goals, expected outcomes
A. Client will have pain controlled
B. Client will understand and comply with dietary restrictions
C. Client will understand and comply with medications
IV. Implementation
A. teach client low purine diet
B. Elevate affected extremity
C. Apply heat or cold as local treatments
D. Administer antigout agents as ordered
E. Teach client about medications
F. Increase fluid intake
V. Evaluations
A. Client recovers from acute attack without complications
B. Client follows dietary and medication regimen

Ruptured or Herniated Intervertebral Disk

I. Assessment
A. Definition/pathophysiology: protrusion of intervertebral disk outside of normal intervertebral space causing pressure on adjacent nerves and nerve roots
B. Incidence: more common in men

TABLE 7–2 Medications to Treat Gout

Example	Action	Use	Common Side Effects	Nursing Implications
Colchicine (Colsalide)	Reduces lactic acid production by leukocytes thereby decreasing uric acid deposition	Relief of pain and inflammation in acute gout	Nausea and vomiting, abdominal pain, diarrhea, hematuria	Warn client about signs of toxicity; discontinue drug when symptoms subside; never give subcutaneously or IM; take with food to reduce GI distress; monitor I & O; maintain high urine output
Probenecid (Benemid)	Reduces renal tubular reabsorption of urates, thereby increasing excretion of uric acid and lowering serum level of uric acid	To treat hyperuricemia associated with gout	GI irritation, rash, headache, increased symptoms of gout at first, diarrhea, frequency, hypersensitivity	Prolongs action of penicillins, cephalosporins, and other drugs; do not give aspirin concurrently; monitor urinary output; give with meals to decrease distress; maintain high fluid intake
Allopurinol (Zyloprim)	Reduces serum uric acid levels through competitive inhibition in the breakdown of purine	To prevent and treat gout or hyperuricemia	Hypersensitivity, diarrhea, GI distress	Warn client about rashes, which may indicate hypersensitivity; perform frequent blood counts; maintain high urine output; thiazide diuretics may interfere with absorption

C. Predisposing/precipitating factors
1. Poor body mechanics
2. Heavy lifting
3. Prolonged sitting, such as that done by long-distance truck drivers
4. Sudden strenuous exercise
5. Trauma

D. Clinical manifestations
1. 95% occur in lumbar spine
2. Pain in lower back radiating down back of leg to foot
3. Pain increases with walking, sneezing, coughing, or straining
4. Pain in arm and hand if cervical injury

E. Diagnostic examinations
1. Myelogram: radiopaque dye injected into spinal column to visualize patency of column
   a. Check for iodine allergy
   b. Client assumes side-lying knee–chest position for lumbar puncture
   c. Force fluids after test to decrease risk of spinal headache
   d. Keep client flat 6 to 12 hours after test to prevent headache
2. X-rays
3. Electromyograms
4. CT scan of spine

F. Medical management
1. Bedrest, firm mattress, semi-Fowler's position with knees slightly gatched (Williams' position)
2. Cervical or pelvic traction
3. Hot packs
4. Medication—muscle relaxants such as methocarbamol (Robaxin) (see Table 7–1)
5. Back braces
6. Special exercises after acute episode

G. Surgical management
1. Laminectomy: removal of portion of vertebra to decrease pressure
2. Spinal fusion: fusion of two or more vertebrae when multiple vertebrae are involved
3. Chemolysis: chymopapain injections to dissolve affected disk

II. Analysis
A. High risk for injury related to development of ruptured disk
B. Knowledge deficit related to prevention, diagnosis, and treatments

III. Planning/goals, expected outcomes
A. Client will not develop ruptured intervertebral disk
B. Client will recover without surgery
C. Client will be physically and psychologically prepared for surgery

D. Client will recover from surgery without complications
E. Client will understand and comply with therapeutic regimen and exercises to prevent recurrence

IV. Implementation
A. Maintain bedrest, client in semi-Fowler's position with knees slightly raised to decrease pressure on spine (Williams' position)
B. Administer medications and treatments as ordered
C. Postoperatively, after laminectomy
1. Log-roll client
2. Use fracture bedpan
3. Allow men to stand to void
4. Encourage client to avoid sitting
5. Prevent constipation
D. Postoperatively, after spinal fusion
1. Maintain complete bedrest
2. Prepare client for application of body cast
E. Teach client discharge care
F. Encourage client to follow exercises and other instructions
G. Teach client good body mechanics

V. Evaluation
A. Ruptured disk does not occur
B. Client recovers without surgery
C. Client recovers from surgery without complications
D. Client understands and follows therapeutic regimen

POST-TEST Musculoskeletal Disorders

Barbara Ryan is a 40-year-old woman with a 15-year history of rheumatoid arthritis.

1. Which of the following is a common clinical manifestation of rheumatoid arthritis?
   ① Presence of Heberden's nodes
   ② Manifestations aggravated by humidity
   ③ Deformity and displacement of proximal joints
   ④ Presence of crepitus over joints

2. Which of the following would NOT be a common laboratory finding in rheumatoid arthritis?
   ① Positive RA factor
   ② Low hemoglobin
   ③ Positive LE prep
   ④ Increased white blood count

3. Mrs. Ryan has been on steroids for about 5 years to control the symptoms of her arthritis. Which of the following is a common side effect of steroid therapy?
   1. Increased blood glucose
   2. Hyponatremia
   3. Hyperkalemia
   4. Protein anabolism

4. Which of the following diets is best suited to decrease the side effects of Mrs. Ryan's steroid therapy?
   1. High carbohydrate, low protein, low sodium
   2. Low carbohydrate, high protein, low potassium
   3. Normal carbohydrate, high protein, high potassium
   4. Low carbohydrate, high protein, high potassium

5. Prior to starting the steroids, Mrs. Ryan was on ibuprofen (Motrin). The main reason to have stopped the ibuprofen once the steroids were started was that:
   1. It was not needed with the steroids
   2. The two together increase the risk of GI bleeding
   3. The ibuprofen would interfere with the action of steroids
   4. The two together would cause severe liver damage

6. Mrs. Ryan tells you that she is going to quit taking her steroids because she just cannot live with the side effects anymore. Your best response to this would be:
   1. "You're right. The side effects can be very distressing. Let's talk about what's bothering you."
   2. "You can't stop taking your steroids. You'll die without them."
   3. "You must have the steroids to control your arthritis. Let's talk to the doctor about other options."
   4. "It is very important for you to take this medication. We can control all the side effects now."

7. Mrs. Ryan is admitted to the hospital for a total hip replacement. Her nursing care after the surgery should include:
   1. Keeping the legs abducted with one pillow
   2. Maintaining bedrest for 2 to 4 days
   3. Turning her from side to side every 4 hours
   4. Getting her up in a wheelchair the first day postoperatively

8. On the first day postoperatively, Mrs. Ryan is diaphoretic, her pulse is rapid, and her blood pressure is slightly lower than usual. There is no evidence of bleeding from her hip. Your best analysis of this situation is that she is:
   1. In severe pain
   2. Suffering from hypovolemic shock
   3. Slightly dehydrated from being NPO
   4. Experiencing Addisonian crisis

9. Your priority action for the above situation is to:
   1. Administer Demerol as ordered
   2. Increase the IV rate and prepare for transfusions
   3. Increase the amount of IV fluids and monitor output
   4. Administer IV hydrocortisone as ordered

10. Which of the following activities would be appropriate for Mrs. Ryan after discharge?
    1. Not lying on her operative side
    2. Sitting only in low chairs
    3. Resuming all normal ADLs as soon as possible
    4. Sitting at least 4 to 6 hours a day

11. The major cause of gout is:
    1. Obesity
    2. Impaired purine metabolism
    3. High urinary output of uric acid
    4. Autoimmune changes in the joints

12. Clinical manifestations that would lead the nurse to suspect the presence of gout include:
    1. Generalized arthritic changes
    2. High urine output
    3. Presence of uric acid renal stones
    4. Lack of systemic symptoms of inflammation

13. Probenecid is given to the client with gout to:
    1. Lower the level of purine in the blood
    2. Increase excretion of purines
    3. Increase the production of uric acid
    4. Increase the urinary excretion of uric acid

14. Important teaching for the client on colchicine (Colsalide) includes telling the client to:
    1. Take the drug with food to decrease GI distress
    2. Restrict fluids to increase the concentration of uric acid
    3. Avoid the use of aspirin at the same time
    4. Stop the drug if diarrhea occurs

POST-TEST Answers and Rationales

1. ③ The proximal joints are most affected in rheumatoid arthritis. All the other symptoms are of osteoarthritis. 2, II. Rheumatoid Arthritis.

2. ③ The LE prep is used to diagnose lupus. All the other options are laboratory tests that do diagnose rheumatoid arthritis, although the low hemoglobin and increased WBC are not specific to RA. 2, II. Rheumatoid Arthritis.

3. ① Gluconeogenesis occurs with steroids, raising the blood sugar. Hypernatremia, hypokalemia, and protein catabolism are other side effects of steroid therapy. 2, II. Steroids.

4. ④ Because steroids cause high blood sugar, protein catabolism, hypokalemia, and hypernatremia, the diet in choice 4 best meets all the client needs. The diets in the other options are inappropriate. 2, II. Steroids.

5. ② Steroids and nonsteroidal anti-inflammatories both cause GI bleeding and together increase the risk of it even more. None of the other options are correct. 2, II. Steroids.

6. ① This response acknowledges her concern and asks her to continue to talk to you. The other responses tend to cut off communication with either threats or false reassurances. 4, II & III. Steroids.

7. ② The client is kept in bed for about 2 to 4 days after a total hip replacement. The legs must be abducted with four pillows for 6 months to a year. The client should only be turned to the unaffected side with the legs kept in abduction. A wheelchair should not be used because it flexes the hip more than 90 degrees. 4, II. Total Hip Replacement.

8. ④ Addisonian crisis occurs when the level of steroids drops because of the stress of surgery. Because the client is steroid-dependent, she is unable to respond to the stress by secreting more hormone. There are no data that any of the other options could be correct. 2, II. Steroids.

9. ④ The only treatment for Addisonian crisis is an increase in steroid hormones. Because she is post op, the best form is IV hydrocortisone. It should reverse the symptoms quickly. 4, II. Steroids.

10. ① In order to prevent dislocation, the client must not flex the hip more than 90 degrees, adduct the leg, or allow internal or external rotation. She must not lie on the operative side, sit in low chairs, or sit excessively. Resuming all ADLs must be done with care and only in ways that prevent excessive hip flexion. ADL assistive devices must be used. 4, I. Total Hip Replacement.

11. ② Faulty metabolism of purine is the cause of gout. When this faulty metabolism occurs, abnormally high amounts of uric acid accumulate in the blood. Although obesity is often associated with it, it is not the cause. The other options are incorrect. 2, II. Gout.

12. ③ Because there are abnormally high amounts of uric acid in the blood, the levels in the urine increase. If urine output is inadequate, stones will occur. Arthritic changes are usually limited but the symptoms of inflammation can be systemic. 2, II. Gout.

13. ④ Probenecid increases the urinary excretion of uric acid to prevent the buildup of it in joints. It does not affect purines, nor the production of uric acid directly. 2, II. Gout.

14. ① Colchicine causes GI irritation. Taking it with food helps to decrease this side effect. The client should increase fluid intake, because diarrhea is a common effect of colchicine. Aspirin does not interact with colchicine. 4, II. Gout.

BIBLIOGRAPHY

MUSCULOSKELETAL DISORDERS

Bird, A. et al. (1985). *Combined care of the rheumatic patient.* New York: Springer.

Black, J., and Matassarin-Jacobs, E., eds. (1993). *Luckmann and Sorensen's medical surgical nursing: A psychophysiologic approach.* Philadelphia: W. B. Saunders.

Harper, C. A. (1985). Initial assessment and management of femoral neck fractures in the elderly. *Orthopedic Nursing* 4: 55–58.

Lewis, S. M., and Collier, I. C. (1987). *Medical-surgical nursing:*

Assessment and management of clinical problems, 2nd ed. New York: McGraw-Hill.

Phipps, W. J., Long, B. C., and Woods, N. F. (1991). *Medical-surgical nursing: Concepts for clinical practice,* 4th ed. St. Louis: C. V. Mosby.

Pigg, J. S., Driscoll, P. W., and Caniff, R. (1985). *Rheumatology nursing: A problem oriented approach.* New York: John Wiley.

Tompkins, J. S., and Brown, M. D. (1985). Dissolving a lifetime of lower back pain with chemonucleolysis. *Nursing 85* 15: 48

8

Metabolism and Elimination in the Adult Client

PRE-TEST Endocrine Disorders

Mrs. Ortega, a 54-year-old housewife, has been diagnosed as having acromegaly. She is scheduled for a hypophysectomy to remove the pituitary gland.

1. You observe Mrs. Ortega and note that she is evidencing which of the following clinical manifestations of acromegaly?
   ① Polyuria and intense thirst
   ② Hypotension and bradycardia
   ③ Coarse facial features and headache
   ④ Blindness and weight loss

2. Mrs. Ortega has returned to the unit, after having had her hypophysectomy. A priority nursing implementation will be to prevent increasing intracranial pressure by:
   ① Maintaining the head of the bed in a flat position
   ② Keeping the client overhydrated
   ③ Giving dexamethasone (Decadron) as prescribed
   ④ Encouraging ambulation

3. Mrs. Miller is attending an endocrine clinic for treatment of her hyperthyroidism. As her nurse, you will teach her about her health regimen, which includes:
   ① A diet with reduced calories
   ② A cool, quiet environment
   ③ A warm, stimulating environment
   ④ Long-term iodine therapy

4. Mr. Jackson has undergone tests which indicate that he has a deficiency of parathormone secretion. Potential complications that Mr. Jackson should be informed about include:
   ① Osteoporosis
   ② Lethargy
   ③ Laryngeal spasms
   ④ Kidney stones

Mrs. Carter is depressed about the changes in her personal appearance that are related to Cushing's disease. Some of these changes may be reversed by surgery.

5. Mrs. Carter is particularly likely to exhibit which of the following changes?
   ① Weight gain, moon facies, and increased facial hair

   ② Hand tremors and nervousness
   ③ Retracted eyelids and increased skin pigmentation
   ④ Muscle atrophy, bruising, and weight loss

6. When teaching Mrs. Carter about her diet, you will describe a diet that is:
   ① High carbohydrate, high protein, high potassium, and high sodium
   ② Low carbohydrate, low protein, low potassium, and low sodium
   ③ High carbohydrate, low protein, low potassium, and high sodium
   ④ Low carbohydrate, high protein, high potassium, and low sodium

Mr. Brown is a 30-year-old diabetic. He is insulin-dependent and under medical supervision.

7. When testing his FBS level with a self-monitoring fingerstick procedure, Mr. Brown will know that serum glucose, in an FBS test, normally falls into the following range:
   ① 30–50 mg/100 mL
   ② 40–80 mg/100 mL
   ③ 80–110 mg/100 mL
   ④ 110–140 mg/100 mL

8. If Mr. Brown takes an injection of NPH insulin at 7:30 a.m., when should he watch for a hypoglycemic reaction?
   ① After breakfast
   ② Before lunch
   ③ Before supper
   ④ At 6:00 a.m. the following day

9. Mr. Brown is admitted to the hospital after missing a scheduled insulin injection and going into diabetic ketoacidosis. He was not eating a full diet, due to the flu. His nurse is especially careful to monitor Mr. Brown for:
   ① High plasma pH level, caused by acidosis
   ② Potassium imbalance, which may affect the heart
   ③ Pulmonary edema
   ④ Circulatory congestion

10. An appropriate nursing implementation as soon as Mr. Brown is admitted into the hospital with ketoacidosis is to:
    ① Obtain blood glucose specimens
    ② Administer NPH insulin intravenously
    ③ Give intravenous glucagon
    ④ Take vital signs every 4 hours

PRE-TEST Answers and Rationales

1. ③ Acromegaly is caused by a tumor, which increases the secretion of hormones. A growth hormone enlarges facial features and the tumor pressure causes a headache. 1, II. Hyperpituitary.

2. ③ Giving steroids helps to prevent increasing intracranial pressure, by decreasing cerebral inflammation. 4, II. Pituitary.

3. ② Because she is nervous and sensitive to heat, teaching her to maintain a cool, quiet environment will make her more comfortable. 3, I & IV. Hyperthyroid.

4. ③ A deficiency in parathormone leads to a decrease in serum calcium, which can cause tetany and laryngeal spasm. 2, I & II. Hypoparathyroid.

5. ① An increase in adrenocorticoids causes the side effects of the body changes listed. 1, II. Cushing's Disease.

6. ④ An increase in adrenocorticoids causes weight gain, sodium retention, and potassium excretion. The diet recommended will help balance these side effects. 3, II. Cushing's Disease.

7. ③ This range is normal for a FBS serum glucose level. 1, II. Diabetes mellitus.

8. ③ NPH is intermediate-acting insulin, so before supper would be a likely time for a hypoglycemic reaction. 1, II. Diabetes Mellitus.

9. ② In serum acidosis, H^+ ions enter the intracellular fluid to be replaced by K^+ ions. When the acidosis is corrected the process reverses itself. Both hypokalemia and hyperkalemia cause cardiac arrhythmias. 1, II. Diabetes Mellitus.

10. ① Information about glucose level is needed to determine the amount of insulin needed. Vital signs would be the next priority. 4, II. Diabetes Mellitus.

NORMAL FUNCTION OF THE ENDOCRINE SYSTEM

I. Overview
  A. Endocrine glands promote homeostasis by means of regulating:
    1. Response to stress and injury
    2. Growth and development
    3. Reproduction
    4. Ionic homeostasis
    5. Energy metabolism
  B. Endocrine glands secrete hormones directly into bloodstream to act on target tissues; these hormones may also have general effect on tissues throughout body; endocrine and autonomic nervous systems work in harmony; autonomic nervous system functions through electrical stimuli to achieve fast action of short duration, endocrine system functions through minute amounts of powerful hormones to achieve a slower action of long duration
  C. Feedback relationships are important in endocrine system functioning
    1. Low level of blood glucose does not stimulate pancreatic secretion of insulin (negative feedback)
    2. Low level of serum calcium stimulates parathyroid secretion of parathormone (positive feedback)
  D. Diseases result when feedback relationships do not work; hypofunction may require lifelong hormone replacement; hyperfunction may require surgery, radiation, or drug therapy (Table 8–1)
  E. Physiologic changes with aging
    1. Endocrine dysfunction secondary to cellular damage due to aging, wearing on endocrine tissue from long-term use, genetically influenced changes
    2. Most common dysfunctions
      a. Decrease in ovarian functioning
      b. Impaired secretion of hypothalamic hormones
      c. Decrease in prolactin
      d. Decrease in growth hormone (GH)
      e. Increase in antidiuretic hormone (ADH) and normal aging of kidneys: hyponatremia and nocturia
      f. Thyroid gland:
        (1) Decreased T_4 secretion and metabolism
        (2) Decreased T_3 levels
        (3) Increased thyroid-stimulating hormone (TSH) levels
        (4) Decreased responsiveness in TSH secretion to thyrotropin-releasing hormone (TRH)
      g. Decreased cortisol secretion from adrenal glands
      h. Impaired glucose tolerance may result in

TABLE 8–1 Endocrine Glands, Hormones, and Their Functions

Gland	Location	Hormone	Function
Hypothalamus	Floor of third ventricle of brain	Antidiuretic hormone	Decreases production of urine (stored and released by posterior pituitary)
		Inhibiting and releasing hormones	Inhibit or stimulate pituitary secretions
Anterior pituitary	Sella turcica of brain	Growth hormone (GH)/somatotropin	Stimulates growth of bones and tissues
		Thyrotropin (TSH)	Stimulates thyroid growth and secretion
		Adrenocorticotropin (ACTH)	Stimulates adrenal cortex
		Melanocyte-stimulating hormone (MSH)	Stimulates skin pigmentation
		Prolactin (LTH)	Stimulates mammary gland lactation, maintains corpus luteum
		Follicle-stimulating hormone (FSH)	Stimulates growth of follicle, estrogen, and spermatogenesis
		Luteinizing (LH) or interstitial cell-stimulating hormone (ICSH)	Stimulates ovulation, luteinization in women, or production of testosterone in men
Posterior pituitary	Sella turcica of brain	ADH (vasopressin)	See hypothalamus above
		Oxytocin	Contracts uterus and aids in expression of milk
Thyroid	Upper part of trachea	Thyroxine (T4)	Stimulates metabolism
		Triiodothyronine (T3)	Stimulates metabolism
		Thyrocalcitonin	Lowers serum calcium level
Parathyroid	Four small glands in thyroid	Parathormone (PTH)	Raises serum calcium level
Adrenal cortex	On top of upper pole of each kidney	Glucocorticoid (cortisol)	Anti-inflammatory, protects during stress
		Mineralcorticoid (aldosterone)	Retains sodium and water, eliminates potassium
		Sex hormones (androgens)	Development of secondary sex characteristics
Adrenal medulla	On top of upper pole of each kidney	Epinephrine	Stimulates "fight or flight" stress response, increases heart rate, dilates bronchi
		Norepinephrine*	Increases peripheral vasoconstriction, elevates blood pressure
Pancreatic islet cells:	Close to duodenum and spleen	Insulin	Stimulate use of carbohydrates
Alpha cells		Somatostatin	Inhibit growth hormone and glucagon
Beta cells		Glucagon	Elevate blood glucose level
Testes	Scrotum	Testosterone	Stimulate development of male sex characteristics and reproductive function
Ovaries	Below uterine tubes	Estrogen	Stimulate development of female sex characteristics and growth of graafian follicle
		Progesterone	Maintains pregnancy
Pineal	Midbrain	Melatonin	? Initiates sexual maturation

* Norepinephrine is present in the blood, but in very minute amounts, so it may be more accurately referred to as a neurotransmitter for the sympathetic nervous system in the adrenal medulla and elsewhere, with a demonstrated local mode of action.

blood glucose values that are slightly higher than normal
  i. Non–insulin-dependent diabetes (NIDDM)

NURSING PROCESS APPLIED TO ADULTS WITH ENDOCRINE DISORDERS

Hypofunction of the Pituitary

I. Assessment
  A. Definition: hyposecretion of anterior pituitary hormones, which normally affect the thyroid, adrenals, and gonads (Simmonds' disease), and of posterior pituitary hormones, oxytocin, and antidiuretic hormone (ADH) (diabetes insipidus)
  B. Etiology
    1. Head trauma
    2. Ischemia
    3. Tumor
    4. Hypothalamic dysfunction
    5. Radiation
    6. Surgery
    7. Drug therapy
  C. Predisposing/precipitating factors
    1. Postpartum hemorrhage or shock (Sheehan's syndrome)
    2. Post-hypophysectomy
  D. Clinical manifestations
    1. Anterior pituitary hormone deficiencies
      a. Impaired growth
        (1) Children: dwarfism
      b. Weight loss (GH)
      c. Lethargy, increased sensitivity to cold (TSH)
      d. Decreased resistance to stress, circulatory collapse, hypoglycemia (ACTH)
      e. Decreased body hair, impaired sexual development (gonadotropins)
      f. Pale skin color in absence of melanocyte stimulating hormone (MSH)
      g. Cessation of menstrual periods, amenorrhea with a deficit of luteinizing hormone (LH)
    2. Posterior pituitary hormone deficiencies
      a. Diminished contraction of smooth muscle of uterus (oxytocin)
      b. Polyuria, polydipsia (ADH); known as diabetes insipidus
  E. Diagnostic examinations
    1. Reduced amounts of hormones present in blood and urine
    2. Water deprivation/ADH test, specific gravity urine low, 1.001 to 1.005
    3. CT scan of sella turcica
    4. MRI of sella turcica

  F. Complications
    1. Coma
    2. Death
  G. Medical management
    1. General: replacement of deficient hormones
    2. Acromegaly/gigantism: possibly pituitary irradiation (with or without surgery)
  H. Surgical management—acromegaly/gigantism: resection of pituitary tumor (hypophysectomy), with or without radiation
II. Analysis
  A. Knowledge deficit related to disease, procedures, treatment, new disease, and new information
  B. Sensory/perceptual alteration: visual related to tumor in cranium causing pressure on CN III, IV, or VI, or optic chiasm
  C. Ineffective individual coping related to uncertainty about cause of problem
III. Planning/goals, expected outcomes
  A. Client will be able to discuss disease, procedures, treatment about hormone deficiency
  B. Client will not suffer any injuries related to visual impairment
  C. Coping will improve as evidenced by the client listing coping strategies helpful in dealing with pertinent stressors
IV. Implementation
  A. Explain to client importance of complying with lifelong hormone replacement therapy under medical supervision
  B. Discuss with client purpose, administration, and side effects of medications—for example, ADH (Pitressin tannate)
  C. Advise client to wear a Medic Alert tag
  D. Instruct client on how to monitor for dehydration or fluid volume excess
    1. Maintain intake and output record
    2. Daily weight
    3. Urine specific gravity
    4. Condition of mucous membranes
V. Evaluation
  A. Client is able to effectively discuss hormone deficiency
  B. Client did not have any injuries
  C. Client states new coping strategies are effective

Hyperfunction of the Pituitary

I. Assessment
  A. Definition/pathophysiology: oversecretion of pituitary hormones, usually due to tumor
    1. Anterior pituitary: long-lasting stimulation by growth hormone affects skeletal growth in adult by enlarging certain bones and tissues (acromegaly)

2. Posterior pituitary: tumor causes syndrome of inappropriate secretion of antidiuretic hormone (SIADH)

B. Etiology
1. Pituitary adenoma, more often of anterior than posterior pituitary
2. Drug therapy
3. Secondary to hypothalamic dysfunction

C. Predisposing/precipitating factors: SIADH—stress of surgery, hyponatremia, malignant pulmonary neoplasms, CNS disorders (tumors, infection, trauma), adrenal insufficiency, anterior pituitary insufficiency, drugs

D. Clinical manifestations
1. Anterior pituitary
  a. Coarse facial features, enlarged hands and feet—acromegaly (GH)
  b. Increased intracranial pressure, due to tumor, and headache and blindness
  c. Obesity, muscular wasting, weakness, slow movements, lethargy, hypertension, hyperglycemia, glycosuria, Cushing's disease (ACTH)
  d. Tachycardia, nervousness (TSH)
  e. Amenorrhea (prolactin)
  f. Virilization of women (increased gonadotropin)
2. Posterior pituitary
  a. Water intoxication, edema—SIADH
  b. Client may develop emotional problems due to changes in body image

E. Diagnostic examinations
1. Serum levels of growth hormone and other hormones will increase
2. Increases in the basal metabolic rate (BMR), blood sugar level, glucose tolerance test (GTT), and serum calcium level
3. Weight gain
4. Decrease in urine output
5. X-rays show changes in jaw, skull, long bones
6. CT scan of sella turcica
7. MRI of sella turcica to demonstrate adenomas
8. Increase in urinary sodium and osmolality; decrease in serum sodium and osmolality (SIADH)

F. Complications
1. Acromegaly
2. Cushing's disease
3. Hyperthyroidism
4. SIADH
5. Hypophysectomy with potential problems postoperatively

G. Medical management
1. Radiation: with or without surgery
2. Pharmacological agents: bromocriptine (Parlodel) to decrease prolactin levels and GH; octreotide (Sandostatin) to decrease GH and manifestations of acromegaly; demeclocycline to block action of ADH on renal tubule and collecting ducts
3. Fluid and electrolyte balance (SIADH)

H. Surgical management: surgical resection—transsphenoidal hypophysectomy

II. Analysis
(for clients with pituitary tumors):
A. Anxiety related to uncertainty about cause of problem and outcome of treatment
B. Knowledge deficit of disorder and treatment related to new diagnoses and new treatment
C. Pain related to headache from intracranial mass
(for clients with prolactin-secreting tumor):
D. Sexual dysfunction related to alteration in menstrual cycle, decreased libido
(for clients with GH secreting tumor):
E. Pain related to pressure on nerves associated with changes in joints and vertebrae associated with abnormal bone growth
(for clients with post-pituitary tumor):
F. Fluid volume deficit related to inadequate amounts of ADH

III. Planning/goals, expected outcomes
A. Client will state less anxiety as client becomes more familiar with causes and treatment responses
B. Client will relate to nurse information learned about diagnoses and treatment
C. Client will state decrease in headaches
D. Client will state improved sexual functions as hormone levels increase
E. Client will state relief of pain
F. Client with SIADH will maintain fluid and electrolyte balance within normal limits

IV. Implementation
A. Discuss alterations in body image
B. Monitor hypophysectomy client postoperatively for signs of infection and hemorrhage, alteration in level of consciousness, hypotension, tachycardia, shock, and diabetes insipidus
C. Monitor transsphenoidal hypophysectomy client postoperatively for nasal leakage of cerebrospinal fluid (glucose positive)
  1. Dipstick for presence of glucose
  2. Look for dark halo around fluid on white dressing
D. Teach client about importance of lifelong medical supervision
E. Teach client about purpose, administration, and side effects of medications
F. Teach client with SIADH to maintain prescribed fluid restriction of under 1000 mL per day and to maintain urine output and weight within normal limits

G. Discuss with client and family changes in sexual function

V. Evaluation

A. Client relates less anxiety

B. Client effectively relates information learned on diagnoses and treatment

C. Client has fewer headaches

D. Client states menstruation and libido are satisfactory

E. Client has relief of pain

F. Client did not develop fluid volume deficit

Hypofunction of the Thyroid

I. Assessment

A. Definition: decreased secretion of thyroid hormones, which may lead to myxedema in adults

B. Etiology

1. Anterior pituitary TSH deficiency
2. Thyroidectomy
3. Radioactive iodine
4. Antithyroid drugs
5. Thyroiditis (autoimmune)

C. Predisposing/precipitating factors

1. Hypothalamic dysfunction inhibiting pituitary
2. Lack of iodine
3. Ingestion of foods, such as cabbage, which inhibit hormone production and lead to compensatory gland enlargement, goiter
4. Age: very underdiagnosed in elderly

D. Clinical manifestations

1. Slow onset of hypothyroidism
   a. Lethargy, fatigue, diminished intellect
   b. Arteriosclerosis, decreased BMR, temperature, pulse, cardiac output, increased intolerance to cold
   c. Facial expression mask-like, dry hair, thickened skin, enlarged tongue, and drooling
   d. Binding water as mucinous edema, constipation, pleural effusion, weight gain
   e. Intolerance of sedatives
2. Myxedema coma: represents the most severe form of hypothyroidism; usually seen in untreated clients with a progressive history of hypothyroidism
   a. Precipitating factors
      (1) Undiagnosed hypothyroidism
      (2) Drugs: sedatives and narcotics
      (3) Exposure to cold
      (4) Surgery
      (5) Infections
   b. Clinical manifestations
      (1) Same as hypothyroidism
      (2) Coma
      (3) Severe hypothermia

(4) Dilutional hyponatremia
   c. Medical management includes supportive care, treatment of underlying cause, and thyroid hormone replacement

E. Diagnostic examinations

1. Decreased serum and urine levels of hormones such as TSH if pituitary problem, thyroid hormones
2. Radioactive iodine uptake (RAIU)
3. BMR
4. Serum protein-bound iodine (PBI) tests
5. Thyroid scan
6. Thyroid ultrasound
7. Thyroid suppression test

F. Complications

1. If thyroid hormone replaced, levothyroxine (Synthroid) given to speed up metabolism; this can lead to angina and heart failure when client has arteriosclerosis
2. Myxedema clients given tranquilizers can go into a coma and die

G. Medical management: pharmacological—thyroid hormone replacement (levothyroxine [Synthroid], liothyronine [Cytomel], thyroid extract) (Table 8–2)

II. Analysis

A. Activity intolerance related to fatigue and muscle weakness, decreased cardiac function

B. Constipation related to decreased peristalsis

C. Body-image disturbance related to weight gain, puffiness, enlarged tongue

D. Hypothermia related to diminished heat production secondary to depressed metabolism

E. Altered nutrition: more than body requirements related to decreased metabolic rate

III. Planning/goals, expected outcomes

A. Client will demonstrate an increase in activity tolerance after therapy has begun

B. Client will return to usual bowel habits after therapy has begun

C. Client will relate causes of physical changes and relate that most changes will reverse with thyroid replacement

D. Client will maintain a normal body temperature

IV. Implementations

A. Teach client to maintain lifelong medical supervision

B. Provide information about purpose, administration, and side effects of medication

1. Avoid sedatives that can cause coma
2. Instruct client to hold thyroid replacement medication and call physician if pulse over 100 beats per minute, or as instructed; be aware of potential reactions with other medications; report angina or shortness of breath

TABLE 8–2 Drugs Used to Treat Thyroid Disorders

Class	Example	Action	Use	Common Side Effects	Nursing Implications
Antithyroid agents	Propylthiouracil (PTU)	Interfere with the uptake of iodine and block the synthesis of thyroxine (T4) and triiodothyronine (T3); do not interfere with release and utilization of stored thyroid; takes days or weeks for effect to be seen; hormone reduction leads to increased TSH, which leads to hyperplasia and increased vascularity of gland; euthyroidism occurs in 6 to 12 weeks	To establish euthyroidism preoperatively and for palliative care of toxic goiter	Nausea and vomiting, diarrhea, loss of taste, skin changes, headache, dizziness, drowsiness, lymphadenopathy, hypersensitivity, agranulocytosis, hypothyroidism	Monitor blood counts; should not be used in the last trimester of pregnancy or during lactation; report any symptoms of infection; urge continued compliance since response slow
	Saturated solution of potassium iodide (SSKI)	Inhibits the secretion of thyroid hormones in thyroid hyperplasia temporarily; effect lasts only 10 to 14 days; during this time, it shrinks the gland and decreases vascularity	To decrease size and vascularity of gland preoperatively	Diarrhea, nausea and vomiting, stomach pain, hypothyroidism, hypersensitivity, iodine poisoning, irregular heartbeat, productive cough	Use with caution in patients with TB, hyperkalemia, acute bronchitis, impaired renal function, or cardiac disease; safety not established in pregnancy, lactation, or childhood; give after meals with fruit juice; monitor potassium level; avoid sudden withdrawal; keep in light-protected bottle; ensure preoperative compliance
Thyroid hormones	Levothyroxine sodium T4 (Synthroid)	Synthetic thyroid preparation of controlled potency; contains T4, which is converted to T3; acts as a replacement for thyroid hormone	To treat hypothyroidism	Rare, hyperthyroidism, tremors, hunger, weight loss	Use with caution in patients with acute MIs, hypertension, renal insufficiency, diabetes, and in elderly or pregnant patients; give a single dose in morning; watch for adverse effects early in treatment; monitor for improvement of symptoms

C. Advise client to avoid outdoor activity in cold weather
D. Discuss diet with adequate fluids and roughage to avoid constipation
E. Encourage more activity to facilitate alertness
V. Evaluation
A. Client demonstrates an increase in activity tolerance
B. Client states that bowel movements have returned to usual pattern

C. Client able to discuss body changes and expects most to reverse
D. Client states that he is comfortable
E. Client's weight is decreasing since therapy has begun

Hyperfunction of the Thyroid

I. Assessment
A. Definition: increase in secretion of thyroid

hormones, which leads to an increase in the metabolic rate of the body

   B. Etiology
      1. Increased TSH from pituitary
      2. Thyroid tumors, benign and malignant
      3. Stress
      4. Graves' disease
      5. Autoimmune factors
   C. Predisposing/precipitating factors
      1. Excess thyroid therapy
      2. Immunoglobulins
      3. Viral infection
   D. Clinical manifestations
      1. Tachycardia, increased systolic BP, increased respirations, dyspnea, increased cardiac output, fatigue, goiter
      2. Nervousness, tremor of hands, emotional lability, insomnia, shortened attention span
      3. Intolerance to heat, profuse perspiration, warm moist skin
      4. Polyphagia, weight loss, increased bowel movements
      5. Retraction of eyelids, exophthalmos
      6. Enlarged thyroid; may feel thyroid "thrill"; auscultate "bruit"
   E. Diagnostic examinations
      1. Same as for hypothyroid, except will show an increase instead of a decrease in hormone levels
      2. Hyperglycemia in GTT
      3. Glycosuria and creatinuria in urine test
   F. Complications
      1. Thyroid storm with severe exacerbation of symptoms of hyperfunction listed above, fever, delirium and coma
      2. Congestive heart failure
      3. Blindness from exophthalmos
      4. Hypoparathyroidism as postoperative complication
   G. Medical management (see Table 8–2)
      1. Radioactive iodine (^{131}I)
      2. Antithyroid drugs; propylthiouracil (PTU), methimazole (Tapazole) to block thyroid hormone synthesis
      3. Iodines: Lugol's solution to block release and synthesis of thyroid hormone
      4. Symptomatic relief for tachycardia, anxiety, etc.
   H. Surgical management: partial or total thyroidectomy

II. Analysis
   A. Altered nutrition: less than body requirements related to increased basal metabolic rate and increased needs
   B. Ineffective individual coping, related to anxiety, emotional lability, excitability, decreased attention span
   C. Knowledge deficit related to new diagnosis
   D. Hyperthermia related to increased heat production from hypermetabolism
   E. Activity intolerance related to fatigued muscles and wasting associated with increased metabolism

III. Planning/goals, expected outcomes
   A. Client will show an increase in weight after dietary intervention has begun
   B. Client will relate and demonstrate improved coping skills
   C. Client will relate the disease process, physical changes, and therapy to the nurse
   D. Client will have a normal body temperature
   E. Client will state an increase in activity tolerance after therapy has been initiated

IV. Implementations
   A. Maintain cool, quiet environment and limit visitors
   B. Provide diet with increased calories (4000), vitamins, carbohydrates, proteins, with supplementary feedings between meals or at bedtime
   C. Teach client purpose, administration, and side effects of medication prescribed—for example, eyedrops for protection if exophthalmos present; Lugol's solution (iodine) given preoperatively to decrease the size and vascularity of the thyroid; digitalis or propranolol for cardiovascular problems
   D. Explain to client importance of lifelong adherence to health regimen, as prescribed by physician
   E. After thyroidectomy, monitor client
      1. Respiratory distress, laryngeal nerve damage, difficulty in speech or swallowing
      2. Hemorrhage; check back of dressing as well as front
      3. Tetany, laryngeal spasm, and muscle twitching due to accidental removal of parathyroids
      4. Thyroid storm or hypothyroidism
      5. Correct positioning; elevate head of bed and do not hyperextend neck

V. Evaluation
   A. Client's weight is increasing
   B. Client effectively uses new coping skills
   C. Client is knowledgeable about the disease process, physical changes, and therapy of hyperthyroidism
   D. Client's body temperature is within normal ranges
   E. Client is able to tolerate an increase in activity since therapy has begun

Hypofunction of the Parathyroid

I. Assessment
  A. Definition: decreased secretion of parathyroid hormones
  B. Etiology
    1. Parathyroidectomy
    2. Postoperative thyroidectomy or radical neck dissection
    3. Idiopathic
  C. Predisposing/precipitating factors
    1. X-ray to neck
    2. Autoimmune factors
    3. Serum alkalosis, which makes symptoms worse because amount of ionized calcium drops
  D. Clinical manifestations
    1. Tetany
      a. Involuntary jerky spasms, circumoral tingling and numbness, muscle cramps
      b. Positive Trousseau's sign: carpopedal spasm when blood flow to arm reduced using a BP cuff for 3 minutes
      c. Chvostek's sign: contraction of facial muscle when angle of jaw tapped
      d. Wheezing
      e. Dyspnea
      f. Laryngeal spasm
      g. Convulsions
    2. Cardiac arrhythmias, prolonged Q-T interval
    3. Calcification cataracts, photophobia, diplopia
    4. Dental abnormalities—depending on age at onset
  E. Diagnostic examinations
    1. Decreased serum calcium
    2. Increased serum phosphate
    3. X-ray shows increased bone density
    4. Low, undetectable levels of PTH
  F. Complications
    1. Cardiac arrhythmias
    2. Cataracts
    3. Tetany
    4. Seizures
    5. Complications of therapy: vitamin D toxicity and renal calculi formation
  G. Medical management
    1. Calcium replacement
    2. Vitamin D supplement
    3. Treat the cause of hypoparathyroidism
    4. Supportive treatment for symptoms until serum calcium within normal range
II. Analysis
  A. Anxiety related to emotional lability and confusion secondary to hypocalcemia

  B. Ineffective breathing patterns related to stridor and laryngeal spasms
  C. Decreased cardiac output related to increased electrical excitability secondary to hypocalcemia
  D. Pain related to muscle spasms and tingling of fingers associated with hypocalcemia
III. Planning/goals, expected outcomes
  A. Client will be less anxious as therapy is initiated
  B. Client's airway will be maintained
  C. Client will not experience any cardiac compromise
  D. Client will state decrease or absence of pain
IV. Implementations
  A. Give calcium gluconate orally or, if emergency, IV for signs and symptoms of tetany
  B. Provide information to client about medication and diet regimen
  C. Teach client about high-calcium, high-vitamin D, low-phosphate diet; will have to limit milk, cheese, and egg yolks because of high phosphate along with calcium
  D. Provide calm, quiet environment; if seizures occur, give sedative such as chloral hydrate
  E. Place on cardiac monitor
  F. Monitor serum calcium and phosphate levels; may need parathormone (PTH) injections in an emergency, but it often causes allergic reactions
  G. Have emergency equipment ready for tracheostomy if laryngeal spasm causes respiratory distress
  H. Monitor client for 4 days post-thyroidectomy to ascertain if tetany occurs; if parathyroid function not regained in 3 weeks, then is probably permanently decreased
V. Evaluation
  A. Client states he or she is less anxious
  B. Client did not experience ineffective airway
  C. Client experienced stable cardiac performance
  D. Client states pain is decreased

Hyperfunction of the Parathyroid

I. Assessment
  A. Definition: oversecretion of parathyroid hormone, parathormone
  B. Etiology
    1. Primary hyperparathyroidism occurs because of tumor development that interrupts PTH secretion
    2. Secondary hyperparathyroidism occurs in renal failure patients and "renal rickets" secondary to phosphorus retention, in-

creased stimulation of parathyroid glands, and increased PTH secretion
  C. Predisposing/precipitating factors
    1. Hypocalcemia due to lack of vitamin D
    2. Calcium deficiency in diet
    3. Kidney disease
  D. Clinical manifestations
    1. Fatigue, weakness, bone pain, fractures
    2. Kidney stones, renal pain, pyelonephritis, polyuria, polydipsia
    3. Anorexia, nausea, vomiting, constipation
    4. Cardiac arrhythmias
    5. Increased incidence of peptic ulcer disease and pancreatitis
  E. Diagnostic examinations
    1. Increased serum calcium
    2. Decreased serum phosphate
    3. Increased PTH level in blood
    4. X-rays reveal bone demineralization
  F. Complications
    1. Cardiac arrhythmias
    2. Fractures
    3. Kidney stones
    4. Digitalis toxicity
  G. Medical management
    1. Pharmacological: IV fluids to promote calcium excretion; phosphate therapy to correct hypophosphatemia and decrease calcium levels by promoting calcium deposit in bone. Plicamycin (Mithracin) is a cytotoxic agent used to decrease hypercalcemia; its mechanism of action is unknown. Cytotoxic agents and dialysis may be used in hypercalcemia emergency.
    2. Low-calcium diet
  H. Surgical management
    1. Partial parathyroidectomy: usually only the diseased glands are removed. If four glands are hyperplastic, $3\frac{1}{2}$ glands are removed. One half gland can maintain normal PTH levels.
II. Analysis
  A. Injury potential related to demineralization of bones resulting in pathologic fractures
  B. Pain related to pathologic bone changes or renal calculi
  C. Altered urinary elimination patterns related to renal involvement secondary to hypercalcemia and hyperphosphaturia
  D. Alteration in bowel elimination: constipation related to adverse effects of hypercalcemia on GI tract
III. Planning/goals, expected outcomes
  A. Client will be free from bone injury
  B. Client will state a decrease or absence of pain
  C. Client will have normal urinary output each shift

  D. Client will have bowel movements three to four times per week
IV. Implementation
  A. Teach client importance of following prescribed diet and medication regimen
    1. Follow a low-calcium diet preoperatively, avoiding milk (too low calcium intake in the presence of a high parathormone level can worsen bone resorption)
    2. High calcium intake postoperatively if insufficient parathyroid tissue left undamaged
  B. Monitor renal function
    1. Encourage high fluid intake (3000 mL per day) and cranberry juice intake to decrease urinary pH
    2. Strain urine for stones
    3. Monitor for hematuria or pain
  C. Encourage ambulation to prevent bone resorption
  D. Prevent falls to avoid fractures of weakened bones
  E. Prevent constipation and fecal impaction with ambulation, fluids, stool softeners, laxatives
  F. Administer nursing care postparathyroidectomy, using guidelines for thyroidectomy and paying particular attention to monitoring for tetany as described under hypoparathyroidism signs and symptoms
V. Evaluation
  A. Client did not sustain any bone injury
  B. Client states he or she is pain-free
  C. Client had normal urinary output
  D. Client is able to move bowels three to four times per week

Hypofunction of the Adrenals

I. Assessment
  A. Definition/pathophysiology: decreased secretion of adrenal hormones; undersecretion of adrenal medulla does not cause health problems, because function taken over by the sympathetic nervous system; undersecretion of the adrenal cortex causes Addison's disease and is life-threatening because of deficiencies of glucocorticoids, mineralocorticoids, and androgens
  B. Etiology
    1. Atrophy
    2. Hemorrhagic necrosis secondary to trauma, sepsis, anticoagulation
    3. Surgical adrenalectomy
    4. Drugs
    5. Hypopituitarism
  C. Predisposing/precipitating factors
    1. Tuberculosis
    2. Autoimmune factors

3. Long-term administration of steroids suppressing secretion of hormones

D. Clinical manifestations
   1. Manifestations may appear when patient is stressed by infection, surgery, trauma, or alcohol withdrawal
   2. Anorexia, nausea, vomiting, diarrhea, abdominal pain, weight loss
   3. Fatigue, muscular weakness
   4. Hypotension, volume depletion, hyponatremia, hypoglycemia, hyperkalemia
   5. Decreased resistance to stress
   6. Hyperpigmentation of skin; bronze color, due to increased melaninocyte stimulating hormone (MSH)

E. Diagnostic examinations
   1. Low levels of adrenocortical hormones in blood and urine; if ACTH injections cause levels to rise to normal, then problem is pituitary deficiency; if not, then problem is adrenal cortex deficiency
   2. Hyponatremia, elevated serum potassium, hypoglycemia

F. Complications
   1. Adrenal crisis: cardiovascular collapse— shock, hypotension, kidney shutdown, tachycardia, rapid respirations, fever, cyanosis
   2. Weakness—due to acute deficiency of adrenal cortex hormones
   3. Side effects due to long-term steroid therapy—see Cushing's disease under hyperfunction of adrenals
   4. Dehydration from electrolyte imbalance

G. Medical management
   1. Lifelong replacement of corticosteroids and mineralocorticosteroids
   2. Supportive treatment of vascular collapse, IV steroids, hydrocortisone, dexamethasone

II. Analysis
   A. Knowledge deficit: disease process, symptoms, treatment related to new diagnosis
   B. Decreased cardiac output related to hypovolemia and hypotension
   C. Activity intolerance related to decreased adrenal hormones producing fatigue, muscular weakness, and hypoglycemia

III. Planning/goals, expected outcomes
   A. Client will be able to discuss disease, symptoms, and lifelong treatment
   B. Client will not be symptomatic of decreased cardiac output
   C. Client will demonstrate an improved tolerance for activity

IV. Implementation

A. Assess client for adrenal crisi shock-like symptoms
B. Advise client to wear a Medic, carry emergency kit containing inje drocortisone
C. Teach client importance of complying wi. lifelong medication regimen of steroid replacement
   1. Do not omit scheduled dose of cortisone; if cannot be taken orally, obtain order for injectable steroid; illness or stress will require an increase in dosage
   2. Fludrocortisone (Florinef) common mineralocorticoid replacement
   3. Monitor for Cushing's syndrome with long-term use of steroids
D. Avoid people with infections; monitor for signs and symptoms of infection
E. Teach client to space rest and activities to reduce stress

V. Evaluation
   A. Client is able to discuss disease, symptoms, and treatment
   B. Client did not experience a decrease in cardiac output
   C. Client is able to demonstrate an improved tolerance for exercise

Hyperfunction of the Adrenals

I. Assessment
   A. Definition: increased secretion of adrenal hormones; increased secretion of the glucocorticoids and mineralocorticoids of cortex leads to Cushing's disease; increased secretion of the catecholamines of the medulla due to tumor called a pheochromocytoma
   B. Etiology
      1. Tumor of adrenals—90% are benign
      2. Excess pituitary secretion of ACTH
      3. Long-term use of steroids
   C. Predisposing/precipitating factors
      1. Stress
      2. Obesity
      3. Steroid therapy
   D. Clinical manifestations
      1. Mineralocorticoids, aldosteronism—hypertension with hypokalemia diagnostic, may also show signs of hypernatremia, polydipsia, polyuria, pyelonephritis
      2. Glucocorticoids, Cushing's disease
         a. Early signs—amenorrhea, weight gain in trunk, thin arms and legs, muscle weakness, osteoporosis, emotional difficulties, decreased libido
         b. Moon face, buffalo hump, bruising, thin skin, stretch marks, acne, hirsutism

c. Low resistance to stress and infection
d. Hypertension, hyperglycemia, hypokalemia, hypernatremia
3. Catecholamines from medulla—pheochromocytoma: increased secretions cause crisis attacks lasting from minutes to an hour
    a. Hypertension, systolic and diastolic elevations
    b. Tachycardia
    c. Headache
    d. Palpitations
    e. Sweating
    f. Chest pain
    g. Nausea and vomiting
    h. Hyperglycemia
    i. Glycosuria
E. Diagnostic examinations
    1. Tests show increased levels of hormones or their metabolites in blood and urine
    2. Mineralocorticoids: increased levels of aldosterone, decreases in serum potassium, renin, low urinary specific gravity, hypernatremia—increased urinary protein
    3. Glucocorticoids: increased plasma cortisol, increased ACTH if pituitary tumor, hyperglycemia, increased 17-hydroxysteroids in urine
    4. Catecholamines—if client symptomatic, metabolites can be found in a 24-hour urine specimen, using the VMA test
F. Complications
    1. Aldosteronism: hypertension, hypokalemia, tetany, alkalosis
    2. Cushing's: hypertension, congestive heart failure, hypofunction/no steroid production secondary to surgery
    3. Pheochromocytoma: angina, congestive heart failure, myocardial infarction, CVA, sudden death
G. Medical management: may or may not be used with surgical management
    1. Aldosteronism: supportive treatment for fluid overload, electrolyte imbalance
    2. Cushing's: radiation therapy, aminoglutethimide to inhibit cholesterol synthesis, mitotane to inhibit cortisol production, metyrapone partially inhibits cortex steroid synthesis
    3. Pheochromocytoma: supportive therapy for hypertension and cardiac involvement; radiation; chemotherapy
H. Surgical management
    1. Aldosteronism: adrenalectomy
    2. Cushing's: because majority of cases are from pituitary tumors, transsphenoidal hypophysectomy is primary choice of treatment; bilateral adrenalectomy

3. Pheochromocytoma: adrenalectomy
II. Analysis
A. Aldosteronism
    1. Activity intolerance related to muscle weakness and fatigue associated with electrolyte imbalance
    2. Fluid volume excess related to abnormal retention of sodium and water
    3. Pain related to headache associated with hypertension
B. Cushing's
    1. Altered skin integrity related to edema, impaired healing, thin, fragile skin
    2. Disturbed body image related to altered physical appearance, impaired sexual functioning, and decrease in activity level
    3. High risk for injury and infection related to altered protein metabolism and inflammatory response
C. Pheochromocytoma
    1. Knowledge deficit: diagnosis, symptoms, treatment, related to new information
    2. Altered tissue perfusion, cerebral, related to hypertension
III. Planning/goals, expected outcomes
A. Aldosteronism
    1. Client will improve tolerance to activity as electrolytes improve
    2. Client will have fluid balance maintained
    3. Client will state absence or decrease of pain
B. Cushing's
    1. Client will be assessed for any interruptions in skin integrity
    2. Client will relate improved body image as evidenced by positive statements about self
    3. Client will be assessed for high-risk injury situations and early signs
C. Pheochromocytoma
    1. Client will be able to relate diagnosis to symptoms and treatment
    2. Client will not experience consequences of uncontrolled hypertension
IV. Implementation
A. Teach client purpose, administration, and side effects of medications
    1. Spironolactone (Aldactone) given as potassium-sparing diuretic preoperatively for aldosteronism
    2. Corticosteroids given for lifelong replacement after bilateral adrenalectomy; partial adrenalectomy not usually performed because problems recur
    3. Pituitary hormone replacement, if hypophysectomy necessary
    4. Antihypertensive and adrenergic-blocking agents preoperatively, for control of crisis attacks of pheochromocytoma

B. Teach client to comply with lifelong medical regimen
   1. Explain to client why surgery is not cure of health problem and medication still needed
   2. Teach client to wear Medic Alert tag and to carry emergency kit with injectable hydrocortisone and to monitor self for signs and symptoms of circulatory collapse of adrenal crisis (see under hypofunction of adrenals)
C. Inform client that thin skin easily damaged and steroids decrease resistance to infection
D. Advise client to reduce stressful activities and postpone nonessential life changes; when under stress, prescribed cortisone must be increased to mimic body's normal mode of secretion; obtain order from physician
E. Assist client and significant others to adjust to changes in body image
F. Follow guidelines for intracranial surgery if hypophysectomy necessary
G. Follow guidelines for abdominal surgery if adrenalectomy necessary
   1. Nursing care will include monitoring for circulatory collapse of adrenal crisis
   2. Keep pressor medications and parenteral corticosteroids ready to administer
   3. Wound infection and slow healing associated with use of steroid medications
H. Advise client with pheochromocytoma to decrease stress and take adrenergic blockers as prescribed to reduce hypertension and other symptoms of crisis attack
V. Evaluation
   A. Aldosteronism
      1. Client is able to tolerate activity
      2. Client's fluid balance is stable
      3. Client states is pain-free

B. Cushing's
   1. Client's skin integrity remained intact
   2. Client states he or she feels better about self
   3. Client did not experience injury or infection
C. Pheochromocytoma
   1. Client is able to discuss disease process and treatment
   2. Client did not experience complication of hypertension

Hypofunction of the Pancreas (Diabetes Mellitus)

I. Assessment
   A. Definition: decreased secretion of pancreatic insulin
      1. Diabetes mellitus made up of a group of disorders manifesting hyperglycemia resulting from lack of insulin or resistance to insulin
      2. Types (Table 8–3)
         a. Insulin-dependent (IDDM), also known as type I
         b. Non–insulin-dependent (NIDDM), also known as type II
   B. Pathophysiology: insulin and glucagon normally balance each other; in diabetes, insulin cannot suppress glucagon and convert excess blood sugar into glycogen; proteins and fats used instead of carbohydrates, for energy, which can lead to ketoacidosis; glycosuria causes loss of fluid due to high osmotic pressure; pancreatic somatostatin, stimulated by rise in glucagon, suppresses both insulin and glucagon, thus offering temporary protection against ketoacidosis

TABLE 8–3 Comparison of Insulin-Dependent Diabetes Mellitus (IDDM) and Non–Insulin-Dependent Diabetes Mellitus (NIDDM)

Characteristic	IDDM	NIDDM
Etiology	Atrophy of islets of Langerhans—failure to produce insulin	Obesity creates insulin demand that cannot be met by amount of circulating insulin present
Predisposing/precipitating factors	Genetic; associated more with Caucasians, than Asians or Africans; viral infection in children; autoimmune factors cause insulin resistance, since insulin binds to serum components instead of circulating freely	Maturity onset, after age 40
Management	Diet, exercise, insulin injections	Weight reduction diet and exercise to reduce obesity may control hyperglycemia; oral hypoglycemics may be necessary, particularly if client is noncompliant with diet
Complications	Diabetic ketoacidosis, hypoglycemia, nephropathy, neuropathy, atherosclerosis, peripheral vascular disease, blindness	Atherosclerosis, peripheral vascular disease, neuropathy, infections; has enough insulin to prevent ketoacidosis but may develop hyperosmolar, hyperglycemic, nonketotic coma

C. Etiology
1. NIDDM—obesity, age
2. IDDM—genetic influence, autoimmune, environmental (i.e., viral infection)
D. Incidence: estimated 6 million people with diagnosed DM; approximately 80 to 90% with NIDDM; another 4 to 6 million people are estimated to have undiagnosed DM
E. Predisposing/precipitating factors
1. Elderly
2. Obese
3. Family history of DM
4. Women who give birth to babies weighing more than 9 lb
F. Clinical manifestations
1. Hyperglycemia, glycosuria
2. Polyuria, polydipsia, polyphagia, weight loss, nausea, and vomiting
3. Fatigue, weakness
4. Blurred vision
5. Atherosclerosis, peripheral vascular changes, gangrene, slow wound healing, susceptibility to infection
G. Diagnostic examinations
1. Fasting blood glucose
2. Two-hour postprandial test
3. Oral glucose tolerance test
4. If client does not wish to do home blood glucose monitoring, can be taught urine testing for glucose and ketones
5. Glycosylated hemoglobin greater than 8%
H. Complications
1. Microangiopathy; includes nephropathy (with or without hypertension), retinopathy
2. Macroangiopathy; includes atherosclerosis, CAD
3. Neuropathy
   a. Sensory changes
   b. Autonomic changes affecting bladder, sexual function, GI system, cardiovascular reflexes
4. Hypoglycemia
5. DKA—diabetic ketoacidosis
6. HHNK—hyperosmolar hyperglycemic non-ketotic coma (for NIDDM patients)
I. Medical management
1. NIDDM: diet, exercise, oral hypoglycemic agent
2. IDDM: diet, exercise, insulin
3. Dietary: 50 to 60% of calories from carbohydrates; 20 to 30% from fat; remaining 12 to 20% from protein
II. Analysis
A. High risk for sensory/perceptual alterations: peripheral related to loss of sensation and circulation associated with long-term hyperglycemia
B. Fluid volume deficit related to hyperglycemia and polyuria, polydipsia
C. High risk for infection related to hyperglycemia, microangiopathy, depressed immune competence
D. Knowledge deficit: disease, goals of care, symptoms, self-monitoring related to new diagnosis
III. Planning/goals, expected outcomes
A. Client will not experience injury
B. Client will not be dehydrated
C. Client will not develop an infection
D. Client will be able to relate disease, goals, symptoms, and self-monitoring techniques
IV. Implementation
A. Assist client to monitor blood levels
1. Blood—use of glucometer
B. Assist client in understanding disease process of diabetes—for example, pathophysiology of why continuous use of an insulin pump with added bolus before meals more physiologically normal for client
C. Discuss with client how to use diabetic exchange lists from American Diabetic Association (ADA) to plan the prescribed diet (Table 8–4)
D. Teach client to modify diet to compensate for changes in exercise or illness
E. Obtain an order for insulin dosage on days when sick and unable to eat
F. Teach client purpose, administration, and side effects of oral hypoglycemics and insulin—for example, large doses of insulin can cause hypoglycemia, which leads to a rebound hyperglycemia (the Somogyi effect); physician will cut back on insulin dosage gradually (Table 8–5)
G. Discuss with client site rotation of injections to avoid lipodystrophy
H. Teach client to recognize signs and symptoms of hyperglycemia or hypoglycemia (Table 8–6)
I. Client will perform self-care safely—for example, safe foot care
1. No heating pads to feet
2. Cut toenails straight across
3. Avoid applying harsh lotions to feet
V. Evaluation
A. Client did not experience injury
B. Client did not experience fluid volume deficit
C. Client did not develop an infection
D. Client states he or she understands disease, treatment, complications

TABLE 8–4 ADA Lists for Meal Planning

Exchange List	Carbohydrates (g)	Protein (g)	Fat (g)	Calories Per Serving
Milk	12	8	Trace	80
Vegetable	5	2	—	25
Fruit	10	—	—	40
Bread (also includes cereal and starchy vegetables)	15	2	—	70
Meat (three lists)				
Lean meat	—	7	3	55
Medium-fat meat	—	7	5	75
High-fat meat	—	7	8	100
Fat	—	—	5	45
Free foods, unlimited amounts: Diet (calorie-free) beverage, coffee, tea, bouillon without fat, unsweetened gelatin, unsweetened pickles				

TABLE 8–5 Hypoglycemics

Example	Onset (hours)	Peak (hours)	Duration (hours)
Oral Agents			
Acetohexamide (Dymelor)	—	—	12–24
Chlorpropamide (Diabinese)	—	—	60
Tolbutamide (Orinase)	—	—	6–12
Tolazamide (Tolinase)	—	—	16
Humulin Insulins			
Rapid-Acting			
Regular insulin zinc suspension	$\frac{1}{2}$–1	2–4	4–6
Prompt (Semilente)	1	6–10	12–16
Humulin Intermediate-Acting			
Isophane insulin suspension (NPH)	1–2	8–12	28–32
Insulin zinc suspension (Lente)	1–2	8–12	28–30
Humulin Long-Acting			
Protamine zinc (PZI)	4–6	16–24	24–36
Extended insulin zinc suspension (Ultralente)	4–6	16–24	>36

Action	Use	Common Side Effects	Nursing Implications
Drugs that act to either stimulate the islet cells in the pancreas to secrete more insulin (oral) or act as insulin replacement when pancreatic function ceases (parenteral)	Treatment of diabetes mellitus	Hypoglycemic reactions, GI distress, neurological symptoms, alcohol intolerance (oral)	Know onset and duration of action for each agent and teach to patient; monitor for and teach patient to monitor for hypoglycemic reactions; stress compliance with total diabetic regimen; check for pork or beef allergy; teach patient insulin self-administration, site rotation, care of equipment, proper storage, self-testing for glucose and urine

TABLE 8–6 Comparison of Hypoglycemic Reaction and Diabetic Ketoacidosis in Diabetes Mellitus

Characteristic	Hypoglycemic Reaction	Diabetic Ketoacidosis
Definition	Blood glucose less than 60 mg/100 mL	Acidosis due to excessive production of ketone bodies; blood sugar over 300 mg/100 mL
Etiology	Too much insulin for food intake	Insufficient insulin for food intake
Predisposing/precipitating factors	Increased physical work or exercise, stress	Decreased exercise, stress, infection, diarrhea and vomiting, injury, surgery, pregnancy
Onset	Sudden if regular insulin, slower if modified insulin, or hypoglycemics given orally	Slow (days, probably because somatostatin suppresses high glucagon level for 48 hours)
Clinical manifestations	Diaphoretic and pale skin, feels cold; looks weak; nervous; trembling; neuroglycopenia; blurred vision; hunger; headache; shallow rapid respirations; numbness, tingling lips, fingers; confusion, slurred speech; glycosuria not usually present, depends upon time last voiding, tachycardia	Hot, dry, flushed skin; dehydration; polydipsia; polyuria; ketonuria; looks very ill; headache; abdominal pain; Kussmaul's respirations, deep and gasping, sweetish odor due to acetone; acidosis; hyperglycemia; glycosuria
Client goal	Client will recognize the signs and symptoms of hypoglycemia and will seek help appropriately	Client will recognize the signs and symptoms of diabetic ketoacidosis and will seek help appropriately
Implementation	Give client a glass of orange juice, soft drink, or hard candy; offer complex carbohydrate and protein to prevent another hypoglycemic reaction; give glucagon parenterally if necessary; investigate cause of hypoglycemic reaction, and teach client to make necessary adjustments in lifestyle or diet, to prevent recurrence	Insert IV and Foley catheter; take blood and urine samples to examine for glucose, ketone bodies, and hypokalemia or hyperkalemia; administer insulin IV (regular); observe cardiac monitor for hypokalemic arrhythmias as acidosis subsides; replace fluid and electrolytes; treat cause of acidosis; teach client how to avoid a recurrence of ketoacidosis by compliance with health regimen and monitoring for hyperglycemia
Evaluation	Client remains free from further hypoglycemic reactions	Client remains free from further episodes of diabetic ketoacidosis

POST-TEST Endocrine Disorders

1. Mrs. Vitt has just been diagnosed with Addison's disease. Which of the following are classic symptoms of this adrenal deficiency?
   1. Anorexia, hyperkalemia, hyperpigmentation, decreased resistance to stress
   2. Moon face, buffalo hump, hypertension, hypokalemia
   3. Sporadic hypertension, tachycardia, headaches, palpitations
   4. Kidney stones, hypercalcemia, bone pain, weakness, increased PTH

2. Mr. Smith is an IDDM diabetic. He is on H. NPH 35 U and H. Reg 10 U subq q a.m. and p.m. Which of the following choices is the best rationale for this insulin prescription?
   1. It is better to divide your total insulin needs in two doses so you don't get hypoglycemic
   2. This insulin coverage is to provide you with good glycemic control for your two meals per day
   3. Your blood sugar is too difficult to control with only one injection

4. This schedule best reflects the insulin peaks your own pancreas would create in response to your daily food intake

---

Mrs. Andrews is admitted to the hospital for a thyroidectomy. She first sought help because of a goiter of the thyroid.

---

3. Mrs. Andrews' preoperative nursing care includes monitoring for clinical manifestations of thyroid storm such as:
   1. Hypothermia and bradycardia
   2. Fever and tachycardia
   3. Hypoglycemia and decreased basal metabolic rate
   4. Weight gain and lethargy

4. After thyroidectomy surgery, a priority nursing implementation for Mrs. Andrews' care is to:
   1. Monitor for hemorrhage by examining the front of the dressing on her neck every 6 hours
   2. Monitor every hour for signs of respiratory distress

③ Check laboratory reports for increased levels of serum calcium

④ Take vital signs every 6 hours

5. When evaluating the treatment of a client with pheochromocytoma, the nurse would expect to see improvement in the control of the following symptoms:

① Weight gain, buffalo hump, and acne

② Hypoglycemia, osteoporosis

③ Hypotension, bradycardia

④ Hypertension attacks, tachycardia, nervousness

6. Mr. James takes oral corticosteroid medication for Addison's disease. He is going for abdominal surgery this morning. A priority nursing implementation is to:

① Discuss the effect of low steroid levels on wound healing

② Ascertain if he has received his corticosteroids by IV this morning

③ Explain the rationale for an NPO order before abdominal surgery

④ Demonstrate deep breathing and coughing techniques

Mrs. Taylor is a 60-year-old, newly diagnosed diabetic. She is 70 lb overweight.

---

7. As a new diabetic, the first topic Mrs. Taylor should be taught about is:

① How to give subcutaneous injections of insulin

② Diabetic exchange lists

③ The nature of the disease process of diabetes mellitus

④ How to test blood for glucose

8. Oral hypoglycemic medication was prescribed for Mrs. Taylor because she:

① Does not want to give herself injections

② Has a pancreas that secretes sufficient insulin when stimulated by medication

③ Has a mild form of diabetes that can be controlled by oral insulin

④ Has brittle diabetes, which is difficult to control

9. Mrs. Taylor demonstrates comprehension of your teaching by accurately selecting which of the following as clinical manifestations of hypoglycemia?

① Sweating, nervousness, dizziness

② Ketonuria, hot dry skin

③ Glycosuria on second voiding, thirst

④ Kussmaul's respirations with acetone odor on breath

10. Mrs. Taylor is put on a 1600-calorie ADA diet. A goal of her diet teaching is that she will choose a diet that:

① Will help her maintain her weight

② Is made up of two meals a day (breakfast and dinner), with complete flexibility as to time of eating and amounts eaten

③ Consists of three regularly scheduled meals plus snacks, to maintain a stable pattern as to time of eating and amounts consumed

④ Is limited to 100 g daily in carbohydrates

POST-TEST Answers and Rationales

1. ① Choice 1 contains the classic symptoms of Addison's disease (hypoadrenalism); 2 contains symptoms of Cushing's syndrome; 3 of pheochromocytoma; and 4 of hyperparathyoidism. 1, II. Hypofunction of the Adrenals.

2. ④ Choice 4 is the best way to control the client's glucose. This is not done to prevent hypoglycemia directly. The diabetic eats three balanced meals, often with two snacks, daily. Choice 3 is true, but not the best reason. 4, I & II. Diabetes Mellitus.

3. ② Thyroid storm (thyrotoxicosis) is an acute exacerbation of hyperthyroidism, so would exhibit the signs and symptoms listed. 1, I. Hyperthyroid.

4. ② Respiratory distress is a potential problem due to local swelling after thyroidectomy, or to tetany as a result of accidental damage to the parathyroid glands. Calcium may be low. 1, I & II. Thyroidectomy/Hypoparathyroid.

5. ④ These are the signs and symptoms of pheochromocytoma. 5, II. Pheochromocytoma.

6. ② A preoperative client on steroid therapy needs an increase in steroid dosage to handle the stress of surgery. If Mr. James misses his scheduled medication, he could go into adrenal crisis. The others are routine preoperative teaching. 4, I & II. Steroids.

7. ③ If Mrs. Taylor understands the disease process of diabetes mellitus, then she will appreciate the rationale for her treatment and comply with it. 4, II. Diabetes Mellitus.

8. ② Oral hypoglycemics stimulate pancreatic secretion of insulin. Elderly obese diabetics are usually non–insulin-dependent. 2, II. Diabetes Mellitus.

9. ① A low blood sugar level stimulates the autonomic nervous system and depresses the central nervous system, causing the listed signs and symptoms. 5, I. Diabetes Mellitus.

10. ③ A daily pattern of regularly scheduled meals with similar amounts of foods maintains a more stable blood sugar level. One goal will be for her to lose weight. 3, I & II. Diabetes Mellitus.

PRE-TEST Gastric/Biliary/Exocrine Pancreas/Lower Intestinal Disorders

Joe Sirgota, aged 25, is admitted to the hospital with right-sided lower abdominal pain. His temperature is 101°F and WBC is 15,000. The admitting orders read bedrest, NPO, IV fluid at 125 mL per hour, no pain medication, and Fleet enema times one.

1. Which of the following clinical manifestations may indicate Joe has a ruptured appendix?
   ① Pain becomes generalized over entire abdomen
   ② Pain becomes localized halfway between right iliac crest and umbilicus
   ③ Projectile vomiting begins
   ④ Joe guards his abdomen during palpation
2. Which of the following orders would the nurse question before implementing?

   ① Bedrest
   ② NPO
   ③ IV fluids at 125 mL per hour
   ④ Fleet enema
3. Joe's abdomen becomes increasingly rigid and his temperature rises to 104°F (40°C). He is taken to surgery for a ruptured appendix. A week after surgery, Joe remains weak, bowel sounds have not returned, and he continues to have a low-grade fever. Total parenteral nutrition (TPN) is started. The purpose of TPN for this client is to:
   ① Allow the bowel longer to rest
   ② Provide adequate nutrition for healing
   ③ Correct the infectious process
   ④ Increase the catabolism of tissue proteins
4. During administration of TPN, Joe complains of thirst and frequent urination. This most likely indicates:
   ① Hypothalamus response to NPO status
   ② Bladder infection
   ③ Increased metabolic rate
   ④ Hyperglycemia

Mary Smith, aged 66, is scheduled for a bowel resection and possible colostomy for cancer of the colon.

5. Which symptom in the early stage of colorectal cancer would Mrs. Smith be LEAST likely to complain of?
   1. Decrease in diameter of stools
   2. Bright red blood in stool
   3. Weakness and fatigue
   4. Continuous lower abdominal pain

6. Which of the following increased Mrs. Smith's chances of developing colorectal cancer?
   1. Her age
   2. High fiber diet
   3. History of peptic ulcer
   4. Sedentary lifestyle

7. Preoperatively, Mrs. Smith is given neomycin 1 g every 4 hours orally for 2 days. This is to:
   1. Decrease bacterial growth in intestine
   2. Decrease inflammation around the tumor
   3. Provide a therapeutic blood level of antibiotic to prevent infection
   4. Maintain normal level of intestinal flora

8. Postoperatively, Mrs. Smith complains of fatigue and requests no visitors. The most appropriate nursing response would be to:
   1. Encourage her to have family and friends visit
   2. Provide time for her to verbalize feelings
   3. Ensure adequate time for privacy while in hospital
   4. Ask her if there are family problems

9. Which of the following statements by Mrs. Smith would be most appropriate regarding care at home?
   1. ''I'll change the colostomy bag three times a week.''
   2. ''I'll follow a bland diet.''
   3. ''I'll provide entertainment for myself at home.''
   4. ''I'll ask the visiting nurse questions about the colostomy.''

James Smith is an obese, 55-year-old construction worker who has been experiencing changes in his bowel habits for 3 months. He is seen as an outpatient for a work-up for colon cancer.

10. Which of the following manifestations is he NOT likely to exhibit if he has rectal cancer?
    1. Bright red blood per rectum
    2. Nausea and vomiting
    3. Pencil-shaped stools
    4. Feeling of rectal fullness

11. The examination Mr. Smith is most likely to have done as an outpatient to definitively diagnose his colon cancer is a:
    1. Digital rectal examination
    2. Stool for occult blood
    3. Sigmoidoscopy and biopsy
    4. CEA level

12. Mr. Smith is diagnosed with rectal cancer and has an abdominal perineal resection with a permanent-end colostomy. Which of the following measures should you teach him to facilitate adherence of the colostomy pouch and decrease skin irritation?
    1. Cleanse the skin surrounding the stoma with mild soap and water and always use some type of skin barrier under the adhesive
    2. Affix the base of the pouch to the skin with tape after painting the skin with tincture of benzoin to toughen it
    3. Don't use a skin barrier, because the drainage is solid; just apply the pouch directly
    4. Do not try to clean off the old adhesive between changes, because this further irritates the skin

13. Postoperative colostomy care teaching should include:
    1. Decreasing the frequency of irrigation to avoid dependency on it
    2. Inserting the irrigation catheter at least 12 inches
    3. Withholding irrigations if diarrhea is present
    4. Irrigating with another 500 mL if there is no fecal return in 1 hour

14. The best time for Mr. Smith to irrigate his colostomy would be:
    1. In the morning
    2. In the evening
    3. Whenever he has about 2 hours of time
    4. When he usually had his normal elimination

PRE-TEST Answers and Rationales

1. ① A ruptured appendix will result in peritonitis, which is manifested by generalized abdominal pain, rigid abdomen, and signs of infection. An inflamed appendix often localizes at McBurney's point, which is halfway between the right iliac crest and the umbilicus. Vomiting may occur, but is generally not projectile. Guarding of the abdomen occurs in both appendicitis and peritonitis. 2, I & II. Appendicitis.

2. ④ An enema is contraindicated in appendicitis. The increased peristalsis may cause rupture of the appendix. The rest are appropriate orders. 4, I & II. Appendicitis.

3. ② An infection and the healing process increase metabolism, thus increasing nutritional need for calories and protein. The body will catabolize body proteins and healing will be delayed. 2, II. Hyperalimentation.

4. ④ A complication of TPN is hyperglycemia, which is caused by the high concentration of glucose being given. Signs and symptoms of hyperglycemia are thirst, polyuria, fatigue, and positive glucose in the urine. 2, I & II. Hyperalimentation.

5. ④ Pain is a late symptom of colorectal cancer. The others are earlier signs and symptoms that should alert the client to seek medical attention for early detection of colorectal cancer. 1, II. Colon Cancer.

6. ① The sixties are a peak age for development of colorectal cancer. A diet low in fiber and high in refined sugar and a history of polyps are other predisposing factors. 1, II. Colon Cancer.

7. ① Preoperatively, the bowel is cleansed of stool and a nonsystemic antibiotic such as neomycin is used to decrease the normal bacterial flora of the intestine. This decreases peritoneal contamination once the bowel is opened in surgery. 4, II. Colon Cancer.

8. ② A colostomy causes a change in body image and often produces a feeling of loss of control. Encouraging the client to express feelings will help clarify the client's perception of the colostomy and allow the nurse to intervene appropriately. 4, III. Colon Cancer.

9. ④ Discharge planning should include information about community resources such as visiting nurse and ostomy associations. The client is demonstrating acceptance of the colostomy and readiness to continue learning by asking questions. The other options are not appropriate. The colostomy bag should be emptied when one half to one third full and changed about every 3 days; the recommended diet includes whatever foods are tolerated, avoiding gaseous and odor-causing foods if necessary. A colostomy should not exclude a client from out-of-the-home activities. 5, IV. Colon Cancer.

10. ② Nausea and vomiting are symptoms of ascending colon cancer, not rectal cancer. The other options are common symptoms of rectal cancer. 2, II. Colon Cancer.

11. ③ The only definitive test is a biopsy and positive cytology, which will require a sigmoidoscopy. The other tests suggest a malignancy but are not definitive. 2, I. Colon Cancer.

12. ① It is very important to clean the area around the stoma well and always use a skin barrier under the adhesive to prevent skin breakdown. None of the other options are appropriate. 4, II. Colostomy.

13. ③ If diarrhea occurs, irrigations must be withheld or severe fluid and electrolyte imbalance could occur. The irrigations should be done on a regular basis to allow for regulation. The catheter should be inserted only about 4 to 6 inches and irrigations should be done only once a day with 500 to 1000 mL. 4, I & II. Colostomy.

14. ④ The best time to irrigate is when the client formerly had bowel movements, because this will help with regulation. The time is highly individualized. 5, II. Colostomy.

NORMAL FUNCTION OF GASTRIC/BILIARY/EXOCRINE PANCREAS/LOWER INTESTINAL SYSTEM

I. Ingestion: intake of foods
   A. Mouth: including lips, tongue, and teeth for lubricating and chewing food
   B. Pharynx and esophagus: involved in swallowing and providing passageway for food into stomach

II. Digestion: breakdown of foods into carbohydrates, fats, and protein
   A. Stomach: stores, mixes, and begins digestion
   B. Small intestine: composed of duodenum, jejunum, and ileum; does major portion of digestion
   C. Enzymes secreted from salivary glands, stomach, small intestine, pancreas, and liver; aid in digestive process

III. Absorption: transfer of usable nutrients across intestinal wall into bloodstream
   A. Small intestine absorbs majority of nutrients
   B. Large intestine absorbs majority of water

IV. Elimination: large intestine (ascending, transverse, descending, and sigmoid) serves as reservoir for waste products until excretion occurs through rectum and anus

V. Control of normal GI function
   A. Appetite center located in hypothalamus promotes ingestion
   B. Parasympathetic nervous system increases peristalsis and secretion of GI enzymes and gastric acid
   C. Sympathetic nervous system decreases peristalsis and secretion of GI enzymes and gastric acid
   D. Hormones released in blood when food enters intestinal system stimulate secretion of enzymes
   E. Reflex action stimulates defecation

NURSING PROCESS APPLIED TO ADULTS WITH GASTRIC/BILIARY/EXOCRINE PANCREAS/LOWER INTESTINAL DISORDERS

Peptic Ulcer Disease

I. Assessment
   A. Definition: a peptic ulcer is a break in the mucosa of the esophagus, stomach, or duodenum that may involve submucosal and muscular layers
   B. Etiology
      1. Gastric ulcers
         a. Break in gastric mucosa secondary to ulcerogenic agent such as aspirin, smoking, corticosteroids
         b. Can occur secondary to back diffusion of acid or pyloric sphincter dysfunction
      2. Duodenal ulcers
         a. Increased hydrochloric acid secretion
         b. Ulcerogenic agents
   C. Incidence: occurs in 5 to 10% of population; detection increasing because of sophisticated diagnosis tools
      1. Gastric: may occur anywhere in stomach
         a. Two times more common in men
         b. Peaks ages 45 to 54
      2. Duodenal
         a. Four times more common in men
         b. Starts between ages 25 and 50
         c. Four times more common than gastric
         d. Peak age: fourth decade
   D. Predisposing/precipitating factors
      1. Smoking
      2. Stress
      3. Ulcerogenic agents such as alcohol
      4. Family history
      5. Poverty, urban living
      6. Diet: exacerbation of symptoms may occur with coffee, spices, fried foods
      7. Drugs: ASA, NSAIDs, high-dose corticosteroids used over a long period
   E. Clinical manifestations
      1. Gastric
         a. Pain in epigastric region
         b. Pain occurs 1 to 2 hours after meals secondary to *hypo*secretion of acid
         c. Described as burning, gaseous, especially after eating
         d. Occasionally no pain or occurs after taking food
         e. Occasional nausea and vomiting
         f. Client usually older than 40
      2. Duodenal
         a. Burning with heartburn, cramp-like pain
         b. Occurs in midepigastric region or back
         c. Pain occurs 2 to 4 hours after meals secondary to *hyper*secretion of acid
         d. Pain usually relieved by food or antacids
         e. ''Pain clusters''—pattern of pain may continue for several weeks, subside, then recur in similar pattern
         f. Occasional nausea and vomiting
         g. Bloating, abdominal distention, intolerance to fatty foods
   F. Diagnostic examinations (Table 8–7)
      1. Upper gastrointestinal (UGI)

TABLE 8–7 Gastrointestinal Diagnostic Tests

GI Tests	Purpose	Pre-Care	Post-Care
X-Ray Studies Flat plate of abdomen	To identify gas, fluid, and growths in abdomen	Remove metal objects	None
UGI series: barium swallow, UGI study	To identify structural or motility changes (obstruction, ulcers, varices, and tumors) in eosphagus and stomach	Explain procedures: will have to swallow barium, a chalky liquid; x-rays taken in various positions; NPO for 8 to 12 hours before; if possible, narcotics and anticholinergics should be avoided because of effect on gastric motility	Encourage fluids; give laxative as ordered to promote elimination of barium; provide for rest; stool may be white for few days but should then return to normal color; observe for constipation or fecal impaction from retained barium
Barium enema: lower GI	To identify presence of lesions, growths, and narrowing in lower GI tract	Should be done before UGI; explain need to retain barium although may experience urge to defecate; may experience cramping; explain that x-rays are taken in various positions; contraindicated in ulcerative colitis, toxic megacolon, perforation and obstruction; enemas are given until clear morning of procedure but not within 3 hours before; clear liquids morning of test; observe for fatigue and provide rest after administration of enemas	Same as UGI
Endoscopy	Allows direct visualization of GI tract utilizing a lighted, flexible hollow tube; biopsy may also be done		
Esophagoscopy	Visualization of esophagus	Obtain consent; explain local anesthetic is used on throat to prevent gag reflex; may sedate before	Keep NPO until gag reflex returns; observe for potential bleeding and perforation
Gastroscopy	Visualization of stomach		
Gastroduodenoscopy	Visualization of duodenum		
EGD—esophagogastroduo-denoscopy	Visualization of esophagus, stomach, and duodenum Provides direct endoscopic visualization and photography of ulcerated areas; tissue samples—cell washings or biopsy; provide local ulcer treatment via laser photocoagulation	Consent needed; no antacids for 6 hours—might obscure ulcer by adhering to mucosa; mild preoperative sedation; local spray anesthetic	Same as for other endoscopies
Proctosigmoidoscopy	Visualization of rectum and sigmoid colon	Enemas until clear before procedure; explain will assume knee-chest or Sims position for procedure; explain may experience cramping	Observe for bleeding after; provide for rest
Colonoscopy	Visualization of ascending, transverse, and descending colon		
Gastric Analysis Tube tests	To measure amount of hydrochloric acid in stomach, either indirectly by checking the pH or directly by analyzing the aspirate	Client NPO for 8 to 10 hours; for tube test: an NG tube is inserted and all gastric contents aspirated, stimulant given and contents aspirated at specific intervals; for tubeless test: have client void, give Diagnex blue tablets and a gastric stimulant, have client void at specific time	For tube test: remove NG tube and feed client; for tubeless test: feed client
Tubeless test			
Oral or IV Cholecystogram	To visualize gallbladder after it fills with radiopaque dye given orally or by injection into bile duct	Check for allergy to iodine before giving radiopaque tablets; fat-free meal evening before; give 6 tablets 5 minutes apart evening	

TABLE 8–7 Gastrointestinal Diagnostic Tests *Continued.*

GI Tests	Purpose	Pre-Care	Post-Care
		before; NPO after ingestion of tablets; laxative may be ordered	
ERCP—Endoscopic Retrograde Cholangiopancreatography	To visualize and x-ray biliary system after a scope is passed through stomach, duodenum, and into the common bile duct	Obtain consent; NPO before procedure; may be given sedative	Observe for signs of infection; keep NPO until gag reflex returns
Ultrasound of Gallbladder, Pancreas	To identify masses and changes in structure	NPO before procedure; encourage fluids for 24 hours before NPO status; 6 to 8 glasses of water before test to distend bladder	None
CT Scan—Computerized Tomography of Gallbladder, Pancreas	To identify masses and changes in structure	NPO 8 to 12 hours before procedure; check for allergies to iodine if contrast material is to be used	None

2. Gastroscopy/EGD
3. Complete blood count (CBC)
4. Stool for occult blood
5. Gastric analysis

G. Complications
   1. Pyloric or duodenal obstruction ("gastric outlet obstruction"): caused by inflammation, edema around ulcer, spasm, or scarring
   2. Hemorrhage: caused by ulcer eroding into blood vessel
   3. Gastric perforation: ulcer perforates all layers of GI tract, allowing gastric/duodenal contents into peritoneal cavity and resulting in peritonitis
   4. Intractable ulcer: ulcer that fails to respond to medical treatment, recurs frequently, with bleeding unable to be controlled
   5. Morbidity and mortality associated with peptic ulcers and their complications are higher for Caucasians than non-Caucasians; may be drug-induced (ASA, NSAIDs, corticosteroids)

H. Medical management
   1. Pharmacologic management: antacids, H_2 receptor antagonists, coating agents, anticholinergic agents
   2. Dietary management: avoidance of foods that exacerbate symptoms

I. Surgical management: for control of severe symptoms/complications:
   1. Gastric—antrectomy
   2. Duodenal—vagotomy
   3. Partial gastrectomy
      a. Billroth I: gastroduodenostomy
      b. Billroth II: gastrojejunostomy

II. Analysis
   A. Knowledge deficit related to risk factors
   B. Pain related to inflamed gastric mucosa
   C. High risk for altered tissue perfusion related to complications (hemorrhage, perforation)
   D. High risk for fluid volume deficit related to development of complications
   E. Anxiety related to preoperative or postoperative events

III. Planning/goals, expected outcomes
   A. Client will identify and alleviate risk factors
   B. Client will be free from pain
   C. Client will not develop complications from peptic ulcer
   D. Client will remain hemodynamically stable if complications occur
   E. Client will have minimal anxiety preoperatively and postoperatively

IV. Implementation
   A. Assist client to identify presence of risk factors
   B. Modify diet to eliminate ulcerogenic substances such as caffeine, alcohol, spices, cola, ASA, steroids, NSAIDs
   C. Stop smoking
   D. Assist client to identify stressful situations and ways to cope effectively such as exercise, meditation, counseling, relaxation, and hobbies
   E. Teach client to eat well-balanced meals in smaller portions and at more frequent, regular intervals
   F. Teach client to avoid foods not well tolerated

G. Teach client to take medications as ordered, not only until pain subsides (Table 8–8)

H. During acute phase, promote quiet, restful environment

I. Observe for and teach client to report signs and symptoms of complications
   1. Pyloric or duodenal obstruction
      a. Distention
      b. Nausea after eating
      c. Anorexia
      d. Weight loss
      e. Obstipation
      f. Vomiting
   2. Hemorrhage
      a. Melena
      b. Hematemesis
      c. Weakness
      d. Shock (hypotension, tachycardia, restlessness)
   3. Gastric perforation
      a. Shock

b. Rigid abdomen
c. Fever

J. Assist and implement measures to maintain stability of client if complications occur
   1. Check vital signs frequently for hemodynamic status
   2. Maintain patency of NG tube
   3. Cold saline lavage as ordered to control bleeding
   4. Give intravenous fluids and blood as ordered to maintain fluid balance
   5. Prepare client for possible surgical procedure
   6. Provide rest

K. Provide preoperative and postoperative care suitable to type of gastric surgery performed and postoperative complications (Table 8–9)
   1. Provide preoperative teaching
   2. Provide pain relief measures as necessary
   3. Observe patency of NG tube but do not

TABLE 8–8 Common Medications Used in Peptic Ulcer Disease

Class	Type	Action and Use	Common Side Effects	Nursing Implications

Antacids	Magnesium and aluminum base
	  Maalox, Maalox Plus, Mylanta, Gelusil, Riopan
	Aluminum base
	  Amphojel
	Calcium base
	  Tums, Alka-2
		Buffers and neutralizes acid in upper GI tract	Aluminum-based antacids cause constipation; calcium-based antacids may cause hypercalcemia and acid rebound; magnesium-based antacids cause diarrhea and hypermagnesemia in patients with renal failure	Give 1 to 3 hours after meal for best effect; chew tablets thoroughly; follow with glass of water; since ulcer generally takes 4 to 6 weeks to heal, should continue to take as long as prescribed not only until symptoms have subsided; observe for constipation or diarrhea; may interfere with absorption of other medications such as tetracycline

Histamine receptor antagonist	Cimetidine (Tagamet), ranitidine (Zantac), famotidine (Pepcid), nizatidine (Axid)	Inhibits gastric acid secretion	Diarrhea, fatigue, dizziness, drowsiness, rash; with cimetidine, may see gynecomastia and confusion in elderly	With cimetidine, give with meals and 1 hour before or after antacids; give single dose at bedtime
Anticholinergics	Atropine, propantheline (Pro-Banthine), atropine and phenobarbital (Donnatol)	Inhibits gastric acid secretion and GI motility	Confusion, tachycardia, angina, dry skin and mouth, urinary hesitancy and retention, mydriasis and blurred vision, nasal congestion	Give 30 minutes before meals and bedtime; increase fluid intake to decrease potential constipation and dry mouth; do not give to client with prostatic hypertrophy, glaucoma, paralytic ileus; use with peptic ulcer uncertain because of side effects
Coating agents	Sucralfate (Carafate)	Forms a barrier at ulcer site	Constipation, dry mouth, skin rash, nausea, dizziness	Give 1 hour before meals; do not give within half an hour of antacid; may interfere with absorption of tetracycline

TABLE 8–9 Gastric Surgeries

- Partial or subtotal gastrectomy: removal of lower portion of stomach
- Vagotomy: total or partial severing of vagus nerves to stomach, which decreases gastric emptying and gastric secretions
- Pyloroplasty: enlarging of pyloric sphincter to make passage of food to duodenum easier, especially after vagotomy
- Billroth I (gastroduodenostomy): removal of distal stomach with anastomosis of gastric stump to duodenum
- Billroth II (gastrojejunostomy): removal of distal stomach with anastomosis of gastric stump to side of jejunum; duodenal stump sutured closed

Complications of Gastric Surgery	Rationale
Hemorrhage	May occur from interruption of the suture line
Atelectasis and pneumonia	More prone to because client often avoids taking deep breaths because of discomfort from high abdominal incision
Thrombophlebitis	Potential postoperative complication because of limited mobility
Infection	May be more prone to if debilitated before surgery
Duodenal stump leakage	Serious complication that typically occurs 3 to 6 days after surgery; leakage of bile and intestinal content results in peritonitis
Gastric retention	Common in first week after surgery resulting from edema, adhesions, or NG tube dysfunction
Dumping syndrome and postprandial hypoglycemia	Common occurrence 1 to 3 weeks after surgery; due to distention of the intestine resulting in increased peristalsis and decrease in plasma volume resulting from an osmotic pull of fluid into the intestine from the highly concentrated food bolus; this food bolus also results initially in hyperglycemia followed by rapid insulin secretion and hypoglycemia 2 hours later
Anemia	Iron deficiency anemia may result from continued GI bleeding or decreased release and absorption of iron; vitamin B_{12} absorption also impaired if intrinsic factor not produced by parietal cells of stomach, resulting in pernicious anemia

reposition or irrigate because of close proximity to suture line
4. Expect NG drainage to be bright red first few hours and dark red by 24 hours
5. Provide mouth care
6. Provide IV fluids as ordered and assess fluid and electrolyte status

7. Encourage coughing and deep breathing every 2 hours
8. Encourage leg exercises and early ambulation
9. Observe for symptoms of dumping syndrome
   a. Abdominal cramps
   b. Diarrhea
   c. Nausea and vomiting
   d. Palpitations
   e. Diaphoresis
   f. Light-headedness
10. Teach client measures to reduce dumping syndrome
    a. Drink fluids between meals, not at mealtime
    b. Eat four to six small meals a day
    c. Avoid large amounts of carbohydrates at one time (Table 8–10)
    d. Increase protein in diet
    e. Lie down after meals on left side
11. Observe and teach client to report signs and symptoms of iron deficiency anemia
V. Evaluation
   A. Client able to identify and alleviate risk factors
   B. Client is pain-free
   C. Client did not develop complications

TABLE 8–10 Fat, Protein, Carbohydrate, and Fiber Content in a Variety of Foods

High Fat	Low Fat	High Protein
Beef, veal pork	Fruit	Milk and milk products—cheese, yogurt, ice cream
Margarine, butter	Vegetables	Meat, poultry, fish
Oils	Lean beef, chicken, fish	Eggs
Bacon		Legumes
Avocado		Nuts
Milk, cheese, ice cream		
Nuts		

High Carbohydrates	Low Carbohydrates	High Fiber/High Residue
Refined sugar products: candy, cookies, cake	Most vegetables	Raw and dried fruits
Bread and cereals	Meats	Raw and cooked vegetables
Pasta	Milk and milk products	Whole grain cereal and breads
Potatoes, rice	Bacon, margarine	Seeds
Corn, lima beans		Nuts
Fruit		Baked beans

D. Client remains hemodynamically stable

E. Client states absence of anxiety

Inflammatory Conditions

Gastritis

I. Assessment

  A. Definition: acute or chronic inflammation of gastric mucosa, which results in edema and degenerative changes in superficial epithelium

  B. Predisposing/precipitating factors

    1. Drugs: alcohol, ASA, digitalis, chemotherapeutic agents, NSAIDs

    2. Foods coarse and extreme in temperature

    3. Foods such as excess coffee, tea, mustard, paprika, cloves, pepper

    4. Medical conditions such as shock, uremia, CNS lesions, cirrhosis, pancreatitis, respiratory disorders, renal failure, trauma

    5. Stress

    6. Radiation

    7. Caustic agents

  C. Clinical manifestations

    1. Epigastric pain

    2. Anorexia

    3. Nausea and vomiting

    4. Full feeling

    5. Eructation

    6. Hematemesis

    7. May be asymptomatic

  D. Diagnostic tests (see Table 8–7)

    1. Gastroscopy

    2. CBC

  E. Complications

    1. Pernicious anemia

    2. Increased risk of gastric carcinoma

    3. Dehydration

    4. Bleeding

  F. Medical management

    1. Pharmacological: mild—antacids, rest; severe—IV fluids, antiemetics, H_2 antagonists, B_{12} (for atrophic gastritis), anticholinergics

    2. Dietary: eliminate or decrease foods that exacerbate symptoms

II. Analysis

  A. Knowledge deficit related to precipitating factors

  B. High risk for fluid volume deficit related to development of complications

  C. Pain related to inflammation of gastric mucosa

III. Planning/goals, expected outcomes

  A. Client will eliminate precipitating factors

B. Client will not develop complications

C. Client will be free from pain

IV. Implementation

  A. Maintain NPO status until vomiting ceases, then encourage bland diet

  B. Give antacids and histamine antagonists as ordered (see Table 8–8)

  C. Teach client causes of gastritis and ways to eliminate

  D. Explore dietary intolerances

  E. Observe for signs and symptoms of dehydration, alkalosis, and loss of electrolytes (K^+, CO^-)

  F. Give antiemetics as ordered

  G. Encourage medical follow-up for cancer screening

V. Evaluation

  A. Client verbalizes ways to reduce causes of gastritis

  B. Client remains free of complications

  C. Client remains free of pain

Pancreatitis

I. Assessment

  A. Definition: acute or chronic inflammation of pancreas, which in chronic pancreatitis results in permanent damage

  B. Pathophysiology: damage to pancreatic tissue believed to be caused by autodigestion of pancreas by pancreatic enzymes that are normally secreted into intestine

  C. Incidence

    1. Most common in middle-aged men and women

    2. Occurs in 0.5% of population

  D. Predisposing/precipitating factors

    1. Alcohol

    2. Gallbladder disease

    3. Viral infection

    4. Trauma

    5. Metabolic disorders such as hyperlipidemia, renal failure, hyperparathyroidism

    6. Drugs

    7. Cystic fibrosis

    8. Idiopathic

  E. Clinical manifestations

    1. Acute

      a. Constant left upper quadrant (LUQ) or midepigastric pain that may radiate to back

      b. Pain ranges from mild to severe

      c. Pain aggravated by eating and lying flat

      d. Rebound tenderness

      e. Nausea and vomiting

      f. Low-grade fever, elevated pulse, tachypnea

g. Corresponding decrease in blood pressure from relative hypovolemia

h. Abdominal distention and tenderness and guarding

i. Bowel sounds decreased or absent

j. Mental confusion may be present

k. Jaundice

l. Elevated serum and urine amylase and serum lipase levels

2. Chronic

a. Recurrent attacks of pain

b. Similar to acute symptoms but may be less severe

c. Steatorrhea

d. Hyperglycemia

e. Often dependence on narcotics

F. Diagnostic examinations (see Table 8–7)

1. Electrolytes—especially calcium

2. Glucose

3. CBC

4. Liver function tests: bilirubin, alkaline phosphatase, prothrombin time (PT)

5. Amylase, lipase

6. Abdominal and chest x-ray

7. Biopsy may be necessary for chronic disease

8. ERCP

9. Hemorrhage

10. Encephalopathy

11. Hypotension

12. Hypoalbuminemia

13. Disseminated intravascular coagulation

G. Complications

1. Fluid and electrolyte disturbances, resulting from vasodilation and loss of fluid into peritoneal space

2. Hypovolemic shock

3. Obstruction of common bile duct, resulting from inflammation

4. Hyperglycemia

5. Hypocalcemia

6. Pseudocyst, abscess, peritonitis

7. Acute renal failure—may result from hypovolemia

8. Respiratory problems such as atelectasis, pleural effusion, dyspnea

9. Peptic ulcer, gastritis

H. Medical management

1. Pharmacological—narcotics, IV fluids, calcium replacement

2. Hemodynamic monitoring

3. Ventilatory management

II. Analysis

A. Knowledge deficit related to causes of pancreatitis

B. Pain related to inflammation of pancreas and/or peritoneum

C. Fluid volume deficit related to vomiting, pancreatic hemorrhage

D. Altered health maintenance related to unhealthy lifestyle pattern, including alcoholism

E. High risk for altered tissue perfusion related to fluid and electrolyte imbalance, hypoalbuminemia, and anemia

III. Planning/goals, expected outcomes

A. Client will identify and alleviate causes of pancreatitis

B. Client will be free from pain

C. Client will have adequate fluid volume as demonstrated by normal blood pressure

D. The client will assume safe and adequate health care practices

E. Client will not develop complications

IV. Implementation

A. Teach client about drugs and foods that should be avoided (for example, rich, fatty stimulating foods) and about not overeating (see Table 8–4)

B. Give pain medications as ordered, avoiding morphine sulfate, which can cause spasm of the sphincter of Oddi

C. Give anticholinergics (for example, atropine) to decrease spasm (see Table 8–8)

D. Encourage side-lying position for relief of pain

E. Maintain NPO status during acute attack

F. Monitor NG tube if utilized during acute attack

G. Monitor I & O, IV fluids, and TPN utilized to maintain fluid, electrolyte, and nutritional status (Table 8–11)

H. After acute attack, encourage diet high in protein and carbohydrates and low in fats (see Table 8–10)

I. Maintain bedrest during acute phase

J. Observe for respiratory complications, dyspnea, atelectasis, adventitious breath sounds

K. Encourage coughing and deep breathing

L. Give antibiotics as ordered to prevent infection, treat abscesses

M. Observe for hyperglycemia, positive glucose in urine, polyuria, and thirst

N. Observe for hypocalcemia, muscle twitching, and irritability

O. Give pancreatic enzymes (pancreatin, pancrelipase) and bile salts with meals to clients who have lost pancreatic function and are unable to digest fatty foods; observe for possible side effects of nausea, diarrhea, and hyperuricemia with these medications

P. Observe for inability to digest fatty foods, steatorrhea, weight loss

TABLE 8–11 Nutritional Feedings

	Enteral Feedings	Total Parenteral Nutrition (Hyperalimentation)
Indications	Clients who are unable to ingest adequate nutrients because of dysphagia, CNS disorders such as unconsciousness, decreased appetite, as in clients having cancer, obstruction of esophagus, increased need, as in clients with severe burns	Clients who are unable to ingest, digest, or absorb adequate nutrients because of: Disorders of GI tract such as obstruction, inflammatory bowel disease, pancreatitis Burns/trauma Cancer Debilitated pre- and postoperative clients
Techniques	Given through nasogastric or gastrostomy tube Tube feedings consist of blenderized food or prepared products providing carbohydrates, fats, protein, and water May be given continuously or intermittently	10 to 15% dextrose solutions can be given in peripheral vein 25 to 70% dextrose solutions given into central vein, which dilutes concentrated solution quickly 2.75 to 5% amino acid solution given 10 to 20% lipid solution given Vitamins and minerals added for total nutrition
Complications	Nausea or vomiting Diarrhea or constipation Regurgitation and aspiration Bacterial contamination Dehydration	Infection Air embolism Hyperglycemia or hypoglycemia Pneumothorax with insertion Fluid and electrolyte imbalances
Nursing Care	Keep head of bed elevated at all times to prevent aspiration Check placement of tube every 4 to 8 hours Check for residual every 4 to 8 hours and hold feeding if more than 150 mL Irrigate tube with water after each feeding to maintain patency Give feedings at room temperature to avoid nausea Do not hang feeding for longer than 8 hours and change feeding bag every 24 hours to avoid contamination Monitor for signs of dehydration: decreased urine output, decreased skin turgor, dry mucous membranes If diarrhea occurs, feeding may be changed or decreased in strength or antidiarrhea agents may be given Administer by use of gravity or infusion pump, depending on cost, need for close regulation, and consistency of feeding	Assist with insertion of catheter Maintain aseptic technique Position client in Trendelenburg position with towel under scapula When catheter being inserted, ask client to perform Valsalva's maneuver to prevent air emboli Place occlusive dressing over site Do not infuse TPN until placement confirmed by x-ray Change TPN dressing three times per week (may be done by special team) Do not use TPN catheter for blood draws or administration of other medications or fluids Gradually increase rate of administration to allow pancreas time to adjust If catheter disconnected, ask client to do Valsalva's maneuver Administer correct rate avoiding over- or underinfusion Monitor weight and I & O daily Monitor electrolytes, glucose, and BUN as ordered Monitor urine for sugar and acetone four times per day Do not hang TPN solution for longer than 24 hours Monitor vital signs, including temperature, every 4 to 8 hours

Q. Assess renal function—a decrease in urine output may result from hypotension and shock

R. Encourage a healthy lifestyle: diet, sobriety, weight reduction

S. Assess for acute abdomen

V. Evaluation

A. Client verbalizes ways to eliminate causes of pancreatitis from diet and lifestyle

B. Client remains free of pain

C. Client does not demonstrate fluid volume deficit

D. Client states he or she will practice healthy lifestyle

E. Client remains free of complications from pancreatitis

Cholecystitis

I. Assessment
  A. Definition: inflammation of the gallbladder, results from a blockage of the cystic duct secondary to stones (cholelithiasis) or blockage of duct secondary to edema and spasm initiated by passage of the gallstone
  B. Incidence
    1. Found in 10 to 20% of adult population
    2. Four times higher in females
    3. Multiparous females
    4. After age 40
    5. Use of birth control pills (BCP)
    6. More common in Caucasians, Native Americans, Mexican Americans
  C. Predisposing/precipitating factors
    1. Obesity
    2. Family history
    3. Sedentary lifestyle
    4. Diabetes
    5. "5 Fs"; fat, fair, female, forty, fertile
  D. Clinical manifestations
    1. Moderate to severe right upper quadrant (RUQ) pain, which may radiate to back and right shoulder
    2. Steady pain often precipitated by recumbent position
    3. Pain occurs frequently several hours before meals or 3 to 6 hours after a heavy meal
    4. Indigestion
    5. Low-grade fever
    6. Leukocytosis
    7. Nausea and vomiting
    8. Diaphoresis and tachycardia
    9. Jaundice
    10. Fat intolerance
  E. Diagnostic examinations (see Table 8–7)
    1. Oral or IV cholecystogram
    2. Ultrasound of gallbladder
    3. WBC, liver enzymes, conjugated s. bilirubin
    4. ERCP
  F. Complications
    1. Choledocholithiasis: stone in common bile duct resulting in obstruction of bile flow
    2. Pancreatitis
    3. Biliary cirrhosis
    4. Peritonitis: resulting from rupture of gallbladder

    5. Prolonged PT with vitamin K disruption
  G. Medical management
    1. Pharmacological—analgesics, IV fluids, vitamin K if prothrombin time is prolonged, dissolution agents
    2. Diet—low fat
    3. Lithotripsy
  H. Surgical management
    1. Cholecystectomy
    2. Laparoscopic laser cholecystectomy (aka: endoscopic cholecystectomy)

II. Analysis
  A. Pain related to inflammation of gallbladder
  B. Altered health maintenance related to unhealthy lifestyle of obesity and high fat intake
  C. High risk for injury related to bleeding from impaired vitamin K deficiency
  D. Altered skin integrity related to surgical incision
  E. High risk for fluid volume deficit related to nausea/vomiting, fever, decreased fluid intake

III. Planning/goals, expected outcomes
  A. Client will be free from pain and discomfort
  B. Client will identify need to maintain optimal weight and pursue lifestyle that includes exercise
  C. Client will not develop bleeding from cholecystitis
  D. Client will not develop complications (infection) from surgical procedures
  E. Client will maintain adequate hydration

IV. Implementation
  A. Give pain medication as ordered; meperidine (Demerol) given over morphine sulfate because of increase in spasm of sphincters with morphine
  B. Give nitroglycerin, amyl nitrate, or anticholinergics as ordered to relax smooth muscle, observe for headache, flushing, and dizziness with nitrates (see Table 4–5)
  C. Maintain NPO status and NG decompression to prevent further stimulation of gallbladder
  D. Teach weight reducing and low-fat diet and/or make referral to dietitian (see Table 8–10)
  E. Monitor fluid and electrolyte status, I & O, skin turgor
  F. Administer IV fluids as necessary
  G. Assist with self-care needs, such as mouth care and hygiene as necessary during acute phase
  H. Reassure client, answer questions, explain procedures
  I. Observe for symptoms of biliary obstruction, jaundice, clay-colored stools, dark, foamy urine, steatorrhea
  J. Give bile salts as ordered to facilitate diges-

tion and fat-soluble vitamin absorption (A, D, E, and K)

K. Provide preoperative teaching for surgical procedure
   1. Cholecystectomy: removal of gallbladder
   2. Choledocholithotomy: removal of stones from common bile duct
   3. Laparoscopic laser cholecystectomy

L. Postoperative care—cholecystectomy
   1. Maintain high Fowler's position to facilitate drainage and provide optimal expansion of lungs
   2. Encourage coughing and deep breathing every 2 hours; high abdominal incision makes deep breathing painful, thus clients tend to not fully expand lung, increasing risk of atelectasis
   3. Provide support to incision with pillow to make deep breathing less painful
   4. Change or reinforce dressing as necessary around Penrose drain and incision; expect heavy drainage first 24 to 48 hours
   5. Maintain NPO status until client begins passing flatus or bowel sounds are present
   6. Monitor fluid and electrolyte status and administer IV fluids as ordered
   7. Care of T-tube: placed after surgery to allow drainage of bile until edema subsides, especially if common duct exploration and/or removal of stones in the duct occurred
     a. Maintain closed gravity drainage system
     b. Observe and measure drainage; normal drainage is 400 mL per day and greenish brown; as swelling decreases, drainage decreases
     c. Protect skin from damage from irritating bile
     d. Clamp tube as ordered before and after meals to allow bile to aid in digestion; assess tolerance and return of normal digestion
     e. When bile drainage continues through T-tube for period of time, it may be ordered to give bile drainage orally or through NG tube to prevent fluid and electrolyte loss and for fat and vitamin absorption, or bile salts may be ordered

M. Postoperative care laparoscopic laser cholecystectomy
   1. NPO until clear liquids tolerated
   2. IV
   3. Analgesics—PO preferred; IM can decrease intestinal motility, cause vomiting and drowsiness
   4. Earlier ambulation
   5. Heating pad for referred shoulder pain
   6. Assess for fever, abdominal distention, vital signs, bleeding, bile leakage

N. Pre-lithotripsy care includes:
   1. Client education
   2. IV
   3. Client lies prone for procedure
   4. Procedure done with ultrasound to locate stone
   5. Light sedation may be used

O. Post-lithotripsy care includes:
   1. Analgesics
   2. Low-fat diet
   3. I & O
   4. Hematuria ×24 hr is acceptable
   5. Assessment of fever, nausea, vomiting

V. Evaluation
A. Client remains free of pain and complications from cholecystitis and surgical procedure
B. Client verbalizes plan to achieve and maintain optimal weight including low-fat diet and exercise
C. Client did not have bleeding secondary to cholecystitis
D. Client did not have complications from surgical procedure
E. Client's hydration maintained

Inflammatory Bowel Disease

I. Assessment
A. Definition: includes both ulcerative colitis and Crohn's disease (regional enteritis), which are chronic disorders that involve inflammation of colon in ulcerative colitis and inflammation of small intestine, ileum, and colon in Crohn's disease; both disorders follow course of remissions and exacerbations
B. Pathophysiology
   1. Ulcerative colitis: mucosa of colon becomes edematous with formation of abscesses and bleeding; disorder tends to start in distal colorectal area and spread upward in continuous pattern
   2. Crohn's: find cobblestone type ulcerations in all layers of bowel wall affecting noncontinuous segments of small bowel, ileum, and colon; ulcers may perforate or form fistulas to colon, vagina, and perirectum
C. Incidence
   1. Ulcerative colitis
     a. Age at onset 15 to 25
     b. Slightly higher in females
     c. More common in people of Jewish origin
     d. Two times more common than Crohn's disease

2. Crohn's disease
   a. Age at onset 15 to 25
   b. More common in people of Jewish origin
   c. Slightly higher in females
D. Predisposing/precipitating factors
   1. Ulcerative colitis
      a. Family history
      b. Psychosocial factors
   2. Crohn's disease—family history
E. Clinical manifestations
   1. Ulcerative colitis
      a. Four to 20 diarrheal stools per day common
      b. Mucus, pus, and occasional blood
      c. Abdominal cramps may occur before diarrhea
      d. Incontinence of stools
      e. Fever
      f. Weight loss
   2. Crohn's disease
      a. Three to four diarrheal stools per day
      b. Mucus and pus in stool, semisolid
      c. Right lower quadrant abdominal pain
      d. Low-grade fever
      e. Abdominal distention
      f. Nausea and vomiting
      g. Weight loss
      h. Adbominal cramps relieved with bowel movement
      i. Leukocytosis
      j. Iron-deficiency anemia
F. Diagnostic examinations (see Table 8–7)
   1. CBC, electrolytes
   2. Stool for occult blood, pus, mucus, fat
   3. Barium enema
   4. Colonoscopy
   5. Sigmoidoscopy
G. Complications
   1. Ulcerative colitis
      a. Bowel obstruction
      b. Increased risk of colorectal cancer
      c. Toxic megacolon
      d. Fluid and electrolyte imbalance (Na^+, K^+, HCO_3, Ca^{++}) from malabsorption
      e. Infection
      f. Bleeding, anemia
      g. Perforation
   2. Crohn's disease
      a. Perirectal and intra-abdominal lesions that may perforate and form abscesses and fistulas
      b. Peritonitis
      c. Minimal/no risk of carcinoma
      d. Malnutrition and fluid and electrolyte imbalance

   e. Fat-soluble vitamin deficiency
   f. Malabsorption, anemia
   g. Strictures
   h. Perianal disease
H. Medical management is primarily supportive during exacerbations:
   1. Pharmacological: corticosteroids, sulfasalazine (Azulfidine), immunosuppressants, antibiotics, bulk hydrophilic agents for diarrhea, vitamin and iron supplements
   2. Diet: TPN, low residue, high calorie, high protein
I. Surgical management
   1. Ulcerative colitis—for complications or poor response to medical management:
      a. Total proctocolectomy with permanent ileostomy
      b. Total proctocolectomy with continent ileostomy
      c. Total colectomy with ileorectal anastomosis
      d. Total colectomy and mucosal proctectomy with ileoanal anastomosis
   2. Crohn's disease—surgery is restricted because of high rate of recurring disease
      a. Indications: bowel obstructions, fistulas, intra-abdominal abscess, relief of symptoms
      b. Surgical options: segmental resection of diseased bowel, bypass of diseased bowel by anastomosis of ileum to colonic area free of disease
II. Analysis
   A. Pain: abdominal and rectal related to bowel disease, diarrhea
   B. Diarrhea related to chronic inflammation
   C. Ineffective individual and family coping related to prolonged disability
   D. Impaired skin integrity related to diarrhea
   E. Fluid volume deficit related to diarrhea, decreased fluid intake
III. Planning/goals, expected outcomes
   A. Client will have minimal pain
   B. Client will have less than four stools a day
   C. Client/family will describe ways to promote the client's independence and cope with feelings regarding client's disease
   D. Client will not develop skin excoriation from incontinence
   E. Client will maintain normal fluid and electrolyte balance
IV. Implementation
   A. Maintain accurate record of amount and consistency of stools
   B. During acute exacerbation, maintain bedrest to promote healing, but avoid letting client become debilitated

C. Maintain bowel rest as ordered to promote healing
   1. Partial: diet free of bulk and fiber, low fat, nutritional, balanced (see Table 8–10)
   2. Total: NPO, use of total parenteral nutrition (see Table 8–11)
D. Give medications as ordered
   1. Sulfasalazine (Azulfidine)
      a. Action: local sulfa antibiotic that reduces bacteria in stool and inhibits prostaglandins that cause diarrhea
      b. Side effects: allergic reactions, nausea and vomiting, anemia, and blood dyscrasias
      c. Nursing implications include providing 2000 mL of fluid daily and observing for side effects
   2. Antidiarrheal (Table 8–12)
   3. Steroids
E. Give support and reassurance
F. Provide consistent approach to client
G. Provide time to spend with client to discuss possible feelings regarding incontinence, weakness, lifestyle changes
H. Keep bedpan or commode close to avoid incontinence
I. Assist client to analyze lifestyle, stressors, coping mechanisms
J. Assist client in development of plan that includes healthy coping mechanisms and reduction of stress
K. Weigh daily, monitor I & O, check electrolytes as ordered
L. Encourage fluids to 2500 mL per day
M. Assess for bowel obstruction, decrease in bowel sounds, abdominal distention
N. Assess for signs of infection
O. Provide skin care if rectal area becomes excoriated
P. Provide measures to prevent skin breakdown for debilitated clients on bedrest such as Eggcrate mattress, massage of bony prominences, frequent change of position
Q. After acute phase, teach client dietary changes—small frequent meals, high protein, high carbohydrate, low residue, nonirritating foods excluding chocolate, citrus foods, carbonated drinks, alcohol, and milk products in general (see Table 8–10)
R. Teach and support client regarding possible need for surgery (Table 8–13)
   1. Ulcerative colitis: bowel resection and/or ileostomy performed for medically unresponsive condition that seriously interferes with normal functioning, or for complications such as bowel obstruction, perforation, toxic megacolon, abscesses
   2. Crohn's disease: bowel resection may be utilized for correction of fistula, perforation, and obstruction; because disease often progresses in noncontinuous pattern in bowel, recurrence after surgery common
V. Evaluation
   A. Client states pain is decreased or absent
   B. Client reports less than four stools per day
   C. Client/family reports they are coping better

TABLE 8–12 Antidiarrheal Medications

Example	Action	Common Side Effects	Nursing Implications
Kaolin & pectin (Kaopectate)	Acts as adsorbent by coating walls of intestine and adsorbing bacteria and toxins	Constipation with continued use	Give after each loose stool; avoid prolonged use
Bismuth subsalicylate (Pepto-Bismol)	May inhibit synthesis of prostaglandins, which increase GI motility; also antimicrobial action and neutralization of intestinal bacteria	Stool and tongue may temporarily turn darker; fecal impaction	Protect from light; avoid prolonged use
Diphenoxylate HCL with atropine (Lomotil)	Decreases motility by inhibiting intestinal smooth muscle	Headache, sedation, tachycardia, nausea and vomiting, dry mouth, rash, mydriasis, urinary retention	Decrease dosage when diarrhea subsides; observe for anticholinergic effects
Loperamide (Imodium)	Inhibits gastric motility	Drowsiness, dizziness, abdominal distention, nausea and vomiting, dry mouth	Avoid prolonged use; observe for side effects
Paregoric (tincture of opium)	Inhibits gastrointestinal motility	Nausea and vomiting, constipation, drowsiness, physical dependence with high dosage	Administer with sufficient water; discontinue promptly when diarrhea ceases

TABLE 8–13 Ostomies

Terminology

Colostomy: opening into ascending, transverse, descending, or sigmoid colon; may be temporary or permanent

Ileostomy: opening into ileum; generally permanent

End colostomy: proximal portion of bowel brought to surface of abdomen and distal portion of bowel removed

Double barrel: both distal and proximal bowel brought to surface forming two stomas

Loop ostomy: loop of bowel brought to surface forming one stoma that opens into distal and proximal colon

Kock pouch: an internal pouch is created from unused portion of ileum; acts as a reservoir for feces and is emptied via catheter four times per day

Reasons for Ostomy	Complications
Cancer	Prolapse
Diverticulitis	Bleeding
Congenital deformities	Stricture
Inflammatory disorders	Necrosis
Obstruction	Skin irritation
Trauma	

Nursing Care

Check stoma for normal dark pink to red color, minimal bleeding and no edema

Empty pouch when one third to one half full

Monitor output; descending and sigmoid colostomy may have formed stool; others will be semi-soft to liquid in consistency

Support client in stage of acceptance; avoid expression of negative feelings when caring for ostomy

Increase client's involvement in care as ready

Observe and respond to potential feelings of anxiety, helplessness, and anger

Provide diet as tolerated; may need to limit hard-to-digest foods such as seeds, corn, and nuts and gas-forming foods such as onions, eggs, cabbage, beer, and some cheeses

Answer questions and fears regarding sexuality

Utilize skin barrier if necessary to protect skin

Appliance opening should be one eighth of an inch larger than stoma opening

Provide deodorants for bag and odor-proof pouches if odor is a problem

May irrigate descending or sigmoid colostomies to stimulate peristalsis and evacuation of bowel contents at a specific time each day

Refer client to ostomy association for support and information

D. Client does not develop skin excoriation

E. Client is normovolemic

Peritonitis

I. Assessment
   A. Definition: inflammation of peritoneum that involves the parietal and visceral surfaces caused by introduction of chemical substance or bacteria either by rupture of an organ or traumatic injury
   B. Pathophysiology: body attempts to wall off inflamed area, potentially resulting in healing, scar, or abscess formation; fluid, electrolytes, and protein accumulate in abdominal cavity, potentially resulting in hypovolemia and shock; peristalsis decreases and bowel obstruction may ensue; as infectious process continues, septic shock may occur
   C. Clinical manifestations
      1. Pain, tenderness over involved area
      2. Muscle rigidity
      3. Abdominal distention
      4. Fever
      5. Leukocytosis
      6. Nausea and vomiting
      7. Diminished or absent bowel sounds
      8. Tachycardia, hypotension
      9. Hypovolemia, hemoconcentration
      10. Metabolic acidosis
      11. Hyperkalemia
   D. Diagnostic examinations (see Table 8–7)
      1. CBC
      2. Abdominal paracentesis
      3. Abdominal x-ray
      4. CT of abdomen
   E. Complications
      1. Sepsis
      2. Paralytic ileus
      3. Adhesions
   F. Medical management
      1. Pharmocologic: IV fluids, antibiotics
      2. Other: nasal gastric tube
   G. Surgical management
      1. Laparotomy to close perforations, drain abscesses

II. Analysis
   A. Pain related to peritoneal inflammation and irritation
   B. Infection related to contamination of intra-abdominal cavity
   C. Altered tissue perfusion: paralytic ileus related to severe peritoneal infection

III. Planning/goals, expected outcomes
   A. Client will be free from pain and discomfort
   B. Client will not develop sepsis
   C. Client will not develop paralytic ileus

IV. Implementation

A. Monitor vital signs every 1 to 2 hours as necessary
B. Give IV fluids as ordered to treat hypovolemic shock
C. Monitor for urine output greater than 30 mL per hour
D. Provide rest and quiet environment
E. Maintain NPO status and patency of NG tube
F. Give antibiotics as ordered
G. Assess for increasing distention
H. Encourage TC and DB exercises
I. Prepare client for surgery for peritoneal lavage, correction of cause, and possible bowel resection

IV. Evaluation
A. Client remains free of pain
B. Infectious process resolves
C. Client remains free of paralytic ileus

Appendicitis

I. Assessment
A. Definition: inflammation of appendix, commonly caused by accumulation of hard feces in appendix
B. Pathophysiology: appendix becomes enlarged and bacterial infection may occur in the wall; appendix may rupture, spilling contents of bowel into abdominal cavity
C. Incidence
1. Peak age 10 to 30 years
2. More common in males
D. Clinical manifestations
1. Persistent, continuous abdominal pain
2. Pain begins in mid-abdomen and progresses to McBurney's point in right lower quadrant (RLQ) halfway between umbilicus and iliac crest
3. Pain elicited upon light palpation with rebound tenderness and muscle rigidity
4. Nausea and anorexia
5. Elevation of temperature
E. Diagnostic examinations (see Table 8–7)
1. WBC
2. Abdominal x-ray
F. Complications
1. Perforation
2. Peritonitis
3. Abscess formation
G. Medical management: observation, rest, IVs, NPO, possibly antibiotics
H. Surgical management: appendectomy

II. Analysis
A. Pain related to inflamed appendix
B. High risk for infection related to rupture and peritonitis
C. Knowledge deficit related to diagnosis and treatment

III. Planning/goals, expected outcomes
A. Client will be free of pain
B. Client will not develop complications
C. Client will verbalize knowledge of surgical procedure

IV. Implementation
A. Avoid laxatives, enemas for clients with acute abdominal pain; increased peristalsis may cause rupture of appendix
B. Observe for signs of rupture and resulting peritonitis
1. Rigidity over entire abdomen as opposed to RLQ may indicate rupture
2. Initially, there is decrease in pain
3. Increase in temperature
C. May use ice for pain relief but never heat, which may cause rupture of appendix
D. Maintain NPO status during acute attack
E. Use alternative measures for pain relief—positioning, distraction; pain medications not used since they may mask symptoms
F. Administer IV fluids as ordered to maintain fluid and electrolyte status
G. Prepare client for appendectomy, which is the surgical removal of the appendix
H. Postoperative care: similar to other abdominal surgery; if appendix has not ruptured, recovery rapid

V. Evaluation
A. Client remains pain-free
B. Client remains free of complications

Chronic Conditions

Constipation

I. Assessment
A. Definition: difficulty or infrequency in passing of stool; constipation is a symptom of an alteration in GI function, not a disease
B. Predisposing/precipitating factors
1. Stress
2. Ignoring urge to defecate
3. Overuse of laxatives
4. Diet low in roughage, bulk fluids
5. Medications such as morphine, codeine, iron
6. Lack of exercise
7. Organic disease
C. Clinical manifestations
1. Small, hard, dry stool
2. Decrease in frequency from normal pattern
3. Difficulty passing stool
4. Abdominal distention, crampy pains, "bloating"
5. Anorexia
D. Diagnostic examinations (see Table 8–7)

1. Flexible sigmoidoscopy
2. LGI
  E. Complications
    1. Fecal impaction
    2. Bowel obstruction
    3. From laxative overuse
      a. Hypokalemia
      b. Hyponatremia
      c. Dehydration
  F. Medical management
    1. Pharmacological: laxatives (Table 8–14)
    2. Diet: increased fiber and fluids
  G. Surgical management (very controversial): recommended for
    1. Hirschsprung's disease
    2. Colonic inertia
    3. Rectocele
    4. Rectal intussusception, prolapse
II. Analysis
  A. Constipation related to precipitating factors
  B. Knowledge deficit related to predisposing factors
III. Planning/goals, expected outcomes
  A. Client will return to normal pattern of defecation
  B. Client will not develop complications
IV. Implementation
  A. Encourage regular time for defecation
  B. Teach client not to ignore urge
  C. Encourage pattern of regular exercise
  D. Teach client ways to minimize stress in lifestyle
  E. Teach client about foods high in bulk and residue, which help retain water in stool (see Table 8–4)
  F. Assess for abuse of laxatives and explain that continued laxative use does not allow the intestine to fill enough for normal defecation reflex to be felt; encourage gradual decrease in laxative use
  G. For hospitalized client, provide as normal a setting as possible: privacy and comfort, sitting position
  H. Implement preventive measures for high-risk clients
  I. Provide minimum of eight glasses of fluid (warm water or fruit juice) per day
  J. Give suppository, laxative, or stool softeners as ordered (see Table 8–14)
V. Evaluation

TABLE 8–14 Laxatives

Class	Example	Action	Common Side Effects	Nursing Implications
Saline laxatives	Magnesium hydroxide (MOM) Magnesium citrate	Osmotic effect pulls water into feces	Abdominal cramps; electrolyte disturbance with long-term use; hypermagnesemia with renal insufficiency	Take with glass of water on empty stomach; expect results in 2 to 6 hours with magnesium citrate and 4 to 8 hours with MOM
Stimulant laxatives	Cascara sagrada	Produce irritation of gastrointestinal mucosa, thus increasing peristalsis	Nausea and vomiting, discoloration of urine, loose stools, hypokalemia, fecal impaction	Administer at bedtime; administer with water on empty stomach; avoid overuse; expect results in 8 to 12 hours
	Bisacodyl (Dulcolax)		Cramping, rectal burning with suppository	Do not crush enteric-coated tablets; results seen in 6 to 12 hours after oral administration and 15 to 60 minutes after suppository
Bulk-forming laxatives	Psyllium hydrophilic mucilloid (Metamucil) Polycarbophil (Mitrolan)	Increase consistency of stool, thus stimulating normal motility and defecation	Abdominal fullness/cramps, intestinal impaction above stricture	Give with adequate fluid; results seen in 12 to 48 hours; crush or chew tablets thoroughly; avoid prolonged use
Lubricant-Emollient laxatives	Mineral oil	Prevent absorption of water from feces	Lipid pneumonia if aspirated; decreases absorption of fat-soluble vitamins; interference with postoperative anorectal wound healing; dependence with prolonged use	Best given in evening; give cold and with juice for easier ingestion; avoid long-term use; do not use to lubricate nasal passages
Stool softeners	Docusate calcium (Surfak) Docusate sodium (Colace)	Encourage fat and water to mix with and soften stool for easier passage	Occasional abdominal cramps	Encourage adequate fluid intake; results take 1 to 3 days

A. Client has normal pattern of bowel movements
B. Client is able to identify precipitating factors and methods to prevent constipation

Bowel Obstruction

I. Assessment
   A. Definition: inability of bowel contents to move through the small or large intestine; may be partial or complete; caused by:
      1. Organic causes—mechanical obstruction such as hernia, twisting of bowel (volvulus), inflammation, adhesions, tumors, impaction (most common)
      2. Paralytic ileus—neurogenic obstruction (decrease in peristalsis)
      3. Infarction—vascular obstruction (interference with blood supply)
   B. Pathophysiology: when bowel obstruction occurs, contents of bowel collect proximal to obstruction, resulting in distention and decreased absorption from the bowel; increased venous pressure may cause fluid to be lost into bowel peritoneal cavity and blood supply may be impaired from edema
   C. Clinical manifestations
      1. Small bowel obstruction
         a. Nausea and vomiting
         b. Mild abdominal distention
         c. Initially, increase in bowel sounds except in neurogenic obstruction
         d. Abdominal pain in rhythmic pattern
         e. Constipation or diarrhea for short period of time, in partial obstruction
      2. Large bowel obstruction
         a. Severe abdominal distention
         b. Mild, steady lower abdominal pain
         c. Constipation
         d. Vomiting rare
   D. Diagnostic examinations (see Table 8–7)
      1. Flat plate of abdomen
      2. CBC, electrolytes, BUN
      3. Barium enema with care
      4. Sigmoidoscopy
   E. Complications
      1. Rupture with peritonitis resulting
      2. Fluid and electrolyte imbalance; may be severe with small bowel obstruction
      3. Hypovolemic shock from fluid loss
      4. Strangulation of bowel with resulting gangrene
      5. Compromised/ischemic blood supply
   F. Medical management—usually for partial obstructions caused by impaired peristalsis: bedrest, NPO, IV fluids, stomach decompression via nasogastric tube, parenteral nutrition
   G. Surgical management—procedure varies with cause and location and condition of involved bowel

II. Analysis
   A. Pain related to abdominal distention
   B. Constipation related to inability of stool to pass through obstructed area
   C. High risk for infection (peritonitis), related to possible rupture
   D. Fluid volume deficit, potential related to nausea, vomiting, anorexia, nasogastric tube

III. Planning/goals, expected outcomes
   A. Client will be free from pain and discomfort
   B. Client will have normal pattern of defecation
   C. Client will not develop complications from bowel obstruction or possible surgical procedure
   D. Client will not develop fluid volume deficit

IV. Implementation
   A. Position client for optimal comfort; semi-Fowler's position may assist with breathing
   B. Give analgesics as ordered avoiding morphine and codeine because of side effect of decreasing intestinal motility
   C. Maintain bedrest and quiet environment
   D. Assist with self-care, including mouth care as needed
   E. Care of client with nasogastric or intestinal tube
      1. Nasogastric
         a. Salem: double-lumen tube, one lumen for suctioning gastric contents and other provides vent to limit pressure on gastric mucosa
         b. Levin: single-lumen tube for suctioning
         c. Ewald: large-diameter, single-lumen tube, generally used for lavage
      2. Intestinal: weighted with mercury at tip to encourage passage to intestine
         a. Cantor tube: single-lumen tube with mercury-filled balloon at tip, which is filled before insertion
         b. Miller-Abbott: double-lumen tube in which mercury inserted into one lumen to balloon tip after insertion
      3. Use: provide decompression of stomach or intestine and relieve obstruction if neurogenic obstruction cause
      4. Insertion
         a. Place rubber tubes in ice water to stiffen for easier insertion; lubricate tip
         b. Encourage client to relax and swallow as tube passes back of throat; intestinal tubes passed 2 inches per hour after in stomach

c. After insertion, tube connected to suction and checked for placement

5. Care
   a. Nasogastric tubes are taped in place, but intestinal tubes are not, to allow for passage into intestine
   b. Mark clearly two different lumens of Miller-Abbott so lumen with mercury is never suctioned
   c. Observe for advancement of tube or advance as ordered, usually 2 inches per hour
   d. Assess for effectiveness of tube, continued drainage, decreased abdominal distention, decreased pain, and return of bowel sounds

F. Assess fluid and electrolyte status, I & O, weight, skin turgor, hypokalemia, hyponatremia

G. Vital signs: an increase may indicate further obstruction, strangulation, or peritonitis

H. Maintain IV fluids as ordered

I. Prepare client for bowel surgery (see nursing care of client with bowel surgery under colorectal cancer)

J. Assess for decrease or return of bowel sounds

K. Measure abdominal girth every 2 to 4 hr

V. Evaluation
   A. Client remains free of pain and complications
   B. Client returns to normal pattern of defecation
   C. Client did not develop peritonitis
   D. Client did not develop fluid volume deficit

Hernia

I. Assessment
   A. Definition: protrusion of abdominal contents through opening or weakness in the abdominal wall (may be inguinal, ventral, umbilical, or hiatal)
      1. Reducible: contents can be manipulated to return to abdominal cavity
      2. Incarcerated or irreducible: segments of bowel caught and cannot be reduced; thus intestinal flow obstructed
      3. Strangulated: blood supply to trapped bowel is cut off
   B. Incidence
      1. Inguinal: increased incidence in men
      2. Ventral (incisional)
         a. Obesity
         b. Multiple abdominal incisions
         c. Malnutrition
      3. Hiatal
         a. Obesity
         b. Increased intra-abdominal pressure
   C. Clinical manifestations

1. Inguinal, ventral, or umbilical—swelling or bump in area of hernia that may always be there or may appear after activity that increases abdominal pressure
2. Hiatal
   a. May have no manifestations
   b. Heartburn
   c. Fullness with eating
   d. Manifestations increase when recumbent

D. Diagnostic examinations—depend on location of hernia (see Table 8–7)
   1. Barium swallow
   2. Esophagoscopy
   3. UGI or barium enema

E. Complications
   1. Inguinal, ventral, or umbilical
      a. Strangulation
      b. Bowel obstruction
   2. Hiatal
      a. Ulceration
      b. Esophagitis, gastritis
      c. Stenosis and obstruction

F. Medical management: hiatal only—antacids, H_2 antagonists

G. Surgical management
   1. Herniorrhaphy
   2. Hernioplasty

II. Analysis
   A. Pain related to protrusion of and pressure on herniated contents; hiatal, heartburn
   B. High risk for altered tissue perfusion: GI related to strangulation
   C. Anxiety related to impending surgery and new information on diagnosis
   D. Knowledge deficit related to proper postoperative body mechanics

III. Planning/goals, expected outcomes
   A. Client states he or she will be free of pain and discomfort
   B. Client will not develop complications from hernia or surgical procedure
   C. Client will have minimal anxiety pre- and post-surgery
   D. Client will demonstrate proper body mechanics

IV. Implementation
   A. Inguinal, ventral, or umbilical
      1. Utilize truss to support hernia from protruding
      2. Assess for ability to reduce hernia
      3. Assess for complications of bowel obstruction or strangulation
      4. Prepare client for surgery
      5. Postoperative care for herniorrhaphy
         a. Encourage client to support incision

when coughing to prevent strain on suture line

  b. Monitor and avoid urinary retention

  c. Utilize ice bags, scrotal support, and elevation for scrotal swelling common after inguinal surgery

  d. Teach to avoid heavy lifting for 6 to 8 weeks

  e. Teach proper body mechanics for lifting to prevent recurrence

  f. Observe for and teach client to report redness, swelling, or pain at incision

  B. Hiatal

    1. Encourage client not to lie down after meals and to eat slowly

    2. Discourage use of girdles or tight clothing

    3. Depending on severity of symptoms, a bland diet may be utilized

    4. Give antacids, H_2 antagonists as ordered

    5. Assist in planning weight reduction diet as needed

    6. Prepare for surgery if symptoms, esophagitis, or ulceration are severe; surgery aimed at restoring the stomach below diaphragm

    7. Care of client post-surgery will be similar to client who underwent gastric surgery or thoracic surgery depending on approach used; will have chest tubes with thoracic approach

V. Evaluation

  A. Client states he or she is free of pain

  B. Client did not develop complication of strangulation

  C. Anxiety is minimal

  D. Client able to demonstrate correct body mechanics

Anorectal Disorders

I. Assessment

  A. Definition

    1. Fissures: small cracks in mucosa of anal canal

    2. Abscess: pocket of bacteria and pus often caused by fissures; an acute manifestation

    3. Fistula: track that forms between anorectal canal and perianal skin; a chronic manifestation, often resulting from an infection

    4. Hemorrhoids: engorged rectal veins that may be internal or external

  B. Predisposing/precipitating factors

    1. Fissures: passing of hard, formed stool; may occur secondarily to underlying disease (inflammatory bowel disease, proctitis, leukemia, carcinoma, immunodeficient states)

    2. Hemorrhoids

      a. Straining with passage of stool

      b. Increases in venous pressure, standing, obesity, and pregnancy

      c. Portal hypertension from cirrhosis

  C. Clinical manifestations

    1. Hemorrhoids: itching, pain, bright red bleeding with defecation

    2. Abscess: foul-smelling pus, pain; if superficial, swelling, redness, tenderness, fever

    3. Anal fissure: painful defecation, burning, scant bleeding

  D. Diagnostic examinations—proctoscopy (see Table 8–7)

  E. Medical management

    1. Pharmacological: bulk-forming agents/laxatives PLUS:

      a. Fissures—topical anesthetics, sitz baths

      b. Hemorrhoids—sitz baths, topical anesthetics, anal hygiene

    2. Diet: high fiber, adequate fluid

  F. Surgical management

    1. Fissures (chronic)—sphincterotomy

    2. Abscess—incision and drainage

    3. Fistulas—fistulectomy

    4. Hemorrhoid—hemorrhoidectomy, external hemorrhoid tag removal with laser therapy, rubber band ligation

II. Analysis

  A. Pain related to irritation, pressure, sensitivity in recto-anal area

  B. Constipation related to ignoring the urge to defecate because of pain during elimination

  C. High risk for injury: bleeding, related to surgical procedure

  D. Anxiety related to impending surgery and embarrassment

III. Planning/goals, expected outcomes

  A. Client will be free from pain

  B. Client will have a minimum of three bowel movements per week

  C. Client will not develop complications from surgery

  D. Client will state decrease in anxiety

IV. Implementation

  A. Teach measures to prevent constipation

  B. Prepare client for surgical procedure

    1. Incision and drainage of abscess

    2. Fistulectomy

    3. Hemorrhoidectomy

  C. Postoperative care for anorectal surgery

    1. Medicate for pain as necessary; hemorrhoids very painful

    2. Encourage positioning that decreases pressure on rectal area

    3. Provide sitz baths as ordered

4. Observe for urinary retention, which is potential complication
5. Observe for potential complication of bleeding, which can occur 7 to 10 days after hemorrhoidectomy
6. Give stool softeners and bulk laxatives as ordered (see Table 8–14)
7. Teach measures to avoid constipation
8. Teach to not avoid urge to defecate after surgery because of fear of pain
9. Expect drainage after incision and drainage

V. Evaluation
   A. Client remains free of pain and discomfort
   B. Client has three bowel movements per week
   C. Client remains free of bleeding from surgical procedures

Malignancies

Oral Cancer

I. Assessment
   A. Definition: cancer of mouth can affect lips, oral cavity, and tongue
   B. Incidence
      1. 4% of cancers in males
      2. 2% of cancers in females
      3. 90% of oral cancers in persons age 45 to 70
      4. Most are squamous cell carcinomas
      5. 75% of oral cancers occur in persons over 60 years old
   C. Predisposing/precipitating factors
      1. Alcoholism
      2. Exposure to sun (lip cancer)
      3. Smoking, chewing tobacco
      4. Lack of oral hygiene
   D. Clinical manifestations
      1. Often asymptomatic until late in disease, painless sore that does not heal
      2. Lesions in mouth may appear initially as fissure or painless ulcer
      3. Lesions on tongue appear as hard, plaque-like ulcerated areas on one side
      4. As cancer progresses: tenderness, difficulty chewing, dysphagia, dysarthria, leukoplakia, erythroplakia
   E. Complications: metastasis to neck common with cancer of the tongue
   F. Diagnostic examinations: biopsy of suggestive lesion
   G. Medical management—may be combined with surgical management
      1. Pharmacological: chemotherapy, radiation
      2. Diet: nutritional support as indicated
   H. Surgical management: resectional surgery
II. Analysis

A. Knowledge deficit related to treatment plan and disease process
B. Altered oral mucus membrane related to pathological changes of surgery, radiation, chemotherapy
C. Altered nutrition: less than body requirements related to dysphagia, painful oral mucosa, anorexia
D. Disturbed body image related to disfigurement from lesion or surgery

III. Planning/goals, expected outcomes
   A. Client will be able to relate treatment plan and disease process to caregiver
   B. Client will learn mouth hygiene
   C. Client will maintain optimal weight and fluid intake
   D. Client will express fears and concerns about disfigurement and ways to cope

IV. Implementation
   A. Prevention: teach client to seek medical attention for any mouth lesion that does not heal within 2 to 3 weeks
   B. Care after mouth surgery
      1. Give pain medications as ordered
      2. Allow client to verbalize feelings about change in body image
      3. Position client either on side or high Fowler's to promote drainage of oral secretions
      4. Provide nonalcohol mouth care/rinses as ordered preventing trauma to suture lines
      5. Provide feedings as ordered depending on extent of surgery
         a. Monitor tube feedings if ordered (see Table 8–11)
         b. Initially, oral feedings may have to be placed in back of mouth with Ascepto syringe
         c. Provide soft diet, limiting hot or cold foods that may be irritating to suture line
         d. Be patient, listen carefully, encourage client to speak slowly, and use other means of communication for possible speech impairment
   C. Care during and after radiation
      1. Maintain patency with radioactive needles in mouth
      2. Provide frequent oral hygiene for symptoms of mouth dryness and mucositis
      3. Encourage brushing of teeth to decrease effects of tooth decay common after radiation therapy
   D. Encourage client to stop smoking
V. Evaluation
   A. Client able to relate disease process and treatment

B. Client able to demonstrate effective oral hygiene

C. Client is maintaining weight and adequate fluid intake

D. Client able to express fears and ways to cope

Cancer of the Esophagus

I. Assessment
  A. Incidence
    1. 2% of all cancer deaths
    2. Twice as high in males
    3. Peak age 60 to 79 years
    4. Most tumors are squamous cell carcinomas
  B. Predisposing/precipitating factors
    1. Alcoholism
    2. Smoking
    3. Achalasia
    4. History of hiatal hernia, strictures
  C. Clinical manifestations
    1. Dysphagia—first with solid foods, then liquids
    2. Regurgitation
    3. Feeling of fullness
    4. Foul-tasting mouth and breath odor
    5. Weight loss—late symptom
  D. Diagnostic tests (see Table 8–7)
    1. Barium swallow
    2. Esophagoscopy
    3. CT scan
  E. Complications
    1. Metastasis
    2. Aspiration pneumonia
    3. Esophageal perforation or fistula formation
  F. Medical management (may or may not be done in combination with surgery)
    1. Radiation
    2. Chemotherapy (see Ch. 6)
    3. Diet: supplements—TPN as indicated (see Table 8–11)
  G. Surgical management
    1. Esophagogastrostomy (removal of lower part of esophagus and part of stomach) and pyloroplasty
    2. YAG laser therapy—for nonresectable tumors
    3. Esophageal stent in esophagus to allow passage of food
II. Analysis
  A. Altered nutrition: less than body requirements, related to dysphagia, anorexia, vomiting
  B. Fluid volume deficit related to nausea, vomiting
  C. Disturbed body image related to postoperative disfigurement
  D. Impaired communication, potential related to treatment of lesion
  E. High risk of infection related to altered immunological responses secondary to chemotherapy and radiation
III. Planning/goals, expected outcomes
  A. Client will attain optimal body weight
  B. Client will be hemodynamically stable
  C. Client will learn to accept surgically induced disfigurement
  D. Client will be able to communicate effectively
  E. Client will not develop an infection
IV. Implementation
  A. Give pain medications as necessary
  B. Provide adequate nutrition, soft or liquid diet as necessary
  C. Provide small feedings in upright position
  D. Observe for respiratory infection
  E. Prepare for possible surgery, which may involve removal of portion of esophagus, replacement of esophagus with portion of colon and partial gastrectomy to reduce reflux of gastric acid into esophagus
  F. Postoperative care
    1. Encourage coughing and deep breathing because of high abdominal or thoracic incision
    2. Head of bed up at all times
    3. Observe for leakage from anastomosis
      a. Inflammation
      b. Low-grade fever
      c. Tachycardia
    4. Encourage expression of feelings
    5. Provide nutritional support as appropriate
      a. Provide gastrostomy feedings and care
      b. Progression of oral feedings slowly from liquids to soft, small feedings
V. Evaluation
  A. Client attains optimal body weight
  B. Client is hemodynamically stable
  C. Client is learning to accept ''new'' appearance
  D. Client communicates effectively
  E. Client did not develop an infection

Gastric Cancer

I. Assessment
  A. Incidence
    1. Twice as common in men (2 : 1)
    2. More common in nonwhite population
    3. Most frequent between ages 50 to 70
  B. Predisposing/precipitating factors
    1. Family history
    2. Environmental
    3. Pernicious anemia

4. 90% are adenocarcinomas of distal curvature

C. Clinical manifestations
1. Often asymptomatic until after metastasis occurs
2. Vague gastric complaints: discomfort, indigestion, eructation, vomiting, "fullness"
3. Anorexia
4. Nausea
5. Weight loss—late symptom
6. Pain—late symptom

D. Diagnostic examinations (see Table 8–7)
1. UGI
2. Endoscopy
3. CEA—elevated in late disease
4. Stomach biopsy

E. Complications: metastasis (see Table 8–3)

F. Medical management
1. Chemotherapy
2. Radiation
3. Dietary supplement as indicated (TPN)

G. Surgical management—depends on location and advancement:
1. Antrectomy and vagotomy, removal of adjacent lymph
2. Total gastrectomy
3. Palliative resection
4. Billroth II

II. Analysis
A. Altered nutrition: less than body requirements related to gastric obstruction, nausea, vomiting
B. Fluid volume deficit related to gastric obstruction or perforation
C. Pain related to pathological process
D. Anticipatory grieving related to diagnosis of cancer
E. Anxiety related to anticipating surgical procedure

III. Planning/goals, expected outcomes
A. Client will attain optimum nutrition
B. Client will maintain normovolemic state
C. Client will state decrease or absence of pain
D. Client will develop outlets to express grief
E. Client will relate an increase in psychological comfort

IV. Implementation
A. See again nursing care for gastric surgery (see Table 8–9)
B. Encourage expression of feelings and explain all procedures
C. Provide diet or feedings to minimize anorexia and promote adequate nutrition
1. Small, more frequent feeding
2. Assess preferences and provide
3. Attractive appearance

V. Evaluation
A. Client attains optimal weight
B. Client maintained normovolemic state
C. Client relates absence of pain
D. Client able to share grief with spouse
E. Client states he or she is less anxious

Colorectal Cancer
I. Assessment
A. Incidence
1. Common type of cancer in men and women
2. Increases after age 40, peaks after age 60
3. Most are adenocarcinomas

B. Predisposing/precipitating factors
1. Family history of polyposis, colorectal cancer
2. Polyps
3. Inflammatory bowel disease
4. Diet high in animal fat, beef, and refined sugars and low in fiber
5. Blood in stool

C. Clinical manifestations
1. Change in shape or consistency of stool (narrowing of stool)
2. Bright red blood in stool
3. Constipation or diarrhea
4. Weakness
5. Anorexia
6. Weight loss and pain—late symptoms
7. Rectal or abdominal pain
8. Feeling of incomplete emptying

D. Diagnostic examinations (see Table 8–7)
1. Rectal examination
2. Stool for occult blood
3. Barium enema
4. Colonoscopy, sigmoidoscopy
5. CEA—used to identify recurrence or spread
6. Biopsy

E. Complications
1. Metastasis
2. Bowel obstruction
3. Perforation with peritonitis

F. Medical management
1. Radiation therapy (see Ch. 6)
2. Chemotherapy (see Ch. 6)
3. Diet: supplemental—TPN as indicated (see Table 8–11)

G. Surgical management—depends on location and size of tumor
1. Bowel resection (for stages I, II, and III colon cancers) and anastomosis:
   a. Anterior rectosigmoid resection
   b. Hemicolectomy, right or left
   c. Abdominoperineal resection with colostomy

II. Analysis
   A. Preoperative
      1. Constipation/diarrhea related to colorectal obstruction by tumor
      2. Anxiety related to new diagnosis of cancer
      3. Pain related to ulceration, obstruction
   B. Postoperative
      1. Knowledge deficit related to colostomy care
      2. Pain related to postoperative swelling and manipulation in surgery
      3. High risk for infection related to bowel surgery

III. Planning/goals, expected outcomes
   A. Preoperative
      1. Client will have relief of constipation/diarrhea
      2. Client will express less anxiety after disease teaching
      3. Client will state a decrease or absence of pain
   B. Postoperative
      1. Client will demonstrate correct colostomy care
      2. Client will state a decrease or absence of pain
      3. Client will not have infection postoperatively

IV. Implementation
   A. Teach American Cancer Society recommendations for early detection of colorectal cancer
      1. Yearly rectal exam after age 40
      2. Fecal occult blood studies after age 50
      3. Flexible sigmoidoscopy every 3 to 5 years after two negative examinations after age 50
   B. Encourage verbalization of feelings
   C. Prepare client for surgery
      1. Right hemicolectomy: removal of tumor in ascending colon and reanastomosis of bowel
      2. Left hemicolectomy: removal of tumor in descending colon with reanastomosis
      3. Abdominoperineal resection: removal of tumor of lower sigmoid colon or rectum with proximal intestine brought to the surface, forming a colostomy and rectum either sutured closed or packed and left open to heal
   D. Provide preoperative bowel preparation as ordered
      1. Give low-residue diet (see Table 8–10 for low-residue diet)
      2. Give enemas and laxatives to cleanse bowel

      3. Give antibiotics that are poorly absorbed in GI tract to decrease intestinal bacteria
         a. Phthalylsulfathiazole (Sulfathalidine)
         b. Kanamycin sulfate (Kantrex)
         c. Neomycin sulfate
         d. Erythromycin
   E. Provide postoperative care to promote normal elimination and healing, decrease pain, and prevent complications of atelectasis, infection, thrombophlebitis, and fluid and electrolyte imbalance
      1. Encourage coughing and deep breathing
      2. Encourage early ambulation and leg exercises
      3. Give pain medications as needed
      4. Maintain patency of NG tube until peristalsis returns
      5. Monitor vital signs, and bowel and lung sounds
      6. Provide necessary assistance with self-care
      7. Administer IV fluids as ordered
      8. Monitor for fluid and electrolyte imbalance—I & O, skin turgor, mucous membranes, laboratory values
      9. Monitor incision for redness, swelling, and discharge
      10. Provide ostomy care and teaching (see Table 8–12)
      11. Perineal wound
         a. Maintain patency of wound drains
         b. Observe and record drainage; initially expect large amount of serosanguineous drainage
         c. Provide irrigation or sitz bath to wound as ordered
         d. Utilize T-binder to secure dressing
      12. Monitor for hemorrhage, shock, and urinary retention after abdominoperineal resection
      13. Observe for and teach client about colostomy complications: prolapse of stoma (usually due to obesity), perforation (due to improper stoma irrigation), stoma retraction, fecal impaction, and skin irritation
   F. Provide support for clients with advanced disease who may also require chemotherapy

V. Evaluation
   A. Preoperative
      1. Constipation resolved (by radiation, chemotherapy, or surgery)
      2. Client states anxiety more manageable after learning about colorectal cancer and treatment
      3. Client states pain is absent
   B. Postoperative

1. Client demonstrates good colostomy care
2. Client did not have infection during post-operative course
3. Client states absence of pain

POST-TEST Gastric/Biliary/Exocrine Pancreas/Lower Intestinal Disorders

Jane Harrison, a 25-year-old computer programmer, is admitted to the hospital with a diagnosis of ulcerative colitis. She is having eight to ten liquid stools per day.

1. Jane calls the nurse and states she has had blood in her stool. The nurse should:
   1. Call the physician for new orders
   2. Explain this commonly occurs with this disorder
   3. Check the stool for occult blood
   4. Check vital signs more frequently
2. An important nursing intervention during the acute phase of the disease is to:
   1. Ambulate client four times a day
   2. Reassure client not to worry
   3. Provide room with nearby bathroom or commode
   4. Encourage coughing and deep breathing
3. Which of the following dietary goals would be LEAST appropriate for Jane after the acute phase?
   1. Increase calories
   2. Increase protein
   3. Increase carbohydrates
   4. Increase fiber

John Rooks, a 34-year-old banker, is admitted to the emergency room because of hematemesis. He has a history of indigestion and stomach pains.

4. Initially, the nurse would want to further assess for signs and symptoms of:
   1. Renal failure
   2. Shock
   3. Infection
   4. Hypoglycemia
5. After vital signs are stabilized, the physician orders a gastroscopy. The nurse explains to the client that:

1. A general anesthetic will be used
2. He will be placed in a knee-chest position
3. He will feel no discomfort
4. His throat will be numbed during the procedure

6. A duodenal ulcer is found. John remains in stable condition. He is started on antacids four times a day orally and ranitidine (Zantac) 150 mg orally four times a day. While taking a history of John's previous abdominal pain, the nurse notes complaints consistent with duodenal ulcers. These would include pain that:
   1. Is relieved by food
   2. Occurs in lower abdomen
   3. Occurs more frequently in recumbent position
   4. Is accompanied by fever and chills
7. An appropriate client goal to prevent ulcer recurrence is to:
   1. Eat three low-fat meals a day
   2. Minimize situations that produce high stress
   3. Use ASA instead of Tylenol for pain relief
   4. Limit coffee to four cups per day
8. Which of the following would demonstrate correct client knowledge regarding administration of medications?
   1. "I'll take antacids half an hour before meals."
   2. "I'll take ranitidine four times a day as needed for stomach pain."
   3. "I'll take medications for entire time ordered."
   4. "I'll expect stool to be white from antacids."
9. John returns to the hospital for a gastric resection after two more bleeding episodes. Initially after surgery, which of the following would be a cause for concern?
   1. Bright red drainage in NG tube
   2. Moderate abdominal pain
   3. Negative bowel sounds
   4. Increasing abdominal distention
10. Two weeks postoperative, John complains of nausea, bloating, sweating, and headaches after meals. This is most likely related to:
    1. Return of ulcer
    2. Infectious process
    3. Rapid entry of food into intestine
    4. Loss of vagal stimulation
11. The nurse would encourage John to do which of the following to relieve the above symptoms?
    1. Eat a high-carbohydrate, high-protein diet
    2. Eat small, more frequent meals
    3. Drink fluids during meals
    4. Remain in sitting position after eating

POST-TEST Answers and Rationales

1. ② The stools of a client with ulcerative colitis in the acute stage may have blood, mucus, and pus in them. This is not cause for alarm, but should be recorded along with the number of stools per day to determine effectiveness of therapy. 4, II. Ulcerative Colitis.

2. ③ A nearby bathroom or commode will potentially ease anxiety and embarrassment and prevent incontinence related to increased urgency of frequent diarrhea stools. The client should be encouraged to rest, not ambulate, and to verbalize feelings. 4, II. Ulcerative Colitis.

3. ④ After the acute stage, a diet that provides calories, carbohydrates, and protein is necessary to maintain or rebuild optimal weight. A high-fiber diet is irritating to the healing of the lower GI tract. 3, II. Ulcerative Colitis.

4. ② The priority concern when treating a client with an actively bleeding ulcer is the loss of blood and possible hypovolemic shock. The other options are not related to ulcers. 1, I & II. Peptic Ulcer Disease.

5. ④ Xylocaine, a local anesthetic, is used to numb the throat to prevent gagging. A sedative may be given, but generally the client is awake in a sitting or recumbent position. A small amount of discomfort may be felt because of the tube in the throat. 4, I & II. Peptic Ulcer Disease.

6. ① Ulcer pain generally is in the epigastric region and relieved by the ingestion of food or antacids. With a gastric ulcer, pain is increased by food. 1, II. Peptic Ulcer Disease.

7. ② Stress, coffee, and aspirin are predisposing/precipitating factors in the development of peptic ulcer disease and should be eliminated. A regular diet, eliminating personal intolerances, is recommended. 3, II. Peptic Ulcer Disease.

8. ③ Medications should be taken as long as prescribed to allow adequate time for ulcer to heal, which is generally 4 to 6 weeks. Antacids are given 1 hour after meals. Ranitidine is taken on a regular basis as ordered, not as needed. Antacids do not turn the stool white. 5, II. Peptic Ulcer Disease.

9. ④ Gastric distention is a serious problem because of potential pressure exerted on the new suture line. The other symptoms are normal in the immediate postoperative period. 2, I. Gastric Resection.

10. ③ The stomach and pyloric valve act as a reservoir and gate allowing small amounts of food into the duodenum. After gastric surgery, food quickly enters the intestine. The highly concentrated food pulls fluid into the intestine, producing a decrease in fluid volume and increase in peristalsis. This and the rapid entry of glucose into the bloodstream and resulting insulin secretion cause the symptoms referred to as dumping syndrome and related postprandial hypoglycemia. 2, I. Dumping Syndrome.

11. ② The symptoms of dumping syndrome can be relieved by eating small frequent meals low in carbohydrates, avoiding fluids during meals, and lying recumbent after eating. 4, I & II. Dumping Syndrome.

PRE-TEST Hepatic Disorders

1. Which of the following disorders poses the most risk of transmission to health care workers?
   ① Hepatitis A
   ② Hepatitis B
   ③ Cirrhosis of the liver
   ④ Hepatitis A and hepatitis B
2. A client who consumed contaminated shellfish would most likely develop:
   ① Hepatitis A
   ② Hepatitis B
   ③ Hepatitis C
   ④ Delta hepatitis

John Smith, a 40-year-old unemployed truck driver, is admitted to your unit. His history includes many years of excessive alcohol abuse. Tomorrow he is scheduled for a liver biopsy and you are assigned to care for him.

3. Prior to his liver biopsy, it is most important for you to:
   1. Assess John's vital signs
   2. Verify that compatible donor blood is available
   3. Verify that hemostasis and blood coagulation tests have been completed and charted
   4. Ensure that John has been NPO since midnight

4. Mr. Jones, a client you have been assigned to, has just been diagnosed with viral hepatitis. When caring for him, the most important nursing precaution/intervention is:
   1. Gowning, gloving, and wearing a mask when caring for him
   2. Good handwashing before, during, and after his care
   3. Utilizing disposable items when caring for him
   4. Calling Mr. Jones's physician to administer the hepatitis vaccine immediately

5. One of your clients has been placed on a 2-g low-sodium diet. Which of the following foods would you advise him to AVOID?
   1. Smoked ham, sausage, or bacon
   2. Canned soup and vegetables
   3. Sauerkraut, tomato juice, creamed vegetables
   4. All of the above

6. One of the nursing measures recommended to protect persons exposed to clients with hepatitis type B is:
   1. Institute blood and body fluid precautions
   2. Institute blood precautions only
   3. Give hepatitis A vaccine
   4. Give hepatitis C vaccine

7. In treating a client with hepatic encephalopathy, the nurse should remember:
   1. That the client will be on a high-protein diet to promote liver regeneration
   2. That neomycin may be administered to increase the ammonia-producing organisms in the GI tract
   3. That clinical manifestations of impending coma include a disorientation to time, place, and person
   4. All of the above

Robert Anderson is admitted to your unit with the diagnosis of Laennec's cirrhosis. You are assigned to care for him.

---

8. In view of Mr. Anderson's diagnosis, you know that sedatives will be contraindicated. Which of the following best explains this rationale?
   1. The liver's ability to synthesize protein is altered
   2. Sedatives may mask the signs of impending coma
   3. The liver's ability to detoxify drugs is decreased
   4. Sedatives may cause mental confusion

9. The suggested diet for Mr. Anderson will be:
   1. High calorie, high protein
   2. High calorie, low protein
   3. Low calorie, high protein
   4. Low calorie, low protein

PRE-TEST Answers and Rationales

1. ② Hepatitis B is the most transmissible to health care workers. It is transmitted by contact with contaminated blood or blood products. 1, I. Hepatitis

2. ① One of the modes of transmission of hepatitis A is through shellfish caught in contaminated water. 1, I. Hepatitis.

3. ③ Hemostasis and coagulation tests are essential to assess for bleeding tendencies related to altered clotting. 1, I & II. Cirrhosis.

4. ② Handwashing is the most important precaution when caring for a client with viral hepatitis. Gowning and gloving are necessary when handling infected material or if soiling is likely. 4, I. Hepatitis.

5. ④ All of the items are foods to avoid on a low-sodium diet. 4, II. Cirrhosis

6. ② Clients with hepatitis B should be placed on blood and body fluid precautions. 4, I. Hepatitis.

7. ③ Clinical manifestations of impending coma include a disorientation to time, place, and person. 1, I & II. Hepatic Encephalopathy.

8. ③ The liver's ability to detoxify drugs is decreased, because the normal liver cells have been replaced by scar tissue. 4, II. Cirrhosis.

9. ① A high-calorie, high-protein diet is recommended for clients with cirrhosis to promote liver cell regeneration. 3 & 4, II. Cirrhosis.

NURSING PROCESS APPLIED TO ADULTS WITH HEPATIC DISORDERS

Infectious Diseases

Viral Hepatitis

I. Assessment
   A. Definition: inflammation of the liver
   B. Pathophysiology (Table 8–15)
      1. Regardless of mode of transmission, pathophysiology is same
      2. Hepatitis virus invades, replicates, and produces widespread inflammation and causes changes in liver cell architecture and liver cell damage
      3. There is proliferation and enlargement of Kupffer's cells, portal duct inflammation with lymphocytes and monocytes, bile stasis, and degeneration and regeneration of the liver cells with eventual necrosis
      4. In most patients, liver cells regenerate with no residual damage
      5. If no complications occur, liver usually resumes normal function and appearance
      6. Degree of impairment depends on amount of liver cell impairment
      7. Most clients recover normal liver function
   C. Types: differ in mode of transmission, incubation period, severity, and virus
      1. Hepatitis A: formerly called infectious hepatitis
      2. Hepatitis B: formerly called serum hepatitis
      3. Hepatitis C: usually with hepatitis B
      4. Delta hepatitis: usually with hepatitis B
   D. Etiology/Incidence
      1. Most common viral infection
      2. Hepatitis A
         a. Most common type of viral hepatitis
         b. Caused by hepatitis A virus (HAV)
         c. Transmitted primarily via fecal–oral route, contaminated water, food, or shellfish caught in contaminated water
         d. After infection, lifelong immunity
         e. Incubation period 15 to 45 days
         f. Abrupt onset
         g. Worldwide prevalence
         h. Most common among young children, middle aged, and individuals living in crowded conditions
         i. Higher during fall and winter months
         j. Short, acute course
         k. Signs and symptoms develop 2 to 7 days before onset of jaundice
         l. New, experimental vaccine
      3. Hepatitis B
         a. Caused by hepatitis B virus (HBV)
         b. Transmitted by infected blood and/or blood products, parenteral drug use, or by direct contact with infected body fluids and contaminated objects
         c. Incubation period 30 to 180 days
         d. Occurs at any age, affects all age groups
         e. Insidious onset

TABLE 8–15 Comparison of Four Types of Hepatitis

Factor	Hepatitis A	Hepatitis B	Hepatitis C	Delta Hepatitis
Incidence	Endemic in areas of poor sanitation, common in fall and early winter	Worldwide, especially in drug addicts, clients and others exposed to blood and blood products; occurs all year	Post-transfusion, those working around blood and blood products; occurs all year	Found in conjunction with hepatitis B
Incubation period	15 to 45 days	28 to 180 days	7 to 8 weeks	Same as hepatitis B
Risk factors	Close personal contact or by handling feces, contaminated wastes	Health care workers in contact with blood and blood products; hemodialysis and post-transfusion clients, homosexually active males and drug abusers	Same as for hepatitis B	Same as hepatitis B
Mode of transmission	Infected feces, fecal–oral route; may be airborne if copious secretions; shellfish from contaminated water; also parenteral	Parenteral, sexual contact, and fecal–oral route	Contact with blood and body fluids	Co-infects with hepatitis B, close personal contact
Severity	Usually not fatal	More serious, may be fatal	Not known	Increased mortality with hepatitis B
Diagnostic tests	IgM positive in acute, IgG positive after infection	HB$_s$AG, HB$_c$AG, and HB$_e$AG positive	Not identified	HD Ag positive
Vaccine	Experimental	Hepatitis B vaccine	None	None

f. Vaccine available (Engerix-B)
g. Worldwide incidence
h. Highest incidence in young adults, parenteral drug users, health care workers, hemodialysis clients, recipients of blood transfusions, sexual partners of infected individuals
i. No seasonal preference
j. More serious than hepatitis A or C
4. Hepatitis C
a. Caused by unidentified virus
b. Transmitted parenterally through blood, personal contact, possible fecal–oral route
c. Most common form of post-transfusion hepatitis
d. Incubation period 7 to 8 weeks
e. Insidious onset
f. Intermediate acute and chronic course of illness
g. Affects all ages
h. Worldwide incidence
i. No seasonal preference
5. Delta hepatitis (see Table 8–15): found with hepatitis B
E. Predisposing/precipitating factors
1. May also be caused by nonviral substances such as alcohol, chemicals, and drugs

2. Hepatitis A
a. Associated with poor sanitation or overcrowding
b. Virus found in blood, feces, saliva, and urine of infected individuals
c. Experimental vaccine for active immunity
d. Once clinical manifestations appear, transmission potential decreases
3. Hepatitis B
a. Virus found in all body fluids and secretions; blood, saliva, semen, and tears
b. Health care workers at high risk due to close contact with blood of carriers
c. Lifetime immunity after infection
d. Vaccine available
4. Hepatitis C
a. Degree of immunity following infection not determined
b. No vaccine available
c. Client becomes carrier after infection
5. Delta hepatitis
a. Same as hepatitis B
b. No vaccine available
F. Clinical manifestations: range from asymptomatic to three phases.
1. Pre-icteric (prodromal phase): period of maximal communicability

a. Precedes jaundice—flu-like symptoms
b. Malaise
c. Weight loss
d. Anorexia—major manifestation
e. Extends from 1 to 21 days
f. Most contagious period
g. Nausea
h. Vomiting
i. Constipation
j. Diarrhea
k. Distaste for cigarettes if smoker
l. Decreased sense of smell
m. Low-grade fever
n. Headache
o. Hepatomegaly
p. Lymphadenopathy
q. Fatty foods intolerance

2. Icteric phase
a. Lasts 4 to 6 weeks
b. Characterized by jaundice as bilirubin metabolism is disrupted
c. Pruritus
d. Fatigue
e. Weight loss
f. Dark, bile-colored urine that foams when shaken
g. Light or clay-colored stools (acholic)
h. Hepatomegaly with tenderness
i. Lymphadenopathy
j. Fever subsides when jaundice occurs
k. Yellow sclerae and skin
l. Hepatitis C not associated with icteric phase

3. Post-icteric phase
a. Convalescent stage
b. Jaundice diappears, but does not mean total recovery
c. Lasts 2 weeks to 4 months
d. Malaise
e. Easily fatigued
f. Hepatomegaly
g. Relapse may occur

G. Diagnostic examinations
1. Client history
2. Blood tests (see Table 8–15)
a. Enzymes
(1) Transaminase (aminotransferase)
(a) SGOT (AST): serum glutamic-oxaloacetic transaminase; alanine aminotransferase elevated
(b) SGPT (ALT): serum glutamic pyruvate transaminase; aspartate aminotransferase elevated; indicates liver cell injury peak at onset and fall during recovery may be more than eight times normal during clinical disease
(2) Alkaline phosphatase; elevated due to impaired excretory function of liver
(3) Lactate dehydrogenase (LDH): elevated in obstructive jaundice; indicates liver cell injury

b. Proteins
(1) Serum albumin: decreased due to impaired hepatic synthesis of albumin
(2) Gamma globulin: increased impaired hepatic synthesis of protein

c. Serum bilirubin (total): elevated, indicates liver cell damage

d. Prothrombin time: increased, due to decreased and impaired vitamin K absorption in the intestine and decreased production of prothrombin by the liver

e. Complete blood count: increased WBC—inflammation; decreased RBC, hemoglobin, hematocrit—liver's inability to store hematopoietic factors

f. Hepatitis serology
(1) Hepatitis A: confirmed by presence of hepatitis A antibodies in the serum (anti-HAV) or stool; antibodies against virus of two types:
(a) IgM: appear early at onset of disease and then taper off; indicate present infection, confirm diagnosis
(b) IgG: remain in blood indefinitely; generally give immunity to client; indicate client does not have acute infection, but has had it in the past
(2) Hepatitis B: presence of hepatitis B surface antigens (HB_sAg) in serum and/or hepatitis B antibodies (anti-HB_s); peaks just before onset of jaundice and disappears by the third month
(3) Hepatitis C: if above tests negative in client with clinical symptoms of viral hepatitis, hepatitis C is suspected; no specific laboratory test at present; diagnosed by excluding hepatitis A and hepatitis B; no antigens or antibodies are found in either A or B virus
(4) Delta hepatitis: hepatitis D surface antigen (HD_sAg) identified

3. Urine tests
a. Urinary bilirubin: elevated due to conjugated bilirubin

    b. Urinary urobilinogen: elevated due to diminished reabsorption of urobilinogen

H. Complications

  1. Most clients recover without complications

  2. Mortality rate low

  3. Higher in older individuals and those with underlying debilitating diseases

  4. Chronic persistent hepatitis

  5. Chronic active or aggressive hepatitis

  6. Fulminant viral hepatitis

  7. Cirrhosis of the liver (postnecrotic cirrhosis)

II. Analysis

A. Fatigue related to impaired liver functioning

B. Altered nutrition: less than required related to decreased appetite

C. High risk for altered skin integrity related to pruritus

D. Fluid volume deficit related to decreased fluid intake

E. Knowledge deficit related to disease, treatments, long-term restrictions

F. Ineffective individual coping related to bedrest and prognosis

III. Planning/goals, expected outcomes

A. Client will achieve adequate rest

B. Client will maintain adequate nutritional intake

C. Client will maintain intact skin

D. Client will maintain adequate hydration

E. Client will cooperate with prescribed treatment

F. Client verbalizes understanding of hepatitis

G. Client verbalizes or expresses feelings and concerns

IV. Implementation

A. Assist client to achieve adequate rest

  1. Maintain bedrest during the acute phase as prescribed

  2. Increase activities as tolerated when feasible

  3. Provide rest periods before and after activities and treatments

  4. Schedule activities and treatments to avoid disturbing rest periods and allow maximum rest

  5. Decrease environmental stimuli

  6. Keep frequently used objects within reach

  7. Promote rest by utilizing comfort measures—for example, give back massage, change linens, adjust position

  8. Assist client in planning specific rest periods

  9. Provide quiet environment

  10. Provide care in unhurried manner

B. Maintain adequate nutrition (Table 8–16)

TABLE 8–16 Dietary Management for the Client with Hepatitis

Objective	To aid in the regeneration of liver tissue, prevent further liver damage, maximize protein utilization
Calories	High caloric intake: 3000 to 4000 per day
Protein	1.5 to 2 g protein per kg of body weight or 100 to 150 g of protein per day needed to promote regeneration of liver cells and to prevent fatty infiltration of liver
Sources	Meat, milk, poultry, eggs, fish, dried beans, cheese, dairy products
Fat	Moderate: if fat content poorly tolerated then decrease amount; 100 to 150 g per day, weight gain more rapid and palatability of diet increased
Sources	Whole milk, cream, butter, margarine, meat, vegetable and palm oil
Carbohydrate	300 to 400 g per day ensures adequate glycogen reserves needed for liver function maintenance, protects against further liver injury, protein-sparing action
Sources	Potatoes, bread, cereal, pasta
Vitamins	Vitamin B supplements may be added to aid in metabolism of carbohydrates, protein, fats, and vitamin B_{12}; vitamin K if there are bleeding tendencies
Special Considerations	No alcohol secondary to toxic effect on liver; abstinence for at least 4 to 6 months recommended; client must be encouraged to eat; serve foods attractively

1. Monitor I & O

2. Check weight daily

3. Monitor serum albumin and electrolyte levels daily

4. Offer and provide frequent mouth care, especially before meals

5. Minimize unpleasant sights and odors near patient

6. Assess and document medications that may be contributing to loss of appetite

7. Provide pleasant surroundings during meals to increase appetite

8. Offer largest meal at breakfast

9. Maintain calorie count

10. Consult with dietitian as needed

11. Avoid very hot or very cold foods

12. Administer antiemetics (nonphenothiazines) one half hour before meals to prevent nausea/vomiting, if allowed

13. Instruct client to avoid alcohol for 6 months

14. Provide supplemental vitamin K or B complex as necessary

15. Encourage family to bring in food if possible
16. Assess food likes and dislikes as allowed
17. Encourage small frequent meals high in calories (2000 to 3000 calories per day), protein (70 to 100 g), and carbohydrates (300 to 400 g) and moderate in fat (100 to 150 g)
18. Parenteral or enteral nutrition if anorexia severe

C. Maintain tissue integrity
1. Maintain clean, dry skin
2. Bathe client with cool water and baking soda
3. If itching severe, may use calamine lotion
4. Provide diversional activities
5. Instruct client on importance of avoiding scratching skin if possible
6. Use antihistamines with caution
7. Avoid use of soap
8. Encourage client to keep nails short and wear gloves at night if necessary
9. Provide frequent skin care with lotion and frequent linen changes
10. Encourage client to wear light clothing
11. Provide cool environment

D. Maintain client comfort
1. Provide adequate rest
2. Use analgesics with caution
3. Avoid ASA and aspirin-containing products because of potential bleeding
4. Provide alternate methods of pain relief
5. Assess for nonverbal cues of pain
6. Convey to client that total comfort may not be achievable
7. Pace care activities appropriately to client's pain level
8. Discuss comfort measures with client
9. Provide diversional activities
10. Assess and document client's response to pain relief measures
11. Assess previous coping mechanisms for pain

E. Maintain adequate hydration
1. Monitor I & O
2. Weigh client daily
3. Initiate parenteral fluids with electrolyte replacement if necessary
4. Monitor lab values, electrolytes, blood urea nitrogen (BUN), creatinine, hemoglobin, hematocrit
5. Monitor for ascites and/or edema formation
6. Offer fluid of client's choice at bedside
7. Encourage fluids to at least 3000 mL per day
8. Assess skin turgor and mucous membranes

F. Prevent infection
1. Establish isolation techniques (Table 8–17)
2. Use meticulous handwashing
3. Place on enteric precautions (hepatitis A) and blood and body fluids (hepatitis B)
4. Do not recap needles to avoid contamination and self-injury
5. Private room if client fecally incontinent or has poor personal hygiene
6. Bag, label, and discard articles contaminated with infected material
7. Teach client importance of handwashing
8. Wear gloves when handling items that may be contaminated with urine or feces, bedpans, linens, instruments, or linens soiled by body excretions
9. Explain isolation protocol; wear gown if in direct contact with the client's blood or feces
10. Prevention
   a. Hepatitis A
      (1) Administration of immune serum globulin (ISG) before or after exposure to type A hepatitis
      (2) Good handwashing practices
      (3) Good personal hygiene
      (4) Enteric precautions and isolation

TABLE 8–17 Isolation Precautions for Hepatitis

	Hepatitis A	Hepatitis B	C and Delta Hepatitis
Mask	No, unless copious respiratory secretions	No	No
Gloves	Yes, for handling infective material	Yes, for handling infective material	Yes, for handling infective material
Private Room	If client's hygiene poor or if incontinent	No	No
Transmission	Feces	Blood and body fluids	Blood and body fluids
Length of Precautions	7 days after onset of jaundice	Until client is HB_gA_g negative	Duration of illness

b. Hepatitis B
   (1) Blood and body fluid precautions
   (2) Practice good handwashing
   (3) Administer hepatitis B vaccine if individual at risk
   (4) Hepatitis B immune globulin (H-BIG) after exposure to hepatitis B antigen-positive blood (needle stick or mucous membranes)
   (5) Dispose of needles properly
   (6) Wear gloves, gown when direct contact anticipated with blood and body fluids, needles, blood specimens
   (7) No blood donation
c. C and delta hepatitis
   (1) Use blood precautions, wash hands, have minimal contact with blood, wear gloves
   (2) Discard needles with caution and place in appropriate containers
   (3) Place blood, feces, or body secretions in sterile containers, and label ''hepatitis''
   (4) Terminal disinfection of areas grossly contaminated with feces or blood of hepatitis client
   (5) Use disposable equipment if possible
   (6) No blood donation
G. Educate client about disease and disease transmission
   1. Emphasize necessity for follow-up treatment and examinations
   2. Avoid nonprescription medications; explain dangers
   3. Explain importance of adequate rest, ingesting a well-balanced meal, and avoiding alcohol
   4. Avoid sharing personal items
   5. Avoid mucous membrane contact with other individuals with hepatitis B
   6. Assess level of understanding of disease process
   7. Explain restrictions for blood donations
   8. Stress importance of good personal hygiene and careful handwashing
   9. Caution client not to engage in sexual contact until serum liver function tests return to normal
H. Help client cope with illness
   1. Support client and encourage to verbalize feelings, concerns, and questions
   2. Encourage client to maintain daily grooming routine
   3. Provide privacy as necessary
   4. Emphasize rationale for isolation

5. Establish trusting and nonjudgmental relationship/attitude
V. Evaluation
   A. Client is well rested
   B. Client's nutritional status balanced with adequate caloric intake; weight maintained
   C. Client's skin integrity maintained and itching relieved
   D. Client verbalizes reasonable comfort, physical appearance of comfort
   E. Client maintains adequate hydration; mucous membranes and skin turgor within normal limits
   F. Client verbalizes reasons for prescribed restrictions, causes of hepatitis, and measures that assist in preventing transmission of hepatitis
   G. Client indicates comprehension of disease process
   H. Client verbalizes concerns about therapy and disease

Cirrhosis

I. Assessment
   A. Definition: chronic, progressive, degenerative disease of the liver in which there are structural changes in liver
   B. Pathophysiology: cirrhosis is end result of pathological changes associated with liver disease; normal liver cells damaged and replaced by scar tissue or fibrosis, decreasing amount of normal liver tissue; this scar tissue distorts normal liver structure and ultimately interferes with flow of blood through liver; with structural changes and loss of normal liver tissue, normal functions altered, leading to liver dysfunction
   C. Types
      1. Laennec's cirrhosis: also called portal, nutritional, or alcoholic cirrhosis
      2. Postnecrotic cirrhosis: also called posthepatitis or toxin-induced cirrhosis
      3. Biliary cirrhosis
      4. Cardiac cirrhosis
   D. Incidence/etiology
      1. Laennec's cirrhosis
         a. Most common in North America, higher incidence among men
         b. Incidence higher among clients with chronic alcohol abuse, malnourished with vitamin and protein deficiency
      2. Postnecrotic cirrhosis: related to scar tissue formation following toxic or viral hepatitis
      3. Biliary cirrhosis: related to prolonged

biliary obstructive jaundice or to an infection

4. Cardiac cirrhosis: related to congestive long-standing heart failure

E. Pathophysiology

1. Alcohol has a direct toxic effect on liver cells
2. Final stage of liver injury
3. Normal liver architecture disrupted
4. Alcohol results in massive disruption of normal liver function and hepatic lobules
5. Liver cell destruction occurs with formation and replacement of fibrotic scar tissue and liver nodules
6. Normal liver tissue replaced by scar tissue with necrosis and regeneration of liver cells
7. Liver nodules distort morphology of liver and obstruct hepatic flow of blood and lymph
8. An increase in fibrous tissue distorts normal structure of hepatic lobules
9. Compresses blood, lymph, and bile channels, altering flow of these fluids through the liver, resulting in severe physiological damage and derangement
10. Obstruction of blood and lymph results in backflow of blood in portal vein, causing increased pressure in portal vein (drains blood from digestive organs) or portal hypertension
11. As normal tissue replaced by scar tissue, blood flow through liver obstructed
12. Increased pressure in portal vein causes increased blood flow around liver and reverse flow of blood
    a. Stasis and eventual enlargement (dilation) of the umbilical, esophageal, and rectal veins, resulting in liver dysfunction, varices and changes in portal circulation
    b. Fluid retention, ascites, accumulation of large quantities of fluid within peritoneal cavity
    c. Insufficient removal of metabolic wastes
13. As disease progresses, various toxic substances are unable to be metabolized by cirrhotic liver and accumulate in brain, resulting in hepatic encephalopathy or coma
14. If disease caught early, early changes characterized by fatty infiltration of liver; disease is reversible if client abstains from alcohol ingestion; if alcohol intake continues, scar tissue forms, eventually causing liver to shrink in size

F. Clinical manifestations

1. Often subtle, insidious
2. Disease may go unrecognized for many years
3. Nonspecific and vague early symptoms
4. Disease progresses slowly
5. Most manifestations related to pathophysiology
6. History of failing health
7. Nausea, vomiting, anorexia, dyspepsia, change in bowel habits, weakness, indigestion, fatigue, flatulence, constipation, abdominal discomfort
8. Hepatomegaly, weight loss, jaundice
9. Edema of extremities, ascites, hemorrhoids, hematemesis, emaciation, splenomegaly, prominent abdominal wall veins (caput medusae), bleeding tendencies, anemia, esophageal varices
10. Spider nevi, angiomas, palmar erythema, altered hair distribution
11. Delirium, changes in thinking and mental function
12. Oliguria

G. Diagnostic examinations

1. Blood tests
    a. Enzymes
        (1) SGOT (AST): serum glutamate oxaloacetic transaminase; alanine aminotransferase elevated, released from damaged liver cells
        (2) SGPT (ALT): serum glutamate pyruvate transaminase, aspartate aminotransferase elevated, released from damaged liver cells
        (3) LDH: lactic dehydrogenase elevated; indicates liver injury
        (4) Alkaline phosphatase: elevated in obstructive jaundice or biliary obstruction, due to reduced excretion in bile
    b. Proteins
        (1) Serum albumin: decreased, due to impaired synthesis of albumin
        (2) Serum globulin: elevated, due to increased synthesis by reticuloendothelial system
        (3) Serum ammonia: elevated, due to impaired liver ability to convert (detoxify) ammonia to urea
    c. Hemostasis
        (1) Prothrombin time: prolonged, due to impaired synthesis of prothrombin and/or impaired vitamin K absorption
        (2) Complete blood count: decreased hemoglobin, hematocrit, platelet count, white blood cells, and red

blood cells due to liver's inability to store hematopoietic factors

d. Lipid and carbohydrate tests
   (1) Serum cholesterol: decreased, reflecting impaired hepatic synthesis
   (2) Serum bilirubin: elevated in jaundice due to regurgitation of conjugated bilirubin into blood from liver cell destruction or obstruction of biliary tract

2. Urine tests
   a. Urinary bilirubin: increased, more urinary excretion of conjugated bilirubin, decreased ability of liver to process bilirubin reduction products
   b. Urinary urobilinogen: increased, more urinary excretion of conjugated bilirubin, decreased ability of liver to process bilirubin reduction products
   c. Urinalysis: dark, bile-colored urine

3. Radiological studies
   a. Esophagoscopy
      (1) Purpose: used to verify presence of esophageal varices and/or bleeding
      (2) Procedure: visual examination, using flexible fiberoptic scope, of lining of esophagus, stomach, and upper duodenum
      (3) Pre-procedure
         (a) Fast for 6 to 12 hours before test
         (b) Inform patient that flexible instrument will be passed through mouth and into esophagus
         (c) Performed by physician; takes about 30 minutes
         (d) Will receive local anesthetic in mouth; may taste bitter and make swallowing difficult
         (e) Will receive sedative before procedure to assist in relaxation
         (f) Consent required
         (g) Need to remove dentures
         (h) Assess client allergies
      (4) Post-procedure
         (a) Observe client for possible perforation; if perforation occurs, client will complain of pain with swallowing and with neck movement
            Thoracic perforation: produces substernal or epigastric pain that increases with breathing

Diaphragmatic perforation: produces shoulder pain and dyspnea
            Gastric perforation: causes abdominal or back pain
         (b) Check vital signs every 15 minutes for 4 hours, every hour for 4 hours, then every 4 hours
         (c) Withhold food and fluid until gag reflex returns
         (d) Inform client of possible sore throat; provide lozenges

   b. Abdominal x-rays: show organ displacement and liver enlargement
   c. Mesenteric angiography: detects area of upper gastrointestinal bleeding
   d. Ultrasound: detects biliary obstruction
   e. Liver scan: decreased uptake in liver from intrahepatic shunts that bypass liver cells
   f. Upper GI (barium contrast esophagography) barium swallow: may show ulcer
      (1) Pre-test
         (a) Nothing by mouth 12 hours before the test
         (b) Takes about 30 minutes
         (c) Instruct client about milkshake consistency and chalky taste of the barium preparation
         (d) Must drink 12 to 14 oz; performed in x-ray lab
      (2) Post-test
         (a) Administer cathartic, if ordered
         (b) Inform patient that stools may be chalky and light colored for 24 to 72 hours
         (c) Notify physician if client has not expelled barium in 2 to 3 days
   g. Liver biopsy
      (1) Procedure: needle aspiration of a segment of liver tissue for histologic analysis
      (2) Purpose: establish definite diagnosis
      (3) Pre-test
         (a) Nothing by mouth for 4 to 8 hours before the test
         (b) Takes about 10 to 15 minutes; consent required
         (c) Check prothrombin time, platelet count

(d) Have client void before test

(e) Local anesthetic used

(f) Instruct client on how to breathe during biopsy; prior to biopsy needle insertion and during biopsy (25 seconds), client must be able to hold breath

(g) Assess client's allergies

(h) Instruct client on avoiding sudden movement or coughing during procedure to avoid trauma

(i) Explain that frequent assessment will be made, including vital signs and biopsy site inspections

(4) Contraindications: thrombocytopenia, prolonged prothrombin time, peritonitis, massive ascites, uncooperative client

(5) Post-procedure

(a) Place client on right side with small pillow or sandbag under costal margin for extra pressure

(b) Maintain bedrest for 24 hours

(c) Assess biopsy site and vital signs every 15 minutes for 1 hour, every 30 minutes for 2 hours, then every hour for 6 hours, then every 4 hours for 24 hours

(d) Report any decreased blood pressure, bleeding at biopsy site, increased temperature, or severe pain at site

(e) Assess for any signs of shock

(f) Client may resume normal diet

(g) Assess for respiratory distress or signs of peritonitis

(h) Document tolerance to procedure and disposition of tissue specimen

II. Analysis

A. Altered nutrition: less than body requirements related to poor appetite and altered taste

B. Activity intolerance related to impaired liver function

C. High risk for altered skin integrity related to pruritus

D. High risk for injury related to bleeding from decreased prothrombin level

E. Fluid volume deficit: Intravascular related to fluid volume excess: ascites

F. High risk for noncompliance related to lifestyle alteration from stopping alcohol

G. High risk for injury related to altered mental status

H. Altered breathing pattern related to ascites

I. Ineffective individual coping related to concern about illness and treatments, need for alteration in lifestyle

III. Planning/goals, expected outcomes

A. Client will improve or maintain adequate nutritional intake

B. Client will achieve adequate rest

C. Client will maintain skin integrity

D. Client will not develop bleeding or exhibit signs of bleeding

E. Client will return to normal fluid volume state

F. Client will comply with prescribed treatment

G. Client's mental status will not deteriorate

H. Client's breathing pattern will remain within normal limits

I. Client will verbalize feelings and concerns about illness and/or treatment modalities

IV. Implementation

A. Provide adequate nutritional intake (Table 8–18)

1. Monitor I & O

2. Weigh client daily

3. Consider client preferences in food choices

4. Assist with meals as necessary

5. Monitor serum albumin and electrolyte levels daily

6. Offer and provide frequent mouth care

7. Encourage small, frequent meals and nourishing snacks

8. Administer vitamin and mineral supplements as ordered

9. Promote bedrest to reduce metabolic demands on liver

10. Encourage client to eat

11. Encourage high calories (3000 calories per day), high carbohydrates (300 to 400 g per day), protein (70 to 100 g per day, if precoma), and moderate fat (100 to 150 g per day), low sodium (500 to 1000 mg/day) (see Table 8–18)

12. Serve meals in an environment conducive to eating

13. Discuss need for nasogastric tube (NG) with physician if needed

14. If hepatic encephalopathy present or serum ammonia levels rise, *limit* dietary protein

15. Soft diet may be necessary if client has esophageal varices

16. If client has edema or ascites, restrict sodium and protein

B. Protect client fom excessive fatigue

1. Maintain bedrest or limit activities; gradu-

TABLE 8–18 Dietary Management for the Client with Cirrhosis

Objective	Liver regeneration occurs if appropriate diet therapy initiated before disease well advanced; adequate intake of food has been replaced by alcohol
Protein	According to tolerance; with increasing liver damage, protein metabolism hindered; intake must be adjusted as disease progresses or improves; 1 to 1.5 g of protein per kg of body weight or 65 to 95 g per day; protein intake restricted to less than 35 g daily if signs of impending coma develop; encourage high biological value proteins
Sources	See Table 8–16
Fat	Malabsorption of fats may occur along with an intolerance to fats; moderate intake; if tolerated poorly, decrease amount; 100 to 150 g per day
Sources	See Table 8–16
Carbohydrate	300 to 400 g per day
Sources	See Table 8–16
Calories	High caloric intake: 3000 calories per day
Vitamins	Malabsorption of fat soluble and B complex vitamins occurs in cirrhosis; vitamin B supplementation may be necessary to replenish liver stores and repair tissue damage
Sodium	Restricted if edema and ascites present; severe restriction of sodium may be necessary for effective removal of excess fluid; low sodium usually restricted to 500 to 1000 mg per day; instruct client to avoid foods processed with salt or sodium-based preservatives; close attention to food selection in order to provide adequate protein intake
Sources	Contain high sodium: canned soups and vegetables, cured meats, crackers, catsup
Special Considerations	No alcohol; reduction in fiber content with provision of soft foods if there are esophageal varices, to prevent rupture and/or bleeding; a liquid diet may also be used; monitor medications for sodium content

ally increase activity as tolerated when condition stabilizes to conserve client strength

2. Promote rest by utilizing comfort measures
3. Provide quiet environment

C. Prevent altered skin integrity
1. Use Eggcrate mattress or sheepskin
2. Reposition every 2 hours
3. Avoid the use of soap and adhesive tape
4. Apply oil-based lotions
5. Massage around reddened areas, bony prominences
6. Maintain good handwashing
7. Assess skin for breakdown
8. Change linens frequently
9. Cut client's fingernails short; client may need to wear gloves to avoid scratching

10. Avoid shearing forces
11. Maintain clean, dry skin; cleanse perianal area after each stool
12. If itching severe, use calamine lotion

D. Provide for client comfort
1. Assess level of pain/discomfort
2. Avoid hepatotoxic drugs; i.e., morphine sulfate, codeine, propoxyphene (Darvon), acetaminophen, phenothiazines
3. Use alternate methods of pain relief
4. Utilize non-narcotic, nonaspirin analgesics
5. Offer emotional support
6. Inform client that total relief of discomfort may not be possible
7. Assess for nonverbal cues of pain
8. Pace care activities appropriately to client's pain level
9. Offer frequent comfort measures; i.e., backrub, turn frequently

E. Prevent bleeding
1. Monitor for signs and symptoms of bleeding
2. Provide soft foods and avoid roughage
3. Monitor lab values (prothrombin time [PT], partial thromboplastin time [PTT], hemoglobin, hematocrit, platelet count)
4. Administer stool softeners as ordered
5. Assess stool for blood
6. Avoid IM injections; if necessary, rotate sites, use small-gauge needles, and apply pressure to site
7. Inspect gums, test urine and emesis for blood
8. Avoid use of razor and toothbrush; use toothettes and electric razor
9. Administer vitamin K as prescribed
10. Report any evidence of bleeding to physician immediately
11. Pad side rails
12. Instruct client to avoid straining at stool, nose blowing, and so on
13. Observe client for signs of bleeding or shock
14. Provide IV fluids as ordered
15. If client has an NG tube, maintain patency
16. Maintain and monitor Sengstaken-Blakemore tube (Figure 8–1)
17. Provide gentle nursing care

F. Maintain fluid balance
1. Monitor I & O
2. Weigh client daily
3. Measure abdominal girth and extremities daily
4. Monitor serum and urine electrolytes
5. Administer diuretics as ordered (see Table 4–1)

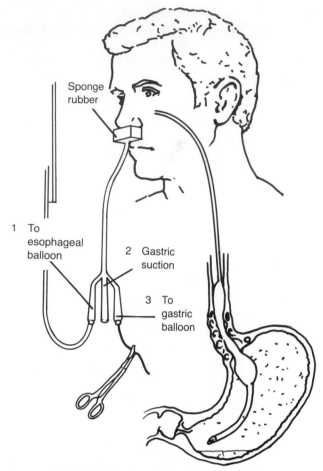

FIGURE 8–1. Sengstaken-Blakemore tube.

Sponge rubber

1 To esophageal balloon

2 Gastric suction

3 To gastric balloon

6. Provide frequent mouth care with nonalcohol mouth washes
7. Assess skin turgor
8. Change position frequently
9. Administer albumin as ordered
10. Use ice chips sparingly
11. Monitor sodium and fluid intake and maintain sodium and fluid restriction if ordered (1000 to 1500 mL per 24 hours)
12. Elevate client's limbs
13. Monitor vital signs
14. Monitor fluid loss; not to exceed 1 kg per day

G. Assist client to comply with prescribed therapy
1. Determine client's pattern of alcohol abuse
2. Stress importance of avoiding alcohol and complying with therapy
3. Emphasize importance of good nutrition
4. Assist client in identifying support persons
5. Emphasize importance of rest
6. Avoid judgmental attitude

7. Assist client with identifying hepatotoxins to avoid
8. Emphasize the importance of taking only medications prescribed by a physician (Table 8–19)
9. Refer client and/or family members to Al-Anon
10. Inform client about physical limitations
11. Emphasize the importance of follow-up care
12. Provide diversional activities of interest to client

H. Monitor for signs of mental deterioration
1. Have client demonstrate signature daily
2. Protect client from injury that can be precipitated by confused state
3. Provide safety measures
4. Assess for fetor hepaticus
5. Avoid use of tranquilizers and sedatives
6. Assess client's orientation to time, place, person
7. Assess for asterixis
8. Supervise ADLs and provide assistance
9. Instruct client not to get out of bed unassisted
10. Side rails up
11. Assess neurological status
12. Administer neomycin, if ordered, if mental status changes (see Table 8–19)
13. Monitor ammonia levels
14. Administer lactulose if ordered (see Table 8–19)
15. Provide continuity of care
16. Monitor protein intake, decrease if necessary (see Table 8–18)
17. Provide adequate hydration
18. Note changes in client's behavior
19. Obtain baseline assessment of client's personality

I. Maintain normal respiratory function
1. Reposition frequently
2. Administer supplemental oxygen as needed
3. Assist abdominal paracentesis as needed
4. Place client in semi- or high Fowler's position
5. Monitor ABGs; notify physician of findings
6. Encourage deep breathing and coughing if secretions present
7. Use incentive spirometer
8. Assess for signs of infection, increased temperature, chills, diaphoresis, adventitious breath sounds
9. Monitor chest x-ray
10. Monitor vital signs, temperature, lung sounds

TABLE 8–19 Medications Used in the Treatment of Cirrhosis

Class	Example	Action	Common Side Effects	Route	Nursing Implications
Blood derivative	Albumin	Blood volume expander; increases plasma oncotic pressure; assists in maintaining intravascular volume by shifting fluid from interstitial spaces to circulation resulting in reabsorption of ascitic fluid and enhanced renal perfusion	Vascular overload after rapid infusion, hypotension, urticaria, chills, fever, dehydration, heart failure	IV infusion	Assess for circulatory overload—signs and symptoms of pulmonary edema or heart failure; STOP infusion immediately if cough, dyspnea, cyanosis, or rales occur; assess for diuresis and decrease in edema; monitor blood pressure and pulse closely; avoid rapid infusion; monitor I & O, weight, protein, hemoglobin, hematocrit, and electrolytes during therapy
Antibiotic, aminoglycoside	Neomycin	Reduces number of bacteria in colon that normally convert urea and amino acids of proteins into ammonia and other toxic metabolites; can reach high antibacterial concentration in colon without causing systemic toxicity; destroys normal bacterial flora of the bowel	Nausea, vomiting, nephrotoxicity, rash, urticaria, lethargy, electrolyte imbalance, hypersensitivity reactions	PO, NG tube, rectal (enema)	Monitor weight; obtain baseline renal functions before therapy; monitor renal function daily (BUN, creatinine, creatinine clearance); notify physician if there are signs of decreased renal function; monitor hearing; notify physician if tinnitus, vertigo, or hearing loss occur; hearing loss may occur several weeks after drug discontinued; may need to administer laxative after dosage
Synthetic posterior-pituitary hormone	Vasopressin (Pitressin)	Reduces portal blood pressure; produces vasoconstriction of mesenteric arteriolar bed; slows blood flow into portal system, decreases variceal bleeding in GI tract	Sweating, hypersensitivity, angina, tremor, bradycardia, abdominal cramping, skin blanching, cardiovascular complications, hypertension	Peripheral intravenous or intra-arterial infusion	Monitor heart rate and blood pressure during infusion; monitor IV site frequently for warmth, pulse, color, if peripheral infusion; monitor I & O; monitor body weight; monitor lab values—prothrombin time, partial thromboplastin time, platelet count, hemoglobin, hematocrit; assess if bleeding has decreased
Ammonia detoxicant, laxative	Lactulose (Cephulac)	Synthetic derivative of the sugar lactose causes a decrease in blood concentration of ammonia in clients with portal-systemic encephalopathy; reaches lower digestive tract without changes or absorption; colonic bacterial enzymes convert it to lactic and acetic acids,	Nausea, vomiting, cramps, flatulence, fluid and electrolyte imbalances, gaseous distention, belching, increase in number of bowel movements per day	PO, NG tube, rectal (enema)	To decrease sweet taste, dilute with water or fruit juice; when administered by NG tube, dilute well to prevent clogging NG tube; administer carefully to diabetic patients due to sugar concentrations; monitor blood sugar levels; monitor serum sodium; acts within 30

Table continued on following page

TABLE 8–19 Medications Used in the Treatment of Cirrhosis *Continued.*

Class	Example	Action	Common Side Effects	Route	Nursing Implications
		which lower colon's pH, making it an acid environment and unfavorable to bacterial growth; acidification of colon's contents converts ammonia to ammonium ion thus reducing concentration of ammonia, allowing more ammonia to diffuse from blood to colon where ammonium ion can be evacuated with feces; laxative action of lactulose speeds this evacuation; reduces serum ammonia levels by 25 to 50%			minutes; report GI distress to physician; assess serum K^+ to evaluate if drug causing further potassium loss; monitor serum ammonia levels; monitor changes in level of consciousness; monitor number and consistency of stools per day
Loop diuretic	Furosemide (Lasix)	Inhibits reabsorption of Na and Cl in ascending loop of Henle, resulting in excretion of Na^+, Cl^-, K^+, and water	Hypokalemia fluid and electrolyte imbalances, hyperglycemia, hearing loss, abdominal discomfort, orthostatic hypotension, fatigue	PO or IV	Monitor blood pressure and heart rate; monitor serum electrolytes; BUN, CO_2; may need to supplement potassium; monitor for signs of hypokalemia; consult with physician to provide high potassium diet; administer in morning to prevent nocturia; administer with meals to avoid GI upset; monitor diabetic patients for signs of hyperglycemia; protect IV dose from light
Thiazide diuretic	Chlorothiazide (Diuril)	Increases urinary excretion of sodium and water by inhibiting sodium, potassium, and water reabsorption in the proximal tubule	Hypokalemia, hyperglycemia, orthostatic hypotension, unusual fatigue, vertigo, photosensitivity	PO or IV	Monitor I & O, weigh client daily; monitor serum electrolytes and glucose, blood urea nitrogen, creatinine daily; consult with physician and dietitian to provide high potassium diet; monitor for signs of hypokalemia (weakness, cramps); administer in the morning to prevent nocturia; monitor vital signs; assist client to sit up slowly; may need to supplement potassium
Diuretic, aldosterone antagonist, potassium-sparing	Spironolactone (Aldactone)	Blocks action of sodium-retaining effects of the hormone aldosterone, which causes sodium and chloride retention; increases excretion of sodium and water but spares potassium	Hyperkalemia, hyponatremia, drowsiness, diarrhea/cramps, lethargy, dry mouth	PO	Monitor blood pressure; potassium supplements are not used with this class of drug; monitor serum potassium levels; monitor I & O; weigh client daily; assess client for tolerance to drug; watch for edema

TABLE 8–19 Medications Used in the Treatment of Cirrhosis *Continued.*

Class	Example	Action	Common Side Effects	Route	Nursing Implications
					and decreased urine output
Vitamin B complex (B_1)	Thiamine	Water-soluble vitamin	Hypersensitivity, pruritus, urticaria, sweating, tightness in throat, weakness	PO or IV	Use parenteral only when PO route not feasible; do not administer IV push; test client's skin before treatment if there is history of hypersensitivity; be prepared to treat anaphylaxis AFTER large parenteral dose; thiamine deficiencies usually require concurrent treatment for multiple deficiencies
Vitamin B complex (B_9)	Folic acid	Required to maintain normal levels of mature red blood cells; stimulates production of red and white blood cells	Flushing of face, sweating, weakness, chills, fever, dizziness, a sense of constriction of chest (usually after IV administration)	PO, SQ, or IM	Monitor prothrombin time to determine dosage effectiveness; assess patient for side effects; use large doses cautiously in clients with severe hepatic disease; store in dark place; inform client that temporary pain or swelling may occur after SQ or IM injection

11. Monitor laboratory values, check for anemia
12. Use sterile technique with all procedures
13. Avoid contact with persons with infections
14. Maintain good handwashing practices
  J. Encourage client to express feelings
    1. Encourage client/family to ask questions
    2. Encourage client to maintain daily grooming
    3. Provide privacy as needed
    4. Establish trusting and nonjudgmental relationship/attitude
    5. Encourage client and family to participate in care
    6. Present accepting attitude
V. Evaluation
  A. Adequate nutrition maintained for metabolic needs
  B. Client well-rested, no demonstration of signs and symptoms of fatigue
  C. Client's skin integrity maintained
  D. Client verbalizes comfort and demonstrates no signs of discomfort
  E. Client does not experience any bleeding

  F. Client's fluid volume adequate; client's abdominal girth and peripheral edema decreases
  G. Client verbalizes importance of adhering to therapy and participates in care
  H. Client oriented to time, place, and person
  I. Client's breathing pattern is within normal limits
  J. Client verbalizes causes of disease and body changes

Complications of Cirrhosis

Portal Hypertension and Esophageal Varices
I. Assessment
  A. Definition: elevated pressure in the portal vein
  B. Pathophysiology: cirrhosis causes structural changes in liver, resulting in obstruction of normal flow of blood through portal system and interruption of blood flow through and out of liver; a rise in portal venous pressure occurs and as a result, portal hypertension develops; blood backs up into spleen and flows through collateral channels that develop to venous system bypassing liver; as portal pressure increases, these vessels dilate, leading to esoph-

ageal, rectal, and abdominal varices; these vessels inadequate to accommodate increased blood flow and may hemorrhage; esophageal varices are dilated, tortuous veins in lower esophagus

C. Etiology: disease processes that alter or damage flow of blood through liver or its major vessels
   1. Alcohol ingestion
   2. Increased abdominal pressure
   3. Nausea, vomiting, straining at stool
   4. Coughing or sneezing, lifting heavy objects

D. Clinical manifestations: result from three pathological changes: splenomegaly, formation of collateral channels, and ascites
   1. Enlarged spleen
   2. Internal hemorrhoids
   3. Ascites
   4. Hematemesis
   5. Melena
   6. Massive hemorrhage
   7. Shock

E. Diagnostic examination
   1. Endoscopy: may demonstrate source of bleeding
   2. Mesenteric angiography: demonstrates collateral circulation or bleeding site
   3. Barium studies

F. Medical management
   1. Pharmacological: vasopressin (Pitressin) therapy constricts splanchnic veins, promotes arteriolar vasoconstriction, decreases portal pressure; may halt hemorrhage but does not prolong life; temporary measure (see Table 8–19)
   2. Local therapy: sclerotherapy
      a. Passage of a fiberoptic endoscope into esophagus
      b. Bleeding site identified, and sclerosing agent (morrhuate sodium) injected or administered directly into varices causing thrombosis and sclerosis
      c. May be repeated as necessary for patients who are poor surgical risks
   3. Sengstaken-Blakemore tube
      a. Temporary measure
      b. Three lumens—gastric, esophageal, and gastric
      c. Two ballons—gastric and esophageal
      d. Applies pressure on bleeding site
      e. Applies direct pressure to bleeding varices in lower esophagus and upper stomach
      f. May also administer iced saline lavage through gastric lumen
      g. May need to suction client, as client unable to swallow saliva
      h. Decompress after 24 hours
      i. Inflation of esophageal balloon to pressure of 20 to 40 mm Hg will compress esophageal varices
      j. Deflate esophageal balloon for 5 to 10 minutes every 8 to 12 hours to prevent esophageal necrosis
      k. Monitor vital signs
      l. Keep head of bed elevated 30 to 45 degrees
      m. Intermittent gastric suctioning

G. Surgical management
   1. Shunts: classified according to influence on portal hemodynamics; reduces portal hypertension by diverting blood and bypassing the liver but allowing adequate liver perfusion; does not prolong life; types:
      a. LeVeen or Denver shunt
      b. Portal systemic shunt
      c. Portal caval shunt

II. Analysis: high risk for injury related to bleeding or shock

III. Planning/goals, expected outcome: client will not develop symptoms and signs of shock or bleeding

IV. Implementation
   A. Assess for signs and symptoms of shock, such as changes in blood pressure, heart rate, respiratory rate; cool, clammy skin; changes in mental status; decreased urine output
   B. Monitor laboratory values, hemoglobin, hematocrit
   C. Administer blood transfusions as ordered
   D. Monitor I & O
   E. Monitor for transfusion reaction
   F. Perform gastric lavage with iced saline as ordered by physician
   G. Advise client to avoid straining at stool
   H. Provide client with soft foods and avoid roughage
   I. Administer lactulose, neomycin as ordered
   J. Maintain patency of NG tube
   K. Assess vital signs, neurological status, respiratory status, fluid and electrolytes, and renal status every 15 to 30 minutes
   L. Administer antacids as ordered
   M. Assist with insertion of Sengstaken-Blakemore tube
   N. Provide IV fluids as ordered
   O. Provide gentle nursing care

V. Evaluation: client shows no manifestations of GI bleeding

Peripheral Edema and Ascites

I. Assessment
   A. Definition: fluid accumulation in the peritoneal or abdominal cavity and peripherally
   B. Pathophysiology: as portal pressure increases within liver, congestion of lymph channels occurs, and plasma proteins (albumin) leak through liver capsule into peritoneal cavity; osmotic pressure of proteins pulls additional fluid into peritoneal cavity, resulting in ascites; hypoalbuminemia also occurs from liver's inability to synthesize albumin, resulting in decreased colloidal osmotic pressure; as a result of damaged liver cells, impaired metabolism of aldosterone occurs, resulting in increased amounts of sodium retained by renal tubules; retention of sodium together with an increase in antidiuretic hormone causes additional water retention; peripheral edema occurs as result of impaired liver synthesis of albumin and increased portal pressure from portal hypertension
   C. Etiology
      1. Portal hypertension
      2. Decreased plasma colloid osmotic pressure
   D. Clinical manifestations
      1. Abdominal distention with weight gain
      2. Bulging flanks
      3. Protruding umbilicus
      4. Abdominal striae
      5. Dehydrated appearance
      6. Sunken eyeballs
      7. Muscle weakness
      8. Dull sound upon percussion of abdomen
      9. Fluid wave upon tapping the abdomen
      10. Ankle and presacral edema
   E. Diagnostic examinations
      1. Abdominal x-rays
      2. Ultrasound
      3. Computed tomography (CT) scan
      4. Paracentesis
         a. Purpose: to assist in determining cause of ascites; to relieve pressure
         b. Procedure: aspiration of fluid from peritoneal space through needle or trocar inserted into the abdominal wall; no more than 1000 to 1500 mL removed at a time; temporary, palliative measure
         c. Pre-test
            (1) Signed consent
            (2) Instruct client to void immediately prior to procedure
            (3) Explain procedure to alleviate anxiety
            (4) Place client in upright position to facilitate removal of fluid
            (5) Emphasize importance of avoiding sudden movement or coughing to prevent trauma to peritoneal organs
            (6) Record baseline vital signs, weight, abdominal girth for post-test comparison
            (7) Assist in making client as comfortable as possible
            (8) Local anesthetic used at site of fluid removal
         d. Post-test
            (1) Apply sterile pressure dressing to site
            (2) Assist client in finding comfortable position
            (3) Monitor client's vital signs every 15 minutes for 1 hour, every 30 minutes for 2 hours, every 1 hour for 4 hours, or more frequently as necessary
            (4) Note color, amount, and character of any drainage
            (5) Monitor dressing for drainage every 15 minutes
            (6) Assess for vertigo, faintness, diaphoresis, pallor, tachycardia, hypotension; if any of these develop, call physician
            (7) Measure client's abdominal girth
            (8) Assess urine output every 1 to 2 hours

II. Analysis: high risk for fluid volume deficit (intravascular) related to fluid volume excess (ascites and extracellular)
III. Planning/goals, expected outcomes: adequate fluid volume maintained
IV. Implementation
   A. Monitor daily weight
   B. Monitor I & O, aim loss at not more than 1 kg per day
   C. Measure abdominal girth and extremities daily
   D. Assess skin turgor
   E. Administer diuretics as ordered
   F. Monitor serum and urine electrolytes
   G. Perform frequent mouth care
   H. Restrict fluid intake if ordered
   I. Restrict sodium (1000 mg per day) and protein (80 to 100 g per day) intake
   J. Administer salt-poor albumin if ordered; in clients with ascites only, not more than 0.5 kg per day
   K. Maintain bedrest, reposition every 2 hours

L. Prepare client for shunt if necessary

V. Evaluation

A. Decrease or absence of peripheral edema

B. Abdominal girth decreases

Hepatic Encephalopathy and Coma (Portal-Systemic Encephalopathy)

I. Assessment

A. Definition: metabolic encephalopathy of brain associated with liver impairment characterized by impaired mentation and altered level of consciousness; cerebral intoxication caused by intestinal contents not being metabolized by liver

B. Pathophysiology: in liver cell damage and necrosis, liver can no longer convert ammonia to urea; as a result of this decreased detoxification ability, blood ammonia rises; ammonia a cerebral toxin; in addition, blood shunted from portal system directly into systemic circulation, bypassing liver; large amounts of ammonia remain in systemic circulation

C. Clinical manifestations

1. Disorientation to time, place, and person

2. Changes in mental and neurological responsiveness

3. Personality changes

4. Confusion

5. Inability to perform self-care activities

6. Asterixis or liver flap, characteristic sign

7. Fetor hepaticus

8. Deterioration in handwriting

9. Can develop rapidly or insidious

10. Slow, slurred speech

11. Sleep–wake reversal pattern

12. Muscle incoordination

13. Impaired intellectual function

14. Coma

15. Hyperventilation with respiratory acidosis

D. Predisposing/precipitating factors

1. Infection

2. GI hemorrhage

3. Hypovolemia

4. Cerebral depressants

5. Paracentesis

6. Fluid and electrolyte disturbance, especially hypokalemia

7. High protein intake

E. Diagnostic examinations

1. Serum arterial ammonia levels: increased

2. Serum electrolytes: decreased potassium, metabolic alkalosis

3. Blood glucose: increased

4. EEG: abnormal

II. Analysis

A. Altered thought process related to increased serum ammonia levels

B. Altered skin integrity related to pruritus

III. Planning/goals, expected outcomes

A. Client will not develop altered thought process from increased serum ammonia

B. Client will maintain skin integrity

IV. Implementation

A. Prevent deterioration of mental status; monitor for changes in level of consciousness, personality, behaviors

B. Record changes and report to physician

C. Assess serial handwriting levels

D. Monitor serum ammonia levels

E. Monitor for signs of hypokalemia and acidosis

F. Protect client from injury, pad side rails, if necessary

G. Encourage family cooperation as necessary

H. Prevent constipation

I. Administer lactulose per NG tube or rectally (see Table 8–19)

J. Reduce dietary protein to decrease ammonia production in intestines; may vary depending on stage (20 to 40 g per day) (Table 8–20)

K. Administer neomycin per NG or rectally

L. Maintain continuity of care

M. Maintain good oral hygiene

TABLE 8–20 Dietary Management for the Client with Hepatic Encephalopathy and Coma

Objective	To reduce protein intake to minimum and decrease amount of ammonia formation
Calories	1500 to 2000 calories needed to prevent breakdown of tissue proteins for energy and hypoglycemia; provided mainly in carbohydrates and fats
Protein	Very low protein diet; protein intake limited to 20 g per day at onset of hepatic failure; must be of high biological value; increases in protein by 10 g per day or maximum of 1 g per day permitted without causing signs and symptoms of hepatic encephalopathy; client must be carefully watched following each increment; with improvement, diets providing 20 to 60 g protein may be introduced
Sources	Toast, cereal, rice, tea, fruit juices
Carbohydrate	300 to 400 g per day
Sodium	May be restricted if edema and ascites persist
Fat	Limited to prevent early satiety
Special Considerations	Serum ammonia determines level of protein intake; may pose problems with feeding secondary to mental status deterioration and changes in behavior patterns; oral tube feedings or intravenous feedings may be necessary

N. Maintain a patent airway

O. Maintain caloric intake, stress importance of low-protein diet

P. Monitor fluid balance

Q. Avoid use of central nervous system depressants

R. Maintain safety measures

V. Evaluation

A. Client's thought processes not impaired

B. Skin integrity maintained

Hepatorenal Syndrome

I. Assessment

A. Definition: sudden renal failure with progressive liver disease

B. Pathophysiology: serious complication of cirrhosis; functional disorder of kidneys without anatomic or cellular changes in kidneys; client usually had previous normal renal functioning

C. Etiology

1. Oliguria

2. Azotemia

3. Abrupt development

4. Anorexia

5. Weakness

6. Fatigue

D. Clinical manifestations

1. Unknown

2. Theories

a. Possible decrease in effective circulating blood volume

b. Shunts in kidneys

c. After diuretic therapy

d. Altered renal hemodynamics

e. Cortical vessel constriction

E. Medical management

1. Salt-poor albumin

2. Sodium and water restriction

3. Diuretics

4. Fluid and electrolyte replacements

F. See Cirrhosis for Planning/goals, expected outcomes, Implementation, and Evaluation

Hepatic Failure

I. Assessment

A. Definition: a syndrome that is a consequence of massive deterioration of liver function; essentially, complete liver failure

B. Pathophysiology

1. Because of various causative factors, hepatic failure often a complex syndrome

2. Because the liver has numerous as well as varied functions, its failure affects every organ system, eventually causing multisystem failure

3. Pathophysiological processes of hepatic failure can be directly correlated with fact that liver unable to perform its more than 400 functions

4. Various disease processes or etiological agents that cause liver dysfunction can eventually lead to widespread replacement of hepatic architecture with fibrous tissue and massive hepatic cell necrosis

5. Continuing necrosis and degeneration of liver cell tissue leads to liver dysfunction and failure

6. Fibrotic and necrotic tissue contribute to liver edema, ultimately obstructing portal system and its own blood supply system, further interfering with important functions of liver

7. Blood flow through hepatic vasculature further reduced, causing additional death to liver cells

8. Various ultrastructural lesions may also be present from excessive lipid accumulation in liver

9. Regardless of the etiological agent, amount of structural change determines degree of liver compromise

C. Predisposing/precipitating factors: any number of factors can precipitate hepatic failure in individual with marginal hepatic reserve

1. Viral or toxic hepatitis

2. GI bleeding

3. Paracentesis

4. Circulatory failure with hypovolemic or septic shock

5. Prolonged periods of hypoxia

6. Failure to follow the prescribed protocol of therapy (i.e., alcohol abuse)

7. Infection

8. May be idiopathic

D. Clinical manifestations: may present insidious onset or can occur suddenly in event of acute overwhelming liver injury; often, signs and symptoms depend on which liver functions primarily affected and to extent affected

1. Jaundice

2. Edema and ascites

3. Anemia

4. Fever and sepsis

5. Muscle wasting

6. Deterioration of health

7. Hemorrhage

8. Encephalopathy

9. Hepatic coma

10. Lethargy

11. Changes in personality

12. Flapping tremors

13. Renal failure

14. Bleeding tendencies
15. Portal hypertension
II. Analysis (see Cirrhosis)
III. Planning/goals, expected outcomes—center on treatment of signs and symptoms: ascites, hepatic encephalopathy, and portal hypertension
IV. Implementation (see Cirrhosis)
V. Evaluation (see Cirrhosis)

POST-TEST Hepatic Disorders

Mr. Timmons, a 35-year-old with Laennec's cirrhosis is admitted to your unit with complications of esophageal varices. You are assigned to care for him.

---

1. Which of the following foods would be appropriate for Mr. Timmons?
   1. Fresh fruits and vegetables
   2. High-protein, high-fiber shredded wheat and breads
   3. Hot chocolate with fresh whole milk
   4. Rice pudding

2. Mr. Timmons' type of cirrhosis is most frequently caused by:
   1. Hepatitis A
   2. Nutritional impairment and chronic alcohol abuse
   3. Chronic congestive heart failure
   4. Blockage of the bile duct

3. In view of Mr. Timmons' esophageal varices, which of the following nursing interventions would be appropriate in your care of him?
   1. Encourage him to continue an exercise routine such as weightlifting
   2. Advise him to limit himself to one drink per day
   3. Advise him to avoid straining at stools
   4. Provide him with hot liquids as desired

4. Hepatic encephalopathy is most likely to occur:
   1. During the early phase of cirrhosis
   2. From elevated serum ammonia levels
   3. From a low protein diet
   4. When about 50% of liver tissue has been destroyed

5. The primary mechanism responsible for causing portal hypertension is:
   1. A decreased resistance to blood flow through the liver
   2. An increased resistance to blood flow through the liver
   3. Ascites and peripheral edema
   4. An increased resistance to bile flow through the liver

Mary Smith, a client with cirrhosis of the liver, is scheduled for a liver biopsy tomorrow.

---

6. Which of the following is an INAPPROPRIATE nursing action in preparing Mary for her biopsy?
   1. Reinforcing the physician's explanation of the procedure
   2. Assessing her coagulation studies and making sure the results are charted
   3. Making certain the consent is properly signed
   4. Withholding vitamin K injections until after the test

7. After her liver biopsy, which of the following positions would be best for Mary?
   1. High Fowler's position to facilitate coughing and deep breathing
   2. Trendelenburg position to prevent post-biopsy shock
   3. A right side-lying position with a pillow or sandbag placed under the right costal margin
   4. A left side-lying position with a pillow or sandbag placed under the left costal margin

8. Nursing interventions used specifically to decrease serum ammonia levels in clients with hepatic encephalopathy include all of the following EXCEPT:
   1. Administering neomycin orally or rectally to reduce bacterial flora in the colon
   2. Administering lactulose orally or rectally to create an acidic environment in the colon
   3. Treating precipitating causes such as GI hemorrhage and hypovolemia
   4. Increasing the amount of protein in the diet orally or by tube feedings

9. Treatment of hepatic encephalopathy includes which of the following?
   1. A high-calorie, high-protein diet
   2. Intravenous penicillin
   3. Oral or rectal neomycin administration
   4. Intravenous or oral administration of steroids

10. Which of the following are NOT characteristic manifestations of hepatic encephalopathy?
    1. Confusion
    2. Increased blood urea nitrogen (BUN)
    3. Deterioration of writing ability
    4. Asterixis

11. You are administering neomycin to your client.

Suddenly, the client complains of tinnitus and vertigo. Your first nursing action is to:
① Inform the client that this is to be expected and will go away soon
② Encourage the client to cough and deep breathe
③ Stop the medication and notify the physician
④ Slow the frequency of administration

12. Late manifestations of hepatic cirrhosis do NOT include which of the following?
① Edema and ascites
② Asterixis
③ Hepatic encephalopathy
④ Enlarged liver

13. Client teaching in the early stages of Laennec's cirrhosis includes:
① Complete bedrest
② A low-protein diet
③ Increased exercise
④ No alcohol

POST-TEST Answers and Rationales

1. ④ Soft foods are generally recommended for the client with esophageal varices because hot or hard foods may cause ruptures. 4, II. Cirrhosis.

2. ② Laennec's cirrhosis is usually associated with chronic, long-term alcohol abuse along with poor nutrition. 1, II. Cirrhosis.

3. ③ Esophageal varices may rupture with increased intra-abdominal pressure such as straining at stools or lifting heavy objects. Drinking alcohol is not recommended and hot liquids may cause bleeding. 4, I & II. Esophageal Varices.

4. ② Hepatic encephalopathy is a terminal complication in liver disease. The main pathological agent involved is nitrogenous ammonia, which is a cerebral toxin. 1, II. Hepatic Encephalopathy.

5. ② Portal hypertension is caused by an obstruction in the normal blood flow through the portal system. Choice 3 is a result of the hypertension. 1, II. Portal Hypertension.

6. ④ Answering any questions she may have about the procedure, reinforcing the physician's explanation, and making certain her coagulation studies were completed and charted all are appropriate actions to prepare the client. Vitamin K is needed to help with clotting and should not be withheld. 4, I & II. Liver Biopsy.

7. ③ The right side-lying position with pressure over the site decreases the risk of hemorrhage or bile leakage. 4, I. Liver Biopsy.

8. ④ Neomycin and lactulose are utilized in treating hepatic encephalopathy. GI hemorrhage and hypovolemia are both precipitating causes of hepatic encephalopathy. Increasing the amount of protein can precipitate, not prevent, increased ammonia levels. 4, II. Hepatic Encephalopathy.

9. ③ Oral or rectal neomycin administration is used in the treatment of hepatic encephalopathy to reduce the bacterial flora of the colon. 4, II. Hepatic Encephalopathy.

10. ② Increased BUN is not a characteristic sign of hepatic encephalopathy, because ammonia is not being converted to urea. 2, II. Hepatic Encephalopathy.

11. ③ Tinnitus and vertigo are not normal side effects and should be reported to the physician immediately. 5, II. Hepatic Encepholopathy.

12. ② Ascites, edema, jaundice, and hepatic encephalopathy are all later signs of hepatic cirrhosis. Ascites is a manifestation of both hepatocellular failure and portal hypertension. Asterixis is a characteristic sign of progressing hepatic coma. An enlarged liver is an early sign, since it later becomes hard and shrunken. 1, II. Cirrhosis.

13. ④ Complete avoidance of alcohol is absolutely necessary in the early stages of Laennec's cirrhosis. Complete bedrest is unnecessary, but too much exercise is contraindicated. A high-protein diet is recommended. 4, I & IV. Cirrhosis.

PRE-TEST Renal/Urinary Disorders

1. Which of the following statements regarding physical assessments of the urinary system is accurate?
   ① An empty bladder is palpated as a small nodule
   ② Auscultation is used to listen to urine in the bladder
   ③ The client lies prone when the kidneys are palpated
   ④ The flank area is percussed with a firm, slow motion

2. An important nursing responsibility following a renal arteriogram is to:
   ① Encourage ambulation 2 to 3 hours after the study
   ② Apply warm wet packs to the insertion site
   ③ Palpate peripheral pulses in the affected leg
   ④ Give the client nothing by mouth for 4 hours after the test

3. Which of the following is a normal constituent of urine?
   ① Ketones

② Creatinine
③ Amino acids
④ Bacteria

4. Which of the following is the minimum urinary output per hour that is acceptable for an adult?
   ① 10 mL
   ② 30 mL
   ③ 50 mL
   ④ 100 mL

5. Clinical manifestations of renal calculi include:
   ① Dribbling at the end of urination and pyuria
   ② Severe flank pain and hematuria
   ③ Frequency of urination and polyuria
   ④ Urgent, uncontrolled urination

6. Which of the following best describes acute renal failure?
   ① Complete absence of renal blood flow
   ② Sudden reduction in renal function
   ③ Rapid increase in urine output with azotemia
   ④ Gradual increase in glomerular filtration rate (GFR)

7. A common complication associated with an internal arteriovenous (AV) fistula is:
   ① Infection
   ② Palpable thrill
   ③ Thrombosis
   ④ Bleeding

8. The most common problem associated with immunosuppressive therapy is:
   ① Anemia
   ② Thrombocytopenia
   ③ Predisposition to infection
   ④ Hypercoaguability

9. Which of the following classes of medication require the client to maintain large fluid intake to prevent complications?
   ① Sulfa drugs
   ② Antihypertensive drugs
   ③ Nitrofurantoin drugs
   ④ Methenamine mandelate drugs

10. Which of the following is NOT a predisposing factor to pyelonephritis?
    ① Pregnancy
    ② Diabetes
    ③ Thrombophlebitis
    ④ Hypertension

11. Three of the four following measures will help prevent the development of urinary tract infections. Which one will NOT help?
    ① Proper perineal hygiene
    ② Restricting fluid intake
    ③ Voiding after intercourse
    ④ Changing infant's soiled diapers frequently

Mr. Rocke, a 30-year-old, has a sudden onset of severe right flank pain. His wife brings him to the hospital, where he is admitted for tests and observation. The preliminary diagnosis is urinary calculi.

---

12. Before receiving Mr. Rocke's medical orders, which of the following nursing actions will have the highest priority?
    ① Ensuring that he remain NPO
    ② Straining his urine through several layers of gauze
    ③ Assessing his grip strength and pupil reactivity
    ④ Obtaining a clean catch urine specimen

13. Mr. Rocke is scheduled to have an IVP. Which of the following information is the most important for the nurse to obtain before he undergoes this procedure?
    ① The date of his last ECG
    ② The time of his last meal
    ③ His response to antibiotics
    ④ His history of allergies

14. The test results confirm that Mr. Rocke has renal calculi. He is started on phenazopyridine hydrochloride (Pyridium) and sulfisoxazole. Which of the following side effects should be explained to him before he starts taking the Pyridium?
    ① Dizziness and lethargy may occur
    ② His urine will become bright red-orange
    ③ His urine will become more dilute
    ④ Urinating will be uncomfortable

15. A long-term goal for Mr. Rocke's treatment is the prevention of further stone formation. Which of the following dietary recommendations, if adhered to, would be most helpful in meeting this goal?
    ① Drink in excess of 3000 mL of fluid per day
    ② Avoid eating milk products, shellfish, and eggs
    ③ Drink at least two glasses of cranberry juice per day
    ④ Eat large amounts of citrus fruits

Arthur Burns is a 60-year-old man who has come into the outpatient surgery for a cystoscopy for continued hematuria that has lasted for over a year. He does not have an

infection, so he is being worked up for either renal or bladder cancer.

---

16. A risk factor that Mr. Burns might have that would make him prone to renal cancer is his:
    ① Use of aspirin products
    ② History of chronic alcohol use
    ③ Smoking two packs of cigarettes per day for 30 years
    ④ Working as a printer for the last 25 years
17. Other than the hematuria, what symptom would further confirm a diagnosis of renal cancer?
    ① Leukocytosis
    ② Costovertebral angle (CVA) mass
    ③ Suprapubic pain
    ④ Pain and burning on urination
18. Which of the folowing diagnostic tests would NOT be useful in confirming the diagnosis of renal cancer?
    ① A cystoscopy
    ② A renal ultrasound
    ③ An intravenous pyelogram (IVP)
    ④ Renal angiography
19. Preparation for an IVP should include:
    ① Clear liquids for 12 hours pre-test
    ② A 24-hour urine prior to the test
    ③ Laxatives before the test
    ④ Enemas after the test

Mark Lee is a 45-year-old man who has just been diagnosed with bladder cancer. He is admitted for a radical cystectomy and an ileal conduit.

---

20. The symptom he was most likely to have exhibited was:
    ① Foul-smelling urine
    ② Gross hematuria
    ③ Flank pain
    ④ Symptoms of a UTI
21. Which of the following in Mr. Lee's history is the most likely risk factor for bladder cancer?
    ① A history of smoking and alcohol ingestion
    ② Chronic use of aspirin
    ③ Recurrent urinary tract infections
    ④ A work history of a sedentary desk job
22. The definitive diagnostic test for bladder cancer is a(n):
    ① Urine for cytology
    ② IVP
    ③ Cystoscopy
    ④ CEA level
23. Mr. Lee is scheduled for blood tests, an IVP, and a cystoscopy. Important nursing care after the cytoscopy includes:
    ① Restricting fluids
    ② Monitoring for fever and sepsis
    ③ Reporting the presence of blood in the urine
    ④ Reporting if the client experiences any pain on voiding
24. The most significant complication of surgery that Mr. Lee should be prepared for is:
    ① Impotence
    ② Lack of urinary control
    ③ Spread of the disease
    ④ Chronic infections
25. Mr. Lee is scheduled for a radical cystectomy and ileal conduit. His postoperative care plan includes the following nursing order: "Observe for edema of stoma." If edema occurs, the nurse would expect:
    ① An elevated temperature
    ② Decreased urine output
    ③ Leukocytosis
    ④ Dark-colored urine

PRE-TEST Answers and Rationales

1. ④ The flank areas are where the lower poles of the kidneys are located. Percussing and palpating over this area can disclose the presence of the kidneys, their size, and whether or not there is any pain. Only a full bladder can be palpated, urine cannot be auscultated, and the client should sit when the kidneys are to be palpated. 1, II. Renal.

2. ③ The most important action following an arteriogram is to assess the blood flow distal to the insertion site. The client remains on bedrest with the leg straight for 24 hours. Warm packs are not applied, although ice may be used. There is no reason for the client to remain NPO. 4, I. Renal Arteriogram.

3. ② Creatinine is a normal constituent of urine. All the rest are abnormal. 2, II. Renal.

4. ② The urine output must remain at least 30 mL per hour for the kidneys to be adequately perfused. If it is lower, then there is inadequate perfusion or other renal problems, 1, I. Renal.

5. ② Renal calculi cause severe flank pain and bleeding. There is no dribbling, frequency, or urgency. The calculi may also stimulate the bowel, causing renal colic. The pain is very severe and clients may require large doses of narcotics to control it. 1, I & II. Renal Calculi.

6. ② Acute renal failure happens when there is a sudden abrupt reduction in renal function. It may or may not be related to a decrease in renal blood flow. It is a decrease in urine output with azotemia plus a decrease in the GFR. 1, II. Renal Failure.

7. ③ An AV fistula is prone to thrombosis because there is a mixing of arterial and venous blood leading to increased turbulence. Infection is unlikely once the initial incision heals. A palpable thrill is normal and bleeding is highly unlikely. 2, I. Renal Failure.

8. ③ The client who is immunosuppressed is less able to mount an inflammatory response or to fight an infection. Anemia, thrombocytopenia, and hypercoagulability do not occur with the immunosuppressed client. 1, I & II. Renal Transplant.

9. ① Sulfa drugs can crystallize if there is insufficient urine to maintain their solubility. None of the other drugs are susceptible to precipitation in low urine output. 1, II. Urinary Tract Infection.

10. ③ Pyelonephritis can be caused by pregnancy, diabetes, hypertension, infections (either systemic or urinary), and other stressors. Thrombophlebitis does not predispose the client to pyelonephritis. 1, II. Pyelonephritis.

11. ② Restricting fluid intake will foster urinary tract infections, not prevent them. The other three options are measures that will help prevent urinary infections. 4, II. Urinary Tract Infection.

12. ② One of the top priorities is to strain the urine so that if the stone is passed, it can be saved for analysis. The client needs to force fluids, not remain NPO. The other options are irrelevant. 4, I & II. Renal Calculi.

13. ④ When a client is going for an IVP, it is important for the nurse to assess the client for an allergy to iodine. It the client is allergic, the IVP can cause fatal anaphylaxis. The other options do not really affect the IVP. 1, I & II. Renal Calculi.

14. ② Pyridium contains an analgesic dye that soothes the bladder mucosa and turns the urine a bright red-orange. It is important to warn the client so that this is not mistaken for bleeding. Urination should be more comfortable. The other options are not correct. 4, II. Renal Calculi.

15. ① The most important intervention to prevent further stone formation regardless of the stone type is to force fluids. Avoiding milk products and maintaining acidic urine can help prevent calcium stones but not uric acid stones. Citrus fruits will alkalinize the urine, which can help prevent uric acid stones but not calcium. 4, I & II. Renal Calculi.

16. ③ Cigarettes are a risk factor for renal cancer. Phenacetin is also a risk factor but alcohol, aspirin, and dyes are not. 1, IV. Renal Cancer.

17. ② The two symptoms other than hematuria are CVA pain and a palpable mass. Pain, burning, suprapubic pain, and leukocytosis are problems only if there is an infection. 1 & 2, II. Renal Cancer.

18. ① A cystoscopy can rule out bladder cancer but it cannot confirm renal cancer. The other tests are done to confirm the

diagnosis of renal cancer. 2, II. Renal Cancer.

19. ③ The bowel must be cleaned out to allow visualization of the kidneys. The client should also be NPO before the test. A 24-hour urine and enemas are not needed. 4, II. Renal Cancer.

20. ② The major symptom of bladder cancer is gross, painless hematuria. None of the other options are symptoms associated with bladder cancer. 1 & 2, II. Bladder Cancer.

21. ① Risk factors for bladder cancer include smoking and alcohol ingestion along with things such as dyes, hydrocarbons, and cyclophosphamide (Cytoxan). None of the other options are risk factors for bladder cancer. 2, IV. Bladder Cancer.

22. ③ Bladder tumors are easily visualized via a cystoscopy because they occur in the lower third of the bladder. Bladder tumors are always malignant or premalignant.

Cytology is not usually positive, an IVP may not be definitive, and a CEA level is inappropriate. 2, II. Bladder Cancer.

23. ② A cystoscopy can cause urinary sepsis. Fluids should be encouraged. Blood in the urine and pain on voiding are normal for a time after the cystoscopy. 4, I & II. Bladder Cancer.

24. ① All of these options are possible, but the most significant outcome of his surgery will be impotence. Sexual counseling should be provided for this client before the surgery. 2, III. Bladder Cancer.

25. ② If there is edema of the stoma, it will be more difficult for urine to be expelled through the edematous stoma. It is important for the nurse to differentiate between the cause since low output can also be from hemorrhage or obstruction. None of the other options would result from edema of the stoma. 1, I. Ileal Conduit.

NORMAL URINARY SYSTEM

I. Anatomy of urinary system (from L/S)
   A. Kidneys
      1. Bean-shaped, paired organs
      2. Left kidney larger and higher than right
      3. In posterior abdominal cavity
      4. Positioned adjacent to vertebral column, costovertebral angle (CVA)
      5. Move down during respiration as diaphragm contracts
      6. Layers: outer is cortex, inner is medulla
      7. Urine collects in pelvis
      8. Functional unit: nephron
         a. Glomerulus: removes filtrate from blood through afferent and efferent arterioles
         b. Bowman's capsule: filtrate through to tubule
         c. Tubule
            (1) Proximal convoluted: reabsorption of Na^+, H^+, H_2O, glucose, K^+, amino acids, Cl^-, HCO_3, PO_4
            (2) Loop of Henle: concentration of urine; Na^+ passively and, Cl^- actively absorbed, Ca^{++} reabsorbed
            (3) Distal convoluted tubule: Na^+, H_2O, Cl^-, HCO_3, K^+ reabsorbed; secretion of H^+, K^+
            (4) Collecting tubule: Na^+, K^+, H^+, NH_3, secreted or reabsorbed
   B. Bladder
      1. Hollow, muscular organ
      2. Lies within pelvic cavity
      3. Normal capacity: 500 mL
      4. Contracts under voluntary and involuntary control
      5. Nerve supply: parasympathetic and sympathetic
   C. Ureters
      1. Anatomy: hollow tubes, 12 inches long
      2. Physiology: propel urine to bladder from kidneys
II. Diagnostic studies
   A. Urine studies (Table 8–21)
      1. Urinalysis
      2. Urine culture and sensitivity
      3. 24-hour excretion tests
         a. Creatinine clearance
         b. Phenolsulfonphthalein (PSP)
   B. Blood studies (see Table 8–21)
      1. Creatinine
      2. Blood urea nitrogen (BUN)
      3. Potassium (K^+)
      4. Osmolality
      5. Albumin
      6. Hematocrit (Hct)
      7. Calcium (Ca^{++})

8. Magnesium (Mg^{++})
9. Phosphate (PO_4^-)
10. Arterial blood gases (ABG) (see Chapter 4)
C. Radiological studies (see Table 8–21)
  1. Abdominal x-ray of kidney, ureter, bladder (KUB)
  2. Cystoscopy
  3. Retrograde pyelogram
  4. Cystourethrogram
  5. Intravenous pyelogram (IVP)
  6. Ultrasound
  7. Computed tomography (CT) scan
  8. Renogram-scan
  9. Renal arteriogram
  10. Renal biopsy

NURSING PROCESS APPLIED TO ADULTS WITH RENAL/URINARY DISORDERS

Infectious Renal/Urinary Disorders

Cystitis

I. Assessment
  A. Definition: inflammation of the bladder wall
  B. Incidence
    1. More common in women; pregnancy; position of urethra, proximity to bowel
    2. High incidence related to indwelling urinary catheters
    3. 90% nosocomial or hospital induced—*Escherichia coli*
  C. Predisposing/precipitating factors
    1. Poor hygiene after urination, defecation
    2. Sexual intercourse
    3. Pregnancy
    4. Urological instrumentation of bladder
    5. Urethral obstruction
    6. Structural or functional urinary abnormality
    7. Chronic health problems such as diabetes, strep throat
    8. Reinfection
    9. Chemotherapy, cyclophosphamide (Cytoxan) induced
  D. Clinical manifestations
    1. 50% may be asymptomatic
    2. Urgency
    3. Frequent urination, both day and night (nocturia)
    4. Burning (dysuria)
    5. Bladder spasms (tenesmus)
    6. Foul-smelling urine (pyuria)
    7. Bloody urine (hematuria)
  E. Diagnostic examinations (see Table 8–21)

    1. Urinalysis: bacterial count more than 10,000/mL
    2. Urine culture and sensitivity; midstream; obtain before starting antibiotics; cleanse urethra; bacterial colonies greater than 100,000/mL
  F. Complications
    1. Reinfection
    2. Retrograde pyelonephritis
  G. Medical management
    1. Medications (guided by culture and sensitivity report)
      a. Single-dose antibiotics when infection localized to bladder and organism antibiotic sensitive; amoxicillin (Augmentin), ampicillin, trimethoprim (Proloprim), co-trimethoxazole (Bactrim, Septra) (Table 8–22)
      b. Antimicrobials, antiseptics for 7 to 14 days; sulfisoxazole (Gantrisin), nitrofurantoin (Furadantin), nalidixic acid (NegGram), methenamine mandelate (Mandelamine) (see Table 8–22)
      c. Combine antiseptics, analgesics; phenazopyridine hydrochloride (Pyridium); stains urine red-orange color (see Table 8–22)

II. Analysis
  A. Altered pattern of urinary elimination: dysuria and frequency related to irritated bladder mucosa
  B. Pain related to irritated bladder mucosa
  C. Knowledge deficit related to treatment and prevention of recurrence

III. Planning/goals, expected outcomes
  A. Client's urinary pattern will return to normal
  B. Client's pain will be relieved or controlled
  C. Client will understand and comply with treatment; recurrence will not occur

IV. Implementation
  A. Assist client in relieving symptoms and preventing recurrence
    1. Diet
      a. Force 3000 mL fluid per day to encourage movement of pathogens out of urinary tract
      b. Cranberry juice in large quantities to lower urine pH, keep acidic
      c. Discourage caffeine products (coffee, tea, and cola) because they exacerbate frequency
    2. Teach client health promotion
      a. Teach to:
        (1) Urinate when urge to void present
        (2) Drink at least eight glasses of water per day
        (3) Cleanse properly after urination and defecation (front to back)

TABLE 8–21 Diagnostic Studies Table

Blood/Urine Studies

Test	Normal Value	Purpose	Nursing Implications
Urinalysis	Color yellow; specific gravity, 1.003 to 1.039; pH 4.5 to 8.0; 1 to 2 L/24 hours	Indicates renal tissue ability to excrete water	Save first morning specimen; examine within 1 hour
Urine culture and sensitivity	<10,000 colonies/mL	Confirm infections, organisms; determine antibiotic	Cleanse external meatus with povidone-iodine or soap and water (midstream catch), sterile container
Creatinine clearance	Women: 85 to 125 mL/min; men: 95 to 140 mL/min	Indicates filtration ability	24-hour collection; draw blood for creatinine at end of test
Phenolsulfonphthalein (PSP)	50% of PSP excreted	Measures tubular secretion rates	Drink 8 to 10 glasses of water: 1 mL PSP dye IV; urine specimens at 15-minute intervals (4 specimens)—mark exact time
Osmolality	300 to 400 Osm/Kg	Measure of the solute concentration in urine	Random specimen; obtain serum osmolality at same time

Serum Studies

Test	Normal Value	Purpose	Nursing Implications
Creatinine	0.4 to 1.2 mg/dL	Specific indicator renal function	Evaluate in relation to baseline
Blood urea nitrogen (BUN)	5 to 25 mg/dL	Less specific indicator renal function, end product of protein metabolism	Less specific than creatinine; affected by fluid volume or high protein diet
Potassium (K^+)	3.5 to 5.0 meq/L	Indicates tubules' ability to excrete	Note if patient on K^+-wasting diuretics
Osmolality	280 to 300 nOsm/L	Measures solute concentration of blood	Depends on hydration
Albumin	3.2 to 5.5 g/dL	To monitor for fluid shifts, wound healing	Relationship to fluid status, wound healing
Hematocrit (Hct)	Women: 36 to 47/dL; men: 40 to 54/dL	Erythropoietin secretion less	Renal failure patients can acclimate and function with an Hct of 20/dL
Calcium (Ca^{++})	4.0 to 5.0 mEq/L or 9.0 to 11.0 mg/dL	Vitamin D not excreted for Ca^+ absorption in the gut	Many renal patients take calcium supplements
Magnesium (Mg^{++})	1.4 to 2.2 mEq/L or 1.7 to 2.7 mg/dL	Renal tubules unable to secrete	Beware of Mg-containing medications; neurological side effects when elevated—seizures
Phosphate (PO_4^-)	3.5 to 5.5 mEq/L	Renal tubules unable to secrete	Aluminum hydroxide medications bind phosphate
pH	7.35 to 7.45	Metabolic acidosis occurs when tubules unable to buffer H^+ ions	From arterial blood gas sample; keep on ice and apply site pressure 5 minutes

Radiological Studies

Test	Procedure	Purpose	Nursing Implications
Abdominal x-ray (KUB)	Flat x-ray plate over abdomen and x-ray taken	Shows calcified deposits or gross renal abnormalities	Painless; may need bowel prep
Cystoscopy	Lighted scope inserted through urethra	Visualization of bladder	May be uncomfortable; post-test: encourage fluids, monitor I & O, character of urine and check for abdominal distention, frequency, fever, and hematuria; pre-test: assess for codeine allergies, cathartics to cleanse bowel

TABLE 8–21 Diagnostic Studies Table *Continued.*

Radiological Studies

Test	Procedure	Purpose	Nursing Implications
Retrograde intravenous pyelogram (IVP)	Contrast dye injected	Outlines the renal pelvis and ureters	
Cystourethrogram	Catheter inserted and radiopaque dye injected, client voids while x-rays taken	X-ray study of bladder and urethra	Same as cystoscopy; check if allergy to iodine
Intravenous pyelogram (IVP)	Dye/contrast material injected IV; as kidney filters and excretes the dye, x-rays are taken	Evaluates function, filling, emptying of urinary tract	Bowel prep; NPO, post-test x-rays; alert for dye reaction: edema, itching, wheezing, dyspnea
Ultrasound	Sound waves passed, computer interprets tissue density in print form	Images obtained by sound waves	No prep; not painful; no post-test follow-up; full bladder, assists in outline studies
CT scan	Dye may be used	To visualize kidneys and renal circulation	If dye used, same as IVP
Renogram-scan	Radioactive isotope with contrast medium injected; a scanning machine is used to trace isotope	Records the radioactivity over the kidneys	Given diagnostic dose of radioactive substance; not harmful and no special precautions
Renal arteriogram	Similar to IVP except dye injected either via translumbar or femoral catheter	Allows visualization of the renal circulation	Same care as IVP; monitor for bleeding and apply pressure dressing; bedrest for 8 hours; vs every 15 minutes × 4 hours
Renal biopsy	X-rays prior; skin marked to indicate lower pole of kidney; position patient prone and bent at diaphragm and holds breath during needle insertion	Kidney tissue obtained by needle aspiration for pathological examination for type and stage of renal pathology	Check coagulation status; post-test: pressure to site 20 minutes, pressure dressing, flat in bed for 24 hours; check for bleeding, hematuria

TABLE 8–22 Drugs Used to Treat Urinary Disorders

Class	Example	Action	Use	Common Side Effects	Nursing Implications
Urinary antiseptics	Nitrofurantoin (Macrodantin)	Act as disinfectants within the urinary tract; concentrated by kidneys and reach therapeutic levels only within the urinary tract	Prevention and treatment of urinary tract infections	Nausea and vomiting, GI upset, diarrhea, hypersensitivity	Maintain adequate I & O; keep urinary pH in acid range with vitamin C and cranberry juice; give with food or antacids; warn patient drugs may discolor urine; watch for hypersensitivity
Analgesics	Methenamine (Mandelamine), Phenazopyridine HCl (Pyridium)	Analgesic action on mucosa	To decrease pain	"	
Sulfonamides	Co-trimoxazole (Bactrim, Septra), sulfisoxazole (Gantrisin), trimethoprim (Proloprim), Septra DS (double strength)	Drugs that are bacteriostatic against both gram-positive and gram-negative organisms; excreted unchanged and undissolved and dissolve well in urine; therefore they are excellent for treating UTIs	To treat bacterial infections	GI distress, allergic reactions, headache, peripheral neuritis, hearing loss, crystalluria, hypoglycemia	Administer with large amounts of fluid; monitor serum glucose levels (may produce false positive urine glucose); monitor for allergies; check I & O; maintain alkaline pH since drugs more soluble in alkaline urine; teach patient to take full course of drugs

(4) Identify causes and signs and symptoms of early urinary tract infections

(5) Take medications for prescribed period, usually 10 to 14 days

(6) Follow up with repeated urine tests, cultures

3. Pain relief measures

a. Encourage client to take warm sitz baths

b. Encourage client to void frequently and completely

V. Evaluation

A. Urine culture and sensitivity negative and bacterial count less than 10,000/mL on follow-up urinalysis

B. No symptoms of urinary tract infection

C. Preventive measures practiced

Pyelonephritis

I. Assessment

A. Definition: inflammation of kidney tissue (renal pelvis, parenchyma)

B. Incidence

1. Most commonly caused by bacterial invasion, for example, *E. coli*

2. Often diagnosed secondary to cystitis when kidney already affected

3. May be retrograde or blood-borne in origin

C. Predisposing/precipitating factors

1. May follow cystitis

2. In children, associated with urinary tract abnormalities (vesicoureteral reflux)

3. In adults, common pre-existing factors are bladder tumors, prostatic hypertrophy, strictures, and urinary stones

4. Instrumentation or trauma to urinary tract

5. Pregnancy

6. Chronic health problems, diabetes, analgesia abuse, polycystic and hypertensive kidney disease

D. Clinical manifestations:

1. Fever

2. Chills

3. Malaise

4. Flank pain

5. Costovertebral (CVA) tenderness

E. Diagnostic examinations (see Table 8–21)

1. Urinalysis: casts, bacteria, large amounts of WBCs, RBCs, pus, high alkaline pH

2. Blood: leukocytosis (elevated WBC), positive cultures

3. IVP: enlargement of involved kidney(s)

4. Renal biopsy: to confirm diagnosis and/or complications

F. Complications

1. Scarring and fibrosis of infected part of kidney

2. Chronic pyelonephritis

3. Chronic renal failure; one third of cases have pyelonephritis as original diagnosis

II. Analysis

A. Altered renal tissue perfusion related to infection

B. Pain related to inflammation

C. Knowledge deficit related to prevention, treatment, and follow-up

III. Planning/goals, expected outcomes

A. Client's underlying cause will be identified and prevented

B. Client will be free of signs and symptoms and verbalize what they are

C. Client will be knowledgeable about treatment regimen, follow-up, and prevention, and will comply with it

IV. Implementation

A. Assist with diagnostic tests to determine underlying cause (see Table 8–21)

B. Monitor urine for appearance, color, and specific gravity; monitor temperature and administer antipyretics; monitor I & O, weight, signs and symptoms of fluid and electrolyte imbalances; provide relief of flank pain with analgesics, rest, massage, and external application of heat

C. Administer orally for 10 to 14 days (if mild) or IV (if severe) antibiotics such as sulfamethoxazole (Bactrim, Septra), tetracycline, ampicillin, cephalosporins (see Tables 4–22, 8–22), teach purpose and side effects, and monitor response

D. Bedrest during acute phase

E. Encourage fluid intake of at least 3 L per day

F. Teach client importance of follow-up urinalysis every 2 weeks for a month, then monthly until urine sterile

G. Teach client to report chills; symptoms of urinary tract infection such as frequency, burning, urgency

V. Evaluation

A. Underlying cause identified

B. Client free from signs and symptoms

C. Client understands potential for and prevention of reinfection

Glomerulonephritis

I. Assessment

A. Definition

1. A group of diseases that damage the renal glomeruli

2. Nonbacterial inflammation of glomeruli

of both kidneys, which involves an antigen-antibody reaction

3. Can be acute or chronic

B. Incidence
   1. Most common in preschool and grade-school aged children
   2. Commonly follows by 1 to 3 weeks a respiratory infection (sore throat or tonsillitis) or skin infection (impetigo)

C. Predisposing/precipitating factors
   1. Frequently follows group A hemolytic streptococcus or *Staphylococcus aureus* infection
   2. Lupus erythematosus
   3. Hypertension
   4. Diabetes mellitus
   5. Disseminated intravascular coagulation (DIC)
   6. Exposure to drugs or immunizations

D. Clinical manifestations
   1. Shortness of breath (SOB)
   2. Headache
   3. Fever, chills
   4. Fatigue, weakness
   5. Anorexia, nausea, vomiting
   6. Rapidly swelling face and feet
   7. Pains in back
   8. Hypertension
   9. Smoky brown urine
   10. Oliguria
   11. Proteinuria
   12. Hematuria

E. Diagnostic examinations (see Table 8–21)
   1. Urinalysis: proteinuria, hematuria, cell debris, high specific gravity
   2. CBC: anemia
   3. Serum BUN, creatinine, albumin
   4. Serum complement studies, ASO titers
   5. Renal biopsy, if indicated

F. Complications
   1. Chronic glomerulonephritis
   2. Congestive heart failure
   3. Pulmonary edema
   4. Renal failure

G. Medical management
   1. Control of hypertension
   2. Antibiotics to control infection

II. Analysis
   A. Altered tissue perfusion: renal related to disease process
   B. High risk for fluid volume excess related to renal failure
   C. High risk for infection related to altered immune status
   D. Altered nutrition: less than body requirements related to low protein intake
   E. Knowledge deficit related to disease, treatment, and life changes

III. Planning/goals, expected outcomes
   A. Client's symptoms will be relieved
   B. Client will maintain bedrest until proteinuria, hematuria, and hypertension subside
   C. Client's edema will be reduced
   D. Client's hypertension will be decreased
   E. Client will eat high calorie diet
   F. Client will understand and comply with medication regimen

IV. Implementation
   A. Relieve symptoms of headache and fever with appropriate analgesics and massage; monitor temperature
   B. Bedrest, for up to several months, until BP normal, and proteinuria, hematuria, and edema subside
   C. Reduce edema by restricting fluids and sodium and by administering diuretics—for example, furosemide (Lasix); measure I & O, monitor weight
   D. Control BP by frequent monitoring and by administration of antihypertensives—for example, clonidine (Catapres), hydralazine (Apresoline), and methyldopa (Aldomet); also, administer diuretics and monitor potassium
   E. Dietary
      1. Na^+ restriction for moderate to severe edema
      2. Protein restriction while oliguria, proteinuria, and elevated BUN/creatinine present to decrease excretory load on kidney
      3. Fluid intake according to urine output
      4. High calories and carbohydrates and fats to prevent the use of tissue proteins for energy
   F. Administer penicillin treatment (check for allergies) for up to 2 months: avoid exposure to infections and activities that could potentiate reinfection
   G. Assist with plasmapheresis (to remove immune complexes)
   H. Teach client health maintenance
      1. Importance of prompt medical treatment for sore throats and upper respiratory or skin infections; cultures to be taken and, when indicated, appropriate antibiotics
      2. Reporting signs and symptoms of hematuria, elevated BP, edema, and headache
      3. Importance of compliance with treatment including medications, bedrest, dietary restrictions

V. Evaluation
   A. Client asymptomatic and feeling well, with normal renal function

B. Client able to discuss need for appropriate rest, medications, dietary compliance
C. Client follows up with BP monitoring, urinalysis, and activities as ordered
D. Client knows how to minimize exposure to infective agents

Obstructive Renal/Urinary Disorders

Renal and Ureteral Calculi
I. Assessment
  A. Definition: mineral crystallization formed around organic matter
    1. Urolithiasis: formation of urinary stones
    2. Nephrolithiasis: formation of kidney stones
  B. Incidence
    1. Half of cases are idiopathic
    2. Three times more common in men
    3. Highest occurrence between ages 20 and 55
    4. More common in Caucasians
    5. 1 per 1000 hospitalized annually for calculi
    6. Associated with obstructions and infections in the United States
    7. Geographical areas of Southeastern United States and Great Lakes region have higher incidence
  C. Predisposing/precipitating factors
    1. Urinary stasis, altered urinary pH
    2. Urinary tract infection (UTI)
    3. Obstructions
    4. Hypercalcemia, hyperparathyroidism
    5. Elevated uric acid, gout
    6. Dehydration
    7. Immobilization
    8. Prolonged catheterization
    9. Deficiency in cystine, vitamin A
    10. Diet high in calcium, oxalate, or purines
    11. Living in mountainous or high temperature climates
    12. Sedentary lifestyle
    13. Family history of stone formation
  D. Clinical manifestations
    1. Pain (renal colic); location depends on location of stone; radiates from flank to abdomen, labia, or scrotum
    2. May have alternating retention (obstruction) and diuresis (stone passage)
    3. Hematuria
    4. Nausea, vomiting
    5. Diaphoresis, restlessness
    6. May have low-grade fever and/or signs of UTI
  E. Diagnostic examinations (see Table 8–21)
    1. History
    2. Urinalysis—hematuria, pH
    3. Urine culture and sensitivity for infection
    4. KUB-IVP for localization
    5. Cystoscopy to rule out tumor
    6. Analysis of stone after passage or removal
    7. Serum level of calcium, phosphorus, and uric acid
    8. Serum and urine creatinine to evaluate renal function (increase in serum and decrease in urine)
    9. CT scan
  F. Complications: recurrence rate about 80%
  G. Medical management
    1. Narcotics and antispasmodics to relieve pain and spasms
    2. Antiemetics to relieve nausea
    3. Antibodies for infection
    4. Dietary management (Table 8-23)
  H. Surgical management (Table 8–24)
II. Analysis
  A. Pain related to calculus or surgical procedure

TABLE 8–23 Food Sources of Inorganic Material Found in Urine to Control Urine pH

Alkaline Ash (increase pH)	Acid Ash (decrease pH)	Neutral Ash Foods for Either
Milk	Eggs	Butter
Fruits (except cranberries, plums, and prunes)	Meat, fish, and poultry	Cream
Rhubarb	Oysters	Sugar
Vegetables	Bread	Tapioca
Small amounts of beef, halibut, veal, trout, and salmon allowed	Cereal	Coffee
	Pastries	Tea
	Pudding	
	Certain fruits and vegetables including cranberries, prunes, plums, tomatoes, and peas	

TABLE 8–24 Common Surgeries for Calculi

Name	Procedure	Nursing Implications
Ureterolithotomy	Incision into ureter to remove stone	Do not irrigate urethral catheter; check incisional Penrose drain and surgical dressing
Nephrolithotomy	Incision into kidney to remove stone	Urethral catheter; incisional Penrose drain; nephrostomy tube; indwelling catheter
Pyelolithotomy	Flank incision into kidney to remove stones from renal pelvis	Incisional Penrose drain; surgical dressing; urethral catheter

    B. Altered patterns of urinary elimination: retention related to calculus

    C. Knowledge deficit related to disease, treatment, and prevention of recurrence

III. Planning/goals, expected outcomes

    A. Client will have pain controlled or relieved

    B. Client will return to normal urinary pattern

    C. Client will have calculus successfully treated and will not develop recurrence

IV. Implementation

    A. Pain management to control renal colic—narcotic analgesics and antispasmodic/anticholinergics (Table 8–25)

    B. Force fluids to 3 L per day

    C. Strain all urine through gauze (two 4 × 4's opened up), as 90% stones pass spontaneously

    D. Monitor I & O, vital signs

    E. If stones are calcium (85% are), put on low-calcium diet, consisting of reduced dairy products and acidify urine with vitamin C

    F. If stones are uric acid, put on low-purine diet, consisting of reduced organ meats, dried beans, and whole grain; administer allopurinol (Zyloprim) (see Table 7–2); alkalinize urine

    G. If stones are cystine, lower intake of oxalate-containing foods such as spinach, tea, chocolate, and nuts and administer penicillamine (Cuprimine)

    H. Follow diet to control pH (see Table 8–23)

    I. Surgical procedures (see Table 8–24)

    J. Extracorporeal shock wave lithotripsy (ESWL) where client submerged in large bath of warm water and ultrasonic waves that "crush" stones are aimed over calculi and passed in urine within a few days

V. Evaluation

    A. Client free of calculi and etiology identified

    B. Client free of pain and infection

    C. Client understands need to increase fluids, take medications, follow dietary restrictions, and strain all urine

Benign Prostatic Hypertrophy (BPH)
(See section on Male Reproductive Disorders, Chapter 3)

Renal Failure

Acute Renal Failure

  I. Assessment

    A. Definition: sudden loss of kidney's ability to excrete urine (oliguria) and nitrogenous waste products (azotemia) and to maintain fluid and pH balance; potentially reversible disease in which 50% recover with conservative management

    B. Incidence

      1. Usually occurs in previously healthy individuals

TABLE 8–25 Anticholinergics

Example	Action	Use	Common Side Effects	Nursing Implications
Atropine, propantheline bromide (Pro-Banthine)	Act as competitive antagonists at cholinergic-receptor sites, thereby blocking the action of acetylcholine	To produce mydriasis; preop to decrease salivation and prevent laryngospasms and bradycardia; decrease GI motility; antiparkinsonian; decrease nasopharyngeal and bronchial secretions	Blurred vision, photophobia, urinary hesitancy, increased intraocular pressure, palpitations, flushing, tachycardia, dry mouth, allergic reactions, restlessness	Contraindicated in patients with glaucoma, GI obstruction, BPH, renal or hepatic disease; caution patient against driving; warn about usual side effects; monitor vital signs; give 30 minutes before meals

2. Follows identifiable trauma or contact with nephrotoxic agent
3. Often follows surgical procedures

C. Precipitating/predisposing factors
1. Prerenal causes are decrease in renal blood flow that may include dehydration, blood loss, shock, trauma, burns
2. Intrarenal causes are those that result from primary damage to kidney, such as glomerulonephritis, pyelonephritis, and blood transfusion reactions
3. Postrenal causes are related to obstructions of urinary tract distal to kidneys, such as calculi or BPH

D. Clinical manifestations
1. Onset stage: time from precipitating event to anuria (urine less than 100 mL per day)
2. Oliguria/anuria stage: lasts 1 to 2 weeks
   a. Decreased skin turgor, petechiae, pruritus
   b. Dried mucous membranes
   c. Pallor, discolored skin
   d. Weight changes, edema
   e. Acidotic breath odor
   f. Anorexia, nausea, vomiting
   g. Drowsiness, lethargy, confusion, coma
   h. Restlessness, tetany, seizures
3. Diuretic, early stage
   a. BUN stops rising
   b. Urine output 400 mL per day
4. Recovery, late stage
   a. BUN starts falling to within normal limits
   b. Urine output 4 to 5 L per day
   c. Increase in both mental and physical activity level
5. Convalescent stage
   a. May take months to recover fully when BUN and urine both within normal limits
   b. May develop chronic renal failure (CRF)

E. Diagnostic examinations (see Table 8–21)
1. Serum tests show elevated BUN, creatinine, potassium, sodium, pH, and CO_2; decreased calcium and RBC
2. Urine tests show output of less than 20 mL per hr; fixed specific gravity of 1.010; excretion of protein, RBCs, WBCs, and casts
3. Microscopic examinations show that basement membrane of tubules destroyed and that glomeruli filter at much slower rate
4. X-rays may show an enlarged or normal-sized kidney on KUB and will rule out obstruction
5. ECG may show peaked T-waves if there is an elevated potassium

F. Complications
1. Cardiac failure
2. Pulmonary edema
3. Septic shock
4. Chronic renal failure

G. Medical treatment
1. Reverse cause
2. Low-protein diet (Table 8–26)
3. Supportive care

II. Analysis
A. Fluid volume excess related to retention secondary to renal failure (oliguric phase)
B. Fluid volume deficit related to diuresis secondary to renal failure (diuretic phase)
C. Activity intolerance related to acute illness
D. Knowledge deficit related to disease, diet, dialysis, and prevention of recurrence
E. High risk for injury and infection related to already weakened renal system

III. Planning/goals, expected outcomes
A. Client will have potential cause determined and recovery promoted
B. In oliguria phase
   1. Client will not suffer from fluid and electrolyte imbalance
   2. Client will maintain protein-sparing diet with restricted fluids
   3. Client will tolerate dialysis
   4. Client will not develop infection
C. In diuretic phase
   1. Client will not become dehydrated

TABLE 8–26 High and Low Protein Foods

Low Protein Foods	High Protein Foods
Fruits, fresh or canned	Meats
Green vegetables	Eggs
Carrots	Fish
Potatoes	Milk
Margarine	Soybeans
Prepared low protein items such as breads	Gelatin
Farina	Protein supplements
Sherbet	Yogurt
Corn starch	Peanut butter
Wheat starch	Cheese
	Legumes
	Protein-fortified cereals

2. Client will maintain fluid and electrolyte balance and adequate nutrition
   D. In convalescent phase
      1. Client will learn preventive habits such as avoiding nephrotoxins and attending promptly to infections
      2. Client will understand and comply with diet, medications, and activity
IV. Implementation
   A. Be alert to conditions that may precipitate renal failure and prevent them
   B. Assist in determining cause of renal failure
   C. Encourage a low-protein diet to decrease work of kidneys; increase calories and carbohydrates, either by mouth or TPN; restrict sodium and potassium according to electrolytes; restrict fluids to equal output
   D. Administer medications to treat symptoms (**Note:** Medications that are primarily excreted by the kidneys require modification of dosage and/or frequency. Dialyzable medications may need to be increased, or held and given after dialysis)
      1. Anti-infectives to treat organisms
      2. Antacids such as Amphojel to bind phosphates to control hyperphosphatemia
      3. Alkalyzers such as $NaHCO_3$ to treat acidosis
      4. Antihypertensives (as previously discussed)
      5. Diuretics (as previously discussed)
      6. Potassium-lowering agents such as insulin, glucose, and $NaHCO_3$ by IV, Kayexalate by NG tube or enema, or dialysis
   E. Supportive care
      1. Strict monitoring of I & O and of weight
      2. Bedrest with side rails up
      3. Oral hygiene
      4. Control for potential infection; skin care for dryness and pruritus
      5. Calm environment
V. Evaluation
   A. Client knows early signs and symptoms of urinary disorder
   B. Client follows diet, medication, fluid, and activity restrictions and knows purpose
   C. Client free of renal disease; continued follow-up

Chronic Renal Failure
I. Assessment
   A. Definition: slow, insidious, irreversible, ongoing deterioration of kidney function resulting in uremia or end-stage renal disease (ESRD) requiring dialysis or kidney transplant to maintain life

   B. Incidence
      1. May follow acute renal failure
      2. More common in women
      3. Often follows glomerulonephritis
   C. Predisposing/precipitating factors
      1. Recurrent infections, exacerbations of nephritis, or obstructions
      2. Destruction of blood vessels from long-standing hypertension or diabetes
      3. Direct insult or trauma to kidney
   D. Clinical manifestations
      1. See Acute Renal Failure
      2. Azotemia symptoms such as lethargy, headache, fatigue, weight loss, irritability, depression
      3. Fluid and electrolyte symptoms such as fluid retention, edema, anorexia, nausea, vomiting, shortness of breath
      4. Alterations in urine output
      5. Hypertension
      6. Increased pigmentation of skin
      7. Muscular twitching
      8. Numbness of feet, legs
   E. Diagnostic examinations
      1. See section on acute renal failure
      2. Hyperuricemia, elevated serum phosphate and calcium
   F. Complications: same as those of acute renal failure
   G. Medical management
      1. Hemodialysis
      2. Peritoneal dialysis
   H. Surgical management: renal transplant
II. Analysis
   A. Knowledge deficit related to disease, diet, dialysis, and long-term problems
   B. Activity intolerance related to fatigue and weakness secondary to anemia and uremia
   C. Altered skin integrity related to pruritus secondary to uremia
III. Planning/goals, expected outcomes
   A. Client will have symptoms relieved
   B. Client will understand and comply with fluid and electrolyte regulation, diet, medications
   C. Client will have treatment for concurrent disorders such as anemia, hypertension, diabetes, infection
   D. Client will undergo successful dialysis
   E. Client will have potential for transplant explored
IV. Implementation
   A. Similar to acute renal failure
   B. Supportive measures: skin care, oral hygiene, rest, calm atmosphere
   C. Fluid and electrolytes

1. Renal dietary restrictions per lab values and signs and symptoms
2. Monitor I & O; weigh client daily
3. Monitor extent of edema
4. Vital signs (VS), including breath sounds
5. Restrict fluids
6. Diet: high in carbohydrates and within prescribed limits for protein, Na^+, K^+, and phosphate
7. Give Basogel or Amphojel to bind phosphate

D. Provide continuous ultrafiltration/hemofiltration for very ill clients unable to tolerate dialysis
E. Provide treatment for underlying concurrent disorders
F. Prevent infection, injury; skin care including anti-itch medications
G. Assist with dialysis (Table 8–27)
  1. To correct fluid and electrolyte problems
  2. To remove waste products and drugs from system
H. Discuss possibilities/ramifications of kidney transplant with client and family
  1. Recipient care similar to any major surgery previously discussed
  2. Donor care as with nephrectomy plus immunosuppression management
    a. Azathioprine (Imuran)
    b. Prednisone
    c. Cyclosporin
  3. Rejection
    a. Acute
      (1) 1 week to 4 months
      (2) Potentially reversible with increased immunosuppression

  b. Chronic
    (1) Months to years after transplant
    (2) Irreversible
    (3) Manage considerably with diet, antihypertensive drugs, dialysis, and search for donor kidney

V. Evaluation
A. Client understands relationships between symptoms, causes, diet, laboratory work, medications, and activities
B. Client follows dietary and drug regimen
C. Client understands need for follow-up treatment
D. Client understands and adheres to dialysis procedures
E. Client prepared for renal transplant if appropriate donor available and adheres to follow-up immunosuppression therapy

Malignancies

Renal Cancer
I. Assessment
A. Incidence
  1. Men 2 : 1
  2. High in Scandinavia and low in Japan
  3. Usually between ages 55 to 60
B. Predisposing/precipitating factors
  1. Cigarette smoking
  2. Analgesics containing phenacetin
C. Clinical manifestations
  1. Gross hematuria, without manifestations of infection
  2. Dull, aching renal pain
  3. Palpable mass
D. Diagnostic examinations
  1. Kidney, ureter, bladder (KUB) x-ray

TABLE 8–27 Comparison of Hemodialysis and Peritoneal Dialysis

	Hemodialysis	Peritoneal Dialysis
Access	AV fistula, external shunt	Teflon or Silastic catheter in the peritoneal cavity
Dialysis Solution	Electrolyte solution similar to that of normal plasma	Similar to hemodialysis
Dialyzer	Artificial kidney machine with semipermeable membrane	Peritoneum dialyzing membrane
Procedure	Blood shunted through dialyzer 3 to 5 hours, 2 to 3 times per week	Repeated cycles that last 36 to 48 hours; catheter cleansed and attached to line leading to peritoneal cavity; dialysate infused into peritoneal cavity to prescribed volume (2 L) in 20 minutes; dialysate then drained from abdomen after prescribed amount of time (30 minutes)
Advantage	Efficient removal of wastes, fluid, K^+; home use possible	Can institute readily; less complicated technically; portable system; home use; useful in clients with vascular access problems; heparinization not necessary; less stress on cardiovascular system
Disadvantages	Vascular access necessary; hepatitis risk; requires heparin; special equipment and staff required	Risk of peritonitis; protein loss into dialysate; contraindicated in recent postoperative abdominal patients or recent trauma; respiratory difficulty

2. Nephrotomogram to differentiate cysts from tumors
3. Intravenous pyelogram (IVP)
   a. Pre-test
      (1) NPO 6 to 8 hours
      (2) Laxatives and enemas to clean out bowels
      (3) Check for iodine allergies
   b. Post-test
      (1) Watch for anaphylaxis
      (2) Maintain good urinary output
4. Retrograde pyelogram
   a. Pre-test same as IVP
   b. Post-test
      (1) Greater risk of sepsis
      (2) Monitor urine output
      (3) Monitor temperature
5. Renal ultrasound to differentiate cysts from tumors
6. CT scans of kidney and of brain, abdomen, and chest for metastasis
   a. Pre-test
      (1) NPO
      (2) Enemas and laxatives to clean bowel
   b. Post-test
      (1) Monitor for headache if contrast media used
7. Renal angiography
   a. Pre-test
      (1) Assess pulses distal to insertion site
      (2) NPO 8 hours
      (3) Check for iodine allergies
      (4) May need enemas or laxatives to clean bowel
      (5) Sedation before test
   b. Post-test
      (1) Check for allergic reactions
      (2) Monitor for bleeding or hematoma at insertion site; use pressure dressing
      (3) Keep flat in bed 8 to 12 hours
      (4) Monitor pulses distal to insertion site
   E. Complications
      1. Lung, bone, and liver metastases
      2. Abnormal endocrine secretions
   F. Medical and surgical treatment
      1. Radical nephrectomy
      2. No effective chemotherapy and tumor's spread usually radioresistant
II. Analysis
   A. Knowledge deficit related to diagnosis and treatment
   B. High risk for infection: respiratory related to high incision for nephrectomy

III. Planning/goals, expected outcomes
   A. Client will be adequately prepared for surgery
   B. Client will recover without complications
   C. Client and significant others will cope with terminal prognosis
IV. Implementation
   A. Support client during diagnostic tests
   B. Monitor renal function carefully
   C. Prevent postoperative complications
      1. Severe pain
         a. Medicate to prevent complications
         b. Turn and reposition frequently
      2. Prevent atelectasis and pneumonia
         a. Medicate
         b. Cough and deep breathe hourly
         c. Use incentive spirometer
      3. Monitor renal function
      4. Monitor for paralytic ileus
      5. Monitor for shock and hemorrhage
   D. Encourage client to verbalize fears and questions
   E. Encourage follow-up care
V. Evaluation
   A. Client recovers from surgery without complications
   B. Client and significant others cope with terminal prognosis

Bladder Cancer
   I. Assessment
   A. Pathophysiology
      1. Tumors usually in trigone region
      2. Tumors always premalignant
      3. Usually multiple tumors that often recur
      4. Early tumors grow on stalk and are noninfiltrating
   B. Incidence
      1. Over age 50
      2. White males
   C. Predisposing/precipitating factors
      1. Exposure to chemicals: benzines, naphtha, phenol
      2. Working with dyes and printing inks
      3. Smoking and alcohol
      4. Taking saccharin, phenacetin, or cyclophosphamide (Cytoxan)
      5. Schistosomiasis
   D. Clinical manifestations
      1. Painless, gross hematuria
      2. Bladder irritability
      3. Symptoms of obstruction with large tumor
      4. Pain and manifestations of metastasis late
   E. Diagnostic examinations
      1. IVP
      2. Cystoscopy
         a. Pre-test

(1) NPO

(2) Mild sedation

(3) Warn client room dark during procedure

b. Post-test

(1) Force fluids

(2) Monitor for first voiding; painful, usually blood-tinged

(3) Monitor for fever and sepsis

3. Urine cytology

4. CEA level as tumor marker

5. Bone, liver, and lung scans

F. Complications

1. Spread by direct extension to ureters, prostate or vagina, and colon

2. Bone, liver, and lung metastases

3. Impotence in men

4. Lower extremity lymphedema after radical pelvic lymph node dissection

G. Medical management

1. Radon seeds

2. Radiation therapy

3. Chemotherapy

H. Surgical management

1. Transurethral resection of bladder (TURB)

2. Partial cystectomy

3. Radical cystectomy and urinary diversion

a. Ureterosigmoidostomy

(1) Disadvantages

(a) Infections into renal pelvis

(b) Hyperchloremic acidosis

(c) Diarrhea

(2) Advantage: continence

b. Cutaneous ureterostomy

(1) Palliative surgery

(2) Two stomas

c. Continent ileal conduit

(1) Similar to Kock pouch or Indiana pouch used for ileostomy

(2) Use catheter to drain urine from pouch

d. Ileal conduit and radical cystectomy

II. Analysis

A. Knowledge deficit related to diagnosis, treatment, and care of urinary diversion

B. High risk for sexual dysfunction related to impotence in men

C. Altered body image related to ostomy

D. High risk for injury related to extensive surgery

III. Planning/goals, expected outcomes

A. Client will understand diagnostic procedures

B. Client will be physically and psychologically prepared for surgery

C. Male clients will adjust to impotence postoperatively

D. Client will recover from surgery without complications

E. Client will demonstrate ability to care for own urinary appliance and will cope effectively

IV. Implementation

A. Preoperatively

1. Low-residue diet, then clear liquid diet

2. Bowel preparation

a. Antibiotics such as neomycin or kanamycin

b. Cathartics

c. Enemas until clear

3. Emotional support and sexual counseling for men

4. Stoma placement same as ileostomy

5. Encourage visit from ostomy visitor

B. Postoperatively: ileal conduit

1. Priority is urine output; must be constant because there is no bladder

2. Shock and hemorrhage possible due to extensive surgery and vascularity of area

3. Pelvic thrombus because of trauma to pelvic region

C. Client teaching: stoma care (see Table 8–13)

1. Tight seal; appliance 1 cm larger than stoma

2. Check skin irritation, non-karaya barrier, change as needed

3. Empty frequently, hook to drainage bag at night to avoid reflux into kidneys

4. Application of appliance and skin care similar to ileostomy

5. Most dangerous complication is reflux and pyelonephritis

6. High fluid intake—acid ash, cranberry juice, and vitamin C

7. Loss of continence, severe body image changes

D. Male impotence: penile implant, counseling

E. Continent ileal conduit: similar to continent ileostomy—emptied at regular intervals through stomal catheterization

V. Evaluation

A. Client adequately prepared for surgery and urinary diversion

B. Male client and significant others adapt to altered sexuality and body image

C. Client recovers from surgery without complications

D. Client cares for own urinary appliance without difficulty

POST-TEST Renal/Urinary Disorders

1. Which of the following diseases is known to be related to renal problems?

① Measles
② Diabetes mellitus
③ Gastric ulcer
④ Jaundice

2. Which of the following is NOT an abnormal finding in a routine urinalysis?
① pH 6.0
② Pus
③ RBCs
④ Protein

3. Which of the following is NOT part of the normal procedure to obtain a urine culture and sensitivity specimen?
① Void 50 mL of urine and discard it
② Clean the external meatus with alcohol-acetone wipes
③ Void remainder of urine into sterile container
④ Refrigerate specimen until sent to laboratory

4. Which of the following complications is NOT usually a concern during a cystoscopy?
① Urinary tract infections
② Urinary retention
③ Perforation of the bladder
④ Renal colic

5. Women who are especially susceptible to urinary tract infections should:
① Take prophylactic sulfonamides for the rest of their lives
② Drink at least 2 to 3 L of fluid per day
③ Take tub baths and bubble baths
④ Cleanse themselves from the rectum to the urethra after voiding

6. Clinical manifestations of acute pyelonephritis include:
① Elevated blood pressure
② Albuminuria and edema
③ Bacteria and white blood cells in the urine
④ Hematuria and polyuria

7. During the diuretic phase of acute renal failure, which of the following serum electrolyte imbalances is most likely to develop?
① Increased K^+ and decreased Na^+
② Increased K^+ and increased Na^+
③ Decreased K^+ and increased Na^+
④ Decreased K^+ and decreased Na^+

8. The following measures are used in the management of chronic renal failure. For which of the following is the correct rationale given?
① Kayexalate to reduce peripheral edema
② Aluminum hydroxide to decrease serum phosphate
③ Calcitrol to decrease serum calcium
④ Methyldopa to increase urine output

9. Common complications of hemodialysis include all of the following EXCEPT:
① Transfusion reactions
② Shock
③ Bleeding from the lines
④ Hepatitis

10. Which of the following conditions does NOT predispose to the development of renal failure?
① Mismatched blood transfusions
② Severe dehydration
③ Septicemia
④ Cerebrovascular accident

11. Nursing care for a client on chronic peritoneal dialysis would NOT include which of the following?
① Encourage protein intake of high biological value
② Decrease the inflow rate if referred shoulder pain is experienced
③ Change the peritoneal catheter every 2 to 3 weeks
④ Instruct client that fluid intake is unrestricted

12. Hyperkalemia can be a fatal complication of electrolyte imbalances because hyperkalemia causes:
① Hypertension and strokes
② Acute dysrhythmias
③ Increased clotting time, which may lead to hemorrhage
④ Seizures

Mr. Rocke, aged 30, has a sudden onset of severe right flank pain. His wife brings him to the hospital, where he is admitted for tests and observation. The preliminary diagnosis is urinary calculi.

---

13. Which of the following explanations most accurately describe the purpose of the IVP?
① The renal pelvis can be observed directly
② Medication can be injected directly into the loop of Henle
③ The entire urinary tract can be visualized under x-ray
④ The ureters and bladder can be visualized for stones

14. After Mr. Rocke undergoes the IVP, he returns to his room very angry and upset, claiming that he was lied to about the nature of the test. Which of the following information had Mr. Rocke probably NOT received that he should have?
    1. The catheter insertion causes fluttery sensations and fainting
    2. The test may cause spasms and abdominal discomfort
    3. The dye injected may cause a hot feeling and nausea
    4. The injection of radiopaque dye may induce chills and shivering

15. Because Mr. Rocke will also receive sulfisoxazole (Gantrisin) twice a day, it will be important for him to increase his fluid intake in order to:
    1. Prevent crystallization in the renal tubules
    2. Prevent severe dehydration from insensible water loss
    3. Promote metabolism of the drug by the liver
    4. Promote sodium excretion

Arthur Burns is a 60-year-old man who has come into outpatient surgery for a cystoscopy for continued hematuria that has lasted for more than a year. He does not have an infection, so he is being worked up for either renal or bladder cancer.

---

16. An important assessment that must be made before renal angiography is:
    1. The presence of bowel sounds
    2. Whether he has a urinary tract infection
    3. If he has had a similar test before
    4. The pulses distal to the insertion site

17. Post-renal angiogram, it is important for the nurse to:
    1. Have the client ambulate and sit in a chair
    2. Withhold fluids for 12 hours after the test
    3. Assess the insertion site for a hematoma or bleeding
    4. Monitor blood pressure every 2 hours

18. The diagnosis of renal cancer is confirmed. Mr. Burns is scheduled for a radical nephrectomy. The most important assessment that must be made before the surgery is:
    1. The degree of function of the unaffected kidney
    2. A baseline estimate of urine output

3. Whether or not the tumor has spread
4. The client's acceptance of his diagnosis

19. Postoperatively, which of the following complications is most likely to occur with this type of surgery?
    1. Phlebitis
    2. Atelectasis and pneumonia
    3. Urinary tract infection
    4. Wound infection

20. Which of the following is a reasonable expected outcome for the client with metastatic renal cancer?
    1. Client recovers with minimal alteration in body image
    2. Client accepts dialysis for the rest of his life
    3. Client recovers with limited renal function
    4. Client copes with terminal diagnosis

Mr. Lee had a radical cystectomy and ileal conduit yesterday to treat his bladder cancer.

---

21. Which of the following symptoms immediately postoperatively would be the most critical?
    1. Lack of urine output for 30 minutes
    2. Respiratory rate of 24
    3. Complaints of severe incisional pain
    4. Some lower extremity edema

22. Mr. Lee needs to be taught to avoid and/or recognize which of the following problems that might result from his ileal conduit?
    1. Recurrent bladder infections
    2. Possible intestinal obstruction
    3. Kidney infections
    4. Dilation of the stoma

23. Mr. Lee needs to be informed that the most common and serious problem that develops if the ileal conduit pouch does not fit properly is:
    1. Infection of the stoma
    2. Skin excoriation
    3. Stricture of the ileal stoma
    4. Mucous drainage from the stoma

24. It is important to teach Mr. Lee to attach the ileal drainage pouch to gravity drainage at night to:
    1. Prevent infection of the stoma because of urinary stasis in the pouch
    2. Prevent leakage of urine from overdistention of the pouch
    3. Facilitate a more normal form of elimination

④ Prevent reflux of the urine back into the renal pelvis

25. Which of the following is an important and realistic goal for Mr. Lee after his surgery?
    ① Client will not develop sexual problems
    ② Client will regain normal urinary control
    ③ Client will care for own urinary appliance
    ④ Client will regain normal bowel function

26. Which of the following is an expected outcome of Mr. Lee's surgery?
    ① Client does not develop sexual problems
    ② Client regains normal urinary control

③ Client is able to care for own urinary appliance
④ Client regains normal bowel function

27. Preoperative physical preparation for the client scheduled for an ileal conduit would NOT include which of the following?
    ① Administering antibiotics such as neomycin
    ② Giving enemas until clear and laxatives
    ③ Marking the skin for stoma placement
    ④ Inserting a Foley catheter

POST-TEST Answers and Rationales

1. ② Diabetes predisposes the client to renal disease. The other options do not affect renal function. 1, II. Renal.

2. ① The normal urine pH should be about 5 to 7. Pus, blood, and protein are all abnormal constituents of urine. 2, II. Renal.

3. ② The client should clean the meatus with soap and water before voiding. The client then voids about 50 mL and discards it, and voids the rest into a sterile container. The specimen should be kept refrigerated until it is sent to the laboratory. 4, II. Renal.

4. ④ A cystoscopy can produce urinary tract infection, retention, and perforation. Renal colic is not a possible effect of a cystoscopy. 2, I. Cystoscopy.

5. ② Forcing fluids is the best way to prevent urinary tract infections, because it helps to wash the bacteria out of the urinary tract. Sometimes antibiotics are used prophylactically after intercourse, but not sulfa drugs. Tub baths and bubble baths increase the risk of infections, as does wiping back to front. 4, I & II. Urinary Tract Infections.

6. ③ Pyelonephritis is an acute infection characterized by bacteria and white blood cells in the urine. The blood pressure is not necessarily elevated. Albumin is not found in the urine and no edema occurs. Hematuria may occur but there is no polyuria. 1, II. Pyelonephritis.

7. ④ Both sodium and potassium are decreased in the diuretic phase of renal failure because they are both washed out with diuresis. 2, II. Renal Failure.

8. ② Aluminum hydroxide binds with phosphorus to lower the serum phosphate level. Kayexalate lowers the serum potassium, calcitrol increases the serum calcium, and methyldopa is an antihypertensive that has no effect on the urine. 4, II. Renal Failure.

9. ① Transfusions are not a normal part of hemodialysis, so transfusion reactions are unlikely. The other options are common potential problems associated with dialysis. 2, I. Hemodialysis.

10. ④ A CVA in no way predisposes to renal failure. The other options do. Mismatched blood causes acute tubular necrosis; dehydration and septicemia are prerenal causes. 2, I. Renal Failure.

11. ③ The peritoneal catheter is changed only as needed, not every few weeks. High biological value protein is important in the diet, there is no fluid restriction, and if pain in the shoulder occurs, the inflow should be slowed. 4, II. Peritoneal Dialysis.

12. ② Potassium levels affect cardiac function and hyperkalemia predisposes the client to potentially life-threatening dysrhythmias. The other options are not caused by hyperkalemia. 2, I. Dialysis.

13. ③ The IVP is useful because the entire urinary tract can be visualized under x-ray. The dye is injected intravenously and picked up by the renal system where it is excreted. Choice 4 is also true, but 3 is more complete. 2, I & II. Renal Calculi.

14. ③ The dye may cause a hot, flushed feeling and many clients complain of nausea immediately after the injection. There is no catheter, and the test does not cause spasms or abdominal discomfort. 4, I & II. Renal Calculi.

15. ① Sulfa drugs have low solubility and can crystallize in the urine if the intake is not sufficient to dilute the urine. There is no abnormal insensible water loss, sodium excretion is not a problem, and the drug does not require extra fluid to metabolize the drug. 4, II. Renal Calculi.

16. ④ The most important assessment are the pulses distal to the insertion site because after the procedure, a sign of problems would be a change in these pulses. The other assessments are important, but not as vital as this one. 1, I. Renal Cancer, Arteriogram.

17. ③ The insertion site must be carefully checked after the procedure to monitor for hemorrhage or interference with circulation. The client should be encouraged to drink fluids and should lie flat for 24 hours. The blood pressure should be checked, but it is not as important as assessing the site. 1, I & II. Renal Cancer, Arteriogram.

18. ① All of the options are assessments that should be made preoperatively, but the function of the remaining kidney is the most vital assessment since it will be the total renal function. 1, I. Renal Cancer.

19. ② Since the kidney is just below the diaphragm and the surgery causes a great deal of pain, atelectasis and pneumonia are a greater risk. All of the other options are possible, but no more likely in this client than any other surgery. 2, I. Renal Cancer.

20. ④ Renal cancer has a very poor prognosis because it is usually not found early. The most reasonable outcome is acceptance of the terminal prognosis. 5, IV. Renal Cancer.

21. ① Urine flow should be continuous as soon as the ureters are attached to the ileum. The low output could mean anything from obstruction to shock. The other options are normal changes postoperatively. 2, I. Ileal Conduit.

22. ③ Pyelonephritis is a serious but real problem that can occur after surgery since nothing can stop urine from refluxing back up into the renal pelvis. There is no bladder to become infected, intestinal obstruction is unlikely, and there is no problem with dilation of the stoma. 2, I & II. Ileal Conduit.

23. ② Urine is very caustic to the skin and if the pouch does not fit properly, severe skin excoriation can occur. Infection is unlikely, as are strictures, and mucous drainage is normal. 4, I & II. Ileal Conduit.

24. ④ Pyelonephritis is a real risk and attaching the drainage bottle to gravity drainage is the best way to prevent it. There is some risk of overfilling of the pouch, but that is not a really serious problem. The stoma will not become infected, and elimination is not normal. 4, IV. Ileal Conduit.

25. ③ It is important for the client to learn to care for his own appliance as soon as possible. It is unrealistic to think that he will not develop some sexual difficulties postoperatively. He will not regain normal urinary control, and there is no reason to think he will have bowel problems. 3, I & IV. Ileal Conduit.

26. ③ Caring for his own appliance is the best outcome that can be expected and shows that the client is adjusting to his stoma. Sexual difficulties are inevitable, bowel function should not be affected, and urinary control is unrealistic. 5, I & IV. Ileal Conduit.

27. ④ Preparation for an ileal conduit includes cleansing the bowel with laxatives, enemas, and antibiotics. It is also important that the stoma be properly marked before surgery. A catheter is not used since it could introduce an infection. 4, I. Ileal Conduit.

BIBLIOGRAPHY

ENDOCRINE DISORDERS

Black, J., and Matassarin-Jacobs, E., eds. (1993). *Luckmann & Sorenson's Medical-surgical nursing: A psychophysiologic approach,* 4th ed. Philadelphia: W. B. Saunders.

Cataldo, C., and Whitney, E. (1991). *Nutrition and diet therapy.* St. Paul: West Publishing.

Davidson, M. (1986). *Diabetes mellitus: Diagnosis and treatment.* New York: John Wiley.

Hahn, A., Oestreich, S., and Barkin, R. (1986). *Mosby's pharmacology in nursing.* St. Louis: C. V. Mosby.

Wilson, J., and Foster, D., eds. (1985). *Williams' textbook of endocrinology.* Philadelphia: W. B. Saunders.

GASTRIC/LOWER INTESTINAL DISORDERS

Belcher, A. (1992). *Cancer nursing.* St. Louis: Mosby-Year Book.

Brodrick, R. (1991). Preventing complications in acute pancreatitis. *Dimensions of Critical Care Nursing* 10 (5): 262–270.

Bryant, G. (1992). When bowel is blocked. *RN* 55 (1): 58–67.

Carpenito, L. J. (1992). *Nursing diagnosis—application to clinical practice,* vol. 4. Philadelphia: J. B. Lippincott.

Cooke, D. (1991). Inflammatory bowel disease: Primary health care management of ulcerative colitis and Crohn's disease. *Nurse Practitioner* 16 (8): 27–39.

Friedmen, G. (1988). Peptic ulcer disease. In *Clinical Symposia 1988 Annual* 40 (5): 2–32. Summit, NJ: Pharmaceutical Division, CIBA-GEIGY Corporation.

Gauwitz, D. (1990). Endoscopic cholecystectomy. *Nursing 90* 20 (12): 58–59.

Jurf, J., Clements, L., and Llorente, J. (1990). Cholecystectomy made easier. *American Journal of Nursing* 90 (12): 36–39.

Phipps, W., Long, B., Woods, N., and Cassemeyer, V. (1991). *Medical surgical nursing: Concepts and clinical practice,* 4th ed. (pp. 1279–1384). St. Louis: Mosby Year Book.

Smeltzer, S., and Bare, B., eds. (1992). *Brunner and Suddarth's textbook of medical–surgical nursing,* 7th ed. Philadelphia: J. B. Lippincott.

Wardell, T. L. (1991). Assessing and managing a gastric ulcer. *Nursing '91* 21 (3): 34–42.

Welch, J. (1990). *Bowel obstruction—Differential diagnosis and clinical management.* Philadelphia: W. B. Saunders.

Yamada, T. (1991). *Textbook of gastroenterology,* vols. 1–2. New York: J. B. Lippincott.

HEPATIC/BILIARY DISORDERS

American Cancer Society. (1992). *Cancer facts and figures.* New York: American Cancer Society.

American Liver Foundation (1986). *Cirrhosis: Many causes.* Cedar Grove, Iowa: American Liver Foundation.

American Liver Foundation (1986). *Viral hepatitis*. Cedar Grove, Iowa: American Liver Foundation.

Anderson, F. D. (1986). Portal-systemic encephalopathy in the chronic alcoholic. *Critical Care Quarterly* 8 (4): 40–50.

Arias, I. M., et al. (1988). *The liver: Biology and pathobiology*. New York: Raven Press.

Axon, A. T. (1989). Endoscopic retrograde cholangiopancreatography in chronic pancreatitis: Cambridge classification. *Radiology Clinics of North America* 27 (1): 39–50.

Balthazar, E. J. (1989). CT diagnosis and staging of acute pancreatitis. *Radiology Clinics of North America* 27 (1): 19–37.

Bayless, T. M. (1989). *Current therapy in gastroenterology and liver disease*, 3rd ed., vol. 3. St. Louis: C. V. Mosby.

Beasley, R. P., and Hwang, H. Y. (1984). Hepatocellular carcinoma and hepatitis B virus. *Seminars in Liver Disease* 4: 113–121.

Black, J., and Matassarin-Jacobs, E., eds. (1993). *Luckmann & Sorensen's Medical-surgical nursing: A psychophysiologic approach, 4th ed. Philadelphia*: W. B. Saunders.

Braunwald, E., Isselbacher, K. J., Petersdorf, R. G., Wilson, J., Martin, J. B., and Fauci, A. S., eds. (1987). *Harrison's principles of internal medicine*, 11th ed. New York: McGraw-Hill.

Clouse, M. E. (1989). Current diagnostic imaging modalities of the liver. *Surgical Clinics of North America* 69 (2): 193–234.

Gillinsky, N. H. (1987). The role of pancreatic function testing in the 1980's. *South African Medical Journal* 71 (4): 235–238.

Gitnick, G., ed. (1989). *Modern concepts of acute and chronic hepatitis*. New York: Plenum.

Gitnick, G., ed. (1988). *Handbook of gastrointestinal emergencies*, 2nd ed. New York: Elsevier Science.

Gitnick, G., et al, eds. (1988). *Principles and practice of gastroenterology and hepatology*. New York: Elsevier Science.

Go, V. L. W., et al. (1986). *The exocrine pancreas: Biology, pathobiology, and disease*. New York: Raven Press.

Grimson, A. E. S., et al. (1986). A randomized trial of vasopressin and vasopressin plus nitroglycerin in the treatment of acute variceal hemorrhage. *Hepatology* 6: 410–413.

Guyton, A. C. (1991). *Textbook of medical physiology*, 8th ed. Philadelphia: W. B. Saunders.

Hayworth, M. F., and Jones, A. L. (1988). *Immunology of the gastrointestinal tract and liver*. New York: Raven Press.

Holland, P., and Hussain, I. (1989). Biliary lithotripsy: Nonsurgical treatment of gallstones. *Society of Gastrointestinal Assistants Journal* 3: 158–162.

Jeffery, R. B. (1989). Sonography in acute pancreatitis. *Radiology Clinics of North America* 27 (1): 5–17.

Johnson, L. R., et al. (1987). *Physiology of the gastrointestinal tract*, 2nd ed. New York: Raven Press.

Keith, J. S. (1985). Hepatic failure: Etiologies, manifestations and management. *Critical Care Nurse* 5 (1): 60–86.

Maloney, J. P. (1986). Surgical interventions in the alcoholic patient with portal hypertension. *Critical Care Quarterly* 8 (4): 63–73.

Marta, M. R. (1987). Endoscopic retrograde cholangiopancreatography: Its role in diagnosis and treatment. *Focus on Critical Care* 14 (5): 62–63.

Mosley, J. W., et al. (1990). Non-A, non-B hepatitis and antibody to hepatitis C virus. *Journal of the American Medical Association* 263: 77–78.

Oberfield, R. A., et al. (1989). Liver cancer. *CA: A Journal for Clinicians* 39: 206–218.

Quinless, F. W. (1985). Severe liver dysfunction. *Focus on Critical Care* 12 (1): 24–32.

Rakel, R. E. (1990). *Conn's current therapy*. Philadelphia: W. B. Saunders.

Ricci, J. A. (1987). Alcohol induced upper GI hemorrhage: Case studies and management. *Critical Care Nurse* 7 (1): 56–65.

Rollins, B. J. (1986). Hepatic veno-occlusive disease. *American Journal of Medicine* 81: 297–306.

Sabiston, D. C. Jr. (1991). *Textbook of surgery: The biologic basis of modern surgical practice*, 14th ed. Philadelphia: W. B. Saunders.

Schiff, L., and Schiff, E. R. (1987). *Diseases of the liver*, 3rd ed. Philadelphia: J. B. Lippincott.

Schindler, M. S., and Eastwood, G. L. (1987). Delta hepatitis: A deadly corollary to hepatitis B. *Journal of Critical Illness* 2: 91–100.

Schroeder, S. A., Krupp, M. A., and Teirney, L. M. (1988). *Current medical diagnosis and treatment*. Norwalk, CT: Appleton & Lange.

Sherlock, S. (1985). *Diseases of the liver and biliary system*. Oxford: Blackwell Scientific.

VanSonneberg, E., et al. (1989). Imaging and interventional radiology for pancreatitis and its complications. *Radiology Clinics of North America* 27 (1): 65–72.

Vyas, G. N., Dienstag, J. L., and Hoofnagle, J. H. (1984). *Viral hepatitis and liver disease*. Orlando: Grune & Stratton.

Widmann, F. (1987). *Goodall's clinical interpretation of laboratory tests*, 10th ed. Philadelphia: F. A. Davis.

Witkin, G. B., et al. (1987). Choosing liver function tests. *Emergency Medicine* 19 (20): 22–46.

Wyngaarden, J. B., and Smith, L. H., eds. (1988). *Cecil textbook of medicine*, 18th ed. Philadelphia: W. B. Saunders.

Zakim, D., and Bayer, T. D., eds. (1990). *Textbook of liver disease*, 2nd ed. Philadelphia: W. B. Saunders.

RENAL/URINARY DISORDERS

American Association of Critical Care Nurses. (1985). *Care curriculum for critical care nursing*. Philadelphia: W. B. Saunders.

Anderson, R. J. (1983). Drug prescribing for patients with renal failure. *Hospital Practice* 19: 145–160.

Andrucci, V. (1984). *Acute renal failure: Pathophysiology, prevention, and treatment*. Boston: Martinus Nijhoff.

Binkley, L. S. (1984). Keeping up with peritoneal dialysis. *American Journal of Nursing* 84: 729–733.

Black, J., and Matassarin-Jacobs, E., eds. (1993). *Luckmann & Sorensen's Medical-surgical nursing: A psychophysiologic approach, 4th ed. Philadelphia*: W. B. Saunders.

Brown, R. O. (1983). Nutritional support in acute renal failure. *American Association of Nephrology Nurses & Technicians Journal* 10: 25.

Brundage, D. (1982). *Nursing management of renal problems*, 2nd ed. St. Louis: C. V. Mosby.

Campbell, M., and Harrison, J. (1985). *Urology*, 5th ed. Philadelphia: W. B. Saunders.

Clifford, C. M. (1982). Urinary tract infection—a brief selective review. *International Journal of Nursing Studies* 19 (4): 213–222.

Curha, B. A. (1982). Nosocomial urinary tract infections: causes, diagnosis, control measures, treatment. *Heart & Lung* 11: 545–551.

Doyle, J., and Reilly, N. (1985). Genitourinary problems. Florence, KY: Medical Economics.

Harwood, C. (1985). Pulverizing kidney stones: what you should know about lithotripsy. *RN* 48 (7): 32–37.

Johnson, D. (1989). Nephrotic syndrome: A nursing care plan based on current pathophysiologic concepts. *Heart & Lung* 18 (1): 85.

Kee, J. L. (1986). *Fluid and electrolytes with clinical applications*, 4th ed. New York: John Wiley.

Kurtzman, N. A. (1982). Chronic renal failure: Metabolic and clinical consequences. *Hospital Practice* 17:107–122.

LaCorte, A., and Pawley, M. (1985). Percutaneous lithotripsy for urinary calculi. *American Journal of Nursing* 22: 722–733.

Levine, D. Z. (1983). *Care of the renal patient*. Philadelphia: W. B. Saunders.

Matheny, N. (1987). *Fluid and electrolyte balance: Nursing considerations*. Philadelphia: J. B. Lippincott.

Matheny, N. (1982). Renal stones and urinary pH. *American Journal of Nursing* 82: 1372–1375.

Montefusci, C. M., Goldsmith, J., and Veith, F. J. (1984). Cyclosporine immunosuppression in organ graft recipients: Nursing implications. *Critical Care Nursing* 4: 117–119.

Norris, M. K. (1982). Nursing care plan for the patient with chronic renal failure. *Critical Care Nursing* 2: 59–63.

Orr, M. L. (1981). Drugs and renal disease. *American Journal of Nursing* 81: 969.

Pagana, K. D., and Pagana, T. J. (1985). *Diagnostic testing and nursing implications*, 2nd ed. St. Louis: C. V. Mosby.

Renal and urologic disorders (1984). Springhouse, PA: Nurse's Clinical Library.

Rodman, M. J., and Smith, D. W. (1985). *Clinical pharmacology in nursing*. Philadelphia: J. B. Lippincott.

Schreiner, G. E. (1983). Past, present and future of transplantation. *Kidney International* 23: 54.

Stark, J. L. (1983). Renal calculi. *Nursing 83* 13: 24.

Stark, J. L. (1982). Acute poststreptococcal glomerulonephritis. *Nursing 82* 12: 114.

Ulrich, B. T. (1989). *Nephrology nursing: Concepts and strategies.* Norwalk CT: Appleton & Lange.

VanStone, J. C. (1983). *Dialysis and treatment of renal insufficiency.* New York: Grune & Stratton.

Whittaker, A. A. (1985). Acute renal dysfunction: Assessment of patients at risk. *Focus on Critical Care* 12: 12–17.

Williams, S. R. (1985). *Nutrition and diet therapy,* 5th ed. St. Louis: C. V. Mosby.

UNIT III

The Pediatric Client

9

Pediatric Growth and Development

PRE-TEST GROWTH AND DEVELOPMENT

1. Sharon, a 15-year-old girl with chronic asthma, has been admitted to the hospital for the third time in 3 months. She seems to be angry and questions every treatment. One of the most important nursing interventions for Sharon is:
   1. Encouraging her autonomy while she is in the hospital
   2. Urging her family to visit frequently
   3. Discussing the schedule of respiratory treatments with her
   4. Using play therapy to channel her aggression

2. Mrs. Johnson tells the nurse that her toddler, Sam, has been eating only peanut butter sandwiches during the past few days. No matter what she tries to give him, he refuses everything else. The nurse's best response to Mrs. Johnson is:
   1. "You need to insist that he eat at least three servings of vegetables and fruits a day."
   2. "You don't need to be too concerned. This is not abnormal for his age."
   3. "Peanut butter sandwiches will provide all the essential nutrients he needs."
   4. "You need to start giving him vitamins to compensate for his poor diet."

3. Mr. Sampson is concerned because his 2-month-old daughter, Sarah, seems to be breathing rapidly. After assessing Sarah for respiratory distress and finding no data to suggest a serious respiratory problem, you can reassure Mr. Sampson that there is no need for concern at this time because:
   1. Sarah probably just has an upper respiratory infection
   2. Every infant has a different physiological respiratory pattern
   3. Sarah's respiratory rate probably decreases to 20 when she is asleep
   4. As Sarah's lungs become more mature and efficient, the rate will decrease

4. Stephen, a 4-year-old, has come to the clinic for his checkup. He tells the nurse that he is Peter Pan and that fairy dust is protecting him from harm. Knowing that he needs to have his finger pricked for hemoglobin and lead testing, the nurse plans to:
   1. Prick his finger first to get it over with, and then do the history and physical measurements
   2. Do the history and physical measurements first, and then explain the procedure step-by-step as it's being done
   3. Tell Stephen he doesn't have to worry, that the fairy dust will protect him from harm
   4. Do the history and physical measurements first, and then tell him that he'll get his finger pricked later

5. One rationale for administering iron-fortified formula to non–breast-fed infants under 1 year of age is that:
   1. Prenatally, infants lack sufficient levels of iron stores
   2. Birth trauma may result in depression of red blood cells
   3. Iron from maternal iron stores is generally depleted by 6 months of age
   4. Bone marrow production of red blood cells is hyperactive for 2 months after birth

6. When assessing 6-month-old Tanika, the nurse might expect to see the following:
   1. Beginning to sit with support, transfers a rattle from one hand to another, babbles
   2. Pulls self up to stand, has pincer movement, says "dada" and "mama"
   3. Head lags when pulled to sit, grasps a rattle, laughs, squeals
   4. Sits unsupported, picks up small objects with the whole hand, plays pat-a-cake and peek-a-boo

7. When planning care for the hospitalized school-age child, the nurse considers which of the following to be most instrumental in the child's understanding of and adjustment to the experience of hospitalization? The school-age child is:
   1. Achieving autonomy according to Erikson
   2. In Piaget's concrete operations stage
   3. Able to take the initiative in planning care
   4. No longer experiencing separation anxiety

8. Eighteen-month-old Angela has arrived at the well-child clinic for her routine physical examination. At her prior visit, her mother had expressed some concern about toilet training. Which of the following statements by Angela's mother would most indicate to the nurse that teaching had been effective?
   1. "I told my mother-in-law that you said Angela was too young to be potty trained."
   2. "I have started to sit Angela on the toilet every morning after breakfast to get her used to it."

③ "I give Angela prune juice in the morning to regulate her bowel movements."

④ "I have put a potty chair in the bathroom, and Angela likes to sit on it fully dressed while I use the bathroom in the morning."

9. Richard, a 6-year-old, is a client on your pediatric unit. He has begun wetting the bed both at night and during the day, although he has been trained for 2 years according to his parents. Because he is ambulatory and has a bathroom in his room, his parents are concerned. A possible nursing diagnosis for Richard is:

① Altered growth and development related to incomplete toilet training

② Ineffective individual coping related to the crisis of hospitalization

③ Urge incontinence related to increased fluid intake

④ Altered patterns of urinary elimination related to lack of privacy in the hospital

10. Thirteen-year-old Daniel is worried because he is one of the shortest boys in his class. Which of the following assessment data indicates that Daniel might be ready to begin his adolescent growth spurt?

① His testes have begun to enlarge

② He has gained a lot of weight recently

③ His father began his growth spurt at age 13

④ His twin sister is 4 in. taller than he

PRE-TEST Answers and Rationales

1. ③ Because Sharon is an adolescent, it is important for her to help plan her treatments and treatment schedule. One of the primary adverse reactions of adolescents to hospitalization is a feeling of loss of independence. Encouraging cooperative care planning can minimize this. The other options are more appropriate for children at younger developmental stages. 4, I & III. Growth and Development.

2. ② Food jags are frequently seen in toddlers. Controlling the type and amount of food that is eaten is one way in which a toddler exerts autonomy. Because jags are usually temporary, lasting only a few days, they do not compromise nutrition. Forcing a child to eat can create nutritional problems later in life. 4, IV. Growth and Development.

3. ④ Because infant lungs have no actual respiratory function before birth, they have proportionately more dead air space in their alveolar sacs at birth and therefore less area for exchange of oxygen and carbon dioxide. This, along with a high metabolic rate, requires increased respirations for adequate gas exchange. As the effective volume of the lungs increases, the respiratory rate will naturally slow. Assessment of the infant has shown no evidence of infection. 2, II. Growth and Development.

4. ② Preschoolers often use magical thinking as a way of coping with perceived threats. Although the nurse can go along with the fantasy to a certain extent, it is important to tell a child truthfully what can be expected. Preparing a preschool child too far in advance of a procedure can inappropriately heighten anxiety. The child should be prepared immediately before the procedure or be told in step-by-step fashion what will happen as it is being done. 3, III. Growth and Development.

5. ③ Prenatally, skeletal erythropoietin, the hormone that regulates red blood cell production, is active, but it becomes relatively hypoactive at birth. At about 2 months, it begins to gradually increase. Until the levels are high enough, infants need extra iron from external sources. At about 6 to 9 months of age, the infant's stores of maternal iron are depleted, requiring an external iron source. Recently, research has indicated that iron deficiency anemia in infancy can contribute to cognitive and developmental problems later in life. 3, II. Growth and Development.

6. ① Six-month-olds usually have good head control, can begin to sit unsupported, and have learned to transfer objects from one hand to another. The other options are more appropriate for older or younger infants. 1, IV. Growth and Development.

7. ② When school-age children are admitted to the hospital, their cognitive level of development makes it easier for them to understand procedures and increases their ability to cope with them. Children at this developmental stage can comprehend time and can relate to the time frame for their hospital stay. School-age children still experience separation anxiety but miss friends nearly as much as family. Achievement of autonomy and initiative are developmental tasks that are not applicable for this age. 2, I. Growth and Development.

8. ④ Children need to be physiologically ready for toilet training. Signs of readiness include the ability to walk well, the ability to communicate the need to use the toilet, parents' understanding of nonverbal behavior, and achievement of some sphincter control. Toilet training should not be started too young and should not be forced. Exposing the child to a potty chair and allowing the child to sit on it at will is a good beginning step. 5, II. Growth and Development.

9. ② Although regression is most commonly seen in toddlers, often a preschooler will regress to cope with a situational crisis. It is not unusual to see previously trained children have toilet accidents when in an unfamiliar environment. Because there is a bathroom readily available, lack of privacy should not be a problem. None of the assessment data given indicate increased fluid intake. 2, II & III. Growth and Development.

10. ① The growth spurt in males usually is preceded by testicular enlargement. Penile length increases as growth progresses.

Although heredity somewhat affects maturational timing, it is not a precise indicator. Weight gain in boys is not a predictor of growth as most weight gain in adolescent boys is related to increasing muscle mass during maturation. 1, II. Growth and Development.

Definitions

I. Growth increase in physical size of body or body part
II. Development: gradual change in function, not size, that results in more complex abilities and skills

INFANCY (1 MONTH TO 1 YEAR)

I. Physical
  A. Height: increases 1 in. a month for 6 months; increases 50% by 1 year
  B. Weight
    1. Neonate loses 5 to 10% of birth weight; regained at 1 to 2 weeks
    2. By 5 months, birth weight doubles
    3. By 1 year, birth weight triples
  C. Head circumference
    1. At birth, head circumference greater than chest, averages 13½ in. (34.3 cm)
    2. By 1 year, head and chest circumference are equal, chest circumference is larger thereafter
  D. Vital signs
    1. Pulse: 140 at birth to 100 at 1 year, varies with activity
    2. Respirations: average 30, obligatory nose breathing until 3 to 4 months
  E. Fontanelles
    1. Posterior closes at 2 to 3 months
    2. Anterior closes at 12 to 18 months
  F. Teeth
    1. Primary teeth erupt at about 6 to 7 months, central incisors first
    2. Approximately six teeth by 1 year
  G. Gross motor skills
    1. Develop cephalocaudal (head to toe)
    2. 2 to 3 months: raises head and chest
    3. 5 months: turns over both ways
    4. 5 to 6 months: sits with support
    5. 7 to 8 months: sits without support
    6. 8 months: pulls to standing position; begins creeping, then crawling
    7. 12 months: stands upright; begins walking
  H. Fine motor skills
    1. Develop proximodistal (trunk to fingers)
    2. 3 months: hands open most of time; swipes at objects but can hold only if placed in hand
    3. 4 months: brings objects to mouth
    4. 6 months: transfers objects
    5. 9 months: pincer grasp
II. Social skills
  A. 1 month: differentiates between object and face
  B. 2 months: begins social smiling
  C. 3 months: interested in environment
  D. 4 months: knows mother/primary caregiver
  E. 6 months: enjoys play
  F. 7 to 8 months: stranger anxiety
  G. 10 to 12 months: separation anxiety
  H. Trust versus mistrust (Erikson)
III. Cognitive development (Piaget): sensorimotor period
  A. 1 month: reflexive
  B. 1 to 4 months: Primary circular reactions
    1. Repetitive and voluntary actions
    2. Beginning stimulus-response
    3. Recognizes familiar faces, objects, and sounds
  C. 4 to 8 months: secondary circular reactions
    1. Beginning to develop object permanence
    2. Imitation begins
    3. Affected by external environment
  D. 8 to 12 months: coordination of secondary schemata
    1. Distinguishes means from end, e.g., search for hidden objects
    2. Begins to anticipate events
IV. Language development
  A. Neonate: crying
  B. 1 to 3 months: cooing; laughing
  C. 4 to 5 months: simple vowel sounds
  D. 6 months: babbling; addition of some consonant sounds, e.g., *g, k, d*
  E. 9 to 12 months: patterned speech, e.g., "mama," "dada"
  F. 12 months: two or three words with meaning
V. Play
  A. Birth to 3 months
    1. Dependent
    2. Social with adult

B. 3 to 6 months
  1. Plays alone with rattle
  2. Soft toys
  3. Interaction increases
  4. Preference for certain toys
  5. Recognizes image in mirror and vocalizes
C. 6 to 8 months
  1. Selective "partners" for play, i.e., parents
  2. Peek-a-boo; pat-a-cake
  3. Verbal repetition
D. 12 months: increased sensorimotor skills, e.g., activity boxes, books, push-pull toys, large ball

VI. Health maintenance
  A. Nutrition
    1. Caloric intake: 100 to 115 kcal per kg per day
    2. Breast feeding or iron-fortified formula for 1 year
      a. Formula fortified with iron is needed because of potential for anemia during various times of infancy, i.e., birth to 2 months, because of hypoactive erythropoietin; 6 to 9 months when stores of maternal iron are depleted
      b. Fluoride supplements; vitamin supplements for breast-fed infants
    3. Introduction of solid foods
      a. 4 to 6 months of age
      b. Introduce one food at a time starting with rice cereal
      c. Continue 3 to 4 days before introducing another
      d. Small quantities to start
      e. Cooked iron-fortified cereals: strained fruits, vegetables, and meats; finger foods (when teething)
    4. Self-feeding
      a. 6 months: begin introducing finger foods, cup
      b. 10 to 12 months: increase self-feeding; introduce spoon
    5. Food allergies
      a. Common foods include egg whites, chocolate, milk, wheat/corn cereals, oranges, tomato, nuts
      b. Hypersensitivity symptoms include urticaria, abdominal pain, nausea and vomiting, respiratory symptoms
      c. Diagnosis: food history, singular addition of food
      d. Treatment: remove causative food(s)
  B. Safety/accidents
    1. Aspiration/suffocation
      a. Keep plastic bags out of reach
      b. No strings/ribbons around neck (for pacifiers)
      c. Keep small objects out of reach
      d. Avoid propping bottles
    2. Falls
      a. Crib rails up at all times
      b. Never leave infant on raised surface unattended
      c. Use infant seat/highchair with restraints
      d. Gate stairways at top and bottom
    3. Motor vehicles
      a. Use approved carseat at all times, rear-facing
      b. Do not allow strollers or playing behind parked cars
    4. Poisons
      a. Assess for lead exposure
        (1) Lives in home built before 1978 with peeling paint or plaster
        (2) Uses older crib or toys
        (3) Family member works with lead or lead solder
        (4) Household member has lead poisoning
      b. Keep plants out of reach, not on floor
      c. Do not store toxic substances in food containers
      d. Place toxic substances on high shelf or in locked cabinet
      e. Use childproof caps on all medications; keep on high shelf or in locked cabinet
      f. Keep poison control number posted near the telephone
      g. Advise parents of proper use of syrup of ipecac
    5. Burns
      a. Check temperature of bath water, warmed formula, food
      b. Keep hot substances out of reach, e.g., coffee, cigarette ashes
      c. Use sun block when in sun; do not stay in sun for long periods
      d. Use flame-retardant pajamas; wash properly
      e. Keep faucets out of reach
      f. Place protective devices in front of heating appliances, fireplaces
      g. Keep electrical wires out of reach
      h. Do not allow infant to play with electrical appliances
  C. Immunizations (Tables 9–1 and 9–2)
    1. Common reactions
      a. Mild fever, malaise, fussiness
      b. Soreness, redness, or swelling at injection site

TABLE 9–1 Immunization Schedule Recommended by the American Academy of Pediatrics

Age	Immunization
Birth	Hepatitis B-1
1 to 2 months	Hepatitis B-2
2 months	DPT-1 (diphtheria, pertussis, tetanus), OPV-1 (oral polio vaccine), HbCV-1 (*Haemophilus influenzae* type b conjugate vaccine)
4 months	DPT-2, OPV-2, HbCV-2
6 months	DPT-3, HbCV-3
6 to 18 months	Hepatitis B-3
15 months	MMR-1 (measles, mumps, rubella), HbCV-4
18 months	DPT-4, OPV-3
4 to 6 years	DPT-5, OPV-4, MMR-2 (optional)
11 to 12 years	MMR-2 (if not given earlier)
14 to 16 years	Td (tetanus and diphtheria), repeat every 10 years

   c. Mild rash or joint stiffness 1 to 2 weeks after immunization (measles, rubella)

  2. Contraindications

    a. Delay immunization if child is sick with anything more serious than a minor illness such as the common cold

    b. Omit immunization if there was an allergic response to a previously administered vaccine within a few hours of administration or if child is allergic to vaccine components, e.g., eggs for measles, mumps, rubella (MMR)

TABLE 9–2 Recommended Immunization Schedule for Infants and Children Not Initially Immunized at Recommended Times

Age	Immunization
Under 7 years, first visit	DPT, OPV MMR, if 15 months (Tb test given at same time) HbCV if younger than 59 months
After first visit	
2 months	DPT, OPV, HbCV (if younger than 15 months for first dose)
4 months	DPT
10 to 16 months	DPT, OPV
4 to 6 years	DPT (not necessary if fourth dose given after age 4), OPV (not necessary if third dose given after age 4), MMR-2 (optional)
11 to 12 years	MMR (if not given earlier)
10 years after last DTP	Td, repeat every 10 years
Over 7 years, first visit	Td, OPV, MMR
After first visit	
2 months	Td, OPV
8 to 14 months	Td, OPV
11 to 12 years	MMR
10 years after last Td	Td, repeat every 10 years

   c. History of convulsions may or may not contraindicate certain vaccines

   d. Possible contraindications to diphtheria, pertussis, tetanus (DPT)

    (1) Inconsolable crying lasting 3 hours or more after immunization, fever 105°F (40.5°C) or higher, high-pitched cry

    (2) Convulsions or shock symptoms within 3 days after immunization

   e. Possible contraindications to oral polio vaccine (OPV)

    (1) Altered immune system in the child or household contact, e.g., leukemia, malignancy, immunosuppressive drug therapy, HIV infection, AIDS

    (2) Inactivated polio vaccine (IPV) can be given instead

   f. Possible contraindications to MMR

    (1) Altered immune system

    (2) Allergy to vaccine components, e.g., eggs, neomycin

    (3) Administration of blood transfusions, gamma globulin in previous 3 months

D. Sleep patterns

  1. Neonate averages 16 hours' sleep daily

  2. Usually sleeps through the night by 5 months

  3. Takes one or two naps by 1 year

E. Screening

  1. 9 months

    a. Tuberculosis skin test

    b. Lead screening if infant at risk

  2. 1 year

    a. Hemoglobin/hematocrit, then yearly

    b. Lead screen if not done previously, repeat yearly until age 4 to 5 years

VII. Hospitalization reactions

  A. Separation anxiety

    1. Assessment

     a. Begins in midinfancy

     b. Crying: clinging to parents

     c. May progress to withdrawal, passivity

    2. Interventions

     a. Rooming-in

     b. No visitation restrictions

     c. Meet needs immediately

     d. Pay attention to information on admission history

     e. Care by a primary nurse

  B. Pain

    1. Assessment

     a. Total body reaction in neonate: increased pulse, crying, irritability, motor activity

b. Offers physical evidence beginning in mid-infancy
2. Interventions
   a. Comfort and hold infant
   b. Have parent available during painful procedures
   c. Use pacifier/bottle after procedure as sucking main source of comfort
   d. Acetaminophen after age 6 weeks

TODDLERHOOD (AGES 1 TO 3)

I. Physical
   A. Height
      1. Gains more in proportion to weight
      2. Boys slightly taller than girls
      3. Estimate adult height by multiplying 2-year length by 2
   B. Weight
      1. Rate of gain declines sharply secondary to decreased appetite, decreased basal metabolic rate (BMR), loss of subcutaneous fat
      2. Gains in spurts
   C. Head circumference
      1. Equal to chest circumference by 1 to 2 years
      2. Anterior fontanelle closes at 12 to 18 months
   D. Chest circumference
      1. Transverse greater than anteroposterior diameter
      2. Exceeds abdominal girth after 2 years
   E. Vital signs
      1. Pulse and respirations decrease with increasing size and age
      2. Pulse: 80 to 120 (ages 1 to 5)
      3. Respirations: 20 to 40 (ages 1 to 5)
   F. Teeth: completion of primary teeth by 2½ to 3 years
   G. Vision
      1. Well-developed by 2 years; 20/40 acuity
      2. Depth perception increasing
   H. Gross motor skills (Table 9-3)
   I. Fine motor skills (Table 9-4)
II. Social skills: Autonomy versus shame and doubt (Erikson)
   A. 15 months
      1. Moves independently
      2. Stranger anxiety decreases
   B. 18 months
      1. Imitates housework
      2. Says "no" frequently
      3. Has temper tantrums
      4. Hugs and kisses familiar people/toys
      5. Begins bedtime rituals
   C. 24 months
      1. Peak age for temper tantrums
      2. Separation anxiety at height
      3. Plays alone and/or parallel play
      4. Passive with toys
      5. Cooperates with toilet training
   D. 30 months
      1. Ritualistic
      2. Resists bedtime
      3. Begins to cope with separations from mother for 3- to 4-hour time spans
      4. "Security" toys
   E. 36 months
      1. Interactive play
      2. Daytime toilet training complete
      3. Fewer temper tantrums and less negative behavior
      4. Imitates adult behavior, e.g., sex-role behavior
III. Cognitive development (Piaget)
   A. Sensorimotor period
      1. 13 to 18 months: tertiary circular reactions
         a. Active experimentation to achieve goals
         b. Increased object permanence
         c. Explores relationships between shapes
         d. Early signs of memory development

TABLE 9–3 Gross Motor Skills, 15 to 36 Months

15 Months	18 Months	24 Months	30 Months	36 Months
Walks alone	Walks sideways and backward	Walks steadily	Walks on tiptoes	Rides a tricycle
Jumps in place; falls		Runs without falling	Walks up stairs with one foot per stair	Balances one foot 2 seconds
Creeps up stairs	Runs, but falls	Jumps with both feet in place	Throws ball 3 to 4 ft	
Comes down backward	Walks up stairs, holding rail	Walks up stairs, both feet on same step	One foot standing/ hopping	
Throws ball; falls	Comes down backward	Walks down holding on		
	Throws overhand	Kicks ball forward		

TABLE 9–4 Fine Motor Skills, 15 to 36 Months

15 Months	18 Months	24 Months	30 Months	36 Months
Holds cup with frequent spills	Drinks with cup	Uses one hand for glass/cup	Pours with spills	Copies circle, cross
Turns spoon upside down when feeding	Fills spoon, but spills trying to eat	No spilling with spoon	Builds tower with seven or eight blocks	Builds bridge of blocks
Takes shoes and socks off	Helps unzip clothes	Can undress self almost totally	Holds crayons in fingers vs. hands	Puts raisins, small pellets into narrow-neck bottle
Helps with washing arms and legs	Helps take off shirt	Begins putting on shirt	Begins drawing	Draws recognizable figures
		Turns page of a book	Imitates a vertical and circular stroke	
		Turns door knobs		

2. 18 to 24 months: invention of new means through mental combinations
   a. Can infer cause from observing or experiencing event; can predict results by observing causes
   b. Object permanence regardless of number of events
   c. Symbolic imitation, "make-believe"
   d. Beginning sense of time
   e. Egocentric in behavior and thought

B. Preoperational stage (ages 2 to 4): preconceptual phase
   1. Symbolism with increased use of language, "magical" thinking
   2. Egocentrism continues
   3. Transductive reasoning; thinks particular to particular, not whole
   4. Animistic thought; animal or human characteristics given to objects, e.g., teddy bears talk
   5. Increased sense of time and space
   6. Field dependency; all aspects of situation important and interrelated

IV. Language development
  A. 15 months
    1. Five to 10 words
    2. Uses expressive jargon
    3. Points to desired objects
    4. Says "no" to all requests
  B. 18 months
    1. 10 to 20 words
    2. Gestures
    3. Understands simple requests
    4. Holophrastic words: whole word equals whole sentence
  C. 24 months
    1. 275 to 300 words
    2. Two- to three-word sentences
    3. Uses "I," "me," and "you"
    4. Uses first name

    5. Understands/obeys simple requests
    6. Vocalizes for drink, food, potty
    7. Talks incessantly
  D. 30 to 36 months
    1. 900 words
    2. Uses first and last names
    3. Uses plurals
    4. Names one color
    5. Uses appropriate pronoun for self
    6. Talks in complete sentences using all parts of speech

V. Play
  A. "Child's work"
  B. Parallel play
  C. Possessive of toys
  D. Encourages socialization
  E. Learn by play
  F. Imitative
  G. Toys
    1. Push-pull toys
    2. Balls
    3. Puzzles with large pieces
    4. Crayons (thick)
    5. Blocks
    6. Musical/talking toys

VI. Health maintenance
  A. Nutrition
    1. Caloric intake: 100 cal per kg per day
    2. Food binges; 3- to 4-day cycles
    3. Voracious appetite one day, nothing the next day
    4. Refusal to eat
      a. Do not force
      b. Let child decide order to eat food
      c. Small portions
    5. Ritualistic eating habits
      a. Feed small portions on child-size dinnerware with child utensils
      b. Have child eat in one place
      c. Let child eat with rest of family if possible

d. Encourage child to "feed" dolls and friends
e. Let child feed self
6. Finger foods
7. Self-feed by 18 to 24 months
8. Vitamin supplements (with iron if necessary)

B. Dental care
1. Have regular checkups beginning at completion of primary dentition
2. Brush teeth with soft bristle brush at least two times per day; begin teaching child
3. If water is not fluoridated, give oral supplements (0.25 to 0.5 mg per day depending on age)
4. Limit between-meal "sweet" snacks
5. Do not allow bottles with milk or juice at nap or bedtime; produces "bottle-mouth caries"

C. Toilet training
1. One of major tasks of toddlerhood
2. Factors influencing must be present
   a. Timing
      (1) Daytime bowel: 18 to 24 months
      (2) Daytime bladder: 2 to 3 years
      (3) Nighttime bladder: 3 to 5 years
   b. Readiness
      (1) Physiological: child walking well: anywhere from 15 to 24 months
      (2) Recognizes urge; ability to walk to bathroom and pull down clothing; must have sphincter control to wait until on "potty"
      (3) Must have ability to communicate need to defecate and urinate
      (4) Mother/caregiver must recognize child's nonverbal behavior

D. Safety (accidents leading cause of death for ages 1 to 5)
1. Aspiration/suffocation
   a. Avoid large pieces of meat
   b. Avoid hard candy and chewing gum
   c. Select toys with large parts; no removable small pieces
   d. Keep doors off old appliances and toy chests
   e. Keep doors closed on washer/dryer at all times
2. Falls
   a. Keep gates at bottom and top of stairs
   b. Keep windows and doors screened or closed
   c. Keep crib/bed rails up at sleep
   d. Supervise at play
   e. Keep clothes and shoes properly cared for and fitted

3. Motor vehicles
   a. Always use carseat, preferably in rear-center, forward facing
   b. Do not allow child to play behind parked cars, on a curb, or in the street
   c. Begin teaching traffic safety
   d. Keep fences closed if play is unsupervised
   e. Supervise tricycle riding and riding small toys such as wagons
4. Poisons (see Infancy)
   a. Administer medications as drugs, not candy
   b. Teach child not to eat anything found outdoors (leaves, berries)
5. Burns
   a. Turn pot handles toward back of stove; remove front knobs on gas stove
   b. Cover electrical outlets with protective caps
   c. Teach child what "hot" means
   d. Keep electrical wires out of reach
   e. Check bath water temperature
   f. Keep faucets out of reach; keep faucet protectors on at all times
6. Drowning
   a. Have swimming pool fence and gates with child-proof locks
   b. Teach swimming and water safety
   c. Do not leave child unsupervised near water, including bath
7. Cuts and stabs
   a. Keep knives and scissors out of reach
   b. Teach safety with sharp objects
   c. Keep dangerous objects out of reach, e.g., guns and power tools

E. Sleep patterns
1. Requires 10 to 14 hours of sleep, including naps
2. May experience nightmares, sleep terrors, sleep walking

F. Screening
1. Hemoglobin/hematocrit yearly
2. Lead screen yearly

VII. Hospitalization reactions
A. Separation anxiety
1. Assessment
   a. Fear of abandonment
   b. Fear of unknown
   c. Crying out for parent
   d. Regression in eating, toileting
2. Intervention
   a. Encourage expression of feelings through doll play
   b. Rooming-in

c. No visitation restrictions

d. Allow child to keep favorite toy from home

B. Pain

1. Assessment: physically resistant to painful or intrusive procedures

2. Interventions

a. Have parents/significant other comfort during procedure

b. Use simple, concrete explanations of procedures that will occur

c. Use play therapy before procedure

C. Loss of autonomy

1. Assessment: major task of toddlerhood altered by hospital rules and routines

2. Interventions

a. Continue routines from home whenever possible

b. Let children assist with all tasks that they can

c. Ask for child's input; let child make decisions whenever possible

RESCHOOL YEARS (AGES 3 TO 6)

I. Physical

A. Height

1. Gains more in proportion to weight

2. Generally occurs more in elongation of legs versus trunk

3. Has erect posture; appears tall

B. Weight

1. Average gain about 5 lb per year

2. Appears thinner than during toddlerhood

C. Gross motor skills (Table 9-5)

D. Fine motor skills (Table 9-6)

II. Social skills

A. Initiative versus guilt (Erikson)

1. Instigates activity

2. Tries new ways to use known skills

3. Is confident when approaching tasks

4. Derives satisfaction from accomplishments

5. Knows that there will be punishment/discipline when behavior morally or socially unacceptable or harmful

B. Sex-role identification

C. Parental support and encouragement

1. Needs opportunities to explore different people and things

2. Parents should praise acceptable behavior and encourage creativity

3. Use verbal limitations rather than physical restraints for discipline

III. Cognitive development (Piaget): preoperational stage

A. Preconceptual phase (refer to section on Toddlerhood)

B. Intuitive phase (ages 4 to 7)

1. Perceptions versus logic

2. Concept of centration: sees parts, not whole

3. Lacks conservation

a. Judges objects only in "static" quality

b. Sees large glass as having more liquid than small glass, even though amounts equal

4. Lacks reversibility: sees pouring liquid from one glass to another glass of different shape as changing amount of liquid

5. Magical/fantasy thinking

6. Time correlates with events, e.g., after nap, before lunch

7. Accepts words in literal sense, e.g., "You are bad" versus "What you did was bad"

IV. Language development

A. 3 years

1. 900 words

2. Three- to four-word sentences

TABLE 9–5 Gross Motor Skills, 3 to 5 Years

3 Years	4 Years	5 Years
Walks backward	Walks down stairs with alternate feet	Backward heel-to-toe walk
Jumps off bottom step	Skips	Skips
Stands on one foot 2 to 3 seconds	Hops on one foot	Hops on alternating feet
Climbs steps using alternate feet	Balances on one foot 5 seconds	Stands on one foot 10 seconds
Rides tricycle	Catches ball without missing	Throws and catches ball well with hands
Catches ball with arms out in front with some misses		Jumps rope
		Uses roller skates

TABLE 9–6 Fine Motor Skills, 3 to 5 Years

3 Years	4 Years	5 Years
Washes hands, feet	Dresses/undresses self, except tying laces and zippers	Dresses without assistance
Undresses self; dresses with help	Buttons clothes	Ties shoelaces
Builds nine- or 10-block tower	Laces shoe without bow	Builds things with boxes; complex
Builds three-block bridge	Brushes teeth	Copies diamond and triangle
Copies circle	Builds gate with blocks	Draws six- to nine-part stick man
Imitates cross	Copies a square	Prints few letters, numbers, words, first name
Names drawings	Draws three-part stick-man	Hand preference
Makes faces in circle	Draws two geometrical shapes	Uses scissors, simple tools well

3. May repeat numbers
4. Uses plurals, pronouns, past tense of verbs

B. 4 years
  1. 1500 words
  2. Four- to five-word sentences
  3. Uses concrete speech
  4. Asks questions
  5. Uses prepositions, adjectives, many verbs
  6. Counts to 5

C. 5 years
  1. 2100 words
  2. Six- to eight-word sentences
  3. Uses all parts of speech correctly with exception of "rule-breakers"
  4. Defines simple objects by color, shape, use
  5. Knows some opposites
  6. Names four or more colors
  7. Counts to 10
  8. Knows coins, e.g., penny, nickel, etc.

D. By age 6, describes objects by composition, e.g., cup made of paper

E. Vocabulary increases 600 words per year

V. Play
A. "Cooperative" play
B. Stimulation of curiosity and exploration
C. Increased use of vocabulary
D. Refinement of gross and fine motor skills
E. Imagination, imitation, and dramatization forms of activities
  1. Dress-up
  2. Doctor-nurse games
  3. Playing house
F. Imaginary playmates
  1. Normal at this age
  2. Provide "friends"
  3. Accomplish what child attempts
  4. Understand child
  5. Disappear when child is more involved

with "real" friends and play and school activities

G. Toys
  1. Playground equipment
  2. Tricycles
  3. Skates
  4. Puzzles
  5. Musical toys
  6. Paints, crayons, clay
  7. Electronic games for learning numbers, spelling
  8. Books, especially large, easy-to-handle books
  9. Dolls with houses; puppets; "communities"
  10. Simple board games
  11. Construction and transport toys

VI. Health maintenance
A. Nutrition
  1. Caloric intake: 90 cal per kg per day
  2. Food preferences remain; can be finicky
  3. Quality more important than quantity
  4. Self-feeder
B. Safety
  1. Emphasis on education for safety and hazards
  2. Parents should set "good" example
  3. Less reckless, less prone to falls than toddler
  4. Motor vehicles
    a. Teach child to wear seat belt
    b. Teach safety on streets
      (1) Look both ways before crossing
      (2) Play in yard rather than street
      (3) Do not chase balls into street
      (4) Avoid strangers
C. Sleep patterns
  1. May give up nap completely
  2. Bedtime fears/nightmares; comfortable in own bed
  3. Resists bedtime

a. Provide quiet time before bedtime
b. Establish consistent bedtime rituals

D. Sex education
1. Aware of anatomical differences between sexes by age 3
2. Curiosity about eliminative function of anatomy of opposite sex; distinct from sexual curiosity
3. Plays "doctor" to explore unknown
4. Imitates "mommy and daddy" roles
5. Masturbation normal and healthy if not excessive
   a. Form of exploration
   b. Parents should not punish
   c. Explanation of privacy of act and its meaning should be done by parents
6. Parents should answer questions ("whys?") about sexuality and birth process openly and honestly but without details
7. Use words understandable to child and use correct names for body parts

E. Preschool/nursery school
1. Provides opportunities for group learning experiences of many types
2. Can increase child's confidence and self-esteem
3. Increases child's interactions with peers
4. "Stepping stone" to regular school
5. Provides learning and stimulation in areas of physical, social, and language development
6. Before starting, parents should prepare child
   a. Talk about activities, children
   b. Take on tour of school
   c. Do not let child see your feelings of anxiety, nervousness
   d. Start school slowly

F. Screening
1. Hemoglobin/hematocrit yearly
2. Lead screen yearly
3. Urinalysis
4. Vision and hearing screen at ages 4 to 6
5. Tuberculosis skin test before kindergarten

VII. Hospitalization reactions
A. Fear of mutilation/body invasion
1. Assessment
   a. Main fear of preschooler
   b. Smiling inappropriately, clinging to parents, anger, crying
2. Interventions
   a. Never threaten child; e.g., never say, "If you don't behave, I'll give you a shot"
   b. Prepare child ahead of time, but immediately before or during a procedure
   c. Explain procedure in understandable terms
   d. Use play therapy
   e. "Cover up" all holes from shots, blood tests

B. Withdrawal
1. Assessment: passive, immobile in "threatening" situations
2. Interventions
   a. Accept behavior
   b. Use play therapy to express fear

C. Aggression
1. Assessment
   a. Preschoolers let feelings show
   b. Cannot control impulses/behavior
2. Interventions
   a. Create safe outlets for aggression, e.g., punching bag, pounding tool sets
   b. Let child know you understand behavior

D. Sleep disturbances
1. Assessment: unable to fall asleep, nightmares or night terrors
2. Interventions
   a. Accommodate bedtime rituals whenever possible
   b. Allow parent(s) to room-in

SCHOOL-AGE YEARS (AGES 6 TO 12)

I. Physical
A. Height
1. Slow, steady growth
2. Average 2 in. per year
3. Boys taller until 10 years, then girls taller until 14 years

B. Weight
1. Average 5 to 7 lb per year
2. Boys somewhat heavier until puberty

C. Other physical changes
1. Head circumference decreases in relation to height
2. Facial changes secondary to face growing faster than skull
3. Increase in leg length related to height
4. Eyes acquire 20/20 vision
5. Permanent teeth acquired
6. Body systems stabilizing and achieving adult capacity
7. Cardiac output increases as rate decreases to approach adult levels
8. May begin development of secondary sex characteristics

D. Gross motor skills

1. Muscular strength doubles
2. Time for refinement and expansion of skills
3. Regular exercise required to develop new muscles
4. Activities
   a. Running games
   b. Swimming
   c. Jump rope
   d. Skating
   e. Bicycling
5. Clumsy, awkward as "growth spurt" begins
E. Fine motor skills
   1. Refines printing, writing, drawing skills
   2. Definite preference for particular hand
   3. Creativity takes over; writes stories, poems
   4. Uses tools more proficiently; engages in craft projects

II. Social skills
A. Industry versus inferiority (Erikson)
B. Interactions with friends most important
C. Group activities
D. Sensitive to social norms
E. Peer pressure
F. Friendships with same-sex peers
G. Parent as adult versus buddy
H. Looks for teacher approval
I. Cooperation increases

III. Cognitive skills (Piaget): concrete operations stage (ages 7 to 11)
A. Organizes, orders, classifies objects concretely experienced
B. Symbolic thinking: able to experience event without seeing or touching it
C. Conservation: able to perceive that quantities remain the same despite changes in appearance
   1. Decentration: able to perceive objects in more than one dimension
   2. Reversibility: able to mentally reverse a process
D. Classification: able to group/sort in logical categories
E. Seriation: able to arrange objects according to one common characteristic, e.g., by increasing or decreasing size
F. Symbol manipulation
G. Time recognition
   1. Clock
   2. Season/months

IV. Language development
A. Rapidly expanding vocabulary
B. Descriptions of objects include size, shape, color
C. Can tell time and use calendar
D. Eager to learn new words and meanings

V. Play
A. Cooperative play
B. Dramatic play
C. Aggressive play, primarily in boys
D. Team sports
E. Fantasy allows child to be anyone and to do anything
F. Play related to sex roles
   1. Boy or girl dolls
   2. Scouts
G. Quiet play important to balance out increased activity; likes collecting things
H. Toys
   1. Bicycles
   2. Sports equipment
   3. Model or craft kits
   4. Art sets
   5. Board games
   6. Computer games
   7. Books

VI. Health maintenance
A. Nutrition
   1. Caloric needs increase—2500 cal per day
   2. "Empty calorie" junk foods prevalent
   3. Childhood obesity incidence increases
   4. Snacking increases
   5. Mass media influences
   6. Education important
B. Dental health
   1. Permanent teeth erupt
   2. Dental caries most prevalent health problem
   3. Teach good oral hygiene
      a. Brushing and flossing
      b. Balanced nutrition; avoid large intake of sweets
      c. 6-month checkups
      d. Continue fluoride
C. Safety
   1. Motor vehicle accidents most common cause of injury and death
      a. Use seat belts
      b. Teach street and bicycle safety including use of helmets
   2. Drowning: teach water safety early
   3. Burns: increased curiosity with fire, matches, guns
   4. Physically active and thus susceptible to minor injuries; teach how to avoid hazards and enforce safety rules
D. Sleep patterns
   1. Amount of sleep needed individualized
   2. Bedtime resistance
   3. Maintain secure bedtime rituals

4. Frequent nightmares
E. Screening every 2 years
   1. Hemoglobin/hematocrit
   2. Urinalysis
   3. Baseline cholesterol (once only)
   4. Scoliosis
F. Self-care/hygiene
   1. Child should assume responsibility
   2. Health education classes
G. Sex education
   1. Sex play in response to normal curiosity
   2. Formal sex education, from parents and school
   3. Discuss myths and misconceptions about sexuality, pregnancy, sexually transmitted diseases
   4. Be open and honest in answering questions
   5. Mass media has both positive and negative influences
H. Drug and alcohol abuse
   1. Parental and school education of utmost importance
   2. Role models
VII. Hospitalization reactions
A. Fear of pain and bodily injury
   1. Assessment
      a. Concerned with looking different from friends
      b. Concerned about death and disability
   2. Interventions
      a. Projective techniques, e.g., doll play, role play, drawings to express fears
      b. Complete explanations of procedures
B. Fear of losing emotional control
   1. Assessment: child believes he or she should be brave, may be defiant
   2. Interventions
      a. Do not say, ''Big boys/girls don't cry''
      b. Plan play activities that encourage release of energy, anger
      c. Allow to participate in planning treatment
C. Separation anxiety
   1. Assessment: misses friends and social activities
   2. Interventions
      a. Encourage friends to call and visit
      b. Arrange for child to keep up with schoolwork
D. Perception of illness as punishment
   1. Assessment: believes being good brings rewards, thus being bad brings punishment, i.e., illness and hospitalization
   2. Intervention: offer reassurance

ADOLESCENT YEARS (AGES 12 TO 20)

I. Physical
A. Height: one fourth of adult height acquired during growth spurt; occurs earlier in girls
B. Weight
   1. Boys gain 15 to 65 lb, increase more in muscle development
   2. Girls gain 15 to 55 lb, increase more in body fat
C. Secondary sex characteristics
   1. Female maturation
      a. Average age menarche 12 to 13 years
      b. Breast development
      c. Pubic and axillary hair growth
      d. Increase in vaginal secretions
      e. Hips widen
   2. Male maturation
      a. Voice changes
      b. Increase in size of penis
      c. Pubic, axillary, facial, chest hair growth
      d. Production of spermatozoa
      e. Shoulders broaden
   3. Other pubescent changes
      a. Increase in perspiration
      b. Acne
      c. Physiological functions becoming those of an adult
II. Social skills
A. Identity versus role confusion (Erikson)
   1. Integrating past social skills with present maturation
   2. Trying various roles searching for a ''fit''
B. ''What do I want to be?'' thinking about career choice
C. Peer relationships integral
D. Needs to be ''just like'' peers
E. Intimate sexual relationships begin to develop in late adolescence
F. May become sexually active
G. Adapts to changes in body image
H. Detaches self from parental supervision
I. Develops close relationships with adults other than parents
III. Cognitive skills (Piaget): formal operations stage (age 11 or older)
A. Thinks abstractly
B. Forms hypotheses
C. Thinks deductively and inductively
D. Exhibits egocentrism (especially in early adolescence)
IV. Recreational activities
A. School dances
B. Boy-girl parties
C. Music and concerts

D. Organized sports
V. Health maintenance
  A. Nutrition
    1. Caloric needs increase with rapid growth; adequate calcium and iron most important
      a. Girls: 2200 cal per day
      b. Boys: 2700 cal per day
    2. Increased intake of fast foods
    3. Snacking prevalent
    4. Skips breakfast
    5. Athletics increase nutritional needs
    6. Anorexia nervosa/adolescent obesity on rise
    7. Education is imperative
  B. Safety
    1. Accidental injuries leading cause of death; educate how to "survive" in expanded environment
    2. Motor vehicle accidents prevalent
      a. Driver's education
      b. Education about drinking and driving
    3. Alcohol and drug abuse
    4. Suicides on rise
  C. Screening every 2 years
    1. Hemoglobin/hematocrit
    2. Urinalysis
    3. Scoliosis
    4. Breast/testicular examination
  D. Self-care/hygiene
    1. Regular physical examinations
    2. Gynecological care for females
    3. Regular eye examinations
    4. Cigarette smoking increases
    5. Proper posture to prevent scoliosis
  E. Sex education classes
    1. Anatomy and physiology
    2. Sexually transmitted diseases
    3. Birth control
    4. Pregnancy
    5. Alternative lifestyles
VI. Hospitalization reactions
  A. Feelings of loss of independence and identity
    1. Assessment
      a. Increased questioning behaviors
      b. Difficulty admitting need for support
    2. Interventions
      a. Plan care with adolescent
      b. Liberal visitation
      c. Hospital-bound teachers
  B. Fear of body image changes
    1. Assessment: any new body changes plus normal changes of adolescence increase vulnerability
      a. Worried about what others think
      b. Lack of cooperation with treatment
    2. Interventions
      a. Preoperative teaching if appropriate
      b. Reassurance of intact body

      c. Allow to visit others who have adjusted to similar procedure
  C. Fear of rejection
    1. Assessment: major fear at this stage, concerned about being teased
    2. Interventions
      a. Encourage peer interaction
      b. Liberal visitation
      c. Access to telephone
  D. Fear of losing control emotionally
    1. Assessment: mood changes common
    2. Interventions
      a. Accept behavior
      b. Do not overreact to outbursts
      c. Do not minimize feelings
      d. Give opportunity to express aggression

POST-TEST Growth and Development

1. Alan is a 4-year-old who has been hospitalized with osteomyelitis. He will need at least 14 days of IV antibiotics. Alan seems to be very afraid of the hospital. Which of the following nursing interventions might most help to relieve his fears?
  ① Place him in a private room and allow him to keep some of his own toys.
  ② Advise his family to stay away.
  ③ Encourage Alan to socialize with other patients.
  ④ Allow Alan's parent to stay with him.

2. Brad is a 16-year-old admitted for acute appendicitis. Which of the following interventions will help him to maintain normal growth and development?
  ① Keep him on bedrest and encourage him to read and rest
  ② Let him participate with other teenagers in activities when his condition permits
  ③ Allow his family to bring in stuffed toys from home
  ④ Let his parents stay the night in his room, sleeping at his bedside until his discharge

3. Nina is a 6-month-old infant admitted to the hospital for placement of ear tubes. After surgery, the nurse who is caring for her observes that she is fussy and restless, her pulse rate is elevated, and she keeps hitting her ears with her hands. Given the assessment data, which of the following is the most likely nursing diagnosis?
  ① Body image disturbance related to diminished hearing
  ② Anxiety related to separation from parents

③ Hyperthermia related to fluid loss during surgery

④ Pain related to the effects of surgery

4. Susan is a 9-year-old who is in the hospital. She is seen by the nurse to be sucking her thumb. The most appropriate nursing intervention is to:
① Quietly remind Susan that she is too old for this activity
② Tell her to stop acting like a baby
③ Talk to her parents and have them tell Susan to stop this
④ Assess the level of stress Susan is under but ignore this regression

5. Ian is a 2-year-old admitted to the hospital for treatment of extensive second-degree burns of his chest and abdomen, which he sustained while trying to drink a cup of hot tea his mother had left on the kitchen table. Which of the following statements by Ian's mother would demonstrate her understanding of safety principles reviewed by the nurse before discharge?
① "I'll have to keep him in the playpen all the time to prevent him from getting into trouble."
② "He will need to learn what 'hot' means so he will not endanger himself again."
③ "I will have to remind my husband and older children that we can't leave hot liquids unattended."
④ "We'll have to keep hot liquids in the kitchen only and gate the door so he can't get in."

6. John is an 8-year-old hospitalized for severe asthma. He requires respiratory inhalation treatments every 4 hours on a 24-hour basis. The nurse notices that he is becoming increasingly irritable and aggressive, is unable to concentrate during the day, and says that he is tired all the time. A likely nursing diagnosis for John is:
① Ineffective individual coping related to separation from peers
② Activity intolerance related to the side effects of his medications
③ Sleep pattern disturbance related to frequency of treatments
④ Diversional activity deficit related to the length of his treatments

7. When planning to meet the developmental needs of the hospitalized adolescent, the nurse understands that achievement of independence and identity are important developmental tasks. Which of the following adaptations to care would help hospitalized adolescents adjust?
① Allow them to wear their own clothes whenever possible
② Permit them to play loud music in the solarium
③ Provide structure through maintaining established routines
④ Let them perform their own treatments and procedures

8. Which of the following behaviors seen in a hospitalized preschooler might cause the nurse concern?
① Crying and clinging to parents
② Aggression in play and toward others
③ Passivity and withdrawal from play activities
④ Nightmares

9. Three-year-old Jamie has been hospitalized for severe croup. Her condition has improved, but she is now refusing to eat. Her parents have brought food from home, and Jamie has been allowed to eat her meals at a table with the other children in the toddler room. Which of the following would be an appropriate evaluation of the situation?
① Despite interventions, Jamie's nutritional needs are not being met.
② Her refusal to eat is developmentally appropriate and not a cause for concern at this time.
③ Jamie is using food as a way to punish her parents for leaving her.
④ Jamie is refusing to eat as a way of getting attention.

10. One-year-old Erik comes to the well-child clinic for a routine physical examination. The nurse notices that he has had two hepatitis B immunizations and two each of DPT, OPV, and HbCV. He also has had a tuberculosis skin test. Which of the following will the nurse plan to do during this visit if he is healthy?
① Hemoglobin, lead screen, MMR, HbCV booster
② Lead screen and hemoglobin only
③ Hepatitis B #3, MMR, HbCV booster
④ DPT #3, HbCV #3, hemoglobin, lead screen

POST-TEST Answers and Rationales

1. ④ Preschoolers are often afraid of the unfamiliar. Although having familiar toys from home is important, a private room is unnecessary. Parents are still more important than peers. Pediatric units are designed to meet the needs of children and parents. Both are often more comfortable if the parents can stay and provide some of the care. Having Alan alone or without family will only increase the stress of hospitalization. 4, III. Growth and Development.

2. ② Giving adolescents the opportunity to participate in age-related activities meets their developmental needs and helps to prevent excessive stress. Bedrest is unnecessary, and choices 3 and 4 might promote regression in the teenager. 4, III. Growth and Development.

3. ④ Although these assessment data could suggest separation anxiety or fever, the fact that she is also hitting her head near the surgical site would suggest that pain is the correct diagnosis. She is too young for body image to be a major factor. 2, II. Growth and Development.

4. ④ Regression is a normal response to stress in the hospitalized child, and the child should not be reprimanded because this will only increase the level of stress. The regression should disappear as soon as the level of stress is lower. 4, III. Growth and Development.

5. ③ Safety principles involve not only teaching children what situations are dangerous to them but also seeing that their environment is safe. Although it is necessary to begin to teach toddlers the meaning of ''hot'' or ''dangerous,'' their cognitive stage of development inhibits the transfer of those principles to other situations. Involving the whole family in keeping the child's environment safe is a better approach than keeping a toddler restrained or assuming he cannot overcome an obstacle such as a gate. 5, I & IV. Growth and Development.

6. ③ Waking children frequently for treatments and procedures interrupts their sleep pattern and can cause signs of irritability, mood changes, and complaints of fatigue. School-age children often stay up late but usually have sleep periods lasting many hours through the night. The data given do not correspond with the other choices, although those are frequently seen in school-age children as well. 2, II. Growth and Development.

7. ① Although adolescents are striving for independence and identity, they still need reasonable limits. Allowing them to play loud music, which might disturb others, is not appropriate. Permitting them to do some of their own treatments is certainly desirable but not if it interferes with achieving therapeutic benefit. Encouraging them to wear their own clothing helps them retain their identity and usually does not interfere with the provision of care. 3, IV. Growth and Development.

8. ③ When a preschool child withdraws quietly, especially from play activities, it is often a sign of hopelessness or despair. The other options given are expected ways preschoolers might respond to stressful situations. 1, III. Growth and Development.

9. ② Although it is appropriate for the nurse to be concerned about the toddler's nutritional intake, interventions have not changed the situation. This does not mean that they have been unsuccessful, however, because toddlers often go through periods of playing with their food and refusing to eat. The other options are probably not applicable to a child in this developmental stage. 5, II & III. Growth and Development.

10. ④ By 1 year, children should have had two OPVs, three DPTs, three HbCVs, two hepatitis B vaccines, and a skin test for tuberculosis. Erik is missing his DPT #3 and HbCV #3. He also should have his hemoglobin and lead levels checked. Giving the third hepatitis vaccination at this age may be appropriate, but it could wait. MMR is not given until after 15 months. 3, II. Growth and Development.

BIBLIOGRAPHY

GROWTH AND DEVELOPMENT

American Academy of Pediatrics, Committee on Nutrition (1989). Iron-fortified infant formulas. *Pediatrics* 84(6): 1114.

American Academy of Pediatrics, Committee on Nutrition (1992). The use of whole cow's milk in infancy. *Pediatrics* 89(6): 1105–1108.

Beal, J. A. (1986). The Brazelton Neonatal Behavioral Assessment Scale: A tool to enhance parental attachment. *Journal of Pediatric Nursing* 1: 170.

Cole, M., and Cole, S. R. (1989). *The development of children.* New York: W. H. Freeman.

Foster, R. L. R., Hunsberger, M. M., and Anderson, J. T. (1989). *Family-centered nursing care of children.* Philadelphia: W. B. Saunders.

Frankenburg, W. K., and Thornton, S. M. (1989). A child development program for a busy office practice. *Contemporary Pediatrics* 6(2): 90–106.

Frankenburg, W. K., Fandal, A. W., and Thornton, S. M. (1987). Revision of the Denver Preschool Screening Developmental Questionnaire. *Journal of Pediatrics* 110:653–657.

Frankenburg, W. K., Thornton, S. M., and Cohrs, M. E., eds. (1981). *Pediatric developmental diagnosis.* New York: Thieme-Stratton, Inc.

Hall, S., ed. (1986). *Nursing assessment and strategies for the family at risk,* 2nd ed. Philadelphia, J. B. Lippincott.

Mott, S. R., James, S. R., and Sperhac, A. M. (1990). *Nursing care of children and families,* 2nd ed. Redwood City, CA: Addison-Wesley.

Pipes, P. L. (1989). *Nutrition in infancy and childhood,* 4th ed. St. Louis: C. V. Mosby.

Universal hepatitis B immunization (1992). *AAP News.* February: 13–15.

Vaughan, V. C., and Litt, I. F. (1990). *Child and adolescent development: Clinical implications.* Philadelphia: W. B. Saunders.

10

Fluid/Gas Transport in the Pediatric Client

PRE-TEST Cardiovascular/Hematological Disorders

1. Angel is a 3-month-old just diagnosed with a small ventricular septal defect (VSD). The nurse might expect to see Angel exhibit which of the following?
   1. Cyanosis, clubbing of the fingers, hypoxic spells
   2. Respiratory distress, extreme fatigue, irritability
   3. Systolic murmur at lower left sternal border, otherwise asymptomatic
   4. Feeding difficulties, cyanosis, continuous diastolic rumble
2. Martha is suffering from poor weight gain secondary to congestive heart failure. When planning Martha's care, the nurse takes into consideration that her failure to thrive is most probably related to:
   1. Inadequate attention from her parents
   2. A vitamin deficiency
   3. Increased urination and diuresis
   4. Fatigue while eating
3. Cardiac catheterization is one of the procedures used most frequently to diagnose children with congenital heart defects. Which of the following postcatheterization interventions would be a priority for the nurse?
   1. Keep the child in bed for 6 hours
   2. Monitor color, temperature, and capillary refill of affected extremity
   3. Limit fluids
   4. Leave the insertion site open to the air

Wendy is a 7-year-old who has recently experienced low-grade afternoon fevers, intermittent hip joint pain, and fatigue. When taking a nursing history, the nurse notes that her ASO titer and erythrocyte sedimentation rate (ESR) are both elevated.

---

4. Which of the following questions is most important for the nurse to ask Wendy?
   1. "Have you injured your leg recently?"
   2. "Have you been able to eat and sleep as usual?"
   3. "Do you know anyone else who has similar symptoms?"
   4. "Have you had a recent sore throat?"
5. Wendy is diagnosed as having acute rheumatic fever and is placed on bedrest for carditis. Which of the following is a potential nursing diagnosis associated with prolonged bedrest in children?
   1. Fluid volume excess
   2. Impaired skin integrity
   3. Diarrhea
   4. Altered nutrition: more than body requirements
6. Wendy is started on aspirin. The rationale behind the administration of aspirin is to:
   1. Decrease her fever
   2. Treat her headache
   3. Reduce her inflammation
   4. Help her relax
7. Wendy is about to be discharged. At this point, she does not appear to have any permanent cardiac damage. Which of the following statements would indicate to the nurse that her parents have understood the discharge teaching?
   1. "Wendy will have to take daily penicillin by mouth until she is 20 years old."
   2. "Wendy will need to have a room of her own to keep her from getting sick."
   3. "Wendy will have to stop playing soccer."
   4. "Wendy will need to take extra vitamins to prevent colds."
8. Andrew is a 2-year-old whose mother brings him to the physician because he is pale and tired all the time. When his height and weight are checked, he falls below the 10th percentile on the growth chart. The physician orders a complete blood count (CBC), and Andrew's hemoglobin reading is 10.0 g/dL. Which of the following would be the most appropriate nursing diagnosis for Andrew?
   1. Altered nutrition: less than body requirements related to inadequate intake of calories
   2. Altered growth and development related to bizarre eating patterns
   3. Altered nutrition: less than body requirements related to inadequate intake of iron
   4. Altered growth and development related to refusal to eat
9. Latoya is a 14-year-old who was diagnosed with sickle cell disease when she was an infant. She is hospitalized with a vaso-occlusive crisis, and her joints are painful. Which of the following nursing interventions would be best to deal with her pain?
   1. Apply cool compresses and administer aspirin
   2. Use hot soaks and encourage activity as tolerated
   3. Apply heat and administer Tylenol with codeine as ordered
   4. Use cold packs and maintain strict bedrest

10. Latoya's parents are concerned about Latoya passing sickle cell disease on to her children. The nurse asks them what they know about how sickle cell disease is transmitted. Which of the following statements indicates that they understand the genetics of sickle cell disease?

  ① "If the father does not have the disease, none of their children will have the disease, but some of them will have the trait."

  ② "If the father does not have the trait or disease, none of their children will have the disease, but all of them will have the trait."

  ③ "If the father has the trait, all of their children will have the disease."

  ④ "If the father has the disease, some of their children will have the disease and some of them will have the trait."

11. Six-year-old Garth has been diagnosed as having acute lymphocytic leukemia, and he is about to undergo chemotherapy. When planning to address his long-term psychosocial needs, which of the following is most appropriate for the nurse to advise his parents to do?

  ① Bring in a stuffed animal from home

  ② Give him a Nerf basketball game to play with later

  ③ Encourage him to wear his favorite baseball cap

  ④ Allow him to choose a decorative bandage to cover the IV line site

PRE-TEST Answers and Rationales

1. ③ VSD is the most commonly seen congenital heart defect in children. It is an acyanotic defect with shunting of oxygenated blood from the stronger left side of the heart to the weaker right side through the abnormal opening. If the defect is small, the child usually is asymptomatic, having only a systolic murmur at the left lower sternal border. 1, II. Congenital Cardiac Disorders.

2. ④ Children who have congestive heart failure do not get the calories they need for growth for a variety of reasons. Their activity tolerance is greatly reduced because of their decreased cardiac output. They become extremely tired during feedings, often falling asleep before nursing adequately or finishing a bottle. When congestive heart failure is severe, respiratory distress also interferes with eating. Congestive heart failure causes fluid retention and decreased urinary output. Parental neglect is a cause of failure to thrive that can be suspected when physiological causes have been ruled out, which is not so in this case. 3, I. Congestive Heart Failure.

3. ② Because thrombus formation, phlebitis, or swelling may occur at the catheter insertion site, obstruction of the blood vessel used is a possibility. Frequent monitoring of the circulatory status of the extremity used for the catheterization is essential to determine decreased circulation and prevent tissue hypoxia. Although the affected extremity should be kept still for several hours following the procedure, this is not as great a priority as monitoring circulatory status. The other two answers are incorrect. 4, I & II. Congenital Cardiac Disorders.

4. ④ Although fever, joint pain, fatigue, and elevated ESR are nonspecific signs of an inflammatory process, an elevated ASO titer is evidence of exposure to recent streptococcal infection. Confirmation of the elevated ASO by history of sore throat would substantiate a diagnosis of acute rheumatic fever. An ongoing sore throat would require immediate culture and probable treatment with antibiotics. Although the other options are usual

questions asked when taking a history, 4 would be considered to be most pertinent. 1, II. Rheumatic Fever.

5. ④ When a child is inactive and faces a long period of bedrest, fewer calories are needed, and if the diet is not carefully monitored, the child can gain excessive weight. Constipation is another potential problem. Skin breakdown and fluid overload are unlikely problems in these children. 2, II. Rheumatic Fever.

6. ③ Aspirin is an anti-inflammatory given to interfere with the inflammatory process of rheumatic fever. Although aspirin can also reduce fever, this is not the primary purpose for which it is given. 3, I. Rheumatic Fever.

7. ① Prophylactic penicillin to prevent streptococcal infections is indicated for all children who have had rheumatic fever. Monthly injections or daily oral doses are necessary until the child is 20 or for at least 5 years after having the disease. None of the other options is either necessary or desirable. 5, III. Rheumatic Fever.

8. ③ A hemoglobin level of 10.0 indicates the child is suffering from iron deficiency anemia, which is usually related to inadequate intake of dietary iron. Inadequate caloric intake could also contribute to slowed growth; however, pallor and fatigue are supporting signs for anemia. Two-year-olds often have periods when they do not eat, followed by periods of eating more than adequate amounts; however, this is normal for the developmental level. 2, II & IV. Anemia.

9. ③ The pain from a vaso-occlusive crisis may require both nonpharmacological and pharmacological relief. Cold can precipitate a crisis by increasing sickling and constricting blood vessels. Heat is a better treatment. Aspirin is not used for pain relief in sickle cell anemia because of its effect on coagulation. Because the pain can be severe, a narcotic analgesic often is required. 4, II. Sickle Cell Anemia.

10. ② Sickle cell disease is the result of an autosomal recessive inheritance pattern. Both parents must pass the gene for disease to occur. Just because the father does not have the disease does not necessarily mean he does not carry the

trait. If he carries the trait, some of the children may have the trait only, and some may have the disease. With both parents having the disease, all of the children will have the disease. If the father has no disease or trait, all of the children will carry the trait, but none will have the disease. 5, I. Sickle Cell Anemia

11. ③ One of the major concerns of school-age children is body image and looking different from friends. Planning ahead for the body changes associated with chemotherapy helps the child cope when alopecia actually begins. The other choices address children of different developmental levels. 3, III. Leukemia.

NORMAL ANATOMY AND PHYSIOLOGY

I. Cardiopulmonary system
  A. Consists of heart, vessels, nose, pharynx, larynx, trachea, bronchi, and lungs; primary purpose is to both supply cells with oxygen for metabolism and remove carbon dioxide; cardiac and pulmonary systems work together to facilitate gas exchange and distribute gases throughout the body
  B. Cardiovascular system circulates oxygenated blood throughout the body via arteries; veins return systemic blood to heart and lungs for oxygenation, then recirculation
  C. Primary responsibility of pulmonary system is to distribute air and exchange gases

NURSING PROCESS APPLIED TO CHILDREN WITH CARDIOVASCULAR DISORDERS

Congenital Cardiac Disorders

I. Assessment
  A. Definition: structural defects that occur during fetal development and cause functional disruption of normal circulation; manifest either acyanotically, where there is no mixing of unoxygenated and oxygenated blood, or cyanotically, where unoxygenated blood mixes with oxygenated blood regardless of whether cyanosis occurs (Table 10-1); defects often associated with *shunting,* the flow of blood from an area of higher pressure to an area of lower pressure through an abnormal opening
  B. Etiology/incidence
    1. Etiology unknown
    2. 10 per 1000 live births
    3. Found in high percentage of stillborns, spontaneous abortions, low-birth-weight infants
    4. Nine common lesions comprise 90% of all anomalies
  C. Predisposing/precipitating factors
    1. Maternal rubella and other viruses during pregnancy
    2. Poor maternal nutrition
    3. Maternal alcoholism
    4. Drugs taken during pregnancy
    5. Maternal age over 40
    6. Maternal insulin-dependent diabetes, PKU, lupus
    7. Prematurity, neonatal hypoxia, respiratory distress syndrome
    8. Parents/sibling with heart disease
    9. Born with other congenital anomalies
    10. Chromosomal defects (e.g., Down's syndrome)
  D. Clinical manifestations (see Table 10-1)
    1. General clinical manifestations: fatigue, feeding difficulties, exercise intolerance, failure to thrive
    2. Atrial septal defect (ASD) (Fig. 10-1A)
      a. Acyanotic
      b. Ostium secundum defect most common
      c. Usually asymptomatic; may have pulmonary hypertension late in life
      d. Split second heart sound (S_2) and systolic ejection murmur at upper left sternal border
    3. Ventricular septal defect (VSD) (Fig. 10-1B)
      a. Acyanotic; most common form of congenital heart disease
      b. Small or moderate openings may be asymptomatic except for systolic murmur heard at lower left sternal border
      c. Large defects
        (1) Loud, harsh murmur best heard at left sternal border radiating throughout precordium
        (2) Right ventricular hypertrophy

TABLE 10–1 Congenital Cardiac Defects

Defect	Incidence/ Frequency	Structural Abnormality	Hemodynamics
Acyanotic			
Atrial septal defect	5 to 10%	Abnormal opening between right and left atria	Left-to-right shunting through atrial opening; volume overload to right heart and pulmonary circulation
Ventricular septal defect	20 to 25%	Abnormal opening between right and left ventricles	Left-to-right shunting due to incomplete closure of septum; pulmonary vascular resistance
Patent ductus arteriosus	5 to 10% excluding premature infants	Communication between pulmonary artery and aorta due to failure of ductus arteriosus to close after birth	Left-to-right shunting; increased pulmonary vascular resistance
Coarctation of the aorta	8%	Narrowing of the aortic lumen; usually bicuspid aortic valve	Left ventricle must generate higher-than-normal pressure to eject adequate stroke volume; reduces systolic pressure distal to coarctation
Pulmonic stenosis	5 to 8%	Obstruction of pulmonary artery; usually at pulmonic valve; often occurs with other cardiac anomalies	Obstruction of flow of blood from right ventricle to lungs; increased pressure in right side of heart; right-sided hypertrophy
Aortic stenosis	5%	Narrowing or malformation of aortic valve	Obstruction of flow of blood from left ventricle to aorta; left-sided hypertrophy; increased oxygen demand; pulmonary vascular congestion
Cyanotic			
Transposition of great vessels	5%	Reversal of anatomic position of aorta and pulmonary artery; aorta originates from right ventricle, pulmonary artery from left ventricle	If not treated immediately, incompatible with extrauterine life; venous blood enters right atrium to right ventricle to aorta and systemic circulation without oxygenation; oxygenated blood from lungs enters left atrium to left ventricle to pulmonary artery and back to lungs without supplying oxygen to body
Tetralogy of Fallot	10%	Four anomalies present: Pulmonic stenosis Ventricular septal defect Aorta overriding ventricular septal defect Right ventricular hypertrophy	Right-to-left shunting decreasing flow to lungs; right-sided hypertrophy; unoxygenated blood to systemic circulation through ventricular septal defect overriding aorta

(3) Cardiac enlargement by radiograph
4. Patent ductus arteriosus (PDA) (Fig. 10-1C)
  a. Acyanotic
  b. Almost continuous machinery-like murmur best heard at upper left sternal border
  c. Diastolic "rumble" with large defects
  d. Widened pulse pressure: difference between systolic and diastolic pressures
  e. May develop signs of congestive heart failure: fatigue, feeding difficulties, increasing respiratory distress
5. Coarctation of the aorta (Fig. 10-1D)
  a. Acyanotic
  b. Episodes of sudden epistaxis
  c. Full, bounding pulses, elevated blood pressure in upper extremities
  d. Weak or absent pulses in lower extremities, blood pressure lower than in upper extremities
  e. Headaches
  f. Leg fatigue and weakness from decreased peripheral circulation
  g. Systolic murmur
  h. If symptomatic in infancy: right ventricular hypertrophy, congestive heart failure, failure to thrive
6. Pulmonic stenosis (Fig. 10-2A)
  a. Acyanotic
  b. Systolic murmur best heard over upper left sternal border
  c. Thrill

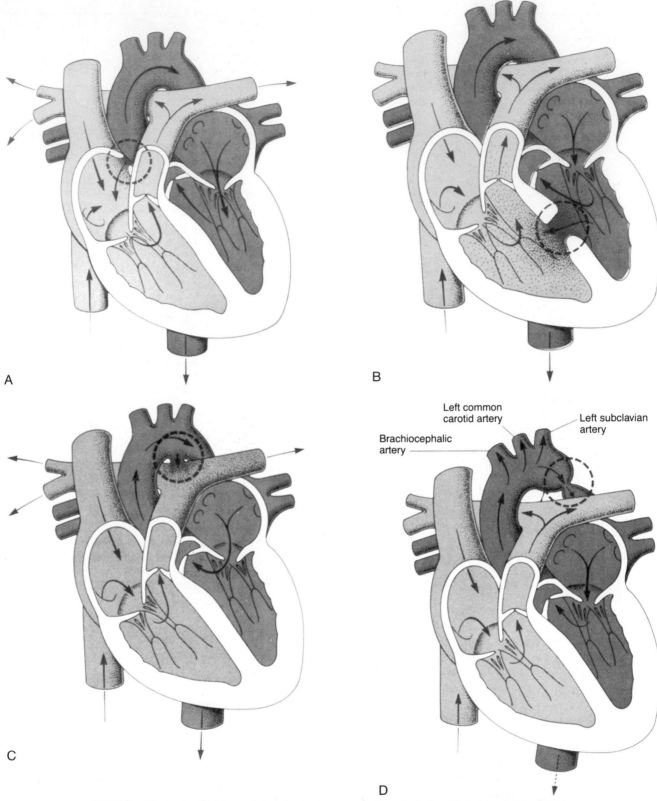

A

B

C

D

Left common
carotid artery

Left subclavian
artery

Brachiocephalic
artery

FIGURE 10–1. *A,* Atrial septal defect. Abnormal flow is left atrium to right atrium. *B,* Ventricular septal defect. Abnormal flow is left ventricle to right ventricle. *C,* Patent ductus arteriosus. The shunt is from aorta to pulmonary artery. *D,* Coarctation of the aorta. Flow is normal but diminished distal to coarctation. Blood pressure is increased in vessels leaving aorta proximal to coarctation. (From Foster, R. L. R., Hunsberger, M. M., and Anderson, J. J. T. (1989). *Family-centered nursing care of children.* Philadelphia: W. B. Saunders.)

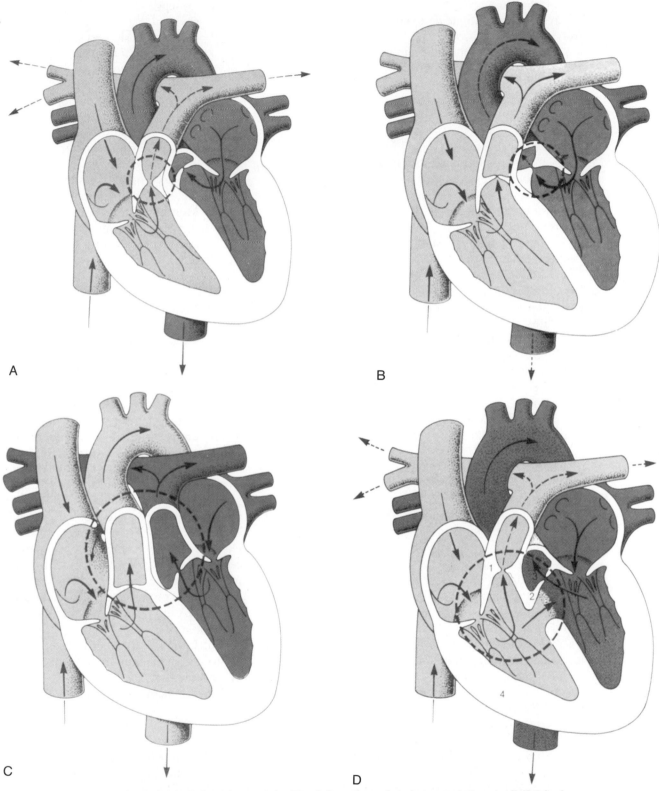

A

B

C

D

FIGURE 10–2. *A,* Pulmonic stenosis. Blood flow through pulmonary artery is diminished. *B,* Aortic stenosis. Flow patterns are normal, but blood flow into aorta is diminished. *C,* Transposition of great vessels. Blood flow exists as two parallel systems—one recirculating oxygenated blood and the other recirculating unoxygenated blood. *D,* Tetralogy of Fallot with pulmonic stenosis, ventricular septal defect, overriding aorta, and right ventricular hypertrophy. Flow is determined by degree of pulmonic stenosis. (From Foster, R. L. R., Hunsberger, M. M., and Anderson, J. J. T. (1989). *Family-centered nursing care of children.* Philadelphia: W. B. Saunders.)

d. Split S$_2$

e. Dyspnea and fatigue if severe

7. Aortic stenosis (Fig. 10-2B)

a. Acyanotic, predominantly in boys

b. Systolic thrill throughout precordium

c. Ejection click

d. Fatigue, exercise intolerance

e. Epigastric/anginal pain

f. Dyspnea

8. Transposition of great vessels (Fig. 10-2C)

a. Cyanotic, predominantly in boys

b. Signs of congestive heart failure

c. Arterial pulses full and bounding

d. Murmur present only if VSD or PDA present

e. Hypoxemia unless communication between right and left atria present or created

9. Tetralogy of Fallot (Fig. 10-2D)

a. Cyanosis appears during first year of life

b. Clubbing of fingers in older infants

c. Hypoxic spells

d. Squatting position after any form of exercise

e. Small for age

f. Harsh, systolic ejection murmur best heard at middle to upper left sternal border

g. Characteristic ''boot-shaped'' heart on radiograph

E. Diagnostic examinations

1. Based on findings of history and physical

2. Chest radiograph to visualize cardiac size and shape

3. ECG measures electrical activity

4. Echocardiogram uses sound waves to obtain structural image

5. Complete blood count (CBC)/arterial blood gases (ABGs)

6. Cardiac catheterization

a. Nursing responsibilities—pre-test

(1) Explain procedure to child and family using visual aids

(2) Baseline assessment of general health status; marking location, strength, and quality of pulses distal to proposed catheter site; peripheral circulatory status

(3) Schedule ECG, x-ray, and blood work before test

(4) NPO for 4 to 6 hours before test

(5) Sedate as ordered

(6) Accompany child to test if possible

b. Nursing responsibilities—post-test

(1) Observe monitor for dysrhythmias

(2) Check vital signs every 15 minutes until stable, then every 2 to 4 hours for 24 to 48 hours

(3) Report tachycardia, bradycardia, dysrhythmias to doctor immediately

(4) Check circulation on involved extremity (e.g., color, temperature, capillary refill)

(5) Observe operative site for bleeding, signs of infection

(6) Monitor hydration status

(7) Pressure dressing at surgical site; keep leg straight for 6 hours

(8) Keep child relatively quiet, side rails up

F. Complications

1. Congestive heart failure (see discussion to follow)

2. Bacterial endocarditis

a. Infection of the endocardium near congenital defects or cardiac lesions

b. Caused by *Streptococcus viridans*, organisms often found in skin or mucous membranes

c. Prevented by administration of amoxicillin (Table 10-2) (erythromycin if penicillin allergic) before and after dental procedures and procedures compromising skin or mucous membranes, particularly if infection is already present

G. Surgical management: depends on specific cardiac disorder, surgical correction often treatment of choice; some children undergo multiple surgical procedures; pharmacological closure of PDA in low-birth-weight infants

II. Analysis

A. Altered nutrition: less than body requirements related to inadequate intake, feeding difficulties, chronic hypoxia

B. Decreased cardiac output related to structural defects

C. Impaired gas exchange related to altered pulmonary blood flow

D. High risk for altered growth and development related to fatigue, multiple hospitalizations, parental overprotection

E. Activity intolerance related to imbalance between oxygen supply and demand

F. High risk for infection related to pulmonary congestion and cardiac disease

G. Anxiety (child and family) related to perception of the disease, its management, prognosis

TABLE 10–2 Antibiotics/Antibacterial Agents

Example	Action	Use	Common Side Effects	Nursing Implications
Penicillin (Amoxicillin, Ampicillin, Augmentin)	Bacteriocidal/bacterio-static drugs that act by interfering with synthesis of bacterial cell wall	Effective against susceptible organisms	Hypersensitivity reactions (i.e., range from mild urticarial rash to anaphylaxis)	Careful history of previous allergic reaction; give oral doses on empty stomach
Erythromycin	Similar to penicillin	Effective when child is allergic to penicillin; used with *Mycoplasma* infections	Nausea, vomiting, epigastric distress	Give oral doses on a full stomach to decrease gastric distress
Cephalosporins (Keflex, Ceclor, Ceftriaxone [IM])	Effective against penicillin-resistant organisms	Infections caused by *Staphylococcus aureus* and penicillin-resistant bacterial strains; can be used when child is allergic to penicillin	Diarrhea, hypersensitivity	Be careful of allergic cross-reactions in children who are penicillin allergic; watch for allergic reactions
Sulfas (Bactrim, Septra, Gantrisin)	Interfere with biosynthesis of substances essential to many bacteria	Primarily for urinary tract infection or otitis media but can be used for persistent respiratory infection	Skin rashes, including erythema multiforme; gastrointestinal irritation; photosensitivity	Usually not given to infants less than 2 months; keep out of the sun; encourage fluids

H. High risk for ineffective individual coping related to chronic condition and multiple surgeries

I. Knowledge deficit about procedures, treatment, and surgery related to unfamiliarity with the appropriate information

III. Planning/goals, expected outcomes
   A. Family will identify possible causes of congenital defect
   B. Family will identify circumstances that aggravate/alleviate dyspnea, fatigue, exercise intolerance, feeding difficulties
   C. Child will be free of complications
   D. Family will identify necessary diagnostic procedures
   E. Family will describe their understanding of surgical procedure, if necessary
   F. Child will be maintained before and after surgery
   G. Family will describe discharge instructions
   H. Family will have emotional support provided
   I. Family will describe need for prenatal care with all subsequent pregnancies

IV. Implementation
   A. Feed small, frequent feedings of breast milk or high-calorie infant formula
   B. Allow frequent rest periods during feeding; use nipple with larger hole
   C. Minimize oxygen requirements with frequent rest periods, anxiety relief, quiet environment, meeting child's needs quickly
   D. Position with head at 30- to 40-degree slant; knee-chest position during hypoxic spells
   E. Administer oxygen as ordered

F. Provide age-appropriate stimulation but modify according to child's energy level

G. Encourage parents to allow child to return to appropriate age–level activities after hospitalization

H. Assist parents in planning for routines that include appropriate play

I. Provide regular rest periods and uninterrupted sleep

J. Help child to limit own activity and increase exercise tolerance gradually

K. Teach family infection-prevention measures

L. Alert family about situations requiring prophylactic antibiotics to prevent bacterial endocarditis

M. Prepare child for all procedures and surgery (Table 10-3)

N. Encourage child and family to ask questions, express feelings

O. Encourage appropriate parenting skills to reduce overprotection

P. Teach principles of medication administration and follow-up care

V. Evaluation
   A. Family can state the signs, symptoms, origins of the child's disease
   B. Child is able to eat with fewer rest periods
   C. Child demonstrates increased tolerance for activity
   D. Family describes play activities appropriate for child's growth and tolerance level
   E. Child demonstrates greater tolerance of procedures and treatments

TABLE 10–3 Preoperative and Postoperative Care for Cardiac Surgery

Preoperative

Goals	Implementations
Practice procedures to be used after surgery	Demonstration—return demonstration of turning, coughing, deep breathing, postural drainage, incentive spirometer
Baseline observations	Monitor vital signs with blood pressure, I & O, height, weight; urinalysis, CBC; usual sleep/wake pattern
Decreased fear	Review what to expect with child and family—chest tubes, monitor, catheter, IV line

Postoperative

Goals	Implementations
Provide rest	Plan activities around sleep/wake pattern
Monitor return of vital signs	Check vital signs with blood pressure; ECG, arterial/venous pressure
Maintenance of respiratory status	Lung assessment; turn, cough, and deep breathe every 1 to 2 hours; percussion/postural drainage every 2 to 4 hours; suction as needed; assess chest tube functioning every 1 to 2 hours; monitor for stasis pneumonia (i.e., decreased/absent breath sounds)
Maintenance of fluid and electrolytes	Strict I & O; check weight daily; specific gravity of void; monitor electrolytes, especially potassium; observe for bleeding
Pain management	Regular administration of ordered analgesics
Infection prevention	Aseptic technique when handling catheters; antibiotics as ordered

F. Family states actions and side effects of medications
G. Family can demonstrate procedures and treatments to be done at home
H. Family plans a routine of care that provides for maximum rest
I. Family seeks appropriate community resources for support

Acute and Chronic Disorders

Congestive Heart Failure

I. Assessment
   A. Definition: inability of heart to pump sufficient amount of blood, thus oxygen and nutrients, to systemic circulation to meet metabolic needs of body
   B. Etiology/incidence
      1. Occurs most frequently secondary to structural abnormalities; results from excessive workload on heart
      2. May occur secondary to systemic disease involving renal or pulmonary systems
      3. Majority affected are infants, often less than 1 month of age
   C. Predisposing/precipitating factors
      1. Increased blood volume
      2. Increased afterload
      3. Ineffective contractions of heart
      4. High cardiac output demand
      5. Dysrhythmias
   D. Clinical manifestations
      1. Cardinal signs
         a. Tachycardia
         b. Cardiomegaly
         c. Tachypnea
         d. Dyspnea and respiratory distress
      2. Gallop rhythm
      3. Weak peripheral pulses
      4. Cool, mottled, or cyanotic extremities
      5. Fatigue and feeding difficulties
      6. Decreased urinary output
      7. Indicators of left-sided heart failure
         a. Dyspnea
         b. Tachypnea
         c. Retractions
         d. Wheezes, rales, hacking cough
         e. Flared nostrils
         f. Orthopnea
      8. Indicators of right-sided heart failure
         a. Hepatomegaly
         b. Distended neck veins
         c. Periorbital edema
         d. Ascites
   E. Diagnostic examinations
      1. Based on clinical manifestations
      2. Must have cardiac manifestations as well as pulmonary manifestations to differentiate from pulmonary congestion
   F. Complications
      1. Can be recurrent depending on cause
      2. May be terminal depending on cause
   G. Medical management
      1. Medications
         a. Cardiac glycosides (Table 10-4)

TABLE 10–4 Cardiac Glycosides

Example	Action	Use	Common Side Effects	Nursing Implications
Digoxin (Lanoxin), digitoxin	Increase force of myocardial contraction; decrease conduction through sinoatrial and atrioventricular nodes; increase cardiac output and slow heart rate	Management of congestive heart failure	Anorexia, nausea, vomiting; bradycardia; dysrhythmias; fatigue	Monitor for signs of toxicity; take apical pulse for 1 minute before giving; withhold if pulse less than minimum rate recommended by physician; monitor serum level of drug, electrolytes, renal function; best given 1 hour before or 2 hours after meals; encourage foods high in potassium

b. Diuretics (Table 10-5)

2. Diet: low sodium, high potassium (Table 10-6)

II. Analysis

  A. Decreased cardiac output related to volume overload and ineffective pumping

  B. Altered peripheral tissue perfusion related to decreased cardiac output

  C. High risk for infection related to increased pulmonary secretions and ineffective airway clearance

  D. Fluid volume excess related to compromised regulatory mechanisms

  E. Activity intolerance related to impaired metabolic functions

  F. Altered nutrition: less than body requirements related to increased metabolic demands and decreased energy level

  G. Altered growth and development related to decreased energy for achieving developmental milestones

  H. Anxiety (parent) related to infant's uncertain health status

  I. Parental role conflict related to the infant's hospitalization

III. Planning/goals, expected outcomes

  A. Child will demonstrate improved cardiac output

  B. Child will rest comfortably

  C. Child will demonstrate decreased respiratory distress and be free of signs of infection

  D. Child will demonstrate adequate fluid balance

  E. Child will gradually increase tolerance to activity and energy expenditure

  F. Child will maintain or gain weight according to appropriate norms

  G. Parents will express feelings of anxiety or fear

  H. Parents will describe therapeutic measures necessary for child's well-being

  I. Parents will describe the need for follow-up care and what it entails

IV. Implementation

  A. Measure vital signs every 1 to 4 hours depending on child's condition

  B. Monitor ECG as ordered

TABLE 10–5 Diuretics (Thiazides, Loop, Potassium-Sparing)

Example	Action	Use	Common Side Effects	Nursing Implications
Hydrochlorothiazide (Hydrodiuril), furosemide (Lasix), spironolactone (Aldactone)	Reduce cardiac workload by decreasing circulating blood volume Increase urinary output through prevention of reabsorption of water from kidney tubules; diuresis Promote sodium excretion without potassium loss	Management of conditions resulting in excess fluid load; hypertension; cardiac condition to reduce preload/afterload	Metabolic alkalosis, hypovolemia, hypokalemia, hyponatremia, headache, ataxia	Monitor electrolytes periodically, especially potassium; monitor fluid status (i.e., I & O, edema, skin turgor); monitor blood pressure; may give with food or milk; administer in morning

TABLE 10–6 Low-Sodium, High-Potassium Diet

Low-Sodium Foods	High-Sodium Foods
Eggs	Lunch meats
Low-sodium meats, cheeses	Shellfish
Skim, 2%, or whole milk	Cheese
Fresh fruits, vegetables	Commercial milk products
Low-sodium bread products	Canned fruits, vegetables
Unsalted butter, margarine	Spinach, carrots
Unsalted nuts	Commercial breads, cereals
	Salted butter, margarine
	Canned soups

Low-Potassium Foods	High-Potassium Foods
Apples, grapes	Fresh fruits, especially bananas
Cabbage, cucumber, onion	Fresh or frozen vegetables, especially green leafy vegetables, potatoes
Oatmeal, dry cereals in restricted amounts	
Beef, poultry in restricted amounts	Whole grain products
	Meats, poultry, fish
	Commercial milk products

General Principles

Objective of diet is to reduce sodium and fluid retention, to replace potassium loss due to diuretics, and to minimize cardiac workload

RDA sodium: 1100 to 3300 mg/day
RDA potassium: 1875 to 5625 mg/day

Normal serum sodium: 132 mEq/L to 145 mEq/L
Normal serum potassium: 3.5 mEq/L to 5.0 mEq/L

C. Administer digoxin as ordered, and teach parents proper administration
D. Observe for signs of digitalis toxicity (see Table 10-2); anorexia may be first sign in infants
E. Maintain child in semi-Fowler position; may use infant seat for short periods
F. Administer oxygen as ordered, and monitor oxygen saturation
G. Provide chest percussion and physiotherapy as ordered; may need to modify according to child's energy level
H. Suction as needed
I. Maintain strict intake and output monitoring; check weight daily (more often depending on condition) on same scale at same time of day; monitor for signs of dehydration
J. Administer diuretics as ordered
K. Monitor electrolyte status, particularly potassium level, and give potassium supplements or sodium-restricted, potassium-rich diet (see Table 10-5) as ordered

L. Maintain normal body temperature with appropriate dress and avoidance of chilling
M. Use soft nipple with larger hole or provide frequent rest periods while feeding
N. Administer small, frequent feedings of breast milk or formula; use high-calorie formula if slow weight gain
O. Encourage play in gradual increments as tolerated; have parents bring familiar toys from home
P. Increase activity level daily as tolerated
Q. Allow parents to express feelings of anxiety or fear; refer to appropriate support group
R. Allow parents to participate in child's care; explain rationales for nursing actions
S. Teach parents home care: medication administration, signs of congestive heart failure, cardiopulmonary resuscitation (CPR) (Table 10-7)

V. Evaluation
   A. Child's cardiac output improved
   B. Child free of infection without respiratory distress
   C. Child has adequate fluid volume
   D. Child's activity tolerance increases
   E. Child's weight falls within norms for age
   F. Parents express feelings of fear or anxiety
   G. Parents understand and describe treatment and follow-up care

Rheumatic Fever

I. Assessment
   A. Definition: acute, systemic inflammatory disease that affects connective tissue of heart, joints, central nervous system, and subcutaneous tissue
   B. Etiology/incidence
      1. Evidence of relationship between group A beta-hemolytic streptococcal infections and subsequent rheumatic fever 1 to 4 weeks after streptococcal infection; probably an autoimmune process
      2. Primarily affects school-age children
      3. Although incidence has decreased in general, it is still the most frequent cause of cardiac disease in children
   C. Predisposing/precipitating factors
      1. Antigen-antibody response to toxin released by group A beta-hemolytic *Streptococcus*
      2. Lower socioeconomic areas, crowded housing, cold humid climates
   D. Clinical manifestations
      1. History of previous streptococcal infection
         a. Sudden onset of sore throat, often as-

TABLE 10–7 Cardiopulmonary Resuscitation in Infants and Children

Definition   A rapid sequence of activities to restore respiratory (ventilation) capabilities and circulation; brought about through mouth-to-mouth/nose resuscitation and closed-chest massage; speed is of utmost importance as irreversible brain damage occurs in adult in 4 to 6 minutes, and it is believed to occur even sooner in children; the smaller the child, the higher the demands of his or her tissues for oxygen

Step	Infants	Children
Airway (A)	Place infant on a flat, hard surface; flick sole of foot	Place child on a flat, hard surface; tap or shake gently
		Place one hand on forehead and fingers of other hand under chin; gently tilt back head
	Look, listen, and feel for breath; if none, proceed to step B	Same as for infant
Breath (B)	Place mouth over infant's mouth and nose, forming airtight seal; give two slow breaths, allowing for exhale between breaths	Place mouth over child's mouth only, pinch nose; if child is small, use mouth and nose approach; give two slow breaths, watching for chest to rise
	Check for spontaneous breathing; check brachial artery for pulse (inner aspect of elbow)	Check for spontaneous breathing; check carotid artery for pulse
	If pulse present but not breathing, continue breaths at rate of one breath every 3 seconds	If pulse present but not breathing, continue breaths at rate of one breath every 4 seconds (child less than 8 years) or one breath every 5 seconds (child more than 8 years)
	If pulse not present, proceed to step C	Same as for infant
Circulation (C)	Place index and middle finger on center of chest, one finger-width below nipple line. Compress ½ to 1 in., 100 to 120 compressions per minutes; give one breath every five compressions; check for pulse and respiration after 1 minute and each several minutes thereafter until functions return or life support takes over	With index finger, follow lower rib cage line to sternum; place middle finger there and index finger above; place heel of one hand above index finger (on child more than 8, place other hand on top). Compress chest 1 to 1½ in. (1½ to 2 in. for child more than 8) at rate of 80 to 100 compressions per minute; give one breath for every 5 compressions (two for every 15 if one rescuer and child more than 8); check for pulse and respirations after 1 minute and each several minutes after that until functions return or life support takes over

sociated with headache or stomach-ache

  b. Febrile

  c. Cervical/mandibular adenitis

  d. Malaise

2. Revised Jones' criteria—two major manifestations or one major and two minor constitute a diagnosis

  a. Major clinical manifestations

    (1) Carditis: most severe manifestation

    (2) Polyarthritis: affects large joints, usually migratory

    (3) Sydenham's chorea/St. Vitus' dance: presence of sudden, aimless, rapid movements of extremities; involuntary facial grimaces; speech disturbances

    (4) Subcutaneous nodules: visible nodules on flexor surfaces of joints

    (5) Erythema marginatum: circular, erythematous lesions

  b. Minor clinical manifestations

    (1) Fever

    (2) Arthralgia

    (3) History of previous rheumatic fever or heart disease

    (4) Elevated ESR (more than 13 mm/hr)

    (5) Elevated C-reactive protein

    (6) Leukocytosis

    (7) Anemia

    (8) Prolonged PR intervals on ECG

    (9) Positive throat culture for group A beta-hemolytic *Streptococcus*

    (10) Elevated ASO titer (more than 333 Todd units)

    (11) Mild anemia

E. Complications: permanent cardiac damage, particularly of the valves, from inflammation-related scarring

F. Medical management

  1. Treatment of active streptococcal infection with injection of long-acting benzanthine penicillin G; 10-day course of oral erythromycin if penicillin allergic (see Table 10-2)

  2. Analgesics to control pain; salicylates (aspirin) in most cases during acute phase

to control inflammation; steroids (prednisone) sometimes necessary for severe carditis (Table 10-8)

3. Bedrest during acute phase: 2 weeks to 3 months depending on extent of cardiac involvement

4. Prophylaxis for preventing recurrent streptococcal infection: penicillin G by either monthly injection or daily oral doses until child is 20 years old or for 5 years after disease in older adolescent (erythromycin for children allergic to penicillin). Later prophylaxis when exposure to streptococcal infection likely (illness episodes or for invasive dental or surgical procedures)

II. Analysis

A. Impaired physical mobility related to imposition of bedrest

B. Pain related to inflammation (polyarthritis, arthralgias)

C. High risk for impaired skin integrity related to prolonged bedrest

D. High risk for diversional activity deficit related to movement limitations

E. High risk for altered nutrition: less than body requirements related to decreased metabolic demands

F. High risk for injury related to choreic episodes

G. High risk for anxiety (child and family) related to perception of the disease and its consequences

H. Knowledge deficit related to incomplete understanding of disease and its complications, home management, prophylaxis

III. Planning/goals, expected outcomes

A. Child will rest comfortably and be free of complications of bedrest

B. Child will be free of pain

C. Child will maintain adequate nutritional intake based on age and weight

D. Child will be free of injury during choreic episodes

E. Child will be free of further episodes of rheumatic fever

F. Child/family will describe necessary actions for proper long-term follow-up care

G. Child/family will receive emotional support

IV. Implementation

A. Encourage bedrest and activity limitations as prescribed

B. Plan daily activities with periods of daily rest

C. Provide diversional activities that do not require excessive movement

D. Encourage peer visitation

E. Administer anti-inflammatory agents or analgesics as prescribed

F. Use bed cradles to prevent linen from causing or aggravating joint pain

G. Position joint on pillows

H. Maintain proper body alignment

I. Measure I & O

J. Maintain daily calorie count

K. Check weight daily

L. Provide small, highly nutritious feedings

M. Encourage fluids, but observe for fluid overload

N. Have side rails up during choreic episodes

O. Assist with ambulation; when allowed to ambulate, protect from injury

P. Teach parents clinical manifestations of streptococcal infections; culture family members

TABLE 10–8 Anti-inflammatory Agents

Example	Action	Use	Common Side Effects	Nursing Implications
Salycilates (aspirin)	Anti-inflammatory; inhibit transmission of pain impulses	Inflammation, pain, and fever management	Gastric irritation, prolonged bleeding; has been associated with development of Reye's syndrome when given to children with viral illnesses (cold, chickenpox, influenza), monitor serum salycilate level	Do not use for children with bleeding disorders or gastric ulcers; never give to children with suspected viral illness
Steroids (prednisone, Decadron)	Adrenal corticosteroid; anti-inflammatory, immunosuppressive	Moderate-to-severe inflammation, immunosuppression	Gastric irritation, bleeding, masking of underlying infection, fluid retention	Administer on a full stomach; monitor vital signs closely; never discontinue abruptly; monitor for signs of infection

Q. Teach family importance of prophylaxis in preventing recurrence of rheumatic fever

R. Teach family importance of antibiotic therapy before any invasive procedures or dental work

S. Encourage family to discuss concerns about possible heart damage

V. Evaluation

  A. Child expresses being comfortable, especially at rest

  B. Child does not complain of pain

  C. Child helps plan nutritious diet and consumes adequate fluids

  D. Child does not sustain injury during choreic episode

  E. Child engages in quiet, age-appropriate recreational activities

  F. Family describes accurately posthospitalization and long-term care, including infection-prevention strategies

NURSING PROCESS APPLIED TO CHILDREN WITH DISEASES OF THE HEMATOLOGICAL SYSTEM

Leukemia

I. Assessment

  A. Definition: broad term given to group of malignant diseases of bone marrow that cause overproduction of immature, nonfunctional white blood cells (blasts), which crowd bone marrow and prevent development of other blood cells (e.g., red blood cells, platelets); most common type of cancer in children

  B. Etiology/incidence

    1. Unknown

    2. 80% have acute lymphocytic leukemia (ALL), overproduction of lymphoblasts of various classes of lymphocytes

      a. Usually diagnosed after 1 year of age, especially 2 to 5 years

      b. More common in boys

    3. 20% develop acute nonlymphocytic leukemia (ANLL), overproduction of immature cells from various cell lines (myeloblasts, monoblasts)

      a. More common in older children

      b. Affects girls and boys equally

  C. Predisposing/precipitating factors

    1. Exposure to ionizing radiation

    2. Exposure to certain viruses

    3. Chromosomal aberrations

    4. Suppressed immune systems

    5. Siblings with leukemia

  D. Clinical manifestations

    1. Effects of bone marrow crowding and failure

      a. Increased immature white blood cells

        (1) Infection from decreased immune function

        (2) Fever

      b. Decreased red blood cells

        (1) Anemia with reduced oxygen to cells

        (2) Pallor

        (3) Fatigue

      c. Decreased platelets

        (1) Petechiae

        (2) Ecchymoses

        (3) Bleeding

    2. Effects of extramedullary infiltrates

      a. Joint pain

      b. Splenomegaly/hepatomegaly

      c. Lymphadenopathy

      d. Anorexia, nausea, vomiting

      e. Central nervous system involvement

    3. Hyperuricemia from cell lysis

  E. Diagnostic examinations

    1. CBC: shows peripheral blast cells, anemia, decreased red blood cells and platelets

    2. Bone marrow aspiration (Table 10-9) shows high percentage of abnormal blast cells; essential for differential diagnosis between ALL and ANLL

    3. Lumbar puncture (Table 10-10) with spinal fluid aspiration to determine central nervous system involvement

    4. Chest radiograph to assess for mediastinal mass

  F. Complications

    1. Extramedullary infiltration of spleen, liver, kidneys, testes, ovaries, and central nervous system

    2. Hemorrhage

TABLE 10–9 Bone Marrow Aspiration

Procedure	Nursing Care
Sterile; area washed with povidone-iodine solution	Explain procedure to child/parent
Local anesthetic (lidocaine) administered	Sedate as per orders
Aspiration taken from posterior or anterior iliac crest (it contains active bone marrow and is easy to locate)	Position prone with pillow under hips
	Restrain as necessary
Aspiration takes less than 1 minute; child may feel a sharp pain	
Specimen sent to laboratory for examination	
Pressure dressing applied to site	

TABLE 10–10 Lumbar Puncture

Procedure	Nursing Care
Sterile; area washed with povidone-iodine solution	Explain procedure to child/parent
Local anesthetic (lidocaine) administered	Position side-lying, knee-chest (this exaggerates curvature of lumbar area)
Subarachnoid space between third and fourth lumbar vertebrae used	Hug child behind neck and knees to maintain position
Spinal needle inserted, and cerebral spinal fluid withdrawn	Keep flat 4 to 6 hours after procedure to avoid headache (secondary to pressure changes)
Specimen sent to laboratory for examination (i.e., cell count, culture, Gram stain)	
Manometer might be used to measure intracranial pressure	
Intrathecal chemotherapeutic agents may be injected	
Needle withdrawn, and dressing applied	

3. Overwhelming infection
4. Effects of chemotherapy: depend on agent used
   a. Acute side effects
      (1) Hypersensitivity: anaphylaxis, urticaria, photosensitivity
      (2) Fever
      (3) Nausea and vomiting
      (4) Extravasation and necrosis at administration site
   b. Intermediate side effects (usually after 1 to several weeks)
      (1) Bone marrow suppression leading to anemia, infection, bleeding
      (2) Alopecia
      (3) Stomatitis
   c. Late-appearing, long-term effects: liver, heart, renal, and neurological toxicity
G. Medical management
   1. Remission induction
      a. Leukemic cells undetectable
      b. Use of chemotherapy protocol, usually vincristine, prednisone, L-asparaginase for ALL; cytosine arabinoside and daunorubicin or doxorubicin used with ANLL (Table 10-11)
      c. Allopurinol to block formation of uric acid
      d. Initial remission achieved in approximately 90 to 98% of children with ALL and approximately 70% of children with ANLL
   2. Central nervous system prophylaxis

a. Necessary because conventional chemotherapy does not pass blood-brain barrier
b. Chemotherapeutic agents, usually methotrexate, cytosine arabinoside, or combination of agents, injected into spinal fluid directly through lumbar puncture (intrathecal administration)
c. Radiotherapy to cranial area also might be used
   3. Maintenance therapy
      a. Continued for approximately 3 years
      b. Usually daily oral 6-mercaptopurine, weekly methotrexate; monthly prednisone and vincristine might be given as well
   4. Bone marrow transplantation considered for repeat relapse
II. Analysis
   A. High risk for infection related to compromised immune system from bone marrow suppression
   B. High risk for injury related to administration of chemotherapy and decreased platelets
   C. Altered oral mucous membranes related to effects of chemotherapy
   D. Altered nutrition: less than body requirements related to nausea, vomiting, altered taste sensation
   E. Activity intolerance related to anemia
   F. High risk for fluid volume deficit related to vomiting
   G. High risk for constipation related to effects of chemotherapy or decreased appetite
   H. Pain related to effects of disease process or treatment given
   I. High risk for body image disturbance related to alopecia, change in health status
   J. Anxiety (child and family) about disease and its prognosis
   K. Knowledge deficit about treatments, procedures, home management related to unfamiliarity or denial
III. Planning/goals, expected outcomes
   A. Child will exhibit no signs and symptoms of infections
   B. Child's environment will be safe, especially when platelet count decreased
   C. Child will increase tolerance to activity and exercise
   D. Child does not exhibit any breaks in skin integrity or mucosa
   E. Child maintains adequate nutritional intake based on age and weight
   F. Child will rest comfortably
   G. Child will be as comfortable as possible after chemotherapy or radiation

TABLE 10–11 Chemotherapeutic Agents

Class	Example	Use	Common Side Effects	Nursing Implications
Antimetabolites	Methotrexate	To treat leukemias and some other cancers	Gastrointestinal ulceration, severe stomatitis, bone marrow depression, nephrotoxicity, diarrhea, hepatotoxicity, anaphylaxis, neurological symptoms with intrethecal administration	Give leucovorin as ordered to prevent toxicity; hydrate well; monitor blood counts closely; watch for Gastrointestinal bleeding
	Cytosine arabinoside (Ara-C, Cytosar)	Leukemias	Nausea and vomiting, bone marrow suppression, fever, stomatitis, hepatotoxicity, rashes	Discard solution if hazy; administer slowly; monitor blood counts; monitor intake and output
	6-Mercaptopurine (6-MP)	Leukemias	Bone marrow suppression, hyperuricemia, hepatotoxicity	Potentiated by allopurinol—may need to decrease usual dose if taking allopurinol; monitor blood counts; provide adequate hydration
Plant alkaloids	Vincristine (Oncovin)	Leukemias	Alopecia, constipation, neurotoxicity and peripheral neuropathy, extravasation at site of administration	Monitor for neurological changes; administer stool softeners; administer IV slowly and monitor carefully for extravasation
Antitumor antibiotics	Doxorubicin (Adriamycin)	Leukemias	Bone marrow suppression, severe necrosis at site of administration, nausea and vomiting, alopecia, stomatitis, red urine, fever, cardiotoxicity, anaphylaxis, hyperuricemia	Avoid and treat extravasation; monitor blood studies and for cardiovascular function; treat stomatitis; provide adequate hydration and monitor urinary output
	Daunorubicin (Daunomycin)	Leukemias	Same as for doxorubicin; myocardiotoxicity is a danger from cumulative effects	Same as for doxorubicin
Enzyme	L-Asparaginase	Acute lymphocytic leukemia	Anaphylaxis, hepatotoxicity, fever, coagulation alterations, hyperglycemia, hyperuricemia, bone marrow suppression	Monitor for allergic reaction; monitor blood work—CBC, liver function, electrolytes, coagulation studies; watch for bleeding
Miscellaneous	Prednisone	Immunosuppressive	See Table 10-8	See Table 10-8
	Allopurinol	Reduces uric acid production	Skin rashes (some severe), nausea, diarrhea, altered liver function	Monitor for reactions, reduce dose of 6-mercaptopurine; encourage increased fluids; monitor renal and liver functions

H. Child will maintain fluid balance

I. Child will be free of pain

J. Child/family express fears and begin to cope effectively

K. Child/family will seek appropriate emotional support

L. Child/family describe therapeutic measures necessary

IV. Implementation

   A. Place child in a private room; keep anyone with an infection out; meticulous hand-washing

   B. Measure vital signs every 4 hours; no rectal temperatures

   C. Monitor potential sites for signs and symptoms of infection

     1. Needle sites

     2. Mucosal areas

   D. Culture sites of suspected infection

   E. Administer antibiotics as ordered (see Table 10-2)

   F. Provide meticulous oral care; frequent oral hygiene with rinses, soft brush, or sponge applicator

G. Avoid IM injections; institute bleeding precautions; keep child away from sharp objects and edges; encourage quiet play

H. Monitor CBC/platelet count

I. Control local bleeding
1. Firm, gentle pressure
2. Tannic acid (dry tea bags) for oral mucosa
3. Ice/cool compresses; avoidance of hot or spicy foods

J. Do not give aspirin or aspirin products

K. Encourage rest periods during day

L. Provide high-calorie, high-protein diet (Table 10-12), small frequent feedings

M. Administer antiemetics (Table 10-13) before chemotherapy treatments or meals if needed

N. Maintain strict I & O; check weight daily

O. Measure urine specific gravity every void; encourage fluids

P. Monitor uric acid levels; give allopurinol as ordered (see Table 10-11)

Q. Administer cytotoxic agents as ordered (see Table 10-11)

R. Administer stool softeners as needed (Table 10-14)

S. Provide sitz baths as needed for rectal ulcers

T. Administer pharmacological pain relief as ordered and nonpharmacological pain relief as needed

U. Prepare child for each diagnostic examination (see Tables 10-9 and 10-10)

V. Help child plan ahead for impact of alopecia: choosing a favorite hat or scarf to wear, purchasing a wig

W. Provide teaching sessions about therapeutic measures and discharge planning, infection prevention including routine immunizations with killed viruses, varicella zoster, immune globulin

X. Encourage family to express fears and concerns; encourage child to attend peer support group

Y. Encourage family to attend support group meetings

V. Evaluation
A. Child is free of signs and symptoms of infection; parents can describe infection-control measures

B. Parents can describe safety modifications to child's environment

C. Child demonstrates gradual return to preillness activity level and interests

D. Child's skin and mucosal integrity remain intact

E. Child eats nutritious diet for growth without nausea and vomiting

F. Child's weight within normal limits for age

G. Child rests comfortably with increasing activity daily

H. Child has no complaints of pain

I. Child's fluid intake is adequate for output

J. Child discusses side effects such as alopecia without anger

K. Parents state diagnostic test regimen accurately

L. Parents state medication regimen accurately

M. Family exhibits less stress and anger daily and with each teaching session

N. Parents talk openly with child and health care team about diagnosis of leukemia

Anemia

I. Assessment
A. Definition: sign of underlying pathological process; reduced red blood cell volume, or hemoglobin concentration below normal level for age

B. Etiology/incidence
1. Increased loss or destruction of red blood cells
2. Impaired or decreased rate of production of red blood cells
3. Nutritional iron-deficiency anemia most common hematological disorder of infancy and childhood
   a. Infants 6 months to 3 years old
   b. Adolescents

C. Predisposing/precipitating factors
1. Blood loss
2. Excessive destruction of red blood cells
3. Impaired or decreased production of red blood cells
4. Nutritional deficit

D. Clinical manifestations
1. Pallor of skin and mucous membranes

TABLE 10–12 High-Calorie, High-Protein Diet

Low-Protein Foods	High-Protein Foods
Fruits	Milk and milk products
Fats	Vegetables
	Meats
	Bread

General Principles

Encourage high-calorie and high-protein foods that children especially like—for example, ice cream, milkshakes, yogurt, peanut butter, tuna, shrimp

RDA: Infants: kg × 2.0 to 2.2 g
Children: 23 to 34 g
Adolescents: 45 to 46 g

TABLE 10–13 Antiemetics

Example	Action	Use	Common Side Effects	Nursing Implications
Hydroxyzine (Vistaril), prochlorperazine (Compazine), promethazine (Phenergan)	Depress chemoreceptor trigger zone and vomiting center	Management of nausea and vomiting	Drowsiness, constipation, dry mouth, blurred vision	Administer 30 minutes before activity that induces nausea and vomiting (e.g., medications); keep client well-hydrated; do not crush capsules; advise client of side effects, restrict activities that require mental alertness; if nauseated at time, give medication by suppository or IM

2. Muscle weakness
3. Fatigue
4. Headache
5. Lightheadedness
6. Irritability
7. Increased pulse
8. Anorexia
9. Cyanosis only if hemoglobin less than 5 g/dL
  E. Diagnostic examinations: CBC (Table 10-15)
  F. Complications
    1. Learning deficits in children anemic in infancy (hemoglobin of 10.0 g/dL or less)
    2. Congestive heart failure
  G. Medical management
    1. Iron-rich diets (Table 10-16)
    2. Iron supplements (Table 10-17)
    3. Transfusion for severe anemia (Table 10-18)
II. Analysis
  A. Altered nutrition: less than body requirements related to dietary practices
  B. High risk for activity intolerance related to inadequate oxygenation of tissue
  C. High risk for knowledge deficit about causes of anemia, treatment, and prevention related to incomplete understanding of principles

  D. High risk for altered growth and development related to inadequate oxygenation of central nervous system tissue
III. Planning/goals, expected outcomes
  A. Child will rest comfortably
  B. Child will not exhibit signs and symptoms of tissue oxygen deprivation
  C. Child will not exhibit signs and symptoms of infection
  D. Child will not exhibit signs and symptoms of transfusion reactions
  E. Child will not develop complications from anemia
  F. Child/family will be prepared for all diagnostic tests and therapeutic procedures
  G. Family will understand prevention of iron deficiency
IV. Implementation
  A. Allow activities as tolerated
  B. Provide diversional activities that are quiet and restful
  C. Use play, music, and art therapy consults
  D. Obtain and check CBC every day if hospitalized
  E. Obtain ABGs as ordered
  F. Check vital signs every 4 hours

TABLE 10–14 Stool Softeners

Example	Action	Use	Common Side Effects	Nursing Implications
Dioctyl sulfosuccinate (Colace, Surfak)	Lower surface tension of stool, allowing it to be penetrated by intestinal fluids	Prevention of constipation, facilitate passage of stool	Mild cramps	Assess abdomen, bowel sounds, bowel function; assess characteristics of stool; encourage alternatives to stimulate bowel elimination (e.g., increase bulk/fluid, exercise)

TABLE 10–15 Complete Blood Count (Specific for Anemia)

Component	Description	Normal Level	Indications
Red blood cells (RBCs)	Number of RBCs per mm^3 of blood	Infant: 2.7 to 5.4/mm^3 Child: 3.9 to 5.3/mm^3 Adolescent: 4.1 to 5.3/mm^3	Indirect estimate of hemoglobin
Hemoglobin	Amount of hemoglobin per deciliter of whole blood	Infant: 9.0 to 14.0 g/dL Child: 11.5 to 15.5 g/dL Adolescent: 12.0 to 16.0 g/dL	Measures oxygen-carrying capacity of blood
Hematocrit	Per cent RBCs in whole blood	Infant: 28 to 42% Child: 35 to 45% Adolescent: 36 to 49%	Assesses per cent of RBCs
Reticulocytes (immature RBCs)	Per cent reticulocytes to RBCs	Infant (1 to 2 months): 0.3±2.2 Older: 0.5±1.5	Indicates mature RBC production in bone marrow; dependent on accurate RBC count
RBC indices	Indicates size and hemoglobin content of RBCs		
Mean corpuscular hemoglobin (MCH)	Average weight of hemoglobin in RBCs	Infant: 23 to 35 pg/cell Child: 24 to 33 pg/cell Adolescent: 25 to 35 pg/cell	Less accurate than MCHC
Mean corpuscular volume (MCV)	Average volume of a single RBC	Infant: 70 to 86 μm^3 Child: 77 to 95 μm^3 Adolescent: 78 to 102 μm^3	Indicates size as well as volume of RBCs
Mean corpuscular hemoglobin concentration (MCHC)	Average concentration of hemoglobin in RBCs	Infant: 29 to 37% Older: 31 to 37%	Ratio of weight of hemoglobin to volume of RBCs

G. Restrict visitors with infectious diseases, such as colds
H. Provide high-iron, high-protein, high–vitamin C diet (see Tables 10-12 and 10-16); administer iron supplements as ordered
I. Transfuse with blood as ordered (see Table 10-18)
J. Explain to child and parents all diagnostic tests to be performed in understandable terms
K. Allow child to "play" through diagnostic procedures
L. Encourage family to express fears and concerns

V. Evaluation
A. Child's activity level increases daily with no signs or symptoms of fatigue
B. Child's tissue oxygenation levels remain within normal limits for age through adequate intake of iron
C. Child is free of signs and symptoms of infection
D. Child has no transfusion reactions
E. Child exhibits no signs and symptoms of congestive heart failure
F. Family can describe appropriate diet and proper administration of iron supplements

TABLE 10–16 Iron-Rich Foods

Iron-Rich Foods

Breast milk
Iron-fortified infant formula
Enriched cereals and breads
Meats, especially red, organ meats
Dark-green, leafy vegetables: spinach, kale, collards
Dried fruits: raisins, prunes, apricots
Legumes/nuts
Other: molasses, egg yolk

General Principles

RDA	Infants: 7.5 to 8 mg/day Toddlers: 8 mg/day Preschoolers: 10 mg/day School age: 12 mg/day Adolescents: 15 mg/day

Sickle Cell Anemia

I. Assessment
A. Definition: autosomal recessive disease in which normal hemoglobin (HbA) is replaced by hemoglobin variant (HbS); causes sickling (crescent shape) of normally round erythrocytes when the hemoglobin releases oxygen;

TABLE 10–17 Iron Supplements

Example	Action	Use	Common Side Effects	Nursing Implications
Imferon	Iron replacement	Severe iron deficiency, when child not able to take oral iron	Staining and tissue damage at site of injection	Give with Z-track technique; change needle between drawing up medication and administration
Feosol (Fer-in-sol)	Iron supplementation or replacement	Iron-deficiency anemia	Nausea, diarrhea or constipation, black stools, staining of teeth	Give with juice high in vitamin C to enhance absorption; give between meals; give by dropper in back of the mouth or through a straw; brush teeth after administration

sickled cells occlude small vessels and capillaries throughout the body, causing obstruction and tissue hypoxia distal to the obstructions; because sickled cells are more fragile, increased hemolysis occurs; children with heterozygous "trait" usually exhibit no symptoms except under conditions of oxygen deprivation: excessive exercise or stress, illness, surgery, areas of low oxygen

B. Etiology/incidence
   1. Primarily affects black population and persons of Mediterranean descent
   2. One in 400 African Americans have sickle cell anemia
   3. One in 10 African Americans have sickle cell trait

C. Predisposing/precipitating factors
   1. Both parents must possess trait for disease to be passed to offspring
   2. Low oxygen concentration begins anemic process
   3. Symptoms usually appear around 6 months of age when maternal iron stores are depleted
   4. Infection, emotional stress, and physical

stress (e.g., exercise, exposure to cold) can cause oxygen concentrations to decrease

D. Clinical manifestations
   1. Chronic anemia
   2. Pallor and jaundice (mucous membranes, nail beds, sclera)
   3. Anorexia, fussiness, recurrent infections often first signs in infants
   4. Fatigue and weakness
   5. Slowed growth and development
   6. Decreased renal function with enuresis
   7. Splenomegaly, hepatomegaly
   8. Crises: precipitated by illness and other factors related to increased oxygen demands
      a. Vaso-occlusive crises (caused by occlusion of capillaries, tissue hypoxia and ischemia): acute abdominal, leg, chest, or flank pain; swelling of joints, especially in the feet and hands; fever; respiratory distress; cerebrovascular accident (stroke)
      b. Splenic sequestration crises (pooling of blood in the spleen): splenomegaly,

TABLE 10–18 Transfusion Reactions

Type of Reaction	Signs and Symptoms	Treatment
Hemolytic (ABO/Rh incompatibility)	Chills, fever, back or chest pain, red or dark urine, signs of respiratory distress	Stop transfusion; keep vein open with normal saline; check vital signs; administer oxygen as needed
Febrile	Mild chills, fever, back pain	Stop transfusion, administer antipyretics as ordered
Allergic	Pruritus, urticaria	Stop transfusion; give antihistamine and/or epinephrine as ordered; monitor for airway obstruction

liver failure; decreased circulating blood volume, shock; usually occurs in children less than 5 years

    c. Aplastic crises (bone marrow shutdown): profound anemia, usually self-limiting

E. Diagnostic examinations
1. CBC
2. Stained blood smear
3. Sickle cell slide prep test
4. Sickledex—most common screening test
5. Hemoglobin electrophoresis
6. Universal newborn screening programs
7. Prenatal screening for those at risk

F. Complications: risk of death greatest in children less than 5 years; pneumococcal infections; leg ulcers

G. Medical management
1. Supportive and symptomatic; aimed at prevention or control of crises
2. Includes: adequate hydration to promote hemodilution; electrolyte replacement; analgesic administration during crises (Table 10-19); energy conservation; antibiotics to treat or prevent infection; oxygen therapy for severe hypoxia; transfusions for severe anemia; ongoing transfusions to prevent stroke

II. Analysis
A. Altered tissue perfusion related to obstruction from sickling of cells
B. High risk for infection related to impairment of splenic function
C. Activity intolerance related to inadequate oxygenation
D. Pain related to tissue hypoxia
E. Altered growth and development related to chronic nature of disease
F. Inefficient family coping related to knowledge of inheritance pattern and chronic nature of the disease

G. Knowledge deficit about recognizing and treating impending crises, preventing and managing infections, complications

III. Planning/goals, expected outcomes
A. Family will participate in screening programs for early detection
B. Child will be diagnosed as soon as possible and monitored closely for indications of crises
C. Child/parents will understand disease and its implications with an emphasis on basic defect and therapeutic regimen to prevent sickling
D. Child will maintain adequate tissue oxygenation
E. Child will be adequately hydrated at all times
F. Child will be free of signs and symptoms of infection
G. Child will be free of pain during crises
H. Child will rest comfortably
I. Child will be free of complications during exchange transfusions, if ordered
J. Child will be free of complications during crises, such as shock, cerebrovascular accident
K. Child/parents will have opportunity to discuss concerns and fears about diagnosis, long-term care
L. Parents will have opportunity to discuss genetic counseling with appropriate personnel

IV. Implementation
A. Participate in community screening programs for sickle cell anemia
B. Encourage high-risk population to seek antepartal care
C. Teach child/parents about disease and its effects on body in general and during crises
D. Teach child/parents to be aware of signs indicating impending crises
1. Fever
2. Pallor
3. Pain, especially in legs

TABLE 10–19 Analgesics

Example	Action	Use	Common Side Effects	Nursing Implications
Nonnarcotic Acetaminophen (Tylenol), ibuprofen (Advil, Motrin)	Inhibits transmission of pain impulses	Mild-to-moderate pain	Side effects rare, occasionally gastric irritation with ibuprofen	Use child-resistant caps; overdosage of acetaminophen can cause liver toxicity
Narcotic Morphine sulfate, meperidine (Demerol), codeine (often given with acetaminophen)	Alters perception of pain	Moderate-to-severe pain	Mood changes, sedation, dizziness, nausea, vomiting, altered pulse rate, depressed respirations, urinary retention	Controlled substance; monitor for effects; institute safety precautions for ambulation; side rails up

E. Teach child/parents ways to ensure proper tissue oxygenation and perfusion
   1. Avoid areas where low levels of oxygen are present (high altitudes, airplanes, scuba diving)
   2. Avoid strenuous activity
   3. Avoid emotional stress; use stress-reduction techniques
   4. Prevent infections
      a. Avoid excessive contact with infected persons
      b. Obtain routine childhood immunizations and pneumococcal vaccine
      c. Take preventive antibiotics as ordered
      d. Seek help immediately for fever
F. Promote increased fluid intake
G. Maintain adequate nutritional intake
H. Medicate with analgesics for pain during crises as ordered (see Table 10-19)
   1. Position child to minimize pain
   2. Apply warm packs to painful areas
   3. If pain severe, use bed cradle for sheets
I. Promote bedrest during crises
J. Administer blood as ordered
K. Monitor for clinical manifestations of transfusion reactions
L. Monitor child for clinical manifestations of shock or cerebrovascular accident
M. Allow child/parents opportunity to discuss with health care team disease process and long-term effects and care
N. Encourage child to participate in normal activities within capabilities
O. Encourage child and parents to seek additional assistance from sickle cell anemia clinics and support groups
P. Emphasize importance to parents of genetic counseling before another pregnancy

V. Evaluation
A. Newborn counseling alerts parents to signs and symptoms of disease
B. Child and parents participate in teaching sessions about disease process, what sickle cell anemia crisis is, and therapeutic management
C. Child free of complications
D. Child takes in 1½ to 2 times normal fluid requirement
E. Child's nutritional status is within normal limits for age
F. Child is able to participate in age-appropriate play activities
G. Child is free of pain during crises
H. Child rests comfortably
I. Child tolerates exchange transfusion without complications
J. Child remains free of infection, and parents describe infection preventions and control

K. Child/parents participate in team conference and express feelings about disease process and long-term care
L. Child/parents begin to cope effectively with diagnosis and care involved and ask for assistance when necessary
M. Parents referred to genetic counselor and have made appointment for immediate future

POST-TEST Cardiovascular/Hematological Disorders

1. Anthony is in the hospital receiving a blood transfusion. While the transfusion is infusing, he suddenly develops urticaria. After stopping the transfusion, the most appropriate nursing measure would be to:
   ① Treat his fever
   ② Send his urine to the laboratory
   ③ Monitor for airway obstruction
   ④ Observe for signs of shock

2. Melinda is a toddler whose mother tells you that she drinks milk all the time and will hardly eat any of the solid foods she is given. Based on this, you know that it is likely that Melinda will develop:
   ① Anemia
   ② Rickets
   ③ Pellagra
   ④ Vitamin D deficiency

3. The physician has ordered an iron supplement for Melinda. In teaching the parents how to administer the iron, which of the following is vital for the nurse to include in her teaching?
   ① Iron can stain the teeth and should be given through a straw
   ② Iron should be given at mealtimes to aid absorption
   ③ Liquid supplements can be put in the bottle for easy administration
   ④ Mix the iron with cereal or other soft food three times a day

---

Jamey, age 4, is admitted to the hospital with a 3-week history of fever, chills, fatigue, and pallor. The bone marrow aspiration shows 75% blast cells and a white blood cell count of 50,000/mm³. Jamey is diagnosed with acute lymphocytic leukemia. Her chemotherapy is to include a remission-induction protocol of vincristine, prednisone, and L-asparaginase.

---

4. Which of the following laboratory data most likely explain Jamey's fatigue and pallor?
   1. Hemoglobin of 6 g/dL
   2. Platelet count of 50,000/mm³
   3. Cerebrospinal fluid with 100 white blood cells
   4. Potassium of 4.1 mEq/L

5. At this stage of Jamey's illness, her parents are visibly upset and ask innumerable questions of the nursing staff. An appropriate nursing diagnosis for them at this time would be:
   1. Knowledge deficit about the prognosis
   2. Anxiety
   3. Ineffective family coping
   4. Altered thought processes

6. After her second cycle of chemotherapy, Jamey's white blood cell count drops to 1200/mm³. Based on this, the nurse should do which of the following?
   1. Encourage no limitations on activity or visitors
   2. Have her stay in her room most of the time and avoid people with infections
   3. Encourage her to play quietly and institute bleeding precautions
   4. Maintain bedrest except for bathroom privileges and administer oxygen as needed

7. Jamey's platelet count is now 27,000/mm³. Which of the following nursing interventions is appropriate for her care?
   1. Maintain strict isolation to prevent infections
   2. Provide a diet high in iron-rich foods to counteract anemia
   3. Encourage frequent periods of rest to avoid fatigue
   4. Encourage quiet play activities to avoid injury

8. Jamey is about to be discharged. When planning for discharge, the nurse considers which of the following goals to be a priority for Jamey?
   1. Jamey will get enough exercise
   2. Jamey will gain weight
   3. Jamey will be free of pain
   4. Jamey will be free of infection

David is a 2-month-old infant who is brought to the pediatrician's office because his mother noticed that he had a cough and irregular breathing. She also thought that he was having trouble swallowing because he was not eating well. When weighed and measured, David was noted to be considerably smaller than his twin brother (below the fifth percentile for length and weight), although they had been approximately equal at birth. The nurse noted that David was pale, his pulse was 160, his respirations were 60 and irregular, and he had slight retractions with an expiratory grunt. The pediatrician palpated an enlarged liver, and a chest radiograph showed cardiac enlargement.

---

9. Which of the following would be the most appropriate nursing diagnosis requiring immediate intervention for David?
   1. Altered nutrition less than body requirements for growth related to fatigue
   2. High risk for infection related to ineffective airway clearance
   3. Decreased cardiac output related to ineffective pumping
   4. Altered growth and development related to poor nutritional intake

10. David is diagnosed as having congestive heart failure secondary to aortic stenosis. The nurse knows that congestive heart failure often is a complication of congenital heart disease because:
    1. Blood is shunted from one side of the heart to the other, decreasing oxygen supply to the heart
    2. The heart is more prone to infection when there is a defect
    3. Interference with the normal circulation in the heart increases the cardiac workload by increasing volume within the heart
    4. Shunting of blood through a defect causes decreased pressure within the chambers of the heart

11. After an aortic valve dilatation, David is placed on digoxin (Lanoxin) and furosemide (Lasix). The nurse teaches David's mother that which of the following are signs of possible digitalis toxicity in an infant:
    1. Anorexia, vomiting, no other signs of illness
    2. Irregular respiratory rate
    3. Apical pulse of less than 120
    4. Increased fluid output

12. Which of the following is the correct number of compressions per minute for external cardiac massage on an infant?
    1. 125
    2. 100
    3. 80
    4. 60

POST-TEST Answers and Rationales

1. ③ Laryngeal edema is a possible effect of an allergic reaction, so it is important for the nurse to check for respiratory distress whenever an allergic reaction is suspected. Choices 1, 2, and 4 are related to other types of transfusion reactions. 4, II. Anemia.

2. ① Milk is not as rich in iron as many other foods, and when toddlers drink excessive amounts of milk, they are unlikely to consume other iron-rich foods. 1, IV. Anemia.

3. ① Oral iron supplements will stain the teeth if in direct contact with them. Giving it through a straw avoids this. Iron absorption is decreased if there is food in the stomach because iron requires an acid environment to facilitate its absorption in the duodenum. 3, I. Anemia.

4. ① A low hemoglobin level indicates anemia; fatigue and pallor are two common signs. None of the other laboratory data would be responsible for these symptoms. 2, II. Leukemia.

5. ② The parents are exhibiting classic signs of anxiety, which is appropriate for this stage of their daughter's illness. Knowledge deficit is a potential problem, but asking repeated questions is more a sign of anxiety and the need for reassurance than it is a sign of inquiry at this point in time. The other diagnoses may be more identifiable as the illness progresses. 2, III. Leukemia.

6. ② Infection is the greatest risk in children with low white blood cell counts. Avoiding individuals with infections is one way of protecting the child. 4, I. Leukemia.

7. ④ With a low platelet count, bleeding is the highest risk. Encouraging quiet play and avoiding injury will help prevent bleeding episodes. Iron, isolation, and avoiding fatigue make no difference with this problem. 4, I. Leukemia.

8. ④ Preventing infection is a priority goal for the child with leukemia. Although the other goals are reasonable, infection can be a most serious complication. 3, II. Leukemia.

9. ③ David is having symptoms of congestive heart failure, which is caused by increased workload of the heart. Although all the diagnoses are appropriate for the child with congestive heart failure, the priority is to intervene to increase cardiac output and prevent death from complete heart failure. 2, II. Congestive Heart Failure.

10. ③ Congenital defects interfere with the usual circulation of blood within the heart and the pulmonary system. Some defects allow for gradually increasing volumes of blood to traverse the heart because shunted blood volume is added to volume returning from the systemic circulation; other defects restrict the outflow of blood from the heart, and therefore more pressure is needed to circulate the blood. Both these mechanisms increase cardiac workload and can contribute to congestive heart failure. 1, II. Congestive Heart Failure.

11. ① Signs of digitalis toxicity include anorexia, nausea, vomiting, bradycardia, and dysrhythmias. Often, anorexia is the first sign in an infant and would be a cause for concern. 3, I. Congestive Heart Failure.

12. ② The compression rate for infants during cardiac resuscitation is 100 to 120 compressions per minute. 4, II. Congestive Heart Failure.

PRE-TEST Pulmonary Disorders

1. Three-year-old Michael wakes in the middle of the night with a tight, brassy-sounding cough. He has a low-grade fever and says it is hard to breathe. What would you advise Michael's parents to do first for Michael?
   ① Give him a dose of cough medicine
   ② Place him in a cool, humid environment
   ③ Give him a glass of milk
   ④ Bring him to the emergency department

2. When assessing a child who is brought to the emergency department complaining of difficulty breathing, which of the following data indicates that the child might have epiglottitis?
   ① Gradual onset of symptoms, low-grade fever, pallor, dry cough
   ② Fever for several days, loose cough, chest pain, fatigue
   ③ Wheezing associated with cough, mild retractions, afebrile, sudden onset of symptoms
   ④ Sore throat, moderately high fever, drooling, sudden onset of symptoms

3. Which of the following is the most common causative agent for bronchiolitis and croup during infancy?
   ① Rhinovirus
   ② Respiratory syncytial virus
   ③ Adenovirus
   ④ Nonspecific virus

4. Ellen, a 2-month-old infant, has been admitted to the hospital for bronchiolitis. She is pale, demonstrates moderate respiratory effort, and has an increased pulse, respirations of 65, decreased PaO_2, and decreased oxygenation saturation. Which of the following nursing diagnoses is most appropriate for Ellen?
   ① Impaired gas exchange
   ② Ineffective breathing patterns
   ③ Ineffective airway clearance
   ④ Anxiety

5. When planning to feed an infant in mild respiratory distress, the nurse knows to feed oral fluids slowly because:
   ① Sick infants tire more easily trying to suck
   ② Tachypneic infants are at risk for aspiration of fluids
   ③ With dehydration, the fluid loss is too great to replace orally
   ④ Hypoxic infants are more likely to develop cyanosis with the exertion of sucking

6. Which of the following is the most likely factor causing the usual clinical manifestations of cystic fibrosis?
   ① Abnormal function of the exocrine glands
   ② Hyperactivity of the parasympathetic nervous system
   ③ Decreased activity of the sweat glands
   ④ Mechanical obstruction of the endocrine glands

7. Which of the following best describes why a child with cystic fibrosis is at risk for respiratory infection?
   ① High levels of sodium in the saliva can irritate the mucous membranes in the nasopharynx
   ② The related cardiac defects and congestive heart failure can cause increased respiratory distress
   ③ Associated neuromuscular irritability can lead to excessive bronchial constriction
   ④ Thick secretions are difficult to clear from the bronchi

8. Zak, a 4-month-old, had been asleep about 3 hours when his parents found him not breathing and unresponsive. His cause of death was determined to be sudden infant death syndrome (SIDS). After receiving counseling and support from a SIDS support group, which of the following explanations by the parents would indicate to you that they understand the cause of SIDS?
   ① Suffocation from bed clothing is the cause of death
   ② SIDS is caused by a genetic defect
   ③ Death is caused by a change in the sleep/wake cycle
   ④ The cause has not been clearly or completely identified

9. Because of the sudden nature of an infant's death from SIDS, an important initial nursing intervention to facilitate the grieving process for parents is to:
   ① Encourage them to agree to an autopsy immediately
   ② Allow them to hold and say good-bye to their infant privately
   ③ Refer them to a SIDS support group
   ④ Take a nursing history about the circumstances of death

10. Which of the following is most likely to trigger an attack in the child with intrinsic asthma?
   ① Cat hair
   ② Spring flowers
   ③ Cold air
   ④ Freshly mowed grass

11. What is an appropriate goal for a child taken to the emergency department having an acute asthma attack? The child will:
   ① Take in copious amounts of clear fluids
   ② Comply with appropriate medication therapy
   ③ Be able to breathe more easily
   ④ Demonstrate stress-reduction exercises

PRE-TEST Answers and Rationales

1. ② Placing a child with croup in a cool, humid environment helps to reduce airway inflammation and prevent obstruction. Using cool mist is helpful, although taking the child into a steamy bathroom or out in the night air also can be helpful if cool mist is not available. Giving fluid is important, but milk would not be the fluid of choice. Taking the child to the emergency department is appropriate only if respiratory distress increases. 4, II. Laryngotracheobronchitis.

2. ④ Epiglottitis is a condition that is a medical emergency and must be differentiated from other respiratory diseases, particularly croup, which is usually more benign. Epiglottitis differs from croup in that its onset is sudden (appears over several hours), fever is moderate, the throat is sore and voice is muffled, and the child usually drools. Choice 1 indicates signs of croup. Other choices describe symptoms of other respiratory dysfunctions. 1, II. Laryngotracheobronchitis.

3. ② Respiratory syncytial virus is responsible for croup and for more than 50% of bronchiolitis during infancy. 1, I. Bronchiolitis.

4. ① Bronchiolitis and hyperinflation lead to air trapping in the alveoli. This combined with edema and excessive mucus production leads to impaired gas exchange. The impaired gas exchange can lead to the other diagnoses. 3, II. Bronchiolitis.

5. ② The rapid respiratory rate of infants with bronchiolitis makes aspiration a risk. The nurse must be very careful to prevent aspiration when feeding the infant. The other options are not wrong, but they are not as important. 3, II. Bronchiolitis.

6. ① The major problem in cystic fibrosis is the abnormal function of the exocrine glands, which leads to the production of thick mucus. This leads to the respiratory symptoms noted in cystic fibrosis. 1, II. Cystic Fibrosis.

7. ④ The thickened secretions from the exocrine glands cause blocking of the bronchioles, which predisposes the child to pneumonia. The other options are incorrect. 3, II. Cystic Fibrosis.

8. ④ SIDS is defined as the sudden, unexpected death of an apparently healthy infant. The cause of SIDS has not been identified, although numerous theories exist. 5, I. SIDS.

9. ② Although all the options are interventions for parents of an infant who died of SIDS, allowing them to hold their infant and say good-bye in private is the most important initial intervention. In the confusion of the child's death, parents would not have had that opportunity to begin the grieving process. Questions and decisions can come later. 4, III. SIDS.

10. ③ Intrinsic asthma results from hyperreactive airways, not direct allergic response, so cold air is the more likely trigger. The other options would trigger an allergic response. 1, I. Asthma.

11. ③ The child experiencing an acute attack of asthma usually presents with difficulty breathing, wheezing, and tight cough. Although there is potential for the child to become dehydrated, opening the airway so the child can breathe more easily is a priority. The other choices are goals for the ongoing care of a child with asthma. 3, II. Asthma.

NURSING PROCESS APPLIED TO CHILDREN WITH PULMONARY DISORDERS

Acute Disorders

Laryngotracheobronchitis (Viral Croup)
  I. Assessment
     A. Definition: inflammatory condition of respiratory tract involving larynx, trachea, and bronchi; most common form of croup
     B. Etiology/incidence
        1. Viral infection, parainfluenza, respiratory syncytial virus, or rhinovirus
        2. Peak incidence, second year of life
        3. Affects children 6 months to 4 years
     C. Predisposing/precipitating factors
        1. Mild upper respiratory infection
        2. Edematous subglottic area
     D. Clinical manifestations: appear over several days, worse in evening
        1. Harsh, brassy cough

2. Slight fever
3. Pallor
4. Signs of increasing respiratory distress: stridor, dyspnea, increased pulse, retractions
   E. Diagnostic examinations
      1. Based on clinical manifestations
      2. Differentiate from signs of epiglottitis
         a. Rapid onset of respiratory distress from inflammation and edema of the epiglottis, causes upper airway obstruction
         b. Peak age 3 to 7 years
         c. Usually caused by *Haemophilus influenzae*
         d. Sore throat with muffled voice, drooling, fever of more than 38.5°C (101.3°F), inspiratory stridor, mild-to-moderate retractions, increased respirations and pulse, paleness or cyanosis, anxiety, insistence on upright position
   F. Complication: respiratory distress
   G. Medical management
      1. Home management
         a. Place child in cool, humid environment (cool mist humidifier, exposure to night air, steam from bathroom shower if cool mist not available)
         b. Monitor for signs of respiratory distress: anxiety, pallor, increasing difficulty breathing
      2. Hospital management
         a. Administer racemic epinephrine (Table 10-20) for severe croup; admit for observation; monitor for rebound
         b. Place in cool, humidified air; provide low concentrations of oxygen for hypoxia
         c. Oral liquids (IV if not able to take orally)
         d. One dose of IM dexamethasone (Decadron) (see Table 10-8) is controversial but may be given in an attempt to shorten course
         e. Intubation for airway obstruction and hypoxia

II. Analysis
   A. Ineffective airway clearance related to edema and inflammation
   B. High risk for impaired gas exchange related to increasing obstructive process
   C. High risk for fluid volume deficit related to fluid loss from increased respirations
   D. Activity intolerance related to increased respiratory effort
   E. Anxiety (child and family) related to respiratory distress and placement in a tent

III. Planning/goals, expected outcomes
   A. Child's airway will remain patent at all times

   B. Child will not exhibit signs and symptoms of respiratory distress
   C. Child will maintain adequate oxygenation
   D. Child will rest comfortably at all times
   E. Child will take in adequate amounts of fluid
   F. Child/parents will have opportunity to ask questions
   G. Child/parents will have opportunity to express concerns about diagnosis and therapeutic regimen

IV. Implementation
   A. Monitor respiratory status every 1 to 2 hours
      1. Rate and quality of respirations
      2. ABGs, if ordered
      3. Skin color/perfusion of extremities
      4. Oxygenation by pulse oximetry
   B. Monitor for signs and symptoms of respiratory distress
      1. Tachypnea
      2. Tachycardia
      3. Restlessness
      4. Dyspnea
      5. Retractions
      6. Cyanosis
   C. Keep emergency tracheostomy/intubation kit nearby; provide appropriate care for intubated child
   D. Administer cool, humidified air and oxygen if ordered through croup tent
      1. Keep sides of tent tucked in to prevent loss of oxygen if oxygen is ordered; keep side rails up
      2. Keep child in tent at all times
      3. Keep child warm and dry
      4. Change linen as needed
   E. Maintain bedrest; elevate head of bed
   F. Provide age-appropriate diversional activities while in tent but avoid toys that might spark and those made of wool; frequent physical contact with child while child is in tent
   G. Administer fluids by mouth or IV line
   H. Teach parents how to assess respiratory status and respiratory distress, home management of croup
   I. Allow parents opportunity to ask questions
   J. Allow parents opportunity to express concerns

V. Evaluation
   A. Child's airway remains patent at all times
   B. Child's respiratory status returns to normal
   C. Child remains in croup tent without complications
   D. Child does not regress developmentally during therapeutic regimen
   E. Child rests comfortably at all times
   F. Child's urinary output adequate at 1 mL/kg/hr; good skin turgor

TABLE 10–20 Medications Used to Treat Respiratory Problems in Children

Example	Action	Use	Common Side Effects	Nursing Implications
Beta$_2$-adrenergic agonists: albuterol, Ventolin, Proventil	Bronchial smooth muscle relaxant	Relief of acute bronchospasm	Tremors, nervousness, dizziness, tachycardia, elevated blood pressure, nausea, headache, rebound bronchospasm	Excitement and nervousness is more common in children ages 2 to 6 years; effects last up to 6 hours, and medication should not be used more frequently than recommended by physician; use of inhaled medication is effective for preventing bronchospasm (especially exercise-induced bronchospasm); teach child use of inhaler; spacer device should be used for young children
Theophylline	Relaxes smooth muscle of bronchial airways, resulting in bronchodilation	Respiratory conditions involving reversible bronchospasm	Gastrointestinal irritation including nausea, vomiting, epigastric pain, headaches, irritability, tachycardia, dysrhythmias	Take on an empty stomach for maximum absorption but take with full glass of water; monitor vital signs; cardiac monitor required during IV administration; theophylline level should be checked regularly and should be less than 20 μg/mL to prevent toxicity; sustained-release preparations used for prevention of acute episodes of bronchospasm
Racemic epinephrine	Bronchodilator, vasoconstrictor	Severe croup	Causes increase in cardiac rate and force of contraction, dizziness, palpitations	Monitor vital signs carefully; be alert for rebound effect; child should be admitted to hospital for observation after receiving racemic epinephrine
Cromolyn sodium (Intal)	Action not clearly understood; inhibits mediators of allergic/inflammatory response	Used prophylactically to prevent asthma and exercise-induced bronchospasm	Throat dryness or irritation, cough, wheeze, nausea, potential for anaphylaxis	Given by nebulizer or inhaler; must be administered regularly as directed and usually in connection with other pharmacological agents (e.g., bronchodilators)

G. Parents participate in teaching session about assessment of respiratory status and respiratory distress

H. Parents cope effectively with therapeutic regimen

Bronchiolitis

I. Assessment

A. Definition: inflammation of bronchioles with excessive mucus production and airway obstruction

B. Etiology/incidence

1. Respiratory syncytial virus predominantly
2. Incidence greater in winter months
3. Highest incidence at 2 to 6 months

C. Predisposing/precipitating factors

1. Mild upper respiratory infection
2. Edema and mucus production in small and medium airways

D. Clinical manifestations

1. Cough, low-grade fever, wheezing
2. Increasing respiratory distress
   a. Rapid, shallow, labored respirations
   b. Nasal flaring

c. Intercostal/subcostal retractions
d. Barrel-shaped chest
e. Fine rales or wheezes (rhonchi) on auscultation
f. Restlessness

E. Diagnostic examinations
1. Based on clinical manifestations
2. Chest x-ray shows hyperinflation and air trapping
3. Nasopharyngeal smear and culture for respiratory syncytial virus

F. Complication: atalectasis, respiratory failure

G. Medical management
1. Oxygen administration for respiratory distress and hypoxia
2. Aerosolized albuterol by nebulizer every 4 hours
3. Increased fluid intake, oral or IV
4. Pulmonary therapy

II. Analysis
A. Ineffective airway clearance related to inflammation and increased secretions
B. Ineffective breathing patterns related to decreased airway clearance
C. High risk for impaired gas exchange related to air trapping and increased secretions
D. High risk for fluid volume deficit related to increased respirations and increased metabolic demands
E. Activity intolerance related to increased respiratory effort
F. High risk for ineffective individual coping related to isolation
G. Anxiety related to increased respiratory distress

III. Planning/goals, expected outcomes
A. Child's airway will remain patent at all times
B. Child's respiratory effort will decrease, and respiratory status will return to normal
C. Child will rest comfortably and increase activity gradually as tolerated
D. Child will take in fluids adequate to prevent dehydration
E. Child will not regress developmentally as a result of isolation
F. Parents will have opportunity to ask questions about therapeutic regimen
G. Parents will have opportunity to express concerns about therapeutic regimen

IV. Implementation
A. Place child in respiratory isolation if respiratory syncytial virus suspected, most common cause of nosocomial infection in hospitalized children
B. Monitor respiratory status every 1 to 2 hours including regular ABGs and oxygen saturation measurement

C. Monitor for signs and symptoms of respiratory distress
D. Teach parents how to assess respiratory status and respiratory distress
E. Administer oxygen therapy through cool, humidified oxygen tent
F. Administer aerosol therapy as ordered
G. Avoid sedation—depresses respiratory effort
H. Suction prn; administer chest physical therapy
I. Maintain bedrest schedule treatments to maximize rest
J. Provide age-appropriate diversional activities while in oxygen tent
K. Administer fluids by mouth or IV; monitor urine output for signs of dehydration
L. Allow parents opportunity to ask questions and to express concerns about therapeutic regimen

V. Evaluation
A. Child's airway is patent at all times
B. Child's respiratory status returns to normal—vital signs are within normal limits
C. Child's ABGs and oxygen saturation return to normal
D. Child does not regress developmentally during course of treatment
E. Child rests comfortably without complaints
F. Child is well hydrated—demonstrates adequate urine output, good skin turgor
G. Parents participate in teaching session about assessment of respiratory status and respiratory distress
H. Parents ask questions
I. Parents cope effectively with therapeutic regimen

Pneumonia
I. Assessment
A. Definition: acute imflammation of lung tissue including alveoli
B. Etiology/incidence
1. Viral (Respiratory Syncytial Virus or influenza), bacterial, (*Streptococcus pneumoniae, Staphylococcus aureus),* or *Mycoplasma*
2. Secondary to infection in other parts of respiratory tract
3. Aspiration of infectious agents from upper respiratory tract
4. Secondary infection in already compromised lung
5. Aspiration of foreign body
6. Most common in children less than 5 years, type varies with age
7. Incidence decreases with age
C. Predisposing/precipitating factors
1. History of minor respiratory infection

2. Infection that disseminates throughout lung parenchyma
D. Clinical manifestations
1. High fever (103° to 104°F, 39.4° to 40°C)
2. Chills
3. Restlessness
4. Dry, hacking cough progressing to productive cough
5. Chest pain
6. Fine rales, wheezing on auscultation
7. Decreased breath sounds over areas of consolidation
8. Elevated white blood cell count
E. Diagnostic examinations
1. Chest x-ray demonstrates consolidation in affected area
2. CBC
F. Complications
1. Pneumothorax
2. Empyema
G. Medical management
1. Antibiotics (see Table 10-2) for bacterial pneumonia or those with viral pneumonia at risk for secondary infection
2. Acetaminophen for its antipyretic action
II. Analysis
A. Ineffective airway clearance related to increased secretions
B. High risk for impaired gas exchange related to inflammatory process in lungs
C. Hyperthermia related to the infectious process
D. High risk for fluid volume deficit related to inadequate intake, increased loss through respiratory effort
E. High risk for pain related to lung inflammation
III. Planning/goals, expected outcomes
A. Child will achieve adequate ventilation and adequate oxygenation
B. Child will not develop complications of pneumonia: pneumothorax or empyema
C. Child's fever will progressively decrease
D. Child will not exhibit signs and symptoms of dehydration
E. Child will rest comfortably
F. Child/parents will have opportunity to ask questions
G. Child/parents will have opportunity to express concerns about therapeutic regimen
IV. Implementation
A. Monitor vital signs and respiratory status every 2 to 4 hours
B. Elevate head of bed
C. Have child lie on affected side to decrease pleural pain
D. Turn, cough, deep breathe every 2 to 4 hours
E. Provide postural drainage and chest physiotherapy

F. Apply cool, humidified oxygen as ordered every 4 hours and as needed and child's energy level permits
G. Monitor for clinical manifestations of respiratory distress
H. Monitor for clinical manifestations of pneumothorax
1. Chest pain
2. Dyspnea
3. Cyanosis
4. Absent breath sounds over affected lung
I. Medicate with acetaminophen for temperature of more than 101°F (38.3°C) as ordered and for pain
J. Medicate with antibiotics as ordered (see Table 10-2)
K. Monitor for signs and symptoms of dehydration
1. Dry mucous membranes
2. Poor skin turgor
3. Decreased to absent tears
4. Decreased urine output
L. Administer fluids by mouth; small frequent amounts, or IV
M. Maintain bedrest and quiet activities as tolerated
N. Provide age-appropriate diversional activities while in tent
O. Teach parents clinical manifestations of respiratory distress, pneumothorax, and dehydration
P. Teach parents importance of medicating child as ordered
Q. Allow child/parents to ask questions about therapeutic regimen
R. Allow parents opportunity to discuss concerns
V. Evaluation
A. Child is able to clear airway effectively
B. Child demonstrates adequate oxygenation; ABGs return to normal
C. Child's respiratory status returns to normal
D. Child is free from complications of pneumonia
E. Child's fever decreases progressively each day of therapy
F. Child demonstrates adequate fluid intake and output appropriate for age and weight
G. Child rests comfortably and expresses relief from pain
H. Child cooperates with oxygen therapy and pulmonary treatments and does not become overly fatigued
I. Parents participate in teaching sessions about assessment of respiratory status; can describe signs of respiratory distress and complications of pneumonia
J. Parents describe correct administration of medications

K. Parents cope effectively with therapeutic regimen
L. Child returns to former level of activity

Sudden Infant Death Syndrome
I. Assessment
  A. Definition: sudden, unexpected death of apparently healthy infant that remains unexplained after complete autopsy
  B. Etiology/incidence
    1. Exact etiology unknown; recent research indicates a relationship between prone sleeping position and incidence of sudden infant death syndrome (SIDS)
    2. Might be related to alteration in cardio-respiratory control
    3. Might be secondary to brain stem not responding to build-up of CO_2
    4. Might be related to apneic spells
    5. Leading cause of death in infants 1 month to 1 year
    6. Two to three per 1000 live births
    7. Peak incidence 2 to 4 months; boys more often; higher incidence in low-birth-weight infants
    8. Siblings of SIDS infant have a fivefold greater risk over normal population
  C. Predisposing/precipitating factors: apneic incident
  D. Clinical manifestations: no warning signs of impending death, death usually occurs during sleep
  E. Diagnostic examination: postmortem autopsy
  F. Complication: death
II. Analysis
  A. High risk for dysfunctional grieving related to the sudden death of a child
  B. High risk for ineffective family coping related to child's death
  C. High risk for altered role performance related to the loss of parenting role
III. Planning/goals, expected outcomes
  A. Parents will receive comfort and support from health care team
  B. Parents will have opportunity to say good-bye to child in private
  C. Parents will express feelings/concerns in own time
  D. Parents will understand autopsy procedure and why it is necessary as soon as possible
  E. Parents will begin to deal appropriately with grief
  F. Parents will seek appropriate education about SIDS at appropriate time
  G. Parents will seek counseling from center specializing in SIDS
IV. Implementation

  A. When child admitted to emergency department, place child in private room; assign primary nurse to shelter them from unnecessary interruptions
  B. Clean child/neaten appearance prior to parents having final viewing
  C. Participate with physician in explaining to parents that child is dead
  D. Assure parents that death was quick and painless for child
  E. Allow parents opportunity to express feelings in private area
  F. Ascertain any needed information from parents using simple, clear, nonthreatening questions
  G. Explain autopsy procedure and importance in simple language
  H. Answer all questions honestly
  I. Refer family to SIDS foundation for follow-up care
  J. In follow-up visit, provide educational materials about SIDS
  K. In follow-up visit, let parents take lead
  L. Provide outlets for family to express grief
V. Evaluation
  A. Parents able to say good-bye to child in private
  B. Parents meet with health care team and child's death explained simply and without blame
  C. Parents sign consent for autopsy after explanation from physician/nurse
  D. Parents express grief and concerns as to what happened
  E. Parents/family talk to social worker and SIDS foundation
  F. Family seeks follow-up care psychologically and educationally
  G. After several weeks with counseling, family begins to cope effectively with infant's death

Chronic Disorders

Asthma
I. Assessment
  A. Definition: chronic pulmonary response to certain biochemical, immunological, and psychological variables resulting in obstructive condition of bronchi/bronchioles; reversible condition
  B. Etiology/incidence
    1. Bronchospasm in response to extrinsic and intrinsic trigger factors
    2. Leading chronic childhood illness
    3. Affects 5% of all children
    4. More than 50% demonstrate symptoms in first 2 years of life
    5. Most cases diagnosed by early school-age years

6. More common in males before 12 years; after that age, equal in males and females
C. Predisposing/precipitating factors
   1. Extrinsic factors: airborne allergens
   2. Intrinsic factors: nonallergens such as cold air
      a. Certain foods (e.g., chocolate, wheat, cow's milk)
      b. Respiratory infections
      c. Rapid temperature changes in atmosphere
      d. Vigorous exercise, fatigue
      e. Emotional stress
D. Clinical manifestations
   1. Acute attack
      a. Gradual or abrupt onset
      b. Tightness of chest, itchiness of throat
      c. Accessory muscles used
      d. Audible wheezing, usually expiratory
      e. Paroxysmal coughing
      f. Rapid, labored respirations with retractions
      g. Rales and expiratory wheeze on auscultation
      h. Diaphoretic
      i. Anxious
      j. Upright position with shoulders hunched forward
   2. Chronic
      a. Barrel-chested
      b. Prominent sternum
      c. Hunched shoulders
E. Diagnostic examinations
   1. Chest x-ray
   2. Sputum smear for eosinophils
   3. CBC and differential may show eosinophilia, immunological assays for increased immunoglobulin E
   4. Blood gases: initially, $PaCO_2$ will decrease secondary to child's hyperventilating
   5. Pulmonary function studies: diminished maximal breathing capacity, tidal volume, and timed vital capacity
   6. Skin testing for allergens
F. Complication: respiratory failure and death
G. Medical management
   1. Mild asthma: inhaled (or nebulized) or oral albuterol (see Table 10-20) every 4 to 6 hours prn for duration of episodes
   2. Moderate asthma: inhaled (or nebulized) albuterol prn for symptom relief up to four times a day and cromolyn sodium (see Table 10-20) by nebulizer or inhaler for prevention up to four times a day *or* albuterol and sustained-released theophylline (goal is serum theophylline of 5 to 15 μg/mL; may use inhaled corticosteroid

instead of cromolyn or theophylline if symptoms persist
   3. Severe asthma: inhaled corticosteroid up to four times a day and inhaled (or nebulized) albuterol prn for symptoms up to every 4 hours, with or without oral sustained-release theophylline; oral corticosteroids should be considered for children whose symptoms are severe
   4. Emergency department management: nebulized albuterol every 20 minutes for up to 1 hour, monitor for improvement, oxygen if needed, begin oral steroids, admit if symptoms persist
   5. Influenza vaccine for child with severe asthma
II. Analysis
A. Ineffective airway clearance related to bronchospasm and increased secretions
B. Impaired gas exchange related to air trapping
C. Activity intolerance related to increased respiratory effort
D. High risk for fluid volume deficit related to increased insensible fluid loss
E. High risk for altered growth and development related to chronic nature of the disease
F. High risk for ineffective family coping related to the seriousness of attacks
G. Knowledge deficit about home care, allergy-proofing, medication administration, and treatments related to incomplete understanding
III. Planning/goals, expected outcomes
A. Emergency care
   1. Family will initiate appropriate interventions to prevent severe attack
   2. Family will recognize signs of worsening respiratory status
   3. Child will be able to breathe with minimal effort
   4. Child will be adequately oxygenated
   5. Child will not exhibit signs and symptoms of dehydration
   6. Child will rest comfortably
B. General, continuous care
   1. Child will resume normal breathing patterns after attack
   2. Child's airway will remain patent at all times
   3. Child will comply with appropriate medication therapy
   4. Child will demonstrate slow breathing and relaxation during impending attack
   5. Child/family will identify precipitating factors and avoid them
   6. Child/parents will describe proper administration of medications at home

7. Child/parents will describe proper administration of moist air through humidifier at home
8. Child/parents will participate in support groups for asthmatics

IV. Implementation
   A. Monitor vital signs and for signs of airway obstruction
   B. Assist with mechanical ventilation if required
   C. Administer emergency drugs as ordered
   D. Provide restful, quiet environment
   E. Administer IV fluids as ordered or encourage oral fluid intake
   F. Provide cool, humidified environment
   G. Administer oxygen therapy as ordered
   H. Monitor ABGs and oxygen saturation as ordered
   I. Assist child/parents in identifying precipitating factors and allergy-proofing the home if required
   J. With health care team, discuss ways that child/parent can avoid exposure to allergens
   K. Teach child/parents proper administration of medications
   L. Teach child/parents proper use of humidifier
   M. Refer child/parents to support group
   N. Emphasize importance of anticipatory care

V. Evaluation
   A. Child demonstrates improved respiratory status—decreased pulse and respirations, normal ABGs
   B. Child's airway is patent at all times and does not require mechanical ventilation
   C. Child tolerates emergency drug therapy without complication
   D. Child's anxiety level decreases, and child is able to obtain sufficient rest
   E. Child takes fluids sufficient to prevent dehydration
   F. Child/parents participate in teaching session identifying possible precipitating factors to attacks
   G. Child/parents can describe health regimen that includes proper nutrition, exercise, rest, and avoidance of emotional stress and other precipitating factors
   H. Parents relate to child in a way that facilitates normal growth and development
   I. Child/parents contact support group for assistance in long-range planning
   J. Child/parents identify necessity for continued follow-up care

Cystic Fibrosis

I. Assessment
   A. Definition: hereditary generalized dysfunction of exocrine glands that results in increased viscosity of mucus and leads to obstruction in digestive and pulmonary systems
   B. Etiology/incidence
      1. Autosomal recessive trait
      2. Cystic fibrosis gene located on chromosome 7, approximately 5% of Caucasian population are carriers
      3. Some evidence suggests that cause is an altered enzyme/protein
      4. One per 1800 to 2000 Caucasian births
      5. Can be diagnosed prenatally by amniocentesis
   C. Predisposing/precipitating factors: mechanical obstruction of multiple organ systems secondary to increased viscosity of mucous gland secretions
   D. Clinical manifestations
      1. Meconium ileus in newborns
      2. Passage of bulky, foul-smelling, fatty stools once feeding begins
      3. Failure to thrive despite healthy appetite
      4. Recurrent respiratory infections
         a. Dry, hacking cough
         b. Wheezing, audible
         c. Dyspnea
         d. Barrel-chested
         e. Clubbing of fingers
         f. Rales, wheezes (rhonchi) on auscultation
      5. "Salty" skin
      6. Elevated sweat chloride test—more than 50 to 60 mEq/L
      7. Absence of pancreatic enzymes
      8. Altered pulmonary function studies
   E. Diagnostic examinations
      1. Accurate history, family history of cystic fibrosis
      2. Sweat chloride test
      3. Chest x-ray—confirms obstructive lung disease
      4. Pancreatic enzymes decreased or absent
      5. Fat absorption studies on stool
      6. Pulmonary function studies demonstrate decreased pulmonary function
      7. ABGs decreased oxygenation
   F. Complications
      1. Chronic obstructive lung disease
      2. Recurrent pulmonary infection, especially *Pseudomonas* and *S. aureus*
      3. Eventually fatal, although with excellent management may live into adulthood
   G. Medical management
      1. Pancreatic enzyme replacement therapy with food
      2. High-protein, high-caloric diet to promote growth, may add medium-chain tri-

glycerides (MCT) to provide additional calories
3. Water-soluble vitamin and iron supplements
4. Aerosol bronchodilators
5. Regular chest physical therapy
6. Antibiotics for infections and often prophylactically
7. Increased salt intake during warm weather and exercise
8. Regular breathing exercises and home pulmonary function monitoring
9. Influenza vaccine

II. Analysis
   A. Ineffective airway clearance related to thickness of secretions
   B. Impaired gas exchange related to narrowed airways
   C. Altered nutrition: less than body requirements related to impaired absorption
   D. High risk for pulmonary infection related to inadequate mobilization of secretions
   E. Anxiety related to perceived health status and its impact
   F. Activity intolerance related to inadequate oxygenation
   G. High risk for body image disturbance related to chronic nature of the disease
   H. Knowledge deficit about the disease, its prognosis, home management
   I. High risk for anticipatory grieving related to potentially fatal disease

III. Planning/goals, expected outcomes
   A. Early diagnosis and intervention will decrease complications
   B. Child will participate in diagnostic procedures without complications
   C. Child/parents will understand diagnosis and treatment regimen
   D. Child will maintain adequate nutrition for growth
   E. Child will maintain pulmonary function
   F. Child will not exhibit signs and symptoms of respiratory infection
   G. Child will gauge activity level on daily basis
   H. Child will not regress developmentally or educationally due to disease process
   I. Child/parents will contact proper home health agency for follow-up care
   J. Child/parents will understand each component of treatment regimen and how to perform it at home
   K. Child/parents will express feelings and concerns about diagnosis and treatment regimen
   L. Child/parents will be referred to support group for cystic fibrosis clients

M. Parents will seek genetic counseling if appropriate

IV. Implementation
   A. Obtain accurate family history
   B. Obtain accurate health history and physical of child with suspected signs and symptoms
   C. Prepare child fully for each diagnostic test
   D. Assist with diagnostic tests
   E. Provide high-calorie, high-protein diet (see Table 10-12)
   F. Administer MCT oil with meals if ordered
   G. Administer extra salt or salt supplements with meals
   H. Administer water-soluble vitamins, iron supplements
   I. Administer pancreatic enzyme supplements with meals and snacks
   J. Administer antacids as needed
   K. Turn, cough, deep breathe every 1 to 2 hours and as needed
   L. Provide postural drainage and chest physiotherapy every 4 hours and as needed
   M. Provide aerosol treatments every 4 hours before chest physiotherapy
   N. Teach child/parents how to perform chest physiotherapy and needed treatments
   O. Administer bronchodilators as ordered (see Table 10-20)
   P. Administer antibiotics as ordered (see Table 10-2)
   Q. Restrict contact with persons who have known respiratory infections
   R. Provide age-appropriate diversional activities during hospitalization
   S. Encourage participation in usual activities on discharge
   T. Provide hospital/home bound teachers if required
   U. Have child/parents participate in teaching session with health care team outlining each facet of care with return demonstration
   V. Arrange for regular follow-up care
   W. Allow child/parents opportunity to express concerns and feelings about diagnosis, treatment regimen, prognosis
   X. Refer to support group

V. Evaluation
   A. Child participates in diagnostic procedures without difficulty
   B. Child maintains or gains weight once diet plan initiated
   C. Child has minimal respiratory infections after beginning treatment
   D. Child participates in respiratory treatments without complications
   E. Child is adequately oxygenated—normal

ABGs, increased oxygen saturation, improved pulmonary function tests
F. Child's activity level increases after beginning treatment
G. Child participates in home bound teacher program until return to school allowed
H. Child/parents participate in teaching sessions about each facet of treatment regimen
I. Child/parents perform return demonstration of each component of care and discuss its importance
J. Child/parents express concerns and feelings about long-term management and prognosis with health care team
K. Child/parents slowly cope effectively with cystic fibrosis and effects on family
L. Child/parents attend support group and begin attending meetings
M. Child/parents participate in follow-up care on regular basis

POST-TEST Pulmonary Disorders

1. Which of the following signs and symptoms are commonly seen in all of the croup syndromes?
   ① Tight cough, wheezing
   ② Brassy cough, stridor
   ③ Sore throat, drooling
   ④ Congested cough, fever
2. Angelica, age 2, is brought to the physician's office with a brassy cough and mild stridor. She is afebrile and not in respiratory distress. The physician diagnoses acute spasmodic croup. Which statement by the father before they leave the office indicates an understanding of the home management of croup?
   ① "I will encourage her to take deep breaths and cough every hour."
   ② "She will need to take the entire course of antibiotics."
   ③ "I will use the cool mist vaporizer in her room at night."
   ④ "I will give her Tylenol for her fever."

Ward, a 7-month-old, is admitted to the hospital for bronchiolitis. His nasopharyngeal smear and culture are positive for respiratory syncytial virus. He appears to be in moderate respiratory distress and is placed in an oxygen tent.

---

3. When auscultating Ward's lungs, the nurse notes the presence of wheezing. The reason wheezing occurs in bronchiolitis is:
   ① The airflow in the bronchioles is increased
   ② There is edema of the narrowed airways
   ③ It is precipitated by paroxysmal coughing
   ④ It is caused by cyanosis and air hunger
4. The nurse encourages Ward's parents to get under the tent with him and to touch him and talk with him frequently. This intervention is directed toward what goal?
   ① Maintaining normal growth and development
   ② Promoting adequate rest
   ③ Facilitating adequate oxygenation
   ④ Increasing tolerance for activity

Four-year-old Timmy is admitted with left lower lobe pneumonia. He is exhibiting the following symptoms: fever of 103.1°F (39.5°C), chest pain, and shallow respirations.

---

5. Given the assessment data, which of the following nursing diagnoses might apply to Timmy?
   ① Hypothermia
   ② Ineffective airway clearance
   ③ Fluid volume deficit
   ④ Impaired gas exchange
6. Which of the following nursing interventions will be appropriate for Timmy?
   ① Administer bronchodilators on a 24-hour basis
   ② Position on left side with head elevated
   ③ Administer IV morphine as ordered for pain
   ④ Provide a high-protein, high-calorie diet
7. Which of the following toys would be most therapeutic for Timmy?
   ① Puzzle
   ② Play action characters
   ③ Stuffed animal
   ④ Toy trumpet

Mandy, age 6, has had asthma since she was 1 year old. She is brought into the emergency department with symptoms of moderate respiratory distress, wheezing, and increased use of accessory muscles.

---

8. Mandy is given albuterol by nebulizer. If the albuterol is effective, what might the nurse see?
   ① Reduced mucosal edema
   ② Decreased mucous secretions

③ Reversal of bronchospasm
④ Liquified mucous secretions

9. Mandy has been on oral theopylline at home. Her theophylline level is found to be 2.5 μg/ml. This is indicative of a need to:
   ① Decrease the amount of theophylline Mandy is receiving
   ② Switch to a different form of aminophylline
   ③ Decrease the administration from three times a day to two times a day
   ④ Check Mandy's weight and ask her mother about current dosage and schedule

10. Mandy is scheduled for discharge on cromolyn sodium. Which of the following statements would indicate that her mother understands the use and administration of this drug?
    ① "If the theophylline doesn't work, I'll give the cromolyn."
    ② "I'll mix it with orange juice to disguise the taste."
    ③ "When she starts to wheeze, I'll give her a dose."
    ④ "I'll have her use it before she goes out to play ball."

11. Mandy's mother expresses concern about letting Mandy participate in sports with her friends. She tells the nurse that she would rather Mandy do something quiet like learn to play a musical instrument. A possible nursing diagnosis might be:
    ① High risk for altered growth and development
    ② Knowledge deficit about medication effects
    ③ High risk for activity intolerance
    ④ High risk for ineffective airway clearance

12. Which of the following data would suggest a diagnosis of cystic fibrosis in an infant who fails to thrive?
    ① Positive stool culture
    ② Positive sputum culture
    ③ Decreased gastric pH
    ④ Elevated sweat chloride

Fourteen-year-old Jason has cystic fibrosis that was diagnosed during infancy and is admitted to the hospital for one of several recent episodes of pneumonia. He demonstrates markedly decreased pulmonary function, is small for his age, and states he is much more tired than usual.

13. Jason's fatigue is probably related to which of the following problems?
    ① Inadequate oxygenation
    ② Decreased hemoglobin and hematocrit
    ③ Inability to obtain sufficient rest
    ④ Too much exercise

14. As Jason is filling out his menu for the day, which of the following snack choices would indicate to you that he understands his dietary recommendations?
    ① French fries with ketchup
    ② Slice of pizza with extra cheese
    ③ Salad with Russian dressing
    ④ Fruit cup with ice cream

15. Jason's mother has become pregnant unexpectedly and is extremely worried that the new baby might have cystic fibrosis. She and her husband are referred to the nurse at the genetic counseling clinic. Knowing the inheritance pattern of cystic fibrosis, the nurse plans to teach which of the following facts?
    ① If the new baby is a boy, the baby will probably inherit cystic fibrosis
    ② Because one child has cystic fibrosis, this baby has a greater chance of inheriting the disease
    ③ There is a 75% chance that the baby will not have the disease but a 50% chance that the baby will carry the gene
    ④ There is a 50% chance that the baby will inherit the disease and a 50% chance that the baby will carry the gene

POST-TEST Answers and Rationales

1. ② Croup is a group of disorders characterized by a brassy, harsh, cough and varying degrees of respiratory stridor. Sore throat and drooling may be signs of epiglottitis, which must be differentiated from croup because it often constitutes a medical emergency. The other responses are characteristic of other types of respiratory disorders. I, IV. Laryngotracheobronchitis.

2. ③ A humidified atmosphere helps to prevent laryngeal spasms. The cool mist is safer than hot mist. The other options are not appropriate in this case. 5, I. Laryngotracheobronchitis.

3. ② When an infant has bronchiolitis, the bronchioles become edematous, and the air moving through these narrowed passages is turbulent, creating the wheezing sound. 1, II. Bronchiolitis.

4. ① Infants admitted to the hospital with respiratory syncytial virus must be placed in respiratory isolation. If in respiratory distress from bronchiolitis, a tent might also be required. Both the tent and the equipment needed to maintain isolation place a barrier between the infant and parent. It is important for parents to maintain verbal and physical contact with the infant to prevent developmental consequences of hospitalization. 3, III. Bronchiolitis.

5. ② Children with pneumonia often have difficulty with effective airway clearance because of consolidation of secretions and limited ability to cough because of chest pain. The assessment data do not suggest impaired gas exchange, although that is a potential problem with children with pneumonia, as is fluid volume deficit. Hypothermia is incorrect. 2, II. Pneumonia.

6. ② Children with respiratory disorders are more comfortable in a semierect position. Lying on the affected side helps prevent pleural pain with breathing. Bronchodilators and morphine are not prescribed for children with pneumonia. High-protein, high-calorie diet is not necessary. 4, II. Pneumonia.

7. ④ Most of the toys listed are age appropriate and do not require much activity; however, the toy trumpet requires respiratory effort to use properly. It would facilitate deep breathing. 4, II. Pneumonia.

8. ③ Albuterol by nebulizer rapidly reverses bronchospasm by relaxing the smooth muscle of the bronchi. It may be given in the emergency department as often as every 20 minutes to obtain relief. 5, II. Asthma.

9. ④ This is a subtherapeutic level of theophylline. You should check with the mother to see how much medication she has been giving Mandy. She may have gained weight since the original dosage was set. 3, II. Asthma.

10. ④ Cromolyn sodium acts to block the release of chemical mediators when the child is exposed to an allergen. It does not produce direct bronchodilation and is not effective once the asthma attack has started. It should always be used preventively. 5, II. Asthma

11. ① Parents often become overly anxious about their children who have asthma and try to overprotect them by restricting activities that promote adequate development. Most often, it is not necessary to restrict sports, and exercise-induced bronchospasm can be effectively prevented by medication. The other diagnoses are applicable to the child with asthma but are not applicable to this particular situation. 2, IV. Asthma.

12. ④ Sweat electrolyte levels are elevated in a child with cystic fibrosis. This along with failure to thrive despite healthy appetite and bulky, foul-smelling stools would suggest cystic fibrosis. 1, II. Cystic Fibrosis.

13. ① Decreased oxygen as a result of impaired gas exchange can lead to activity intolerance and fatigue. Children with cystic fibrosis have thick secretions, which can narrow airways and prevent adequate oxygenation. Although the other choices can cause fatigue, it is likely that decreased oxygenation is the cause in this situation. 2, II. Cystic Fibrosis.

14. ② Children with cystic fibrosis need to be on a high-protein, high-calorie diet to obtain enough nutrients for growth. Pizza with additional cheese provides more protein than any of the other choices. 5, IV. Cystic Fibrosis.

15. ③ Cystic fibrosis is inherited by autosomal recessive inheritance pattern; therefore, with each pregnancy there is a 25% chance that the child will inherit the disease, a 50% chance that the child will carry the gene but not have the disease, and a 25% chance that the child will neither have the disease nor carry the gene. 3, I. Cystic Fibrosis.

PRE-TEST Fluid/Electrolyte Disorders

1. Which of the following would you expect to see in a 6-month-old with a 2-day history of vomiting and diarrhea?
   ① Weight loss, bulging fontanelles, decreased urine specific gravity
   ② Dry oral mucous membranes, poor skin turgor, elevated urine specific gravity
   ③ Periorbital edema, weight gain, lack of tears
   ④ Increased urination, weight loss, normal urine specific gravity

2. Before giving advice to a parent who calls and is upset because a child is vomiting, the nurse first needs to determine the child's:
   ① Weight
   ② Diet
   ③ Age
   ④ General health status

3. A major cause of edema in children is:
   ① Underlying system dysfunction
   ② Excessive fluid intake
   ③ Decreased sodium retention
   ④ Increased urination

4. Interventions for a child experiencing edema include:
   ① Placing child in a flat position to facilitate venous return
   ② Starting an IV line for sodium and fluid replacement
   ③ Ambulating child frequently to promote circulation
   ④ Strictly monitoring input, output, and weight

PRE-TEST Answers and Rationales

1. ② Two days of diarrhea and vomiting can cause severe dehydration in an infant. When an infant is experiencing dehydration, the urine output drops and becomes very concentrated, the mucous membranes become dry, weight is lost, and the fontanelles are depressed. The other options contain incorrect signs. 1, II. Dehydration.

2. ③ Because of their fluid status, infants and young children are more vulnerable to dehydration. The nurse should first determine the child's age before giving advice. 1, II. Dehydration.

3. ① Underlying dysfunction of the heart, kidney, or liver is the most common cause of edema in children. Excessive fluid intake in the absence of fluid output is much less common. 2, II. Edema.

4. ④ Monitoring intake, output, and weight is a primary nursing intervention for any child with a fluid imbalance. Fluid restriction, which is a common treatment for an edematous child, makes monitoring intake especially important. Decreasing weight and increasing urinary output are signs that edema is resolving. 4, II. Edema.

NURSING PROCESS APPLIED TO CHILDREN WITH FLUID/ELECTROLYTE DISORDERS

Dehydration

I. Assessment
   A. Definition: occurs when total output of fluid exceeds total intake, regardless of underlying cause; defined as isotonic, hypotonic, or hypertonic depending on fluid loss in relation to sodium loss
   B. Etiology/incidence
      1. Lack of oral intake
      2. Abnormal loss of fluid and electrolytes
      3. Isotonic dehydration is one of most common body fluid disturbances in infancy/childhood
   C. Predisposing/precipitating factors
      1. Vomiting
      2. Diarrhea
      3. Other causes—hemorrhage, burns, fever, tachypnea
      4. Cessation of fluid intake
   D. Clinical manifestations
      1. Mild dehydration
         a. Weight loss: 5%
         b. Skin: pale, cool, dry, slightly dry mucous membranes
         c. Urine: output slightly decreased, slightly increased specific gravity
         d. Vital signs: pulse begins to increase
         e. Supporting signs: thirst in older child
      2. Moderate dehydration
         a. Weight loss: 10%
         b. Skin: gray, cool, decreased skin turgor; dry mucous membranes
         c. Urine: oliguria, increased specific gravity
         d. Vital signs: increased pulse, blood pressure begins to decrease
         e. Supporting signs: absence of tears (child older than 3 months), depressed fontanelles (child under 18 months), sunken eyes, listlessness
      3. Severe dehydration
         a. Weight loss: 15%
         b. Skin: mottled with poor peripheral circulation, cool poor turgor with tenting, parched mucous membranes
         c. Urine: anuria
         d. Vital signs: tachycardia, thready pulse, low blood pressure, signs of impending shock
         e. Supporting signs: sunken fontanelles, markedly sunken eyes, azotemia
      4. Infants and children more vulnerable because of higher percentage of fluid in relation to total body weight and higher percentage of fluid in extracellular space
   E. Diagnostic examinations
      1. Urine specific gravity—usually increased
      2. Serum electrolytes, particularly sodium, potassium, CO_2, blood urea nitrogen
      3. Hemoglobin, hematocrit—elevated in fluid volume loss
   F. Complication: shock
   G. Medical management
      1. Rehydration by oral or IV fluid replacement

2. Replacement of any lost electrolytes

II. Analysis
   A. Fluid volume deficit related to condition causing fluid loss
   B. High risk for decreased cardiac output related to decreased circulating volume
   C. Altered patterns of urinary elimination related to dehydration

III. Planning/goals, expected outcomes
   A. Child will regain fluid balance within 24 hours (48 hours for hypertonic dehydration)
   B. Child's vital signs will improve within 2 to 4 hours
   C. Child will begin to regain electrolyte balance within 24 hours and will be corrected within 2 days
   D. Child's output will increase to at least 1 mL/kg/hr within 12 to 24 hours
   E. Child will begin to gain weight within 24 hours
   F. Child will not exhibit signs and symptoms of shock
   G. Child/parents will have opportunity to discuss diagnosis, underlying cause, therapeutic regimen

IV. Implementation
   A. Monitor for signs and symptoms of dehydration
   B. Vital signs every 1 to 2 hours
   C. Check peripheral circulation every 2 hours
   D. Check specific gravity every void
   E. Maintain strict I & O measurement, weigh diapers
   F. Check weight daily—same time, same clothes, same scale
   G. Administer oral rehydration or IV therapy as ordered
   H. Monitor electrolyte levels
   I. Monitor for signs and symptoms of shock
      1. Confusion
      2. Thready, weak pulse
      3. Tachypnea, progressing to Cheyne-Stokes
      4. Pale extremities
      5. Poor capillary filling
      6. Hypotension
   J. Teach parents principles of preventing fluid and electrolyte loss
      1. Keep NPO, if vomiting, until vomiting stops; then begin fluids with electrolyte solution (e.g., Pedialyte, Ricelyte, Lytrin)
      2. Introduce fluids gradually—1 oz/hr—to facilitate retention
      3. Notify physician for signs of dehydration
   K. Allow child/parents opportunity to ask questions about therapeutic regimen
   L. Allow child/parents opportunity to express concerns about diagnosis and therapeutic regimen

V. Evaluation
   A. Child demonstrates improvement in hydration as evidenced by increasing skin turgor, increasing urinary output, stabilizing vital signs
   B. Child's sodium and potassium levels return to within normal limits if altered by dehydration
   C. Child's blood urea nitrogen decreases to within normal limits 48 hours after treatment begins
   D. Child's output increases to at least 1 mL/kg/hr after treatment begins, urine specific gravity decreases to 1.010 or less
   E. Child shows steady weight gain, even if diarrhea continues
   F. Child does not exhibit signs and symptoms of shock
   G. Child/parents participate in teaching session about diagnosis and therapeutic regimen

Edema

I. Assessment
   A. Definition: presence of excess fluid in interstitial spaces; may be localized or generalized; usually symptom of one of many underlying causes
   B. Etiology/incidence
      1. Increased capillary hydrostatic pressure
      2. Damage to capillary walls and increased permeability
      3. Decreased plasma proteins
      4. Lymphatic obstruction
      5. Excessive concentration of sodium in extracellular fluid
      6. Incidence varies with underlying cause
   C. Predisposing/precipitating factors
      1. Kidney disease, nephrotic syndrome
      2. Starvation, malnutrition
      3. Liver disease, hepatic failure
      4. Congestive heart failure
      5. Trauma, burns
   D. Clinical manifestations
      1. Puffy eyes, face, ankles
      2. Bulging fontanelles (up to 18 months)
      3. Bulging eyes
      4. Weight gain
      5. Dyspnea, cough, rales
      6. Abdominal distention
      7. Normal or decreased urine output depending on underlying renal status
      8. Distended neck veins
      9. Hypertension, rapid bounding pulse
   E. Diagnostic examinations
      1. Daily weight usually increases

2. Serum electrolyte levels may demonstrate sodium alterations
3. Intake and output
F. Complications: vary with underlying cause and organs involved
G. Medical management
   1. Fluid restriction
   2. Diuretic therapy (see Table 10-5)
   3. Sodium restriction
   4. Treatment of underlying dysfunction

II. Analysis
   A. Fluid volume excess related to underlying condition or electrolyte imbalance
   B. High risk for ineffective breathing pattern related to pulmonary fluid overload
   C. High risk for impaired skin integrity related to edema
   D. High risk for sensory/perceptual alterations (kinesthetic) related to cerebral response to fluid shift

III. Planning/goals, expected outcomes
   A. Child will demonstrate return to fluid balance
   B. Child's underlying cause of edema will be diagnosed as soon as possible
   C. Child's electrolyte imbalances will return to normal
   D. Child's weight will not increase and will return to "normal" subsequent to treatment
   E. Child will not exhibit signs and symptoms of complications inherent with underlying cause
   F. Child/parents will understand diagnosis, underlying cause, therapeutic regimen
   G. Child/parents will express feelings and concerns

IV. Implementation
   A. Monitor for signs and symptoms of increasing edema
   B. Maintain accurate history of changes in fluid retention
   C. Elevate head of bed 15 to 30 degrees, turn frequently
   D. Elevate legs on pillows
   E. Monitor pulses, especially in lower extremities
   F. Do neurovascular checks every 2 to 4 hours—sensation, color, capillary refill
   G. Monitor electrolytes, especially potassium, hematocrit, protein
   H. Restrict fluids and sodium as ordered; use creativity to distract child during fluid restriction
   I. Administer diuretics as ordered (see Table 10-5)
   J. Maintain strict I & O, monitor urine specific gravity
   K. Check weight daily—same time, same clothes, same scale
   L. Take vital signs every 2 to 4 hours, monitor depth and quality of respirations, breath sounds
   M. Monitor for changes in status that would signal impending complications
   N. Allow child/parents to ask questions about diagnosis and therapeutic regimen
   O. Allow child/parents opportunity to discuss fears and concerns with health care team

V. Evaluation
   A. Child demonstrates return to fluid and electrolyte balance as underlying condition permits—decreased edema, normal urine output and specific gravity, stable vital signs
   B. Child's weight gain reduced
   C. Child's output returns to an average of 1 mL/kg/hr after treatment begins
   D. Child maintains fluid and sodium restricted diet as long as necessary
   E. Child does not exhibit signs and symptoms of complications
   F. Child/parents discuss diagnosis, therapeutic regimen, concerns with health care team

POST-TEST Fluid/Electrolyte Disorders

Javier is a 9-month-old infant whose father calls because he has been vomiting for 1 day and has had diarrhea. When Javier arrives at the office, the nurse notes that his weight has decreased by 5% from his weight at his physical examination 3 days before.

---

1. What additional signs might the nurse note when assessing Javier?
   ① Puffiness of the eyelids, decreased urinary output, full and bounding pulse
   ② Mottled skin, no wet diapers for 6 hours, sunken fontanelles, dry mucous membranes
   ③ Depressed fontanelles, increased pulse, absence of tears, tenting
   ④ Dry skin and mucous membranes, pulse slightly increased, only one wet diaper the past 6 hours

2. The doctor orders oral feedings with Pedialyte to begin in the office. The nurse explains to Javier's mother that the major goal is to:
   ① Decrease the diarrhea
   ② Replace the lost fluid
   ③ Stop the vomiting
   ④ Increase the calories

3. When Javier's father asks how the baby could

become dehydrated that fast, the nurse's best response is that one of the reasons babies can lose body fluid faster than adults is:

① They don't drink as much during the day
② Their urine output is much higher
③ Their body temperature is generally lower
④ Their body fluid is not stored as well

4. Javier is sent home after 2 hours, and his parents are told to call the doctor in 2 more hours to report on his condition. Which of the following would best indicate Javier is responding to treatment?

① He has had two wet diapers since returning home
② He is drowsy but not fussy
③ His vomiting has stopped, but diarrhea continues
④ He seems to be hungry

5. In addition to fluid volume excess, which of the following potential nursing diagnoses may be identified in a child with edema?

① Infection
② Impaired skin integrity
③ Altered nutrition: less than body requirements
④ Altered oral mucous membranes

POST-TEST Answers and Rationales

1. ④ A 5% weight loss from fluid loss is categorized as mild dehydration. Symptoms associated with mild dehydration include pale dry skin, dry mucous membranes, slightly decreased urine output, and increasing pulse. The other choices describe different states of hydration. 1, II. Dehydration.

2. ② An electrolyte solution can be fed slowly to infants who are mildly dehydrated to replace lost fluids and prevent further dehydration. The other choices are not goals for fluid therapy. 3, II. Dehydration.

3. ④ A major reason why infants dehydrate more quickly than older children or adults is because a higher proportion of body fluid is stored in the extracellular space, which is more vulnerable to fluid shifts. The other choices are incorrect. 4, IV. Dehydration.

4. ① Although all of the choices would indicate that Javier is feeling better, increasing urinary output is one of the first signs that dehydration is beginning to resolve. 5, II. Dehydration.

5. ② Edema can create excessive pressure on certain body parts and decreasing oxygenation to the tissue. The result is skin breakdown. The nursing diagnosis "potential for impaired skin integrity" is the correct answer. The other choices usually are not associated with the edematous child. 2, I. Edema.

BIBLIOGRAPHY

FLUID/GAS TRANSPORT

Albano, E. A., and Pizzo, P. A. (1988). Infectious complications in childhood acute leukemias. *Pediatric Clinics of North America* 35 (4): 873–901.

American Academy of Pediatrics (1991). Prevention of bacterial endocarditis. *Report of the Committee on Infectious Diseases*. Elk Grove: American Academy of Pediatrics.

Balfour, I. C., Drimmer, A. M., Nouri, S., et al (1991). Pediatric cardiac rehabilitation. *American Journal of Diseases of Children* 145 (6): 627–629.

Callow, L. B. (1992). Current strategies in the nursing care of infants with hypoplastic left heart syndrome undergoing first-stage palliation with the Norwood operation. *Heart and Lung* 21 (5): 463–470.

Cooke, D. M. (1992). Shielding your patient from digitalis toxicity. *Nursing '92* 22 (7): 44–47.

Driscoll, D. (1990). Evaluation of the cyanotic newborn. *Pediatric Clinics of North America* 37 (1): 1–23.

Ellis, J. (1991). How adolescents cope with cancer and its treatment. *MCN* 16 (3): 157.

Foster, R. L. R., Hunsberger, M. M., and Anderson, J. J. T. (1989). *Family-centered nursing care of children and families*. Philadelphia: W. B. Saunders.

Gloe, D. (1991). Common reactions to transfusions. *Heart and Lung* 20 (5): 506–512.

Green, J. (1992). Recognizing epiglottitis. *Nursing '92* 22 (8): 33.

Hoffman, J. I. E. (1990). Congenital heart disease. *Pediatric Clinics of North America* 37 (1): 25–43.

Kallen, R. J. (1990). The management of diarrheal dehydration in infants using parenteral fluids. *Pediatric Clinics of North America* 37 (2): 265–286.

Lampkin, B. C., et al (1988). Biologic characteristics and treatment of acute non-lymphocytic leukemia in children. *Pediatric Clinics of North America* 35 (4): 743–760.

Lozoff, B., Jiminez, E., and Wolf, A. W. (1991). Long-term developmental outcome of infants with iron deficiency. *New England Journal of Medicine* 325: 687–694.

Marino, B. L., and Lipshitz, M. (1991). Temperament in infants and toddlers with cardiac disease. *Pediatric Nursing* 17 (5): 445.

Mott, S., James, S. R., and Sperhac, A. (1990). *Nursing care of children and families*, 2nd ed. Redwood City: Benjamin Cummings.

National Asthma Education Program (1991). *Executive summary: Guidelines for the diagnosis and management of asthma*. U.S. Department of Health and Human Services, publication No. 91-3042A.

Park, M. K. (1991). *The pediatric cardiology handbook*. St. Louis: Mosby-Year Book.

Pediatric Oncology Group (1992). Progress against childhood cancer: The Pediatric Oncology Group experience. *Pediatrics* 89 (4): 597–600.

Pegelow, C. H., et al (1991). Experience with the use of prophylactic penicillin in children with sickle cell anemia. *Journal of Pediatrics* 118 (5): 736–738.

Pigott, J. D. (1991). The evolution of surgical treatment for heart disease. *American Journal of Diseases of Children* 145 (12): 1362–1363.

Pinsky, W. W., and Arciniegas, E. (1990). Tetralogy of Fallot. *Pediatric Clinics of North America* 37 (1): 179–192.

Polacek, T. L., Barth, L., Mestad, P., et al (1992). The effect of positioning on arterial oxygenation in children with atelectasis after cardiac surgery. *Heart and Lung* 21 (5): 457–462.

Poplack, D. G., and Reaman, G. (1988). Acute lymphoblastic leukemia in childhood. *Pediatric Clinics of North America* 35 (4): 903–932.

Resar, L. M., and Oski, F. A. (1991). Cold water exposure and vaso-occlusive crises in sickle cell anemia. *Journal of Pediatrics* 118 (3): 407–409.

Shaw, K. N., Bell, L., and Sherman, N. H. (1991). Outpatient assessment of infants with bronchiolitis. *American Journal of Diseases of Children* 145 (2): 151–155.

Wang, W. C., et al (1991). High risk of recurrent stroke after discontinuance of five to twelve years of transfusion therapy in patients with sickle cell disease. *Journal of Pediatrics* 118 (3): 377–382.

Zangwill, K. M., Wald, E. R., and Londino, A. V. (1991). Acute rheumatic fever in western Pennsylvania: A persistent problem into the 1990s. *Journal of Pediatrics* 118 (4): 561–562.

11

Sensory/Perceptual Functions in the Pediatric Client

PRE-TEST Neurological Disorders

1. Corky, aged 4 months, has been recovering from acute nasopharyngitis. He has become listless and lethargic, and he is refusing to eat. He is admitted to the hospital with a diagnosis of meningitis. Which of the following *initial* nursing interventions is appropriate?
   ① Monitor vital signs, and maintain adequate hydration
   ② Place him in isolation, and obtain baseline vitals
   ③ Do not allow visitors at bedside, and administer oxygen per tent
   ④ Maintain enteric isolation, and monitor for seizure activity

2. Reye's syndrome must be diagnosed rapidly. Which of the following should the nurse teach parents to do?
   ① Monitor your child carefully after viral illnesses, especially in warmer months
   ② Call the physician if your child, recovering from a viral illness, suddenly begins to vomit
   ③ Watch for the development of Reye's syndrome because even though it is a self-limiting illness, it can cause liver failure
   ④ If aspirin given during a febrile illness is effective in lowering the temperature, don't worry

3. When assisting with a lumbar puncture on a young child, which of the following goals is a priority?
   ① Pain relief
   ② Education of the parents
   ③ Proper positioning
   ④ Providing anesthesia

4. Which of the following signs might the nurse expect to see in an infant with hydrocephalus?
   ① Elevated blood pressure, severe headache, vomiting
   ② Feeding difficulties, irritability, large head
   ③ Fever, bulging fontanelles, sunset eyes
   ④ Decreased consciousness, irritability, small fontanelles

5. Jenny was admitted to the hospital 2 days ago after being hit by a car when riding her bike. She suffered a closed-head injury, and the graphic sheet shows an increase in her systolic blood pressure and a decrease in her diastolic pressure. The nurse interprets this to be a sign of:
   ① Increased intracranial pressure
   ② Decreased intracranial pressure
   ③ Increased hypercapnia
   ④ Resolving cerebral edema

6. Which of the following is most likely to experience a typical febrile seizure?
   ① A 1-year-old with otitis and a fever of 104°F
   ② A 2-month-old with bulging fontanelles and unequal pupils
   ③ A 10-year-old with a fever of 102°F who is on Dilantin for epilepsy
   ④ A 6-year-old who has meningitis

7. Which of the following would a 6-month-old suspected of having cerebral palsy be most likely to exhibit?
   ① Delay or failure to control head movement or to roll over
   ② Frequent episodes of seizure activity
   ③ Visual or hearing deficits
   ④ Frequent upper respiratory infections

8. Which of the following statements by the parent of the abovementioned child indicates an understanding of the potential seriousness of the child's disability?
   ① "With early and vigorous physical therapy, my child may have only mild problems."
   ② "It's hard to tell so early in the disease, but some degree of mental retardation is likely."
   ③ "The severity of the symptoms varies, but my child should be able to be helped with treatment."
   ④ "It's hard to tell how much disability there will be until my child starts school."

9. Nora has recently been diagnosed with a medulloblastoma. Which of the following symptoms could the nurse expect her to exhibit?
   ① Vomiting and headaches
   ② Gait disturbances
   ③ Diplopia
   ④ Dysphagia

10. Nora is scheduled for a craniotomy for partial excision of her tumor. When planning for care after surgery, which of the following would be a priority goal? The child will:
    ① Remain pain free
    ② Resume normal activities for her age
    ③ Show no evidence of infection
    ④ Show no indication of decreased cerebral perfusion

11. Which of the following actions *most* indicates appropriate adjustment in the family of an infant with spina bifida?
    ① Parents state this will be the last baby they will have
    ② Family sends out a Christmas card featuring a picture of the new baby

③ Parents state they will have no trouble affording the expense of the baby's care

④ Parents and siblings don't talk about the baby with friends

12. Which of the following nursing interventions is most appropriate in the care of a child during a tonic-clonic seizure?

① Restrain the child to prevent injury

② Insert an airway into the mouth to prevent tongue biting

③ Note the time, duration, and activity of the seizure

④ Turn the child to a prone position

PRE-TEST Answers and Rationales

1. ② When a child is admitted with the diagnosis of meningitis, isolation must be a priority to prevent possible spread. Baseline vitals and maintaining a close watch on hydration are also priorities. 4, I. Meningitis.

2. ② Vomiting following a mild viral illness is an early sign of Reye's syndrome. Parents should be taught this as an early symptom to watch for. 4, IV. Reye's Syndrome.

3. ③ It is vitally important that the child not move during a lumbar puncture because this could cause injury. Proper side-lying, knee-chest positioning allows for maximum control. Although teaching and support are important, they are not the priority. 3, I. Lumbar Puncture.

4. ② An enlarged head is one of the first suspicious signs of hydrocephalus in an infant. Signs of increased intracranial pressure in infants include feeding difficulties and irritability. Answer #1 delineates signs of increased intracranial pressure in the older child; neither fever nor small fontanelles are associated with hydrocephalus. 1, II. Hydrocephalus.

5. ① A widening pulse pressure is a major indication of the presence of increased intracranial pressure. The pressure may be caused by increasing cerebral edema. 2, II. Increased Intracranial Pressure.

6. ① A febrile seizure occurs when an infant has a high fever. It is not related to any disease state such as epilepsy or trauma. 2, II. Seizures.

7. ① Gross motor skill milestones are usually delayed in the child with cerebral palsy. Seizures are not common, nor are sensory or hearing deficits or respiratory infections. 1, IV. Cerebral Palsy.

8. ③ Cerebral palsy varies greatly from mild to severe, so it is impossible to tell the parents at this stage that the disease will be mild or that the severe form will occur. 5, II. Cerebral Palsy.

9. ② A medulloblastoma is a rapidly growing common tumor found in the cerebellum and invading the fourth ventricle. Symptoms often include clumsy gait and difficulties in sitting and standing unsupported. 1, II. Brain Tumor.

10. ④ Preventing decreased cerebral perfusion, which would lead to cerebral edema and increased intracranial pressure, is a priority goal for nursing care after neurosurgery. The other options are postoperative goals but are of lesser priority. 3, II. Brain Tumor.

11. ② One of the signs of beginning adjustment to an infant with a long-term disability is the ability to focus on the infant's positive aspects. Refusing to talk about a baby's problems with friends may be a sign of denial. Making a decision about future childbearing during the adjustment to a new family member is inappropriate. Deciding that financial help isn't necessary before fully understanding the impact of the child's medical care on family resources may be premature. 5, III. Spina Bifida.

12. ③ It is important that the nurse note the time duration and actual pattern of the seizure. The nurse should not force anything into the child's mouth. 4, II. Seizures.

NORMAL NERVOUS SYSTEM

I. Normal nervous system: nervous system is composed of central nervous system (CNS), peripheral nervous system (PNS), and autonomic nervous system (ANS); CNS is made up of brain and spinal cord; PNS is made up of cranial nerves and spinal nerves, both controlling motor and sensory functions; ANS is made up of sympathetic and parasympathetic systems responsible for automatic control of body's vital functions; nervous system is "life" of human body.

NURSING PROCESS APPLIED TO CHILDREN WITH NEUROLOGICAL DISORDERS

Congenital Disorders

Hydrocephalus

I. Assessment
   A. Definition: excessive accumulation of cerebral spinal fluid (CSF) within ventricles of brain
   B. Etiology/incidence

1. Choroid plexus—excessive production of CSF
2. Inadequate circulation or reabsorption of CSF in subarachnoid space (communicating)
3. Obstruction of circulation of CSF from ventricle to subarachnoid space (noncommunicating)
4. Three or four per 1000 live births

C. Predisposing/precipitating factors
1. Congenital malformation—most common cause
2. Infection
3. Tumor
4. Head trauma or birth injury

D. Clinical manifestations
1. Bulging fontanelles
2. Dilated scalp veins
3. Shiny scalp
4. Sunset eyes
5. Enlarged head circumference
6. Opisthotonos
7. Irritability
8. High-pitched cry
9. Feeding difficulties

E. Diagnostic examinations
1. Ultrasound in utero
2. Large head size at birth (more than 95th percentile) or abnormal increase in serial head circumference measurements (more than 2 cm per month for first 3 months)
3. Signs and symptoms of increased intracranial pressure (Table 11-1)
4. CT scan, MRI
5. Transillumination of scalp

F. Complications
1. Untreated—death or severe developmental delay
2. Treated—long-term consequences related

to underlying disease process, prognosis in uncomplicated treated hydrocephalus generally good
3. Postsurgical treatment
   a. Infections
   b. Blocked shunts
   c. Seizures

G. Surgical management
1. Shunting procedure to bypass obstruction or remove excess fluid (Fig. 11-1)
   a. Atrioventricular shunt: lateral ventricle to right atrium
   b. Ventriculoperitoneal shunt: lateral ventricle to peritoneal cavity

II. Analysis
A. Preoperative
1. Altered cerebral tissue perfusion related to increased intracranial pressure
2. High risk for impaired skin integrity related to pressure from enlarged head
3. High risk for altered nutrition: less than body requirements related to feeding problems or vomiting
4. Anxiety (family) related to child's condition and prognosis

TABLE 11–1 Signs of Increased Intracranial Pressure in Children

Child Under Age 2 Years	Child Over Age 2 Years
Tense, bulging fontanelle	Headache
Head enlargement with separation of cranial sutures	Double vision, papilledema
Irritability, altered behavior	Irritability, altered behavior
Poor feeding, vomiting	Nausea, vomiting
Delayed development	Change in neurological signs
	Elevated blood pressure, decreased pulse, widening pulse pressure
	Motor or sensory alterations, seizures
	Increasing lethargy, stupor, coma

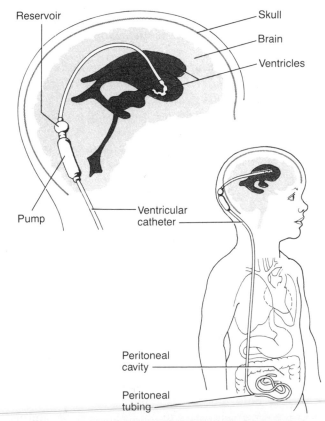

FIGURE 11–1. Placement of the ventriculoperitoneal shunt. (From Foster, R. L. R., Hunsberger, M. M., and Anderson, J. J. T. (1989). *Family-centered nursing care of children.* Philadelphia: W. B. Saunders.)

5. Knowledge deficit about surgery and postoperative care related to unfamiliarity with the condition
   B. Postoperative
   1. High risk for altered cerebral tissue perfusion related to malfunction of shunt or postoperative edema
   2. High risk for fluid volume deficit related to NPO status and volume losses during surgery
   3. Pain related to surgery
   4. High risk for infection related to shunt placement and altered skin integrity
   5. Knowledge deficit about home management related to unfamiliarity with information
III. Planning/goals, expected outcomes
   A. Child's neurological status will improve or remain stable
   B. Child will eat and retain fluids and nutrients appropriate for age
   C. Child's skin integrity will remain intact and free of infection
   D. Child will rest with minimal discomfort
   E. Child will remain free of postoperative complications
   F. Family members will express feelings of anxiety and concerns
   G. Parents will understand the surgical procedure, postoperative management, and home management
IV. Implementation
   A. Preoperative
   1. Monitor neurological status and vital signs frequently (Table 11-2); elevate head of bed 30 degrees
   2. Measure head circumference daily
   3. Provide meticulous skin care to head
      a. Turn every 2 hours
      b. Use sheepskin protectors under head
      c. Provide air mattress/Eggcrate mattress
   4. Administer small, frequent feedings or IV feedings as ordered
      a. Hold when feeding, with head elevated
      b. Maintain strict I & O
      c. Provide rest periods after feeding
   5. Provide tactile stimulation
   6. Encourage parental involvement
      a. Feeding
      b. Physical contact such as bathing, cuddling
   7. Explain all diagnostic procedures to parents in terms they understand
   8. Prepare parents for surgery—shunting procedure to bypass obstruction or remove excess fluids
      a. Atrioventricular shunt
      b. Ventriculoperitoneal shunt
   9. Prepare parents for appearance of child and child's postoperative needs
   B. Postoperative
   1. Position on nonoperative side with head flat or slightly elevated
   2. Turn every 2 hours except onto operative side
   3. Perform neurological check every 15 minutes and extend gradually to every 1 to 2 hours when stable
   4. Monitor operative site for bleeding and infection
   5. Monitor child for signs of CNS infection (fever, irritability, vomiting, altered level of consciousness, signs of increased intracranial pressure)
   6. Measure head circumference daily and watch for signs of shunt malfunction (enlarging head size, signs of increased intracranial pressure)
   7. Strict maintenance of fluid intake as ordered; strict monitoring of I & O, urine specific gravity, serum electrolytes

TABLE 11–2 Neurological Status Assessment

Vital signs	Temperature, pulse, respiration, blood pressure
Pupils	*Size*—normal, constricted, dilated
	2 3 4 5 6 7 8 9 mm
	Equal or unequal size
	Reaction to light—brisk, sluggish, no reaction
Extremities	*Movement*—normal, weak, paralysis
	Strength—equal or unequal
Fontanelle	Normal, bulging, sunken
Level of Consciousness	*Alert*—interacts appropriately for age, eyes open, moves on command (older child)
	Confused—older child responds verbally but may be confused, infant has variety of verbal responses depending on age (smiles, babbles) but response may be diminished, eyes open spontaneously, tries to avoid painful stimulus
	Restless—older child uses inappropriate verbal responses, infant recognizes familiar faces or stares and cries depending on age, eyes open to sounds or speech, abnormal flexion in response to painful stimulus
	Semicomatose—speech incomprehensible in older child, infant cries when stimulated, eyes open to pain, abnormal extension in response to painful stimulus
	Comatose—no response

8. Administer pharmacological pain relief measures as ordered
9. Administer antibiotics as ordered to prevent infection from shunt

C. Encourage parents to discuss concerns about diagnosis and therapeutic regimen
D. Teach parents about home management, including care of incision, signs of shunt malformation or infection, encouraging normal growth and development within activity guidelines recommended, administration of prophylactic antibiotics if ordered
E. Refer to home health agency for follow-up care

V. Evaluation
A. Child's neurological status remains stable
B. Child tolerates small, frequent feedings of formula or foods
C. Child's skin on scalp remains intact, shows no evidence of decubitus ulcers
D. Child rests without evidence of discomfort
E. Postoperatively, child does not exhibit signs and symptoms of infection; neurological function returns to normal; no signs and symptoms of increased cranial pressure
F. Parents express fears about diagnosis and surgery and begin to cope effectively with help of health care team
G. Parents accurately state discharge instructions including describing signs of shunt malfunction or infection
H. Parents contact visiting nurses association for follow-up care

Spina Bifida (Myelodysplasia)
I. Assessment
A. Definition: congenital defect of neural tube; incomplete closure of vertebral column accompanied by varying degrees of protrusion of CNS contents through bony defect (Fig. 11-2)
 1. Spina bifida occulta: anomaly not visible externally, except possibly by dimple or hair tuft; seldom creates health problem
 2. Meningocele: sac-like cyst containing meninges and spinal fluid that protrudes through bony defect
 3. Myelomeningocele: herniated sac of meninges, spinal fluid, and portion of spinal cord and its nerves that protrudes through defect in vertebral column; most commonly occurs in lumbosacral region
B. Etiology/incidence
 1. Occurs in fourth week of embryonic development
 2. Exact cause unknown, possibly multifactorial inheritance pattern
 3. Familial incidence higher than general population
 4. Incidence highest in Great Britain
 5. One per 1000 live births in the United States
C. Predisposing/precipitating factors
 1. Environmental factors—poor nutrition, maternal age (younger than 20 or older than 35)

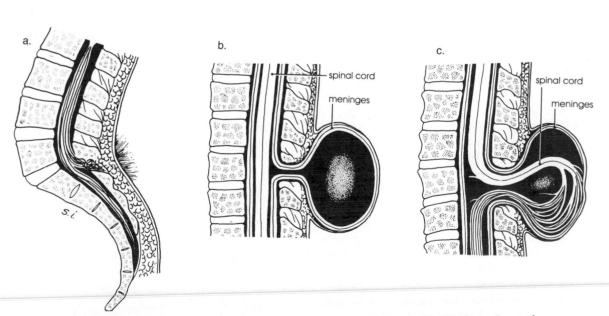

FIGURE 11–2. Spina bifida. *A*, Spina bifida occulta. *B*, Meningocele. *C*, Myelomeningocele. (From Marlow, D. R., and Redding, B. A. (1988). *Textbook of pediatric nursing*, 6th ed. Philadelphia: W. B. Saunders.)

2. Hereditary factors—first-born children at higher risk

D. Clinical manifestations
   1. Meningocele
      a. Sac-like structure located at any point on spinal column
      b. Positive transillumination
      c. Neurological function rarely interrupted
      d. Associated hydrocephalus may occur
   2. Myelomeningocele
      a. Sac-like structure located at any point on spinal column
      b. Flaccid paralysis of lower extremities with skeletal deformities of spine and lower extremities
      c. Varying degrees of motor, sensory, reflex, and sphincter dysfunction depending on location and severity of defect
      d. Associated hydrocephalus subsequent to Chiari type II malformation—downward displacement of cerebellum, medulla oblongata, and fourth ventricle, causing obstruction of CSF outflow

E. Diagnostic examinations
   1. Prenatal detection
      a. Ultrasound
      b. Alpha-fetoprotein elevations at 16 to 18 weeks' gestation
   2. Inspection of meningeal sac
   3. Identification of associated clinical findings—head circumference, motor and sensation, bowel-bladder function
   4. X-ray of spine
   5. CT scan, MRI

F. Complications
   1. Potential cognitive, perceptual, or attention deficits
   2. Impaired bowel/bladder control
   3. Partial or complete motor impairment
   4. Kyphosis, scoliosis
   5. Obesity

G. Medical management
   1. Orthopedic—may include exercises, casts, braces, surgical correction
   2. Urological—regular assisted bladder emptying (usually through clean, intermittent catheterization), medication to improve bladder tone and prevent incontinence, antibiotic treatment of urinary tract infection
   3. Bowel—dietary measures, stool softeners or suppositories
   4. Referral to multidisciplinary agency for management

H. Surgical management
   1. Closure of defect, possibly with skin grafts
   2. Placement of a shunt for hydrocephalus

II. Analysis
   A. Preoperative
      1. High risk for infection related to compromised integrity of sac
      2. High risk for altered cerebral perfusion related to hydrocephalus
      3. High risk for impaired skin integrity related to fragility of the sac
      4. High risk for altered nutrition: less than body requirements related to difficulty feeding
      5. Anticipatory grieving (parents) related to perceived loss of child's health
   B. Ongoing
      1. Impaired physical mobility related to neuromuscular deficits
      2. Altered patterns of urinary elimination related to absent or decreased bladder innervation
      3. Constipation related to neurological deficits
      4. High risk for infection: urinary tract related to urinary retention
      5. High risk for impaired skin integrity related to sensory deficits and immobility
      6. High risk for infection: CNS related to shunt placement
      7. Altered growth and development related to the effects of disability
      8. High risk for body image disturbance related to disability and chronic medical problems
      9. High risk for altered nutrition: more than body requirements related to decreased metabolic demands
      10. Altered family processes related to effects of child's disability

III. Planning/goals, expected outcomes
   A. Child will be free of infection
   B. Child will rest comfortably
   C. Child will not exhibit signs and symptoms of skin breakdown either preoperatively or postoperatively
   D. Child will have adequate nutrition and hydration for age
   E. Child will not exhibit signs and symptoms of increased intracranial pressure
   F. Child will be free of urinary tract infections
   G. Child will not exhibit lower extremity contractures
   H. Postoperatively, child will not exhibit signs and symptoms of infection at operative site,

increased intracranial pressure, or wound leakage

I. Parents will discuss fears and concerns about diagnosis, surgery, and long-term effects of disorder

J. Parents will understand home care before discharge

K. Parents will discuss fears and concerns about their future childbearing

L. Parents will contact home health agency for follow-up care

IV. Implementation

A. Inspect site for tears, leaking of CSF, and signs and symptoms of infection

B. Apply sterile saline-soaked dressing to the site; keep moist with periodic applications of additional saline; use barrier drape to protect site from stool or urine

C. Administer ordered antibiotics

D. Position off site
1. Turn every 2 hours side-prone-side
2. Place cloth rolls under hips to facilitate lower head position when prone
3. Place pads between legs for hip abduction and small roll under ankles to maintain neutral position when prone

E. Teach parents to handle child with care

F. Keep diaper off until site has been repaired and healed

G. Provide meticulous skin care; apply lotion to other areas of skin three times a day; inspect bony prominences for skin breakdown

H. Maintain strict I & O

I. Feed with head turned to the side; touch frequently during feeding

J. Encourage parents to express feelings of anger or grief; emphasize child's positive aspects; encourage parents to participate in child's care

K. Measure head circumference daily

L. Inspect fontanelles for fullness/bulging

M. Observe for signs and symptoms of increased intracranial pressure (see Table 11-1)

N. Empty bladder through intermittent catheterization

O. Provide passive range of motion every 4 hours; teach parents range of motion exercises

P. Explain to parents surgical procedure and possible effects
1. Skin grafting over sac
2. Shunting if associated hydrocephalus

Q. Prepare parents for developmental progress and where delays may occur

R. Teach parents about home care
1. Signs and symptoms of complications
2. Maintaining developmental progress

3. General care
a. Regular skin care with attention to pressure areas from braces or shoes
b. Clean intermittent catheterization
c. Facilitate mobility initially using a board or low casters, assistive ambulatory devices, wheelchair
d. Bowel elimination program
e. Protect from injury, particularly to lower extremities
f. Dietary restriction if indicated
g. Address emotional and developmental concerns

S. Refer to special agencies as needed, including genetic counselor

V. Evaluation

A. Child does not exhibit signs and symptoms of tears or infection at sac site

B. Child rests comfortably without signs and symptoms of discomfort

C. Child does not exhibit signs and symptoms of skin breakdown at bony prominence sites

D. Child's I & O essentially equal

E. Child tolerates small, frequent feedings of formula

F. Child's neurological status does not deteriorate preoperatively

G. Child does not exhibit signs and symptoms of urinary tract infection at any time (adequate urination, clear urine, not malodorous)

H. Child maintains adequate muscle tone and flexibility, no contractures

I. Parents can describe signs of shunt malfunction, CNS infection, urinary tract infection

J. Child maintains desirable weight

K. Child demonstrates appropriate achievement of developmental milestones within limits of disability

L. Parents discuss fears and concerns about diagnosis, surgery, and long-term effects of disorder and begin to cope effectively

M. Parents consult with genetic counselor

N. Parents contact appropriate support group and agencies for ongoing care

Seizure Disorders

I. Assessment

A. Definition: disturbance(s) of normal function of nerve cells; uncontrolled, spontaneous electrical activity of brain, which may cause loss of consciousness, altered body movements, or disturbances of sensation and behavior; chronic, recurrent seizures are referred to as epilepsy
1. Partial, focal seizures—electrical activity usually limited to one cerebral hemisphere

a. Simple partial seizures (motor, sensory, autonomic, or psychic symptoms)—child does not lose consciousness

b. Complex partial seizures—child loses consciousness secondary to simple partial seizure, or loses consciousness at start of seizure; may be preceded by an aura

c. Partial seizures, secondarily generalized

2. Generalized seizures—usually involve both hemispheres; bilateral motor symptoms; may involve loss of consciousness

a. Absence seizures—momentary loss of motor activity and awareness

b. Myoclonic—brief jerking of muscle groups

c. Clonic, tonic, or tonic-clonic—loss of consciousness followed by rigidity and extension of muscle groups (tonic), violent jerking (clonic), relaxation (postictal)

d. Atonic—unexpected loss of muscle tone and consciousness

B. Etiology/incidence
1. Most common in first 2 years of life, different causes more common at different ages
2. Perinatal hypoxia, birth trauma
3. Congenital malformations
4. Infection or metabolic disorders
5. Trauma, tumor, toxins (lead, drugs)
6. Cause unknown for most seizures after age 3
7. Occurs in 2% of general population under age 20
8. Febrile seizures—usually in children under 5 years; precipitated by moderate fever; neurologically benign

C. Predisposing/precipitating factors
1. Cellular dehydration
2. Hypoglycemia, hyperglycemia
3. Electrolyte imbalances
4. Fatigue
5. Emotional or physical stress
6. Endocrine changes

D. Clinical manifestations
1. Vary with seizures
2. Aura: unusual sensation that precedes seizure
3. Eye movement changes, staring in infants
4. Tonic and/or clonic movements bilaterally or unilaterally
5. Loss of consciousness
6. Incontinence

7. Postictal sleep, confusion, weakness or inactivity

E. Diagnostic examinations
1. Health history, physical examination, and description of seizure activity
2. EEG
3. Skull x-rays
4. CT scan, MRI
5. Lumbar puncture (see Table 10-10) for infants, children with suspected meningitis
6. Serum electrolytes
7. Blood glucose

F. Complications
1. Fractures, dislocations
2. Hypoxia
3. Acidosis
4. Increased intracranial pressure
5. Status epilepticus—prolonged seizures, no consciousness between

G. Medical management
1. Pharmacological—daily anticonvulsant therapy (Table 11-3) until 2 years after cessation of seizures; begin with one drug in gradually increasing doses until seizures stop or child experiences adverse effects, add others only if necessary; regular serum drug levels
2. Ketogenic (high fat) diet for intractable absence or myoclonic seizures
3. Status epilepticus
   a. IV diazepam (Valium) to stop seizures
   b. Respiratory support and oxygen if needed
   c. Treatment of underlying metabolic alterations

II. Analysis
A. High risk for injury related to involuntary muscle movements
B. Knowledge deficit about seizures and home management related to inadequate information
C. High risk for ineffective individual coping related to embarrassment, anxiety
D. High risk for altered family processes related to chronic nature of condition
E. High risk for altered growth and development related to parental overprotectiveness

III. Planning/goals, expected outcomes
A. Parent or child able to describe seizure activity
B. Child will not progress to status epilepticus
C. Child will not incur injury during seizure activity
D. Child's respiratory function will remain stable during seizure activity
E. Child will rest comfortably after seizure

TABLE 11–3 Medications Used to Treat Seizures

Example	Action	Use	Common Side Effects	Nursing Implications
Phenobarbital	Raises seizure threshold by increasing the threshold for electrical stimulation of the cortex	Status epilepticus, febrile seizures, tonic-clonic, simple partial motor seizures	Drowsiness, hyperactivity in young children, behavior alterations, altered cognitive and motor performance, rare allergic rash or blood dyscrasia	Monitor child for adverse reactions, encourage routine medication compliance to maintain steady serum level, has additive effect with other CNS depressants, toleration develops with continued use
Primidone (Mysoline)	Same as phenobarbital	Same as phenobarbital	Same as phenobarbital	Potentiates action of phenobarbital; dose should be increased slowly; CBC and liver functions every 6 months
Phenytoin (Dilantin)	Limitation of seizure propagation by alteration of sodium ion transport across neurons in the motor cortex	Tonic-clonic, complex partial	Ataxia, slurred speech, decreased coordination, nystagmus, gastrointestinal discomfort, rashes, rarely Stevens-Johnson syndrome or blood dyscrasias, connective tissue alterations including gingival hyperplasia, lymphadenopathy	Action may be altered by other drugs including phenobarbital and valproic acid, can interfere with effect of vitamin D and contraceptives, meticulous oral hygiene required, routine serum levels, call physician for any sign of adverse effects
Diazepam (Valium), clonazepam (Klonopin)	Sedative effect in limbic system, thalamus, and hypothalamus; fast acting when administered parenterally	Status epilepticus (diazepam), mixed seizure disorder (clonazepam)	Drowsiness, ataxia, confusion, hypotension, gastrointestinal irritation, urinary retention, rare skin rashes, abnormal liver function and blood dyscrasias when administered long-term	IV solution administered slowly—no faster than 1 ml/min; monitor for local irritation and phlebitis; caution when using with other anticonvulsants; frequent CBC and liver functions
Carbamazepine (Tegretol)	Anticonvulsant, exact mechanism unknown	Simple partial, complex partial, secondarily generalized tonic-clonic	Bone marrow depression possible, transient neutropenia frequently seen, allergic rashes, dizziness, drowsiness, nausea, vomiting	Complete blood studies before initiating drug; weekly during first 3 months, monthly thereafter; warn patient about signs of bone marrow depression; protect from infection

Table continued on following page

TABLE 11–3 Medications Used to Treat Seizures (*Continued*)

Example	Action	Use	Common Side Effects	Nursing Implications
Valproic acid (Depakene), divalproex sodium (Depakote)	Exact mechanism unknown	Absence, myoclonic, atonic, tonic-clonic, and mixed seizures	Alopecia, increased appetite with weight gain, rare hepatic toxicity and abnormal coagulation	Can potentiate effect of phenobarbital and alter serum levels of other seizure medications; perform liver function and coagulation studies before initiating drug and frequently thereafter
Ethosuximide (Zarontin)	Depresses motor cortex and suppresses electrical activity associated with lapses of consciousness	Absence seizures	Gastrointestinal irritation, headaches, hiccups, drowsiness, rare allergic skin rashes and blood dyscrasias	CBC and liver functions frequently; may increase tonic-clonic seizures

F. Child's seizure activity will be controlled by anticonvulsant drug therapy or other treatment modality

G. Child/parents will understand proper method of administering drug therapy

H. Child/parents will participate in teaching session on long-term therapy and problems associated with seizures

I. Parents will contact appropriate agency for support and follow-up care

IV. Implementation

A. Maintain accurate history and observation list of all seizure activity

1. Onset, including time, behaviors before and at time of seizure, loss of consciousness

2. Movement during seizure

3. Changes in facial appearance

4. Eye movement

5. Respirations

6. Incontinence

7. Postictal activities, including end time, state of consciousness, motor activities, memory

B. Protect child during seizure

1. DO NOT leave alone at any time

2. Place flat on floor if standing

3. Remove objects that might cause injury

4. Loosen restrictive clothing

5. Use padded side rails if bedridden

6. DO NOT use padded tongue blade if jaw clenched

C. Provide quiet environment during and after seizure

D. Maintain patent airway at all times

1. Turn head to side during seizure

2. Keep oxygen, suction set-up in room or at home at all times

E. Administer anticonvulsants as ordered (see Table 11-3)

F. Administer ketogenic diet if ordered

1. Restrictive of protein and carbohydrate intake

2. 80% caloric requirements in fat

G. Instruct child/parents in proper administration of drug and diet therapy

H. Coordinate multidisciplinary meeting with family to discuss home care and long-term care

I. Instruct parents to schedule conference with school teachers about particular type of seizure, what to expect, what to do and not to do; encourage parents to promote appropriate developmental activities

J. Provide opportunity for child/parents to express fears and concerns

K. Refer to local chapter of National Epilepsy Foundation

V. Evaluation

A. Parents give accurate description of seizure

B. Child's seizures recorded accurately by parents at home

C. Child free of injury during seizure activity

D. Child does not exhibit signs and symptoms of respiratory difficulties during seizure activity

E. Child rests comfortably after seizure activity

F. Child's seizure activity remains controlled

G. Child/parents give return demonstration of medication administration before discharge and describe any diet modifications

H. Family participates in teaching session on seizures and long-term effects and is beginning to cope effectively

I. Family participates in support group initiated and run by National Epilepsy Foundation

Infectious Disorders

Bacterial Meningitis

I. Assessment

A. Definition: inflammation of meninges; potentially fatal disease that can follow infection from anywhere in body

B. Etiology/incidence

1. *Hemophilus influenzae, Streptococcus pneumoniae,* or *Neisseria meningitidis* causative agents in 95% of cases in children older than 2 months

2. Highest incidence in ages 6 to 12 months

3. Males have greater incidence than females

C. Predisposing/precipitating factors

1. Premature rupture of membranes (maternal)

2. Maternal infection during last weeks of pregnancy

3. Prolonged labor

4. Excessive manipulation during labor

5. Immunoglobulin deficiencies in child

6. Sickle cell anemia

7. Primary infections in body

8. CNS anomalies

9. Inadequate vaccination against *H. influenzae*

D. Clinical manifestations

1. Neonates
   a. Poor sucking reflex
   b. Feeding difficulties
   c. Diarrhea
   d. Vomiting
   e. Decreased movement
   f. Poor temperature control

2. Infants/young children
   a. Fever
   b. Poor feeding, resistance to being held
   c. Vomiting
   d. Irritability, cries when legs lifted for diaper change
   e. Bulging fontanelles
   f. Nuchal rigidity
   g. Lethargy
   h. Seizures

3. Childhood/adolescence
   a. Fever
   b. Headache
   c. Vomiting
   d. Seizures
   e. Photophobia
   f. Drowsiness
   g. Agitation
   h. Nuchal rigidity, opisthotonos posture
   i. Positive Kernig's sign—resistance to knee extension in supine position
   j. Positive Brudzinski's sign—flexion of knees and hips when neck is flexed
   k. Rash with meningococcal meningitis

E. Diagnostic examinations

1. Lumbar puncture shows increased CSF pressure (more than 160 mm H_2O); cloudy fluid with increased white blood cells, primarily polymorphonuclear (1000 to 10,000/mm^3); decreased glucose

2. CSF Gram-stain for organisms

3. Blood culture, complete blood count, electrolytes

4. CT scan for complications

F. Complications

1. Peripheral circulatory collapse (Waterhouse-Friderichsen syndrome)

2. Intravascular coagulation with marked thrombocytopenia

3. CSF obstruction

4. Inappropriate ADH secretion

5. Seizures

6. Long-term cognitive, perceptual, language, attention deficits

7. Death

G. Medical management

1. Respiratory isolation for 24 to 48 hours after starting antibiotics

2. Dexamethasone (anti-inflammatory) given immediately after diagnosis and before antibiotics

3. IV antibiotics for 5 to 10 days depending on causative organism—ampicillin or cefotaxime for infants younger than 3 months, ceftriaxone or cefotaxime for children older than 3 months

4. Fever and fluid management

5. Treatment of seizures (see Table 11-3)

6. Prophylactic treatment of contacts if indicated (e.g., rifampin for *H. influenzae*)
7. Follow-up developmental testing

II. Analysis
   A. Pain related to inflammation
   B. Fluid volume deficit or excess related to vomiting or inappropriate ADH secretion
   C. Hyperthermia related to infectious process
   D. Sensory/perceptual alterations related to neurological disease
   E. High risk for injury related to seizures or complications of disease
   F. Fear/anxiety related to seriousness of the condition
   G. High risk for altered growth and development related to neurological deficits

III. Planning/goals, expected outcomes
   A. Child will not transmit disease to others
   B. Child will maintain stable neurological status
   C. Child will not regress developmentally during course of treatment
   D. Child will be free of complications
   E. Child will have adequate nutrition and hydration for age
   F. Child will be free of injury if seizures occur
   G. Child/parents will discuss diagnosis and therapeutic regimen
   H. Child/parents will express concerns about diagnosis and therapeutic regimen

IV. Implementation
   A. Obtain accurate history of presenting signs and symptoms; take baseline head circumference on infants and daily thereafter
   B. Assist with diagnostic procedures
   C. Assist with lumbar puncture (see Table 10-10)
   D. Administer antibiotics as ordered (see Table 10-2)
   E. Maintain respiratory isolation; touch and talk to child frequently
   F. Perform neurological checks every 30 minutes to 1 hour initially and every 2 to 4 hours subsequently
   G. Observe for signs of increasing intracranial pressure
   H. Maintain quiet environment, acetaminophen for pain relief
   I. Monitor for signs and symptoms of shock (decreasing blood pressure, increasing pulse, thirst)
   J. Maintain strict I & O
   K. Check weight daily
   L. Maintain NPO initially, then advance diet as tolerated
   M. Administer IV fluids as ordered
   N. Observe for seizures, maintain seizure precautions, if applicable
      1. Padded side rails
      2. Oxygen at bedside
      3. Suction set-up at bedside
      4. No padded tongue blades
   O. Explain all diagnostic/therapeutic procedures to child/parents
   P. Allow child/parents opportunity to express feelings about diagnosis and therapeutic regimen
   Q. Refer for follow-up developmental evaluation

V. Evaluation
   A. Child demonstrates age-appropriate behaviors while isolated
   B. Child's neurological status remains within normal limits without deterioration
   C. Child rests comfortably with minimal pain
   D. Child does not regress developmentally during course of treatment
   E. Child does not exhibit signs and symptoms of complications
   F. Child resumes normal diet
   G. Child's I & O essentially equal
   H. Child does not exhibit signs and symptoms of seizure activity
   I. Child/parents express concerns about diagnosis and demonstrate effective coping with course of treatment provided and prognosis

Reye's Syndrome

I. Assessment
   A. Definition: acute, toxic encephalopathy with fatty degeneration of viscera
   B. Etiology/incidence
      1. Toxin-viral reaction theory
      2. Hepatic failure with ammonia intoxication theory
      3. Peak incidence between 6 and 11 years
      4. Peak incidence from November to March
   C. Predisposing/precipitating factors
      1. Antecedent influenza or chickenpox outbreak; child appears to recover, then symptoms begin with protracted vomiting and rapid deterioration
      2. Salicylate (aspirin) ingestion during viral infection
   D. Clinical manifestations
      1. Stage I: drowsiness, vomiting, lethargy
      2. Stage II: disorientation, aggressiveness, combativeness, hyperreactive reflexes, hyperventilation, stupor
      3. Stage III: coma, decorticate posturing, dilated pupils
      4. Stage IV: deepening coma, decerebrate posturing; dilated, fixed pupils
      5. Stage V: cessation of respirations, seizures, flaccidity, flat EEG
   E. Diagnostic examinations

1. Elevated SGOT (normal, 8 to 20 U/L), SGPT (normal, 8 to 20 U/L), LDH (normal, 60 to 170 U/L)
   2. Serum ammonia elevated above 125 to 150 μg/dL
   3. Prothrombin time prolonged
   4. Serum glucose decreased
   5. CT scan
   6. EEG becomes slow and dysrhythmic
F. Complications: long-term neurological deficits, mortality related to stage at diagnosis and treatment
G. Medical management
   1. Varies with stage of illness, usually in intensive care unit
   2. Includes controlling cerebral edema with fluid restriction and osmotic diuretics, correcting metabolic imbalances, IV glucose for hypoglycemia, anticonvulsants (Table 11-3) for seizures

II. Analysis
A. Altered cerebral perfusion related to cerebral edema
B. Sensory/perceptual alterations related to elevated serum ammonia and cerebral edema
C. High risk for injury related to altered clotting and seizures
D. Anxiety/fear related to seriousness of disease, unfamiliarity with intensive care unit equipment or routines
E. High risk for altered growth and development related to neurological sequelae

III. Planning/goals, expected outcomes
A. Child's symptoms will be recognized immediately
B. Family will understand the necessity for intensive care
C. Child will rest comfortably and not be frightened by intensive care unit equipment or routines
D. Child's neurological status will remain stable or improve
E. Child will not sustain any injury
F. Child will maintain adequate nutrition and hydration for age
G. Child will demonstrate adequate oxygenation
H. Child/parents will understand diagnosis, therapeutic regimen, and prognosis
I. Child/parents will express fears and concerns about diagnosis and prognosis

IV. Implementation
A. Assist with diagnosis by accurate history and physical examination
B. Move to intensive care unit immediately
C. Assist with necessary procedures, i.e., intubation
D. Perform neurological checks every hour and as needed
E. Monitor for signs and symptoms of increased intracranial pressure, elevate head of bed slightly, disturb child as little as possible, place on hypothermia pad if ordered
F. Maintain seizure precautions, if applicable
G. Auscultate lungs every 2 hours
H. Maintain patent airway/respiratory function at all times
I. Maintain strict I & O
J. Administer and monitor IV fluids closely
K. Keep child NPO
L. Administer feedings via nasogastric tube as ordered
M. Measure specific gravity, sugar, and acetone every void
N. Measure intracranial pressure every 2 hours
O. Re-orient recovering child gradually
   1. Encourage parents to bring to intensive care unit favorite toy, photo, or tape player, or radio with soothing music or quiet story read in familiar voices
   2. If not comatose, schedule activities around sleep-wake patterns
P. Allow parents opportunity to discuss diagnosis, therapeutic regimen, and prognosis with health care team
Q. Consult social worker for discharge plans

V. Evaluation
A. Child demonstrates minimal anxiety, coping responses appropriate for age
B. Child rests comfortably without complaints of pain
C. Child recovers without sequelae as a result of early diagnosis and management
D. Child does not exhibit signs and symptoms of increased intracranial pressure or cerebral edema
E. Child does not exhibit signs and symptoms of seizure activity
F. Child maintains adequate oxygenation, blood gases, and oxygen saturation within normal limits
G. Child's nutritional requirements met for age
H. Child's fluid balance maintained without complications
I. Parents verbalize feelings about diagnosis and prognosis and begin to cope effectively
J. Parents participate in counseling sessions with social worker until child out of danger

Craniocerebral Trauma

I. Assessment
A. Definition: any pathological process or injury involving scalp, skull, meninges, or brain as

result of some mechanical force; may be localized or generalized
B. Etiology/incidence
1. Birth injuries
2. Falls
3. Motor vehicle accidents
4. Sports injuries
5. Physical abuse
6. Approximately 200,000 children admitted
yearly to hospital for neurological work-
up secondary to head trauma
7. Motor vehicle accidents highest cause of
fatal head injury in all age groups
8. Highest incidence in adolescents
9. 2 : 1 male to female ratio
C. Predisposing/precipitating factors
1. Age
2. Level of activity
3. Knowledge of safety recommendations
D. Clinical manifestations
1. Vary according to injury
a. Resiliency of skull
b. Area of primary injury
c. Extent of secondary injury (cerebral
edema, increased intracranial pressure, post-traumatic sequelae)
d. Time manifestations appear, e.g., rapidly with concussion, gradually with
subdural hematoma
2. Loss of consciousness varying in degree
from brief to prolonged
3. Memory loss of events before and after
injury
4. Headache
5. Pallor
6. Nausea, vomiting
7. Irritability, confusion
8. Cranial nerve deficits
9. Increased intracranial pressure
10. Weakness in extremities
11. Changes in vital signs
12. Changes in pupils
13. Outward bleeding from site, ears, nose;
clear drainage from ears or nose
E. Diagnostic examinations
1. Accurate neurological assessment, including vital signs, level of consciousness, neurological signs (see Table 11-2),
balance, assessment of cranial nerve
function
2. Skull x-ray
3. Echoencephalography
4. CT scan, MRI
5. Cerebral angiography
6. Subdural tap
F. Complications
1. Cerebral hemorrhage

2. Infection
3. Cerebral edema
4. Tentorial herniation
5. Seizures
G. Medical/surgical management: dependent on
type and extent of injury but directed toward
controlling cerebral edema, maintaining life
functions, preventing increased intracranial
pressure
II. Analysis
A. Altered cerebral perfusion related to edema
and inflammatory process
B. High risk for sensory/perceptual alterations
related to injury
C. High risk for altered growth and development related to residual neurological deficits
D. Anxiety related to the seriousness of the
trauma
E. Knowledge deficit about accident prevention
and post-traumatic sequelae related to unfa-
miliarity with information
III. Planning/goals, expected outcomes
A. Child will maintain adequate cerebral per-
fusion
B. Child will be free of bodily harm secondary
to manifestations of head trauma
C. Child will not exhibit deterioration of neuro-
logical status
D. Child will have no complaints of pain
E. Child will rest comfortably at all times
F. Child's nutritional status will be stable
G. Child will not exhibit signs and symptoms of
dehydration or overhydration
H. Child will not exhibit signs and symptoms of
complications
I. Child/parents will express feelings of anxiety
or concern
J. Child/parents will understand signs and
symptoms of complications, pertinent prin-
ciples of injury prevention
IV. Implementation
A. Monitor neurological status every 30 minutes
initially, then every 1 to 2 hours and as
needed (see Table 11-2)
B. Prepare child and assist with diagnostic pro-
cedures
C. Maintain bedrest with head of bed flat to ele-
vated 30 degrees; provide quiet environment
with minimal stimulation
D. Keep side rails up at all times
E. Monitor vital signs and neurological status
every 1 to 2 hours
F. Maintain patent airway at all times; turn and
reposition every 2 hours
G. Monitor for seizure activity
H. Monitor for behavioral changes

I. Check drainage from orifices with Dextrostix for presence of CSF (glucose positive)
J. Maintain NPO initially, then advance diet as tolerated
K. Maintain strict I & O
L. Measure specific gravity, sugar, and acetone every void
M. Check weight daily
N. Administer and monitor IV therapy as ordered
O. Medicate for pain as ordered (see Table 10-19) without altering level of consciousness; avoid respiratory depressants such as morphine sulfate
P. Obtain CBC, electrolytes, and blood gases as needed
Q. Monitor for signs and symptoms of infection at wound site, shock, increased intracranial pressure or cerebral edema
R. Administer corticosteroids as ordered (see Table 10-8)
S. Allow child/parents opportunity to express concerns and fears about injury and therapeutic regimen
T. Teach parents how to assess neurological status and proper administration of medications
U. Arrange for follow-up care; review principles of accident prevention

V. Evaluation
A. Child demonstrates stable neurological status, no cerebral edema or increased intracranial pressure
B. Child remains quiet and calm
C. Child remains appropriately oxygenated—normal blood gases and oxygen saturation
D. Child does not complain of pain
E. Child rests comfortably at all times
F. Child's diet advances daily without complications
G. Child does not exhibit signs and symptoms of dehydration or overhydration
H. Child does not develop complications secondary to head trauma
I. Parents cope effectively with accident and course of treatment
J. Child/parents accurately state discharge instructions
K. Parents arrange for follow-up care with private physician

Brain Tumors

I. Assessment
A. Definition: masses of cells that proliferate abnormally; may be benign or malignant
   1. Astrocytoma: located in cerebellum; slow-growing; generally can be excised if well defined
   2. Medulloblastoma: located in cerebellum; fast-growing malignancy; complete excision usually not possible; along with astrocytoma, the most common of childhood brain tumors
   3. Brain stem glioma: located in brain stem; cannot be excised due to surrounding vital centers of brain; affects cranial nerves
B. Etiology/incidence
   1. Proliferation of cancer cells that can originate in nerve cells, neuroepithelium, glia, cranial nerves, blood vessels, pineal gland, and hypophysis
   2. Up to 65% located posterior fossa (infratentorial)
   3. Supratentorial tumors, relatively rare in children, include craniopharyngioma, optic glioma
   4. Male/female ratio varies in relation to specific tumors
   5. Diagnosis most frequently made between ages 5 and 10, but can occur at any age
   6. Second only to leukemia as cause of illness-related deaths in children
C. Predisposing/precipitating factors
   1. Genetic syndromes such as neurofibromatosis
   2. Exposure of parents to carcinogens before conception or during pregnancy
   3. Environmental exposures such as radiation, industrial pollutants, drugs
D. Clinical manifestations vary with location and size of tumor
   1. Headaches
   2. Diplopia, nystagmus, papilledema, signs of cranial nerve involvement
   3. Nausea and vomiting
   4. Ataxia, loss of balance, muscle weakness
   5. Behavioral changes
   6. Irritability, restlessness
   7. Signs and symptoms of increased intracranial pressure
   8. Seizures
   9. Cranial enlargement (up to 18 months)
E. Diagnostic examinations
   1. Complete neurological assessment, including EEG
   2. Fundoscopic examination
   3. CT scan, MRI
   4. Angiography
   5. Myelography
   6. Tissue biopsy, surgical exploration
F. Complications
   1. Generally poor prognosis for 5-year survival except when tumor can be com-

pletely excised, or for medulloblastoma (77%)

2. With radiation or chemotherapy, improved survival, but adverse effects (see Chapter 10)

3. Long-term neurological deficits

G. Medical/surgical management: surgical removal of tumor followed in most cases by radiation and/or chemotherapy

II. Analysis

A. Preoperative

1. Altered cerebral perfusion related to internal pressure of growing tumor

2. High risk for sensory/perceptual alterations related to location of tumor

3. High risk for injury related to sensory/perceptual alterations or seizure activity

4. High risk for altered growth and development related to residual neurological deficits

5. Anxiety related to the seriousness of the prognosis

6. Knowledge deficit about condition, diagnostic studies, and treatment related to unfamiliarity with information

B. Postoperative—related to neurosurgical procedure

1. High risk for altered cerebral tissue perfusion related to edema from neurosurgical insult

2. Pain related to surgery

3. High risk for fluid volume deficit or excess related to fluid losses during surgery or inappropriate secretion of ADH

4. High risk for injury related to altered consciousness or seizures

5. High risk for infection related to operative access to CNS

6. High risk for body image disturbance related to change in appearance

7. Knowledge deficit about home management and additional treatment related to anxiety and unfamiliarity with information

8. High risk for anticipatory grieving related to perceived loss of child

9. High risk for altered growth and development related to long-term neurological deficits

III. Planning/goals, expected outcomes

A. Child will remain free of injury

B. Child/parents will understand all diagnostic procedures

C. Child's neurological status will not deteriorate

D. Child's fluid balances will remain stable

E. Child/parents will understand the need for craniotomy, if required

F. Child's neurological status will remain stable postoperatively, without complications

G. Child/parents will accept the need for radiation or chemotherapy, if applicable

H. Child/parents will understand instructions for discharge and follow-up care

I. Child will resume normal activities within limitations

J. Child will resume educational activities at home or school

K. If prognosis poor, family will seek emotional support before discharge

L. Family will contact appropriate resources for home care or hospice care

IV. Implementation

A. Perform accurate neurological assessment, with neurological checks every 2 to 4 hours

B. Prepare child for diagnostic tests as ordered

C. Obtain consents as necessary

D. Monitor for signs and symptoms of increased intracranial pressure

E. Maintain strict I & O

F. Obtain specific gravity, sugar, and acetone every void

G. Administer and monitor IV fluids closely

H. Prepare for craniotomy

1. Shaving of head

2. Bandaged head postoperatively

I. Postoperative care

1. Perform vital signs and neurological checks every 30 minutes initially, then every hour

2. Report any changes immediately

3. Observe dressing for drainage

4. DO NOT change dressing

5. Keep flat in bed to slight elevation depending on type of surgery and location of tumor

6. Turn every 2 hours, avoiding operative side

7. Deep breathe every 1 to 2 hours

8. NPO to clear liquids to advance diet as tolerated

9. Monitor IV fluids

10. Maintain strict I & O; weigh child daily

11. Maintain quiet, restful environment

12. Monitor for signs of CNS infection (see section on meningitis) or increased intracranial pressure

13. Administer analgesics as ordered

J. Administer chemotherapy as ordered (see Table 10-11)

K. Teach child/parents discharge home care

L. Refer to appropriate agencies for follow-up care

M. Provide emotional support

N. Assist family in developing coping mechanisms to handle inevitable death of child, if applicable

O. Assist family in grieving process

V. Evaluation

A. Child does not exhibit signs of increased intracranial pressure or neurological deficits

B. Child/parents accurately describe procedures and preparation necessary

C. Child rests quietly with minimal discomfort

D. Child does not exhibit signs and symptoms of dehydration or overhydration; urinary output 1 mL per kg per hour, normal specific gravity

E. Child/parents accurately state purpose of surgery and expectations postoperatively

F. Child's neurological status remains stable postoperatively

G. Child does not show signs of infection

H. Child does not exhibit signs and symptoms of complications postoperatively

I. Child/parents accurately state purposes of radiation or chemotherapy and ask questions when necessary

J. Child/parents accurately describe home care and follow-up regimen

K. Child scheduled to have home-bound teacher for 1 month, then return to school

L. Child/family participate in death/dying sessions and begin to cope effectively with child's prognosis, if applicable

Cerebral Palsy

I. Assessment

A. Definition: collective term describing group of nonprogressive disabilities characterized by spastic/involuntary movements, abnormal muscle tone, and incoordination

1. Spastic: most common type; upper motor neuron involvement; hypertonicity of various muscle groups, most commonly hemiplegia, quadriplegia, diplegia

2. Dyskinetic/athetoid: abnormal, involuntary, slow, writhing movements; aggravated by stress, disappear in sleep

3. Ataxic: least common type; balance disturbances

4. Wide range of intellectual function from superior intelligence to moderately impaired

B. Etiology/incidence

1. Two per 1000 live births

2. Most common developmental disability in childhood

C. Predisposing/precipitating factors

1. Prematurity, low birth weight

2. Developmental brain anomalies

3. Difficult labor/birth resulting in perinatal asphyxia

4. Birth trauma or injury

5. Encephalitis, meningitis

6. Prenatal infection or metabolic disturbance

D. Clinical manifestations

1. Developmental delays, particularly in gross and fine motor skills

2. Spasticity, may be noticed first when diapering infant

3. Clumsiness, lack of coordination

4. Abnormal posturing, scissoring of legs, flexion of extremities

5. Irritability

6. Poor sucking reflex, persistent tongue thrust causing feeding difficulties

7. Persistence of infantile reflexes

8. Facial grimacing, abnormal writhing movements

9. Seizures

E. Diagnostic examinations

1. No specific tests

2. Based on physical findings of muscle tone and accurate prenatal, perinatal, neonatal history

F. Complications

1. Debilitating respiratory disease

2. Contractures in severe forms

G. Medical/surgical management

1. Goals: provide optimal motor and communication skills, prevent and correct associated disabilities, facilitate independence in self-care activities

2. Approaches: physical, occupational, and speech therapy; use of orthopedic and mobilizing devices, surgery to correct contractures; nutritional support; seizure control if needed

II. Analysis

A. Impaired physical mobility related to neuromuscular deficit

B. Altered growth and development related to physical disability

C. Altered nutrition: less than body requirements related to feeding difficulties

D. High risk for impaired verbal communication related to poor oromotor control or underlying neurological processing deficit

E. High risk for aspiration related to impaired swallowing or gag reflexes

F. Altered family processes related to child's long-term disability

G. High risk for self-esteem disturbance related to altered function

H. Knowledge deficit about condition and its management related to lack of information

III. Planning/goals, expected outcomes
A. Child will respond well to early intervention
B. Parents will express positive feelings about child and adjustment to diagnosis
C. Child/parents will seek appropriate agencies as required
D. Child will begin to achieve independence within age and physical limitations
E. Child will maintain optimal nutrition at all times
F. Child will not develop contractures
G. Child will not incur injury secondary to motor disabilities
H. Child will have intact skin and remain free of skin breakdown
I. Child's speech patterns will develop normally or child able to use auxiliary form of communication
J. Child will demonstrate adequate respiratory function
K. Parents will demonstrate therapy techniques
L. Child/parents will seek counseling for long-term effects of cerebral palsy

IV. Implementation
A. Obtain accurate developmental history
B. Arrange for multidisciplinary meeting with parents to discuss diagnosis, treatment, prognosis
C. Arrange occupational therapy, physical therapy, speech therapy, and ophthalmological and hearing consultation
D. Coordinate all activities for family
E. Teach parents child's limitations and encourage them to allow child independence within these limitations; focus on child's positive attributes
F. Provide dietary consultation
G. Maintain calorie count and I & O daily
H. Feed slowly
I. Modify feeding technique to compensate tongue thrust
J. Use specially designed eating utensils
K. Apply braces as ordered; provide meticulous skin care
L. Use proper body alignment when positioning
M. Provide range of motion exercises three times a day and as needed
N. Provide assistive devices for movement as required
O. Use safety precautions and equipment when ambulating
P. Encourage parents to demonstrate how to facilitate child's communication patterns
Q. Refer to appropriate agencies such as Easter Seals for long-term counseling

V. Evaluation
A. Parents bring child for regular well care and can identify child's positive attributes
B. Child/parents participate in multidisciplinary meeting discussing feeling and fears about diagnosis and long-term care
C. Child/parents seek assistance from appropriate therapists
D. Child begins to participate in self-care and self-feeding when appropriate developmentally
E. Child's growth appropriate for age
F. Child does not exhibit contractures
G. Child free of injuries secondary to ambulation
H. Child's skin integrity maintained
I. Child's speech develops appropriately or child becomes adept at alternate means of communication
J. Child does not experience problems related to hearing or vision deficits
K. Family enrolls in support group for children with cerebral palsy

POST-TEST Neurological Disorders

Newborn Sean is transferred to the children's unit from the nursery shortly after birth because he was born with myelomeningocele diagnosed during his mother's pregnancy. Sean's father accompanied him to the children's unit but cannot stay because he needs to return home to care for 2-year-old Cathy. When Sean's mother is released from the hospital, she will stay with Sean.

---

1. When assessing Sean, his nurse notes that he has a protruding sac in his lumbosacral area. He is alert and crying; he is moving upper, but not lower, extremities. His head circumference is above the 95th percentile, and his vital signs are within normal limits for a newborn. He is placed in an isolette. Which of the following diagnoses might the nurse consider a priority for intervention?
   ① Pain
   ② High risk for altered nutrition: less than body requirements
   ③ High risk for infection
   ④ High risk for injury

2. Which of the following would have suggested to the obstetrician that Sean's mother might be carrying an infant with spina bifida?
   ① Elevated alpha-fetoprotein, abnormal ultrasound

② Decreased alpha-fetoprotein, normal ultrasound

③ Abnormal chromosome analysis, normal ultrasound

④ Abnormal ultrasound, abnormal chromosome analysis

3. Which of the following would NOT be part of the nursing care for an infant with a myelomeningocele?
   ① Turn infant every 2 hours side-prone-side
   ② Measure head circumference daily
   ③ Inspect sac frequently for tears or redness
   ④ Apply a soft diaper to cover the site

4. Sean is found to have an associated hydrocephalus, from a Chiari type II malformation, and a decision is made to implant a ventriculoperitoneal shunt at the same time as closure of the sac. Which of the following clinical manifestations postoperatively might indicate a malfunctioning shunt?
   ① Irritability, opisthotonos posture, high fever
   ② Bulging fontanelle, seizures, feeding difficulties
   ③ Lethargy, sunset eyes, increased pulse
   ④ Feeding difficulties, irritability, tense fontanelle

5. Because Sean's parents were prepared ahead of time for Sean's diagnosis, they were able to prepare Cathy for Sean's problems. Which of the following explanations to Cathy would indicate an accurate understanding and acceptance of Sean's disabilities?
   ① "The baby is very sick and is never going to get much better, but we will love him anyway."
   ② "The baby might not be able to run and do everything you can, but we are going to help him play and do things his way."
   ③ "We can't let him do too many things because we do not want him to hurt himself trying things he can't do."
   ④ "We don't need to worry much about the baby's problems because he looks just like any other beautiful baby."

A 16-year-old girl was brought to the hospital emergency department by a passing motorist after having fallen off her bike. She was responding but seemed confused and didn't remember much about the accident. She tells the nurse her name is Lucia, but she doesn't remember her last name.

6. The nurse performs an initial neurological check on Lucia and notes the following: opens eyes to look around although seems confused; blood pressure is 120/70 mm Hg; pulse, 86; temperature, 99.2°F; vomited once; slight headache. Which of the following might indicate worsening of Lucia's condition?
   ① Continued vomiting, increased pulse, opening eyes on command
   ② Restlessness, widening pulse pressure, garbled speech
   ③ Irritability, decreased blood pressure and pulse, constricted pupils
   ④ Fever, continued vomiting, dizziness

7. Lucia is admitted to the pediatric unit and her parents are finally located. Her condition improves and stabilizes after 48 hours, and she is ready to be discharged. Expected goals for Lucia and her parents are that they will be able to:
   ① Describe signs of post-traumatic syndrome and bicycle safety principles
   ② Watch for signs of infection, and administer medication safely
   ③ Perform a complete neurological check, and help Lucia remember details of the accident
   ④ Manage seizures, and limit Lucia's participation in sports

8. Mrs. Karl has brought her 18-month-old daughter to the emergency department after the child suffered a seizure at home. The child's temperature is 104°F, and the diagnosis is a febrile seizure. Which of the following should the nurse teach Mrs. Karl concerning fever control?
   ① Give the child aspirin every 4 hours for temperature over 101°F
   ② Bathe the child with cold water mixed with alcohol for high fevers
   ③ Dress the child in lightweight clothes that allow evaporation
   ④ Continue sponge baths for at least 1 hour

9. Altered nutrition with less than body requirements is a nursing diagnosis often made for children with cerebral palsy. Which of the following etiological factors support this diagnosis?
   ① Difficulty controlling muscles for chewing and swallowing
   ② Change in sensation of taste that makes them picky eaters
   ③ Gastrointestinal impairments that decrease absorption of nutrients
   ④ Frequent periods of vomiting caused by muscle spasm

10. Which of the following information would it be most important for the nurse to obtain from the parents of a child admitted with cerebral palsy?
    ① Whether they use restraints at home for the tremors
    ② Methods and utensils best used for feeding
    ③ Whether the child needs someone at the bedside continually
    ④ Special instructions related to skin care

Jaamal is a 7-year-old boy who was admitted to the hospital for status epilepticus. He is treated and stabilized in the emergency department and transferred to the pediatric unit for further evaluation of his seizure disorder.

---

11. Which of the following is an appropriate nursing intervention for the child who has just experienced a tonic-clonic seizure?
    ① Encourage coughing and deep breathing
    ② Increase fluid intake
    ③ Provide reduced environmental stimuli
    ④ Administer a 10% glucose solution as ordered

12. Which of the following would be an appropriate plan for Jaamal before his scheduled EEG?
    ① Limit the amount of sleep before the test
    ② Increase oral fluids before the test
    ③ Administer laxatives before the test
    ④ Shave sections of his head for the test

13. Jaamal is discharged from the hospital with instructions for taking phenobarbital and phenytoin (Dilantin) to control his seizures. He is being monitored at the outpatient clinic. Which of the following indicates that the discharge instructions are being followed?
    ① His serum levels vary widely at each visit
    ② His oral mucous membranes are intact
    ③ He avoids contact with children who are sick
    ④ His diet is high in fiber

14. What is a primary method of preventing and controlling the incidence of bacterial meningitis in infants and children?
    ① Keeping infants and young children away from crowded places
    ② Administering antimeningitis vaccines during outbreaks
    ③ Immediately isolating all children suspected of having meningitis
    ④ Routinely giving infants *H. influenzae* vaccine

15. Children in stage I of Reye's syndrome may exhibit vomiting, lethargy, and sleepiness. In light of the mild nature of these symptoms, the rationale for their admission to the intensive care unit is that:
    ① Supportive care in the intensive care unit can ensure rapid treatment when the disease progresses rapidly
    ② Need to maintain fluid levels to one and a half maintenance fluid levels
    ③ Central venous pressure and intracranial pressure monitoring must be started as soon as the diagnosis is made
    ④ Stage I is the most dangerous stage, and continuous monitoring is needed for the child

POST-TEST Answers and Rationales

1. ③ Because the cystic sac in children with myelomeningocele includes meninges, spinal cord and nerves, and CSF, any compromise to the sac would give an entry point into the central nervous system for infectious organisms. The potential for infection is of primary concern. Infants with myelomeningocele in the lumbosacral region usually have sensory deficits, so pain is not a priority. The others are potential problems for these infants, but lower in priority than infection. 2, II. Spina Bifida.

2. ① An elevated alpha-fetoprotein level at 14 to 16 weeks of pregnancy combined with an abnormal prenatal ultrasound showing an alteration in the spinal area are reasonably diagnostic. Children with spina bifida usually do not have chromosome abnormalities. 3, II. Spina Bifida.

3. ④ It is very important to avoid irritation to the delicate tissue over the spinal nerves in the myelomeningocele. The other options are appropriate actions when caring for the infant. 4, II. Spina Bifida.

4. ④ The first signs of increased intracranial pressure related to shunt malformation in an infant include feeding difficulties, irritable behavior, and tensing of the fontanelle. Fever is not usually associated with increased intracranial pressure, although it is often present after surgery. The other symptoms are more applicable to a hydrocephalus that has been present for a period of time. 1, II. Hydrocephalus.

5. ② Explaining about a sibling's problems to a 2-year-old is difficult and should be related to her own experience. Explaining things in nonthreatening terms and without overwhelming with too much information is the goal. Two-year-olds can understand and relate to play and activity. Recognizing that a child with spina bifida will not be able to do everything as other children would but can do many things in different ways is an important step toward acceptance. 5, III. Spina Bifida.

6. ② Restlessness and garbled speech indicate a deterioration in level of consciousness, whereas widening pulse pressure suggests increasing intracranial pressure. Vomiting, headache, dizziness, elevated blood pressure, and irritability are signs of cranial trauma and may be signs of increased intracranial pressure but do not necessarily indicate a worsening of her status. 5, II. Craniocerebral Trauma.

7. ① Having parents understand and monitor for signs of post-traumatic syndrome, which may occur several months after an injury, and principles of injury prevention are appropriate goals for discharge planning for any child with craniocerebral trauma. The other goals are not appropriate for the condition or the child's age. 3, IV. Craniocerebral Trauma.

8. ③ The best way to control fever is to encourage evaporation so that heat is lost instead of held in. A sponge bath should be given for only about 20 minutes, and tepid water rather than alcohol should be used. Aspirin should not be given, only acetaminophen. 4, I. Seizures.

9. ① Persistent oral reflexes, poor breathing patterns, tongue thrust, excessive opening of the mouth, and drooling make it difficult for the child with cerebral palsy to eat well. 2, I. Cerebral Palsy.

10. ② It is important for the nurse to ascertain methods the family has used for feeding the child. The nurse should also find out if any special utensils are used so that the child's nutritional status will not suffer during the hospitalization. 1, I. Cerebral Palsy.

11. ③ It is important to decrease environmental stimuli so that the child can rest after the seizure. After regaining consciousness, the child may sleep for several hours. The other options are inappropriate. 4, II. Seizures.

12. ① Sleep deprivation may lower threshold for seizure activity and make it easier to identify abnormalities on an EEG. Epileptiform discharges especially occur during the transition between sleep and wakefulness. The other options are inappropriate for this test. 3, II. Seizures.

13. ② A common side effect of Dilantin is gum hyperplasia and gingival overgrowth, so oral care is of extreme importance. The other problems are not side effects of Dilantin. 5, II. Seizures.

14. ④ *H. influenzae* is one of the most common causes of bacterial meningitis in infants and young children. Routine vaccination of

infants will decrease and control the number of cases seen. 4, IV. Bacterial Meningitis.

15. ① Because the disease can progress rapidly,

it is important for the child to be closely monitored so that complications can be prevented. 2, II. Reye's Syndrome.

PRE-TEST Vision, Hearing, and Speech Disorders

1. Which of the following is a cause of sensorineural hearing loss?
   ① Excessive ear wax
   ② Otitis media
   ③ Cochlear damage
   ④ Perforated eardrum

2. Cathy, who is 9 months old, awakens with a fever of 102°F, crying with pain, and pulling at her ear. What is the likely cause of these symptoms?
   ① Serous otitis media
   ② Acute otitis media
   ③ Chronic otitis media
   ④ Acute nasopharyngitis

3. Mr. and Mrs. Harold have a 5-year-old with multisensory deprivation. They are attempting to use behavior modification to reinforce proper behavior at the dinner table. Which of the following is a good example of this method?
   ① Provide hugs if the child doesn't spill
   ② Spank the child for misbehavior
   ③ Feed the child until the child starts self-feeding
   ④ Send the child to bed for misbehavior

4. Which of the following should the parents of toddlers with delayed language skills be encouraged to do?
   ① Enroll them in special education classes
   ② Have them interact with older children
   ③ Read to them on a daily basis
   ④ Punish them for not using the proper word

5. Which of the following evaluation criteria for discharge teaching is most appropriate for an adolescent boy who has been hospitalized for blunt trauma to the eye?
   ① He administers his antibiotics appropriately
   ② He can describe the use of proper protective sports equipment
   ③ He returns to normal activities without complications
   ④ He refrains from sports for 6 months after injury

PRE-TEST Answers and Rationales

1. ③ Cochlear damage results in a sensorineural hearing loss. The other options cause conductive hearing loss. 1, II. Hearing Loss.

2. ② Acute otitis media is a fulminant, either viral or bacterial, infection that increases the pressure within the ear, causing increased irritability, fever, and pain in the child. The child often pulls at the ear as an early sign. 2, II. Otitis Media.

3. ① Behavioral modification provides reinforcement through praise and rewards for acceptable behavior. 4, III. Multisensory Deprivation.

4. ③ Continually speaking and reading to the child encourages understanding of semantics and syntax and enhances word acquisition. 4, III. Delayed Language Skills.

5. ② An important goal for children with eye injury is to teach principles of eye safety before discharge. Describing the use of protective equipment would indicate that the adolescent has understood an important safety principle. Although returning to normal activities without complications is a goal, it is not directly related to discharge teaching. The other answers are incorrect. 5, I. Eye Trauma.

NURSING PROCESS APPLIED TO CHILDREN WITH VISION, HEARING, AND SPEECH DISORDERS

Conjunctivitis

I. Assessment
   A. Definition: inflammation of conjunctiva with or without purulent discharge
   B. Etiology/incidence
      1. Bacterial, viral, or allergic in nature
      2. Most commonly seen in children 2 years old and older
      3. Eye discharge in infants or children less than 2 years old may result from blocked tear duct, underlying otitis media
   C. Predisposing/precipitating factors
      1. Primary or secondary infection
      2. Allergy
      3. Irritation from foreign body, including contact lens
      4. Drug reaction
   D. Clinical manifestations
      1. Conjunctival redness
      2. Edema
      3. Tearing
      4. Mucopurulent discharge
      5. Light sensitivity
      6. Itching (allergic conjunctivitis)
      7. Bacterial conjunctivitis extremely contagious
   E. Diagnostic examinations—positive culture of discharge or conjunctiva
   F. Complications
      1. Orbital cellulitis
         a. Caused by eye infection or injury or underlying infection such as sinusitis
         b. Area surrounding eye is red, swollen, hot, painful; orb displaced anteriorly; fever and signs of infection by complete blood count
         c. Needs vigorous treatment with hospitalization and IV antibiotics to prevent spread to brain
      2. Scarring
      3. Loss of vision
   G. Medical management
      1. Antibiotics (see Table 10-2) if underlying infection suspected
      2. Topical broad-spectrum antibiotic ointment (e.g., polymixin-bacitracin, erythromycin, or tobramycin ophthalmic) or drops for bacterial infection

II. Analysis
   A. High risk for sensory/perceptual alterations related to impaired vision
   B. High risk for injury related to impaired vision
   C. High risk for infection in others related to contagiousness of condition

III. Planning/goals, expected outcomes
   A. Child will follow therapy as prescribed
   B. Child will not develop complications secondary to conjunctivitis
   C. Family members and contacts remain free of infection

IV. Implementation
   A. Instruct child/parent to keep hands away from eye(s); emphasize meticulous hand washing

  B. Separate towels for child and for each eye if unilateral
  C. Teach proper cleansing of eyes
  D. Teach parents correct administration of antibiotic eye ointment or drops
    1. Ointment for younger child
    2. Drops for older child
  E. Instruct parents to complete prescribed therapy
  F. Refer for follow-up visit once therapy completed
V. Evaluation
  A. Underlying problems are identified, e.g., foreign body, allergy, underlying illness
  B. Child completes prescribed therapy with positive results
  C. Child does not develop secondary complications
  D. No other contact contracts infection

Eye Trauma

I. Assessment
  A. Definition: any injury, either penetrating (penetrates into interior eye) or nonpenetrating (e.g., blunt trauma to eye or head) that causes insult to eye structures
  B. Etiology/incidence
    1. Most common in early to middle childhood
    2. Blunt trauma seen more frequently in school-age children and adolescents
  C. Predisposing/precipitating factors
    1. Penetrating—projectiles such as sticks, rocks, pencils, scissors, sharp pieces of toys, poking fingers, knives
    2. Nonpenetrating—balls, sports equipment, motor vehicle accidents, blows from fighting
  D. Clinical management
    1. Pain
    2. Hyphema—presence of blood in anterior chamber of eye
    3. Active bleeding
    4. Edema, bruising
    5. Increased intraocular pressure
  E. Diagnostic examinations
    1. Meticulous examination of affected eye— may require anesthesia
    2. Measurement of intraocular pressure
  F. Complications
    1. Retinal detachment
    2. Acute glaucoma
    3. Permanent loss of vision in affected eye
  G. Medical/surgical management
    1. Surgical repair of lacerations
    2. Patching of affected and unaffected eye

    3. Strict bedrest with medication for pain and sedation if needed
    4. Ophthalmic topical medications to prevent infection
II. Analysis
  A. Sensory/perceptual alterations related to patching
  B. Pain related to injury
  C. Anxiety related to uncertainty of prognosis
  D. High risk for injury related to vision impairment
  E. High risk for knowledge deficit about safety principles related to incomplete understanding of information
III. Planning/goals, expected outcomes
  A. Child will not experience any disorientation related to patching or visual impairment
  B. Child will remain free of complications
  C. Child will maintain bedrest with minimal discomfort
  D. Child will remain free of additional injury
  E. Child and parents will understand principles of eye safety
IV. Implementation
  A. Monitor vital signs and neurological signs frequently
  B. Keep both eyes patched
  C. Maintain strict bedrest with quiet environment; caution child against any sudden movement
  D. Administer pain medications or sedatives as ordered
  E. Assist child with activities of daily living— feeding, elimination, bathing, dressing; explain how to obtain assistance when needed
  F. Speak softly and reassuringly to child; explain all actions; describe in terms with which child is familiar; orient child frequently to time
  G. Plan nursing care to allow for maximum rest and minimal disturbance
  H. Provide quiet diversional activities as child is recovering; e.g., soft music, story-telling, memory games
  I. Allow child and family to express feelings of anxiety or guilt; provide reassurance
  J. Monitor for signs of complications: sudden pain in eye, flashing lights, severe headache, vomiting
  K. Review or teach principles of eye safety
V. Evaluation
  A. Child states that pain is decreasing, rests comfortably
  B. Child able to accomplish activities of daily living with help or independently
  C. Child expresses interest in surroundings and increasing desire for diversional activities

D. Child and family express feelings of anxiety and make positive steps toward coping

E. Child and family can describe symptoms of complications and state circumstances when physician should be notified immediately

F. Child and family list principles of eye safety

Otitis Media

I. Assessment

A. Definition: inflammation and infection of middle ear; may be acute or chronic; with or without effusion (collection of fluid in middle ear)

B. Etiology/incidence
1. Most frequent cause *H. influenzae* or *S. pneumoniae*
2. Peak incidence in infancy, but occurs commonly in children less than 5 years old
3. One of most common illnesses of infancy and early childhood
4. Boys affected more than girls
5. Incidence significantly higher in children in day care
6. Incidence higher in winter

C. Predisposing/precipitating factors
1. Short, wide, straight eustachian tubes in young children
2. Undeveloped cartilage lining
3. Large amount of lymphoid tissue of pharynx
4. Immature humoral defenses
5. Lying down position of infancy, prop feeding

D. Clinical manifestations
1. Purulent drainage accumulation of middle ear
2. Pain/irritability, decreased appetite, night waking
3. Fever
4. Often preceded by upper respiratory infection
5. Poking or batting at ear in infants

E. Diagnostic examinations
1. Otoscopy
a. Inflamed, bulging tympanic membrane
b. Absent light reflex
c. Decreased visual landmarks of middle ear
d. Decreased membrane mobility
2. Tympanometry: measures air pressure in external auditory canal

F. Complications
1. Conductive hearing loss
2. Speech/language, cognitive delay

G. Medical management
1. Ten-day course of oral antibiotics (see Table 10-2)
a. Amoxicillin drug of choice in non–penicillin-allergic children
b. Other agents include sulfamethoxazole-trimethoprim (Bactrim/Septra), cefaclor (Ceclor), erythromycin-sulfisoxazole (Pediazole), and amoxicillin-clavulanate (Augmentin)
2. Recurrent infections prevented with low-dose daily antibiotic prophylaxis using sulfisoxazole (Gantrisin) or amoxicillin

H. Surgical management: myringotomy/tympanostomy with placement of pressure equalizer tubes considered after one or more episodes of prophylaxis failure

II. Analysis
A. Hyperthermia related to infection
B. Pain related to inflammation and increased pressure
C. Sleep pattern disturbance related to pain
D. High risk for altered growth and development (speech/language/cognitive) related to decreased hearing

III. Planning/goals, expected outcomes
A. Child will maintain normal body temperature
B. Child/parents will follow prescribed therapy for its full course
C. Child will be free of pain and will rest comfortably
D. Child will not develop secondary complications
E. If persistent, child/parents will understand surgical procedure, myringotomy, and care of tubes
F. Child will not develop complications secondary to surgical intervention

IV. Implementation
A. Obtain accurate history of signs and symptoms of otitis media
B. Teach parents correct administration of antibiotics
1. Amoxicillin drug of choice for acute episodes
2. Ear drops not used because they obscure view of tympanic membrane
3. Encourage follow-up at end of antibiotic course
C. Administer analgesics as needed for pain (see Table 10-19)
D. Apply heat to ear as needed to decrease pain
E. Have child lie on affected side
F. Speak slowly and clearly to accommodate diminished hearing
G. Teach parents about myringotomy tube appearance, ear wicks, sterile gauze after surgery

H. Teach preventive measures: no propping of bottles, decreasing environmental smoke, avoiding colds, routine hearing screening
V. Evaluation
   A. Incidence of ear infections is reduced
   B. Child completes prescribed therapy with positive results
   C. Child has minimal pain
   D. Child does not develop secondary complications

Hearing Impairment/Deafness

I. Assessment
   A. Definition: loss of hearing ranging from mild to profound; classified as conductive, sensorineural, or mixed
      1. Conductive: hearing loss caused by interruption in passage of sound waves from external ear through middle ear
      2. Sensorineural: perceptive or nerve deafness caused by alteration in cochlear cells or auditory nerve
      3. Mixed: middle ear loss with interference of transmission along neural pathways
   B. Etiology/incidence
      1. May be congenital, hereditary, or acquired
      2. Precise etiology unknown in 30% of cases
      3. Most common disability in United States
      4. Many children have associated disabilities
   C. Predisposing/precipitating factors
      1. Hereditary—family history, particularly sensorineural
      2. Prenatal
         a. Maternal infection (rubella, cytomegalovirus, toxoplasmosis, herpes)
         b. Teratogenic medications
         c. Toxemia
      3. Prematurity, birth trauma, blood incompatibility
      4. Associated diseases or conditions—recurrent otitis media, cerebral palsy, Down syndrome, meningitis, mumps
      5. Ototoxic drugs
      6. Exposure to loud noise
   D. Clinical manifestations
      1. Infant does not respond in age-appropriate manner to loud noises
      2. Delayed speech development, unintelligible speech
      3. Inattentiveness, fails to follow verbal commands or requests
      4. More responsive to movement than to sound, use of gestures to communicate
      5. Asks to have statements repeated or to have volume of sounds increased
      6. Avoids social interactions
      7. Talks more loudly than usual
   E. Diagnostic examinations
      1. Otoscopy
      2. Audiometry
      3. Tympanometry
      4. Evoked response testing
   F. Complications: hearing loss may progress to complete deafness
   G. Medical management: hearing aid, referral for specialized educational services, and speech therapy as appropriate; cochlear implantation helpful for some deaf children
II. Analysis
   A. Sensory/perceptual alterations (auditory) related to hearing impairment
   B. High risk for impaired verbal communication related to hearing loss
   C. High risk for injury related to inability to hear and respond to sounds in environment
   D. Altered growth and development related to speech/language delay and cognitive difficulties because of impaired communication
   E. High risk for self-esteem disturbance related to social consequences of being hearing impaired
   F. Altered family processes related to the child's chronic disability
III. Planning/goals, expected outcomes
   A. Early identification will prevent complications
   B. Parents will understand need for routine hearing screening for all children in the family
   C. Family/child will learn about long-term management and educational implications
   D. Parents/child will voice concerns about diagnosis, prognosis, and long-term impact
   E. Child/parent/family relationship will develop appropriately through means other than hearing (touch, nonverbal expression, visual communication patterns)
   F. Child/family will communicate effectively
   G. Child's residual hearing will be maximized
   H. Child/parents will be educated in use of a hearing aid, if applicable
   I. Child will be independent in self-care needs
   J. Child will progress developmentally and educationally appropriate for age
IV. Implementation
   A. Identify pregnant women at risk
   B. Provide prenatal counseling/care
   C. Perform accurate assessment of hearing at birth and at subsequent checkups
   D. Teach parents about otitis media and compliance with treatment
   E. Assist with hearing tests

F. Provide parents opportunity to discuss fears and concerns

G. Encourage parents to communicate with visual aids and tactile stimulation

H. Discuss with parents advantages and disadvantages of hearing aids, if applicable

I. Gain child's attention before speaking; speak slowly and clearly

J. Refer family to appropriate resource for learning sign language or lip reading

K. Teach family importance of allowing child to be "normal" in activities

L. Provide devices that foster child's independence, e.g., signaling devices for telephone

M. Teach parents to select toys that make use of other senses

N. Encourage child to socialize with both hearing and deaf children

O. Encourage parents to send child to regular school

P. Refer to appropriate agencies for follow-up care and assistance

Q. Encourage participation in support group

V. Evaluation

A. Child's hearing deficit detected in infancy at routine checkup

B. Child/parents discuss fears and concerns

C. Child/parents participate in educational session about hearing impairment and its long-term effects

D. Family communicates effectively with child through sign language and lip reading

E. Child wears hearing aid

F. Parents participate in educational session on hearing aids

G. Child begins to become somewhat independent in self-care

H. Child progresses developmentally and educationally as appropriate for age

Speech/Language Disorders

I. Assessment

A. Definition: any of assorted dysfunctions in the understanding or verbal expression of language that adversely affect the child's ability to communicate

 1. Receptive language disorder—difficulties decoding information or understanding and processing concepts

 2. Expressive language disorder—difficulties formulating words or speaking in grammatically correct format; inability to correctly articulate sounds

B. Etiology/incidence

 1. Incidence highest in preschool child, when

speech development usually is relatively advanced

 2. Some dysfluencies (stuttering, lisps) resolve spontaneously if no undue pressure is placed on child

 3. Incidence of expressive fluency disorders higher in boys

C. Predisposing/precipitating factors

 1. Structural or neurological deficits

 2. Impaired hearing

 3. Impaired cognitive skills

 4. Emotional stress or illness

 5. Decreased environmental stimuli

D. Clinical management

 1. Delayed verbalizations

 2. Inability to understand language or process ideas

 3. Abnormal variations in pitch or tone

 4. Problems with clarity of sounds (lisps)

 5. Dysfluency (stuttering, hesitancies, repetitions)

E. Diagnostic examinations

 1. Routine assessment for language development during infancy and childhood

 2. Denver Articulation Screening Examination (DASE)

 3. Early Language Milestone (ELM) Scale

 4. Hearing screening tests

F. Complications: persistent speech problems

G. Medical management

 1. Accurate history and physical examination for associated health problems

 2. Referral for hearing and language evaluation

 3. Speech/language therapy if problem persists beyond normal age for disappearance

II. Analysis

A. Impaired verbal communication related to underlying disorder

B. High risk for impaired social interaction related to difficulty communicating

C. High risk for self-esteem disturbance related to embarrassment

III. Planning/goals, expected outcomes

A. Parents will understand normal developing speech and language skills

B. Parents will report problems as they occur

C. Child's speech and language development will improve

D. Child will feel comfortable with communication and social interactions

IV. Implementation

A. Monitor child's language development at every well-child visit and refer for delay

B. Tell parents that some children develop verbal speech later than others; normal receptive language in a toddler is reassuring

C. Advise parents that some speech problems are normal and will disappear spontaneously if the child is not under pressure

D. Demonstrate to parents enjoyable ways of stimulating their child's speech—word games, verbalizing familiar objects, singing songs, or reciting poetry

E. Break down concepts into simple ideas for the child who has trouble processing

F. Allow child to complete sentences; ignore dysfluencies

V. Evaluation

A. Parents can describe patterns of developing speech and identify problems as they occur

B. Parents can state ways of stimulating child's speech development

C. Parents/child seek appropriate intervention for any abnormalities

D. Child speaks more clearly

E. Child appears more comfortable and less anxious in social situations

POST-TEST Vision, Hearing, and Speech Disorders

1. Which of the following is the most characteristic finding in infants and children with hearing deficits?
   1. Delayed speech development
   2. Behavioral problems
   3. Excessive nighttime fears
   4. Hyperactivity

2. When a nurse is working with parents of an infant with multisensory deprivation, a major goal would be to assist them to:
   1. Find institutional placement
   2. Develop alternative communication
   3. Limit environmental stimulation
   4. Learn special feeding techniques

3. Which of the following is the rationale for the occurrence of functional obstruction of the eustachian tube in infants?
   1. The eustachian tube lies laterally and is very flexible
   2. The eustachian tube is wide and short; it lies horizontally; and it is not flexible
   3. The eustachian tube is responsible for equalizing pressure on both sides of the mastoid process
   4. There is little difference between the eustachian tubes of infants and adults

4. Sandra, a 6-year-old who has conjunctivitis, is attending overnight camp. In addition to administering the antibiotic ointment, which of the following directions to Sandra will most help prevent the spread of infection to the other campers?
   1. "Make sure you don't rub your eyes."
   2. "Use a different washcloth for each eye."
   3. "Don't take a shower for 3 days."
   4. "Don't play 'guess who' with your hands."

5. Nine-month-old Kyle is being seen for a follow-up after his sixth episode of acute otitis media. He is being placed on prophylactic amoxicillin. Which of the following indicates that Kyle's father understands the concept of prophylaxis?
   1. "He should take the medicine every day to reduce the number of infections he's getting."
   2. "He will be taking the medicine daily for 2 weeks and will need a follow-up again in a month."
   3. "I don't need to worry if he gets a cold while he's on the medicine because he won't get another ear infection."
   4. "I can automatically discontinue the medicine if he goes 1 month without an infection."

POST-TEST Answers and Rationales

1. ① Developing speech patterns are reinforced when children repeat phrases they have heard. If a child misses speech sounds, language acquisition is delayed, and speech deficits can occur. 2, II. Hearing Loss.

2. ② Initially, parent-infant bonding may be difficult if the infant cannot look at the parents' faces or hear their voices. It is important for the nurse to help the parents develop an alternative form of communication so that bonding and development can occur. 3, II. Multisensory Deficit.

3. ② Disorders in the middle ear are common during infancy because the eustachian tubes are more horizontal, wider, straighter, and less flexible than those of older children or adults. Functional obstructions of the drainage system commonly occur. 2, II. Otitis Media.

4. ④ Preventing the spread of conjunctivitis is important because it is easily contagious. Covering another child's eyes in the game of "guess who" can spread the organisms from the infected child's hands. The other interventions reduce the spread from one eye to the other. Option 3 is incorrect. 4, I. Conjunctivitis.

5. ① Antibiotic prophylaxis involves taking a low dose of the prescribed medication daily. Prophylaxis usually lasts for several months during the winter season when the incidence of otitis is highest. The parent shouldn't discontinue the medication without physician recommendation. Prophylaxis may not be completely effective, so parents need to be vigilant about recognizing signs of otitis even when the child is on antibiotic prophylaxis. 5, II. Otitis Media.

BIBLIOGRAPHY

SENSORY/PERCEPTUAL FUNCTIONS

Bogdasarian, R. S. (1991). Q&A on tympanostomy tubes. *Contemporary Pediatrics* 8 (May): 99–101.

Carlin, S. A., Marchant, C. D., et al (1991). Host factors and early therapeutic response in acute otitis media. *Journal of Pediatrics* 118 (2): 178–183.

Dodson, W. E. (1989). Medical treatment and pharmacology of antiepileptic drugs. *Pediatric Clinics of North America* 36 (2): 421–433.

Dreifuss, F. E. (1989). Classification of epileptic seizures and the epilepsies. *Pediatric Clinics of North America* 36 (2): 265–279.

Duhaime, A. C., Alario, A. J., et al (1992). Head injury in very young children: Mechanisms, injury types, and ophthalmologic findings in 100 hospitalized patients younger than 2 years of age. *Pediatrics* 90 (2): 179–185.

Foster, R. L., Hunsberger, M. M., and Anderson, J. T. (1989). *Family-centered nursing care of children.* Philadelphia: W. B. Saunders.

Kennedy, W. A., Hoyt, M. J., and McCracken, G. H. (1991). The role of corticosteroid therapy in children with pneumococcal meningitis. *American Journal of Diseases of Children* 145 (12): 1374–1378.

Marks, M. I. (1991). Early detection and initial management of bacterial meningitis. Lecture, May 1991, for *Practical Reviews in Pediatrics.*

Millchap, J. G., and Colliver, J. A. (1991). Management of febrile seizures: Survey of current practice and phenobarbital usage. *Pediatric Neurology* 7: 243–248.

Mott, S. R., James, S. R., and Sperhac, A. M. (1990). *Nursing care of children and families,* 2nd ed. Redwood City, CA: Addison-Wesley.

Patterson, R. J., Brown, G. W., et al (1992). Head injury in the conscious child. *American Journal of Nursing* 92 (8): 22–27.

Pellock, J. M. (1989). Efficacy and adverse effects of antiepileptic drugs. *Pediatric Clinics of North America* 36 (2): 435–448.

Report of the 102nd Ross Conference on Pediatric Research (1992). *Hearing loss in childhood: A primer.* Columbus: Ross Laboratories.

Reynolds, E. A. (1992). Controversies in caring for the child with a head injury. *Maternal—Child Nursing* 17(Sept/Oct): 246–251.

Teele, D. W. (1991). Strategies to control recurrent acute otitis media in infants and children. *Pediatric Annals* 20 (11): 610–616.

Torfs, C. P., Van den Berg, B. J., et al (1990). Prenatal and perinatal factors in the etiology of cerebral palsy. *Journal of Pediatrics* 116 (April): 615–619.

Whaley, L. F. and Wong, D. L. (1991). *Nursing care of infants and children,* 4th ed. St. Louis: Mosby Year Book.

Yager, J. Y., Johnston, B., et al (1990). Coma scales in pediatric practice. *American Journal of Diseases of Children* 144 (10): 1088–1091.

12

Protective Functions in the Pediatric Client

PRE-TEST Protective Functions

1. Mark is a toddler who was brought to the emergency department after he ingested 10 Children's Tylenol. He was given ipecac immediately in the emergency department. After a period of observation to ensure his safety, he was discharged home. Which of the following is a priority for the nurse to teach his parents?
   ① Clinical manifestations of liver toxicity
   ② Methods for ensuring that Mark coughs and deep breathes hourly at home
   ③ Ways to prevent repeated episodes of dangerous medication ingestion
   ④ Rationale for using aspirin to treat his fever in the future

2. The first action when assessing a child suspected of being poisoned is:
   ① Determining the type of poison
   ② Calling the poison control center
   ③ Checking for airway, breathing, and circulation
   ④ Determining time since exposure

Emma, age 18 months, was admitted to the burn unit after being burned over 35% of her body with partial- and full-thickness burns in a house fire.

---

3. Which of the following interventions is a priority in the nursing care for Emma immediately after her admission to the unit?
   ① Restrict IV fluids to decrease the amount of edema
   ② Institute nasogastric high-calorie feedings to meet increased metabolic demands
   ③ Heavily sedate with narcotics to relieve pain
   ④ Insert a Foley catheter to measure hourly output

4. One of the primary goals when caring for Emma during the burn treatment phase is:
   ① Preventing infection
   ② Preventing pain
   ③ Maintaining a patent airway
   ④ Restoring fluid balance

5. Emma is discharged after many weeks and multiple skin grafts. Several areas on her arm are not completely healed and are still granulating. Her mother will continue to apply Silvadene and sterile dressings to the areas. Which of the following might be an applicable nursing diagnosis for Emma?
   ① Impaired physical mobility related to unhealed tissue
   ② High risk for infection related to impaired skin integrity
   ③ High risk for injury related to normal activity of the toddler
   ④ Body image disturbances related to appearance of the skin

6. Which of the following would be INAPPROPRIATE instructions for the nurse to give the mother of a child with varicella?
   ① Administer aspirin for a fever of more than 102°F (38.9°C)
   ② Keep fingernails short and clean
   ③ Apply Calamine lotion for pruritus
   ④ Encourage liberal amounts of liquids

7. Shari has varicella. To prevent its spread to other children in the hospital, the nurse should:
   ① Keep Shari in bed at all times and out of contact with others
   ② Place Shari in a private room with the door closed and limit visitors
   ③ Wear a mask whenever caring for Shari and have visitors wear one
   ④ Instruct all the children who play with Shari to wash their hands carefully

8. Adam, age 4, has not been immunized and is seen in the clinic with a moderate fever, a raised red rash that began on his face, runny nose, and photophobia. Adam is probably exhibiting signs of:
   ① Rubeola
   ② Rubella
   ③ Roseola
   ④ Varicella

9. If Adam had been immunized, how old would he have been when he received the appropriate immunization?
   ① 9 months
   ② 12 months
   ③ 15 months
   ④ 18 months

10. Bert is a 16-year-old who is admitted to the adolescent unit after an emergency appendectomy. He is in pain, and he has a nasogastric tube in place and draining well. There are three other teenagers in the room staring at him. What is your priority nursing intervention for Bert?
    ① Introduce him to the other young men and encourage interaction
    ② Screen him from the other teenagers and administer an injection of pain medication
    ③ Tell the other children to leave him alone and go to bed
    ④ Explain to the other boys what Bert has been through

11. Which of the following best describes the pathophysiological response to human immunodeficiency virus (HIV)?
    1. HIV, a herpes virus, invades genital tissue, causing vesicle formation that turns into painful ulcers
    2. HIV, a spirochete, causes small, indurated sores on the body
    3. HIV, a retrovirus, causes lymphocyte dysfunction and immune failure
    4. HIV, a rotavirus, causes vulvular edema and profuse discharge

12. Six-year-old Jenna has been living in a foster home subsequent to a hospital admission for injuries sustained when her father beat her with a baseball bat. Which of the following statements by her father would indicate Jenna might soon be able to return home?
    1. "I understand that as upset as I can get about Jenna's behavior at times, I must remember she's only a child."
    2. "I'm so sorry about what I did to Jenna, and I know it won't happen again."
    3. "The reason I abused Jenna was because my parents did that to me when I was a child."
    4. "I know Jenna will need to be disciplined, but I now am beginning to control my temper."

13. Yetta has a rash for which the doctor has prescribed a topical steroid cream. As the nurse, what instructions should you give the parents about the application and use of this medication?
    1. Apply the cream daily to the rash until the tube is empty
    2. Use thick layers of cream to enhance the healing process
    3. Apply a thin layer of cream and gradually decrease its use as the rash heals
    4. Apply the cream at least three times a day for 1 week

PRE-TEST Answers and Rationales

1. ③ It is a priority that the nurse uses this opportunity to teach the parents ways to prevent poisoning in children. For example, it is important to instruct parents not to refer to medicine as candy, which could increase the child's risk of taking it. 4, IV. Poisoning.

2. ③ Although data such as the type of poison, route of exposure, time since exposure, and age and weight of the child are important, checking for airway, breathing, and circulation is the first and most critical assessment. 1, I. Poisoning.

3. ④ Fluid imbalance and shock are very likely after burns. The child will have to receive a large volume of fluid, and urine output is a major way of monitoring that balance. The child will be NPO because paralytic ileus is common after severe burns. Pain medication will be needed, but only in sufficient quantities to control the severe pain and help prevent shock without depressing the central nervous system. 4, II. Burns.

4. ① Preventing infection is a priority goal in the burn treatment phase. The other choices are more applicable to the acute phase. Pain relief also is a goal during the treatment phase, but pain during this phase is associated more with dressing changes. 3, II. Burns.

5. ② As long as burn tissue remains unhealed, there is potential for infection. The other issues are areas of concern, but the data given do not support any of the other choices. 2, II. Burns.

6. ① Aspirin should not be given during a viral illness because of the high risk of Reye's syndrome developing. The other options are appropriate interventions to teach the mother. 4, I. Communicable Diseases, Varicella.

7. ② Varicella is spread through droplets by either direct or indirect contact, so a private room with limited visitors is important to prevent the spread. 4, I. Communicable Diseases, Varicella.

8. ① Coryza, conjunctivitis, photophobia, and a rash of macules changing to papules that begins on the face are manifestations consistent with a diagnosis of rubeola. 2, II. Communicable diseases, Rubeola.

9. ③ Measles, mumps, and rubella immunization is given at age 15 months, and a booster dose is given at entrance to middle school. 3, IV. Immunizations.

10. ② An adolescent needs privacy to cope with pain and stress. He also needs to have his pain relieved without appearing weak in front of the other youths. 4, II & III. Postoperative Care.

11. ③ HIV is a retrovirus that causes failure of the human immune system, which leads to decreased and dysfunctional T-lymphocytes and failure of T-cell–mediated immunity. 2, II. Communicable diseases, AIDS.

12. ① Only choice 1 acknowledges both the root of the problem and a plan to begin to deal with it. Choice 2 is inappropriate because although many abusers feel remorse after an abusive incident, remorse is not sufficient to prevent future occurrences. The other two choices are inappropriate because they do not indicate progress toward prevention. 5, III. Child Abuse.

13. ③ Thin layers of topical steroids should be used to enhance healing. Steroid use should be gradually tapered off, not just stopped, since the rash can ''rebound'' if the medication is stopped suddenly. 4, I. Skin Disorders.

NORMAL PROTECTIVE FUNCTIONS

I. Immune system: composed of humoral (antibody/antigen) and cellular (T-lymphocytes) immunities, which protect the body from invasion by infectious organisms and other foreign substances and control overgrowth of tumor cells within the body; has recognition and memory abilities; is the basic system activated in childhood immunization

II. Skin is largest organ in body; serves not only as body's covering but also as protector to all it covers; skin provides impermeable surface; protects essential constituents from being lost to environment and the interior body from entrance of environmental chemicals, toxins, or organisms;

heat and some fluid regulation controlled by skin as well as sensations of touch, pain, and cold; skin basically composed of epidermis, dermis, and subcutaneous tissue; these components can be broadened to include eccrine glands and apocrine glands; skin of infants and children is more susceptible to irritants, bacterial infections, and maceration secondary to sweat retention because it is thinner than adult skin and contains fewer sebaceous glands

NURSING PROCESS APPLIED TO CHILDREN WITH ALTERATIONS IN IMMUNE PROTECTIVE FUNCTIONS

Immunization

I. See Tables 9-1 and 9-2

Communicable Diseases

I. Assessment
   A. Definition: an illness/disease caused by specific infectious agent or toxic product transmitted directly, from human to human, or indirectly through contaminated articles
   B. Etiology/incidence
      1. Etiology varies with disease
      2. Infectious agent usually viral in nature
      3. Incidence decreased drastically with advent of immunizations
   C. Predisposing/precipitating factors
      1. Exposure to infected person or contaminated articles
      2. No immunization given or available; improper immunization or immunizing agent
   D. Clinical manifestations
      1. Chicken pox (varicella zoster)
         a. Pruritus
         b. Fever
         c. Macule, papule, vesicle, crust sequencing
         d. Distribution primarily on face, trunk, and proximal extremities
         e. Incubation 14 to 21 days; communicable 1 day before lesion eruption to 6 days after; all lesions must be crusted
         f. Prodrome of headache, vomiting, frequently seen before lesions appear
      2. Measles (rubeola, viral)
         a. Fever
         b. Coryza, cough
         c. Koplik's spots on buccal mucosa 2 days before rash, along with fever, malaise
         d. Conjunctivitis, photosensitivity
         e. Maculopapular rash on face and spreading downward, lasting 3 to 4 days
         f. Incubation 10 to 20 days; communicable 4 days before rash appears to 5 days after
      3. Mumps (paramyxovirus)
         a. Fever
         b. Earache aggravated by chewing
         c. Parotitis by third day (unilateral/bilateral)
         d. Incubation 14 to 21 days; communicable before and after swelling begins
      4. German measles (rubella virus)
         a. Blotchy, maculopapular rash on face and spreading rapidly downward, lymphadenopathy (usually posterior cervical)
         b. Lasts only 2 to 3 days
         c. Incubation 14 to 21 days; communicable 7 days before rash appears to 5 days after
      5. Roseola (exanthema subitum, human herpes virus 6)
         a. High fever for 3 to 4 days
         b. Rosy-pink macular rash on trunk, then on face and extremities
         c. Rash appears with disappearance of fever
         d. Lasts 1 to 2 days
         e. Incubation and communicability unknown
      6. Fifth disease (erythema infectiosum, human parvovirus B19)
         a. Low-grade fever, sore throat, headache
         b. Rash appears after 1 week; begins as "slapped cheek" appearance on face, spreads to extremities and trunk; "lacy" appearance that gets worse with heat
         c. Usually lasts 3 to 7 days; rash may appear, disappear, and reappear
         d. Incubation 4 to 20 days; communicable before rash appears
      7. Hand, foot, mouth disease (coxsackie virus)
         a. Vesicular lesions on dorsal surfaces of hands and feet as well as on palms and soles, oral ulcerative lesions on tongue and mucosa causing severe stomatitis
         b. Incidence high in late summer, early fall
         c. Lasts approximately 1 week
         d. Incubation 4 to 6 days; communicability until lesions dry
   E. Diagnostic examinations

1. No specific tests
2. Based on physical findings

F. Complications
1. Chickenpox
   a. Secondary bacterial infection
   b. Reye's syndrome
2. Measles
   a. Otitis media
   b. Respiratory infections
   c. Encephalitis
3. Mumps
   a. Orchitis with possible sterility in males after puberty
   b. Sensorineural deafness
   c. Encephalitis
4. German measles
   a. Rare in children
   b. Teratogenic effects on fetus in first trimester
5. Roseola: febrile seizures
6. Fifth disease
   a. Aplastic crisis in children with hemolytic conditions or immunosuppression
   b. Rarely, stillbirths in women infected during pregnancy

G. Medical management: dependent on infection

II. Analysis
A. Hyperthermia related to increased metabolic demands of illness
B. High risk for impaired skin integrity related to scratching or open lesions
C. High risk for infection related to communicability of disease
D. High risk for sleep pattern disturbance related to discomfort
E. High risk for impaired social interaction related to isolation

III. Planning/goals, expected outcomes
A. Child's disease will not spread to other persons
B. Child/parents will understand the need for any isolation procedures
C. Child will be free of pain and discomfort
D. Child will have adequate nutrition and hydration for age to compensate disease process
E. Child will not develop secondary complications
F. Family and public will understand importance of immunizations

IV. Implementation
A. Accurately monitor presenting signs and symptoms
B. Maintain respiratory isolation (if hospitalized) for chicken pox, measles, mumps, and rubella
C. Teach family proper isolation procedures for home care

D. Keep other children away from infected child; have friends communicate with child by letter or telephone
E. Explain reason for isolation to child/parents
F. Teach parents to provide age-appropriate diversional activities
G. Explain to parents that child's feelings of anger, boredom, and so on are to be expected
H. Discontinue isolation after period of communicability
I. Administer antipyretics/analgesics as needed for pain and discomfort (see Table 10-19); do not administer aspirin to a child with varicella because of the possible connection between aspirin and Reye's syndrome
J. Maintain bedrest or quiet activity
K. Provide tepid baths for pruritus; may add small amount of baking soda or colloidal oatmeal
L. Keep skin and eyes clean
M. Keep nails short and clean
N. Use humidifier as needed
O. Provide good oral care, frequent cool rinses for stomatitis
P. Use heat or cold therapy for pain of mumps
Q. Give fluids frequently
R. Provide soft, bland diet and advance as tolerated
S. Teach child/parents importance of compliance to prevent complications
T. Teach parents signs and symptoms of complications to watch for if not hospitalized
U. Participate in community education programs on immunization

V. Evaluation
A. Parents accurately describe child's symptoms and take steps to protect other family members or friends
B. Child remains in isolation without resistance
C. Family free of other outbreaks of illness
D. Family accurately states isolation precautions to follow and complies with them
E. Child rests comfortably with minimal itching and pain
F. Child consumes adequate fluid and nutrients for age
G. Child's skin remains intact; no secondary infection
H. Child does not develop secondary complications
I. Parents accurately state importance of immunization and comply with schedule

Human Immunodeficiency Virus Infection (Acquired Immunodeficiency Syndrome)

I. Assessment
A. Definition: chronic, potentially life-threaten-

ing disease that affects both cellular and humoral immune responses and results in recurrent viral and bacterial illnesses as well as symptoms related to viral presence in various body systems; primarily interferes with the immune capability of CD4 receptor–bearing T-lymphocytes (helper cells)

B. Etiology/incidence
1. Caused by infection with human immunedeficiency virus (HIV), a retrovirus
2. More than 4000 children and adolescents infected with acquired immunodeficiency syndrome (AIDS) in the United States; does not include those infected with HIV who do not manifest symptoms of AIDS
3. Primary incidence of HIV infection in children occurs in infants born to HIV-infected mothers
4. Important cause of death in children aged 1 to 4 years

C. Predisposing/precipitating factors
1. Perinatal transmission from mother to infant (80% of cases)
   a. Many infants born to HIV-infected mothers exhibit presence of passive HIV antibodies at birth, but between 13 and 40% of infants of HIV-infected mothers actually are infected; the remainder serorevert to HIV-negative status by 24 months of age
   b. Transmission rate seems highest for infants of women who were recently infected with HIV or who are symptomatic for AIDS
   c. Rarely transmitted through breast milk
2. Transmitted through contaminated blood products (15%)
3. Sexually transmitted (1%)
4. Remainder unknown—*not* transmitted by casual contact

D. Clinical manifestations
1. Fifty per cent of infected infants demonstrate clinical manifestations by 12 months of age, 75% develop clinical manifestations by 24 months
2. Centers for Disease Control and Prevention (CDC) classifications
   a. For HIV-exposed infants:
      P_0—status unknown—less than 15 months old, born of infected mothers, asymptomatic
      P_1—known to be infected (more than 15 months and still seropositive), asymptomatic
      P_2—known to be infected, symptomatic

P_3—born to HIV-infected mother, asymptomatic, seroreverted
   b. For diagnosis of AIDS:
      Infants less than 15 months old—positive detection of the virus or HIV antibody, evidence of both cellular and humoral deficiencies not attributable to any other underlying cause, symptoms of nonspecific and specific signs as described by the CDC
      Children more than 15 months old—presence of virus in the blood or tissues, or positive antibody screening, clinical manifestations of AIDS as described by the CDC
3. Initial nonspecific manifestations: lymphadenopathy, hepatosplenomegaly, enlargement of the salivary glands, oral candidiasis, developmental delay; recurrent bacterial infections, particularly otitis media and infections caused by *Streptococcus pneumoniae*, *Hemophilus influenzae*, and *Staphylococcus aureus*
4. Acute opportunistic infections: *Pneumocystis carinii* pneumonia (appears as early as 2 months of age), lymphoid interstitial pneumonitis, persistent esophageal candidiasis
5. Encephalopathy with progressive neurological disease, cognitive/developmental deficits
6. Secondary cancers
7. Other manifestations: fever, chronic diarrhea, failure to thrive or unexplained weight loss

E. Diagnostic examinations
1. Screening—positive antibody to HIV through enzyme-linked immunosorbent assay (ELISA) or immunoblot (Western blot), not positively diagnostic in children less than 24 months old
2. Positive whole virus cell culture, HIV, DNA polymerase chain reaction (PCR), and HIV-specific immunoglobin A can establish diagnosis in infants, but access to tests is difficult
3. CD4 T-cell count decreased, CD4/CD8 (helper/suppressor) ratio decreased
4. Immune globulin levels
5. CT scan for encephalopathy
6. Chest x-ray for pneumonia or tuberculosis

F. Complications
1. Overwhelming infection
2. Tumor development
3. Cardiomyopathy or renal disease
4. Death from complications

G. Medical management

1. Candidiasis—topical or systemic antifungal preparations
2. *P. carinii* prophylaxis
   a. Sulfamethoxazole/trimethoprim (see Table 10-2) for infants and children 1 month to 5 years old, aerosolized pentamidine (antiprotozoal agent) by nebulizer for children more than 5 years old
   b. Begin prophylaxis at 1 month for CD4 count of 1500/mm^3 or less, at 12 to 23 months for CD4 count of 750/mm^3 or less, at 24 to 72 months for CD4 count of 500/mm^3 or less, and at more than 72 months for CD4 count of 200/mm^3 or less; some recommend prophylaxis for all proven HIV-infected infants 1 to 12 months old regardless of CD4 count
3. Consider monthly IV immunoglobulin (IVIG) for children with recurrent bacterial infections and low CD4 counts
4. Zidovudine (AZT) (antiretroviral agent) may be given to HIV-infected infants and children with CD4 count of less than 500/mm^3, whether asymptomatic or symptomatic
5. Nutritional support if needed; routine well care, and immunizations (use inactivated polio vaccine [IPV] instead of oral polio vaccine for child and household members); other infection-prevention measures as needed (e.g., influenza and pneumococcal vaccines, postexposure prophylaxis to varicella)

II. Analysis
   A. High risk for infection related to altered immune system functioning
   B. High risk for altered nutrition: less than body requirements related to altered mucous membranes, anorexia
   C. Diarrhea related to immune deficiency
   D. High risk for activity intolerance related to effects of underlying disease process
   E. High risk for altered growth and development related to neurological deficits or failure to thrive
   F. High risk for impaired social interaction related to inadequate understanding of disease transmission by others
   G. Anticipatory grieving related to potential death of the child
   H. High risk for altered family processes related to impact of illness on child and family
   I. Health-seeking behaviors about disease transmission related to inadequate understanding

III. Planning/goals, expected outcomes

   A. Parents/caregivers/child will understand and follow principles of infection prevention
   B. Child maintains nutritional and hydration status appropriate for age
   C. Child will participate in usual activities
   D. Child will not regress developmentally or educationally
   E. Child will attend school or day care as appropriate
   F. Child will be free of complications
   G. Parents will express feelings, fears, questions at own pace
   H. Child/parents will seek emotional support as necessary
   I. Family will contact appropriate community resources for long-term management and psychological support

IV. Implementation
   A. Obtain history of risk factors in parent or child
   B. Obtain accurate history of presenting signs and symptoms
   C. If adolescent positive for HIV, encourage notifying contacts, not having unprotected sex, not sharing needles
   D. Maintain meticulous handwashing and universal precautions for all children
   E. Maintain meticulous oral hygiene and skin care
   F. Administer medications as ordered, monitor frequently for side effects (e.g., bone marrow depression and liver toxicity with AZT and pentamidine require initial hematological monitoring every 2 weeks, then monthly)
   G. Provide small, frequent feedings high in protein and calories (see Table 10-12); liquids for children irritated by oral candidiasis; infant may need high-calorie formula
   H. Encourage participation in age-appropriate activities as tolerance allows; encourage attendance at school; educate school personnel and others about AIDS
   I. Monitor child's development at routine well-child visits; refer as appropriate for early intervention programs, occupational or physical therapy
   J. Help family find appropriate support group in the community; establish consistent communication with family members, including siblings, to reduce their fears
   K. Encourage parents of HIV-infected infant to hold and cuddle infant as much as possible; emphasize positive parenting behaviors
   L. Teach family/child infection-prevention measures
      1. Meticulous handwashing at all times, par-

ticularly after any contact with infected child's blood

2. Use of universal precautions in the home
3. Cleaning blood spills with bleach solution (1 part bleach to 10 parts water); launder blood-contaminated clothing separately from regular wash
4. Encourage compliance with medications prescribed; teach side effects; facilitate monitoring for complications
5. Advise parents to notify physician immediately if child exhibits any signs of infection; minimize contact with others known to be ill
6. Routine well-child care with appropriate immunizations

M. Refer to private and public health agencies for continued physical, psychological, and home management support
N. Become actively involved with AIDS education in the community and schools

V. Evaluation

A. Parents/caregivers/child describe infection-prevention methods for the home
B. Parents describe signs of infection and notify physician appropriately if child experiences signs of infection or adverse effects of medications
C. Child gains weight according to age and normal growth curve and achieves appropriate developmental milestones
D. Family participates in multidisciplinary support group and begins to express feelings and fears
E. Child develops and maintains appropriate contacts with peers

Disorders of Impaired Skin Integrity

I. Assessment

A. Definition: any of a number of disorders that results in skin lesions of various types, which potentially breach the skin's protective function
B. Etiology/incidence: most commonly seen health problems of infancy and childhood
C. Predisposing/precipitating factors
1. Age of child: certain conditions more prevalent at specific age groups (e.g., diaper dermatitis)
2. Invasion of infectious organisms through skin break
3. Contact with irritant: chemicals, plant poisons, allergens
4. Trauma
5. Infestation
6. Skin manifestations of underlying disease

D. Clinical manifestations
1. Dermatitis
   a. Inflammatory changes in the skin causing erythema, papules, vesicles with oozing and crusting, localized edema, pruritis
   b. Contact dermatitis—caused by irritant (e.g., ammonia causes diaper dermatitis), harsh detergents, plant irritants, irritating clothing, cosmetics
   c. Atopic dermatitis (eczema)—associated with allergy or genetic predisposition, can be exacerbated by stress, can resolve spontaneously (infantile eczema) or continue throughout life
2. Impetigo
   a. Secondary infection caused by streptococcal or staphylococcal organisms entering through skin lesions from bites, trauma, or scratched skin
   b. Pustular or bullous lesions with "honey-colored" crusts that spread from initial site
   c. Highly contagious
3. Pediculosis capitis (head lice)
   a. Parasitis infestation that causes severe itching and bite marks, particularly behind the ears and back of neck
   b. Presence of nits, usually ¼ in. from scalp; live adults can be seen
4. Lyme disease
   a. Caused by a spirochete transmitted through the bite of an infected deer tick
   b. Manifestations appear in three stages (usually over the course of 6 weeks)
      (1) Enlarging circular skin lesion with clearing center; may get to be plate sized; may be followed by small annular lesions, headache, generalized lymphadenopathy, fatigue, joint pain, anorexia, splenomegaly, other nonspecific signs
      (2) Systemic neurological, cardiac, and musculoskeletal manifestations
      (3) Pauciarticular arthritis

E. Diagnostic examinations
1. Accurate history and examination of lesions and affected areas
2. Cultures of infected lesions
3. CBC, erythrocyte sedimentation rate (ESR), Lyme titer for Lyme disease
F. Complications
1. Secondary infection from scratching
2. Chronic systemic problems from Lyme disease
G. Medical management
1. Dermatitis

   a. Eliminate irritant; keep skin clean and hydrated; topical therapy with ointments, creams, lotions, or oils to relieve irritation, protect from additional irritation, promote healing, ensure hydration
   b. Topical steroids (see Table 10-8) for nonoozing lesions to reduce inflammation
   c. Antihistamine to reduce itching
   2. Impetigo: topical or systemic (penicillin, erythromycin) antibiotic therapy (see Table 10-2), depending on extent of condition
   3. Pediculosis: pediculocide shampoos or rinses—permethrin (NIX), pyrethrin (A-200, RID), lindane (Kwell) followed by nit removal
   4. Lyme disease: tetracycline (children more than 9 years old), amoxicillin, or penicillin (see Table 10-2), anti-inflammatories (see Table 10-8) for relief of symptoms
II. Analysis
   A. Impaired skin integrity related to irritants, allergen, infection, infestation, or trauma
   B. High risk for infection related to secondary invasion of infectious organisms
   C. High risk for body image disturbance related to altered appearance
III. Planning/goals, expected outcomes
   A. Child's skin will remain intact and well hydrated
   B. Child will remain free of secondary infection
   C. Child will maintain a positive self-image
   D. Child will remain comfortable
IV. Implementation
   A. Take accurate history to help parents identify and remove causative and risk factors
   B. Relieve pruritis with nonpharmacological methods: cool compresses, baking soda or colloidal oatmeal baths, light clothing
   C. Relieve discomfort as ordered with anti-inflammatory agents or analgesics for pain, antihistamine for itching
   D. Keep child's hands and skin clean, fingernails short; apply covering to hands if severe scratching is a problem
   E. Keep skin well hydrated by applying moisturizers or oil to wet skin after bathing
   F. Protect skin from excoriation as needed using occlusive ointments
   G. Administer antibiotics or other therapies as ordered
   H. Teach family infection control and preventive measures: handwashing, avoiding sources of infection or infestation (e.g., not sharing clothing, brushes, and combs; avoiding areas with ticks, wearing long clothing when tick exposure likely)
   I. Encourage parents to continue hugging child, emphasizing child's positive attributes, de-emphasizing appearance of skin
V. Evaluation
   A. Child shows no sign of redness, irritation, or other signs of skin breakdown
   B. Child remains free of secondary infection
   C. Child and parents describe skin care methods including application of topical preparations
   D. Child rests comfortably without expressing discomfort from itching or pain
   E. Child interacts with family and friends appropriately, participates in care if age-appropriate, helps determine ways of emphasizing positive aspects of appearance

SAFETY PROBLEMS

Poisoning

I. Prevention: see Growth and Development, Safety and Accidents, Chapter 9
II. Nursing management
   A. History: child's condition (airway, breathing, circulation), age and approximate weight of child, type of substance, route of exposure (ingestion, ocular, topical, inhalation), time since exposure, and symptoms if any
   B. Immediate actions if child at home:
   1. Child not breathing: call fire or rescue squad
   2. Prevent further absorption of substance
      a. Ocular: flush eyes with copious amounts of water for minimum of 15 minutes
      b. Topical: Remove contaminated clothing, flush with copious amounts of water, wash with soap and water
      c. Inhalation: bring child to fresh air
      d. Ingestion: remove residual substance from mouth, and call poison control center for further instructions for dilution
   3. Call poison control center and follow directions given
   C. Additional management
   1. Remove the poison: syrup of ipecac as directed, gastric lavage, activated charcoal after gastric emptying to further limit absorption of poison, or administration of cathartics, depending on the type of poison and seriousness of the incident
   2. Provide supportive medical care if necessary

3. Review poison prevention principles with parents

Burns

I. Burn prevention and management: see Growth and Development, Safety and Accidents, Chapter 9, Chapter 6
II. Adaptations for children
  A. Estimating extent of burn: Figure 12-1 estimates percentage of burn allowing for developmental differences according to age
  B. Seriousness of burn
    1. Minor burn: generally no need to admit, partial thickness covering less than 10% body surface; full thickness covering less than 1%; children less than 2 years old may need hospitalization
    2. Moderate burn: may be admitted to local hospital; partial thickness covering 10 to 20%; full thickness covering less than 5%; young children (less than 4 years old) with full-thickness burns and those with burns involving hands, feet, face, genital area may need care at a burn center
    3. Major burn: admit to burn center; partial-thickness covering 20% or more; full thickness covering more than 5%; child less than 4 years old; burns involving hands, feet, face, genital area; children with burns complicated by respiratory tract injury or other injuries or illnesses; children with electrical burns
  C. Medical management
    1. Immediate: Table 12-1
    2. Fluid and electrolyte replacement
      a. Critical in child because of more unstable fluid balance

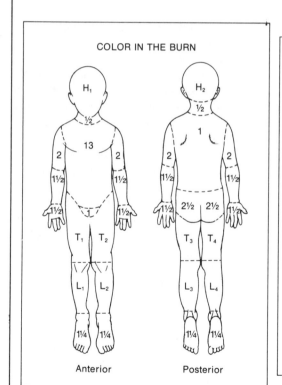

COLOR IN THE BURN

Anterior

Posterior

CALCULATE EXTENT OF BURN

	Anterior	Posterior
	H₁	H₁
Head		
Neck		
Rt. Arm		
Rt. Forearm		
Rt. Hand		
Lt. Arm		
Lt. Forearm		
Lt. Hand		
Trunk		
Buttock	(R)	(L)
Perineum		
Rt. Thigh	T₁	T₄
Rt. Leg.	L₁	L₄
Rt. Foot		
Lt. Thigh	T₂	T₃
Lt. Leg.	L₂	L₃
Lt. Foot		
Subtotal		
% Total Area Burned		%

CIRCLE AGE FACTOR

	Percentage of Areas Affected by Growth Age					
	0	1	5	10	15	Adult
H(1 or 2) = ½ of the Head	9½	8½	6½	5½	4½	3½
T(1,2,3, or 4) = ½ of a Thigh	2¾	3¼	4	4¼	4½	4¾
L(1,2,3, or 4) = ½ of a Leg	2½	2½	2¾	3	3¼	3½

FIGURE 12–1. Estimation of size of burn by per cent. 1, Shade in the diagram to represent the extent of burn, as viewed anteriorly and posteriorly. 2, Circle age closest to that of the patient and use those percentages for the head, thigh, and leg to calculate extent of burn. 3, The percentage of total body surface is printed on the diagram for those areas that do not vary with age. The areas that do vary with age are marked with H (head), T (thigh), and L (leg). The extent of the burn is calculated by adding the percentages of each affected area. If a portion of a body part is burned, an approximate fraction of the percentage should be used. (Redrawn from Feller, I., and Jones, C. A. *Emergency care of the burn victim.* Ann Arbor, Michigan: National Institute for Burn Medicine, 1977.) In Foster, R. L. R., et al. *Family-Centered Nursing Care of Children.* Philadelphia: W. B. Saunders, 1989, p. 2079.)

TABLE 12–1 What to Do if a Burn Accident Happens

Stop the Damage!
- Put out the fire the fastest way you can. Time is critical.
- Stop child from running.
- Pull off burned clothes.
- Wrap the victim in a rug or blanket, if available, and roll to smother flames. Use water, if available, to help extinguish flames.

Immediate Care of Burns
- When a scald burn occurs, flood with cold tap water and remove clothing carefully.
- If a chemical burn occurs, flood with water and remove clothing.
- If a large area is burned, wrap the victim in a clean sheet or towel and take him or her immediately to the nearest hospital emergency department.
- If a small area is burned, wash it with cool water and soap. Do not use ice. Rinse thoroughly and dry gently. Cover with a sterile gauze bandage.
- If you have *any doubt* about what to do, call your family physician or nearest hospital emergency department and ask for advice.
- Contact a physician for a tetanus booster if tetanus immunization is not up to date.

Later Care of Minor Burns
- Cleanse once or twice a day with soap and water; rinse thoroughly and dry. Cover with a sterile dressing.
- Do not break blisters; they provide a sterile cover over the wound.
- Watch for any signs of inflammation: redness, pain, heat, or swelling. If they occur, call a doctor or take victim to the nearest hospital emergency department.

  b. Fluid chosen for replacement depends on child's condition, usually is lactated Ringer's solution, various formulas used to determine replacement amount
  c. Goal is urine output of 1 to 2 mL/kg body wt/hr in child less than 30 kg, 30 to 50 mL/hr in child more than 30 kg
  d. Use of colloids (e.g., albumin) is controversial
 3. Pain management
  a. Initially, IV morphine titrated to provide some sedation, but keep child responsive for assessment of neurological status
  b. Use of pain-rating scale to assess intensity of pain
  c. Administer pain medication 30 minutes before dressing changes
  d. Nonpharmacological measures
   (1) Verbal comfort, tactile comfort to unburned areas
   (2) Distraction: imagery, relaxation breathing, music or story-telling
   (3) Predictability: specific series of events signal when to expect pain
   (4) Control: child included in plan (e.g., helps remove dressings, helps plan time for dressing changes)
 4. Nutritional management
  a. Burned children have nutritional/metabolic requirements 30 to 60%

above normal, higher in the more severely burned child
  b. Diet must be high in protein and calories with foods child likes; increased calories from carbohydrates rather than fat; IV glucose may be necessary; enteral feeding may be required if child unable to tolerate oral feedings or if bowel sounds have not returned

Abuse

 I. Assessment
  A. Definition: eclectic term that encompasses physical abuse or neglect, emotional abuse or neglect, and sexual abuse
  B. Etiology/incidence
   1. Exact cause unknown
   2. Approximately 2 million cases reported per year
  C. Predisposing/precipitating factors
   1. Characteristics of parents
    a. Severely punished as child
    b. Little knowledge of normal development or expectations
    c. Lack of knowledge of parenting skills, low self-esteem
    d. Lack of basic trust
    e. Socially isolated
   2. Characteristics of child
    a. Focus of abuse usually on only one child in family
    b. Product of difficult pregnancy, labor, or delivery
    c. Physically ill child
    d. Temperament of child performing ordinary tasks
   3. Environmental characteristics
    a. Chronic stress, divorce, financial stress
    b. Absence of adequate support system
    c. Socioeconomic level may influence
  D. Clinical manifestations
   1. Physical abuse
    a. Bruises, welts, lacerations, particularly on places that are hard to see
    b. Burns, particularly those with a regular shape
    c. Fractures, dislocations
    d. Poisoning
    e. Withdrawal
    f. Inappropriate reactions
    g. Conflicting accounts of how child sustained injury
    h. Story inconsistent with child's developmental level
   2. Physical neglect

a. Failure to thrive, malnutrition
b. Poor hygiene, inappropriate dress
c. Passive, restless
d. Poor health care
e. Repeated minor injuries
3. Emotional abuse, neglect
a. Failure to thrive, feeding disorders
b. Sleep disorders
c. Sucking fingers, biting nails
d. Withdrawal
e. Fearfulness
f. Delayed language development
4. Sexual abuse
a. Bruises, bleeding, or edema of genitalia
b. Pain on urination
c. Vaginal or penile discharge
d. Sexually transmitted disease, pregnancy
e. Withdrawal
f. Sudden behavioral changes
g. Avoidance of peer relationships
E. Diagnostic examinations: accurate history and physical findings
F. Complications
1. Further abuse
2. Severe psychological disorders
3. Death
G. Medical management
1. Identification and mandatory reporting of suspected abuse
2. Management of injuries or emotional distress
3. Intervention with the family

II. Analysis
A. High risk for injury related to risk factors for abuse
B. High risk for self-esteem disturbance related to continued abuse or neglect
C. High risk for altered growth and development related to neglect
D. High risk for infection related to sexual abuse
E. Altered parenting related to presence of risk factors in parents, child, or environment
F. Altered family processes related to family dysfunction
G. Rape-trauma syndrome related to sexual abuse

III. Planning/goals, expected outcomes
A. Family risk factors will be identified early
B. Child will recover from injury without long-term complications
C. Child will not be abused again
D. Child expresses feelings about abuse, family situation, self-worth
E. Nonabusing parent will express feelings about abuse

F. Family will cooperate with investigation
G. Parent/abuser will seek counseling
H. Family will seek support of social services or other appropriate agency

IV. Implementation
A. Participate in community agencies providing education in parenting and childrearing practices
B. Identify families at risk
C. Report suspicions of abuse to appropriate authorities
D. Keep accurate records of physical, emotional, and behavioral state
E. Protect child once hospitalized
F. Provide consistency in care, primary nurses
G. Use play therapy to help child work through feelings
H. Obtain social work, psychiatric consultation
I. Treat child as normal
J. Do not avoid discussing parents (if abusers); use positive terminology
K. Provide age-appropriate education and diversion
L. Participate in multidisciplinary meeting with parents focusing on abuse as problem not characteristic of parental deficiency
M. Prepare for discharge as applicable
1. Home: arrange for follow-up, counseling
2. Foster care: have child see parents before discharge, explain to child that this is not a punishment
3. Removal from parents permanently: arrange for long-term counseling, allow grief over loss
N. Refer parents to Parents Anonymous, support groups
O. Refer visiting nurse or social worker to perform "home study" for assessing surroundings
P. Educate parents on a continual basis on parenting: arrange for participation in role-modeling sessions

V. Evaluation
A. Child identified immediately after abuse occurs
B. Child abuse does not recur after identified
C. Child's injuries resolve
D. Child in a positive relationship with one nurse in hospital who acts as primary caregiver
E. Child participates in children's support group while in hospital
F. Parents participate in counseling sessions
G. Parents demonstrate positive parenting actions
H. Parents accurately describe behaviors expected at child's developmental level

I. Family cooperates with social worker and outside counselor
J. Home assessed before discharge and appropriate changes made
K. Family followed on a weekly basis immediately after discharge

SURGICAL THERAPY

Preoperative Preparation

I. Nursing goals
   A. Ensure tolerance of procedure
   B. Prevent postoperative complications
   C. Minimize emotional trauma
   D. Prevent regression in developmental, educational process
II. Psychosocial preparation
   A. Check to be sure consent has been obtained
   B. Explain all preparatory tests and surgical procedures in terms that child will understand
      1. Pictures
      2. Stories
      3. Play therapy using dolls
   C. Before surgery, give child a tour and explanation of operating room (OR)/recovery room (RR), if possible
   D. Encourage parents to stay with child until entrance to OR suite
   E. Allow child to take favorite security object to OR, if possible
   F. Have parents at RR when child brought in
III. Physical preparation
   A. Urinalysis
   B. CBC, clotting times, type, and cross-match, as applicable
   C. X-rays, if applicable
   D. ECG, if applicable
   E. Anesthesia check
   F. Assess for signs and symptoms of infections that would delay surgery
   G. NPO 4 to 8 hours before surgery depending on age of the child; give liquids liberally before this time
   H. Baseline vital signs
   I. Void before sedation
   J. Shave and prep site as ordered
   K. Check for loose teeth
   L. Sedate as ordered, based on weight (Table 12-2) (see Table 10-19 for morphine and meperidine)
   M. Explain effects of sedation to parents/child, use least traumatic route possible: rectal, IV, oral if permitted
   N. ID band and allergy band

TABLE 12–2 Common Preoperative Medications

Drug	Purpose	Usual Dosage
Atropine	Inhibits vagal reflex; dries pharyngeal secretions	0.02 mg/kg to maximum of 0.6 mg
Meperidine	See Table 10-19	1 to 2 mg/kg to maximum of 100 mg
Morphine	See Table 10-19	0.05 to 0.2 mg/kg to maximum of 10 mg
Fentanyl	Sedation, analgesia	2 to 3 μg/kg
Methohexital	Ultrashort-acting anesthetic	Individualized according to child's response and length of effect desired

   O. Side rails up at all times, especially after sedation
   P. Do not leave child unattended after sedation

Postoperative Care

I. Nursing diagnoses for the child undergoing surgery
   A. Knowledge deficit about surgery and its effects related to incomplete information and extent of prior experience
   B. Anxiety related to the unfamiliar experience
   C. Pain related to surgical procedure
   D. High risk for infection related to incision
   E. High risk for ineffective breathing pattern related to effects of anesthesia, sedation, pain
   F. High risk for altered patterns of urinary elimination (e.g., incontinence, retention) related to the surgery and medications
   G. High risk for fluid volume deficit related to NPO status and fluid loss during surgery
   H. High risk for injury related to sedation
II. Psychosocial implementation
   A. Communicate caring and security through touch
   B. Emphasize "things" child did right, assisted with
   C. Use play therapy to allow child to express feelings, frustration, autonomy
   D. Encourage "normal" routines, activities, school work as tolerated
   E. Encourage "exploration" of hospital, surgical experience through stories, collections, scrapbooks
   F. Allow child to participate in as much of care as

possible within age, disease process limitations

III. Physical implementation
   A. Vital signs as ordered
   B. Evaluate effects of anesthesia
   C. Assess operative site
   D. Monitor for signs/symptoms of complications
   E. Administer and monitor IV fluids
   F. Advance diet as tolerated
   G. Assess voiding patterns; catheterize if no void 8 hours after surgery
   H. Assess respiratory patterns; turn, cough, and deep breathe every 2 hours
   I. Medicate for pain as needed
   J. Allow parents to participate as much as possible in care

POST-TEST Protective Functions

1. What is the rationale for administering activated charcoal to children who have ingested foreign substances?
   ① To induce vomiting
   ② To reduce absorption of the foreign substance
   ③ To increase the movement of the substance through the gastrointestinal tract
   ④ To prevent excretion through the feces

2. Which of the following reflects the prioritized goals of the immediate management of the child who has ingested poison?
   ① Diluting the poison, removing the poison, restoring vital life functions
   ② Restoring vital life functions, preventing further absorption, removing the poison
   ③ Diluting the poison, removing the poison, preventing further absorption
   ④ Preventing further absorption, providing supportive medical care, teaching preventive principles

3. Mrs. Jackson brings her 2-month-old daughter to the clinic for her first set of immunizations. Before giving the oral polio vaccine, which of the following questions is it important for the nurse to ask Mrs. Jackson?
   ① "Has she recently been checked for anemia?"
   ② "Does anyone in your immediate family have AIDS?"
   ③ "Will a pregnant relative be coming in close contact with her?"
   ④ "Has anyone from a foreign country visited lately?"

Three-year-old Chase is admitted to the hospital with partial-thickness burns over 20% of his body, sustained when he pulled a pan of boiling water off the stove onto himself. He is awake and crying. His parents are with him and seem upset and agitated. His blood pressure is 88/48 mm Hg; pulse, 100; and respirations, approximately 30. His temperature is slightly elevated. An IV line of lactated Ringer's solution is started, and he is given morphine to control the pain.

4. Which of the following nursing interventions would have the highest priority for his immediate care?
   ① Daily dressing changes, pain control, high protein intake
   ② Applying Silvadene, daily dressing changes, physical therapy
   ③ Establishing an airway, inserting a nasogastric tube, monitoring vital signs
   ④ Fluid replacement, strict intake and output, pain control

5. Which of the following diagnoses may be applicable to Chase's parents at the time of his admission?
   ① Anticipatory grieving related to the potential loss of their child
   ② Anxiety related to the accident and hospitalization of their child
   ③ Altered parenting related to potential separation from the child
   ④ Knowledge deficit about safety principles related to incomplete information

6. Which of the following is most likely to be Chase's perception of the nursing interventions and medical treatment?
   ① The nurses are helping him to get better
   ② The nurses will make the pain go away
   ③ The nurses are punishing him for being bad
   ④ The nurses are his friends, but the doctors are not

7. Chase has daily dressing changes where he kicks and screams, remaining upset for some time afterward. Which of the following nursing interventions could help Chase to cope with these dressing changes?
   ① Explain the procedure to him before starting and how it will heal his skin
   ② Let Chase watch another child having the dressing changed
   ③ Let Chase decide the time of day his dressing changes should be done
   ④ Have Chase do dressing changes on a doll

8. As Chase is recovering, which of the following meals that his parents select for him would most show they understand his needs?
   ① Fried chicken fingers, french fries, milk
   ② Hamburger, salad, chips, juice
   ③ Vegetable soup, bagel, chocolate milk
   ④ Peanut butter and jelly sandwich, ice cream, milk

9. Philip is a 4-month-old who had open-heart surgery 2 days ago. You are assessing him for postoperative pain. How will you know if he is experiencing pain?
   ① By the second postoperative day, he should not have any pain
   ② He will cry, refuse food, and be inconsolable if he is in pain
   ③ His mother will be the best judge of his pain
   ④ Infants always experience less pain than adults

10. Which of the following is true about pediculosis capitis?
   ① It is a real health and safety hazard for children
   ② It is most likely to occur in lower socioeconomic groups
   ③ When children are infected, they often exhibit gastrointestinal upset
   ④ Transmission is primarily through personal articles and human contact

11. Which of the following would help promote optimal growth and development in a 14-year-old boy hospitalized with appendicitis?
   ① Maintain bedrest with quiet library activities
   ② Allow participation in activities with other adolescents as soon as condition allows
   ③ Allow parents to bring him clothes from home to wear instead of a hospital gown
   ④ Let his parents sleep at his bedside

12. Beth is an 8-year-old girl with atopic dermatitis, predominantly on her face, elbow, and knee creases. Which of the following would be an appropriate goal for Beth?
   ① Preventing the spread of infection to others
   ② Maintaining intact, well-hydrated skin
   ③ Maintaining intact oral mucous membranes
   ④ Controlling pain

13. A nursing diagnosis most appropriate for Beth might be:
   ① Altered growth and development related to her chronic condition
   ② Sensory/perceptual alterations (tactile) related to skin alteration
   ③ High risk for body image disturbance related to skin appearance
   ④ Sleep pattern disturbance related to discomfort

Four-year-old Brittni is brought to the pediatrician's office by her mother. Visibly upset, the mother tells the nurse that she thinks Brittni was sexually abused by her father's brother during a visit to her father's house over the weekend. Brittni seems to be behaving like a normal 4-year-old, but she describes actions by her uncle that are suggestive of sexual abuse.

14. After obtaining the history suggestive of sexual abuse and a physical examination that appears to be within normal limits, which action should the nurse take next?
   ① Make plans to have Brittni removed from her home
   ② Recommend that Brittni and her mother receive counseling
   ③ Make a verbal report to child protective services
   ④ Wait until more evidence of sexual abuse has occurred

15. Several weeks later, Brittni returns to the office accompanied by her grandmother. Her grandmother reports that Brittni's behavior has changed. She is not sleeping well, has become very aggressive with peers, and cries frequently. Brittni is most likely suffering from:
   ① Body image disturbance
   ② Rape-trauma syndrome
   ③ Sleep pattern disturbance
   ④ Impaired social interaction

One-month-old Chantal is brought to the well-child clinic for her first check-up. While giving the history, her mother begins to cry and tells the nurse that Chantal's father has recently been diagnosed with AIDS. The mother reports that she is HIV positive and is extremely concerned about Chantal.

16. The nurse encourages Chantal's mother to have her screened for HIV antibody. The nurse knows that:
   ① It is probable that Chantal will have a positive antibody for HIV
   ② The majority of children of HIV positive mothers are infected with HIV
   ③ It is unlikely that Chantal will have a positive HIV antibody
   ④ HIV is not likely to be transmitted unless the mother has AIDS

17. Chantal's mother agrees to have the screening test done. While waiting for results, which of the following actions by Chantal's mother indicates an understanding of the transmission of HIV?
    1 She keeps Chantal away from her father
    2 She wears gloves while changing Chantal's diapers
    3 She wears a mask whenever she has a cough
    4 She stops breast-feeding
18. Chantal tests positive for HIV antibody and is monitored closely at every well-child visit. Which of the following signs and symptoms might lead the nurse to believe that Chantal is infected with HIV?
    1 Two episodes of otitis media, increased T-lymphocyte count, thrush
    2 Delayed gross motor development, adequate weight gain, eczema
    3 Lymphadenopathy, persistent oral thrush, failure to thrive
    4 Loose stools, fever, increased fussiness

POST-TEST Answers and Rationales

1. ② Activated charcoal binds with many poisonous substances to reduce or prevent their absorption. 2, II. Poisoning.

2. ② Restoring airway, breathing, and circulation is the first priority if vital functions have been lost. This should be followed by preventing further absorption of the substance by removing it from the mouth and gastric emptying by the method recommended by the poison control center. 3, II. Poisoning.

3. ② Oral polio vaccine is contraindicated in children living with a person whose immune system is depressed. Because oral polio vaccine is a live vaccine, theoretically it is possible for the virus to be present in the feces. 1, IV. Immunizations.

4. ④ Fluid replacement is a priority for any child with a moderate burn to prevent hypovolemic shock. Strictly monitoring intake and output gives the nurse data for evaluating the success of the fluid replacements. Pain control also is a priority. The other choices are more applicable to a child with a flame burn (3) or a child in a more convalescent phase of burn treatment. 4, II. Burns.

5. ② Anxiety would be the overriding feeling by both parents at the time of admission. Crying and agitation are both signs of anxiety, and anxiety is a normal reaction by parents to the injury and hospitalization of a child. The other options are diagnoses that might be made as the child begins to recover. 2, III. Burns.

6. ③ Young children often feel that they are being punished for something when they are sent to the hospital or when they are ill. This is even more the case when the injury is a result of doing something the child knows is wrong. 1, III. Burns.

7. ④ Children this age need the opportunity to "play out" their experiences and fears related to the hospital treatment. He is not old enough to understand the explanation and not able to choose a time for his dressing change. 4, II. Burns.

8. ④ Children with burns need a diet high in protein and calories (particularly carbohydrates) to meet the high metabolic demands of healing. Milk, peanut butter, bread, ice cream, meats, and vegetables are highest in protein and calories. 5, II. Burns.

9. ② Infants experiencing pain will often exhibit irritability, crying, excessive stools, and inability to eat. You should rely on your observations of his behavior, although asking his mother is sometimes useful. 1, II. Postoperative Care.

10. ④ Head lice are commonly transmitted through clothing, combs, caps, and human contact. It is common in school in colder weather when children share caps and combs. 2, II. Communicable Diseases, Lice.

11. ② Adolescents need the opportunity to participate in age-related group activities to help eliminate the stress of hospitalization. 4, IV. Postoperative Care.

12. ② Maintaining skin integrity is a primary goal with any child with atopic dermatitis. Scratching can irritate the skin, leaving it open to invasion by organisms. The other choices are not applicable to a child with atopic dermatitis. 2, II. Atopic Dermatitis.

13. ③ A primary concern of the school-age child is looking different from friends. Chronic atopic dermatitis can alter the appearance of the skin, causing the child to feel self-conscious. Without intervention, the child may experience a disturbance in body image. 2, II. Atopic Dermatitis.

14. ③ Even though a 4-year-old can be somewhat of a poor historian, if abuse is even suspected, a report to child protective services or to the police is mandatory in most states for health care workers. Often, there is nothing in the physical examination that would confirm actual abuse, but suspicion is sufficient for reporting. 4, I. Abuse.

15. ② Although sudden behavior changes such as crying, increased aggressiveness, and disturbances of sleep can happen in 4-year-olds, the history of alleged sexual abuse would suggest Brittni might be suffering from rape-trauma syndrome. Manifestations often do not occur until several weeks or months after a rape has occurred. 2, III. Abuse.

16. ① Nearly all infants born to HIV-infected mothers demonstrate positive antibodies to HIV by screening. This does not mean that the child is infected with HIV,

because the screening test responds to passively transmitted antibodies. At 15 to 18 months, the majority of children serorevert to negative status. 1, II. AIDS.

17. ④ Rarely, HIV can be transmitted through breast milk. It is the recommendation in the United States that HIV-positive women not breast-feed their infants. The other choices are not applicable to the transmission of HIV. 5, I. AIDS.

18. ③ Initial symptoms of infection in HIV-positive infants include lymphadenopathy, fever, persistent oral candidiasis, failure to thrive or unexplained weight loss, delay in achieving developmental milestones, and recurrent bacterial infections. Although loose stools, fever, and fussiness are symptoms of HIV, one episode is more suggestive of a minor gastrointestinal infection. 4, II. AIDS.

BIBLIOGRAPHY

PROTECTIVE FUNCTIONS

American Academy of Pediatrics Committee on Child Abuse and Neglect (1991). Guidelines for the evaluation of sexual abuse of children. *Pediatrics* 87 (2): 254–259.

Aylward, E. H., et al (1992). Cognitive and motor development in infants at risk for human immunodeficiency virus. *American Journal of Diseases of Children* 146 (2): 218–222.

Barnett, E. D., et al (1992). Otitis media in children born to human immunodeficiency virus-infected mothers. *Pediatric Infectious Disease Journal* 11 (5): 360–364.

Chu, S. Y., et al (1991): Impact of the human immunodeficiency virus epidemic on mortality in children, United States. *Pediatrics* 87 (6): 806–810.

Connor, E. (1991). Advances in early diagnosis of perinatal HIV infection. *JAMA* 266 (12): 3474–3475.

Foster, R. L. R., Hunsberger, M. M., and Anderson, J. T. (1989). *Family-centered nursing care of children.* Philadelphia: W. B. Saunders.

Haller, J. O., et al (1991). Diagnostic imaging of child abuse. *Pediatrics* 87 (2): 265–266.

Hein, K. (1991). Risky business: Adolescents and human immunodeficiency virus. *Pediatrics* 88 (5): 1052–1054.

Hutto, C., et al (1991). A hospital-based prospective study of perinatal infection with human immunodeficiency virus type 1. *Journal of Pediatrics* 118 (3): 347–353.

Kline, M. W., and Shearer, W. T. (1991). A national survey on the care of infants and children with human immunodeficiency virus infection. *Journal of Pediatrics* 118 (5): 817–821.

Krugman, R. D. (1991). Child abuse and neglect: Critical first steps in response to a national emergency. *American Journal of Diseases of Children* 145 (5): 513–515.

Mack, R. B. (1992). Toxic plants—winners of our discontent. *Contemporary Pediatrics* 9 (3): 133–141.

Mansson, M. E., Fredrikzon, B., and Rosberg, B. (1992). Comparison of preparation and narcotic-sedative premedication in children undergoing surgery. *Pediatric Nursing* 18 (4): 337–342.

Mott, S. R., James, S. R., and Sperhac, A. M. (1990). *Nursing care of children and families,* 2nd ed. Redwood City: Addison-Wesley.

Orcutt, T. A., and Godwin, C. R. (1992). Aerosolized pentamidine: A well-tolerated mode of prophylaxis against *Pneumocystis carinii* pneumonia in older children with human immunodeficiency virus infection. *Pediatric Infectious Disease Journal* 11 (4): 290–294.

Pelton, S. I. (1992). Pediatric HIV infection. *Clinical care manual for HIV infection.* Presented at Infectious Disease Conference sponsored by Boston University School of Medicine, March 28, 1992.

Quinn, T. C., et al (1991). Early diagnosis of perinatal HIV infection by detection of viral-specific IgA antibodies. *JAMA* 266 (12): 3439–3442.

Ricci, L. R. (1991). Photographing the physically abused child. *American Journal of Diseases of Children* 145 (3): 275–281.

Ross, T., and Dickson, E. J. (1992). Vertical transmission of HIV and HBV. *MCN* 17 (4): 192–195.

Rutstein, R. M. (1991). Predicting risk of *Pneumocystis carinii* pneumonia in human immunodeficiency virus-infected children. *American Journal of Diseases of Children* 145 (8): 922–924.

Thomas, S. A., and Rosenfield, N. S. (1991). Long-bone fractures in young children: Distinguishing accidental injuries from child abuse. *Pediatrics* 88 (3): 471–476.

Trowbridge, G. L., et al (1991): HIV: Recognizing and managing the infant at risk. *Contemporary Pediatrics* 8 (10): 118–134.

Whaley, L. F., and Wong, D. L. (1991). *Nursing care of infants and children,* 4th ed. St. Louis: Mosby-Year Book.

13

Mobility in the Pediatric Client

PRE-TEST Musculoskeletal Disorders

1. Antonio is a newborn admitted to the nursery. On initial assessment, the nurse notes that both his feet turn in. When attempting range of motion, the nurse finds that both feet move relatively freely in all directions. Antonio most likely has:
   ① Clubfoot
   ② Congenital hip dysplasia
   ③ Metatarsus adductus
   ④ Tibial torsion

2. Which of the following will Antonio's mother need to demonstrate before she leaves the hospital?
   ① Foot range of motion exercises to be done after each feeding
   ② Proper foot insertion into Denis Browne splint at night
   ③ Cast care and maintenance
   ④ Application of the Pavlik harness

3. Nine-year-old Susan is admitted to the hospital for closed reduction of fractures of the tibia and fibula sustained when she fell off her bike. A plaster cast is applied, and she is to stay overnight for observation. Which of the following interventions is of primary importance?
   ① Maintaining adequate intake and output
   ② Petaling the cast edges to prevent skin breakdown
   ③ Checking circulation, sensation, and motion of her toes
   ④ Monitoring the cast for signs of hemorrhage

4. In addition to helping Susan and her parents understand cast care and proper nutrition for healing, an important goal for Susan's care is to:
   ① Prevent infection
   ② Assist with developmental regression
   ③ Ensure adequate fluid intake
   ④ Prevent injury

5. Which of the following is an appropriate goal for the child being treated for osteomyelitis?
   ① Preventing injury to the bone
   ② Maintaining a patent IV line
   ③ Prohibiting activities
   ④ Encouraging a high-iron diet

6. Which of the following best describes the condition of Legg-Calvé-Perthes disease?
   ① Dislocation of the head of the humerus
   ② Avascular necrosis of the femoral head
   ③ Evulsion of the tibial tuberosity
   ④ Pain around the brachial plexus

7. As a school nurse, you should be able to screen for idiopathic scoliosis in students. Which of the following would be the best way to screen for this problem?
   ① Observe students touching their toes in a physical education class
   ② Observe a physical education class to see if any students have a waddling gait
   ③ Advise students with knee pain to see a physician for x-ray follow-up
   ④ Observe a physical education class to see if any students have prominent buttocks

8. A nursing diagnosis most applicable to the teenager with scoliosis is:
   ① High risk for body image disturbance
   ② Fear of permanent disability
   ③ Altered nutrition: more than body requirements
   ④ Altered growth and development

9. You determine that one of the students, Emily, has idiopathic scoliosis. She is worried about how long the treatment for this is going to last. The nurse should tell her that the treatment will last:
   ① For the rest of her life
   ② Until the curvature is less than 10 degrees
   ③ Until her body has reached bone maturity
   ④ About 2 to 3 years

10. It is recommended that Emily have a Harrington rod insertion and spinal fusion. The nurse will monitor neurological status closely. Which of the following is another important goal?
   ① Maintaining the teenagers' need for privacy
   ② Preventing postoperative pain
   ③ Ensuring adequate nutrition
   ④ Limiting the number of visitors each day

PRE-TEST Answers and Rationales

1. ③ Clubfoot is a condition in which there is rigid, nonflexible toeing-in of one or both feet. Because this child's feet are flexible, metatarsus adductus is the probable cause. 1, II. Clubfoot.

2. ① Children with metatarsus adductus usually are treated with range of motion exercises. For convenience, exercises are often done in conjunction with meals. 5, II. Clubfoot.

3. ③ Monitoring circulation, sensation, and motion of casted extremity is of primary importance in recognizing circulatory impairment from cast restriction. Petaling the cast and ensuring adequate intake should be done but are of lesser importance. Hemorrhage is unlikely when a closed reduction is done. 4, II. Fractures.

4. ④ Preventing injury from imbalance or inexperience with crutch walking is an important goal. Reviewing safety principles associated with bicycling would be also important for Susan's safety as her injury occurred while bicycling. The extent of her injury should not interfere with fluid intake, making that choice not applicable. 3, II. Fractures.

5. ② Children with osteomyelitis are treated with long-term IV antibiotics. Maintenance of the IV site and monitoring for complications such as phlebitis or infiltration are important goals. A diet high in iron is not necessary, nor is complete restriction of activity. 3, I. Osteomyelitis.

6. ② This disease is characterized by avascular necrosis of the head of the femur. It is not an infection but is related to impairment of the blood supply. 1, II. Avascular Necrosis.

7. ① Children with scoliosis will have unlevel hips when they bend at the waist to touch their toes. The nurse should be able to screen easily for this problem by simply watching students in a physical education class. 1, II. Scoliosis.

8. ① Teenagers with scoliosis have the potential for body image disturbance related to their appearance or the appearance of any corrective devices. Rarely does scoliosis cause permanent disability, and the other choices do not apply. 2, III. Scoliosis.

9. ③ Scoliosis treatment must continue until the bones have reached their maximum growth and maturity is reached. As long as the bones are growing, treatment must continue. 4, II. Scoliosis.

10. ② Controlling pain is important because of the extensive nature of the surgery and the need for movement and exercise such as coughing and deep breathing. Unless the pain is controlled, other postoperative complications are likely to occur. 3, I. Scoliosis.

NORMAL MUSCULOSKELETAL SYSTEM

I. Composed of the skeletal (bones), articular (joints), and muscular (muscles) systems; functions of skeletal system include protection of vital organs, support of surrounding tissue, manufacture of red blood cells, storage of mineral salts, and assistance with body movement; bones classified as either long, short, flat, irregular, or sesamoid; union of two or more bones constitutes a joint; movement does not necessarily need to occur for this area to be considered a joint; joints classified as synarthroses, where no movement occurs; amphiarthroses, where slight movement occurs; and diarthroses, where free movement occurs with the assistance of synovial fluid; muscular system makes up 40 to 50% of a person's body weight; muscles can be classified as cardiac, smooth, or skeletal (see Chapter 7 for Hazards of Immobility).

NURSING PROCESS APPLIED TO CHILDREN WITH MUSCULOSKELETAL DISORDERS

Congenital Disorders

Clubfoot

I. Assessment
   A. Definition: deformity of muscles and bones of foot that prevent it from being manipulated into normal position
   B. Etiology/incidence
      1. Exact etiology unknown; probably multifactorial inheritance

2. Incidence highest in families who already have one child with clubfoot
3. One per 1000 live births
4. Male-to-female ratio of 2 : 1
5. Unilateral slightly more common than bilateral

C. Predisposing/precipitating factors
1. Abnormal positioning or restricted movement in utero
2. Arrested or anomalous embryonic development
3. Often associated with other congenital anomalies (e.g., spina bifida)

D. Clinical manifestations (Fig. 13-1A)
1. Foot twists inward—varus
2. Forefoot adducted
3. Foot plantar flexed—equinus

E. Diagnostic examinations: readily apparent by inspection, needs to be differentiated from other causes of toeing-in, such as tibial torsion, femoral torsion, metatarsus adductus (flexible, nonrigid inwardly turned foot that can be corrected with exercises)

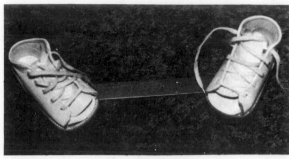

B

FIGURE 13–1B. The Denis Browne splint used for correction of clubfoot. Note the reversal of the shoes on the splint. (From Marlow, D. R., and Redding, B. A. (1988). *Textbook of pediatric nursing,* 6th ed. Philadelphia: W.B. Saunders.)

F. Complications: if not corrected, child can have permanent functional disability
G. Medical management: correct position of foot maintained by serial casting or splinting
H. Surgical management: surgery for children not improved by casting

II. Analysis
A. Impaired physical mobility related to cast
B. High risk for altered growth and development related to impaired mobility
C. High risk for altered peripheral tissue perfusion related to constriction from cast
D. High risk for impaired skin integrity related to cast
E. High risk for injury related to child attempting normal activities
F. Knowledge deficit about cast and home care related to incomplete information

III. Planning/goals, expected outcomes
A. Child will demonstrate adequate gross motor activity of unaffected extremities
B. Child will not experience complications from casting
C. Child's skin integrity will remain intact
D. Child's extremity will remain neurovascularly intact
E. Child will not regress developmentally during treatment period
F. Parents will understand and carry out treatment at home with follow-up care

IV. Implementation
A. Inspect extremities at birth/newborn nursery for clubfoot
B. Differentiate true clubfoot versus positional deformity; true clubfoot cannot be passively manipulated to overcorrected position, whereas positional deformities can be passively corrected or overcorrected
C. Do range of motion exercises every shift to unaffected extremities

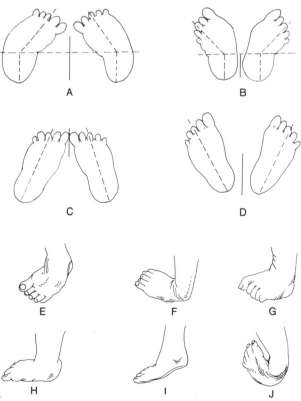

FIGURE 13–1A. Abnormal positions of the feet. *A,* Metatarsus varus; *B,* metatarsus valgus; *C,* pes varus; *D,* pes valgus; *E,* talipes equinovarus; *F,* talipes calcaneovalgus; *G,* talipes varus; *H,* talipes valgus; *I,* talipes equinovalgus; and *J,* talipes calcaneovarus. (From Marlow, D. R., and Redding, B. A. (1988). *Textbook of pediatric nursing,* 6th ed. Philadelphia: W. B. Saunders.)

D. Instruct parents in how to perform range of motion exercises
E. Maintain limb(s) in cast
  1. Serial casting usually treatment of choice
  2. Begins immediately after birth and continues until overcorrection achieved
  3. Adduction deformity corrected first, then inversion deformity, then plantar flexion
  4. Weekly manipulations/cast changes required to accommodate rapid growth
  5. Cast care (Table 13-1)
F. Instruct parents in cast care
G. If splints or appliances necessary, instruct parents in use of Denis Browne splint (Fig. 13-1B)
  1. Shoes affixed to metal crossbar with direction of shoes opposite the norm to counteract adduction
  2. Enhances infant's kicking movements, thus accelerating correction process
H. Assess areas around cast/splint for skin breakdown
I. Turn every 2 hours

TABLE 13–1 Cast Care

Responsibilities	Outcome
Elevate, casted extremity; check circulation, sensation, movement every 1 to 2 hours; check for tightness; handle with palms of both hands; do not pick up spica cast by the crossbar	Circulatory impairment prevented
Observe respiratory effort, chest expansion; observe behavioral changes	Respiratory status maintained (spica or body cast)
Smell cast for foul odor; monitor vital signs	Infection prevented or caught early
Circle any stained areas with pencil or pen to monitor bleeding	Hemorrhage caught early
Petal cast edges; keep food away from cast, cast edges; avoid placing "scratching" objects such as hanger inside cast; monitor skin integrity around cast; protect cast from soiling	Skin integrity maintained
Ambulate if possible; range of motion exercises to unaffected areas; support casted area	Muscle atrophy prevented in unaffected areas
Positional changes as tolerated; position casted area with sling, sandbags, pillows; avoid powder, lotion around cast	Comfort maintained
Teach parents/caregiver proper cast management at home; return demonstration; accurately state care before discharge	Postdischarge complications prevented

J. Provide skin care every shift
K. Do neurovascular checks to affected extremity every 4 hours
  1. Toe nail beds blanch and refill briskly
  2. Toes warm to touch
  3. Sensation of touch is felt on toes (infant demonstrates movement in response)
  4. Wiggling toes
L. Provide age-appropriate diversional activities, particularly those that promote motion of upper extremities and unaffected extremity

V. Evaluation
A. Child's foot exhibits improved position as a result of intervention
B. Child demonstrates strength and flexibility in unaffected extremities
C. Child shows no evidence of skin breakdown; skin intact, well-hydrated, smooth
D. Child demonstrates adequate capillary refill in casted extremity
E. Child achieves appropriate developmental milestones within limits of the cast
F. Parents accurately describe responsibilities of cast care and follow-up

Congenital Hip Dysplasia (Congenital Dislocated Hip)

I. Assessment
A. Definition: broad term applied to malformation of hip present at birth; various degrees of hip joint instability
  1. Acetabular dysplasia (preluxation): mildest form; femoral head remains in acetabulum; apparent delay in acetabular development, unstable hip can be manually dislocated
  2. Subluxation: largest percentage of hip dysplasias; femoral head remains in contact with acetabulum, but is partially displaced
  3. Dislocation: femoral head loses contact with acetabulum; lies laterally and superiorly to acetabulum; results in incomplete formation of the acetabulum and flattening of femoral head
B. Etiology/incidence
  1. Etiology unknown
  2. One per 500 to 1000 live births
  3. Female-to-male ratio of 7 : 1
  4. 25% bilateral hip involvement
  5. Highest incidence among Navajo Indians and Eskimos, who tightly swaddle infants with hips adducted
  6. Lowest incidence in Far East, where infants are carried with legs widely abducted

C. Predisposing/precipitating factors
   1. Familial tendency
   2. Laxity of hip joint capsule and associated ligaments secondary to maternal secretion of estrogen toward end of pregnancy
   3. Breech position at birth
   4. Postnatal positioning
D. Clinical manifestations
   1. Infant (Fig. 13-2)
      a. Positive Ortolani's click: clicking when affected leg abducted, caused by femoral head slipping over acetabulum
      b. Restricted abduction of affected hip
      c. Shortening of limb on affected side
      d. Asymmetrical thigh and gluteal folds
      e. Broadening of perineum (bilateral dislocation)
   2. Older child
      a. Limp on affected side
      b. Positive Trendelenburg's sign: while standing on affected leg, pelvis tilts downward on unaffected side instead of upward
      c. Flattening of buttock on affected side
      d. Affected leg is shorter
E. Diagnostic examinations
   1. Assessment techniques (e.g., inspection, palpation)

2. X-rays in older child
F. Complications
   1. Abnormal gait when walking begins
   2. Total hip replacement in young adulthood if treatment not completed in childhood
G. Medical and surgical management
   1. Corrective devices to maintain full abduction
      a. Newborn: double or triple diapering for preluxation
      b. Infant
         (1) Pavlik harness (Fig. 13-3) or Frejka pillow worn continuously until hip stability is achieved
         (2) Plaster hip spica cast, cast from waist down with hips abducted and knees usually flexed
         (3) Removable abduction brace
      c. Toddler
         (1) Traction followed by hip spica cast
         (2) Open reduction followed by hip spica cast
      d. Older child (4 to 6 years)
         (1) Combination of traction, tenotomy of contracted muscles, osteotomy, casting
         (2) More difficult due to secondary adaptive changes in hip joint

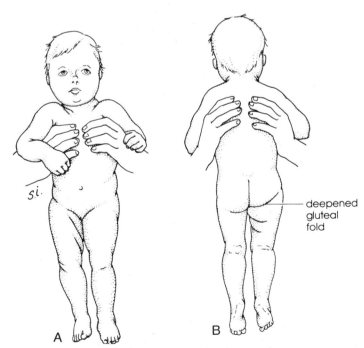

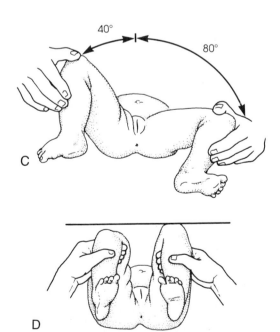

deepened gluteal fold

40°   80°

FIGURE 13–2. Congenital hip dislocation. Physical findings in congenital dislocation of right hip. *A* and *B,* Asymmetry of the thigh folds and gluteal creases, with apparent shortening of the right extremity. *C,* Limited abduction of the right hip. *D,* Allis's sign—apparent shortening of the femur as shown by the difference of the knee levels with the hips and knees flexed at right angles and the child lying on a firm table. (From Marlow, D. R., and Redding, B. A. (1988). *Textbook of pediatric nursing,* 6th ed. Philadelphia: W.B. Saunders.)

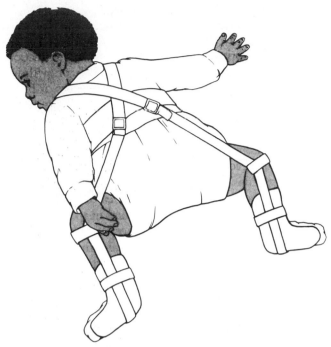

FIGURE 13–3. The child in a Pavlik harness. (From *Nursing Care of Children and Families,* Second Edition, by S. Mott, S. James, and A. Sperhac. Copyright © 1990 by Addison-Wesley Nursing. Reprinted by permission.)

    2. More than 6 years
       a. Total hip replacement
       b. Severe shortening and contracture of muscles in addition to femoral/acetabular deformities make other treatments inadvisable
 II. Analysis: nursing diagnoses are similar to those listed under Clubfoot discussed earlier; add those listed under Pain if surgery is performed
III. Planning/goals, expected outcomes
   A. Child's hip will remain in corrective position
   B. Child's skin integrity will remain intact
   C. Child will demonstrate adequate tissue perfusion
   D. Child will be free of pain
   E. Child will not regress developmentally during treatment period
   F. Parents will understand principles of care at home
   G. Parents will carry out treatment at home with follow-up care
IV. Implementation
   A. Examine every infant for congenital hip dysplasia while in newborn nursery and at follow-up visits
   B. Maintain cast, if applicable (see Table 13-1)
   C. Do range of motion exercises to unaffected extremities at least three times a day
   D. Monitor areas around corrective device for skin breakdown

   E. Turn every 2 hours
   F. Do skin care every shift; keep skin dry and clean; promote adequate circulation
   G. Check circulation, sensation, and motion every 4 hours
   H. Give analgesics as per physician's orders (see Table 10-19)
   I. Provide age-appropriate diversional activities, particularly directed toward exercising unaffected extremities
   J. Instruct parents in care of cast and of corrective device
      1. Pavlik harness
        a. Instruct not to remove Pavlik harness without physician's permission
        b. Mark straps with indelible ink at correct position
        c. Keep areas under straps clean and dry
        d. Give child sponge bath; clean harness with soap and water by sponge
      2. Spica cast
        a. Modify infant car seat to accommodate spica cast
        b. Place disposable diaper covering perineal opening with edges under cast; cover with another diaper or hold on with Velcro closure diaper cover
        c. If cast is tight, use plastic wrap placed under and taped over cast edges before putting diaper over all
        d. Feed child in upright position with legs straddling upper thigh, or use adapted infant seat
        e. Provide mobiles or activity boxes for infants; older toddlers can propel themselves on a scooter board on the floor
 V. Evaluation
   A. Child regains full use of affected extremity
   B. Child's hip maintained in full abduction with proper corrective device at all times
   C. Child's skin shows no evidence of breakdown
   D. Child's neurovascular functions to affected extremity remain intact
   E. Child does not complain of pain
   F. Child achieves developmental milestones within limitations of corrective device
   G. Parents describe responsibilities to maintain corrective device and follow-up care accurately

Fractures

 I. Assessment
   A. Definition: injury to bone that occurs when resistance of bone against stress being

exerted on it yields to that stress; occur relatively close to epiphyseal plate (Table 13-2 and Fig. 13-4)

B. Etiology/incidence
   1. Accidents
   2. Birth injuries
   3. Child abuse
   4. Incidence and type of fracture vary with age
   5. Children's bones more easily susceptible to fracturing than those of adults because their bones are not as strong
   6. Most common sites: long bones of arm and leg

C. Predisposing/precipitating factors
   1. Lack of safety precautions specific to age group
   2. Excessive stress on bone
   3. Participation in activities that place stress on bones (e.g., sports)

D. Clinical manifestations
   1. Edema
   2. Pain
   3. Tenderness
   4. Diminished function of affected area
   5. Obvious deformity
   6. Ecchymosis
   7. Crepitus
   8. Muscle spasms
   9. Paresthesia distal to fracture site
   10. Decreased or absent pulse of affected area

E. Diagnostic examinations
   1. Accurate account of injury, if possible
   2. X-rays
   3. Alkaline phosphatase, LDH, SGOT blood tests—measure muscle enzymes released with muscle damage

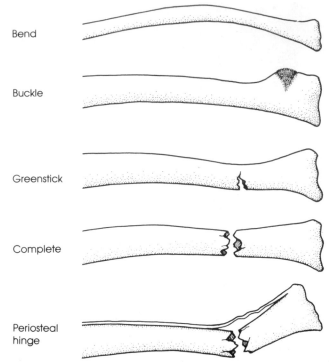

FIGURE 13–4. Types of childhood fractures. Children's bones are more easily injured than adult bones, but since they are more porous, they tend to bend, buckle, or break in a greenstick manner, rather than to fracture completely. A greenstick fracture occurs when the compressed side of the bone bends and the side under tension gives way, resulting in an incomplete fracture. In a complete fracture, the bone fragments are divided, although they may be superficially linked by the periosteal hinge. (From Marlow, S. R., and Redding, B. A. (1988). *Textbook of pediatric nursing*, 6th ed. Philadelphia: W. B. Saunders.)

F. Complications
   1. Emboli
      a. Fat emboli: occur within first 24 to 72 hours after fracture, especially of the femur
      b. Emboli occur secondary to immobility and incorrectly applied casts or traction
   2. Nerve damage
      a. Secondary to fracture itself
      b. Secondary to impaired circulation from tight-fitting cast or traction
   3. Compartment syndrome/contractures
      a. Interference with blood flow to portion of an extremity when joint space fills with blood or edema
      b. Secondary to trauma of fracture, hemorrhage, tight-fitting cast, traction; usually occurs several days after fracture
   4. Bone growth failure with epiphyseal plate injury

TABLE 13–2 Types of Fractures Commonly Seen in Children

Fracture	Definition
Bend/bow	Not true fracture; child's bone will bend as much as 45 degrees before breaking; most common in ulna, fibula
Buckle	Compression of porous bone; bulging projection at fracture site
Complete	Bone, periosteum completely separated from remainder of bone
Greenstick	Incomplete fracture; caused by compression force in long axis of bone
Simple	Closed fracture; muscle, fascia not involved
Compound	Open fracture; muscle, fascia, and skin involved

G. Medical/surgical management
1. Traction (see Chapter 7)
2. Open or closed reduction
3. Casting (Fig. 13-5)

II. Analysis
A. Impaired physical mobility related to application of immobilizing device
B. Fear related to the injury and the presence of immobilizing device
C. Pain related to trauma and associated tissue injury from fracture
D. High risk for altered peripheral tissue perfusion related to cast or traction
E. High risk for infection related to surgery, open fracture, or skeletal traction insertion sites
F. High risk for impaired skin integrity related to immobilizing device or to immobility
G. High risk for constipation related to immobility
H. High risk for altered patterns of urinary elimination related to immobility
I. High risk for sleep pattern disturbance related to presence of immobilizing device or strange environment
J. High risk for activity intolerance related to immobility
K. High risk for altered growth and development related to prolonged immobilization
L. High risk for injury related to imbalance caused by cast or unfamiliarity with crutch walking

III. Planning/goals, expected outcomes
A. Child will not sustain additional injury at fracture site
B. Child will adapt well to immobilizing device

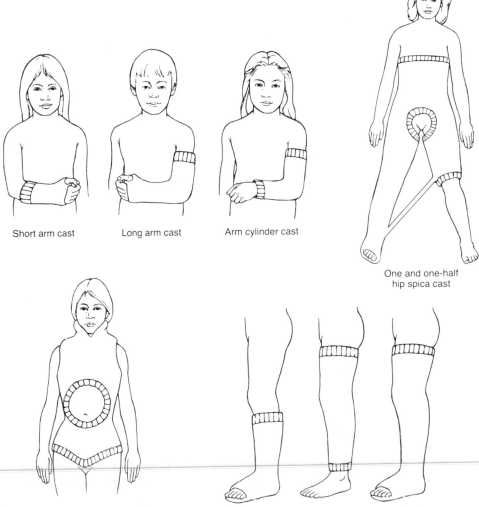

FIGURE 13–5. Types of casts used for children. (From Foster, R. L. R., Hunsberger, M. M., and Anderson, J. T. (1989). *Family-centered nursing care of children*. Philadelphia: W. B. Saunders.)

Short arm cast

Long arm cast

Arm cylinder cast

One and one-half hip spica cast

Risser localizer cast

Short leg cast

Leg cylinder cast

Long leg cast

C. Child will rest comfortably

D. Child will be free of pain

E. Child's skin integrity will be maintained

F. Child's neurovascular function will remain intact

G. Child's fracture site will be free of infection

H. Child will not experience any of the hazards of immobility

I. Child's fracture will heal in proper alignment and without complications

J. Child will maintain range of motion in unaffected areas

K. Child will not regress developmentally or educationally during treatment and rehabilitation period

L. Parents will understand about cast care and traction maintenance

M. Parents will understand home care and follow-up care

IV. Implementation

A. Inspect and immobilize fracture site as soon as possible

B. Assist in application of cast

   1. Types of casts (see Fig. 13-5)
      a. Short/long arm
      b. Short/long leg
      c. Hip spica
      d. Body

   2. Petaling a cast (Fig. 13-6)

C. Assist in application of traction

   1. Skin traction (Table 13-3)
      a. Direct pull to skin surface/indirect pull to skeletal structures by use of ace bandages
      b. Bryant's traction: hips flexed at 90-degree angle: legs, buttocks suspended; child under 30 lb
      c. Buck's extension: lower extremity traction for short-term use (see Fig. 7-2A)
      d. Russel traction: immobilizes hip and knee through skin traction on lower leg and sling under knee (see Fig. 7-3)

   2. Skeletal traction (see Table 13-3)
      a. Direct pull to skeletal structures by use of pins, wires, or tongs inserted into bone distal to fracture
      b. Halo-femoral: metal rings inserted into skull and pins inserted into femur; two-directional traction
      c. Balance supension: two-directional traction wherein leg suspended with hip flexed slightly

D. Prevent complications of immobility (for complications of immobility and nursing care summary, see Chapter 7)

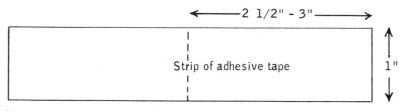

← 2 1/2" - 3" →

Strip of adhesive tape

1"

A   Strip of adhesive tape 1" in width.

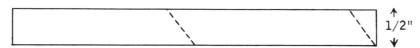

↑ 1/2"

B   Strip of adhesive folded in half with the adhesive side out. Cuts are made as indicated by the broken lines approximately every 2-1/2 " to 3" apart. Petals may be longer depending on the thickness of the cast.

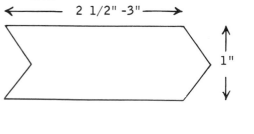

← 2 1/2" -3" →

1"

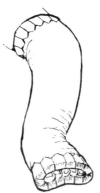

C   Completed petal. Petals are placed over the edge of the cast as shown.

FIGURE 13–6. Petaling a cast. Method of applying adhesive petals around the edges of a cast to prevent the plaster from irritating the skin. *A,* Strip of adhesive tape 1 inch in width. *B,* Strip of adhesive folded in half with the adhesive side out. Cuts are made as indicated by the broken lines approximately every 2½ to 3 inches apart. Petals may be longer, depending on the thickness of the cast. *C,* Completed petal. Petals are placed over the edge of the cast as shown. (From Marlow, D. R., and Redding, B. A. (1988). *Textbook of pediatric nursing,* 6th ed. Philadelphia: W. B. Saunders.)

TABLE 13–3 Traction Care

Responsibilities	Outcome

Knowledge of purpose and function of traction; check functioning of each part of traction
   Pulleys: in place between wheels
   Ropes: knots secured, no fraying
   Weights: hanging freely, proper amount of weight
	Traction properly maintained (in general)

Assess bandages to ensure proper application, make sure they are smooth and unwrinkled, monitor for tightness	Skin traction maintained
Assess pin sites every 2 hours; pin care every shift if ordered; assess pull of traction on pin; should be even	Skeletal traction
Circulation, sensation, movement checks every 2 hours; position changes within limitations every 2 hours; position without disrupting traction alignment; sheepskin, eggcrate mattress	Circulatory impairment prevented
Range of motion exercises to unaffected areas; provide footboard if traction not disrupted	Muscle atrophy, contractures prevented
Force fluids; monitor bowel movements; administer stool softeners, laxatives; assist with fracture bedpan	Constipation prevented
Position with pillows, bedrolls, sandbags; encourage age-appropriate diversional activities	Comfort maintained Growth and development maintained

E. Provide analgesics as per physician's orders (see Table 10-19)
F. Monitor areas around cast/traction for skin breakdown
G. Turn every 2 hours if in a cast; reposition child in traction
H. Give skin care every shift
I. Do neurovascular checks every 4 hours and prn
J. Take vital signs every 4 hours
K. Maintain affected area in proper alignment
L. Provide range of motion exercises to unaffected areas every shift; encourage child to exercise while playing
M. Provide age-appropriate diversional activities (e.g., beanbag toss, Nerf basketball, activities to exercise unaffected extremities)
N. Provide hospital or home bound teachers as appropriate
O. Instruct parents in cast care or traction maintenance
P. Instruct parents/child in home care and follow-up care, including any required physical therapy, teaching about safety principles, crutch walking

V. Evaluation
   A. Child's fracture immobilized immediately after injury
   B. Child does not incur any permanent injury secondary to fracture
   C. Child rests comfortably
   D. Child has no complaints of pain
   E. Child's skin integrity intact with no sign of breakdown
   F. Child exhibits warm, pink extremity distal to fracture; brisk capillary refill; no numbness or tingling
   G. Child's fracture site shows no evidence of infection
   H. Child urinates adequately at least 1 mL/kg/hr
   I. Child has bowel movements according to regular pattern
   J. Child obtains adequate sleep and is alert during wake periods
   K. Child actively participates in play within limitations of immobilizing device
   L. Child does not experience any developmental regression, keeps up with school work
   M. Child maintains contacts with friends
   N. Parents/caregivers describe appropriate home care
   O. Child resumes normal activities slowly and regains muscle strength

Other Disorders

Osteomyelitis

I. Assessment
   A. Definition: infection of the bone, usually femur or tibia
   B. Etiology/incidence
      1. Peak age of occurrence is 5 to 14 years
      2. More common in boys
      3. Causative organisms most often *Staphylococcus aureus*, *Hemophilus influenzae*, *Pseudomonas aeruginosa* (puncture wounds—especially through sneakers), *Salmonella* (seen in children with sickle cell disease)
   C. Predisposing/precipitating factors
      1. Invasion of organisms through the skin directly to the bone (exogenous)
      2. Infection from spread of organisms from an infection in another part of the body (hematogenous)
   D. Clinical manifestations
      1. Redness, swelling, tenderness, and warmth over affected area
      2. Unwillingness to move affected area
      3. Pain
      4. Systemic symptoms: fever, vomiting, irritability, dehydration

E. Diagnostic examinations
1. History of trauma or existing infection elsewhere in body
2. Elevated white blood cell count and erythrocyte sedimentation rate (ESR), positive blood culture for causative organism
3. CT scan may show bone changes
4. X-ray may indicate bone regrowth after 1 to 2 weeks

F. Complications
1. Septicemia
2. Chronic osteomyelitis

G. Medical management
1. IV antibiotics according to causative organisms (see Table 10-2) for at least 4 weeks
2. Immobilization of affected area by splinting or casting

H. Surgical management: surgical decompression if infection does not respond to IV antibiotics

II. Analysis
A. Pain related to tissue injury
B. High risk for fluid volume deficit related to vomiting during acute illness
C. Knowledge deficit about home care related to anxiety and lack of information
D. Other diagnoses related to immobility or cast care may apply

III. Planning/goals, expected outcomes
A. Child will be free of pain
B. Child will take in adequate amount of fluids for age and weight
C. Infection will not spread to others
D. Parent/caregiver understands principles of home management
E. Child does not experience hazards of immobility or complications related to prolonged IV therapy

IV. Implementation
A. Place child on wound drainage precautions
B. Keep child on bedrest; turn slowly, being careful not to jar affected area
C. Maintain splint or cast (see care of child in cast)
D. Monitor IV line carefully; inspect IV site frequently for signs of phlebitis or infiltration
E. Provide adequate fluids that the child likes; monitor urine output
F. Provide age-appropriate diversional activities when child feels better; child can be moved into playroom on a stretcher
G. Teach principles of home management
1. Care and maintenance of IV equipment
2. Proper mixing and administration of antibiotics
3. Cast or splint care
4. Activity limitations
5. Infection prevention including proper disposal of dressings, if used
H. Refer to home health agency for supportive care

V. Evaluation
A. Child rests comfortably and does not complain of pain
B. Child takes in fluids according to preference and demonstrates adequate urinary output of 1 mL/kg/hr
C. Parent/caregiver describes home management and demonstrates medication administration, cast/splint care, turning and repositioning, infection-prevention techniques
D. Child demonstrates adequate elimination, good muscle tone in unaffected extremities, activity tolerance within limits, no regression in development or schooling

Conditions Affecting the Femoral Head

I. Assessment
A. Definition
1. Slipped femoral capital epiphysis (SFCE): displacement of the head (capital epiphysis) from the neck of the femur along the proximal epiphyseal line
2. Legg-Calvé-Perthes disease: avascularity and necrosis of femoral head, which results in incompatibility between femoral head and acetabulum

B. Etiology/incidence
1. SFCE
a. Usually develops immediately before onset of puberty
b. Boys affected more often than girls
c. Usually seen in obese children or tall children who have sustained a rapid growth spurt
d. Bilateral involvement in approximately 25%, with one side following the other
2. Legg-Calvé-Perthes
a. Usually seen in children 4 to 8 years old
b. Boys-to-girl ratio of 5 : 1
c. Bilateral involvement in approximately 15%

C. Predisposing/precipitating factors
1. SFCE: cause unknown; probably precipitated by hormone changes related to puberty; may or may not be related to trauma
2. Legg-Calvé-Perthes
a. Circulatory impairment to epiphysis and acetabulum causes decreased cir-

culation to femoral head, resulting in ischemia and bone necrosis

    b. Course of the disease is prolonged, lasting from 1 to several years before bone revascularization and reossification occur

D. Clinical manifestations

    1. Hip, thigh, or knee pain, either constant or intermittent

    2. Limp

    3. Joint limitation on the affected side

E. Diagnostic examinations

    1. Accurate history combined with knowledge of etiological factors

    2. X-ray confirms diagnosis

F. Complications: permanent dysfunction of affected hip with varying degrees of disability

G. Medical and surgical management

    1. SFCE: varies with degree of displacement; usually involves traction followed by surgical internal fixation

    2. Legg-Calvé-Perthes

        a. Placement and containment of the head of the femur within the acetabulum to preserve femoral head shape

        b. Bedrest and/or traction followed by abduction braces, or casts designed to keep femoral head in acetabulum but allow some weight-bearing

        c. Treatment usually continues for 2 to 4 years, or until reossification occurs

        d. Surgical treatment becoming more acceptable alternative to conservative treatment

II. Analysis: nursing diagnoses are similar to those for any child in traction or cast or the child undergoing surgery; high risk for altered growth and development is of particular concern for the child with Legg-Calvé-Perthes

III. Planning/goals, expected outcomes, Implementation, Evaluation (see sections on caring for the child in traction or cast)

Scoliosis

I. Assessment

A. Definition: lateral curvature of spine, usually associated with rotary deformity; leads to physiological and cosmetic changes to spine, chest, pelvis; may be functional or structural

B. Etiology/incidence

    1. Etiology depends on type

        a. Congenital: congenital malformations of vertebral column

        b. Neuromuscular: neuropathic and myopathic diseases such as cerebral palsy; paralysis of paraspinal/trunk muscles

        c. Idiopathic: unknown etiology; may be multifactorial or autosomal dominant inheritance pattern

        d. Functional: secondary to another abnormality or result of poor posture

    2. 70% cases idiopathic

    3. Female-to-male ratio of 7 : 1 when onset in adolescence

    4. Most common occurrence during adolescent growth spurt

C. Predisposing/precipitating factors

    1. Familial tendency

    2. Adolescent growth spurt

D. Clinical manifestations

    1. Uneven shoulder height, standing

    2. Uneven hip level, standing

    3. Waistline uneven, standing

    4. Obvious curvature of spine, standing, bending

    5. Prominent shoulder blade, standing

    6. Unequal arm lengths, standing

    7. Protrusion/rib hump on one side upper back, bending

    8. Flank asymmetry, bending

    9. Uneven hem lengths

E. Diagnostic examinations

    1. Inspection

    2. Standing x-ray of spine

F. Complications

    1. Respiratory system compromised

    2. Cardiac system compromised

    3. Complications of immobility after surgery, if applicable

G. Medical management: depends on extent of curvature

    1. Exercises

    2. Milwaukee brace or Silastic jacket brace

    3. Electrical stimulation

H. Surgical management: spinal fusion and stabilization by instrumentation

II. Analysis

A. Knowledge deficit about scoliosis, treatment plan, and long-term implications related to inadequate information

B. High risk for body image disturbance related to altered appearance from the condition or the brace

C. High risk for impaired skin integrity related to pressure from the brace

D. High risk for activity intolerance related to immobility and limitations of usual activities from bracing

E. High risk for diversional activity deficit related to bracing or fusion

F. High risk for noncompliance with treatment regimen related to embarrassment or inability to perform usual activities

In addition to usual postoperative diagnoses (see Chapter 12), the following may apply:

    G. Impaired physical mobility related to surgery

    H. High risk for injury to fusion related to maintenance of body alignment

    I. High risk for altered peripheral perfusion related to surgical manipulation

    J. High risk for self-care deficits (activities of daily living) related to immobility

    K. Anxiety related to treatment regimen and long-term prognosis

III. Planning/goals, expected outcomes

    A. Child will be diagnosed early through screening program at school

    B. Parent/child will understand and cooperate with treatment plan

    C. Child will participate in usual activities within limitations of bracing

    D. Child's skin will remain intact

    E. Child will cope with changes in body image

    F. If surgery required, child/parents will be instructed in surgical procedure and postoperative care

    G. Child/parents will be able to express fears and concerns regarding prescribed surgical treatment

    H. Child will be free of postoperative complications
        1. Respiratory infection
        2. Hemorrhage
        3. Neurovascular disfunction
        4. Disorder of skin integrity
        5. Pain
        6. Urinary tract infections
        7. Constipation
        8. Wound infection

    I. Child's nutritional status will be adequate for age and weight

    J. Child will not regress developmentally or educationally during treatment period

    K. Parents will be instructed in home care and follow-up care before discharge

IV. Implementation

    A. Participate in early screening programs for scoliosis in community

    B. Screen child yearly from ages 10 to 13
        1. Clothes do not fit properly
        2. Hems/inseams uneven
        3. Shoulder levels uneven
        4. Hip level uneven
        5. Waistline uneven
        6. Obvious deformity
        7. Prominent shoulder blade
        8. Rib hump
        9. Flank asymmetry

    C. Refer child with positive signs to orthopedic physician

    D. Assist in prescribed treatment regimen
        1. Curve of 0 to 20 degrees: regimen of muscle-strengthening exercises
            a. Pelvic tilts
            b. Abdominal exercises, such as sit-ups
            c. Back-strengthening muscle exercises
        2. Curve of 20 to 40 degrees: bracing and exercise regimen
            a. Milwaukee brace, which fits from under chin to hips, or fiberglass brace with Velcro binding fitting from below breasts to above pubic region
            b. Worn 23 hours per day
            c. Removed only for hygiene
            d. Electrical stimulation (ESO) may be used in conjunction with exercise/brace regimen or alone
            e. ESO consists of surface stimulation to back muscles, which leads to arresting/correction of curvature
            f. ESO used only during sleep
        3. Curve of 40 degrees or more: spinal fusion and instrumentation (Cotrel-Dubousset instrumentation, Harrington rods, Dwyer's procedure)
            a. Most common procedure—spinal fusion with rod instrumentation
            b. Provides stabilization and corrects twisting of vertebrae by derotation and bone graft

    E. Instruct child/parents in prescribed treatment
        1. Meticulous skin care daily
        2. Exercise regimen
        3. Maintenance of brace
        4. ESO operation

    F. Allow child to express feelings/concerns about body changes secondary to brace/casting

    G. Instruct child/parents how to enhance positive body image (e.g., adapting fashionable clothing, emphasizing other positive features)

    H. Encourage child to participate in support groups with other adolescents with scoliosis

    I. Emphasize long-term effects of treatment

    J. If surgery required, instruct child/parent preoperatively on surgical procedure and traction required

    K. Allow child/parents to express fears and concerns about surgery

    L. Instruct child/parents on postoperative care

    M. Turn, cough, and deep breathe every 2 to 4 hours; auscultate lungs every 2 hours; vital signs every 2 to 4 hours

    N. Monitor bandage/bottom sheet for drainage every 2 to 4 hours

O. Obtain CBC daily; hemoglobin and hematocrit may not change for 48 to 72 hours after surgery

P. Do neurovascular checks to lower extremities every 2 hours initially, then every 4 hours

Q. Log-roll every 2 hours; maintain proper alignment at all times

R. Administer narcotic analgesics as per doctor's orders for 3 days, then nonnarcotic analgesics (see Table 10-19)

S. Maintain strict I & O; if no void in 8 hours, catheterize as per orders

T. Administer stool softeners as per orders (see Table 10-14)

U. Monitor incision for signs and symptoms of bleeding or infection

V. Increase diet from fluids to regular as tolerated

W. Provide diversional activities; allow peer visitation; home bound teachers at discharge

X. Instruct child/parents in home care and follow-up care before discharge

Y. Encourage participation in scoliosis support group; give child opportunity to express concerns before discharge

V. Evaluation

A. Child diagnosed by an early screening program

B. Child sought medical care and able to be treated by exercise or bracing

C. Child/parents state responsibilities of treatment regimen and follow-up care

D. Child complies with treatment of bracing/exercise

E. Child free of complications secondary to bracing (e.g., skin remains intact, child deals well with altered appearance)

F. Child/parent describe surgery and postoperative care

G. Postoperatively, child shows no signs and symptoms of complications
1. No respiratory infection or pneumonia
2. Minimal drainage from surgical site
3. Neurovascular status intact to lower extremities
4. No areas of skin breakdown
5. Pain decreases daily
6. Voiding without difficulty
7. Constipation does not develop
8. No signs or symptoms of infection at incisional site
9. Appetite increases daily
10. Child maintains age-appropriate development and educational status
11. Child expresses concerns about body changes and is coping effectively

H. Postoperatively, child/parents describe necessary home care and follow-up care

POST-TEST Musculoskeletal Disorders

1. The goal of treatment for slipped capital femoral epiphysis is to:
   ① Stabilize or improve the position of the femoral head
   ② Maintain the femur in position to encourage growth
   ③ Straighten the curve in the capitis
   ④ Reossify the head of the femur

2. Roberta is suffering from clubfoot and is placed in a Denis Browne splint for discharge. Which of the following would *not* be included in your discharge instructions?
   ① Prevent Roberta from moving her legs
   ② Assess Roberta's feet regularly for signs of redness
   ③ Make sure that Roberta always wears socks with her shoes
   ④ Maintain proper positioning within the splint

3. The Ortolani maneuver and Barlow test are best described as measures that assess:
   ① Muscle spasticity
   ② Hip joint stability
   ③ Degree of joint mobility
   ④ Tendon reflexes and flexibility

Four-year-old Evan fractured his femur after falling off the roof of the porch. He is admitted to the children's unit of the local hospital and immediately placed in skeletal traction. When he arrives on the unit, he is crying but alert. His father is with him.

---

4. Which of the following would be a priority goal for Evan's immediate care?
   ① Ensuring adequate rest
   ② Maintaining fluid balance
   ③ Preventing injury
   ④ Maintaining peripheral perfusion

5. Which of the following complications should the nurse watch for closely during the first few days after the fracture?
   ① Compartment syndrome and ischemia
   ② Fat embolus
   ③ Thrombophlebitis with pulmonary emboli
   ④ Muscle spasms

6. Which of the following would NOT be a part of Evan's routine care after his condition is stable?
   ① Cleaning pin sites and applying antibacterial ointment daily
   ② Wheeling his bed to the playroom daily
   ③ Monitoring circulation, sensation, and motion each shift
   ④ Turning him from his back to unaffected side frequently

7. Which of the following actions demonstrates to the nurse that Evan's father understands the needs of a 4-year-old in traction?
   ① He performs all activities of daily living for Evan
   ② He allows Evan to be directive and to talk back to him
   ③ He agrees to play beanbag toss after Evan takes a rest
   ④ He removes the weights before repositioning Evan

8. After several weeks, Even is placed in a hip spica cast. He complains of itching under his cast. Which of the following nursing interventions would help to relieve this?
   ① Administer an oral antipruritic
   ② Sprinkle powder down the cast daily
   ③ Allow him to insert a padded coat hanger under the cast
   ④ Pour alcohol down the cast

9. Evan is about to be discharged in the spica cast. Which of the following is a priority nursing diagnosis that will need to be addressed in discharge teaching?
   ① High risk for infection related to the fracture
   ② High risk for injury related to the child's developmental stage
   ③ Functional incontinence related to the cast
   ④ Impaired social interaction related to prolonged casting

10. Which of the following would best assist the adolescent placed in a brace for treatment of idiopathic scoliosis to maintain independence in activities of daily living?
    ① Teaching transfer methods to get from bed to chair
    ② Cutting long hair short for easier washing
    ③ Modifying all clothing to be put on feet first
    ④ Providing a flexible straw for dental hygiene

POST-TEST Answers and Rationales

1. ① The goal of treatment is to stop the slipping of the epiphysis and prevent permanent damage by stabilization through internal fixation. Treatment involves maintaining a non–weight-bearing state and surgical correction. 3, II. Slipped Epiphysis.

2. ① The Denis Browne splint is designed so that as the infant kicks, the feet are automatically moved into alignment. Limiting the child's kicking could delay development. The other options are correct interventions. 4, II. Clubfoot.

3. ② These tests are done to evaluate the stability of the hip joint to determine whether the head of the femur can be displaced from the acetabulum and then returned to its normal position. 1, II. Congenital Hip Dislocation.

4. ④ Traction, like casting, can cause circulatory compromise to the affected extremity and result in neurological damage if not corrected quickly. An important nursing goal is to prevent circulatory compromise by recognizing signs and symptoms quickly. 3, II. Fractures.

5. ② Fat embolus is a potential complication of a fracture of a long bone. It occurs usually within the first 24 hours after the injury. Compartment syndrome and ischemia are potential complications; however, they occur after several days. Muscle spasm is not unexpected in a child being treated for fractured femur. 1, II. Fractures.

6. ④ When a client is in skeletal traction, it is important to maintain the pull of the traction without disruption. It is impossible to turn the client without disrupting the skeletal traction. The other options are

appropriate nursing interventions for this client. 4, I & II. Fractures, Traction.

7. ③ Preschool-age children need to exert some control over their environment, even while hospitalized. Performing all activities for the child limits control, especially in a child who normally performs activities of daily living independently at home. Understanding aggressive behavior is important, but accepting it is not. Allowing for an appropriate outlet for the aggression (beanbag toss or other active exercise of upper extremities) within the child's hospital routine helps the child cope with the experience. 5, III. Fractures, Traction.

8. ① Oral antipruritics and distraction are the safest ways to treat itching under a cast. Nothing should ever be inserted into the cast or poured down it. 4. I. Fractures, Cast.

9. ② Four-year-olds usually are particularly active and impulsive. For this reason, their injury potential is high. The parent must be sure that the child is prevented from accidentally falling out of bed while attempting to obtain something out of reach; that the child does not attempt to insert anything into the cast, such as small pieces of toys; and that the child understands activity limitations. 2, I. Fractures, Cast.

10. ④ Adolescents immobilized in a brace for scoliosis are unable to bend from the waist. Because the brace usually can be off for 1 hour a day, bathing and hair-washing can be done then with no need for modification. However, brushing teeth is done several times a day. The adolescent cannot bend over the sink, so a flexible straw, which curves outward from the mouth and then down, facilitates rinsing after brushing with no need to bend. 4, IV. Scoliosis.

BIBLIOGRAPHY

MOBILITY

Alemzadeh, R., et al (1992). Is there compensated hypothyroidism in infancy? *Pediatrics* 90 (2): 207–211.

Corbett, D. (1988). Information needs of parents of a child in a Pavlik harness. *Orthopedic Nursing* 7 (2): 20–22.

Drass, J. (1992). What you need to know about insulin injections. *American Journal of Nursing* 92 (11): 40–43.

Foster, R. L. R., Hunsberger, M. M., and Anderson, J. T. (1989). *Family-centered nursing care of children.* Philadelphia: W. B. Saunders.

Gamron, R. (1988). Taking the pressure out of compartment syndrome. *American Journal of Nursing* 88 (8): 1076–1080.

Jacobs-Zacny, J. M., and Horn, M. J. (1988). Nursing care of adolescents having posterior spinal fusion with Cotrel-Dubousset instrumentation. *Orthopedic Nursing* 7 (1): 17–21.

Jewler, D. (1988). Diabetes costs: Up, up, and away. *Diabetes Forecast* 41 (10): 23–26.

LaFranchi, S., Hanna, C. E., and Mandel, S. H. (1991). Constitutional delay of growth: Expected versus final adult height. *Pediatrics* 87 (1): 82–87.

Ledwith, C. A., and Fleisher, G. R. (1992). Slipped capital femoral epiphysis without hip pain leads to missed diagnosis. *Pediatrics* 89 (4): 660–662.

Lieber, M. T., and Taub, A. S. (1988). Common foot deformities and what they mean for parents. *MCN* 13 (Jan/Feb): 47–50.

MacLean, W. E., et al (1989). Stress and coping with scoliosis: Psychological effects on adolescents and their families. *Journal of Pediatric Orthopedics* 9: 257–261.

Mellick, L. B., et al (1988). Tibial fractures of young children. *Pediatric Emergency Care* 4 (June): 97–101.

Mott, S. R., James, S. R., and Sperhac, A. M. (1990). *Nursing care of children and families,* 2nd ed. Redwood City, CA: Addison-Wesley.

North, B., North C., and Lee, J. (1992). Living in a halo. *American Journal of Nursing* 92 (4): 55–56.

Speers, A. T., and Speers, M. (1992). Care of the infant in a Pavlik harness. *Pediatric Nursing* 18 (3): 229–232.

Thomas, S. A., et al (1991). Long-bone fractures in young children: Distinguishing accidental injuries from child abuse. *Pediatrics* 88 (9): 471–476.

Tonnis, D., et al (1990). Results of newborn screening for CDH with and without sonography and correlation of risk factors. *Journal of Pediatric Orthopedics* 10: 145–152.

Volta, C., et al (1991). Effectiveness of growth-promoting therapies: Comparison among growth hormone, clonidine, and levo-dopa. *American Journal of Diseases of Children* 145 (2): 168–171.

Walter, R. S., et al (1992). Ultrasound screening of high-risk infants: A method to increase early detection of congenital dysplasia of the hip. *American Journal of Diseases of Children* 146 (2): 230–234.

Whaley, L. F., and Wong, D. L. (1991). *Nursing care of infants and children,* 4th ed. St. Louis: Mosby-Year Book.

14

Metabolism and Elimination in the Pediatric Client

PRE-TEST Endocrine Disorders

1. It is vitally important that congenital hypothyroidism be diagnosed in infancy because:
   1. Early intervention means that it can be cured
   2. Long-term side effects will be minimized
   3. Mental retardation can be arrested
   4. Growth will be enhanced

2. Harriet is a 9-year-old who is admitted to the intensive care unit in severe ketoacidosis with a blood sugar level of 600 mg. The cause of this is most likely:
   1. Dehydration
   2. Metabolic alkalosis
   3. Insulin deficiency
   4. Gluconeogenesis

3. Which of the following would NOT be a part of the nursing management of Harriet's ketoacidosis while she is in the unit?
   1. Teaching her insulin administration
   2. Measuring I & O hourly
   3. Monitoring her cardiac status
   4. Monitoring the IV insulin rate

4. Which of the following would NOT be a classic sign or symptom of insulin-dependent diabetes mellitus (IDDM)?
   1. Polyuria
   2. Obesity
   3. Polydipsia
   4. Polyphagia

5. Which of the following would Harriet need to be taught, along with her parents, about when her nutritional requirements would increase?
   1. When her blood glucose level is 140 mg/dL
   2. If she forgets her morning dose of insulin
   3. When she goes through a growth spurt
   4. If she maintains a regular exercise pattern

6. Which of the following statements by Harriet indicates that she has an understanding of her diet?
   1. "I can't have a birthday cake again."
   2. "I need to plan with my mom what I can eat at McDonald's."
   3. "Candy is okay to eat if I only eat it once in a while."
   4. "I can eat as many foods as I want as long as I exercise."

7. Which of the following manifestations would indicate that a child is suffering from diabetes insipidus rather than diabetes mellitus?
   1. Polydipsia
   2. Polyuria
   3. Low urine specific gravity
   4. Ketonuria

8. Which of the following nursing diagnoses might be appropriate for the child with hypopituitarism?
   1. Diversional activity deficit
   2. Altered nutrition: more than body requirements
   3. Activity intolerance
   4. Body image disturbance

9. Activity intolerance in the child with acquired hypothyroidism is generally related to:
   1. Decreased metabolic rate
   2. Inadequate intake of iron
   3. Inadequate oxygenation
   4. Excessive intake of iodine

10. Which of the following diagnostic test results would NOT be associated with hypothyroidism?
    1. Low T_3 and T_4 levels
    2. Low growth hormone levels
    3. High thyroid-stimulating hormone levels
    4. Bone x-rays indicating growth retardation

PRE-TEST Answers and Rationales

1. ③ Congenital hypothyroidism is a common but preventable cause of mental retardation when it is discovered early. Although lifetime replacement of thyroid hormone is required, it will prevent any problems resulting from the disease. 5, II. Hypothyroidism.

2. ③ When there is not enough insulin, diabetic ketoacidosis develops. This is a catabolic state that results in energy production ketoacidosis. 2, II. Diabetes Mellitus.

3. ① Although Harriet will eventually need to learn self-administration of insulin, it is currently a very low priority. Such teaching can begin when she is stable. At this time, the other options are the priority nursing interventions. 4, II. Diabetes Mellitus.

4. ② Weight loss plus the other options are the classic signs of insulin-dependent diabetes; obesity is associated with non–insulin-dependent diabetes. 1, II. Diabetes Mellitus.

5. ③ Growth spurts in children affect caloric requirements, which increases the need for calories to support the growth. After a time, the need decreases again, but during the spurts, children will need more food. 3, II. Diabetes Mellitus.

6. ② Children with diabetes need to avoid concentrated sweets like candy, and their diet should reflect a balance of calories, protein, carbohydrates, and fat regardless of the amount of exercise. Working foods that the child likes into the diet is important for compliance. Children can still eat at fast-food restaurants, so long as they include the food in their dietary plan. 5, III. Diabetes Mellitus.

7. ③ The symptoms of diabetes insipidus are similar to those of diabetes mellitus—polydipsia, polyuria, and polyphagia. In diabetes insipidus, large volumes of urine have low specific gravity and do not test positive for glucose. 1, II. Diabetes Insipidus.

8. ④ The child with hypopituitarism manifests a deficiency in growth hormone, which limits linear growth if not properly treated. Children who are significantly smaller than peers can experience difficulties with body image and self-esteem. 2, III. Diabetes Insipidus.

9. ① Children with acquired hypothyroidism demonstrate a decreased metabolic rate as a result of thyroxine deficiency. They experience fatigue and find it difficult to participate in strenuous activity. 2, II. Hypothyroidism.

10. ② Hypothyroidism may be manifested by altered thyroid hormone levels, increased thyroid-stimulating hormones, and evidence of growth retardation on bone x-rays. Growth hormone levels are not affected. 1, II. Hypothyroidism.

NORMAL ENDOCRINE SYSTEM

I. Responsible for growth, maturation, reproduction, and metabolic processes
   A. Basic components of system
      1. Endocrine cell, which delivers chemical message by means of a hormone
      2. Target cell or end organ, which receives message
      3. Environment through which information is transported
   B. Main endocrine gland is pituitary gland, also known as master gland
      1. Pituitary controlled by hypothalamus
      2. Central nervous system sends message to hypothalamus, resulting in secretion of releasing factors and, ultimately, secretion of tropic hormones
   C. Not all hormones in body dependent on other hormones for release (e.g., insulin production)
   D. Endocrine glands
      1. Pituitary (see Chapter 8, Endocrine, for normal function of glands)
      2. Thyroid
      3. Parathyroid
      4. Adrenal
      5. Islets of Langerhans
      6. Ovaries
      7. Testes

NURSING PROCESS APPLIED TO CHILDREN WITH ENDOCRINE DISORDERS

Hypopituitarism

I. Assessment
   A. Definition: deficiency in growth hormone, specifically somatotropin, which causes delayed linear growth; associated hormone deficiencies may cause altered metabolism, delayed sexual maturation, and fluid and electrolyte imbalance
   B. Etiology/incidence
      1. Etiology unknown for infantile growth hormone deficiency
      2. Insidious onset in late infancy
      3. Brain tumor most common cause in older child
   C. Predisposing/precipitating factors
      1. Reduced secretion of somatotropin resulting in deficient synthesis of somatomedin, which is necessary for bone growth
      2. Possible reduced synthesis of other hormones: ACTH, gonadotropins, thyroid-stimulating, antidiuretic
   D. Clinical manifestations
      1. Hypoglycemia often the first manifestation
      2. Short stature
         a. Slowed growth begins late in first year of life
         b. Height delayed more than weight
      3. Immature appearance for age
      4. Delayed sexual development, although normal fertility
      5. Delayed eruption of permanent teeth
      6. Retarded epiphyseal maturation
      7. Associated hypothyroidism, dehydration, anorexia, and weight loss if other hormones affected
   E. Diagnostic examinations
      1. Accurate history and growth monitoring to rule out familial short stature or other cause of growth delay
      2. Serum somatomedin level
      3. Provocation tests for level of growth hormone
      4. Skeletal x-rays, including wrist, for determination of bone age
      5. CT scan to detect tumor
   F. Complications: psychological adjustment problems due to lack of adult height; complications associated with related hormone deficiencies
   G. Medical and surgical management
      1. Administration of synthetic growth hormone several times weekly until growth plates fuse
      2. Removal of pituitary tumor, if present
II. Analysis
   A. Altered growth and development related to growth hormone deficiency
   B. High risk for altered nutrition: less than body requirements related to altered glucose metabolism
   C. High risk for body image disturbance related to appearance
   D. High risk for self-esteem disturbance related to inability to keep up with peers or peer reaction to appearance
   E. Knowledge deficit about dysfunction and home management related to unfamiliarity with information
   F. High risk for altered family processes related to expense of growth hormone and long-term nature of the disease
III. Planning/goals, expected outcomes
   A. Child's growth delay will be recognized and referred as a result of periodic screening
   B. Parents/caregivers will understand prognosis and treatment regimen
   C. Parents/child will begin to express concerns and feelings about diagnosis
   D. Child will come to accept body size
   E. Child will acquire a positive self-image
   F. Family will not experience undo stress as a result of the child's treatment
IV. Implementation
   A. Accurately measure height and weight
   B. Monitor signs of delayed growth at each checkup
   C. Obtain accurate history about manifestations that might indicate alternate cause of delayed growth
   D. Participate in health team conference with parents and explain hormone therapy and its effects
   E. Provide parents opportunity to ask questions
   F. Allow child to discuss concerns about size
   G. Provide alternative activities that do not rely on height, e.g., swimming, tennis, drama, dance, art
   H. Teach parent/caregiver about growth hormone administration
      1. Do not shake vial of hormone; rotate gently to mix
      2. Do not inject solution if cloudy
      3. Use sterile equipment for injection
      4. Store excess in refrigerator

V. Evaluation
   A. Child's delayed growth pattern diagnosed early, and referral made to endocrinologist
   B. Parents able to describe diagnosis and possible effects of hormone therapy
   C. Child able to discuss concerns openly or through play therapy
   D. Child develops positive self-image, interacts well socially, participates in age-appropriate activities, demonstrates self-confidence

Hypothyroidism

I. Assessment
   A. Definition: congenital deficiency of thyroid hormone, which often leads to central nervous system impairment
   B. Etiology/incidence
      1. Usually results from failure of embryonic development of thyroid gland
      2. May also result from inborn enzymatic defects in the synthesis of thyroxine
      3. One per 4000 live births
      4. May be transient or permanent
      5. More common in girls
      6. Acquired from inadequate dietary intake of iodine or from conditions affecting the thyroid
   C. Predisposing/precipitating factors
      1. Lack of development or total absence of thyroid gland
      2. Deficiency of thyroid hormone
   D. Clinical manifestations
      1. Manifests itself earlier in bottle-fed babies
      2. Usually apparent by age 3 to 6 months, delay due to passive transfer of maternal thyroid hormone
      3. Severity depends on amount of thyroid tissue present, if any
      4. Prolonged physiological jaundice
      5. Lethargy, inactivity, infant sleeps more than expected
      6. Feeding difficulties
      7. Low-pitched, grunt-like cry
      8. Wide, puffy eyes
      9. Coarse, dry skin and hair
      10. Large, protruding tongue
      11. Protruding abdomen
      12. Constipation
      13. Hypothermia and hypotension
   E. Diagnostic examinations
      1. T_3 and T_4 blood levels low, thyroid-stimulating hormone blood levels high
      2. Bone age x-rays reveal growth retardation
      3. Routine newborn screening assisted by evaluation of the basal metabolic rate

(BMR) can identify affected infants before symptoms appear
   F. Complication: permanent mental retardation if not treated early
   G. Medical management: lifetime thyroid hormone replacement

II. Analysis
   A. High risk for altered growth and development related to hormone deficiency
   B. Constipation related to decreased gastric motility
   C. Altered nutrition: less than body requirements related to feeding difficulties (congenital condition)
   D. Activity intolerance related to decreased metabolic rate
   E. Hypothermia related to decreased metabolic rate
   F. Knowledge deficit about condition and home management related to incomplete information

III. Planning/goals, expected outcomes
   A. Child will have diagnosis made as early in life as possible
   B. Child will comply with hormone therapy
   C. Parents will understand diagnosis and treatment regimen
   D. Parents will discuss realistic expectations of child's development
   E. Parents will understand medication regimen and possible side effects or toxic effects to be aware of
   F. Parents will implement treatment at home with follow-up care
   G. Child will develop normally

IV. Implementation
   A. Monitor newborn in nursery for earliest signs of hypothyroidism; obtain blood for routine screening
   B. Obtain accurate history of infant's behavior in follow-up visits to pediatrician
   C. Feed infant slowly; allow to swallow small amounts at a time
   D. Dress to maintain body temperature
   E. Encourage age-appropriate exercise, but allow for adequate rest
   F. Participate in administration of hormone therapy, which begins as soon as diagnosis made
   G. Monitor infant closely for manifestations of overdose
      1. Hypertension
      2. Weight loss
      3. Tachycardia
      4. Dyspnea
      5. Irritability
      6. Insomnia

H. Instruct parents in medication regimen and potential overdose symptoms

I. Teach parents how to manage constipation (high fiber, increased fluids, stool softeners for older child)

J. Give parents opportunity to discuss fears and concerns about diagnosis and prognosis

K. Present realistic expectations to parents about child's development
1. Child will need to take medication for rest of life
2. Some children who receive hormone therapy will develop normally; others will have a variety of impairments, including mental retardation

V. Evaluation
A. Child's condition recognized and treated early
B. Child's hormone therapy is being tolerated without complications
C. Parents describe accurately responsibilities of medication regimen and toxic side effects
D. Parents participate in health team conference and discuss openly their concerns
E. Parents cope effectively with prognosis and seek assistance as needed
F. Child achieves developmental milestones at appropriate time
G. Child participates in age-appropriate activities without fatigue

Diabetes Insipidus

I. Assessment
A. Definition: most frequently occurring disorder of posterior pituitary gland; hyposecretion of antidiuretic hormone (ADH); state of uncontrolled diuresis
B. Etiology/incidence
1. Genetic transmission
2. Central nervous system tumor or infection
3. Congenital malformations of the central nervous system
4. Idiopathic
5. May develop at any age
C. Predisposing/precipitating factor: insufficiency in production of ADH
D. Clinical manifestations
1. Polyuria
2. Polydipsia
3. Weight loss
4. First indication may be enuresis
E. Diagnostic examinations
1. Fluid deprivation test; must be done in hospital setting
a. NPO for 8 hours
b. Changes should occur in urine volume

and concentration (large urine volume independent of intake, low concentration)
2. Specific gravity of less than 1.005
3. Urine osmolality of less than 150 mOsm/kg
4. Serum osmolality elevated
5. Serum sodium elevated
6. Kidney function studies
7. Skull x-ray to detect pituitary tumor
F. Complications
1. Severe dehydration if unrecognized or medication not given
2. None if treatment continued throughout life
G. Medical management: lifetime replacement of ADH through daily injections of vasopressin or twice-daily desmopressin acetate (DDAVP) by nasal spray

II. Analysis
A. High risk for fluid volume deficit related to deficiency of ADH
B. Knowledge deficit about condition and long-term management related to incomplete information

III. Planning/goals, expected outcomes
A. Child will maintain adequate fluid and electrolyte balance
B. Child/parents will understand all diagnostic examinations
C. Parents will participate in teaching sessions about diagnosis and definition of diabetes insipidus (i.e., how it differs from diabetes mellitus)
D. Child will comply with medication regimen
E. Parents will understand correct preparation and administration of drug
F. When child is old enough, child will learn responsibilities of medication administration

IV. Implementation
A. Obtain accurate history of child's toileting habits at each well-child checkup
B. Obtain accurate history of unusual fluid demands at each checkup
C. Accurately measure weight
D. Maintain strict I & O; maintain IV line if ordered for fluid replacement
E. Measure specific gravity at every void during diagnostic period
F. Assist with fluid deprivation test
G. Teach parents about diagnosis and differences between diabetes insipidus and diabetes mellitus
H. Teach child/parents preparation and administration of vasopressin (Pitressin)
1. Administered IM

2. Injections last longer but painful because of thick oil base
3. Must be adequately mixed before administration
4. Medication taken for rest of life
5. Medication should always be on hand in case of increasing urination
 I. Alternatively, teach administration of DDAVP
    1. Prime pump
    2. Insert in nostril and depress pump once
    3. Store in refrigerator
 V. Evaluation
    A. Child diagnosed during routine checkup through accurate history
    B. Child participates in diagnostic tests without complications
    C. Parents accurately explain differences between diabetes insipidus and diabetes mellitus
    D. Parents state and demonstrate correct preparation and administration of medication

Diabetes Mellitus

 I. Assessment
    A. Definition: deficiency in insulin production; multisystem disorder in which carbohydrate, fat, and protein metabolism altered and cardiovascular, renal, ophthalmic, and neurological complications common
    B. Classifications
       1. Insulin-dependent diabetes mellitus (IDDM), or Type I; old name juvenile or brittle diabetes; onset in childhood and adolescence often; ketosis-prone without insulin replacement therapy
       2. Non–insulin-dependent diabetes mellitus (NIDDM), or Type II; old name adult-onset or maturity-onset; ketosis develops rarely
       3. Maturity-onset diabetes of youth (MODY); symptoms similar to NIDDM; develops during adolescence
    C. Etiology/incidence
       1. Multifactorial inherited disorder
          a. 100% of adults whose parents both have NIDDM will develop disorder
          b. 45 to 60% of offspring of both parents who have IDDM will develop disorder
          c. MODY can occur in adolescents with strong family history of NIDDM
       2. Most frequent endocrine disorder in children
       3. One to two per 1000 children

4. Male-to-female ratio of 1 : 1
5. One of four families with history of diabetes
6. IDDM uncommon in African Americans
    D. Predisposing/precipitating factors
       1. IDDM
          a. Reduction in islet cell mass
          b. Destruction of islets
          c. Viruses: attack susceptible pancreas in predisposed individuals; autoimmune reaction
       2. NIDDM
          a. Decreased insulin secretory response in pancreas
          b. Increased insulin requirements
          c. Interference with use of insulin
    E. Clinical manifestations
       1. Polyuria
       2. Polydipsia
       3. Polyphagia
       4. Weight loss
       5. Hyperglycemia, blood sugar level of more than 140 mg/dL; can be as high as 1000 mg/dL
       6. Glycosuria
       7. Ketonuria
       8. Irritability
       9. Recurrent yeast infections
      10. Abdominal discomfort, thirst, nocturnal enuresis
    F. Diagnostic examinations
       1. Routine screening for glycosuria
       2. Fasting blood sugar
       3. Glycosylated hemoglobin to determine glucose concentration in erythrocytes over time
       4. Glucose tolerance tests
    G. Complications
       1. Diabetic ketoacidosis (see Chapter 8; see Table 8–6)
       2. Hypoglycemia
       3. Retinopathy
       4. Kidney disease
       5. Neurological disease
       6. Circulatory disorders
    H. Medical management
       1. Treatment of ketoacidosis
          a. Administration of IV fluids and electrolytes to restore balance
          b. Continuous IV infusion of low-dose insulin
       2. Administration of insulin (oral hypoglycemics for NIDDM) (see Table 8–5)
       3. Diet appropriate for age and growth requirements, insulin requirements, amount of exercise

a. No concentrated sweets

b. Consistent calories, protein, fat, and carbohydrates daily

c. Fast-foods may be incorporated into diet

d. May use American Diabetic Association exchange system, or point system if preferred

4. Exercise normal for age and developmental level

II. Analysis

A. Acute care

1. Fluid volume deficit related to altered metabolism and electrolyte imbalance

2. Altered patterns of urinary elimination: frequency related to osmotic diuresis

3. High risk for impaired gas exchange and ineffective breathing pattern related to underlying metabolic dysfunction

4. Sensory/perceptual alterations related to electrolyte imbalance

5. Anxiety related to severity of the illness

B. Ongoing care

1. Altered nutrition: less than body requirements for growth related to inappropriate metabolism of glucose

2. High risk for ineffective individual or family coping related to effects of chronic condition

3. High risk for body image disturbance related to perceived difference from peers

4. Knowledge deficit about diabetes management related to unfamiliarity with information or incomplete understanding of principles of care

5. High risk for noncompliance with treatment related to body image disturbance

III. Planning/goals, expected outcomes

A. Child will be diagnosed as early as possible as a result of routine screening

B. Child/parents will understand diagnostic tests

C. Child/parents will understand diagnosis, including all facets of disorder and treatment regimen

D. Child's vital signs will remain stable in acute phase

E. Child's fluid and electrolyte balance will remain stable

F. Child will not develop clinical manifestations of hypoglycemia, hyperglycemia, or ketoacidosis

G. Child will maintain adequate nutrition and exercise for age

H. Child/parents will understand:

1. Preparation and administration of insulin

2. Glucose monitoring

3. Nutritional alterations

4. Exercise regimen

5. Modification of insulin dose based on blood/glucose results, changes in diet or exercise, presence of illness

6. Signs/symptoms of hyperglycemia, hypoglycemia, ketoacidosis

I. Child will not develop complications of diabetes:

1. Renal failure

2. Circulatory impairment, especially peripheral vascular disease

3. Altered skin integrity

4. Infections

5. Visual changes

J. Child/parents will cope effectively with altered life-style

IV. Implementation

A. Monitor for clinical manifestations of diabetes during routine examinations

B. Assist with 4- or 6-hour glucose tolerance testing

1. Collect urine before test begins and withdraw blood every hour

2. Assist child in drinking glucagon

3. Ensure that child remains NPO except for water to encourage void

C. Explain to child/parents nature of disease, impact on life, possible treatment regimen

D. Provide child/parents with literature on disease in language they understand (pamphlets from American Diabetic Association)

E. Monitor vital signs frequently during acute phases of disease

F. Monitor I & O; maintain IV line and IV insulin as ordered

G. Monitor blood/urine glucose as ordered

H. Observe for clinical manifestations of hypoglycemia and report immediately

1. Irritability

2. Shaky feeling

3. Headache

4. Hunger

I. If hypoglycemia occurs, administer carbohydrates (fruit juice if conscious) immediately

J. Observe for clinical manifestations of hyperglycemia

1. Thirst

2. Hunger

3. Diuresis

K. Provide and teach prescribed diet, usually three meals a day plus one or two snacks

L. Teach child to avoid concentrated carbohydrates

M. Provide exchange lists and help with home

menu planning; be sure to include foods child likes and make adjustments for adolescent preferences

N. Encourage regular exercise

O. Administer insulin as ordered

P. Instruct child/parents in preparation and administration of insulin
   1. Basic injection technique using orange
   2. Return demonstration for all who will be involved
   3. How to rotate sites, using same body part 1 in. apart for 1 week before changing site
   4. Preparation of insulin injection
   5. Storage of insulin and care of equipment

Q. Monitor child for breaks in skin integrity and continue to reinforce good skin care

R. Teach other aspects of care
   1. Blood glucose monitoring
   2. Urine to test glucose and ketones when child is ill
   3. Hygiene and health maintenance
   4. Wearing a medical alert bracelet or tag

S. Have child take part in age-appropriate diabetic classes

T. Allow child/parents opportunities to discuss feelings and concerns about disease

U. Teach child how to make independent, intelligent choices

V. Help family find least expensive equipment alternatives for their lifestyle

V. Evaluation

A. Child's diabetes diagnosed during routine checkup

B. Child participates in diagnostic tests without complications

C. Child/parents participate in teaching sessions about diagnosis and treatment regimen

D. Child's glycosuria and hyperglycemia brought under control

E. Child/parent can describe signs of hypoglycemia or ketoacidosis

F. Child/parents accurately demonstrate home management techniques

G. Child maintains adequate age-appropriate nutrition

H. Child/parents begin to cope with life changes caused by disease and continue to ask for help when needed

POST-TEST Endocrine Disorders

1. Ruth is a 15-year-old newly diagnosed diabetic. She must learn a new way of life that incorporates a nutritious diet with an exercise regimen. Which of the following is the best approach to achieve this goal?
   1. Emphasize the serious long-term complications of diabetes that will occur if she does not comply
   2. Provide her with detailed menus and an exact schedule for her exercise regimen
   3. Work with Ruth to set mutually acceptable goals for her diet and exercise
   4. Teach Ruth's parents how to plan the meals and the exercise schedule

2. Mr. and Mrs. Spano express concern about their infant son, who is a very pleasant child. They tell you that he sleeps all the time and cries very rarely and that his skin has a yellowish tinge. Biliary atresia has been ruled out. What other condition might be suspected?
   1. Phenylketonuria
   2. Congenital hypothyroidism
   3. Congenital hyperthyroidism
   4. Tay-Sachs disease

3. Roger is an 8-year-old diabetic. Which of the following components of his diabetic care will NOT be included in your teaching?
   1. Teaching him to give his own insulin
   2. Teaching him to monitor his blood glucose weekly
   3. Helping him to select foods based on an exchange list
   4. Assisting him to learn to rotate his insulin sites

4. Which of the following best describes the pathophysiology of diabetes insipidus?
   1. Insufficient production of ADH
   2. Increased secretion of cortisol
   3. Increased aldosterone secretion
   4. Decreased secretion of insulin

5. Which of the following is the treatment of choice for diabetes insipidus?
   1. Transsphenoidal hypophysectomy
   2. Administration of growth hormone if epiphyses open
   3. Administration of glucose for low blood sugar
   4. Administration of Pitressin IM or nasally

6. Which of the following diagnostic results is NOT initially indicative of diabetes mellitus?
   1. Ketosis
   2. Glycosuria
   3. Hyperglycemia
   4. High insulin levels

7. The best indicator that IDDM is in good control is:
   1. No episodes of glycosuria
   2. Normal daily blood sugar levels
   3. High serum insulin levels
   4. Frequent episodes of hypoglycemia

8. Maria, a 12-year-old Type I diabetic, has been

exhibiting signs of weakness, irritability, hunger, and recurring headache. Which of the following recommendations might take care of these symptoms?

① Increase her daily insulin dose
② Decrease the amount of exercise she does
③ Decrease her daily insulin dose
④ Have her take her insulin after breakfast instead of before

9. If Maria was on a combination of regular and NPH insulin every morning before breakfast, when should the nurse tell her to watch for an insulin reaction?

① After breakfast and after lunch
② After lunch and before dinner
③ Before dinner and at bedtime
④ Before lunch and before dinner

10. Nat is a 1-year-old who was diagnosed with hypothyroidism when he was 4 months old. He has been on Synthroid since diagnosis. Which of the following would NOT be a symptom of medication toxicity?

① Protruding abdomen
② Hypertension
③ Weight loss
④ Irritability

POST-TEST Answers and Rationales

1. ③ The adolescent is very likely to resent dependency, and with a disease like diabetes that requires a change in lifestyle, it is important that the client agree with the goals. If Ruth is expected to comply with her plan of care, she intimately must be involved in the establishment of goals and plans. 3 & 4, I. Diabetes Mellitus.

2. ② The diagnosis of congenital hypothyroidism is supported by the parents' description of a child as pleasant, rarely crying, and sleeping most of the time. The presence of prolonged physiological jaundice with these other symptoms indicates hypothyroidism. Most infants with congenital hypothyroidism are identified through newborn screening programs. 2, II. Hypothyroidism.

3. ② The glucose level must be monitored more often than weekly in a newly diagnosed insulin-dependent diabetic because glucose levels may vary until control is established. The other options are elements that must be included in the teaching. 4, II. Diabetes Mellitus.

4. ① Diabetes insipidus results when the posterior pituitary production of ADH is affected, causing uncontrolled diuresis unless replacement hormones are administered. 1, II. Diabetes Insipidus.

5. ④ As stated above, ADH must be replaced artificially, and Pitressin, either IM in oil or nasally, must be administered until the condition is reversed or for life. 4, II. Diabetes Insipidus.

6. ④ Diabetes mellitus is associated with lower-than-normal levels of insulin, not increased levels. The other options contain results characteristic of diabetes. 2, II. Diabetes Mellitus.

7. ② Keeping the blood sugar stable and within the normal range for the child is a goal of diabetes management. Regular urine testing is not done because it is not as accurate as blood glucose testing for determining glucose levels, and for some children a small amount of glycosuria is acceptable to prevent episodes of hypoglycemia. Insulin levels usually are not measured. 3, II. Diabetes Mellitus.

8. ③ The symptoms Maria is exhibiting are characteristic of hypoglycemia or excessive amounts of insulin. All of the other actions would further increase her hypoglycemia. 5, II. Diabetes Mellitus.

9. ④ Regular insulin peaks in 2 to 4 hours, and the blood sugar level is lower before lunch. NPH peaks in about 8 to 10 hours, and the blood sugar level is lower before dinner. 5, I. Diabetes Mellitus.

10. ① A protruding abdomen or ascites is not associated with hyperthyroidism, which is what Synthroid toxicity would look like. The other options are commonly associated with Synthroid toxicity. 1, II. Hypothyroidism.

PRE-TEST Gastrointestinal and Liver/Biliary Disorders

Sarita is a 1-month-old who was brought to the clinic for her well-child checkup. Her mother reports that she has always been a difficult child to feed because she is constantly "spitting up" her formula. Occasionally, she even gags and turns blue after she eats. She has been fussy and difficult to console.

1. When the nurse weighs Sarita, she discovers that her weight percentile has dropped from the 75th at birth to the 25th. After asking Sarita's mother about her pattern of eating and quantity of formula consumed, the nurse should elicit:
   ① What vitamin supplements Sarita is taking
   ② Her usual position when she sleeps
   ③ A description of her vomiting
   ④ How often she has a bowel movement

2. The nurse determines that Sarita appears well hydrated and that her vomiting pattern is not projectile. Which of the following should she suggest that Sarita's mother try for the next week?
   ① Give Sarita smaller, more frequent feedings; burp her frequently; place her in prone position with head slightly elevated after feeding

② Change Sarita's formula to 30 cal/oz; give her larger feedings; add one more feeding per day

③ Use formula without iron supplementation; burp Sarita after every bottle; place her in flat, side-lying position after feeding

④ Feed Sarita with her sitting in an infant seat; begin feeding rice cereal by spoon; give no more than 2 oz of formula at a time

---

Harry is a 4-year-old who is admitted to the children's unit with a diagnosis of Hirschsprung's disease. He is admitted for surgical resection of the aganglionic portion of bowel with possible temporary colostomy.

---

3. Because Harry has been constipated chronically, the physician orders enemas until clear. Which of the following would the nurse be likely to administer until clear?
   ① Adult Fleet enemas
   ② Tap water enemas
   ③ Pediatric soap-suds enemas
   ④ Isotonic saline enemas

4. Which of the following would be an important goal for Harry after surgery?
   ① Achievement of bowel control
   ② Increased weight gain
   ③ Prevention of diarrhea
   ④ Acceptance of permanent disability

5. Harry returns from surgery with a temporary colostomy. A liquid skin barrier is used on the peristomal skin around a colostomy to:
   ① Protect the skin from irritation
   ② Facilitate the drainage of stool
   ③ Improve adhesiveness of the appliance
   ④ Provide for client comfort

6. Nona is suspected of having an intussusception and is scheduled for a barium enema. The major rationale for the enema is to:
   ① Diagnose the type of obstruction
   ② Reduce the telescoping by hydrostatic pressure
   ③ Provide a means for fecal evacuation
   ④ Promote water reabsorption in the large intestine

7. Brian is a newborn who is admitted to the special care nursery after having surgery for tracheoesophageal fistula. Gastrostomy feedings are ordered. Why should Brian be given a pacifier during gastrostomy feedings?

① It will satisfy his need to suck during feedings
② It will prevent regurgitation through his mouth
③ It will help prevent aspiration pneumonia
④ It will substitute for not being held

8. Why are medium-chain triglyceride formulas such as Portagen and Pregestimil used for children with biliary atresia?
   ① To help decrease the severity of jaundice
   ② To prevent extreme weight loss caused by steatorrhea
   ③ Because supplements of vitamins A, D, and E are required
   ④ To provide dietary fats that can be digested without bile

9. Which of the following potential nursing diagnoses might be appropriate for a 15-month-old with a not-yet-repaired cleft palate?
   ① Altered nutrition: less than body requirements related to feeding difficulties
   ② Altered parenting related to the child's physical impairment
   ③ Body image disturbance related to feelings about being different
   ④ High risk for impaired verbal communication related to presence of a defect

10. Which of the following is the likely cause of abrupt lower right quadrant abdominal pain, vomiting, and lack of bowel sounds in an adolescent?
    ① Psychosomatic school phobia
    ② Diverticulosis
    ③ Appendicitis
    ④ Inflammatory bowel disease

11. What would be the desired long-term outcome for a child who has had a pull-through procedure for imperforate anus?
    ① Child/parents able to describe colostomy care
    ② Child achieves bowel control at the appropriate age
    ③ Child's skin remains intact and free from irritation
    ④ Child remains free of infection

12. The manifestations of ulcerative colitis and Crohn's disease differ in which of the following ways?
    ① Crohn's disease has a more insidious onset
    ② Children with ulcerative colitis manifest severe growth retardation
    ③ Frequent, extensive diarrhea is classic for Crohn's disease
    ④ Children with ulcerative colitis can have inflammatory eye disease

13. Which of the following statements best describes the relationship between inflammatory bowel disease and stress?
    ① Teenagers who experience acute stress are more likely to develop inflammatory bowel disease
    ② Stress probably does not cause but may exacerbate inflammatory bowel disease
    ③ Avoidance of stress will prevent inflammatory bowel disease in genetically predisposed children
    ④ There is no relationship between stress and inflammatory bowel disease

14. Adam is a 16-year-old who has been on total parenteral nutrition for 1 week for the treatment of nutritional deficit due to inflammatory bowel disease. He has suddenly developed a fever of 102°F (38.9°C). What is the most likely source of his infection?
    ① The solution is a likely source for the infection
    ② There probably has been trauma to the central IV line
    ③ It is possible that there has been an occlusion in the central IV line
    ④ The fever may be due to excessive amounts of hyperalimentation in the body

15. What is the best long-term prevention strategy against the spread of Type B hepatitis?
    ① Adequate cooking of all shellfish
    ② Universal infant immunization
    ③ Passive immunization of all contacts
    ④ Universal precautions in hospital settings

PRE-TEST Answers and Rationales

1. ③ Eliciting a description of the pattern and type of vomiting is essential for assessing the type of condition the child might have and would have priority over the other choices. For example, a description of projectile vomiting increases suspicion for pyloric stenosis, whereas regurgitation after feedings is probably benign. In Sarita's case, the data already given—vomiting associated with gagging, cyanotic spells, and weight loss—suggest reflux. 1, II. Gastroesophageal Reflux.

2. ① Because the child's symptoms are suggestive of reflux, choice 1 is most appropriate to try for a short period of time. Many cases of reflux resolve on their own and can be managed with modifications in feeding. The other choices are inappropriate for a child with reflux. 4, II. Gastroesophageal Reflux.

3. ④ It is important that an isotonic solution be used in children's enemas as there is the danger of water intoxication and electrolyte imbalances if water is used. 4, II. Hirschsprung's Disease.

4. ② Older children diagnosed with Hirschsprung's disease often are malnourished and anemic. The goal of improving nutritional status to result in increased weight gain is important. Achieving normal bowel control is an appropriate goal for an infant or younger child, but a 4-year-old is more likely to have already achieved bowel control. Children who have had bowel resections do not necessarily experience diarrhea after surgery. 3, II. Hirschsprung's Disease.

5. ① The skin barrier is used to protect the skin from fecal material that could leak out onto the skin. It also helps protect the skin from the actual adhesive on the pouch. 3, II. Colostomy.

6. ② Clinical manifestations of intussusception are fairly classic, with ''currant-jelly'' stools, abrupt onset of painful intestinal spasms, and ''sausage-shaped'' mass. The major purpose of the barium enema is not diagnostic but rather therapeutic. The barium forces the telescoped bowel to return to its normal shape and possibly avoids surgical intervention. 3, II. Intussusception.

7. ① An infant needs to satisfy the need for sucking and should begin to associate sucking with a full stomach. A pacifier exercises the jaw muscles and promotes relaxation, which are associated with normal feeding. 4, III. Esophageal Atresia/Tracheoesophageal Fistula.

8. ④ Biliary atresia means that the intrahepatic and/or extrahepatic ducts that excrete bile are absent. Fat is not digested in the absence of bile, so predigested fat, such as that in these formulas, is required. 3, II. Biliary Atresia.

9. ④ All of the listed nursing diagnoses might be applicable to the child with cleft palate at various stages of development. Because language development is most important for a 15-month-old, the potential for impaired verbal communication is the appropriate choice. 2, IV. Cleft Palate.

10. ③ The clinical manifestations probably are related to appendicitis. The other disorders would have different symptoms or would be unlikely to occur in that age group. 2, II. Appendicitis.

11. ② The successful long-term outcome after surgical repair of imperforate anus is achievement of appropriate bowel control. This is achieved in most cases with varying degrees of success. The other choices are short-term evaluation criteria. 5, II. Imperforate Anus.

12. ① Crohn's disease has a more insidious onset than the abrupt onset of ulcerative colitis. The other choices are incorrect. 2, II. Inflammatory Bowel Disease.

13. ② The relationship between stress and inflammatory bowel disease is not firmly established, but it is generally accepted that although stress probably does not cause the disease, it can exacerbate symptoms. For this reason, teaching affected children stress-reduction exercises is helpful for symptom control. 2, III. Inflammatory Bowel Disease.

14. ③ Infections are the greatest source of fever in this type of client. Because of its high glucose and protein content, hyperalimentation solution is an excellent environment for bacteria. 5, II. Hyperalimentation.

15. ② Inadequately cooked shellfish is a cause of hepatitis A. The other choices are preventive strategies, but the best long-term prevention strategy is universal vaccination of all infants against hepatitis

B. Universal precautions should be used in *all* settings where exposure to blood or infected body fluids is likely. 4, IV. Hepatitis.

NORMAL ELIMINATION

I. Elimination system can be broken down into two separate entities
   A. Gastrointestinal system
   B. Urinary system

Gastrointestinal System

I. Composed of pharynx and its structures, esophagus, stomach, duodenum, liver, spleen, pancreas, gallbladder, small intestine, appendix, large intestine, and rectum
   A. Gastrointestinal system responsible for process of digestion, absorption, and elimination of food components
   B. Digestion occurs mechanically and chemically
   C. Various enzymes present in digestive juices catalyze chemical changes in food
   D. Absorption takes place actively and passively
   E. Elimination occurs secondary to mass peristalsis in large intestine

Urinary System

I. Composed of kidneys, ureters, bladder, urethra, and associated arteries and veins
   A. Kidney's primary function to maintain composition and volume of body's fluids at constant level
   B. Kidney also removes wastes from body, secretes hormones, and plays integral role in metabolism
   C. End product of kidney's proper functioning is urine
   D. Essential process in urine formation includes glomerular filtration, tubular reabsorption of water and solutes, and tubular secretion of solutes
   E. Processes take place in functional unit of kidney—the nephron and its associated tubules

NURSING PROCESS APPLIED TO CHILDREN WITH GASTROINTESTINAL DISORDERS

Congenital Disorders

Cleft Lip/Palate
I. Assessment
   A. Definition: facial malformation including lip and/or palate (Fig. 14-1)
   B. Etiology/incidence
      1. Cleft lip
         a. Defective development of embryonic primary palate, resulting in failure of the lip to fuse at midline; may or may not be associated with cleft palate
         b. Occurs seventh to eighth week of fetal life
         c. One per 1000 Caucasian live births
         d. 50% less prevalent in African Americans; higher incidence in Orientals
         e. Higher male-to-female ratio
      2. Cleft palate
         a. Defective development of embryonic secondary palate (hard and soft palates); may occur with cleft lip or alone (isolated)
         b. Occurs seventh to 12th week of fetal life
         c. One per 2500 Caucasian live births
         d. 50% less prevalent in African Americans; higher incidence in Orientals
         e. Greater female-to-male ratio in isolated cleft palate
      3. Higher incidence in identical twins
   C. Predisposing/precipitating factors: multifactorial inherited disorder; may be associated with other genetic abnormalities or chromosome disorders
   D. Clinical manifestations
      1. Cleft lip

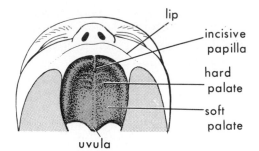

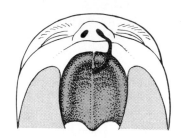

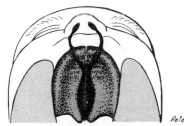

FIGURE 14–1. Drawings of various types of cleft lip and cleft palate. *A,* Normal lip and palate. *B,* Complete unilateral cleft of the lip and alveolar process of the maxilla with a unilateral cleft of the anterior or primary palate. *C,* Complete bilateral cleft of the lip and alveolar processes of the maxillae with complete bilateral cleft of the anterior and posterior plate. (From Foster, R. L. R., Hunsberger, M. M., and Anderson, J. J. T. [1989]. *Family-centered nursing care of children,* Philadelphia: W. B. Saunders.)

a. Obvious at birth
b. Unilateral or bilateral
c. Notch to separation extending to floor of nose
2. Cleft palate
   a. Only visible through mouth inspection and digital examination of the palate
   b. Hard palate continuous opening to extension through nasal cavity
   c. Cannot create suction with mouth
   d. Difficulty swallowing
E. Diagnostic examinations: based on physical findings
F. Complications
   1. Speech disturbances
   2. Hearing loss from frequent episodes of otitis media
   3. Malposition of teeth, arches
G. Surgical management: surgical repair with possible plastic surgery later in life
   1. Cleft lip: repaired either immediately or at 6 to 12 weeks, when infant's condition is stable and infant weighs at least 10 lb
   2. Cleft palate: repaired usually at 1 to 2 years, before altered speech patterns develop; may be done in stages depending on severity of defect; dental plate assists articulation while waiting for surgery in older child

II. Analysis
A. Altered nutrition: less than body requirements related to feeding difficulties
B. High risk for body image disturbance related to feelings about physical appearance and reactions of others
C. High risk for infection related to opening from oral to nasal cavity and eustachian tubes
D. Impaired swallowing related to defect of palate
E. High risk for aspiration related to oral defect and impaired swallowing
F. High risk for altered parenting related to child's physical impairment
G. Impaired verbal communication related to oral defect
H. High risk for sensory/perceptual alterations (auditory) related to repeated ear infections
I. High risk for injury to surgical site related to child's age and comprehension
J. High risk for altered growth and development related to speech/language delay
K. High risk for altered family processes related to need for long-term intervention
L. Knowledge deficit about feeding, home management, and long-term consequences of care related to incomplete information

III. Planning/goals, expected outcomes
A. Preoperative
   1. Infant will not experience problems with attachment
   2. Parents will develop a positive relationship with the infant
   3. Parents will understand cause and short-term and long-term care
   4. Child will be maintained nutritionally according to age
   5. Child will be able to feed appropriately
   6. Child/parents will understand surgical repair

7. Child will develop appropriate speech
8. Child will remain free from infection

B. Postoperative
1. Child will maintain suture line without trauma
2. Child will be free of infection along suture line
3. Child's airway will be patent at all times
4. Child will be free of discomfort and pain
5. Child will be maintained nutritionally according to age
6. Child will not regress developmentally during recovery
7. Parents will express fears and concerns about infant and care
8. Parents will learn immediate and long-term care of infant
9. Parents will contact appropriate outside agencies for follow-up and support

IV. Implementation
A. Preoperative
1. Accurately and thoroughly inspect mouth at birth or in newborn nursery
2. Provide opportunity for parents to participate in multidisciplinary meeting to discuss short-term and long-term care
3. Feed every 3 to 4 hours slowly and carefully; burp frequently
4. Encourage breast-feeding (passive antibodies help prevent infection)
5. Feed in upright position
6. Feed with special nipple
   a. Cleft palate nipple
   b. Large soft nipple with large hole
   c. Crosscut regular nipple
   d. Asepto syringe
   e. Rubber-tipped medicine dropper
   f. Spoon feed
   g. Use of artificial palate
7. Prepare parents for surgical procedures and process of repair; accustom child to feeding method and positioning to be used after surgery

B. Postoperative
1. Maintain Logan bow (metal arch taped to the cheeks) or other protective device over suture line for lip repair
2. Position on back/side (lip), abdomen (palate)
3. Restrain arms at elbows; release at least every 2 hours with supervision at all times
4. Clean suture line as ordered after feedings and as needed; use mild soap and water or diluted H_2O_2
5. Keep suture line dry
6. Monitor for excess mucus production

7. Medicate with Tylenol as ordered (see Table 10-19)
8. Encourage parents to hold and rock child
9. Feed according to surgeon's protocol; avoid spoon or other objects in mouth if palate repair
10. Provide tactile/visual stimulation appropriate for age
11. Give parents opportunity to express fears and concerns
12. Involve parents in care of infant
13. Teach parents care of suture line before discharge
14. Teach principles of home management
    a. Care of suture line
    b. Feeding method
    c. Use and removal of restraints
    d. Facilitating normal development through frequent tactile/visual stimulation
    e. Handling questions and comments from others
15. Refer for follow-up care to visiting nurse or appropriate multidisciplinary agency
    a. Speech therapist
    b. Audiologist
    c. Dentist/orthodontist
    d. Social services if needed

V. Evaluation
A. Parents participate in multidisciplinary sessions and able to discuss fears and concerns over care before and after surgery
B. Child fed effectively
C. Child tolerates surgical repair without complications
D. Child's suture line heals without infection or trauma
E. Child's airway patent at all times
F. Child's pain relieved
G. Child's nutritional status maintained appropriately for age
H. Child does not regress developmentally
I. Parents describe and demonstrate feeding, care of suture line, follow-up, and long-term care before discharge
J. Parents referred to visiting nurse for follow-up care and long-term management

Esophageal Atresia/Tracheoesophageal Fistula
I. Assessment
A. Definition: malformation that results from failure of esophagus to develop and/or failure of esophagus to completely separate from trachea (Fig. 14-2)
B. Etiology/incidence

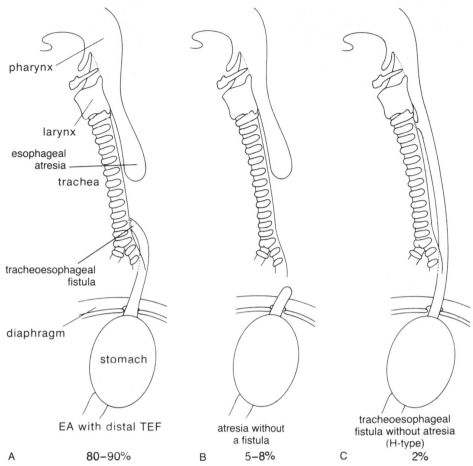

FIGURE 14–2. The three most common types of esophageal atresia and tracheoesophageal fistula. *A,* Esophageal atresia with a distal fistula constitutes 80 to 90% of all cases. *B,* Atresia without a fistula—5 to 8%. *C,* Isolated tracheoesophageal fistula without esophageal atresia (H type)—2%. (From Foster, R. L. R., Hunsberger, M. M., and Anderson, J. J. T. [1989]. *Family-centered nursing care of children,* Philadelphia: W. B. Saunders.)

1. Defective embryonic development of foregut during fourth to fifth week of gestation
2. 85 to 95% of cases involve proximal part of esophagus ending in closed pouch and distal part communicating with trachea at bifurcation
3. One per 800 to one per 5000 live births; true incidence unknown
4. Female-to-male ratio of 1 : 1

C. Predisposing/precipitating factors
   1. Low birth weight
   2. Prematurity
   3. Presence of associated anomalies
      a. Congenital heart defects
      b. Genitourinary defects
      c. Anorectal malformations
   4. Maternal polyhydramnios

D. Clinical manifestations
   1. Excessive drooling
   2. Choking, coughing, sneezing
   3. Excessive salivation, mucus
   4. After feeding, normal swallow followed by sudden cough, struggle, then regurgitation through nose or mouth
   5. Cyanosis, apnea
   6. Distended abdomen

E. Diagnostic examinations
   1. Passage of radiopaque catheter into esophagus; failure to pass into stomach indicative of positive diagnosis
   2. X-rays

F. Complications
   1. Reflux pneumonitis
   2. Respiratory distress/failure
   3. Esophageal strictures

G. Surgical management
   1. Gastrostomy tube temporarily
   2. Surgical repair
      a. Single- or multiple-stage procedure

b. Esophagostomy for drainage of esophageal pouch; gastrostomy
c. Thoracotomy with anastamosis of esophagus and ligation of fistula
d. Esophageal replacement of segments not easily anastamosed

II. Analysis
   A. High risk for aspiration related to opening to trachea
   B. Ineffective airway clearance related to excessive secretions
   C. Impaired swallowing related to excessive secretions and esophageal pouch
   D. Altered nutrition: less than body requirements related to esophageal atresia
   E. High risk for infection related to reflux of stomach contents into trachea
   F. Anxiety of parents related to condition of the child
   G. Knowledge deficit about the defect and its implications related to incomplete information
   H. Other diagnoses appropriate for any child undergoing surgery

III. Planning/goals, expected outcomes
   A. Child will be diagnosed before complications occur
   B. Child will have patent airway at all times before and after surgery
   C. Child will not develop complications before surgery
   D. Child's nutritional status will be maintained before and after surgery
   E. Child will not develop infection after surgery
   F. Child's gastrostomy tube will remain patent
   G. Child will not develop respiratory infection after surgery
   H. Child will be free from pain and discomfort
   I. Parents will learn home care
   J. Parents will seek follow-up care

IV. Implementation
   A. Preoperative
      1. Accurately monitor and report excessive salivation, choking, coughing, cyanosis; first newborn feeding should be sterile water
      2. Suction as ordered or maintain continuous suction
      3. Place in isolette or under radiant warmer
      4. Position to prevent aspiration; head of bed elevated 30 degrees or place in infant seat
      5. Monitor for signs of respiratory distress
      6. Maintain NPO status
      7. Maintain patency of gastrostomy tube; attach to gravity drainage
      8. Administer and monitor IV fluids as ordered
   B. Postoperative
      1. Maintain strict aseptic technique to surgical site
      2. Monitor for signs/symptoms of infection
      3. Maintain strict I & O
      4. Check weight daily
      5. Administer gastrostomy tube feedings as tolerated; give infant pacifier during feeding to satisfy sucking needs and associate sucking with stomach fullness
      6. Measure and record gastrostomy tube drainage
      7. Progress to oral feedings when condition warrants, about 10 to 14 days after surgery
      8. Feed slowly and monitor closely for choking
      9. Administer oxygen as ordered; suction with premeasured, marked catheter
      10. Administer antibiotics as ordered (see Table 10-2)
      11. Encourage parents to hold, rock infant
      12. Teach parents home care
         a. Clinical manifestations of respiratory distress
         b. Suctioning
         c. Feeding techniques
         d. Skin care for esophagostomy
         e. Manifestations of stricture formation: gagging on solids, refusal to eat, excessive drooling, choking related to swallowing
      13. Refer to home health agency for follow-up care

V. Evaluation
   A. Symptoms recognized before or at first feeding
   B. Child has patent airway at all times
   C. Child free of respiratory complications
   D. Child's nutritional and hydration status maintained; child gains weight appropriately
   E. Child shows no signs/symptoms of infection
   F. Child's gastrostomy tube patent and functional
   G. Child has minimal pain, discomfort
   H. Parents accurately describe home care and participate in return demonstration of procedures
   I. Parents obtain home health follow-up care

Imperforate Anus
I. Assessment
   A. Definition: an anorectal malformation; may vary from blindly ending rectum to presence

of fistula; may be complete or incomplete obliteration of anal membrane (Fig. 14-3)
B. Etiology/incidence
   1. Abnormal division of the caudal hindgut (cloaca) and/or persistence of anal membrane during eighth week of gestation
   2. One per 5000 live births
   3. 75 to 80% agenesis type (high and low), 80 to 90% have fistulas as well
   4. Female-to-male ratio of 1 : 1
   5. Higher incidence in Caucasians
C. Predisposing/precipitating factor: associated congenital anomalies
   1. Esophageal atresia
   2. Genitourinary abnormalities
D. Clinical manifestations
   1. Newborn who does not pass meconium in first 24 hours
   2. Absence of anal opening
   3. Thin, translucent anal membrane
   4. Rectal stenosis
   5. Difficult defecation, inability to defecate
   6. Abdominal distention
   7. Ribbon-like stools
   8. Meconium or stool passed through fistula
E. Diagnostic examinations
   1. X-rays (Wangensteen-Rice method)
      a. Infant inverted while abdomen x-rayed
      b. Gas in colon rises to reveal pouch in relation to anal membrane
   2. Ultrasound or tomography
   3. Associated renal studies
F. Complications: with surgical correction some anal stricture, delayed bowel control (depends on level of defect)
G. Surgical management: surgical pull-through operation with or without temporary colostomy and anoplasty
II. Analysis
A. Anxiety related to child's condition and need for surgery
B. Impaired skin integrity related to continuous passage of stool through reconstructed anus or colostomy
C. High risk for infection related to incision
D. Knowledge deficit about surgery, colostomy, or home management related to incomplete information
E. High risk for altered growth and development—delayed achievement of bowel control—related to the defect or need for colostomy
F. High risk for body image disturbance related

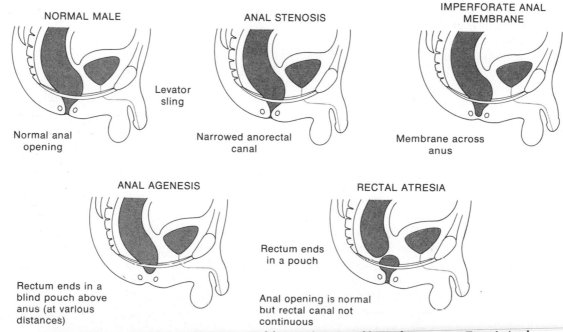

NORMAL MALE

Levator sling

Normal anal opening

ANAL STENOSIS

Narrowed anorectal canal

IMPERFORATE ANAL MEMBRANE

Membrane across anus

ANAL AGENESIS

Rectum ends in a blind pouch above anus (at various distances)

RECTAL ATRESIA

Rectum ends in a pouch

Anal opening is normal but rectal canal not continuous

FIGURE 14–3. Normal anal anatomy and four main types of imperforate anus. Type I, Anal stenosis. Type II, Imperforate anal membrane. Type III, Anal agenesis (this is the most common type occurring in about 80% of cases of imperforate anus). Type IV, Rectal atresia. (From Foster, R. L. R., Hunsberger, M. M., and Anderson, J. J. T. [1989]. *Family-centered nursing care of children*, Philadelphia: W. B. Saunders.)

to reactions to colostomy or bowel difficulties

III. Planning/goals, expected outcomes
  A. Child's symptoms will be recognized and reported
  B. Parents will understand surgical procedure, colostomy if applicable
  C. Child will not exhibit signs/symptoms of infection after surgery
  D. Child's nutritional and hydration status will be maintained
  E. Child's colostomy will function normally
  F. Child will not suffer from developmental delays while in hospital
  G. Parents will learn proper colostomy care before discharge
  H. Parents will have opportunity to discuss treatment and long-term care
  I. Parents will seek follow-up care
  J. Parents will seek advice on toilet training when appropriate
IV. Implementation
  A. Accurately observe for and record passage of meconium stool in first 24 hours of life
  B. Assist with diagnostic procedures
  C. Prepare parents for surgical procedure and presence of temporary colostomy if applicable
    1. Pull-through procedure with anoplasty
    2. Colostomy followed in 6 to 12 months by pull-through procedure
  D. Maintain strict aseptic perirectal care with anoplasty or pull-through procedure
  E. With pull-through, begin oral feedings slowly after peristalsis returns
  F. With colostomy, begin oral feedings slowly once stool passes
  G. Administer and monitor IV fluids as ordered
  H. Maintain strict I & O
  I. Check weight daily
  J. Maintain patency of colostomy
  K. Empty and change pouch as needed
  L. Provide age-appropriate tactile/visual stimulation
  M. Teach parents colostomy care if applicable
    1. Empty pouch as needed
    2. Change pouch every few days as needed
    3. Cleanse peristomal skin with mild soap and water, dry thoroughly, and reapply pouch
    4. Use skin barrier to prevent skin irritation
  N. Provide psychological support to parents
  O. Refer for follow-up procedures, care
V. Evaluation
  A. Parents express feelings and concerns
  B. Parents can describe surgical procedure, colostomy if applicable

C. Child does not exhibit signs/symptoms of infection after surgery
D. Child takes in nutrients adequate to gain weight
E. Child's colostomy functions normally
F. Child does not suffer from developmental delays while in hospital
G. Parents understand and demonstrate proper colostomy or skin care before discharge
H. Parents discuss treatment and long-term care and begin to cope
I. Parents scheduled for follow-up care
J. Parents seek advice on toilet training when appropriate

Obstructive Disorders

Pyloric Stenosis
I. Assessment
  A. Definition: obstruction of pyloric sphincter secondary to combination of hypertrophy and hyperplasia of muscular layer around pylorus (Fig. 14-4)
  B. Etiology/incidence
    1. Obstructing lesion at level of pylorus
    2. Although hypertrophy usually present at

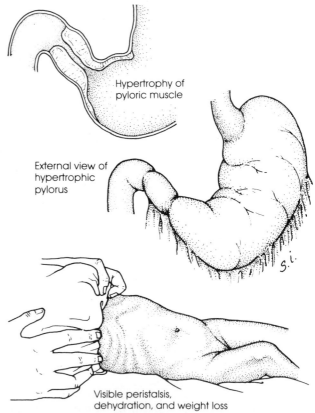

Hypertrophy of pyloric muscle

External view of hypertrophic pylorus

Visible peristalsis, dehydration, and weight loss

FIGURE 14–4. Pyloric stenosis. (From Marlow, D. R., and Redding, B. A. [1988]. *Textbook of pediatric nursing,* **6th ed. Philadelphia: W. B. Saunders.)**

birth, classified as congenital; symptoms usually appear by 4 to 6 weeks of age
    3. Exact etiology unknown
    4. One per 500 live births
    5. Male-to-female ratio of 4 to 5 : 1
    6. Higher incidence among Caucasians
  C. Predisposing/precipitating factors
    1. First-born children
    2. Monozygotic twins
  D. Clinical manifestations
    1. Projectile vomiting, usually shortly after feeding
    2. Dehydration
    3. Failure to thrive
    4. Decreased number of stools
    5. Abdominal distention
    6. "Hungry" behavior
    7. Visible gastric peristalsis in a left-to-right direction
    8. Palpable olive pit–shaped tumor to right of umbilicus
  E. Diagnostic examinations
    1. Physical examination and history
    2. Upper GI series demonstrates delayed gastric emptying and elongated pyloric channel
    3. Serum electrolytes demonstrate signs of metabolic alterations
  F. Complications
    1. Metabolic alkalosis
    2. Hypovolemic shock
  G. Surgical management: pyloromyotomy when child's fluid and electrolyte status stabilized
II. Analysis
  A. Fluid volume deficit related to vomiting
  B. Altered nutrition: less than body requirements related to vomiting
  C. Anxiety related to the necessity for surgery
  D. High risk for altered parenting related to feeding difficulties
  E. Knowledge deficit about condition and surgical management related to lack of prior information
  F. Other nursing diagnoses associated with routine postoperative care
III. Planning/goals, expected outcomes
  A. Child's symptoms will be recognized quickly
  B. Child's episodes of vomiting will decrease
  C. Child's fluid and electrolyte balance remains stable both before and after surgery
  D. Child's nutritional status improves subsequent to intervention
  E. Child will be free of complications
  F. Child will be free of infection
  G. Child will not experience pain, discomfort
  H. Child will not regress developmentally during illness

  I. Parents will express concerns about diagnosis and treatment
  J. Parents will understand home care
  K. Parents will seek appropriate follow-up care
IV. Implementation
  A. Preoperative
    1. Obtain accurate history of presenting signs/symptoms
    2. Monitor fluid and electrolyte status and observe for signs of dehydration
    3. Maintain IV line and nasogastric tube as ordered
  B. Postoperative
    1. Keep NPO until postoperative vomiting stops (usually several hours)
    2. Maintain IV line and accurate I & O, nasogastric tube if ordered
    3. Begin oral feedings as directed starting with small amounts of electrolyte solution or glucose water; advance to diluted breast milk or formula, then to full strength as tolerated
    4. Feed in an upright position; burp frequently
    5. Monitor surgical site for bleeding or infection
    6. Encourage parents to hold and rock child
    7. Provide age-appropriate stimulation
    8. Allow parents to express concerns about treatment and follow-up care
    9. Teach parents home care
      a. Feeding
      b. Clinical manifestations of complications
    10. Refer to home health agency for follow-up care
V. Evaluation
  A. Child eats amounts sufficient to maintain growth
  B. Child's fluid and electrolyte balance maintained, retaining fluids, urinary output 1 mL/kg/hr
  C. Child free of complications
  D. Child free of infection
  E. Child has no pain, discomfort
  F. Child does not regress developmentally during illness
  G. Parents discuss concerns about diagnosis and treatment
  H. Parents describe care required at home
  I. Parents seek follow-up care if needed

Intussusception
I. Assessment
  A. Definition: condition in which there is a telescoping of the intestine at any of a number of locations along the intestinal tract; results in

intestinal obstruction and interference with the passage of intestinal contents

B. Etiology/incidence
 1. Most common location is ileocecal valve
 2. Most frequent cause of intestinal obstruction in infancy because of hyperactivity of digestive tract, although can occur in older children
 3. Average age of onset 3 to 12 months
 4. Male-to-female ratio of 3 : 1

C. Predisposing/precipitating factors
 1. Cause is generally unknown
 2. Associated with cystic fibrosis, celiac disease, intestinal polyps, tumors

D. Clinical manifestations
 1. Abrupt onset of intestinal pain in previously healthy child; spasmodic pain manifested by screaming, drawing knees up to chest; child comfortable between spasms
 2. Vomiting, which gets progressively worse
 3. Passage of "currant-jelly" stools
 4. Abdominal distention with "sausage-shaped" mass felt in upper right quadrant
 5. Manifestations of progressive acute illness, including fever, prostration, shock

E. Diagnostic examinations
 1. Accurate history of clinical manifestations
 2. Barium enema

F. Complications: peritonitis, shock, death if not treated quickly

G. Medical management
 1. Hydrostatic reduction by barium or saline enema
 2. Reduction by air pressure insufflation

H. Surgical management: surgical intervention if previous methods unsuccessful, if condition present more than 24 hours, or if child experiencing signs of peritonitis or shock

II. Analysis
A. Pain related to underlying condition
B. High risk for fluid volume deficit related to vomiting
C. High risk for infection related to intestinal perforation
D. Anxiety related to seriousness of child's condition
E. Knowledge deficit about the condition, treatment, home management, and chances for recurrence related to lack of previous experience
F. Other diagnoses related to care of the child having surgery

III. Planning/goals, expected outcomes
A. Child's symptoms will be recognized and reported immediately
B. Child will maintain stable fluid and electrolyte status
C. Child will not experience signs of infection
D. Parents/caregivers will understand the condition and its management
E. Parents will cope effectively with the experience

IV. Implementation
A. Obtain accurate history from parents
B. Monitor vital signs, electrolyte levels, stool and urine output
C. Explain condition to parents; may use a surgical glove to demonstrate invagination and hydrostatic reduction
D. Observe for passage of stool or barium after hydrostatic reduction
E. Usual postoperative care; carefully monitor for return of bowel sounds, passage of stool, electrolyte status, manifestations of recurring obstruction
F. Allow parents to express feelings of concern and anxiety

V. Evaluation
A. Child's discomfort is reduced as condition is resolved: child rests comfortably, is able to participate in usual activities
B. Child begins to pass normal stools
C. Child shows no manifestations of dehydration or fluid volume loss, urinates adequately (1 mL/kg/hr), has good skin turgor
D. Child's vital signs within normal limits; no fever or signs of infection
E. Parents describe home management of child who has had surgery, can describe signs of recurring intestinal obstruction, state necessity of gaining help immediately if condition reoccurs

Hirschsprung's Disease
(Aganglionic Megacolon)

I. Assessment
A. Definition: mechanical obstruction of bowel secondary to inadequate motility; may be acute or chronic (Fig. 14-5)
B. Etiology/incidence
 1. Absence of autonomic parasympathetic ganglion cells of submucosal and myenteric plexus in colon (aganglionic)
 2. Deficit in innervation causes absence of propulsive movements/peristalsis (megacolon) in affected segments of colon
 3. Male-to-female ratio of 4 : 1
 4. Most commonly seen in rectosigmoid area only
C. Predisposing/precipitating factors
 1. Familial
 2. Down's syndrome

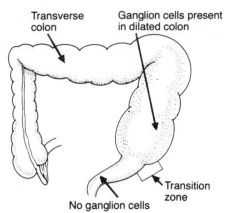

FIGURE 14–5. Hirschsprung's disease. Lack of ganglion cells in a segment of colon prevents transmission of normal peristaltic waves and results in intestinal obstruction. (From Foster, R. L. R., Hunsberger, M. M., and Anderson, J. J. T. [1989]. *Family-centered nursing care of children,* Philadelphia: W. B. Saunders.)

D. Clinical manifestations
  1. Newborn
    a. Failure to pass meconium stool in 24 to 48 hours after birth
    b. Feeding difficulties
    c. Bile-stained vomitus
    d. Abdominal distention
  2. Infants
    a. Failure to thrive
    b. Chronic constipation
    c. Explosive diarrhea
    d. Vomiting
    e. Abdominal distention
  3. Childhood
    a. Chronic constipation
    b. Ribbon-like, foul-smelling stools
    c. Abdominal distention
    d. Visible peristalsis
    e. Palpable fecal masses, usually felt in lower left quadrant, with empty rectal vault
    f. Poorly nourished
    g. Anemia
E. Diagnostic examinations
  1. Physical examination and history
  2. Barium enema shows enlarged proximal colon and narrowed distal segment; not accurate in infants
  3. Abdominal x-ray
  4. Manometric studies
    a. Insert balloons into rectum and inflate
    b. External sphincter contracts; no relaxation of internal sphincter
  5. Rectal biopsy confirms aganglionic tissue
F. Complications
  1. Enterocolitis
  2. Death secondary to enterocolitis (severe inflammation of the colon)

G. Surgical management: surgical removal of affected colon segment, usually with temporary colostomy; usually done when child reaches 20 lb
II. Analysis
  A. Constipation related to absence of peristalsis
  B. High risk for fluid volume deficit related to vomiting
  C. High risk for altered growth and development related to malabsorption
  D. Anxiety related to child's condition, surgery, and long-term management
  E. Knowledge deficit about condition, treatment, and home management related to incomplete knowledge base
  F. High risk for altered growth and development (bowel training) related to colostomy and surgery
  G. High risk for body image disturbance related to colostomy appearance
  H. High risk for impaired skin integrity related to colostomy or acidic stools after surgery
  I. Other diagnoses applicable for the child undergoing abdominal surgery
III. Planning/goals, expected outcomes
  A. Parents will describe child's elimination pattern and express concerns at each well-child visit
  B. Child will maintain adequate caloric and fluid intake for age
  C. Child will gain weight appropriately
  D. Parents will understand the condition, surgical management, and home management
  E. Parents will express concerns and ask appropriate questions about child's care
  F. Skin around colostomy and surgical site will remain intact
  G. Parents will view the child in a positive manner, and child will develop a healthy self-concept
  H. Child will remain free of infection
  I. Child will achieve bowel control at appropriate time
IV. Implementation
  A. Monitor bowel function accurately in newborn nursery
  B. Explain disorder and care to parents
  C. Prepare parents for surgical procedure
  D. Emphasize to parents that colostomy temporary
  E. Administer low-residue, high-calorie, high-protein diet (Table 14-1; see Table 10-12)
  F. Administer isotonic enemas daily for bowel cleansing as ordered
  G. Administer stool softeners as ordered (see Table 10-14)
  H. Prepare child for surgery/colostomy with play therapy if appropriate

TABLE 14–1 Residue Diets

Low-Residue Foods	High-Residue Foods
Spaghetti	Whole grain breads, cereals
Lean broiled hamburger	Pancakes, waffles
Broiled chicken	Fatty or fried meats
Vanilla or chocolate ice cream	Fruit ice cream
Plain cookies	Yogurt
Plain crackers	Fried or sautéed vegetables
	Raw fruits, vegetables
	Spices

General Principles

Objective of diet: provide foods to prevent constipation; select easily digestible foods; provide in conjunction with protein/calories; maintain well-balanced diet

I. Monitor for clinical manifestations of entero-colitis
   1. Explosive diarrhea
   2. High fever
J. Monitor incision site for manifestations of infection
K. Keep incision site clean and dry
L. Take vital signs every 2 to 4 hours
M. Monitor bowel sounds
N. Maintain NPO until bowel sounds return; advance diet slowly as tolerated
O. Maintain nasogastric tube to low Gomco suction; maintain patency and irrigate as ordered
P. Monitor I & O
Q. Monitor for abdominal distention and return of bowel movements; measure abdominal girth daily both before and after surgery
R. Observe for proper functioning of colostomy
S. Teach parents colostomy care (see Imperforate Anus)
T. Encourage parents to participate in child's care
U. Administer and monitor IV fluids as ordered
V. Monitor serum electrolytes
W. Administer analgesics as ordered (see Table 10-19)
X. Encourage parents to rock and to hold infant
Y. Monitor for clinical manifestations of respiratory complications; turn, cough, and deep breathe every 2 hours
Z. Provide information to parents on subsequent surgery and answer their questions
V. Evaluation
  A. Child's clinical manifestations are recognized and reported promptly
  B. Parents describe disease and demonstrate care involved
  C. Parents describe surgery and what is expected after surgery
  D. Child's nutritional and hydration status maintained as evidenced by appropriate weight gain, no signs of dehydration
  E. Child's diet sufficient to accommodate disease process before surgery
  F. Child able, if old enough, to describe surgery/colostomy
  G. Child expresses feelings appropriately through play
  H. Child does not develop any complications before or after surgery
  I. Child free of infection after surgery; normal body temperature, CBC; no signs of inflammation
  J. Child's abdominal/bowel status returns to normal after surgery
  K. Child's colostomy functions normally
  L. Child/parents describe and demonstrate proper colostomy care
  M. Child free from pain/discomfort and rests comfortably
  N. Child does not regress developmentally during illness
  O. Parents discuss subsequent surgical procedure and long-term follow-up
  P. Parents seek advice on toilet training when appropriate

Acute Disorders

Gastroesophageal Reflux (Chalasia)
I. Assessment
  A. Definition: backing up (reflux) of gastric contents into lower esophagus
  B. Etiology/incidence
    1. Etiology unknown; possibly results from maturational delay of lower esophageal function
    2. 95% of infants symptomatic by 6 weeks
  C. Predisposing/precipitating factors
    1. Relaxed or incompetent cardiac sphincter (at lower end of esophagus)
    2. Associated with hiatal hernia
    3. Seen more frequently in child with neurological deficits
  D. Clinical manifestations
    1. Excessive vomiting
    2. Respiratory manifestations: apneic episodes, cyanosis, pneumonia
    3. Slowed weight gain
    4. Irritability
    5. Iron-deficiency anemia
    6. Esophagitis with bleeding
  E. Diagnostic examinations

1. Accurate history and observation of feeding difficulties or vomiting episodes
2. Gastric pH monitoring by probe
3. Barium esophagography
F. Complications
   1. Esophageal strictures
   2. Pneumonia
   3. Failure to thrive
G. Medical management
   1. Often resolves on its own
   2. Small, frequent feedings; burp often; thickened feedings may or may not help, but make reflux more mechanically difficult
   3. Position prone (if infant old enough) with head of bed slightly elevated; maintain position with sling-type harness
   4. Give bethanechol (Urecholine) or metoclopramide hydrochloride (Reglan) before feeding to increase peristalsis or relax pyloric sphincter
H. Surgical management for severe cases
II. Analysis
A. Altered nutrition: less than body requirements related to vomiting
B. Altered growth and development related to inadequate nutrients
C. Anxiety of parents related to child's feeding difficulties
D. High risk for infection related to aspiration
E. High risk for altered sleep patterns related to fussiness and discomfort
III. Planning/goals, expected outcomes
A. Child will consume nutrients sufficient to allow for growth and normal activity
B. Parents/caregivers will understand the condition and adjust feeding schedule to compensate
C. Child will not aspirate as a result of vomiting
D. Child will remain free of infection or complications
E. Child will achieve sleep pattern normal for age and level of development
IV. Implementation
A. Demonstrate proper positioning to parents/caregivers; show how to adapt child's bed accordingly, appropriate application and use of harness
B. Reassure parents that condition usually self-limiting
C. Teach how to adapt feeding schedule for child
   1. If nursing, feed for shorter periods, more frequently
   2. Thicken formula with small amount of rice cereal

3. Enlarge nipple slightly to accommodate thickened formula
4. Feed smaller amounts more frequently
5. Burp every half ounce
D. Encourage parents to facilitate regular sleep periods; reassure that crying will not exacerbate reflux
E. Teach parents proper medication administration if prescribed
F. Prepare parents/child for surgery if indicated
V. Evaluation
A. Child's vomiting episodes decrease; child retains appropriate amounts of breast milk or formula
B. Child remains free of respiratory infection; no manifestations of fever, apnea, cyanosis
C. Child maintains growth velocity
D. Parents demonstrate feeding, positioning, and medication-administration techniques

Appendicitis
I. Assessment
A. Definition: inflammation of vermiform appendix
B. Etiology/incidence
   1. Exact etiology unknown
   2. Rare in children less than 2 years
   3. Most common reason for abdominal surgery in childhood
C. Predisposing/precipitating factors
   1. Obstruction of appendiceal lumen
   2. Bowel infections
   3. Diet: low fiber, low residue
   4. Parasitic infestation
   5. Lymphoid hyperplasia
D. Clinical manifestations
   1. Abdominal pain, generalized then localized in right lower quadrant (McBurney's point)
   2. Abdominal rigidity
   3. Guarding
   4. Fever
   5. Rebound tenderness
   6. Decreased or absent bowel sounds
   7. Vomiting
E. Diagnostic examinations
   1. Based on history and physical findings
   2. WBC; usually elevated as high as $20,000/mm^3$
   3. Abdominal x-ray not often diagnostic; may show associated problems
F. Complications
   1. Perforation, rupture
   2. Peritonitis
      a. High fever
      b. Sudden relief of pain, then subsequent increase in diffuse pain

c. Rigid abdomen
d. Abdominal distention
e. Tachycardia
G. Medical management: antibiotics and bowel rest
H. Surgical management: appendectomy
II. Analysis
A. Pain related to inflammation
B. Hyperthermia related to underlying infection
C. High risk for fluid volume deficit related to vomiting
D. Anxiety related to impending surgery
E. Other diagnoses applicable for the child undergoing abdominal surgery
III. Planning/goals, expected outcomes
A. Child's signs/symptoms will be recognized and reported quickly
B. Child will rest comfortably before surgery
C. Child/parents will be prepared for surgical procedure
D. Child will be free of complications
E. Child will tolerate surgery without problems
F. Child will be infection free after surgery
G. Child's bowel function will return to normal after surgery without complications
H. Child's nutritional and hydration status will be stable
I. Child will be free of pain and discomfort
J. Child's respiratory status will remain stable
K. Child will not regress developmentally or emotionally during hospitalization
IV. Implementation
A. Preoperative
1. Take and record accurate history and presenting symptoms, especially pattern of pain
2. Complete bedrest in comfortable position before surgery; place in Fowler's position if perforation is suspected
3. Maintain NPO status
4. Prepare child and parent for surgery
5. Maintain IV line and accurate output recording
6. Monitor for signs and symptoms of rupture or peritonitis: abrupt cessation of pain followed by increasing pain, rising temperature, resistance to being moved, irritability
B. Postoperative
1. Monitor vital signs frequently
2. Inspect incision for manifestations of infection; monitor drainage from wound or drain site; maintain wound drainage precautions if ruptured
3. Administer antibiotics and analgesics as ordered (see Tables 10-2 and 10-19)

4. Maintain IV line, nasogastric tube to low suction as ordered
5. Accurate I & O
6. Monitor for return of bowel sounds
7. Turn, cough, and deep breathe every 2 hours; ambulate on first postoperative day
8. Provide therapeutic play for child to "work out" surgical experience
9. Provide opportunities for parent/child to ask questions or verbalize concerns
V. Evaluation
A. Child recovers from surgery without complications and returns to normal activities
B. Child/parents describe what to look for after surgery and when child returns home
C. Child shows no clinical manifestations of infection: temperature returns to normal, incision intact, no signs of respiratory complications
D. Child is well hydrated: good skin turgor, urinating adequately
E. Child returns to regular diet and elimination pattern
F. Child is free of pain

Inflammatory Bowel Disease
I. Assessment
A. Definition: inflammatory changes in mucosa and submucosa of various segments of digestive tract; broad term that encompasses ulcerative colitis and Crohn's disease; may be acute or chronic
B. Etiology/incidence
1. Ulcerative colitis
a. Unknown etiology, possibly autoimmune
b. Peak onset ages 10 to 19 years
c. Male-to-female ratio of 1 : 1
2. Crohn's disease
a. Unknown etiology, possibly autoimmune
b. Rare in children less than 6 years old
c. Most prevalent onset in adolescents
d. Male-to-female ratio of 1 : 1
C. Predisposing/precipitating factors
1. Familial tendency
2. Stress, probably does not cause but can exacerbate disease
3. Immunological/autoimmune disease in genetically susceptible children
4. Jewish
5. Caucasians, upper-socioeconomic groups
D. Clinical management, diagnostic examinations, complications (Table 14-2)
E. Medical management

TABLE 14–2 Comparison of Ulcerative Colitis and Crohn's Disease

	Ulcerative Colitis	Crohn's Disease
Primary Area Involved	Superficial ulcerations of colon, rectum	Deep ulcers and fissures of terminal ileum and anus
Clinical Manifestations	Abrupt onset of extensive and frequent diarrhea (sometimes bloody), colicky pain, rectal bleeding, anorexia, anemia, low-grade fever, mild growth retardation, arthralgia/arthritis usually of large joints	Insidious onset of crampy pain becoming persistent and often localized to right lower quadrant, absent-to-moderate diarrhea, fatigue, anorexia, fever, often severe growth retardation, perianal abscesses and/or fistulas, oral ulcers, skin lesions, associated renal problems and inflammatory eye disease
Diagnostic Examinations	Barium enema usually normal except shows "lead pipe" colon in chronic disease; superficial ulcerations by endoscopy; stool may show occult or frank blood; CBC shows elevated WBC, decreased hemoglobin and hematocrit	GI series shows abnormal segments; stool tests to rule out malabsorption syndromes; elevated WBC, ESR, C-reactive protein; endoscopy shows ulcerations and fistulas; rectal biopsy
Complications	May become chronic, predisposes to colon cancer, malnutrition, fluid and electrolyte imbalance	May become chronic, no real cancer risk, malnutrition, abscess and fistula formation

1. Pharmacological management
   a. Sulfasalazine (Azulfidine) or corticosteroids (see Table 10-8) for anti-inflammatory action
   b. Immunosuppressants (e.g., cyclosporine) with steroids to reduce autoimmune response
2. Dietary management
   a. High-protein and -calorie, low-fat and -fiber diet
   b. Elemental, via nasogastric tube, or parenteral feedings to restore nutritional balance and promote weight gain
   F. Surgical management (ulcerative colitis only)
   1. Resection of diseased segment
   2. Total colectomy and ileostomy
II. Analysis
   A. Diarrhea related to underlying inflammation and subsequent malabsorption
   B. Pain related to inflammation
   C. Altered nutrition: less than body requirements related to anorexia and underlying malabsorption
   D. High risk for fluid volume deficit related to diarrhea
   E. Activity intolerance related to anemia
   F. Altered growth and development related to malnutrition
   G. High risk for impaired skin integrity related to diarrhea
   H. High risk for ineffective individual coping related to effects of chronic illness

   I. High risk for altered family processes related to long-term nature of illness
   J. Knowledge deficit about disease and its management related to incomplete knowledge base
III. Planning/goals, expected outcomes
   A. Child's bowel status will be stabilized and managed without surgery
   B. Child will be free of pain and discomfort
   C. Child will regain optimal nutritional status
   D. Child will remain well hydrated
   E. Child will be able to participate in activities normal for age
   F. Child will maintain rate of growth normal for age
   G. Child's skin will remain intact
   H. Child will develop positive self-concept and ability to manage stress
   I. Child/parents will express concerns and seek appropriate help from supporting agencies
   J. Child and family will understand condition, home management, and surgery if required
IV. Implementation
   A. Obtain accurate history and physical examination
   B. Discuss with child/parents disease process and therapeutic regimen
   C. Allow child/parents to ask questions and verbalize understanding
   D. Maintain NPO as ordered until acute phase controlled
   E. Provide high-calorie, high-protein, low-residue diet for chronic phase (see Tables

10-12 and 14-1); teach child/parent dietary principles; include child in menu planning; weigh daily

F. Administer medications as ordered; teach child/parents about side effects and modifications (e.g., need to take vitamin supplements)

G. Monitor for complications
1. Abscess formation
2. Fluid and electrolyte imbalance
3. Malabsorption and malnutrition
4. Secondary infection, such as respiratory, because of debilitation

H. Administer and monitor IV fluids and parenteral nutrition if ordered (see Table 8–11)

I. Provide meticulous perirectal care; wash thoroughly, keep area dry, use protective skin barrier if needed

J. Maintain nonstressful, quiet environment; teach child stress-reduction exercises

K. Provide quiet, age-appropriate diversional and educational activities; encourage child to participate in activities with peers whenever possible and to increase level of activity gradually as condition improves

L. Explain surgical procedure to parents/child including colostomy if appropriate

M. Teach care of ostomy to child/parents (see Imperforate Anus)

N. Allow child/parents to express feelings about ostomy or long-term regimen; encourage to maintain positive attitude during exacerbations

O. Refer to home health agency for follow-up as needed and to local support group

V. Evaluation
A. Episodes of diarrhea decrease, and condition managed without surgery
B. Child appears comfortable and does not complain of pain
C. Child/parents describe disease and therapeutic regimen
D. Child begins to gain weight appropriately
E. Child appears well hydrated; good skin turgor, adequate urine output
F. Child's skin remains intact
G. Child remains free of complications; participates in age-appropriate activities
H. Child/parents describe surgery if applicable
I. Child/parents express feelings of concern about disease or its treatment
J. Child/parents describe long-term management, including pharmacological and dietary principles, stress reduction, ostomy care if applicable

Chronic Disorders: Celiac Disease

I. Assessment
A. Definition: malabsorptive disorder; broad term describing several diseases with same symptomatic complex; gluten-induced enteropathy of the small intestine
B. Etiology/incidence
1. Exact etiology unknown; probably genetic predisposition
2. Generally rare
3. Incidence declined recently, possibly as a result of increased breast-feeding with delayed introduction of solid foods
C. Predisposing/precipitating factors
1. Onset subsequent to introduction of solid foods, usually 9 to 18 months; onset usually insidious
2. Immunological alteration
3. Inborn error of metabolism
D. Clinical manifestations
1. Malnutrition, wasted appearance, hypoproteinemia
2. Steatorrhea: bulky, fatty stools
3. Abdominal distention, pain
4. Vitamin deficiencies result in anemia, clotting difficulties, osteomalacia
5. Irritability
6. Uncooperativeness
7. Vomiting
E. Diagnostic examinations
1. Stools for fecal fat collected for 72 hours, keep on ice
2. CBC often with nutritional anemia
3. Prothrombin time, prolonged
4. Low serum protein, iron, folic acid, vitamin B_{12} levels
5. Altered immunoglobulins
6. GI series
7. Sweat test to rule out cystic fibrosis
8. Bone age studies
9. Jejunal biopsy demonstrates atrophied villae
F. Complication: celiac crisis
1. Profuse diarrhea, vomiting, dehydration, metabolic acidosis
2. Triggered by illness, ingestion of gluten, medications with anticholinergic agents (e.g., preoperative medications, some antihistamines)
3. Can cause shock and death
G. Medical management
1. Gluten-free diet (Table 14-3) and vitamin supplements
2. Steroids and management of fluid and electrolyte imbalance for celiac crisis

TABLE 14–3 Gluten-Free Diet

Foods to Avoid (gluten present in some form)

Cereals and grains (wheat, rye, barley, oats)
Bread
Cake, cookies, crackers, doughnuts, pies
Spaghetti
Pizza
Canned or instant soup
Hot dogs
Luncheon meats
Some chocolate
Many prepared and ready-to-eat foods

General Principles

Objective of diet: to remove gluten products, hydrolyzed vegetable protein (hidden source of gluten) from diet; impossible to remove every source of protein (gluten), so diet is actually low gluten; corn/rice become basic substitute for grain products

II. Analysis
  A. Altered nutrition: less than body requirements related to restricted diet and underlying malabsorption
  B. High risk for altered growth and development related to malabsorption of nutrients
  C. High risk for fluid volume deficit related to celiac crisis
  D. High risk for body-image disturbance related to perception of being different from peers
  E. High risk for altered family processes related to long-term nature of condition and dietary modifications required
  F. Knowledge deficit about disease and management related to incomplete knowledge base
III. Planning/goals, expected outcomes
  A. Child's clinical manifestations will be recognized and reported quickly
  B. Child will adjust to necessary diet modifications
  C. Parents will learn about disease, gluten and its effects on child, dietary management, long-term care
  D. Child will participate in diet therapy without complications
  E. Child will not develop celiac crisis and its complications
  F. Parents/child will cope with condition and its implications
  G. Parents will seek appropriate agencies for long-term follow-up care
  H. Child will not regress developmentally or educationally secondary to disease process

  I. Child will develop positive body image and relationships with peers
IV. Implementation
  A. Obtain accurate history of signs/symptoms and what foods and activities immediately precede them
  B. Allow parents opportunity to discuss concerns or questions about disease and therapeutic management
  C. Teach gluten-free diet (see Table 14-3); obtain dietary consult if needed; advise parent/child to read all labels; modify diet as much as possible to fit child's lifestyle; help locate inexpensive sources of allowed foods
  D. Protect child from people with infections
  E. Protect child from people with infections
  F. Instruct parents to always inform health care providers of child's celiac disease
  G. Monitor for clinical manifestations of metabolic acidosis
    1. Irritability
    2. Weakness
    3. Changes in level of consciousness
    4. Hyperventilation
  H. Treat child immediately for celiac crisis
    1. Administer and monitor IV fluids
    2. Maintain child NPO
    3. Nasogastric tube to low Gomco, irrigate as needed and monitor drainage
    4. Administer steroids as ordered (see Table 10-8)
  I. Allow parents/child to express feeling fears
  J. Present positive outlook with proper dietary management; give extra support to adolescent
  K. Refer to home health agency
  L. Encourage child to continue peer interactions, schoolwork
  M. Encourage parents not to overprotect child and to treat "normally" with dietary restrictions
V. Evaluation
  A. Child consumes diet adequate for growth within dietary limits
  B. Parents can describe disease, gluten and its effects on child, dietary management, long-term care
  C. Child participates in diet therapy and continues therapy when well
  D. Child does not develop celiac crisis and its complications
  E. Child/family express concerns appropriately
  F. Parents seek appropriate agencies for long-term follow-up care
  G. Child does not regress developmentally or educationally secondary to disease process

NURSING PROCESS APPLIED TO CHILDREN WITH LIVER/BILIARY DISORDERS

Congenital Disorders: Biliary Atresia

I. Assessment
   A. Definition: obstruction of bile flow from fibrotic or absent bile ducts
      1. Intrahepatic: within liver
      2. Extrahepatic: main bile passages outside liver (most common site)
   B. Etiology/incidence
      1. Etiology unknown; considered to be part of a continuum of neonatal hepatic manifestations
      2. One per 8000 to 20,000 live births
   C. Predisposing/precipitating factors
      1. Infectious process in utero or during immediate postnatal period
      2. Chemical insult in utero
      3. Vascular insult in utero
   D. Clinical manifestations
      1. Persistent jaundice after 2 to 3 weeks of extrauterine life
      2. Direct and indirect bilirubin levels elevated
      3. Clay-colored stools, putty-like consistency, dark-colored urine
      4. Abdominal distention
      5. Hepatomegaly
      6. Generalized failure to thrive from impaired absorption of fats
   E. Diagnostic examinations
      1. Based on physical findings
      2. Elevated serum bilirubin and liver function levels
      3. Liver biopsy confirms diagnosis
   F. Complications
      1. Cirrhosis
      2. Portal hypertension
      3. Hepatic coma
      4. Death
   G. Surgical management
      1. Liver transplant
      2. Jejunal segment to liver to double-barrel stoma if diagnosed within the first 2 months of life
II. Analysis
   A. Knowledge deficit about condition, treatment, and home management related to incomplete knowledge base
   B. High risk for sleep pattern disturbance related to discomfort
   C. High risk for injury related to clotting disturbance from decreased vitamin K
   D. High risk for altered growth and development related to chronic and severe nature of the condition
   E. High risk for altered parenting related to severity of the condition
   F. Anticipatory grieving related to potential death of the child
   G. Other diagnoses similar to child undergoing abdominal surgery and ostomy care
III. Planning/goals, expected outcomes
   A. Child's clinical manifestations will be recognized and reported quickly
   B. Parents will understand disease, expected outcomes
   C. Parents will express fears and concerns
   D. Child will not regress develomentally
   E. Child will rest comfortably at all times
   F. Parents will understand all diagnostic, surgical procedures
   G. Parents will understand stoma, ostomy care, if applicable
   H. Child will be free of infection at all times
   I. Child's hydration and nutritional status will remain stable
   J. Child will be free of bleeding episodes
   K. Child will be free of respiratory complications
   L. Parents will accept option of liver transplant, if necessary
   M. Parents will be allowed to grieve at own pace
IV. Implementation
   A. Obtain accurate history, physical at two-week check-up for jaundice
   B. Clarify disease, management, expected outcomes to parents; refer to transplant center if appropriate
   C. Allow parents opportunity to ventilate feelings, fears, grief at own pace
   D. Provide age-appropriate visual, tactile stimulus
   E. Encourage bonding process
   F. Allow uninterrupted periods of sleep
   G. Apply tepid or cool compresses for itching
   H. Explain all diagnostic and surgical procedures
   I. Teach parents ostomy care, encourage participation in ostomy care, if needed
   J. Replace bile drainage from proximal stoma to distal stoma (into intestines)
   K. Monitor for clinical manifestations of infection at surgical site
   L. Administer antibiotics as ordered (see Table 10-2)
   M. Feed Portagen or Pregestimil formula every 2 to 4 hours; do not require bile to digest
   N. Administer water-soluble vitamins and vitamin K as ordered
   O. Measure abdominal girth and weigh daily
   P. Elevate head of bed 30 degrees or use infant seat

Q. Monitor for clinical manifestations of respiratory distress

R. Discuss liver transplant with multidisciplinary team

S. Refer to outside agencies for support

V. Evaluation

  A. Parents describe disease, expected outcomes

  B. Parents seek appropriate emotional support and assistance with grieving

  C. Child progresses developmentally

  D. Child rests comfortably at all times

  E. Parents can describe diagnostic, surgical procedures

  F. Parents demonstrate care of stoma, ostomy care

  G. Child is free of infection at all times

  H. Child remains well hydrated, eats sufficiently to maintain growth

  I. Child is free of bleeding episodes

  J. Child is free of respiratory complications

  K. Parents accept option of liver transplant if required

  L. Parents grieve at own pace

Acute Disorders: Hepatitis

I. Assessment

  A. Definition: inflammation of liver caused by any of a number of different viruses

  B. Etiology/incidence (Table 14-4)

  C. Predisposing/precipitating factors (see Table 14-4)

D. Clinical manifestations

  1. Nausea and vomiting

  2. Extreme anorexia

  3. Malaise

  4. Fatigue

  5. Slight-to-moderate fever

  6. Abdominal pain upper right quadrant

  7. Irritability

  8. Liver tenderness

  9. Hepatomegaly

  10. Jaundice at 5 to 7 days (icteric phase) with dark urine, "clay-colored" stools

E. Diagnostic examinations

  1. History of clinical manifestations and contacts, physical findings

  2. Serum anti–hepatitis A virus (HAV), hepatitis B surface antigen (HBsAg), anti–hepatitis C virus (HCV), anti–hepatitis D virus (HDV), anti–hepatitis E virus (HEV)

  3. Abnormal liver function tests: SGOT/SGPT, bilirubin, alkaline phosphatase

  4. Blood ammonia elevated

  5. Urine bilirubin and urobilinogen elevated

F. Complications

  1. Progressive liver destruction

  2. Acute, fulminating hepatitis with hepatic coma

G. Medical management

  1. Rest while liver repairs itself, supportive

  2. Prevention

    a. Postexposure prophylaxis

TABLE 14–4 Etiology and Predisposing Factors for Hepatitis

	Hepatitis A	Hepatitis B	Hepatitis C	Hepatitis D	Enteric Non-A, Non-B
Etiology/ Incidence	Hepatitis A virus (HAV)	Hepatitis B virus (HBV)	Hepatitis C virus (HCV)	Hepatitis D virus (HDV)	Small RNA virus
	Most common in young adults	Seen in IV drug users, immigrants from HBV endemic areas (Asia, Africa), infants of infected mothers, health care workers, residents and workers in residential programs for the developmentally disabled, patients on chronic hemodialysis	Parenteral drug users, persons in frequent contact with blood, infrequent in children less than 15 years	Seen only in those infected with HBV	Most common in adults, especially from under-developed countries
	Incubation: 15 to 50 days	Incubation: 45 to 160 days	Incubation: 7 to 9 weeks	Incubation: 4 to 8 weeks	Incubation: 15 to 60 days
Predisposing/ Precipitating Factors	Fecal/oral transmission, spreads readily in day care settings	Parenteral and sexual transmission, skin or mucous membrane contact, perinatal transmission	Parenteral transmission, rarely sexual	Similar to HBV transmission, perinatal uncommon	Fecal/oral route, usually by contaminated water
	Contaminated shellfish or other foods	Virus survives for 1 month in dried state			
	Rare parenteral transmission				

b. Specific immune globulin for household and sexual contacts
c. Prenatal screening for HBsAg
d. Administration of hepatitis B vaccine series to newborns (see Table 9-1)

II. Analysis
  A. High risk for altered nutrition: less than body requirements related to anorexia, nausea, or vomiting
  B. Activity intolerance related to decreased metabolism of nutrients
  C. Hyperthermia related to underlying infectious process
  D. High risk for infection of others related to disease transmission
  E. High risk for altered growth and development related to fatigue and inability to attend school
  F. Knowledge deficit about the disease, its transmission, and long-term consequences related to incomplete information or denial of social problems

III. Planning/goals, expected outcomes
  A. Child will maintain adequate nutritional intake without undue strain on the liver
  B. Child will rest comfortably and increase activity as tolerated
  C. Child's temperature will return to normal
  D. Child will not transmit the disease to others
  E. Child/parents will express concerns
  F. Child/parents will understand disease transmission and prevention
  G. Child will not experience developmental or educational regression
  H. Child will be free of complications

IV. Implementation
  A. Accurately monitor clinical manifestations
  B. Obtain accurate history of risk factors
  C. Maintain quiet activity
  D. Advance activity as tolerated after icteric stage
  E. Provide tepid baths as needed to relieve itching
  F. Administer diphenhydramine (Benadryl) as ordered during icteric phase for pruritis
  G. Provide small, frequent meals with snacks
  H. Do not force-feed
  I. Monitor vital signs every 2 to 4 hours
  J. Maintain universal precautions with meticulous handwashing technique
  K. Discard all soiled items in specially marked bags
  L. Clean eating utensils properly
  M. Do not allow sharing of items, such as toothbrush, that could be contaminated
  N. Caution against intimate contact while infected
  O. Teach family preventive measures, home

management, avoidance of medications such as Tylenol
  P. Monitor for behavior changes
  Q. Refer to home health agency for follow-up and to social services as needed

V. Evaluation
  A. Child consumes nutrients sufficient for growth
  B. Child rests comfortably at all times and participates in quiet diversional activity
  C. Child's temperature returns to normal
  D. Child's skin free of itching, breaks in integrity
  E. Child/family practice proper preventive measures, and no other members contract disease
  F. Child does not develop secondary complications
  G. Parents seek social service support or home care as needed

POST-TEST Gastrointestinal and Liver/Biliary Disorders

Clint, a 7-week-old, has been admitted with the diagnosis of pyloric stenosis. He is scheduled for a pyloromyotomy.

1. Which of the following is the most characteristic symptom of pyloric stenosis?
   ① Weight loss
   ② Dehydration
   ③ Projectile vomiting
   ④ Mass in lower right quadrant

2. Which two of the following nursing diagnoses are frequently made after assessing a child with pyloric stenosis?
   ① Constipation and altered growth and development
   ② Fluid volume deficit and altered nutrition: less than body requirements
   ③ Impaired skin integrity and potential for infection
   ④ Potential for aspiration and diarrhea

3. About 8 hours after Clint's pyloromyotomy, which of the following might be expected?
   ① Presence of an olive-shaped mass in the upper right quadrant
   ② Tolerance of small oral feedings of clear liquids
   ③ Presence of burping after taking formula or breast milk
   ④ Bile-stained drainage from the nasogastric tube

4. Which of the following is a priority goal for the child who has recently had surgery for imperforate anus?
   ① Promoting a positive body image

② Achieving bowel continence
③ Preventing developmental delay
④ Maintaining skin integrity

5. Which of the following is the usual rationale behind the use of total parenteral nutrition?
   ① To maintain adequate levels of fluid
   ② As a vehicle for medication administration
   ③ To maintain a child's body weight
   ④ To supply needed protein, fat, and calories

Ian, a 13-month-old child with severe bilateral cleft lip and palate, is a new patient at the cleft palate clinic. He is an active child who seems to be growing and developing normally. He has just learned to walk and babbles constantly. He had his lip repaired soon after birth and is to be scheduled for his cleft palate repair when he is 15 months old.

---

6. What is one of the most frequently seen health problems in children with cleft palate?
   ① Aspiration pneumonia
   ② Repeated otitis media
   ③ Nutritional deficits
   ④ Dental caries

7. Ian's father has been bottle-feeding him fluids, using a cleft palate nipple. After his surgery, which of the following feeding methods will most likely be used for fluids during his immediate postoperative period?
   ① Cup
   ② Straw
   ③ Bottle with cleft palate nipple
   ④ Side of soup spoon

8. Which of the following statements made by Ian's father best indicates an appropriate understanding of Ian's long-term needs?
   ① "He will need a diet of high-calorie foods because it will take him too long to consume enough at each meal."
   ② "He may have to have speech therapy, beginning a few weeks after his surgery."
   ③ "He may need orthodontic work when he gets a little older."
   ④ "It's nice to have the surgery over with so we don't have to keep coming to the clinic so regularly."

9. Which of the following increases the incidence of intussusception in infants?
   ① They lack the dietary roughage that adults have
   ② Their gastrointestinal tracts are hypermotile
   ③ They swallow a great deal of air while feeding
   ④ They are able to take only small, frequent feedings

10. Which of the following would be expected assessment data in an infant with intussusception?
    ① Paroxysmal pain and high fever
    ② Clay-colored diarrhea
    ③ "Sausage-shaped" mass in epigastric area
    ④ Hypoglycemia and altered urinary pH

11. Which of the following is the expected goal of thickened feedings to treat the infant with gastroesophageal reflux?
    ① Fewer feedings will be required
    ② Increased caloric needs will be met
    ③ It will be more difficult for reflux to occur
    ④ The infant's appetite will decrease

12. Marlowe, age 3 months, has celiac disease. Which of the following statements is true regarding the difference between celiac disease and inflammatory bowel disease?
    ① Inflammatory bowel disease decreases absorption of nutrients within the bowel, and celiac disease does not
    ② The occurrence of symptoms in celiac disease results directly from the ingestion of certain foods
    ③ The onset of inflammatory bowel disease is most common in children less than 6 years old, and celiac disease is most common in adolescents.
    ④ There is no difference because celiac disease is classified as inflammatory bowel disease.

13. Which of the following choices of breakfast food would indicate that Marlowe's parents understand his diet?
    ① Cheerios
    ② Waffles
    ③ Puffed rice
    ④ Raisin bran

14. What is the primary rationale behind the use of a colostomy to treat children with Hirschsprung's disease?
    ① It will allow the jejunum time to heal
    ② It will enable the colon to return to its original size
    ③ It will enhance the absorption of fat-soluble vitamins
    ④ It will facilitate the passage of fecal material

15. Which of the following would be a nursing diagnosis for an infant with biliary atresia?
    ① High risk for injury related to underlying clotting dysfunction
    ② High risk for infection related to impaired immunity
    ③ Constipation related to impaired bile excretion
    ④ Altered patterns of urinary elimination related to inadequate fluids

16. What is a major secondary preventive intervention for stopping the spread of hepatitis?
    ① Universal vaccination of infants
    ② Passive immunization of contacts
    ③ Isolation of infected clients
    ④ Universal precautions

17. Which of the following is the most likely complication of the most common type of tracheoesophageal fistula?
    ① Reflux pneumonitis
    ② Aspiration pneumonia
    ③ Esophageal varices
    ④ Permanent gastrostomy

POST-TEST Answers and Rationales

1. ③ Projectile vomiting is the characteristic symptom of pyloric stenosis. Choices 1 and 2 are characteristic of almost any gastrointestinal disorder, and choice 4 is a symptom of megacolon. 1, II. Pyloric Stenosis.

2. ② Fluid loss associated with vomiting is frequently seen in infants with pyloric stenosis, and their fluid balance must be corrected before surgery. The infant who is vomiting frequently may experience altered nutrition as well, depending on how soon after eating the vomiting occurs. The other choices are not applicable to infants with this problem. 2, II. Pyloric Stenosis.

3. ② Oral feedings can be started within 8 hours after surgery as long as the infant has stopped vomiting, because the obstruction has been relieved. Oral feedings begin with sterile electrolyte solution and gradually advance. Formula or breast milk is not given initially. 5, II. Pyloric Stenosis.

4. ④ Whether the child has had one-stage pull-through surgery or the placement of a temporary colostomy, preserving skin integrity is a priority for postoperative care. The acidic nature of stool can cause skin breakdown at the site of the anoplasty or surrounding the colostomy. The other choices are less immediate goals. 3, II. Anus.

5. ④ Total parenteral nutrition provides total nutritional replacement for children who are unable to take in normal feedings through the gastrointestinal tract. It contains all protein, calories, and fat needed for growth. 2, II. Hyperalimentation.

6. ② Because of the opening between the palate and the nasopharyngeal area, children with cleft palate can experience repeated episodes of otitis media, which often lead to permanent hearing loss. 1, IV. Cleft Palate.

7. ④ Giving fluids out of the side of a soup spoon and cup-feeding for a child who drinks from a cup are the preferred methods of feeding after cleft-palate surgery. Because Ian had been bottle-fed before surgery, the side of the spoon is a better choice. Care must be taken not to insert the spoon into the mouth so as not to disrupt the suture line. 4, II. Cleft Palate.

8. ③ Although language delay can be a problem in children with cleft palate, surgery before the development of speech usually can minimize that problem. Speech therapy, if needed, would be initiated if articulation difficulties appeared. The child with cleft palate usually needs continuous follow-up care even after surgery to correct any dental problems or developing speech or hearing problems. 5, I. Cleft Palate.

9. ② The intestinal tract in infants is freely moveable, and the hyperactivity of peristalsis may lead to invagination of the bowel onto itself. This condition is referred to as intussusception. 2, II. Intussusception.

10. ① Infants with intussusception exhibit periods of severe, paroxysmal pain manifested by crying and drawing up the legs. This can be accompanied by fever and the presence of ''currant-jelly'' stools. Often, a ''sausage-shaped'' mass is felt in the upper right quadrant of the abdomen. 1, II. Intussusception.

11. ③ Thickened infant formula, one approach to treating gastroesophageal reflux, makes it mechanically more difficult for reflux to occur. Another method of avoiding reflux is to place the infant prone after feedings with the head of the bed elevated. 3, I. Gastroesophageal Reflux.

12. ② In celiac disease, the mucosa of the small intestine responds adversely to the introduction in the diet of certain gluten-containing foods. Its onset usually is during infancy or early childhood after the introduction of solid foods. It is not classified as inflammatory bowel disease, which usually is caused by an autoimmune reaction in the body that results in temporary or permanent inflammatory changes in the bowel. 1, II. Celiac Disease and Inflammatory Bowel Disease.

13. ③ In celiac disease, the mucosa of the small intestine atrophies as a result of the toxic response to dietary wheat, rye, barley, and oats. The only safe breakfast food on the list of possible answers to this question is puffed rice. 5, I. Celiac Disease.

14. ② Treatment of Hirschsprung's disease is done in several stages, the first being a loop or temporary colostomy that allows time for the bowel to rest and return to its original tone and size. 2, II. Hirschsprung's Disease.

15. ① High risk for injury is a nursing diagnosis applicable for infants with biliary atresia because the absorption of fat-soluble vitamin K is decreased, resulting in impaired coagulation. 2, I. Biliary Atresia.

16. ④ Universal precautions with meticulous handwashing is the single most effective method of preventing the spread of

hepatitis. Choice 1 is a primary preventive strategy against the spread of hepatitis B. 4, IV. Hepatitis.

17. ① The most common type of tracheoesophageal fistula has a blind esophageal pouch and a lower esophageal communication from the stomach to the trachea. This results in mechanical reflux of gastric contents into the trachea, causing a pneumonitis. 2, II. Tracheoesophageal Fistula.

PRE-TEST Renal/Urinary Disorders

1. Timmy, who is 18 months old, has bilateral cryptorchidism and is scheduled for an orchidopexy. Which of the following should be included in the preoperative information you give his parents?
   ① It is unlikely that sterility of the undescended testes will occur
   ② Long-term hormonal therapy is necessary to maintain the position of the testes
   ③ There is no increase in testicular cancer in boys with cryptorchidism
   ④ Inguinal hernias commonly occur along with cryptorchidism

2. Before catheterizing 9-year-old Adrienne to obtain a specimen for urine culture, the nurse should obtain what information?
   ① How much residual urine is left in the bladder
   ② Whether Adrienne understands the procedure
   ③ Whether Adrienne has started her menses
   ④ Whether Adrienne's mother will be with her

3. Adrienne is diagnosed as having a urinary tract infection. What would be the most common explanation for the occurrence of urinary tract infection in a child of her age?
   ① Urinary stasis as a result of impaired bladder innervation
   ② Structural abnormality of the urinary tract
   ③ Anatomically short urethra
   ④ High urine acidity

4. There are several forms of chronic dialysis available for clients with renal failure. Which offers the adolescent client the best chance of achieving a normal lifestyle, and why?

① Hemodialysis at home is best because adolescents can set their own schedule
② Hemodialysis in the hospital lets parents share the burden of monitoring side effects
③ Continuous ambulatory peritoneal dialysis is less painful and allows a more liberal diet
④ Intermittent peritoneal dialysis in the hospital uses no needles and can be done while the adolescent sleeps

---

Jack, aged 6, had strep throat 2 weeks ago and now is experiencing periorbital edema, decreased urine output, and headache. He is admitted to the hospital with a diagnosis of poststreptococcal glomerulonephritis.

---

5. Jack is in his room watching television. You notice he is rubbing his eyes and complains of a headache. Which of the following is the most appropriate nursing intervention?
   ① Turn off the television
   ② Check his blood pressure immediately
   ③ Ask the physician for an eye consultation
   ④ Administer Tylenol for his headache

6. What will Jack's urinalysis probably show?
   ① "Cola-colored" urine
   ② Markedly elevated protein
   ③ Specific gravity of 1.005 or lower
   ④ Elevated leukocyte count

7. Which of the following statements by Jack's mother indicates an understanding of Jack's prognosis?
   ① "Most children with this disorder recover without renal damage."

② "He will probably require life-long medication to control his blood pressure."

③ "He will be prone to recurrence of the disease for the rest of his life."

④ "Permanent renal damage may still occur, and he must be retested next year."

8. What is the treatment of choice for the child with nephrotic syndrome?

① Complete bedrest until the glomerular lesions heal

② Administration of antihypertensives and diuretics

③ Low-fat, low-sodium, and low-protein diet

④ Corticosteroids until remission is induced

9. Which of the following is the most appropriate goal for the child with hypospadias?

① Achievement of normal urinary function

② Prevention of infection

③ Acceptable cosmetic appearance

④ Adjustment to external urinary device

10. Which of the following would be a most appropriate nursing diagnosis for a child with enuresis?

① High risk for infection

② High risk for self-esteem disturbance

③ Fluid volume excess

④ Fatigue

PRE-TEST Answers and Rationales

1. ④ Undescended testicles are commonly associated with inguinal hernias. Cancer of the testicle is of higher risk in young men who have had undescended testicles. The risk of sterility would be unknown before surgery. 4, I. Cryptorchidism.

2. ③ The client's understanding of the procedure is top priority. Because a 9-year-old is capable of understanding what is going on, she also is capable of understanding how she can assist so that some degree of independence can be maintained. 1, III. Urinary Tract Infection.

3. ③ An anatomically short urethra, which allows for faster transit of organisms from the perineum into the bladder, is the most frequent cause of urinary tract infection in girls of this age. 2, II. Urinary Tract Infection.

4. ③ Continuous ambulatory peritoneal dialysis offers the adolescent more freedom, allows a more liberal diet, is relatively pain free, and allows the teenager to feel more a part of his or her peer group. 5, II & IV. Chronic Renal Failure.

5. ② When the blood pressure is elevated, headache and diplopia are common symptoms. Acute glomerulonephritis can cause severe hypertension. 4, II. Acute Glomerulonephritis.

6. ① With glomerulonephritis, the urine typically is dark, usually resulting from the presence of blood. It is very concentrated with high specific gravity. Although there may be mild proteinuria, urine protein would not be markedly elevated. 1, II. Acute Glomerulonephritis.

7. ① Poststreptococcal glomerulonephritis usually does not cause permanent renal damage or any residual effect. With proper care, the child will have no residual damage and should recover completely. 5, II. Acute Glomerulonephritis.

8. ④ The administration of corticosteroids to induce remission is the treatment of choice for the child with nephrotic syndrome. Occasionally, steroid therapy is continued if the child is susceptible to relapse. Nephrotic syndrome usually does not cause hypertension. Dietary modification would include a high-protein and -calorie diet composed of the foods the child likes. 4, II. Nephrosis.

9. ① Achievement of normal urinary and reproductive function is a priority goal for the child with hypospadias. Although appearance is important, it is secondary to function. Improving the function will also somewhat normalize appearance. 3, II. Hypospadias.

10. ② Children with enuresis often have to endure the teasing of others and the frustration that they cannot accomplish a developmental task appropriate for their age. These can lead to a self-esteem disturbance if not handled appropriately by parents and supports. 2, III. Enuresis.

NURSING PROCESS APPLIED TO CHILDREN WITH RENAL/URINARY DISORDERS

Congenital Disorders

Hypospadias/Epispadias

I. Assessment

  A. Definition: condition where urethral meatus abnormally located on the penile shaft

    1. Hypospadias: meatus behind glans penis or on ventral surface; often associated with chordee—downward curvature of penis

    2. Epispadias: meatus on dorsal surface; usually associated with exstrophy of the bladder

  B. Etiology/incidence

    1. Etiology unknown

    2. Five per 1000 live births for hypospadias; epispadias much more rare

  C. Predisposing/precipitating factor: familial tendency

  D. Clinical manifestations

    1. Meatus position varies from slightly off center to perineum between two scrotal halves

    2. Downward, crooked appearance of penis (with chordee)

3. Absence of foreskin vertically
4. Altered direction of urine stream
5. Bladder exstrophy
E. Diagnostic examinations: based on physical findings
F. Complication: if located far enough down shaft and not corrected, may lead to later reproductive problems
G. Surgical management
   1. No treatment if minor and still on glans and no chordee
   2. Surgical repair, straightening of chordee, urethroplasty if severe

II. Analysis
A. Altered patterns of urinary elimination related to defect
B. High risk for sexual dysfunction related to extent of defect
C. High risk for body image disturbance related to perception of being different from peers
D. High risk for altered growth and development related to difficulties with toilet training
E. Fear of mutilation related to incomplete understanding of surgical procedure
F. Knowledge deficit about surgery, home management, and possible need for additional surgery related to incomplete knowledge base
G. Other diagnoses appropriate for child undergoing surgery

III. Planning/goals, expected outcomes
A. Child's clinical manifestations will be recognized in newborn nursery
B. Child will not experience altered urinary or sexual function
C. Parents/child (if old enough) will express concerns and fears
D. Parents will understand surgery and treatment regimen
E. Child will be free of complications after surgery
   1. Will not develop bladder spasms
   2. Will not develop infection
F. Child's catheter or stent will remain patent
G. Parents will understand care of catheter or stent
H. Child will have normal urinary function after surgical site heals
I. Child will develop positive body image
J. Parents will understand the condition and potential consequences

IV. Implementation
A. Accurately observe penis and urethra in newborn nursery
B. Explain nature of disorder and treatment to parents/child
C. Prepare parents/child for surgical procedure, postoperative care; reassure that surgery will improve function and appearance; however, appearance will not be completely normal
D. Monitor for bladder spasms; administer antispasmodics as ordered
E. Monitor for signs and symptoms of infection; administer antibiotics as ordered (see Table 10-2)
F. Maintain catheter for straight drainage; ensure patency
G. Maintain restraints if necessary to protect surgical site
H. Encourage high fluid intake
I. Provide guidance for toilet training
J. Refer for home care as needed

V. Evaluation
A. Child's symptoms recognized in nursery and referred for treatment
B. Parents/child describe surgery and what to expect after surgery
C. Parents/child express and deal with fears appropriately
D. Child remains free of postoperative complications
E. Child's catheter remains patent
F. Parents understand and demonstrate care of catheter
G. Child incorporates appearance appropriately in body image development
H. Child achieves normal urinary function after surgical site healed

Exstrophy of Bladder
I. Assessment
A. Definition: serious congenital defect involving failure of abdominal wall and underlying structures/bladder to fuse
B. Etiology/incidence
   1. Etiology unknown
   2. Nonfamilial
   3. Male-to-female ratio of 3 : 1
C. Predisposing/precipitating factor: presence of other congenital anomalies such as undescended testicles, epispadias, and inguinal hernia
D. Clinical manifestations
   1. Exposure of bladder on abdominal wall
   2. Remnants of endodermal tissue (from which bladder derived)
   3. Abnormal urethral outlets
   4. External meatus
   5. Incontinence
   6. Waddling gait (secondary to separation of pubic bones)

E. Diagnostic examinations: based on physical findings

F. Complications
1. Sexual dysfunction after puberty
2. Infection resulting in renal damage/failure

G. Surgical management
1. Bilateral nephrostomies temporarily
2. Ileal conduit
3. Coverage with skin grafts if minimal

II. Analysis
A. High risk for infection related to exposed tissue
B. Other diagnoses similar to child with hypospadias/epispadias

III. Planning/goals, expected outcomes
A. Parents will express disbelief, fears
B. Parents will understand immediate and long-term care
C. Parents will understand and accept surgery
D. Child will be free of urinary tract infection before and after surgery
E. Child's incontinence will resolve after surgery
F. Child will be free of skin infection, ulceration
G. Parents will understand care of ileal conduit or ureterostomy if applicable
H. Child/parents will seek home care follow-up

IV. Implementation
A. Perform accurate examination at birth
B. Arrange for social service consult
C. Allow parents opportunities to express openly grief and fears
D. When ready, teach parents about immediate care and encourage participation and bonding
E. Use strict sterile technique when changing dressings
F. Cover bladder with sterile petrolatum gauze as ordered
G. Change diaper frequently
H. Avoid binding items such as rubber pants
I. Administer sponge baths only
J. Monitor for clinical manifestations of urinary tract infections: fever, foul-smelling urine
K. Keep skin around bladder area clean and dry; use protective skin barrier if needed
L. Prepare parents for surgery, ileal conduit, and expected outcomes
M. Change abdominal dressing as ordered and as needed
N. Monitor abdominal dressing for urinary leakage
O. Apply dressing to stoma if applicable
P. Maintain appliance to stoma as soon as possible
Q. Obtain urine culture and sensitivity before and after surgery

R. Monitor for clinical manifestations of infection
1. Urinary tract
2. Skin/wound

S. Administer antibiotics as ordered (see Table 10-2)

T. Refer to home health agency prior to discharge

U. Continue follow-up care as needed

V. Evaluation
A. Parents demonstrate positive relationship with child
B. Parents able to express disbelief, fears
C. Parents actively seek emotional support when needed
D. Parents describe and demonstrate immediate and long-term care
E. Parents describe what to expect from surgery
F. Child free of urinary tract infection before and after surgery
G. Child's incontinence resolves after surgery
H. Child free of skin infection, ulceration
I. Parents understand care of ileal conduit or ureterostomy if applicable
J. Child/parents seek home care follow-up

Cryptorchidism (Undescended Testicles)

I. Assessment
A. Description: failure of testes to descend into the scrotum during fetal development; may be unilateral or bilateral; often accompanied by inguinal hernia
B. Etiology/incidence
1. Etiology unknown
2. Affects 3 to 4% of full-term male infants
C. Predisposing/precipitating factors: unknown, possibly related to altered hormone function
D. Clinical manifestations: testes not palpable in scrotal sac
E. Diagnostic examinations: palpation of testes during routine well-child care; differentiate true undescended testicle from retractile testes
F. Complications
1. Increased risk of testicular cancer in undescended testicle
2. Increased risk of reproductive damage to undescended testicle
G. Medical management: observation: testicles often descend spontaneously
H. Surgical management: surgery (orchidopexy) before child is 2 years
1. Testes brought down and sutured in position; more complicated surgery may involve temporary placement of external device to keep testes in position
2. Usually done in day surgery

II. Analysis
   A. High risk for sexual dysfunction related to reproductive damage to testicle
   B. Other nursing diagnoses similar to those for any child undergoing surgery
III. Planning/goals, expected outcomes
   A. Child will not experience permanent damage to undescended testicle
   B. Child will have uneventful postoperative course
IV. Implementation
   A. Examine scrotum for presence of testes during well-child checkups
   B. Provide routine postoperative care
   C. Keep surgical site clean of stool or urine
   D. Advise parents how to tell child if future fertility is affected
   E. Teach child testicular examination at appropriate age
V. Evaluation
   A. Child recovers from surgery without complications
   B. Child does not experience long-term complications

Acute Disorders

Urinary Tract Infections

I. Assessment
   A. Definition: infection or bacteriuria, symptomatic or asymptomatic, involving the bladder, kidneys, or associated structures; may or may not be associated with urinary tract abnormalities
   B. Etiology/incidence
      1. Bacterial growth, invasion of any urinary tract structures normally sterile
      2. Exact incidence unknown
      3. Peak incidence at 2 to 6 years (nonstructural)
      4. Female-to-male ratio of 10 to 30 : 1; males more often in infant infection
   C. Predisposing/precipitating factors
      1. Anatomically short urethra in girls
      2. Urine excellent medium for bacterial growth
      3. Structural abnormalities
         a. Vesicoureteral reflux—reflux of urine from bladder into ureters, usually from abnormal placement of ureters in bladder
         b. Neurogenic bladder causing urinary stasis
         c. Hydronephrosis—obstruction of the ureter with collection of urine in renal pelvis and calix
      4. Constipation
      5. Decreased fluid intake
      6. Urinary pH of more than 5 (alkaline)
      7. More common in uncircumcised male infants
      8. Agents that irritate urethra or vaginal area (e.g., bubble bath)
   D. Clinical management
      1. Urinary frequency and urgency
      2. Dysuria
      3. Lower abdominal pain; flank pain for upper urinary tract infection
      4. Irritability
      5. Foul-smelling urine
      6. Fever; may be accompanied by chills in upper urinary tract infection (pyelonephritis)
      7. Incontinence in previously continent child
      8. Nonspecific manifestations in infants: fever, irritability, feeding difficulties, persistent diaper rash, sepsis
   E. Diagnostic examinations
      1. Urinalysis shows cloudy urine, presence of leukocytes, blood
      2. Urine culture and sensitivity grows more than 100,000/mm³ colonies of bacteria; usual organisms *Escherichia coli, Proteus, Pseudomonas;* catheterized specimen or suprapubic aspiration (children less than 2 years) more accurate than clean-catch urine
      3. Tests for structural abnormalities
         a. Renal ultrasound
         b. Voiding cystourethrogram (VCUG)
         c. IV pyelogram (IVP)
   F. Complications: progressive renal injury, damage with numerous recurrent infections
   G. Medical management
      1. Antibiotics based on culture and sensitivity for 10 to 14 days; usually amoxicillin or trimethoprim-sulfamethoxazole (see Table 10-2)
      2. Repeat culture after antibiotic course
      3. Follow-up studies for structural abnormalities recommended after first documented urinary tract infection in all children except adolescent girls
      4. Prophylactic antibiotics for children with structural defects; surgery for severe defects not expected to resolve spontaneously
II. Analysis
   A. Altered patterns of urinary elimination related to infection
   B. Hyperthermia related to underlying infection
   C. Pain related to bladder inflammation
   D. High risk for injury (to urinary tract) related

to inadequate treatment or unrecognized symptoms

E. Knowledge deficit about condition, treatment, or follow-up related to inadequate knowledge base

III. Planning

A. Child's clinical manifestations will be recognized and reported quickly

B. Child's urinary patterns will return to normal

C. Child's body temperature will return to normal within 48 hours of treatment

D. Child/parents will understand all diagnostic procedures

E. Child will not complain of discomfort

F. Child will adhere to therapeutic regimen without difficulty

G. Child will be free of complications, recurrence

H. Parents/child will understand preventive measures

IV. Implementation

A. Obtain accurate history of clinical manifestations

B. Obtain urinalysis, culture, and sensitivity; store urine in refrigerator while waiting for transport to laboratory

C. Prepare for diagnostic examinations
1. Drawings
2. Dolls/play therapy

D. Assure child that urinary tract separate from sexual function if age appropriate

E. Administer antibiotics; child with upper urinary tract infection may need IV antibiotics

F. Teach parents proper administration of medications; emphasize need to take full course

G. Teach parents preventive measures
1. Hygiene; wipe front to back (females)
2. Avoid or limit tub baths (females)
3. Use cotton rather than nylon underpants (females)
4. Empty bladder frequently
5. Complete emptying of bladder; do not rush off toilet
6. Force fluids, especially water, juices

V. Evaluation

A. Child diagnosed and treatment begun as soon as clinical manifestations begin and are identified

B. Child/parents cooperate with all diagnostic procedures

C. Child adheres to therapeutic regimen without difficulty

D. Child free of complications and recurrence

E. Parents/child accurately state preventive measures

Enuresis

I. Assessment

A. Definition: incontinence of urine at an age beyond which urinary continence should have been achieved; usually nocturnal (night bedwetting); can occur in previously continent children

B. Etiology/incidence
1. Increased incidence in relatives
2. More common in boys
3. More frequent in children of low socioeconomic status

C. Predisposing/precipitating factors
1. Tense, worried children
2. Afraid of the dark
3. Situational crisis
4. Associated with personality disorder
5. Associated with sound sleep

D. Clinical manifestations
1. Inadequate bladder control
2. Bed-wetting, often more than once a night
3. Occasional urinary frequency and urgency

E. Diagnostic examinations
1. Urinalysis and urine culture to rule out infection or diabetes
2. Renal studies to rule out organic structural cause

F. Complications: decreased self-esteem, social isolation

G. Medical management
1. Usually involves combined approach
2. Training to increase bladder capacity
3. Positive reinforcement for remaining dry
4. Conditioning therapy: devices to wake child at beginning of urination
5. Pharmacological
   a. Imipramine (Tofranil) to lighten sleep
   b. Desmopressin (DDAVP) nasal spray (see Diabetes Insipidus)
6. Counseling for underlying psychological problems

II. Analysis

A. Functional incontinence related to immature bladder function

B. High risk for self-esteem disturbance related to teasing by others

C. High risk for social isolation related to inadequate hygiene

III. Planning/goals, expected outcomes

A. Child will achieve continence

B. Child will develop positive self-image

C. Child will develop positive relationships with peers

IV. Implementation

A. Explore with child/parents most appropriate approaches

B. Teach proper administration of medications if applicable

C. Encourage parents to involve child in the program and provide positive reinforcement for success

D. Encourage child to keep clean, change clothes as often as necessary

V. Evaluation

A. Episodes of incontinence decrease and eventually resolve

B. Child becomes actively involved in approach chosen

C. Child demonstrates positive attitude that condition will resolve

D. Child maintains friendships and deals well with any teasing

Acute Poststreptococcal Glomerulonephritis

I. Assessment

A. Definition: inflammation of glomeruli; immune complex disease; usually after infection

B. Etiology/incidence

1. Antigen-antibody response to antecedent group A beta-hemolytic streptococcal infection, limited strains

2. Occurs approximately 10 to 14 days after streptococcal infection

3. Peak incidence in preschool or early school-age years

4. Male-to-female ratio of 2 : 1

C. Predisposing/precipitating factors: antecedent streptococcal infection depends on time of year

1. Pharyngitis precedes winter/spring

2. Impetigo in late summer

D. Clinical manifestations (Table 14-5)

E. Diagnostic examinations (see Table 14-5)

F. Complications

1. Hypertensive encephalopathy

2. Acute cardiac decompensation

TABLE 14–5 Differences Between Poststreptococcal Acute Glomerulonephritis and Nephrosis

	Acute Glomerulonephritis	Nephrotic Syndrome
Cause	Antecedent *Streptococcus* infection that precipitates an immune reaction that deposits immune complexes in the glomeruli; peak incidence in early school-aged children	Ideopathic in most cases; majority of children have minimal change nephrotic syndrome; alteration in the glomerular basement membrane allows increased permeability to protein and results in protein loss from serum to urine; peak incidence in preschool-aged children
Clinical Manifestations	Abrupt appearance of periorbital edema; dark, "cola-colored" urine with increased specific gravity, mild proteinuria, and frank or occult blood; decreased urinary output; anorexia; elevated blood pressure; pallor and listlessness	Insidious weight gain and progressively worsening edema; edema may be severe and is generalized; urine dark and "foamy" with markedly elevated protein, occasionally microscopic blood; decreased urinary output; hypoproteinemia, increased serum lipids; anorexia; normal blood pressure; severe pallor and fatigue; increased susceptibility to infection
Diagnostic Examinations	Urinalysis; serum protein; blood urea nitrogen and creatinine may be elevated; throat culture for *Streptococcus*; anti-streptolysin (ASO) titer to determine exposure to strep; CBC may show decreased hemoglobin and hematocrit; elevated erythrocyte sedimentation rate; C_3 complement component—index of total complement activity (in immune complex disease)	Urinalysis for proteinuria; increased specific gravity; serum protein (decreased); CBC usually normal except for elevated platelets; serum electrolytes (low sodium); renal biopsy
Clinical Course	Acutely symptomatic for approximately 2 weeks; recovery signaled by increasing urinary output, decreasing blood pressure, resolution of hematuria	Resolution of proteinuria with therapy usually takes 1 to 3 weeks; diuresis signals beginning of resolution; many children relapse, requiring continuing treatment
Medical Management and Prognosis	Supportive; antibiotic treatment of any positive *Streptococcus* infection; voluntary activity restriction; monitoring fluid and electrolyte balance; sodium restriction and antihypertensives (Table 14-6) with diuretics for high blood pressure; resolves spontaneously	Administration of corticosteroids (see Table 10-8), usually oral prednisone, until urine protein negative; bedrest during active edematous phase; long-term QOD doses of steroid for those who do not respond initially or who relapse; other immunosuppressants for those not responding to steroids alone or for whom steroids contraindicated

3. Acute renal failure

G. Medical management (see Table 14-5)

II. Analysis

A. Fluid volume excess related to decreased glomerular filtration

B. Altered patterns of urinary dysfunction related to glomerular dysfunction

C. Activity intolerance related to edema and possible anemia

D. Anxiety of child/parents related to seriousness of condition

E. Knowledge deficit about disease, home management, and prognosis related to incomplete knowledge base

III. Planning/goals, expected outcomes

A. Child's clinical manifestations will be recognized and reported quickly

B. Child's vital signs will remain within normal limits, especially blood pressure

C. Child's fluid and electrolyte balance will remain stable

D. Child's edema will resolve

E. Child will rest comfortably at all times and participate in activities as tolerated

F. Child's nutritional status will be appropriate for age

G. Child will be free of secondary complications

H. Child will not regress developmentally or educationally during course of illness

I. Child/parents will express concerns

J. Parents will understand home care and follow-up management

IV. Implementation

A. Obtain accurate history of preceding illnesses

B. Obtain accurate history of presenting clinical manifestations

C. Measure vital signs, including blood pressure, every 2 hours

D. Maintain activity restriction during acute phase of disease; provide opportunities for quiet diversional activity

E. Administer diuretics as ordered (see Table 10-5)

F. Administer antihypertensives as ordered (Table 14-6)

G. Maintain strict I & O measurement

H. Check weight daily

I. Measure specific gravity every void

J. Limit fluids as ordered for severe edema

K. Monitor serum electrolytes

L. Maintain no-added-salt diet, small frequent meals; restrict sodium if child hypertensive

M. Monitor for any significant changes in physical, emotional behavior (e.g., headache, dizziness, irritability)

N. Provide age-appropriate diversional activities

O. Encourage peer visitation (noninfectious)

P. Provide home bound teacher if at home or in hospital more than 2 weeks

Q. Teach parents how to check blood pressure, measure urine for blood or protein, monitor for worsening condition

R. Refer to home health agency after discharge

V. Evaluation

A. Child's vital signs remain within normal limits, especially blood pressure

B. Child's urine output at least 1 mL/kg/hr

C. Child's edema decreases as evidenced by decreasing weight

D. Child rests comfortably at all times

E. Child's nutritional status maintained according to age and growth

F. Child does not exhibit secondary complications

G. Child does not regress developmentally or educationally during course of illness

H. Parents accurately perform home care and follow-up management, testing

I. Parents in contact with home health agency

Chronic Disorders

Nephrosis (Nephrotic Syndrome)

I. Assessment

A. Definition: chronic renal condition that may develop during course of several pathological conditions; increased permeability of glomerular membrane to plasma protein, resulting in massive protein loss

B. Etiology/incidence

TABLE 14-6 Antihypertensives

Example	Action	Use	Common Side Effects	Nursing Implications
Vasodilator: hydralazine; adrenergic blocker: methyldopa (Aldomet); beta-adrenergic blocker: propranolol (Inderal)	Act in multiple ways, including decreasing sympathetic nervous system activity, to lower blood pressure directly by acting on peripheral arteriolar vasodilation; decreases cardiac output	Treatment of high blood pressure in combination with diuretics	Sedation, nasal stuffiness, gastrointestinal disturbances, orthostatic hypotension, hemolytic anemia and liver dysfunction (methyldopa)	Monitor blood pressure frequently; strict I & O; instruct on importance of continuing medication even if feeling better; monitor for side effects; teach to change positions slowly

1. Etiology obscure
2. 80% of cases are minimal change nephrotic syndrome (MCNS)
3. Peak age 2 to 3 years
4. Two to three per 100,000 Caucasian children
5. 60% of cases male
C. Predisposing/precipitating factors
   1. Viral upper respiratory infection 4 to 8 days prior
   2. Majority of cases idiopathic, but result in dramatic alterations of glomerular basement membrane
D. Clinical manifestations (see Table 14-5)
E. Diagnostic examinations (see Table 14-5)
F. Complications
   1. Pleural effusion
   2. Ascites
   3. Chronic renal failure
G. Medical management (see Table 14-5)

II. Analysis
A. Fluid volume excess related to decreased oncotic pressure
B. Altered patterns of urinary elimination related to fluid shift
C. High risk for impaired skin integrity related to pressure from edema
D. Activity intolerance related to fluid overload
E. High risk for altered nutrition: less than body requirements related to protein loss and decreased appetite
F. High risk for infection related to anti-inflammatory treatment
G. High risk for altered family processes related to chronic nature of illness
H. Knowledge deficit about condition, prognosis, and home management

III. Planning/goals, expected outcomes
A. Child's clinical manifestations will be recognized and reported quickly
B. Child's fluid and electrolyte balance will remain stable
C. Child will rest comfortably during periods of exacerbation
D. Child's skin will remain intact
E. Child will be free of infectious process
F. Child will receive adequate nutrients according to age
G. Child will be free of secondary complications
H. Child will not regress developmentally or educationally during course of illness
I. Parents/child will express concerns about any exacerbations and their impact
J. Parents will understand home care and follow-up management

IV. Implementation
A. Obtain accurate history and physical examination of presenting clinical manifestations and course of onset
B. Obtain accurate history of preceding illnesses
C. Measure vital signs every 2 hours, including blood pressure
D. Administer corticosteroids as ordered (see Table 10-8)
E. Keep on no-added-salt diet during edematous phase
F. Check weight daily
G. Measure abdominal girth daily
H. Maintain strict I & O; measure specific gravity every void
I. Check urine for protein
J. Monitor serum electrolytes, protein
K. Maintain high-protein, high-carbohydrate diet (see Table 10-12) unless there is azotemia or renal failure, then maintain LOW-protein diet
L. Offer small, frequent meals with foods that appeal to child
M. Maintain bedrest initially, then ambulate as tolerated
N. Provide meticulous skin care
O. Provide support for edematous organs, good positioning
P. Avoid contact with persons with infections
Q. Administer antibiotics for infection as ordered (see Table 10-2)
R. Monitor for any significant changes in physical or emotional behavior
S. Provide quiet age-appropriate diversional, educational activities and encourage peer interactions
T. Provide home bound teacher when appropriate
U. Teach parents home care
   1. Testing urine for protein
   2. Medication administration
   3. Prevention of infection
   4. Strict adherence to regimen
V. Allow parents/child to ventilate fears and feelings
W. Refer to home health agency for follow-up

V. Evaluation
A. Child achieves remission with appropriate treatment; no manifestations of proteinuria or edema
B. Child's fluid and electrolyte balance returns to normal as evidenced by urinary output at least 1 mL/kg/hr, decreased edema
C. Child rests comfortably during periods of exacerbation and increases activity to normal for age during remission
D. Child's skin integrity maintained at all times
E. Child free of infectious process
F. Child demonstrates adequate nutritional in-

take for age; normal weight maintained after edema resolves

G. Child is free of secondary complications

H. Child does not regress developmentally or educationally during course of illness

I. Parents accurately demonstrate home care and follow-up management

Chronic Renal Failure

I. Assessment

  A. Definition: when disease process inhibits normal renal function; point at which more than 50% of functional renal capacity destroyed by disease, injury

  B. Etiology/incidence: progressive renal, nephron destruction

  C. Predisposing/precipitating factors

    1. Congenital renal, urinary tract malformations

    2. Vesicoureteral reflux

    3. Chronic pyelonephritis

    4. Chronic glomerulonephritis

    5. Systemic disease such as lupus erythematosus

    6. Hereditary disorders

  D. Clinical manifestations

    1. Increased fatigue on exertion

    2. Decreased interest in activity, eating

    3. Change in urinary pattern

    4. Compensatory fluid intake

    5. Pallor and bleeding tendencies from anemia and decreased platelet function; urochrome pigmentation

    6. Headache

    7. Muscle cramps

    8. Impaired growth with bone demineralization

    9. Uremic syndrome

      a. Anorexia, nausea and vomiting

      b. Constant itching

      c. "Uremic frost" on skin

      d. "Uremic" breath

      e. Hypertension

      f. Pulmonary edema

      g. Clinical manifestations of metabolic acidosis

      h. Progressive confusion

      i. Coma

  E. Diagnostic examinations

    1. History and physical findings

    2. Blood urea nitrogen elevated

    3. Creatinine elevated; more accurate indicator than blood urea nitrogen

    4. CBC

    5. Abnormal blood chemistries

    6. Renal function studies to determine cause

    7. Renal biopsy

  F. Complication: death

  G. Medical management

    1. Dietary management: restricted protein and phosphorus, low-sodium and -potassium diet if electrolytes altered

    2. Administration of phosphorus-binding agent, vitamin D, and calcium

    3. Blood transfusions for anemia

    4. Antihypertensives and diuretics for hypertension; antibiotics for infections

    5. Peritoneal dialysis or hemodialysis (see Chapter 8 and Table 8–27); continuous ambulatory peritoneal dialysis (CAPD) most appropriate for home treatment of the child

  H. Surgical management—renal transplantation

II. Analysis

  A. Altered patterns of urinary elimination related to fluid imbalances

  B. Altered growth and development related to bone abnormalities, repeated hospitalizations, interrupted schooling

  C. Altered nutrition: less or more than body requirements related to demands of changing condition

  D. High risk for injury related to disturbances in clotting

  E. High risk for infection related to increased susceptibility

  F. Activity intolerance related to anemia

  G. Altered family processes related to long-term nature and expense of condition

  H. Anticipatory grieving related to fear of impending death

  I. Knowledge deficit about condition, home management, and prognosis related to incomplete knowledge base and anxiety

III. Planning/goals, expected outcomes

  A. Child's manifestations of impending renal failure will be recognized as early as possible

  B. Child's renal function will remain stable without further deterioration

  C. Child will not regress developmentally

  D. Child will maintain a diet sufficient for growth within dietary restrictions

  E. Child's fluid and electrolyte status will stabilize

  F. Child/family will understand injury prevention

  G. Child will remain free of infection

  H. Child/family will understand principles and procedure of dialysis if applicable

  I. Child/family will understand need for renal transplantation if required

J. Family will seek assistance from appropriate supporting agencies

K. Parents/child/family members will express feelings/concerns and go through grieving process at own pace

IV. Implementation

A. Monitor for clinical manifestations of renal failure

B. Teach parents clinical manifestations of renal failure to look for and to report immediately

C. Make continuous assessment of vital signs, new or changing clinical manifestations

D. Allow time for parents/family to express feelings and questions and to grieve

E. Assist parents in all aspects of home management including home dialysis if applicable

F. Maintain activity as tolerated

G. Encourage peer interaction

H. Encourage schooling or tutoring as tolerated

I. Avoid contact with infectious persons

J. Use strict handwashing techniques

K. Administer appropriate medications as ordered: antibiotics, antihypertensives, diuretics, phosphorus-binding agents

L. Maintain strict I & O

M. Check weight daily

N. Check blood pressure, vital signs every 4 hours and as needed

O. Measure specific gravity every void

P. Limit protein intake, provide proteins high in essential amino acids, follow other dietary restrictions as ordered

Q. Administer iron supplements

R. Use multidisciplinary approach to explaining dialysis, transplantation

S. Refer family to National Kidney Foundation

T. Refer to appropriate agencies for counseling, support services, and financial assistance

V. Evaluation

A. Child's condition is stabilized

B. Child's renal function maintained at home on outpatient basis

C. Parents/family able to express feelings

D. Child/parents/family members participate in support group and express themselves with hope, not denial

E. Child participates in activities as tolerated

F. Child remains infection free

G. Child's fluid and electrolyte balance stabilized

H. Child's nutritional status adequate for growth

I. Child/family describe and demonstrate dialysis if applicable

J. Child/family state the need for transplantation if applicable

K. Family sees outside agency for specialized support

POST-TEST Renal/Urinary Disorders

Julio is a newborn diagnosed in the nursery as having hypospadias with a moderate degree of chordee. His parents are upset because they have been told that more than one surgical procedure probably will be required.

1. Surgical repair of hypospadias usually begins when the child is between 6 and 18 months. Which of the following best describes why this is the most appropriate time for surgery?
   ① The child is too old to experience any major complications
   ② The wait gives the parents time to get used to the appearance of the penis
   ③ The child is young enough not to be embarrassed by manipulation of the area
   ④ The child is young enough not to have any severe body image concerns

2. Julio is seen in the clinic for his follow-up visit after surgery. Which of the following statements by Julio's father indicates an INCOMPLETE understanding of Julio's condition?
   ① "Julio will be able to stand to urinate, and his penis will remain straight."
   ② "The appearance of his penis will improve so that it will look completely normal."
   ③ "We need to continue to watch him for signs of a urinary tract infection."
   ④ "He will have normal sexual function when he is older."

3. Which of the following is an appropriate nursing diagnosis for the infant with exstrophy of the bladder?
   ① High risk for infection related to exposed tissue
   ② Fluid volume deficit related to seepage of urine
   ③ Anticipatory grieving related to impending death of the child
   ④ Impaired physical mobility related to decreased bladder innervation

Ryanne is a 6-week-old who was brought into the pediatrician's office with unexplained fever of more than 101°F (37.3°C) for the past 24 hours. The nurse obtains the following assessment data from the history: no recent upper respiratory infection or known illness, not sleeping as well as usual, fussy most of the time with a moaning cry, not eating, and not urinating adequately. When the mother

changes Ryanne's diaper, the nurse notes a diaper rash and an obvious strong odor of urine.

___

4. The nurse bags Ryanne for a clean-catch urine specimen. Which of the following best describes the rationale for this action?
   1. Urinary tract infection is more frequently seen in infant girls than in infant boys
   2. It is likely that the mother missed an antecedent streptococcal infection
   3. Nonspecific symptoms and sepsis are common indicators of urinary tract infection in infants
   4. Routine collection of urine for urinalysis is done in the pediatrician's office

5. After performing a septic work-up on Ryanne, the physician admits her to the hospital and prescribes an injection of IM ceftriaxone while waiting for the results of the cultures. Which of the following would be most indicative of a urinary tract infection?
   1. Blood culture growing *E. coli*
   2. Elevated urine protein
   3. More than 100,000 mm^3 colony count
   4. Increased sedimentation rate

6. Ryanne's physician orders a renal ultrasound and VCUG to be done on Ryanne after her infection is resolved. Ryanne's mother questions the necessity for this. The nurse's best response would be:
   1. "This is just routine. The likelihood of there being a problem is very slim."
   2. "Follow-up is extremely important because the occurrence of a structural problem is far higher in infant girls."
   3. "Ruling out a structural problem is important for preventing future kidney damage."
   4. "The treatment of future urinary tract infections will depend on the type of structural problem involved."

7. Which of the following best describes cryptorchidism?
   1. Developmental failure of one or both testes to descend into the scrotum
   2. Engorged varicose veins of the testicles
   3. A collection of fluid in the tunica vaginalis of the testicle
   4. A protrusion of abdominal contents through the inguinal ring into the scrotum

___

Gareth, 3 years old, is admitted with a 3-week history of periorbital edema and decreasing urine output. He is diagnosed with idiopathic nephrotic syndrome.

___

8. Which of the following laboratory values would the nurse expect to find?
   1. Decreased urine specific gravity
   2. 4+ protein level per urinalysis
   3. Severe anemia
   4. Elevated serum protein

9. Which of the following would you include in your nursing care of Gareth?
   1. Maintain a low-protein, low-sodium diet
   2. Encourage him to play ball in the playroom
   3. Provide meticulous skin care and position changes
   4. Force fluids to prevent fluid volume deficit

10. Which of the following accurately describes an important difference between nephrotic syndrome and acute glomerulonephritis?
    1. Nephrotic syndrome is a response to an autoimmune inflammatory process in the glomeruli, whereas the etiology of glomerulonephritis is idiopathic
    2. Nephrotic syndrome is a self-limiting disease, whereas glomerulonephritis is marked by remissions and relapses
    3. The onset of nephrotic syndrome is acute, and it is insidious in glomerulonephritis
    4. Nephrotic syndrome alters the glomerular basement membrane, whereas glomerulonephritis is marked by deposition of immune complexes

11. Which of the following data would NOT be as important when taking a history from the mother of an 8-year-old girl with enuresis?
    1. Type and amount of fluids she drinks at night
    2. The location of the bathroom in proximity to her room
    3. Relationship with her sister and schoolmates
    4. Foods and snacks eaten on a daily basis

12. Which of the following would suggest successful nursing intervention for the child newly diagnosed to be in chronic renal failure?
    1. Weight gain and growth appropriate for age
    2. Urinary elimination of less than 1 mL/kg/hr
    3. Intact skin and reduced itching
    4. Complete resumption of usual activity

POST-TEST Answers and Rationales

1. ④ Surgical repair is done at this time because the child will have time for the penis to grow, making repair somewhat easier, but primarily because it is before the developmental stage where the child is fearful of mutilation. Doing it at this time also precedes toilet training, which would be difficult if the defect were not repaired sufficiently to allow the child to stand to urinate. 2, II & IV. Hypospadias.

2. ② The appearance of the penis after surgery is straighter but not completely normal. It is unlikely that the child with severe hypospadias will have a completely normal-appearing penis, but normal urinary, sexual, and reproductive functions are expected. 5, II. Hypospadias.

3. ① Infection is an ongoing concern in the infant with exstrophy of the bladder because the internal bladder and lower genitourinary tract mucosa are exposed. Meticulous protection of the exposed area is necessary to prevent infection. 2, II. Exstrophy of the Bladder.

4. ③ Infants with urinary tract infections often present with symptoms of sepsis from no known cause. Foul-smelling urine along with persistent diaper rash in an infant is suggestive of urinary tract infection when accompanied by other symptoms. Urine collection often is done in the pediatrician's office, but choice 3 provides a more specific rationale based on data collected. 2, II. Urinary Tract Infection.

5. ③ Growth of organisms in urine of more than 100,000 mm^3 colonies is diagnostic of urinary tract infection. The choice of antibiotics is based on the sensitivity of the particular organism. 1, II. Urinary Tract Infection.

6. ③ Although follow-up to identify structural problems has become routine after a first urinary tract infection in infants, choice 3 best states the rationale to help the mother understand the consequences of not having the follow-up done. 4, I. Urinary Tract Infection.

7. ① Cryptorchidism is a developmental defect where one or both testes remain outside of the scrotum at the time of birth. They either pass into the scrotum after birth or must be surgically manipulated into the correct position. 1, II. Cryptorchidism.

8. ② Protein in the urine along with a decreased serum level is the common finding in children with nephrotic syndrome. Specific gravity will be high, and anemia is a late symptom. 1, II. Nephrosis.

9. ③ It is important during the acute phase to maintain rest, preferably in bed, with frequent position changes. Quiet activities should be encouraged and are important for a usually active 3-year-old. Meticulous skin care is most important along with position changes to maintain skin integrity, which is subject to compromise in the edematous child. The diet usually is normal, and no sodium restriction is necessary. 4, I. Nephrosis.

10. ④ Glomerulonephritis is inflammation of the glomeruli from the deposition of immune complexes. Nephrotic syndrome results from massive loss of protein through the glomerular basement membrane, which is altered by some unknown process. The onset of glomerulonephritis is acute. Nephrosis appears over time and may be characterized by remission and relapse after treatment. 1, II. Acute Glomerulonephritis.

11. ④ Enuresis is often due to environmental factors such as a dark hallway or a long trip to the bathroom at night. Daytime snacks are not important, but the nurse should check nighttime intake of fluids. Occasionally, enuresis causes stress in peer relationships, and this needs to be investigated. 1, II. Enuresis.

12. ① Dietary management that provides nutrients sufficient for growth within restrictions imposed by kidney impairment is the major goal for children newly diagnosed with chronic renal failure. Urine output should be at least 1 mL/kg/hr for adequate fluid balance. The child can resume activities but usually does not participate fully because of decreased energy level or the potential for injury from underlying clotting disturbances. Itching is a sign of progressive end-stage renal disease. 5, II. Chronic Renal Failure.

BIBLIOGRAPHY

ELIMINATION

Andze, G. O., et al (1991). Diagnosis and treatment of gastroesophageal reflux in 500 children with respiratory symptoms: The value of pH monitoring. *Journal of Pediatric Surgery* 26 (3): 295–300.

Barnett, E. (1992). After the UTI: The pediatrician and the radiologist. Presented at Recent Advances in Diagnosis and Management of Infectious Diseases in Children, March 28, 1992, Boston, Mass.

Dagan, R., et al (1992). Once daily cefixime compared with twice daily trimethoprim/sulfamethoxazole for treatment of urinary tract infection in infants and children. *Pediatric Infectious Disease Journal* 11 (March): 198–203.

Fergusson, D. M., et al (1986). Factors related to the age of attainment of nocturnal bladder control: An 8-year longitudinal study. *Pediatrics* 78 (November): 884–890.

Foster, R. L. R., Hunsberger, M. M., and Anderson, J. T. (1989). *Family-centered nursing care of children.* Philadelphia: W. B. Saunders.

Guo, J. Z., et al (1986). Results of air pressure enema reduction of intussusception: 6,396 cases in 13 years. *Journal of Pediatric Surgery* 21 (12): 1201–1203.

Hoberman, A., et al (1991). Prevalence of urinary tract infection (UTI) in febrile infants. *Pediatric Research* 29 (April): 119A.

Kirschner, B. S. (1991). When to suspect inflammatory bowel disease. *Practical Reviews in Pediatrics* 14–16: audio tape.

Mott, S. R., James, S. R., and Sperhac, A. M. (1990). *Nursing care of children and families,* 2nd ed. Redwood City, Calif., Addison-Wesley.

Orenstein, S. R. (1992). Crying does not exacerbate gastroesophageal reflux in infants. *Journal of Pediatric Gastroenterology and Nutrition* 14: 34–37.

Oski, F. A., et al (1992). UTI controversies: Circumcision, reflux, and more. *Contemporary Pediatrics* 9 (3): 75–101.

Sacher, D. B. (1989). Cyclosporine treatment for inflammatory bowel disease: A step backward or a leap forward? *New England Journal of Medicine* 321: 894–895.

Schmitt, B. D. (1990). Nocturnal enuresis: Finding the treatment that fits the child. *Contemporary Pediatrics* 7 (9): 70–97.

Shaw, K. N., et al (1991). Clinical evaluation of a rapid screening test for urinary tract infections in children. *Journal of Pediatrics* 118 (5): 733–736.

Steinhart, J. M., et al (1988). Ultrasound screening of healthy infants for urinary tract abnormalities. *Pediatrics* 82 (October): 609–614.

Taxman, T. L., et al (1986). How useful is the barium enema in the diagnosis of infantile Hirschsprung's disease? *American Journal of the Diseases of Children* 140 (9): 881–884.

Whaley, L. F., and Wong, D. L. (1991). *Nursing care of infants and children,* 4th ed. St. Louis: Mosby-Year Book.

UNIT IV

The Childbearing Family

15

Prenatal Period

PRE-TEST Psychological and Physiological Changes During Pregnancy and Embryonic and Fetal Development

1. Which of the following would occur first in the process of fetal development?
   ① Appearance of vernix caseosa
   ② Muscle contraction
   ③ Increased subcutaneous fat deposits
   ④ Secretion of urine by the kidneys

2. During intrauterine life, the fetus receives oxygen and excretes its wastes through:
   ① The amniotic fluid
   ② Two umbilical arteries and one umbilical vein
   ③ One umbilical artery and two umbilical veins
   ④ The placenta

3. Maternal perception of first fetal movement is referred to as:
   ① Lightening
   ② Quickening
   ③ Involution
   ④ Contractions

4. Fetal movements are first experienced:
   ① Two weeks before delivery
   ② At about 8 weeks
   ③ Within the first week after conception
   ④ Between 16 and 20 weeks of gestation

5. Normal changes that are experienced during pregnancy include:
   ① An increase in vaginal discharge
   ② Persistent vomiting for the first trimester
   ③ Headaches and vertigo
   ④ Edema of fingers and ankles first thing in the morning

6. Hemoglobin and hematocrit counts vary during the pregnancy. The normal variations include:
   ① A decrease in both, due to the increased blood volume
   ② An increase in both, due to the decreased blood volume
   ③ An increase in the hemoglobin and a decrease in the hematocrit
   ④ Neither actually varies consistently during pregnancy

7. Clinical manifestations of placenta previa would include:
   ① Spotting in the early months of pregnancy
   ② Painless bleeding in the last months of pregnancy
   ③ Sharp abdominal pains in the absence of bleeding
   ④ Watery vaginal discharge before birth

8. Your client is admitted with a diagnosis of hyperemesis gravidarum. Your nursing interventions will include:
   ① Encouraging fluids before and with meals
   ② Measuring I & O accurately
   ③ Identifying foods especially nauseating to your client
   ④ Spending a minimal amount of time with her so she can get plenty of rest

PRE-TEST Answers and Rationales

1. ④ The kidneys begin to secrete urine as early as the 12th week after conception. Vernix caseosa and muscle contractions occur later, and subcutaneous fat increases just before birth. 1, IV. Fetal Development.

2. ② The normal umbilical cord contains two arteries and one vein. It is responsible for the oxygenation of the fetus and the removal of waste products. This occurs via the placenta, but the cord itself is responsible. 1, IV. Fetal Development.

3. ② The first fetal movement is called quickening. The other options refer to maternal changes. 1, IV. Fetal Development.

4. ④ Quickening, the first fetal movements, usually occurs between weeks 16 and 20. 1, IV. Prenatal Care.

5. ① Increased vaginal discharge is normal and quite common. All other options are signs of potential abnormalities and require that the physician be notified. 1 & 2, IV. Maternal Physiological Development.

6. ① As the blood volume increases, the relative levels of the hemoglobin and hematocrit are lowered in the mother. The actual values are unchanged, but since both are dilutional values, they appear to be lower. 1 & 2, IV. Maternal Physiological Development.

7. ② Because the placenta is located on or near the cervical os, as the cervix dilates in preparation for birth, painless bleeding occurs. Spotting is not always abnormal early in pregnancy. Sharp pains may be contractions, and a watery discharge may be the rupture of the amniotic membranes. 1 & 2, IV. Placenta Previa.

8. ② Measuring I & O is very important to make sure that the client is not developing a severe fluid imbalance. Food should not be discussed because that often increases the nausea. The client may require professional counseling, so leaving her alone is wrong. Fluids should be discouraged before and with meals as they overdistend the stomach. 4, IV. Hyperemesis.

YOUNG ADULT GROWTH AND DEVELOPMENT

Female Physiological Development

I. Anatomy
   A. External genitalia
      1. Mons pubis
      2. Glans clitoris
      3. Urethral meatus
      4. Labia majora
      5. Labia minora
      6. Hymen
      7. Posterior commissure
      8. Perineum
   B. Internal genitalia
      1. Vestibule
      2. Bartholin's gland
      3. Skene's duct
      4. Vagina
      5. Cervix
      6. Uterus
      7. Round, broad, and ovarian ligaments
      8. Fallopian tube
      9. Gartner's duct
      10. Ovary
   C. Female pelvis (see Intrapartal Care, Chapter 16)
II. Reproductive system matures at puberty
   A. Hormonal influence
   B. Secondary sexual characteristics develop
III. Physiological
   A. Estrogen: secreted by maturing ovarian follicle
      1. Responsible for growth and development of ovaries, uterus, vagina, and breasts
      2. Develops secondary sexual characteristics
      3. Aids in growth of skeleton, resulting in cessation of bone growth
   B. Progesterone: secreted by corpus luteum or, if pregnancy occurs, by placenta
      1. Prepares lining of uterus for implantation of embryo
      2. Decreases rapidly with estrogen if fertilization does not occur
   C. Menstruation
      1. Begins at puberty, ends at menopause
      2. Usually 28-day cycle
      3. Five phases of cycle (Fig. 15-1)
         a. Menstruation phase
            (1) Lasts 4 to 6 days; endometrial lining is shed

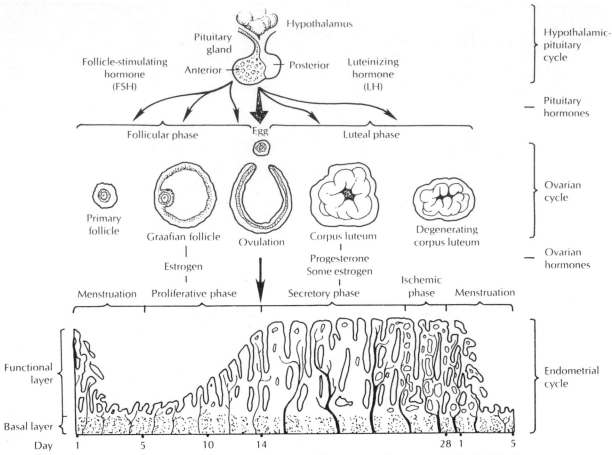

FIGURE 15–1. The menstrual cycle. (From Bobak, I. M., and Jensen, M. D. (1987). *Essentials of maternity nursing: The nurse and the childbearing family,* **2nd ed. St. Louis: C. V. Mosby.)**

(2) Luteinizing hormone (LH), estrogen, and progesterone at lowest levels

(3) Follicle-stimulating hormone (FSH) rises, enabling graafian follicle to begin maturation

b. Proliferative phase

(1) Lasts about 9 days

(2) Uterine lining grows and thickens eight- to 10-fold; changes level off at ovulation

(3) Three to 4 days before ovulation, glands develop and vascularity increases

(4) Estrogen stimulation–dependent phase

c. Ovulation occurs between day 12 and day 16

(1) Estrogen high and progesterone low

(2) Cervical mucus stretchable; important sign of ovulation (Spinnbarkeit)

d. Secretory or luteal phase

(1) Lasts about 12 days

(2) Initiated by ovulation in response to surge of LH

(3) Corpus luteum produces large quantities of progesterone and estrogen

(4) Uterine lining matures to receive and nourish fertilized ovum

(5) If fertilization occurs

(a) Implantation occurs 7 to 10 days after fertilization

(b) Trophoblast produces human chorionic gonadotropin (HCG)

e. Premenstrual or ischemic phase

(1) Lasts 3 to 5 days

(2) Occurs when there is no fertilization

(3) Progesterone and estrogen decrease

(4) Endometrial arteries constrict; uterine lining shrinks and dies

Male Physiological Development

I. Anatomy
   A. External genitalia
      1. Glans penis
      2. Prepuce
      3. Penile shaft
      4. Urethra
      5. Scrotum
   B. Internal genitalia
      1. Cowper's gland
      2. Prostate
      3. Seminal vesicle
      4. Vas deferens
      5. Epididymis
      6. Testes
II. Male organs mature at puberty
   A. Testosterone: produced by interstitial cells in testes
      1. Responsible for production of sex drive and potency
      2. Growth of scrotum and penis
      3. Sperm production by seminiferous tubules of testes
      4. Development of secondary sexual characteristics
         a. Height
         b. Size and number of muscles
         c. Cessation of bone growth

Psychosocial Development

I. Major developmental tasks of young adulthood (Erikson, Havighurst)
   A. Achievement of relative independence from parental figures and development of sense of responsibility for own life
   B. Development of awareness and acceptance of body image, including male and female role
   C. Achievement of more mature relationships with peers of both sexes
   D. Increased self-development and achievement of appropriate roles and positions in society
   E. Beginning development of personal lifestyle away from home; beginning of work life
   F. Development of parenting behaviors
   G. Integration of personal values with career development and societal constraints

PSYCHOLOGICAL AND PHYSIOLOGICAL CHANGES DURING PREGNANCY

Developmental Tasks of Pregnancy

I. Validation: first trimester
   A. Shock, denial, and ambivalence often at first
   B. Introversion begins and lasts 7 to 8 months; encouraged by weight gain and other outward signs of pregnancy
II. Fetal embodiment: second trimester
   A. Attempts to incorporate fetus into body image as integral part of self
   B. Readjusts to life roles
   C. Develops feeling of inner strength
   D. Appears to be time of maturation
III. Fetal distinction: second trimester
   A. Encouraged by quickening
   B. Fetus becomes distinct and apart from self
   C. Daydreams about baby and self as mother, often unrealistic dreams
IV. Role transition: third trimester
   A. Separates fetus from self and makes concrete plans
   B. Becomes more irritable and wants end of pregnancy

Physiological Changes in Mother

I. Reproductive changes
   A. Amenorrhea occurs; ovulation inhibited by increased progesterone and estrogen levels
   B. Goodell's sign (cervical softening) due to increased blood supply
   C. Hegar's sign (softening of lower segment of uterus)
   D. Chadwick's sign (purplish hue to vaginal mucosa)
   E. Uterus enlarges
   F. Leukorrhea; secretions of vaginal cells increase; act as body's first line of defense against infection
II. Endocrine changes
   A. Fatigue from increased hormonal levels leading to sodium and water retention
   B. HCG produced by 14th day; secreted by trophoblastic tissue of conceptus; critical to corpus luteum and tested for in pregnancy testing
   C. Melanocyte-stimulating hormone (MSH) leads to increased pigmentation in localized areas
   D. Estrogen produced by corpus luteum first 5 weeks; levels rise throughout pregnancy
      1. Increases growth of uterine muscles and ability of uterine muscles to contract
      2. Aids in development of breast ducts and secretory system to prepare for lactation
   E. Progesterone produced by corpus luteum for first 5 weeks, then by placenta
      1. Decreases contractility of the uterus, thus preventing spontaneous abortion
      2. Slightly increases basal metabolic rate
      3. Causes smooth muscles to relax
      4. Causes uterine muscle to relax
   F. Aldosterone increases

III. Oxygenation changes
 A. Cardiovascular system
  1. Delivers blood to uterine vessels at pressures adequate to fulfill requirements of placental circulation
  2. Effects physical, chemical, and cellular changes in blood to provide adequate oxygen exchange between mother and fetus
 B. Heart enlarges
 C. Cardiac output increases 30 to 50%
 D. Rate and stroke volume increase
 E. Blood volume increases 30 to 50%
 F. Potential for varicose veins increases
 G. Minute volume of air increases
 H. Increased alveolar ventilation and perfusion
 I. Exchange of CO_2 and O_2 at cellular level improved
IV. Renal changes
 A. Renal blood and plasma flow increase
 B. Glomerular filtration rate and efficiency of clearance increase
 V. Metabolic changes
 A. Appetite and thirst increase
 B. Nutritional requirements increase
 C. Gastric acids and pepsin levels decrease
 D. Heartburn caused by esophageal reflux
 E. Decreased bowel transit time leads to increased absorption of water and constipation
 F. Delayed gastric emptying time results in better absorption of nutrients, especially glucose and iron

Signs of Pregnancy

 I. Presumptive signs
 A. Subjective signs
  1. Amenorrhea
  2. Nausea and vomiting
  3. Breast sensitivity
  4. Urinary frequency
  5. Constipation
  6. Quickening
 B. Objective signs
  1. Breast changes
  2. Integument changes
  3. Abdominal enlargement
  4. Pelvic changes
 II. Probable signs
 A. Uterine enlargement
 B. Hegar's sign
 C. Goodell's sign
 D. Chadwick's sign
 E. Ballottement (rebounding of fetus against examiner's fingers on palpation)
 F. Braxton Hicks's uterine contractions
 G. Positive pregnancy test measuring HCG; reliable 90 to 98% of time

III. Positive signs
 A. Fetal heart tones
 B. Fetal movements palpable
 C. Ultrasound or x-ray of fetus (at 6 to 8 weeks)

EMBRYONIC AND FETAL DEVELOPMENT

Embryonic Stage (Conception to 12 Weeks)

 I. 4 weeks (Fig. 15-2)
 A. Length about 0.5 cm, weight less than 0.5 g
 B. Heart developed and beating
 C. Some gastrointestinal structures present
 D. Lung and ureteral buds present
 II. 8 weeks
 A. Length about 2.5 cm
 B. Body more formed
 C. Eyes, ears, nose, and mouth recognizable
 D. Fetus capable of some movement
 E. Enucleated RBCs in blood
 F. Gastrointestinal, renal, and respiratory systems continue to develop
III. 12 weeks
 A. Nails appearing
 B. Resembles human being
 C. Head erect but enlarged
 D. Length 6 to 9 cm, weight about 19 g
 E. Bones well outlined
 F. Blood forming in marrow
 G. Sucking present
 H. Bile secreted
 I. Kidneys able to secrete urine
 J. Genitalia apparent

Fetal Period (Third Month to Gestation)

 I. 16 weeks
 A. Face begins to look human
 B. Scalp hair appears
 C. Muscle movements detected
 D. Blood formed in spleen
 E. Meconium in bowel, anus open
 F. Bronchioles appear
 II. 20 weeks
 A. Brain grossly formed
 B. Vernix caseosa and lanugo appear
 C. Mother feels fetal movements
 D. Nostrils open
 E. Primitive respiratory movements begin
III. 24 weeks
 A. Body fairly well proportioned
 B. Skin red and wrinkled
 C. Hearing begins
 D. Length about 23 cm, weight about 600 g
 E. Blood formation increases in marrow

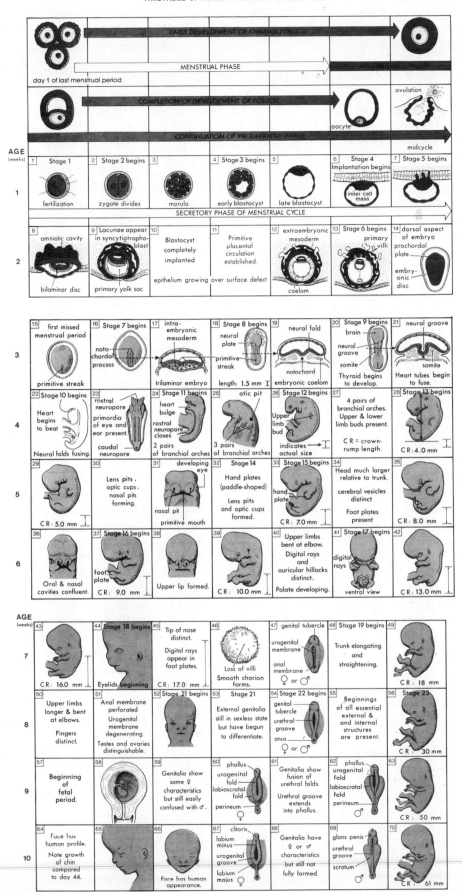

FIGURE 15–2. Timetable of prenatal development (weeks 1 through 10). (From Moore, K. L. (1987). *The developing human: Clinically oriented embryology*, 2nd ed. Philadelphia: W. B. Saunders.)

IV. 28 weeks
    A. Body lean, less wrinkled
    B. Weak sucking reflex
    C. Eyes open; pupils capable of reacting to light
    D. Length 27 cm, weight 1100 g
    E. Surfactant forming

V. 32 weeks
    A. Subcutaneous fat beginning
    B. More rounded appearance
    C. In position for delivery
    D. Turns head side to side
    E. Sense of taste present

VI. 36 weeks
    A. Body plump
    B. Turns and elevates head
    C. Nephron formation ceases

VII. 40 weeks
    A. Skin smooth and pink
    B. Vernix caseosa absent
    C. Lanugo scant
    D. Active, sustained movement
    E. Pulmonary branching two thirds complete
    F. Myelinization of brain begins

Development of Fetal Circulation

I. Placenta supplies oxygen and nutrients to fetus and removes wastes. Responsible for:
    A. Metabolism: fetal digestive tract
    B. Transfer: fetal lungs and kidneys
    C. Endocrine secretions: major endocrine gland

II. Umbilical cord contains two arteries and one vein

III. Major bypasses in fetal circulation
    A. Foramen ovale, opening between right and left atria of heart, bypassing lungs
    B. Ductus arteriosus, connecting pulmonary artery to aorta, bypassing lungs
    C. Ductus venosus, connecting umbilical vein and ascending vena cava, bypassing fetal liver

POST-TEST Psychological and Physiological Changes During Pregnancy and Embryonic and Fetal Development

1. Fetal embodiment occurs during the second trimester. A common sign of this process would be:
    ① Introversion
    ② An attempt to incorporate fetus into body image as a part of self
    ③ Daydreaming about self as mother and about the baby
    ④ Shock and denial

2. Endocrine changes associated with pregnancy include:
    ① Decreased estrogen
    ② Decreased MSH
    ③ Decreased HCG level
    ④ Increased aldosterone

3. Which of the following is a change in oxygenation associated with pregnancy?
    ① Decrease in heart rate
    ② Increase in cardiac output
    ③ Decrease in blood volume
    ④ Increase in blood pressure

4. Which of the following is NOT a metabolic change associated with pregnancy?
    ① Gastric acids and pepsin levels increase
    ② Nutritional requirement increases
    ③ Heartburn from esophageal reflux increases
    ④ Better absorption of nutrients with delayed gastric transit time

5. Which of the following is considered a presumptive sign of pregnancy?
    ① Ballottement
    ② Uterine enlargement
    ③ Positive pregnancy test
    ④ Amenorrhea

6. Which of the following is a probable sign of pregnancy?
    ① Braxton Hicks's contractions
    ② Breast sensitivity
    ③ Nausea and vomiting
    ④ Quickening

7. Which of the following is a positive sign of pregnancy?
    ① Positive pregnancy test
    ② Uterine enlargement
    ③ Palpable fetal movements
    ④ Quickening

8. At what stage of fetal development does the fetus begin to develop subcutaneous fat?
    ① 12 weeks
    ② 28 weeks
    ③ 32 weeks
    ④ 36 weeks

POST-TEST Answers and Rationales

1. ② One of the activities of fetal embodiment is the incorporation of the fetus into the mother's self. Choice 4 is part of the first trimester's psychosocial development, and choice 3 is part of the third. 1 & 2, IV. Psychosocial Changes During Pregnancy.

2. ④ The aldosterone level increases in pregnancy, causing the retention of water. The other options are not physiological changes that occur during pregnancy. 1 & 2, IV. Physiological Changes During Pregnancy.

3. ② Cardiac output increases during pregnancy because the workload on the heart is greater. The other options are not normal physiological changes associated with pregnancy. 1 & 2, IV. Physiological Changes During Pregnancy.

4. ① Gastric acid and pepsin levels decrease during pregnancy. The other options are metabolic changes that do occur during pregnancy. 1 & 2, IV. Physiological Changes During Pregnancy.

5. ④ Presumptive signs of pregnancy are not positive. Amenorrhea is a presumptive sign. The other signs listed are probable signs. 1 & 2, IV. Physiological Changes During Pregnancy.

6. ① Braxton Hicks's contractions are considered probably signs of pregnancy. The other options listed represent presumptive signs of pregnancy. 1 & 2, IV. Physiological Changes During Pregnancy.

7. ③ Palpable fetal movements are one of the positive signs of pregnancy. The other options are either presumptive or probable signs. 1 & 2, IV. Physiological Changes During Pregnancy.

8. ③ Subcutaneous fat—one of the last things to develop in the fetus—starts to increase at about 32 weeks. 1 & 2, IV. Fetal Development.

PRE-TEST Prenatal Period

Sandy Peters, aged 20, first visits a clinic in the 28th week of her pregnancy. Assessments reveal that she is overweight for her height and stature and there is slight edema of her feet and ankles.

1. In addition to emphasizing regular visits for the remainder of the pregnancy, which goal is a priority for Sandy?
   ① Reporting cramping
   ② Including roughage in her diet
   ③ Notifying the clinic of headaches
   ④ Sleeping in left lateral position

2. At Sandy's next visit 2 weeks later, her urine is negative for protein, her blood pressure has increased from 110/70 to 115/75 mm Hg, and she has gained 5 lb. She has some shortness of breath when sleeping on her back and reports that the fetus is very active at night. Which assessment is most indicative of potential problems?
   ① Blood pressure changes
   ② Weight gain
   ③ Respiratory problems
   ④ Fetal activity

3. When discussing health habits with Sandy, you review diet, exercise, and use of over-the-counter medications. Which of the following should be avoided considering her present condition?
   ① Use of bicarbonate of soda for heartburn
   ② Apple slices as snacks
   ③ Brisk walking as exercise
   ④ Skim milk with meals

4. Sandy's symptoms become more severe as pregnancy advances. At a routine visit in the 36th week, it is noted that her urine is 3+ for protein, her blood pressure is 140/110 mm Hg, and there is facial edema. She is hospitalized on strict bedrest. Magnesium sulfate is ordered. Which of the following assessments are critical while administering this medication intravenously?
   ① Respirations and deep tendon reflexes
   ② Blood pressure and temperature
   ③ State of consciousness and blood sugar
   ④ Fetal heart rate (FHR) and apical pulse

5. In addition to monitoring Sandy's condition closely, which of the following nursing measures is most important?
   ① Maintaining a quiet environment
   ② Providing sufficient oral fluids
   ③ Encouraging ambulation
   ④ Promoting diversional activities

6. Which of the following is a priority goal for the client with severe pregnancy-induced hypertension?
   ① Complying with diet modifications
   ② Reporting visual changes
   ③ Remaining on bedrest
   ④ Communicating her feelings

7. Several hours after treatment with magnesium sulfate is begun, each of the following observations is noted. Which one indicates that the treatment is effective?
   ① Hourly output is 50 mL
   ② Blood pressure is 150/110 mm Hg
   ③ Reflexes are hypotonic
   ④ No seizures have occurred

8. Sandy awakens from sleep complaining of sudden sharp abdominal pain. Assessments reveal that the uterus is hard and tender to touch. FHR is 90. Maternal pulse is 130, blood pressure is 100/60 mm Hg, skin is cold and moist to the touch, and moderate vaginal bleeding is noted. The physician determines that abruptio placentae has occurred and prepares for an emergency cesarean delivery. This problem is directly related to:
   ① Infarcts caused by vasoconstriction
   ② High magnesium blood levels
   ③ Abnormal placental position
   ④ Pregnancy-induced hypertension

Tina Dobson, aged 30, visits the antepartal clinic with her husband after missing two menstrual periods. Physical assessment, date of last menstrual period (LMP), and urine analysis for HCG indicate that she is probably 7 weeks pregnant. History includes the information that this is her first pregnancy, her health has been excellent, she is employed as a secretary, and she is a nonsmoker.

---

9. Which of the following is an appropriate long-term goal for Tina?
   ① She will work reduced hours throughout her pregnancy
   ② She will comply with a regular prenatal visit schedule
   ③ She will omit sodium and fat from her daily diet
   ④ She will begin an aerobic exercise program

10. At the second prenatal visit 1 month later, Tina reports that she is experiencing occasional nausea that is relieved with dry foods. She also is feeling very tired, and she has urinary frequency and periods of weeping. In reviewing the assessment data, the nurse identifies which of the following as a potential problem?
    ① Laboratory data show a hematocrit of 36 with a hemoglobin of 12
    ② Urinalysis reveals a trace of glucose with negative bacteria
    ③ Interview reveals mixed feelings about the pregnancy
    ④ Twenty-four–hour diet recall: high-carbohydrate, high-fiber, vegetarian diet

11. Tina feels much better at the 22nd week. She expresses surprise that the physician has ordered a glucose tolerance test. Which explanation is appropriate for this order?
    ① "Because you are vegetarian, it is necessary to check carbohydrate metabolism."
    ② "Since there was sugar in your urine at your second visit, the blood test is a precaution."
    ③ "Because you have little regular exercise, your metabolism may be very slow."
    ④ "This test of blood sugar levels is now routine to identify gestational diabetes."

12. The results of the test show an elevated blood sugar. The problem is diagnosed as gestational diabetes. Health teaching would NOT include which of the following?
    ① Review her understanding of basic four food sources
    ② Emphasize adequate protein and vitamin intake
    ③ Caution her to eliminate all carbohydrates
    ④ Suggest that she eat four small meals each day

13. Tina follows all dietary suggestions and increases regular mild exercise. She feels well, but the blood sugar levels remain elevated. The physician orders regular insulin on a sliding scale appropriate to daily glucose levels. Which statement made by the client shows that she understands the problem?
    ① "I resent that I now face a lifetime on insulin."
    ② "My vegetarian diet must have caused this diabetes."
    ③ "This temporary condition is frustrating to control."
    ④ "My grandmother has diabetes, so I guess it is inevitable."

14. In the 36th week, a nonstress test is ordered. The result is reactive. Select an appropriate explanation of this result that could be given to a nursing student who observed the diagnostic procedure.
    ① "The result shows fetal response to contractions."
    ② "The fetal heart rate increased with activity."
    ③ "The absence of decelerations shows good oxygenation."

④ "The heart rate variability is more than 15 beats."

Martha is admitted with preeclampsia in the 32nd week of pregnancy. Her blood pressure is 160/110 mm Hg, she has 3+ albumin in her urine, and she is complaining of severe headaches.

---

15. Which of the following has the greatest priority in your care of Martha?
    ① Having a support person at the bedside
    ② Monitoring the fetal heart tones every 4 hours
    ③ Checking her blood pressure every 30 minutes
    ④ Measuring I & O accurately

16. The physician orders that IV magnesium sulfate be given. Nursing interventions required while Martha is receiving this medication must include:
    ① Monitoring respirations and patellar reflexes
    ② Administering calcium gluconate concurrently
    ③ Encouraging her to ambulate
    ④ Avoiding blood pressure measurements until after medication has infused

17. Martha begins to experience convulsions. Your priority nursing intervention will be to:
    ① Leave and get help immediately
    ② Put on the call light and ask for help
    ③ Yell for help
    ④ Ask her roommate to get help

18. Which of the following nursing interventions would be INAPPROPRIATE for the nurse to implement with a pregnant client during a convulsion?
    ① Place a tongue blade between her unclenched jaws
    ② Put a blanket over the side rails to protect her
    ③ Monitor the FHR
    ④ Raise the side rails to prevent falling

19. Which of the following expectant mothers would be at the greatest risk for developing toxemia?
    ① A 22-year-old Rh-negative multigravida
    ② A 17-year-old primigravida with a low-protein diet
    ③ A 25-year-old anemic primigravida
    ④ A 28-year-old slightly obese primigravida

Gail Warren is a 26-year-old white woman who has registered at the clinic for prenatal care for her pregnancy.

---

20. In eliciting her health history, the nurse discovers that Gail's last normal menstrual period was July 10, 1987. Which of the following dates would be the appropriate estimated date of confinement (EDC)?
    ① April 3, 1988
    ② April 10, 1988
    ③ April 17, 1988
    ④ April 20, 1988

21. Gail provides a maternal history, including the following data: one healthy female delivered at term; one miscarriage at 8 weeks, one stillborn male delivered at term; one therapeutic abortion at 6 weeks, one premature male delivered at 32 weeks. During this pregnancy, Gail would be considered as:
    ① Gravida vi, para iii
    ② Gravida v, para ii
    ③ Gravida v, para iii
    ④ Gravida vi, para ii

22. Which of the following assessment findings reflects Gail's normal physiological response to the pregnancy?
    ① Augmented peristalsis
    ② Decreased glomerular filtration rate
    ③ Increased cardiac output
    ④ Increased respirations

23. A complete blood count is done in the clinic laboratory. The results indicate that Gail's hematocrit level is 33%. Which of the following possibilities most likely explains this finding?
    ① Pregnancy-induced decreased vitamin B_{12} levels
    ② The presence of iron deficiency anemia
    ③ Depressed bone marrow function
    ④ Hemodilution of pregnancy

24. What other essential screening tests should be conducted during the course of Gail's pregnancy?
    ① Blood typing
    ② Sickle cell screen
    ③ Chest x-ray
    ④ Serological test for gonorrhea

PRE-TEST Answers and Rationales

1. ③ A priority goal is early detection of worsening pregnancy-induced hypertension. Headache is often an early warning of seizure. All other responses are correct but not the *priority*. 3, IV. Prenatal, Preeclampsia.

2. ② Weight changes and edema in a 2-week period indicate risk factors for this woman. Choice 3 is expected at this stage of pregnancy. Choice 1 is a borderline change. An active fetus indicates good placental oxygenation. 1 & 2, IV. Prenatal, Preeclampsia.

3. ① *No pregnant woman should use this home remedy for heartburn!* This additional sodium is even more dangerous considering Sandy's problems. All other responses are good health practices. 4, IV. Prenatal, Preeclampsia.

4. ① Priority assessments while giving magnesium sulfate include respirations, urine output, blood pressure, and level of consciousness. Other choices include one important observation, but only choice 1 consists of two priority assessments. 1, II & IV. Eclampsia.

5. ① Reduced stimuli may reduce the risk of eclampsia. None of the other options are appropriate. 4, I & IV. Eclampsia.

6. ② While all of the goals are appropriate, it is essential that the woman report visual changes, headache, and epigastric pain that often precede seizures. 3, IV. Eclampsia.

7. ④ The central nervous system depressant is administered to prevent eclampsia. Choice 1 is adequate output; the blood pressure is relatively unchanged; and hypotonic reflexes may indicate that the drug dose is excessive (magnesium blood levels should be drawn). 5, II & IV. Eclampsia.

8. ① The hypertensive woman is especially susceptible to this third trimester bleeding disorder because of vascular changes. Choice 3 refers to placenta previa, a painless bleeding condition. Choices 2 and 4 are incorrect. 2, IV. Vascular Disorders of Pregnancy.

9. ② A goal of health maintenance throughout pregnancy is essential for *physiological and psychological integrity*. Choice 1 is not appropriate because many women

safely continue employment during pregnancy. Choice 3 is not based on current knowledge. Active aerobic exercise during pregnancy is controversial. 3, IV. Prenatal Care.

10. ④ The client's recall indicates a diet lacking in essential nutrients and protein for fetal growth. All other responses are normal for early pregnancy. 2, IV. Prenatal Care.

11. ④ Recent research has led physicians to recommend this test for all pregnant clients to identify a possible risk factor of gestational diabetes. Choice 2 is a normal finding in urine of a pregnant woman. Choices 1 and 3 are incorrect. 2 & 4, II & IV. Prenatal Care.

12. ③ All responses *except* elimination of carbohydrates are a part of health promotion for this client. Carbohydrates are needed for energy so that protein is available for growth. 4, II. Prenatal, Diabetes.

13. ③ Understanding the client's need for *psychosocial* adaptation, the nurse recognizes the frustration experienced by the pregnant diabetic. Gestational diabetes is usually confined to the period of gestation and is not caused by diet habits or heredity. However, the client may develop diabetes later in adult life. 5, II. Prenatal. Nutrition.

14. ② A reactive nonstress test and an active fetus are good signs of placental oxygenation. Because there are usually no contractions or labor stimulation, choices 1 and 3 are incorrect. A variability of 5 to 15 beats per minute is optimal. 2, II & IV. Prenatal Care.

15. ③ Blood pressure must be monitored closely as it relates directly to the maternal condition and uterine blood flow to the fetus. The other options are standard nursing interventions for this client and are not of greatest priority. 4, IV. Preeclampsia.

16. ① Magnesium sulfate is a central nervous system depressant, and the nurse must monitor the reflexes continually along with respiratory function. The blood pressure must be closely monitored and the client must be on bedrest during the infusion. 4, II & IV. Preeclampsia.

17. ② The nurse must remain with the client experiencing convulsions, protecting her

from injury. Yelling may needlessly upset other clients and family. The call light should be answered immediately. 4, IV. Preeclampsia.

18. ③ During the convulsion, the mother's protection must be the priority. The fetal heart tone can be monitored as soon as the convulsion is over. The other options are nursing care measures that are done. 4, IV. Preeclampsia.

19. ② Younger clients are always at higher risk, and the rollover test is usually accurate in detecting women at risk for toxemia. 2, IV. Preeclampsia.

20. ③ The formula for determining EDC using Nagele's rule is as follows: add 7 days to the first day of the last menstrual period; then subtract 3 months and add 1 year. 2, IV. Prenatal Care.

21. ① Gravida is defined as total number of pregnancies, and para is defined as the number of pregnancies delivered after the period of viability whether they are alive or stillborn. Abortions and miscarriages are not counted in para. Because the client is currently pregnant, she is gravida vi, para iii. 2, IV. Prenatal Care.

22. ③ Normal physiological findings during pregnancy include decreased peristalsis, increased glomerular filtration rate, increased cardiac output, and no change in respiratory rate. 1, II & IV. Prenatal Care.

23. ④ Decreased hematocrit levels during pregnancy are related to the increased amount of fluid present in the vascular tree (hemodilution). Pregnancy does not induce a decrease in vitamin B_{12} level; iron deficiency anemia would be reflected in a lower hemoglobin level; and there is no evidence that there is any depression of bone marrow function related to pregnancy. 2, I & IV. Prenatal Care.

24. ① Screening tests that would be appropriate for this individual client would be blood type only. A sickle cell screen is not appropriate for a white woman; a chest x-ray is contraindicated during pregnancy; and serological tests are for syphilis, not gonorrhea. 1, I & IV. Prenatal Care.

NURSING PROCESS APPLIED TO NORMAL PREGNANCY

I. Assessment
  A. Definite diagnosis of pregnancy
  B. Complete history and physical examination
  C. Ability to tolerate pregnancy
    1. Obstetrical history
    2. Family situation
      a. Meaning of baby
      b. Relationships among the family
      c. Supports available to mother
      d. Cultural differences during pregnancy (Table 15-1)
  D. Presence of health problems
  E. Estimated date of confinement (EDC)— Nagele's rule: add 7 days to the first day of last menstrual period (LMP), subtract 3 months and add 1 year, or EDC = [(LMP + 7 days) − 3 months] + 1 year; assumes 28-day cycle
  F. Pelvic measurements
  G. Vital signs

TABLE 15–1 Cultural Differences During Pregnancy

Culture	Activity	Significance
Mexican-American	Use of spearmint, Benedictine, or sassafras tea	Self-treatment for morning sickness
	Use of cathartics during the last trimester	Thought to ensure a healthy birth
	Avoids looking at the full moon	Looking thought to cripple or deform the unborn
African American	Use of castor oil, vinegar, baking soda, and Epsom salts	Self-treatment for constipation, heartburn, and edema
	Avoids reaching hands above head	Thought to wrap the umbilical cord above the infant's head
	Emotional fright	Will give the baby a birthmark

1. Blood pressure: upper limits of increase, 10/15 mm Hg systolic/diastolic above normal baseline
2. Pulse: 60 to 90
3. Respirations: 16 to 24
4. Temperature: 97° to 100°F (36.2° to 37.6°C)

H. Weight
1. 20 to 30 lb approximately (varies with client, prenatal weight, and health care provider's advice)
2. 2 to 4 lb first trimester
3. 11 to 14 lb second trimester
4. 8 to 11 lb third trimester

I. Fetal development—McDonald's rule
1. Height of fundus in cm × 2/7 = duration of pregnancy in lunar months
2. Height of fundus in cm × 8/7 = duration of pregnancy in weeks

J. Nutritional status

K. Diagnostic examinations
1. Ultrasound: identifies fetal and maternal structures
   a. Nursing interventions
      (1) Explain test to client
      (2) Tell client to drink six to eight glasses of water before test and not to void; test is done with full bladder
      (3) Tell client that there are no known risks to test
2. Alpha-fetoprotein screening (AFP): assesses the quantity of fetal serum proteins that if elevated is associated with open neural tube defects
   a. Nursing interventions: explain that this parameter is assessed by single maternal blood sample drawn at 15 to 18 weeks' gestation
   b. Results
      (1) If elevated and the gestation is less than 18 weeks, a second sample is drawn
      (2) Level II ultrasound performed for elevated levels to rule out fetal abnormalities, multiple gestation, or fetal demise
3. Chorionic villus sampling (CVS): aspiration of a small sample of chorionic villus tissue at 8 to 12 weeks' gestation for the purpose of detecting genetic abnormalities
   a. Nursing interventions
      (1) Explain test to client
      (2) Tell client to fill bladder before procedure to aid in position of the uterus for catheter insertion
      (3) Instruct client to report bleeding,

infection, or leakage of fluid after procedure
      (4) Inform client results are generally available in 2 to 14 days
      (5) Rh-negative women are given Rho-Gam to cover the risks of immunization from the procedure
4. Daily fetal monitor count (DFMC): assesses active and passive states of fetus
   a. Nursing interventions
      (1) Explain that this is noninvasive test that may be done by client
      (2) Tell client that fetal cycle varies normally
      (3) Three or more movements per hour when client lying down is usual
      (4) Teach client to report marked decrease in fetal activity
5. Nonstress test (NST): evaluates fetal heart rate (FHR) in response to fetal movement to determine fetal well-being; done to assess placental function and oxygenation
   a. Nursing interventions
      (1) Requires indirect external monitoring to measure FHR and to trace fetal activity
      (2) Record baseline blood pressure
      (3) Client in semi-Fowler's turned slightly to left side
      (4) May take up to 50 minutes
   b. Results
      (1) Reactive (normal): two FHR accelerations (more than 15 beats per minute) above baseline for 15 seconds or more with fetal movement in a 10- to 20-minute period
      (2) Nonreactive (abnormal): zero to one FHR acceleration above baseline for 15 seconds or more with fetal movement in a 10-minute period or accelerations less than 15 beats per minute or lasting less than 15 seconds
      (3) Uninterpretable results, repeat test or do oxytocin challenge test (OCT)
6. OCT or stress test: determines fetal well-being and fetal ability to withstand stress of labor; done for abnormal NST or at-risk fetus; assesses placental oxygenation and function
   a. Nursing interventions
      (1) Tell client monitoring and positioning are same as for NST, but IV oxytocin may be used

(2) Baseline and frequent maternal blood pressure readings taken

(3) Test takes 1 to 3 hours

(4) Monitor closely while increasing doses of oxytocin are given until contractions occur

b. Results

(1) Negative (normal): absence of late decelerations of FHR with each of three contractions; negative window

(2) Positive (abnormal): presence of late deceleration of FHR with three contractions during 10-minute period; positive window

(3) Equivocal or suspicious: absence of positive or negative window

(4) Unsatisfactory: inadequate contractions or tracings

(5) High-risk pregnancies continue with weekly negative tests

7. Amniocentesis: determines genetic disorders, sex, and fetal maturity by aspiration of amniotic fluid for analysis; done from 14th week on

a. Nursing interventions

(1) Explain risks to client: maternal hemorrhage, infection, Rh isoimmunization, abruptio placentae, labor; fetal death, infection, hemorrhage, injury from needle (less than 1% overall)

(2) Have client empty bladder before procedure

(3) Ultrasound performed to locate placenta

(4) Baseline vital signs and FHR, then checked every 15 minutes

(5) Positioned supine with abdominal scrub

(6) Support client while needle passed into amniotic sac

(7) Instruct client to report any side effects: chills, fever, leakage of fluid, decreased fetal movement, uterine contractions

L. Risk factors (Fig. 15-3)

1. German measles: can cause congenital defects in fetus if contracted during first trimester

2. Sexually transmitted diseases

a. Syphilis

(1) May cross the placenta; usually leads to spontaneous abortions

(2) Increased incidence of mental subnormality and physical deformities

(3) Effects prevented if treated early in pregnancy

b. Genital herpes

(1) May cross placenta

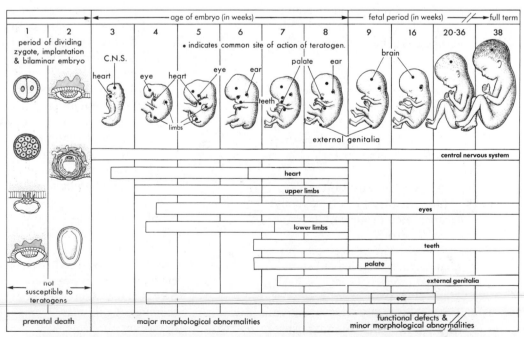

FIGURE 15–3. Sensitivity to teratogens. (From Moore, K. L. (1987). *The developing human: Clinically oriented embryology,* 2nd ed. Philadelphia: W. B. Saunders.)

(2) Fetus contaminated after membranes rupture or with vaginal delivery

(3) Generalized herpes results in 100% neonatal mortality

c. Gonorrhea

(1) Fetus contaminated at the time of delivery

(2) May result in postpartum infection

(3) Risks to the neonate: ophthalmia neonatorum, pneumonia, sepsis

(4) Effects prevented if treatment instituted before delivery

(5) Sexual partner also requires treatment and follow-up

d. Human papilloma virus (HPV)

(1) Virus transmitted through sexual contact

(2) May be transmitted to the fetus at delivery

(3) Virus responsible for the growth of genital warts (vagina, vulva, anus, cervix)

(4) May result in abnormal Pap smear screening results

e. Chlamydia

(1) Intercellular bacterium transmitted through sexual contact

(2) Identification through cervical culture

(3) May be transmitted to the fetus at delivery

(4) May cause conjunctivitis and pneumonia in the newborn

f. Human immunodeficiency virus (HIV)

(1) Virus transmitted through blood, blood products, and other bodily fluids such as urine, semen, vaginal fluid

(2) Affects T cells, thereby decreasing the body's immune response and increasing susceptibility to opportunistic organisms

(3) Centers for Disease Control recommends screening for HIV (1989) women who:

(a) Engage in prostitution

(b) Have a history of sexually transmitted diseases

(c) Use IV drugs

(d) Have current or previous sexual partners who have been bisexual, abused IV drugs, have hemophilia

(4) Individuals usually test positive within 2 to 12 weeks after exposure and usually remain asymptomatic for 5 to 7 years

(5) AIDS is diagnosed when severe infection develops; usually pneumocystis pneumonia or Kaposi's sarcoma

(6) Risk of transmission of HIV to the neonate is estimated to be approximately 30 to 75%

(7) Infants are usually asymptomatic at birth; median age for onset of symptoms is 9 months

(8) Azidothymidine (AZT) may be given to the HIV-positive pregnant client, although safety during pregnancy has not been established

(9) Prenatally HIV-positive clients need to be monitored for normal fetal growth patterns, weight gain, signs of fatigue, weakness, recurrent diarrhea, pallor, and night sweats

3. Drugs/alcohol/tobacco

a. Because many drugs cross placenta, no drugs, including over-the-counter medications, should be taken unless prescribed by physician

b. Substance abuse

(1) Drugs commonly abused include alcohol, cocaine, crack, marijuana, amphetamines, barbiturates, and heroin

(2) Abuse of drugs threatens normal fetal growth and successful term completion of the pregnancy

(3) Physical signs of drug abuse may include dilated or contracted pupils, fatigue, track marks, skin abscesses, inflamed nasal mucosa, and inappropriate behavior

(4) Substance abuse places the pregnancy at risk for fetal growth retardation, abruptio placentae, and fetal bradycardia

c. Alcohol during pregnancy may lead to fetal alcohol syndrome

(1) Physical abnormalities

(2) Congenital anomalies

(3) Growth deficits

(4) Jitteriness

d. Smoking leads to low birth weights, higher incidence of birth defects, and stillbirths

4. Radiation exposure increases risk of miscarriage and physical deformities

5. Stress causes increased activity in fetus in response to increased epinephrine levels in mother

6. Women over 35 have greater risk of chromosomal abnormalities

7. Adolescents under 15 have greater risk of stillbirths, miscarriages, and premature births
8. Parity over vi higher risk for mother
9. Past obstetrical problems
   a. Abortions
   b. Premature births
   c. Lack of antepartal care
   d. Previous fetal death
   e. Pregnancy-induced hypertension
   f. Vaginal bleeding
10. Low socioeconomic status
    a. Asian and African-American women at higher risk for small-for-gestational-age newborns
    b. Inadequate prenatal care
11. Malnutrition

M. Discomforts of pregnancy
   1. First trimester
      a. Nausea and vomiting due to elevated HCG levels and changes in carbohydrate metabolism
      b. Urinary urgency and frequency due to pressure of fundus on bladder
      c. Breast tenderness from increased levels of estrogen and progesterone
      d. Increased vaginal discharge from hyperplasia of mucosa and increased mucus production
      e. Nasal stuffiness and epistaxis from elevated estrogen levels
      f. Fatigue from hormonal changes
   2. Second and third trimesters
      a. Heartburn from esophageal reflux
      b. Ankle edema from venous stasis
      c. Headaches from changes in blood volume and vascular tone
      d. Varicose veins from weakening walls of veins or faulty valves
      e. Hemorrhoids from increased venous pressure and/or constipation
      f. Constipation from displaced intestines and iron supplements
      g. Skin changes due to increased hormone levels
      h. Backache from exaggerated lumbosacral curve due to enlarged uterus
      i. Leg cramps from low calcium, pressure of uterus on nerves, or fatigue
      j. Orthostatic changes
      k. Shortness of breath from pressure on diaphragm

II. Analysis
   A. Knowledge deficit related to prenatal care, normal discomforts of pregnancy, nutritional needs, and childbirth

   B. High risk for ineffective individual coping related to lack of preparation for childbirth

III. Planning/goals, expected outcomes
   A. Client will progress through pregnancy without complications
   B. Client will understand and comply with prenatal care
   C. Client will be aware of usual discomforts of pregnancy and know how to safely cope with them
   D. Client will understand and comply with nutritional needs throughout prenatal period
   E. Client and family will be prepared educationally for childbirth

IV. Implementation
   A. Encourage regular prenatal visits
      1. Every 4 weeks first 32 weeks
      2. Every 2 weeks from 32 to 36 weeks
      3. Every week from 36 to 40 weeks
   B. Intervene as necessary based on assessments
   C. Help client find appropriate treatments for discomforts of pregnancy
      1. Nausea and vomiting
         a. Dry crackers before arising
         b. Small, frequent, low-fat meals during day
         c. Drink liquids between meals
         d. Avoid all antiemetics throughout pregnancy
      2. Urinary frequency
         a. Sleep on side at night
         b. Limit fluid intake in evening
         c. Void at regular intervals
      3. Vaginal discharge
         a. Consult physician if infection suspected
         b. Wash carefully and keep dry
         c. Use yogurt for vulvular itch
         d. Avoid use of Flagyl throughout pregnancy
         e. Use nystatin vaginal tablets or Monistat as ordered
      4. Fatigue
         a. Get regular exercise
         b. Sleep as much as needed; nap during day
         c. Avoid stimulants (e.g., too much caffeine) throughout pregnancy
      5. Heartburn
         a. Drink milk between meals
         b. Small, frequent meals
         c. Avoid antacids such as calcium carbonate, Gaviscon, baking soda, and histamine receptor antagonists such as Tagamet throughout pregnancy
         d. Can use Maalox or Mylanta occasionally

6. Ankle edema
   a. Elevate legs at least twice a day
   b. Sleep on left side
   c. Avoid use of diuretics
7. Headaches
   a. Change position slowly
   b. Apply cool cloth to forehead
   c. Drinking milk or eating a small snack helps some women
   d. Avoid use of aspirin, nonsteroidal anti-inflammatories, or tranquilizers during pregnancy
   e. Use Tylenol sparingly
8. Varicose veins
   a. Elevate feet when sitting
   b. Use support hose
   c. Avoid pressure on lower thighs
9. Hemorrhoids
   a. Soak in warm sitz bath
   b. Sit on soft pillows
   c. Eat high-fiber diet, and drink sufficient fluid
   d. Use local hemorrhoidal ointment such as Anusol
10. Constipation
    a. Eat high-roughage foods, such as fresh fruits, vegetables, and bran
    b. Drink plenty of fluids
    c. Exercise regularly
    d. Avoid mineral oil or castor oil during pregnancy
    e. Use Metamucil, Senokot, or 1 teaspoon milk of magnesia at bedtime sparingly
11. Backache
    a. Perform back exercises, such as pelvic tilt
    b. Wear low-heeled shoes or flats
    c. Avoid heavy lifting
    d. Avoid aspirin, nonsteroidal anti-inflammatories, or codeine during pregnancy
    e. Use Tylenol sparingly
12. Leg cramps
    a. Get regular exercise, especially walking
    b. Elevate feet and dorsiflex feet when resting
    c. Increase milk intake
13. Orthostatic changes
    a. Sit with feet up
    b. Change position slowly
    c. Avoid use of alcohol
14. Shortness of breath
    a. Sleep with head elevated or on side
    b. Do not overexert
    c. Allow frequent rest periods
D. Teach client proper nutrition, and encourage approriate intake

1. A gain of 24 to 30 lb average (will vary with prepregnancy weight and other factors)
2. Assess current dietary intake
3. Increase calories, protein, vitamins, calcium, and other minerals as needed
4. Drink at least eight glasses of water a day
5. Sodium not restricted unless specifically ordered
6. Choose from four basic food groups
7. Refer to dietician if needed
8. Influences on nutrition (Table 15-2)
E. Explain need for childbirth education to client
   1. Refer to Lamaze or other appropriate resource
   2. Encourage involvement of family or significant other
V. Evaluation
   A. Client delivers healthy baby without complications
   B. Client understands and complies with prenatal care
   C. Client aware of usual discomforts of pregnancy and safely copes with them
   D. Client maintains adequate nutrition throughout pregnancy
   E. Client and family adequately educated and prepared for childbirth

NURSING PROCESS APPLIED TO COMPLICATIONS OF PREGNANCY

Pregnancy-Induced Hypertension

I. Assessment
   A. Definition: group of disorders characterized by presence of hypertension; onset early in pregnancy; symptoms during last trimester of pregnancy

TABLE 15–2 Cultural, Religious, and Ethnic Influences on Nutritional Practices During Pregnancy

Group	Nutritional Practices
Asian	Seafood, rice, vegetables, and fresh fruits are staple diet items. Milk and cheese are used infrequently.
Jewish (Orthodox)	Poultry and some meat of cattle, sheep, goats, and deer are permissible; pork and pork products are not. Milk and cheese may not be eaten with or within 6 hours of a meat meal.
Mexican	Staple food items include corn, chili peppers, and beans. Milk is used infrequently.

B. Incidence/etiology
   1. One of three leading causes of maternal mortality, and high cause of fetal death
   2. 6 to 7% of all pregnancies
   3. Cause unknown
      a. Underlying mechanism believed to be vasospasm and ischemia
      b. Placental function impaired by vasospasm
      c. Leads to hypoxia and malnutrition to fetus
      d. Maternal degenerative changes may occur in kidneys or brain
C. Predisposing/precipitating factors
   1. Age: less than 17 or more than 35 years
   2. Primiparity
   3. Low socioeconomic status
   4. Little or no prenatal care
   5. Protein malnourishment
   6. Diabetes
   7. Previous history of hypertension
D. Types
   1. Toxemia
      a. Preeclampsia
      b. Eclampsia
   2. Chronic essential hypertension
      a. Present before pregnancy
      b. Combines with preeclampsia
E. Clinical manifestations
   1. Mild preeclampsia
      a. Hypertension of 15 to 30 mm Hg above baseline
      b. Weight gain of 1 lb or more per week in last trimester
      c. Mild generalized edema
      d. Proteinuria, 1+ (about 1 g per 24 hours)
   2. Severe preeclampsia
      a. Severe hypertension, 30 to 40 mm Hg while on bedrest
      b. Massive, generalized edema and weight gain
      c. Proteinuria, 4+ (5 g per 24 hours or more)
      d. Less than 400 mL output in 24 hours
      e. Severe headache
      f. Dizziness
      g. Blurred vision and spots before eyes
      h. Nausea and vomiting
      i. Epigastric pain
      j. Irritability
   3. Eclampsia
      a. All changes of preeclampsia
      b. Tonic and clonic convulsions or coma
      c. Hypertensive crisis
   4. HELLP syndrome: characterized by hemolysis of RBCs, elevated liver enzymes, and low platelet count related to severe vasospasm and developing disseminated intravascular coagulation (DIC)
      a. Mortality rate 0 to 24%
      b. Perinatal mortality 8 to 60%
      c. Platelet and RBC transfusions often are given; coagulation factors are closely monitored
      d. Labor may be induced if more than 32 weeks; cesarean section if less than 32 weeks
   5. DIC: abnormal overstimulation of the coagulation process. Occurs secondary to an underlying disease (abruptio placentae, fetal demise, severe pregnancy-induced hypertension, retained products of conception)
      a. Clinical manifestations of DIC include varying degrees of bleeding from oozing to generalized hemorrhage, purpura, and petechiae
      b. Coagulation factors: platelet, fibrinogen levels, and fibrin split products are monitored closely and replaced as necessary
      c. Treatment of the underlying cause frequently resolves DIC
F. Medical management
   1. Only real cure is end of pregnancy
   2. Bedrest
   3. High-protein, low-salt diet
II. Analysis
   A. Fluid volume deficit related to fluid shift from intravascular to extravascular space secondary to vasospasm
   B. Knowledge deficit related to pregnancy-induced hypertension, its treatment, and the implications for the fetus
   C. High risk for injury: convulsions secondary to cerebral edema
III. Planning/goals, expected outcomes
   A. Client will have symptoms of preeclampsia noted early
   B. Client's blood pressure will be controlled
   C. Client will continue pregnancy as long as possible
   D. Client will not suffer injury
   E. Client will deliver healthy baby
IV. Implementation
   A. Monitor blood pressure and weight closely
   B. Encourage regular prenatal visits
   C. Teach client signs of preeclampsia and to call if they occur
   D. Teach dietary regimen, including sodium restrictions if needed
   E. Maintain bedrest if symptoms occur
   F. Administer magnesium sulfate as ordered (Table 15-3)
   G. Administer antihypertensives as ordered to

TABLE 15–3 Anticonvulsants

Example	Action	Use	Common Side Effects	Nursing Implications
Magnesium sulfate	Decreases amount of acetylcholine liberated with nerve impulses; relaxes smooth muscle; decreases cerebral edema; central nervous system depressant; lowers blood pressure	To prevent seizures in women with severe preeclampsia or eclampsia	Maternal: severe central nervous system depression, hyporeflexia, confusion, flushing; fetal: increased FHR, hypoglycemia, hypocalcemia, hypermagnesemia	Contraindicated with renal disease; monitor for seizure activity; watch for signs of central nervous system depression; stop IV if respirations less than 12, reflexes hypotonic, urine output less than 20 to 30 mL/hr, client becomes lethargic; monitor FHR; keep antagonist, calcium gluconate, available

prevent cerebrovascular accident (see Table 4–1)
H. Monitor for seizure activity
I. Protect mother from injury
J. Administer O$_2$ as needed
K. Monitor FHR
L. Prepare mother and family for early induction of labor
V. Evaluation
A. Client's preeclampsia caught early
B. Client's blood pressure controlled
C. Pregnancy continues until fetus viable
D. Client suffers no injury before or 48 hours after delivery
E. Client delivers healthy baby

Hyperemesis Gravidarum

I. Assessment
A. Definition: persistent, excessive vomiting that causes dehydration and starvation
B. Incidence/etiology: cause unclear but may be related to psychological factors, hormonal factors, multiple pregnancy, or hydatidiform mole
C. Clinical manifestations
1. Uncontrolled vomiting
2. Metabolic alkalosis from loss of deep gastrointestinal contents
3. Starvation with hypoproteinemia and hypovitaminosis
4. Fetus, and even mother, may die
D. Medical management
1. Hospitalization with fluid, electrolyte, vitamin, and mineral replacement
2. Rest and quiet environment
3. Treat for dehydration and malnutrition
4. Recommend referral to counselor if severe
E. Surgical management: if uncontrollable, may have to terminate pregnancy

II. Analysis
A. Altered nutrition: less than body requirements, related to persistent vomiting
B. Fear related to effects of persistent vomiting on fetal growth
III. Planning/goals, expected outcomes
A. Client's emesis will be controlled
B. Client will not develop dehydration or starvation
C. Client will deliver healthy baby
IV. Implementation
A. Monitor amount of vomitus
B. Maintain absolutely accurate intake and output records
C. Check weight daily
D. Assess client's affect and emotional state
E. Maintain patent IV line with sufficient replacements
F. Encourage client to express concerns and fears
G. Provide meticulous hygiene
H. Provide clean, odor-free environment
I. Monitor fetus and report signs of distress
V. Evaluation
A. Client's emesis is controlled
B. Client does not develop dehydration or starvation
C. Client delivers healthy baby

Abortion

I. Assessment
A. Definition: termination of pregnancy before fetus viable, 20 weeks or weight of 500 g; may be elective procedure or reproductive problem (most occur in second or third month)
B. Predisposing/precipitating factors
1. Often unknown for about 20 to 25%
2. Embryonic or fetal problems for about 50 to 60%

a. Chromosomal defects
b. Faulty placental development
3. Maternal problems for about 15 to 20%
   a. Infection
   b. Hyperemesis
   c. Trauma
   d. Disease
   e. Incompetent cervical os
C. Types
  1. Spontaneous: pregnancy ends of natural causes
  2. Induced: therapeutic or elective reasons for terminating pregnancy
  3. Threatened: developing spontaneous abortion
  4. Inevitable: threatened loss that cannot be prevented
  5. Incomplete: loss of some products of conception and retention of others
  6. Complete: loss of all products of conception
  7. Missed: retention of products of conception in utero after fetal death
  8. Habitual: spontaneous abortions in three or more successive pregnancies
D. Clinical manifestations
  1. Spontaneous vaginal bleeding
  2. Uterine cramping
  3. Contractions
  4. Hemorrhage and shock
E. Medical management: bedrest to try to prevent abortion
F. Surgical management: D & C for incomplete abortion

II. Analysis
A. Fear related to possible pregnancy loss
B. Pain related to uterine cramping
C. Anticipatory grieving related to expected loss of pregnancy

III. Planning/goals, expected outcomes
A. Client will not develop spontaneous abortion
B. Client will not develop complications associated with abortion

IV. Implementation
A. Monitor for and rapidly identify symptoms
B. Monitor vital signs closely
C. Count perineal pads to evaluate blood loss
D. Provide fluids to prevent shock
E. Monitor for tissue loss and save tissue for examination
F. Prepare for D & C if incomplete or missed
G. Provide emotional support

V. Evaluation
A. Client does not develop spontaneous abortion
B. Client develops no complications associated with abortion
C. Client has D & C without complications

Ectopic Pregnancy

I. Assessment
A. Definition: a pregnancy that occurs in extra-uterine area with implantation usually occurring in ampulla of fallopian tubes (about 90%)
B. Incidence/etiology
  1. One in 200 pregnancies
  2. 75% diagnosed in first trimester
  3. Maternal morbidity about one in 800, especially in late diagnosis
  4. 10% recur; 50% achieve normal pregnancy
C. Predisposing/precipitating factors
  1. Pelvic inflammatory disease
  2. Endometriosis
  3. Prolonged use of IUD
  4. Congenital defects
D. Clinical manifestations
  1. Pain unilaterally, cramping and tenderness before rupture
  2. Mass in the adnexa or cul-de-sac
  3. Nausea and vomiting occasional before rupture, frequent after
  4. Slight dark vaginal bleeding
  5. Fever around 100°F (37.7°C)
  6. Tachycardia
  7. Leukocytosis, low hemoglobin and hematocrit, elevated ESR
  8. Profound shock if ruptures
E. Diagnostic examinations
  1. Laparoscopy to determine presence of ruptured tube
  2. Ultrasound
F. Complications
  1. Fetal death
  2. Maternal death
  3. Residual scarring
  4. Infertility
G. Surgical management
  1. Laparotomy and removal of pregnancy and tube, if necessary, or repair of tube
  2. May be emergency if tube ruptures

II. Analysis
A. Pain related to abdominal bleeding secondary to rupture of fallopian tube
B. Anticipatory grieving related to loss of pregnancy
C. High risk for fluid volume deficit related to acute blood loss
D. Knowledge deficit related to treatment of ectopic pregnancy and future pregnancy success

III. Planning/goals, expected outcomes
A. Client will have ectopic pregnancy diagnosed before complications occur
B. Client will have safe termination of pregnancy
C. Client will have successful future pregnancy

IV. Implementation

A. Recognize assessment data rapidly, and initiate preventive measures against shock
B. Monitor for bleeding
C. Obtain blood for type and cross-match
D. Prepare client for surgery including explanations and physical preparation
E. Follow up after surgery with emotional support
F. Administer antibiotics and RhoGam as needed
G. Encourage follow-up care and counseling for future pregnancies

V. Evaluation
A. Client's ectopic pregnancy is diagnosed, and no complications occur
B. Client has safe termination of pregnancy
C. Client has successful future pregnancy

Hydatidiform Mole

I. Assessment
A. Definition: rare condition of abnormal development of placental villi into grape-like cysts filled with viscid material
B. Incidence/etiology
   1. About one in 2000 pregnancies
   2. More common in Asian women, older women, and after induction of ovulation with clomiphene therapy
C. Clinical manifestations
   1. Initially normal pregnancy
   2. Uterus larger than expected for gestational age
   3. Soft and full lower uterine segment on palpation
   4. Hyperemesis
   5. Brown vaginal discharge usually around 12th week
   6. Hypertension
D. Diagnostic examinations
   1. High HCG level
   2. No FHR or palpable fetal parts
   3. Ultrasound shows no fetal skeleton
E. Complications
   1. May be malignant, choriocarcinoma
   2. May require hysterectomy, resulting in sterility
F. Surgical management
   1. Surgical removal as soon as possible
   2. May require total hysterectomy

II. Analysis
A. Knowledge deficit related to treatment of hydatidiform mole and need for regular monitoring of HCG levels
B. Fear related to possible development of choriocarcinoma

III. Planning/goals, expected outcomes
A. Client will have hydatidiform mole diagnosed early

B. Client will have mole removed successfully

IV. Implementation
A. Recognize symptoms quickly
B. Administer fluids and blood as needed to prevent shock
C. Prepare client for surgery
D. Teach client that 1-year follow-up is absolute minimum
   1. HCG levels
   2. Potential of development of choriocarcinoma
E. Maintain contraception for 1 year

V. Evaluation
A. Client's hydatidiform mole diagnosed early
B. Client's mole successfully treated

Placenta Previa

I. Assessment
A. Definition: improperly implanted placenta in lower uterine segment
B. Incidence/etiology
   1. One in 150 to 200 pregnancies
   2. Most common cause of bleeding late in pregnancy
C. Predisposing/precipitating factors
   1. Multiparity
   2. Failure of upper segment to have required vascularity
   3. Presence of myomas
D. Classification
   1. Complete, total, or central: internal os covered by placenta when cervix fully dilated
   2. Partial: incomplete coverage of os
   3. Marginal or low lying: only edge of placenta approaches internal os
E. Clinical manifestations
   1. Anemia
   2. Mild bleeding to hemorrhage
   3. Painless bleeding as early as 7 months
   4. Soft uterus
F. Diagnostic examinations
   1. Ultrasound
   2. Measurement of fetal position
   3. Hemoglobin and hematocrit
   4. Sterile vaginal examination deferred unless double set-up available
G. Complications
   1. Maternal shock and hemorrhage
   2. Fetal prematurity and death
   3. Sepsis

II. Analysis
A. Altered tissue perfusion related to excessive blood loss
B. Impaired gas exchange related to decreased blood volume

C. Fear related to concern for personal and fetal safety

III. Planning/goals, expected outcomes
   A. Client will have placenta previa diagnosed early
   B. Client will not develop hemorrhage or shock
   C. Client will be prepared for surgical intervention
   D. Client and fetus will survive

IV. Implementation
   A. Assess bleeding—amount and quality
   B. Maintain bedrest
   C. Avoid vaginal examination if bleeding is occurring
   D. Monitor maternal vital signs and FHR
   E. Treat shock if it develops
   F. Provide psychological support as needed
   G. Prepare mother for premature birth or cesarean section

V. Evaluation
   A. Placenta previa diagnosed early
   B. Client does not develop hemorrhage or shock
   C. Client prepared for cesarean section
   D. Mother and baby survive and are healthy

Abruptio Placentae

I. Assessment
   A. Definition: premature separation of placenta from uterine wall
   B. Incidence/etiology
      1. About 15% of all perinatal deaths
      2. About one third of infants die
      3. Correction of symptoms promptly decreases perinatal death drastically
   C. Predisposing/precipitating factors
      1. Most common in older gravidas
      2. Hypertension
      3. Fibrin defects
      4. History of previous placental separation
   D. Clinical manifestations
      1. Classic manifestation in third trimester is painful vaginal bleeding; degree of bleeding does not always reflect severity of condition
      2. Uterus hypertonic to tetanic
      3. Enlarged uterus
      4. Manifestations of shock
      5. Manifestations of coagulopathy (DIC)
   E. Diagnostic examinations
      1. Decreased hemoglobin and hematocrit
      2. Increased clot retraction
      3. Ultrasound normal
   F. Complications
      1. Hypovolemic shock
      2. Fetal death
      3. DIC
      4. Bleeding into myometrium

G. Surgical management: deliver fetus by cesarean section

II. Analysis
   A. Pain related to increased uterine tonus
   B. Impaired gas exchange related to blood loss
   C. High risk for infection related to decreased hemoglobin
   D. Fear related to unknown outcome for self and fetus

III. Planning/goals, expected outcomes
   A. Client will have abruptio placentae diagnosed early
   B. Client will be prepared for emergency delivery or cesarean section
   C. Client will not develop coagulopathy
   D. Client will deliver healthy fetus

IV. Implementation
   A. Assess for early symptoms
   B. Maintain bedrest
   C. Monitor and report any uterine activity
   D. Monitor maternal vital signs and FHR closely
   E. Assess blood loss and abdominal pain
   F. Replace blood and fluids to prevent shock
   G. Treat manifestations of shock appropriately
   H. Prepare for emergency cesarean section
   I. Provide emotional support for mother
   J. Observe postpartum for signs of DIC

V. Evaluation
   A. Client has abruptio placentae diagnosed early
   B. Client prepared for emergency delivery or cesarean section
   C. Client does not develop coagulopathy
   D. Client delivers healthy baby

Diabetes Mellitus

I. Assessment
   A. Definition/pathophysiology: inherited metabolic disorder caused by insulin deficiency
      1. Maternal effects
         a. Uteroplacental insufficiency
         b. Increased risk of dystocia
         c. Hydramnios: amniotic fluid of more than 2000 mL
      2. Effects on fetus
         a. Increased fetal mortality
         b. Increased risk of congenital abnormalities
         c. Increased hypoxia
         d. Large-for-gestational-age infant
         e. Neonatal hypoglycemia
      3. Effects of pregnancy on diabetes
         a. Development of insulin resistance (occurs in all pregnancies, but major problem in pregnant diabetics)
         b. Changing insulin needs and difficulty controlling blood sugar
         c. Insulin shock more common

B. Incidence/etiology
1. One to two in 100 pregnancies
2. 30 to 40% of gestational diabetics become diabetics
C. White's classification: considers age at onset, duration and presence of vascular or renal changes
1. Class A: gestational diabetes, abnormal glucose tolerance test, diet controlled, insulin may be needed
2. Class B: onset after age 20, 0 to 9 years' duration, no vascular disease
3. Class C: onset between ages 10 and 19, 10 to 19 years' duration, no vascular disease
4. Class D: onset under age 10, 20 years' or more duration, vascular disease (retinitis and calcification in legs)
5. Class E: calcified pelvic vessels
6. Class F: characteristics of Class E plus retinopathy and nephropathy
D. Clinical manifestations
1. Clinical manifestations of hypoglycemia or hyperglycemia (see Chapter 8, Diabetes)
2. Indications of hydramnios, infection, preeclampsia
E. Diagnostic examinations
1. Two-hour-postprandial blood sugar (screening now recommended for all women during second trimester)
2. Four-hour glucose tolerance test (GTT)
3. Fasting blood sugar
4. Fetal tests: NST, fetal activity determination, contraction stress test
F. Complications
1. Large-for-gestational-age fetus
2. Fetal death
3. Maternal hypoglycemia or hyperglycemia
G. Medical management
1. Careful monitoring and strict dietary control
2. Home monitoring and reporting of glucose levels
3. Observe for clinical manifestations of hypoglycemia and hyperglycemia
4. Insulin requirements will steadily increase in the second and third trimesters in response to human placental lactogen (HPL) levels
5. Oral hypoglycemics are contraindicated during pregnancy
6. Evaluation of fetal status by ultrasound, serial NST, measurement of lecithin-to-sphingomyelin ratio and PG for fetal lung maturity and biophysical profile
7. Anticipation of early delivery related to decreased uteroplacental functioning

II. Analysis
A. Altered nutrition: greater than body require-ments related to imbalance of nutrient intake and available insulin
B. High risk for injury related to hypoglycemia and hyperglycemia
C. High risk for infection: urinary tract related to glycosuria
D. Knowledge deficit related to the disease, treatment, and implications for mother and fetus
E. Altered family processes related to recurrent need for periodic hospitalization of diabetic mother

III. Planning/goals, expected outcomes
A. Client has gestational diabetes diagnosed and treated early
B. Client follows therapeutic regimen to control diabetes
C. Client is able to carry fetus as long as possible without difficulties
D. Client will not suffer long-term complications from diabetes
E. Client will deliver healthy baby

IV. Implementation
A. Assess presence of diabetes early
B. Stress importance of continuing prenatal care
C. Teach client about disease and how to control it (see Chapter 8, Diabetes)
D. Prevent infection and teach client preventive measures
E. Encourage client and family to verbalize fears and concerns
F. Initiate ophthalmological referral
G. Prepare client for early or cesarean delivery

V. Evaluation
A. Client's gestational diabetes diagnosed and treated early
B. Client's diabetes controlled without complications
C. Client carries fetus to delivery without problems
D. Client suffers no long-term complications from diabetes
E. Client delivers healthy baby

Cardiac Disease

I. Assessment
A. Definition/pathophysiology
1. Inability to cope with added volume and increased cardiac output
2. Includes large number of diseases and defects (see Chapter 4, CHF)
3. Classification according to New York Heart Association's functional classification of organic heart disease
a. Class I: no symptoms of insufficiency, no limits of physical activity
b. Class II: slight limitations of activity,

dyspnea, fatigue, palpitations, and angina with ordinary activity

c. Class III: considerable limitation of activity, less-than-normal activity produces symptoms

d. Class IV: inability to perform any physical activity without discomfort; symptoms of insufficiency present at rest

4. Prognosis

a. Depends on extent of disease, functional capacity of heart, presence of other diseases, quality of health care

b. Risk increases from Class I to Class IV

c. Class I and Class II may carry to term

d. Class III and Class IV may require therapeutic abortion

B. Incidence/etiology

1. About 0.5 to 2 per 100 pregnancies

2. Maternal mortality 1 to 3%; fourth cause of maternal death

3. Perinatal mortality about 50%

C. Predisposing/precipitating factors

1. Congenital heart disease

2. Rheumatic heart disease

3. Syphilis

4. Atherosclerosis

5. Pulmonary or renal disorders

D. Clinical manifestations: if progressive, indicate CHF

1. Cardiac enlargement

2. Cardiac murmurs

3. Severe dysrhythmias

4. Edema, peripheral and possibly pulmonary

5. Angina

6. Dyspnea and fatigue

7. Frequent cough and rales

8. Palpitations and tachycardia

E. Diagnostic examinations

1. Cardiac work-up

2. Physical examination

3. Chest x-ray

F. Medical management

1. Treatment of heart disease, including rest, antibiotics to prevent infections, and treatment of CHF (see Chapter 4, CHF)

2. Hospitalization may be required before delivery

II. Analysis

A. Impaired air exchange related to pulmonary edema

B. Knowledge deficit related to cardiac conditions and self-care activities

C. Fear related to the effects of cardiac condition on fetal development

III. Planning/goals, expected outcomes

A. Client's cardiac disease will be diagnosed early

B. Client will understand and comply with therapeutic regimen

C. Client will not experience complications of cardiac disease during pregnancy

D. Client will deliver healthy infant

IV. Implementation

A. Stress importance of continuing prenatal care

B. Teach client necessary restrictions, and urge compliance with therapy

C. Encourage adequate nutrition

D. Prevent anemia

E. Stress need for sufficient rest

F. Avoid exposure to infections, especially upper respiratory

G. Administer antibiotics as ordered

H. Monitor mother's vital signs and condition of fetus

I. Administer cardiac medications as ordered

J. Maintain bedrest for client as needed during last weeks of pregnancy

K. Allow client and family to express concerns and fears

L. Prepare client for normal vaginal delivery, preferably with forceps, under regional nerve block

V. Evaluation

A. Client's cardiac disease diagnosed early

B. Client understands and complies with therapeutic regimen

C. Client does not experience complications of cardiac disease during pregnancy

D. Client delivers healthy baby

Anemia

I. Assessment

A. Definition/pathophysiology: decrease in RBCs in the blood leading to a decrease in oxygen-carrying capacity of blood

B. Types

1. Iron deficiency

2. Folic acid deficiency

3. Hemoglobinopathies such as sickle cell anemia or thalassemia

C. Incidence/etiology

1. About 20% of all pregnancies

2. Most common in adolescent pregnancies

3. Usually iron deficiency from low intake or poor iron stores

D. Predisposing/precipitating factors

1. Low intake of iron

2. Frequent pregnancies resulting in low iron stores

3. Adolescent pregnancy with low iron stores and poor intake

E. Clinical manifestations

1. Fatigue

2. Shortness of breath, if severe

3. Activity intolerance

4. Pallor

F. Diagnostic examinations
1. Hemoglobin and hematocrit low
2. Serum iron levels low
3. Serum folic acid levels low
4. Total iron-binding capacity (TIBC) low
G. Medical management
1. Iron supplements
2. High-iron diet
3. Folic acid supplements
II. Analysis
A. Knowledge deficit related to need for increased iron
B. Altered nutrition: less than body requirements related to low-iron diet and/or nausea
III. Planning/goals, expected outcomes
A. Client will have anemia diagnosed and treated early
B. Client will comply with dietary and therapeutic regimen
C. Client will have anemia corrected
IV. Implementation
A. Monitor hemoglobin and hematocrit with each prenatal visit
B. Provide dietary counseling, including iron-rich foods
C. Administer iron supplements as ordered (Table 15-4)
D. Administer folic acid supplements as ordered, about 5 mg per day
E. Monitor for hemolytic crisis in clients with hemoglobinopathies
V. Evaluation
A. Client's anemia diagnosed and treated early
B. Client complies with dietary and therapeutic regimen
C. Client's anemia corrected

Infections

I. Assessment
A. Definition: a wide variety of infectious agents affecting mother and fetus, with increased morbidity and mortality
B. Types
1. TORCH complex: *T*oxoplasmosis, *O*ther, *R*ubella, *C*ytomegalovirus, *H*erpes
a. Toxoplasmosis (protozoa)
(1) Transmitted through raw meat, handling cat litter of infected cats
(2) Symptoms of acute flu-like infection in mother
(3) Organism passes through placenta
(4) Spontaneous abortion likely early in pregnancy

TABLE 15–4 Medications Associated with Childbirth

Type	Therapeutic Outcome	Method	Common Side Effects	Nursing Implications
Oxytocics				
Methyl ergonovine maleate (Methergine)	Prevention and treatment of postpartum hemorrhage	PO, IM	Nausea and vomiting, vertigo, hypertension, headache, tinnitus, palpitations	Contraindicated in prenatal and hypertension states
Antianemic Agents				
Iron: ferrocholinate, ferrous and ferric salts, iron dextran injection (Imferon)	Prevention and treatment of anemias specifically resulting from iron deficiency	PO, IM (Z-track)	Nausea and vomiting, cramps, diarrhea, dark green stools, constipation	Stools may turn greenish black; medication may be taken with citrus juice to minimize gastric discomfort; Imferon should be given by Z-track injection
Generic				
Rho(D) immune globulin (human) (Gamulin Rh, HypRho-D, RhoGAM)	To prevent sensitization in a subsequent pregnancy to the Rho(D) factor in an Rh-negative mother who has given birth to an Rh-positive infant. To prevent Rho(D) sensitization in Rh-negative clients accidentally transfused with Rh-positive blood	IM	Discomfort at injection site, slight fever	Give within 72 hours after delivery, miscarriage, or abortion

b. Other: streptococcal infections, syphilis, gonorrhea, hepatitis
   (1) Spread in usual manner (see Chapter 6, STDs)
   (2) Increased risk of spontaneous abortions, stillbirths
c. Rubella
   (1) Extremely teratogenic in first trimester
   (2) Transmitted across placenta
   (3) Congenital defects of eyes, heart, ears, and brain
   (4) Women with low titers should be vaccinated at least 2 months before becoming pregnant
d. Cytomegalovirus (CMV)
   (1) Flu-like or mononucleosis-like symptoms
   (2) Transmitted through respiratory or sexual route
   (3) Crosses placenta or may be infected through birth canal
   (4) No effective treatment available
   (5) May cause fetal death, retardation, heart defects, deafness
e. Herpes simplex virus type 2 (genital herpes)
   (1) Sexually transmitted disease with painful blisters on genitalia
   (2) May cross placenta; usually transmitted with passage through birth canal
   (3) High infant mortality
   (4) Fetus delivered by cesarean section if herpes active
C. Clinical manifestations: typical for each infectious disease
D. Diagnostic examinations
   1. Serological studies for venereal disease
   2. Rubella titer
   3. Virological studies
   4. Vaginal smears
E. Medical management: varies with each infectious disease
II. Analysis
A. High risk for infection related to knowledge deficit
B. High risk for injury related to threat of infection to fetus
C. Fear related to TORCH infection risk to fetus
III. Planning/goals, expected outcomes
A. Client will not contract infectious disease during pregnancy
B. Client's infectious disease will be diagnosed early
C. Client will have infectious disease treated effectively

D. Client and fetus will not develop complications
E. Client will deliver healthy fetus
IV. Implementation
A. Teach client precautions to minimize risk for developing infection
B. Monitor client during prenatal visits for manifestations of infection
C. Administer medications as ordered
D. Stress importance of client following therapeutic regimen
V. Evaluation
A. Client does not contract an infectious disease during pregnancy
B. Client's infectious disease diagnosed early
C. Client's and partner's infectious disease treated effectively
D. Client and fetus do not develop complications
E. Client delivers healthy baby

Adolescent Pregnancy

I. Assessment
A. Definition: pregnancy in client under age 17
B. Incidence: worldwide about 1 million teenage pregnancies a year, one third of all births, 10% of all teenagers
C. Predisposing/precipitating factors
   1. Early onset of menarche
   2. Changing sexual behaviors
   3. Faulty family development
   4. Poverty
   5. Lack of knowledge of reproduction and birth control
D. Clinical manifestations
   1. Poor nutritional status
   2. Emotional/behavioral difficulties
   3. Lack of support systems
   4. Lack of knowledge about reproductive process
E. Prognosis
   1. Increased risk of stillbirth, low-birth-weight infants, fetal mortality, cephalo-pelvic disproportion in clients under 15 years
   2. Increased risk of maternal complications such as hypertension, anemia, prolonged labor, and infections
II. Analysis
A. Knowledge deficit related to appropriate pregnancy self-care behaviors
B. Anxiety related to parental reaction to unplanned pregnancy
C. Altered nutrition: less than body requirements related to inadequate nutrient intake to meet pregnancy demand
III. Planning/goals, expected outcomes

A. Client will seek and receive adequate prenatal care
B. Client will understand and comply with additional nutritional needs
C. Client will be prepared physically and emotionally for infant's birth
D. Client will achieve normal developmental tasks of adolescence
E. Client will deliver healthy baby

IV. Implementation
A. Stress importance of comprehensive prenatal care
B. Provide dietary teaching
1. Well-balanced meals
2. High-iron foods
3. Food preparation for high-protein, -iron, and -calcium foods
C. Encourage client to express fears and concerns
D. Help client understand unrealistic nature of some expectations
E. Assist client in own development
F. Educate client for childbirth
G. Assess support systems
H. Recommend follow-up parenting classes
I. Discuss family planning with client

V. Evaluation
A. Client seeks and receives adequate prenatal care
B. Client understands and meets additional nutritional needs
C. Client is physically and emotionally prepared for infant's birth
D. Client achieves normal developmental tasks of adolescence
E. Client delivers healthy baby

POST-TEST Prenatal Period

1. Martha's last menstrual period started on October 1, 1987. Using Nagele's rule, her expected date of confinement will be:
   ① July 1, 1988
   ② July 8, 1988
   ③ August 1, 1988
   ④ July 28, 1988

2. Martha is scheduled for an ultrasound to confirm her pregnancy. Nursing care to prepare her for this test would include:
   ① Administering enemas until clear
   ② Keeping her NPO for 12 hours
   ③ Starting an IV line to maintain hydration
   ④ Having her drink eight glasses of water and not void

3. Martha has an NST done. The results are found to be nonreactive. Based on this, the nurse knows that which of the following must have occurred during the test?
   ① Two FHR accelerations above baseline for 15 seconds
   ② Acceleration less than 15 beats per minute
   ③ Fetal movement in a 10- to 20-minute period
   ④ FHR acceleration more than 15 beats per minute

4. Because of the results of the NST, Martha is scheduled for an OCT. The results show the presence of late deceleration of FHR with three contractions during a 10-minute period; positive window. This test would be reported as:
   ① Positive
   ② Negative
   ③ Suspicious
   ④ Unsatisfactory

5. The risks of amniocentesis would include which of the following?
   ① Delayed fetal growth
   ② Infection
   ③ Delayed fetal lung maturity
   ④ Chromosomal damage

6. Which of the following treatments would be INAPPROPRIATE for the pregnant client who is suffering from nausea and vomiting?
   ① Eat small, frequent meals
   ② Maintain a low-fat diet
   ③ Take antiemetics before arising
   ④ Drink liquids between meals

7. Which of the following is CONTRAINDICATED in the pregnant client who is suffering from heartburn?
   ① Take Gaviscon for the problem
   ② Drink milk between meals
   ③ Sit up after meals
   ④ Take Maalox occasionally

8. Many pregnant clients suffer from headaches during pregnancy. Which of the following is CONTRAINDICATED in treating those headaches?
   ① Change positions slowly
   ② Apply cool cloths to the forehead
   ③ Take aspirin sparingly
   ④ Take Tylenol sparingly

9. Many women have leg cramps during pregnancy. Which of the following would be an appropriate way to treat leg cramps?
   ① Wear knee-high support hose
   ② Dorsiflex the foot
   ③ Maintain bedrest when cramps are severe
   ④ Increase caloric intake

10. Which of the following statements is true about most abortions?
    1. They are usually caused by maternal infections
    2. The cause of most abortions is unknown
    3. An incompetent maternal cervical os is the common cause
    4. Most are the result of fetal abnormalities

11. When some of the products of conception remain in utero after fetal death, it is referred to as:
    1. Spontaneous abortion
    2. Missed abortion
    3. Incomplete abortion
    4. Inevitable abortion

12. Which of the following is considered a typical sign of an ectopic pregnancy?
    1. Nausea and vomiting, especially after rupture
    2. Bradycardia
    3. Respiratory distress
    4. Heavy, bright-red vaginal bleeding

13. Which of the following is a typical sign or symptom of a hydatidiform mole?
    1. Brownish vaginal discharge around week 12
    2. Hypotension
    3. Uterus small for estimated gestational age
    4. Hard, distended lower uterine segment

14. Which of the following is a predisposing factor for abruptio placentae?
    1. Young primigravida
    2. Hypertension
    3. Multiparity
    4. Presence of myomas

15. Using White's classification, the presence of vascular disease in a client who became diabetic at age 8 and has been a diabetic for 21 years places the client in:
    1. Class B
    2. Class C
    3. Class D
    4. Class E

16. Which of the following women should be screened for diabetes during their second trimester with a 2-hour postprandial blood sugar?
    1. Obese women
    2. Older women
    3. Adolescents
    4. All women

17. Mary is a 38-year-old multigravida with a history of rheumatic heart disease. She has been classified as Class II. Which of the following clinical manifestations would you expect her to exhibit?
    1. Dyspnea, fatigue, and angina with normal activity
    2. Manifestations of cardiac insufficiency at rest
    3. No manifestations with normal activities
    4. Dyspnea, fatigue, and angina with less-than-normal activity

18. Which of the following is INCORRECT concerning rubella and pregnancy?
    1. Women with low titers should be vaccinated 2 months before pregnancy
    2. Rubella is extremely teratogenic in the first trimester
    3. The rubella virus does not cross the placenta
    4. All women should have rubella titers before their first pregnancy

---

Gail Warren is a 26-year-old white woman who has registered at the clinic for prenatal care for her pregnancy.

---

19. Gail reports feelings of fatigue as well as constipation and nausea. The hormone that most likely contributes to these symptoms is:
    1. Chorionic gonadotropin
    2. Relaxin
    3. Prolactin
    4. Progesterone

20. A change in vaginal mucosal color from pink to violet is recorded on Gail's chart. This is referred to as:
    1. Goodell's sign
    2. Chadwick's sign
    3. Hegar's sign
    4. Montgomery's sign

21. When Gail's pregnancy has reached the last trimester, the nurse conducts Leopold's maneuvers during the course of a prenatal examination. Which step in this maneuver assists in locating the fetal head?
    1. First
    2. Second
    3. Third
    4. Fourth

22. McDonald's measurements indicate that Gail's fundal height is 31 cm. Which gestational age is compatible with this assessment?
    1. 28 weeks
    2. 32 weeks
    3. 35 weeks
    4. 39 weeks

23. Which of the following statements should guide the nurse's understanding in preparing a teaching plan for Gail?

① Fetal needs for calcium cause demineralization and loss of maternal teeth during pregnancy

② Calories must be regulated to 1800 calories per day to prevent excess weight gain and difficult labor

③ Ambivalence about the pregnancy and mood swings are evidence of rejection of the pregnancy

④ Uterine muscle activity known as Braxton Hicks's contractions occurs throughout the pregnancy

POST-TEST Answers and Rationales

1. ② Using Nagele's rule, the expected date of confinement is calculated by adding 7 days to the start of the last menstrual period and then subtracting 3 months and adding 1 year. Using this formula, July 8 is the correct answer. 4, IV. Prenatal Care.

2. ④ Preparation for the ultrasound requires the client to drink six to eight glasses of water and not to void so that the bladder is distended for the test. The bladder is used as a landmark. None of the actions in the other options are appropriate. 4, IV. Prenatal Care.

3. ② An abnormal or nonreactive stress test has results of zero to one FHR accelerations above the baseline for 15 seconds or more with fetal movement in a 10-minute period or accelerations less than 15 beats per minute or lasting less than 15 seconds. 2, IV. Prenatal Care.

4. ① The results describe a positive or abnormal OCT. A normal OCT is negative with a negative window, a suspicious or equivocal OCT is without a definite positive or negative window, and an unsatisfactory OCT means inadequate contractions or tracings. 2 & 5, II & IV. Prenatal Care.

5. ② Amniocentesis carries some risk of intrauterine infection. Chromosome damage, delayed fetal growth, and maturity are not caused by amniocentesis. 2, IV. Prenatal Care.

6. ③ When a client is pregnant, any medication may potentially cross the placenta and damage the fetus. There are no antiemetics that are considered safe for the pregnant client. The other options contain effective treatments for nausea. 4, IV. Prenatal Care/Discomforts of Pregnancy.

7. ① Gaviscon may upset the acid-base balance of the pregnant client, so it should not be used. The other options contain treatments that can be used with the pregnant client. 4, IV. Prenatal Care/Discomforts of Pregnancy.

8. ③ Aspirin should not be taken during pregnancy and especially toward the last trimester because it can predispose bleeding and other adverse effects. The other options are appropriate treatments. 4, IV. Prenatal Care/Discomforts of Pregnancy.

9. ② Dorsiflexion of the foot relieves acute spasm. The other options are not appropriate treatments, 4. IV. Prenatal Care/Discomforts of Pregnancy.

10. ④ Fetal abnormalities are the most common cause of spontaneous abortions. The others may be causes, but they are not as common. 2, IV. Complications of Pregnancy/Abortions.

11. ② By definition, a missed abortion is one in which some of the products of conception remain in utero after the death of the fetus. 2, IV. Complications of Pregnancy/Abortions.

12. ① An ectopic pregnancy is characterized by nausea and vomiting after rupture. Bleeding associated with it is usually slight and dark. Bradycardia and respiratory distress are not common findings. 1 & 2, IV. Complications of Pregnancy.

13. ① A typical sign of a hydatidiform mole is brownish vaginal drainage at about 12 weeks. The other options are not signs of the mole. 4, IV. Complications of Pregnancy/Hydatidiform Mole.

14. ② A risk factor for abruptio placentae is hypertension. None of the other options are risk factors. 1, IV. Complications of Pregnancy/Abruptio Placentae.

15. ③ White's classification of diabetes states that a woman who has been a diabetic for more than 20 years and has vascular disease is classified as Class D. Class E means there is more severe vascular damage; Class B and Class C are less serious and apply to clients who have been diabetics for less time. 2, IV. Complications of Pregnancy/Diabetes.

16. ④ It is recommended now that all pregnant women should be screened for diabetes with a 2-hour postprandial blood sugar during the second trimester. 4, IV. Complications of Pregnancy/Diabetes.

17. ① In Class II cardiac disease, the client has activity intolerance and symptoms with normal activity. The other options refer to other classes of cardiac disease. 1, IV. Complications of Pregnancy/Cardiac Disease.

18. ③ Rubella can cross the placenta, and during the first trimester it is especially likely to cause congenital abnormalities in the fetus.

The other options are correct concerning pregnancy and rubella. 2, IV. Complications of Pregnancy/Infections.

19. ② Fatigue during pregnancy is related to the ovarian hormone relaxin. Chorionic gonadotropin, prolactin, and progesterone are all hormones that are present during pregnancy, but each has a function unrelated to the feeling of fatigue. 1, II & IV. Prenatal Care.

20. ② Color change in the vaginal mucosa is known as Chadwick's sign. Goodell's sign and Hegar's sign have to do with softening of the cervix and its isthmus, respectively. Montgomery's sign refers to development of breast changes. 1, II & IV. Prenatal Care.

21. ③ There are four Leopold's maneuvers. The first maneuver determines what part of the fetus is present in the uterine fundus; the second determines which side of the uterus contains the fetal back; the third determines whether the fetal head is present over the symphysis pubis, and the fourth determines the amount of descent into the pelvis. 1, II & IV. Prenatal Care.

22. ③ McDonald's measurements are conducted to estimate fetal gestational age in weeks. The procedure for determining this parameter is to measure the height of the fundus in centimeters from the top of the pubis to the top of the fundus; multiply this number by 8, and divide the product by 7. 1, IV. Prenatal Care.

23. ④ The teaching plan can be guided by the nurse's knowledge that because the uterus is a muscle, uterine contractions are present throughout the course of the pregnancy. Including this information in the teaching plan will help the client to understand how her body works and will prepare her to deal with such changes. There is no evidence that the fetus causes demineralization or loss of maternal teeth; caloric intake should be between 2000 and 2200 per day to meet the needs of fetus and mother. Ambivalence and mood swings are normal emotional responses to pregnancy. 3, I & IV. Prenatal Care.

16

Intrapartum Period

PRE-TEST Labor and Delivery

1. Fetal descent into the pelvis 2 weeks before delivery is referred to as:
   ① Quickening
   ② Lightening
   ③ Braxton Hicks's contractions
   ④ False labor

2. Which of the following is one of the prodromes to labor?
   ① Breast enlargement and tenderness
   ② Brownish or bloody show
   ③ Sudden gain of 2 to 3 lb from fluid shifts
   ④ Uterine round ligament pain

3. Which of the following characteristics is typical of false labor?
   ① An increase in the force and frequency of contractions when walking
   ② Contractions that do not produce dilation, effacement, or descent
   ③ Descent of the presenting part into the pelvis
   ④ Heartburn; increased gastric reflux

4. During the latent phase of the first stage of labor, the mother often complains of cramps and backache. Nursing measures to decrease these symptoms include:
   ① Medicate with Demerol as ordered
   ② Encourage the client to lie on her back
   ③ Provide a pillow for client's back
   ④ Have the client bear down with contractions

5. During the transitional phase of the first stage of labor, the client is often nauseated, hot, and sweaty. Which of the following nursing interventions is appropriate for the client at this time?
   ① Administer antiemetics as ordered
   ② Provide the client with cool liquids to drink
   ③ Encourage open-mouthed deep breathing
   ④ Set up a fan in the room to cool the client

6. Which of the following characteristics is typical of the second stage of labor?
   ① Moderately increased pain
   ② Severe rectal pressure
   ③ Circumoral pallor
   ④ Decreased bloody show

Sandy is a 20-year-old overweight primigravida who suffers from pregnancy-induced hypertension.

---

7. Immediately after the cesarean birth under general anesthesia of a 4-lb infant, Sandy is monitored closely. Which nursing care activity has priority?
   ① Administer transfusions and IV fluids
   ② Monitor hematocrit and fibrinogen levels closely
   ③ Allow family and clergy to remain at bedside
   ④ Monitor skin color, respiratory rate and depth

8. The disturbed father is concerned about the health of mother and the infant in intensive care. Which of the following statements meets his needs at this time?
   ① "Don't worry; the doctors are doing all they can."
   ② "Let's talk about what you are feeling now."
   ③ "It won't help your loved ones to be so upset."
   ④ "You must remain strong to support your family."

9. Sandy's condition remains critical for several hours. Postoperative bleeding is excessive but eventually controlled with transfusions and administration of oxytocic drugs.
   Which of the following assessments is essential while the client receives IV Pitocin postpartum?
   ① Report strong contractions
   ② Measure I & O
   ③ Observe any discomfort
   ④ Note behavioral changes

10. During a discharge teaching session, Sandy asks the nurse how long she can expect her bleeding to continue. The nurse's response is:
    ① 1 week
    ② 3 weeks
    ③ 5 weeks
    ④ 8 weeks

PRE-TEST Answers and Rationales

1. ② The movement of the fetus is known as lightening. This usually occurs about 2 weeks before delivery. The other options are incorrect. 2, IV. Normal Labor and Delivery.
2. ② Bloody show is a prodromal sign of labor. Breast enlargement and uterine ligament pain are common discomforts of pregnancy. 2, IV. Normal Labor and Delivery.
3. ② With false labor, progressive dilation, effacement, and descent do not occur. The other options are typical characteristics of labor. 2, IV. Normal Labor and Delivery.
4. ③ Providing a pillow and rubbing the client's back are the best ways to treat the client's cramps and backache. The other options arc dangerous in the latent phase. 4, IV. Normal Labor and Delivery.
5. ③ Antiemetics are not given, and all liquids are avoided in case the client requires anesthesia later in the labor. A fan can cause excessive chilling of the client. Encouraging slow, open-mouthed deep

breathing will help the client's nausea. 4, IV. Normal Labor and Delivery.
6. ② During the second stage of labor, the fetus moves down the birth canal for delivery. The client will feel an increase in rectal pressure at this time. The other options are incorrect for the second stage. 2, IV. Normal Labor and Delivery.
7. ④ Cardiac and respiratory function are priority nursing assessments in the immediate postoperative period. Other nursing actions are of lesser importance. 4, I & IV. Postpartum, Cesarean Section.
8. ② Allow the father to express his feelings during this time of crisis. Other options are blocks to therapeutic communication. 4, IV. Postpartum, Cesarean Section.
9. ② Because Pitocin has an antidiuretic effect, this assessment is critical. Strong, painful contractions are expected as the medication acts as intended. Choice 4 is not expected with this drug. 1 & 2, II & IV. Postpartum.
10. ② Lochia can normally be expected to persist for 2 to 3 weeks postpartum. 4, I & IV. Postpartum, Cesarean Section.

NORMAL LABOR AND DELIVERY

Overall Assessment

I. Labor: coordinated sequence of involuntary uterine contractions resulting in effacement and dilation of cervix, followed by expulsion of products of conception

II. Delivery: actual event of birth

III. Essential factors in labor: the "five P's"—passenger, passageway, powers, person, psychological response

A. Passenger: the fetus
1. Attitude (habitus or posture): relationship of fetal body parts to each other; normal intrauterine posture is completely flexed
2. Lie: relationship of spine of fetus to spine of mother
   a. Longitudinal or vertical
      (1) Fetus parallel with mother's spine
      (2) Either cephalic or sacral presentation
   b. Transverse or horizontal
      (1) Fetus is at right angle to mother's spine

(2) Presenting part is shoulder
3. Presentation: portion of fetus that enters pelvis first; presenting part
   a. Cephalic most common, 96%
   b. Breech
      (1) Frank: sacrum
      (2) Footling: foot
4. Position: relationship of fetal reference point or landmark to one of four quadrants or sides of mother's pelvis such as right occiput anterior (ROA) (Fig. 16-1)
   a. Maternal pclvis side
      (1) L—left
      (2) R—right
   b. Fetal reference point
      (1) O—occiput
      (2) M—mentum
      (3) B—brow
      (4) S—sacrum
      (5) Sc—scapula
   c. Maternal pelvis quadrant
      (1) A—anterior
      (2) T—transverse
      (3) P—posterior

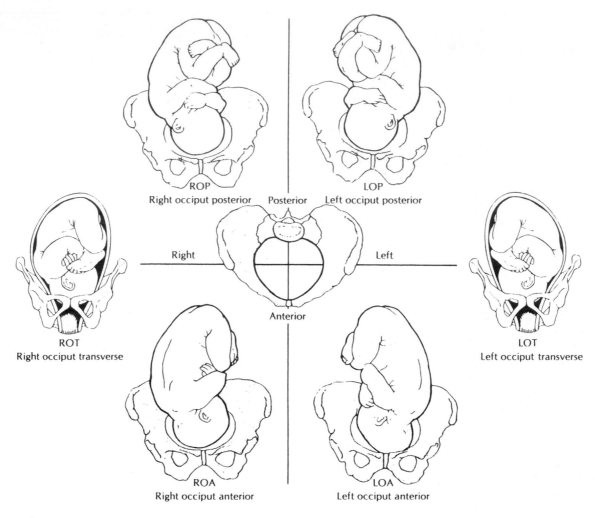

ROP
Right occiput posterior

Posterior

LOP
Left occiput posterior

Right

Left

ROT
Right occiput transverse

LOT
Left occiput transverse

Anterior

ROA
Right occiput anterior

LOA
Left occiput anterior

Lie: Longitudinal or vertical
Presentation: vertex
Reference point: occiput
Attitude: complete flexion

FIGURE 16–1. Fetal vertex presentations. (From Bobak, I. M., and Jensen, M. D. [1991]. *Essentials of maternity nursing: The nurse and the childbearing family,* **3rd ed. St. Louis: C. V. Mosby.)**

5. Station: degree of engagement measured in centimeters above or below midplane from presenting part to ischial spines (Fig. 16-2)
   a. Station 0—at ischial spine
   b. Minus station—above spines
   c. Plus station—below spines
B. Passageway
   1. Pelvis
      a. Types
         (1) Gynecoid, about 50%
             (a) Slightly ovoid or transversely rounded
             (b) Vaginal delivery in (OA) position usual
         (2) Android, about 20%

         (a) Heart shaped or angulated; resembles male shape
         (b) Vaginal delivery difficult with forceps, usually cesarean
      (3) Anthropoid
         (a) Oval, wider anteroposterior diameter
         (b) Vaginal delivery with forceps or spontaneous, OP or OA position
      (4) Platypelloid
         (a) Flattened anteroposterior, wide transversely
         (b) Spontaneous vaginal delivery usually
   b. Planes of true pelvis

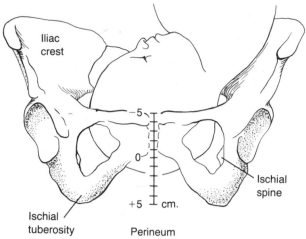

FIGURE 16–2. Degree of fetal descent.

  (1) Plane of inlet
  (2) Midplane—greatest dimension
  (3) Plane of outlet—least dimension
  2. Soft tissues: lower uterine segment, cervix, vagina, and introitus
C. Powers: forces acting to expel fetus
  1. Primary: involuntary uterine contractions
  2. Secondary: voluntary bearing down
  3. Function of uterine contractions
    a. Effacement: shortening and thinning of cervix during first stage of labor
    b. Dilation: enlargement of cervical os and cervical canal during first stage of labor
D. Person/psychological response
  1. Response to contractions
  2. Perceptions and beliefs about labor and delivery
  3. Prenatal care and education
  4. Support systems
  5. Ability to communicate with others

Process of Labor

I. Prodromes to labor
  A. Lightening or dropping: fetus descends into the pelvis about 2 weeks preterm
    1. Easier to breathe
    2. More pressure on bladder
    3. In multiparas, may not occur until true labor in progress
    4. Persistent low back pain from relaxation of pelvic joints
  B. Braxton Hicks's contractions increase

C. Show
  1. Vaginal mucosa congested and vaginal mucus increases
  2. Brownish or blood-tinged cervical mucus passed
D. Cervix ripens, becomes soft, partly effaced, and may begin to dilate
E. Sudden burst of energy, "nesting instinct"
F. Loss of 1 to 3 lb from water loss resulting from fluid shifts produced by changes in progesterone and estrogen levels
G. Spontaneous rupture of membranes (SROM)
II. False labor
  A. Exaggeration of normal contractions
  B. Does not produce dilation, effacement, or descent
  C. Contractions irregular without progression
  D. Walking has no effect on contractions; often relieves false labor
  E. Absence of bloody show
III. Onset of labor
  A. No single cause
  B. Hormonal changes
    1. Oxytocin stimulation
    2. Progesterone withdrawal
    3. Estrogen stimulation
    4. Prostaglandin secretion
    5. Fetal secretion of cortical steroids
  C. Distention of uterus: increasing intrauterine pressure
  D. Aging of placenta: associated with increasing myometrial irritability
IV. Physiological changes
  A. Dilation of cervix to 10 cm
  B. Effacement of cervix
  C. Physiological retraction ring: separation of upper and lower uterine segments
V. Mechanisms of labor
  A. Engagement: when presenting part of fetus becomes fixed in true pelvis
  B. Descent: progression of presenting part through pelvis: station, degree of descent (see Fig. 16-2)
  C. Flexion: when descending head meets pelvic floor; chin brought down to chest
  D. Internal rotation: fetal head rotates from transverse diameter to anteroposterior diameter to facilitate movement through pelvis
  E. Extension: when fetal head reaches perineum, it extends to be born
  F. Restitution: after delivery of head, it rotates back to position prior to engagement
  G. External rotation: shoulders engage and move similarly to head
  H. Expulsion: entire infant emerges from mother

Stages of Labor (Table 16-1)

NURSING PROCESS APPLIED TO NORMAL LABOR AND DELIVERY

I. Assessment
   A. State of labor
      1. Presence of prodromes
      2. Signs and symptoms of true labor
      3. Stage/phase of labor

B. Uterine contractions
   1. Duration
   2. Frequency
   3. Intensity
   4. Tonus
C. Fetal monitoring
   1. Periodic auscultation, count for 1 full minute
   2. Electronic monitoring
      a. External mode
         (1) Tocotransducer: pressure-sensing device applied to maternal abdo-

TABLE 16–1 Stages of Labor

	Phase		
	Latent	**Active**	**Transition**
First stage: onset of regular contractions to full dilatation			
Dilatation	0 to 3 cm	4 to 7 cm	8 cm to complete
Duration	8.5 hours for primigravida, 3 to 5 hours for multipara	4 hours for primigravida, 2 hours for multipara	1 hour for primigravida, 10 to 15 minutes for multipara
Contractions	Frequency, every 15 to 20 minutes; duration, 30 to 40 seconds; mild intensity	Frequency, every 2 to 4 minutes; duration, 30 to 40 seconds; moderate intensity	Frequency, every 2 to 4 minutes; duration, 45 to 90 seconds; strong intensity
Manifestations	Abdominal cramps, bloody show, backache, excitement, need for control	Moderately increased pain, serious fear of losing control, skin warm and flushed	Irritable, panicky, loss of control, fear of tearing, nausea, sweating, rectal pressure
Nursing Interventions	Monitor vital signs and fetal heart rate every hour; encourage position of comfort; provide backrubs; encourage support from significant other	Monitor vital signs and fetal heart rate every 30 minutes; monitor contractions; encourage left lateral position and use of accelerated-decelerated breathing techniques; inform patient of labor's progress	Monitor vital signs and fetal heart rate every 15 minutes; do not leave alone; encourage pant-blow breathing; keep perineal area clean and dry; inform patient of labor's progress and praise for efforts

	Duration	**Contractions**	**Manifestations**	**Nursing Interventions**
Second stage: time from full dilatation to delivery of infant	30 to 60 minutes for primigravida 20 minutes for multipara	Frequency, every 2 to 3 minutes; duration, 60 to 90 seconds; intensity, strong	Rectal pressure, urge to bear down, increased bloody show, excitement and exhaustion, bulging perineum	Encourage effective pushing with contractions; offer praise and support for labor's efforts; closely monitor maternal vital signs and fetal heart rate
Third stage: time from delivery of infant to delivery of placenta	5 to 30 minutes		Gush of blood; visible lengthening of the cord; uterus assumes a globular shape; feeling of relief at completion of delivery; intense focus on newborn	Encourage mother to bear down to aid in the delivery of the placenta; inform parents of newborn status
Fourth stage: time from delivery of placenta to homeostasis.	First hour postpartum		Uterus firm at the midline; two fingerbreaths below the umbilicus, small-to-moderate rubra lochia; initial encounter with newborn; bonding begins; newborn first period of reactivity	Assess vital signs every 5 to 15 minutes; assess fundus height, consistency, and location; assess amount and character of lochia; assess and support bonding behaviors: eye-to-eye contact, en face position, fingertip touching, palmar massage

men to monitor frequency and duration of contractions

(2) Ultrasound transducer: continuous monitor of FHR, which can be interpreted in relation to contractions

(3) Phonotransducer and abdominal electrodes: fetal electrocardiography

b. Internal mode

(1) Spiral electrode: applied to fetal presenting part; provides continuous measurement of FHR, baseline variability, and periodic changes

(2) Intrauterine catheter: pressure transducer inserted beyond presenting part; measures frequency, duration, and intensity of contractions

3. FHR

a. Baseline: without contractions, usually 120 to 160 per minute

b. Baseline variability: variation in FHR in response to fetal sleep/wake states, medications, hypoxia

c. Acceleration: transient rise more than 15 beats per minute for more than 15 seconds

(1) May or may not be related to uterine contractions

(2) Marked (more than 180 beats per minute) may be related to prematurity, maternal fever, hypoxia, fetal infection, or drugs

d. Decelerations: transient decrease in FHR (Fig. 16-3, Table 16-2)

4. Fetal scalp sampling: a small sample of fetal blood is taken from a puncture wound made into the fetal scalp to test for the presence of fetal acidosis

a. Laboratory analysis of fetal pH is done

b. Normal values range from 7.25 to 7.35

c. A reported value of 7.20 or below indicates fetal acidosis

D. Maternal discomfort

1. Assess pain with each stage/phase of labor

2. Plan for use of analgesics as needed

E. Diagnostic examinations

1. Routine blood work

FIGURE 16–3. Fetal heart rate stress patterns. (From Burroughs, A. [1992]. *Maternity nursing: An introductory text,* 6th ed., p. 146. Philadelphia, W. B. Saunders.)

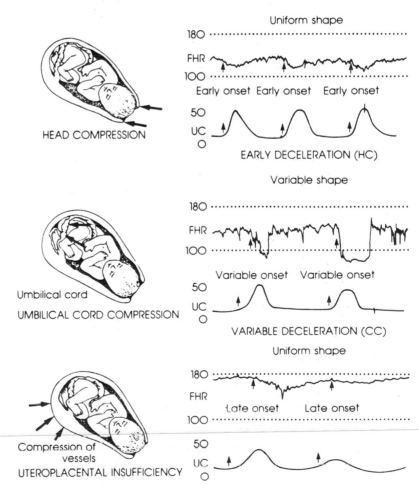

TABLE 16–2 Fetal Heart Rate Patterns (Deceleration)

Pattern	Shape	Cause	Nursing Interactions
Type I (early deceleration)	Uniform shape mirrors the contraction; decreases with the onset of the contraction; returns to baseline as the contraction ends	Head compression	Continue to monitor fetal heart rate
Type II (late deceleration)	Uniform shape; fetal heart rate decreases after the onset of the contraction and persists beyond the completion of the contraction	Uteroplacental insufficiency	Turn patient to left lateral position, give oxygen at 6 to 10 L/min via mask; discontinue oxytocin if in use; notify physician
Type III (variable deceleration)	Nonuniform shape; deceleration is V or U shaped; fetal heart rate decreases during or between contractions	Umbilical cord compression	Change patient position; give oxygen at 6 to 10 L/min via mask; notify physician

2. Urinalysis
3. Cultures if indicated by history
4. Ultrasound
5. Fetal monitoring
6. Maternal monitoring
7. Arterial blood gases on cord blood

F. Analgesics
  1. Narcotics
    a. Can slow labor and depress neonatal respirations
    b. Given during active labor for pain
  2. Tranquilizers
    a. Produce sedation and relaxation
    b. No analgesic effect
  3. Amnesiacs (rarely used)
    a. Produce sedation and memory loss
    b. May cause dysrhythmias and fetal tachycardia
    c. Example: scopolamine
  4. Sedatives
    a. Produce sedation
    b. May depress fetus
    c. May be used very early in labor
  5. Anesthetics
    a. General
      (1) Induces sleep
      (2) May depress fetus
      (3) May cause uterine atony
      (4) Cannot use if mother has eaten because of risk of aspiration
    b. Regional
      (1) Xylocaine, local anesthetic
        (a) Local used for blocking pain during episiotomy
        (b) No effect on fetus
      (2) Paracervical block
        (a) Used in first stage
        (b) Rapid block of uterine pain
        (c) No effect on perineal area

        (d) No effect on ability to bear down
        (e) May cause fetal bradycardia
      (3) Pudendal block
        (a) Used in second stage
        (b) Blocks perineal area for about 30 minutes
        (c) No effects on contractions or fetus
      (4) Peridural block
        (a) Used in first or second stage
        (b) Rapid relief of uterine and perineal pain
        (c) Single dose or continuous
        (d) Epidural: may cause maternal hypotension
        (e) Caudal: same side effects
      (5) Intradural blocks
        (a) Spinal
          (i) Relieves uterine and perineal pain rapidly
          (ii) May cause maternal hypotension
          (iii) Client must lie flat 8 to 12 hours
        (b) Saddle block
          (i) Used for forceps delivery
          (ii) Client must lie flat 8 to 12 hours

II. Analysis
  A. High risk for injury related to labor and delivery
  B. Family process, potential for growth related to healthy infant bonding
III. Planning/goals, expected outcomes
  A. Client will be properly monitored throughout labor and delivery
  B. Client and fetus will safely complete first stage of labor

C. Client will deliver healthy infant

D. Client will complete third phase of labor with expulsion of placenta

E. Client will bond with infant

F. Client will complete recovery period without complications

IV. Implementation

  A. First stage

    1. Monitor client for stage of labor on admission

    2. Review setting and procedures for expectant family

    3. Assess client's level of knowledge

    4. Obtain baseline vital signs, FHR, contraction frequency and duration

    5. Perform Leopold's maneuver (Fig. 16-4) after having client empty bladder and flex knees

      a. Palpate fundus, note presentation

      b. Palpate for back and small parts of fetus

      c. Palpate above pubic symphysis for position and mobility of presenting part

      d. Identify the degree of flexion or extension of the fetal head

    6. Administer enema and prep as ordered

    7. Prepare client for and assist with vaginal examinations

    8. Note color, amount, consistency, and presence of meconium in amniotic fluid

    9. Determine time of last meal

   10. Have client empty bladder

   11. Start IV line

   12. Maintain bedrest if membranes ruptured

   13. Monitor fetal status

      a. Monitor FHR both audibly and with monitors every 30 minutes early to every 5 minutes late

      b. Monitor uterine contractions through palpation and monitors every 30 minutes early to every 5 minutes late

      c. Check for prolapse of cord (Fig. 16-5)

        (1) If prolapsed

          (a) Place mother in Trendelenburg's or knee-chest position

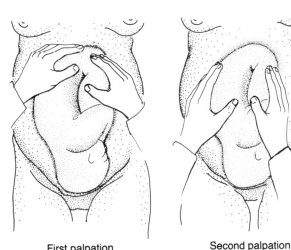

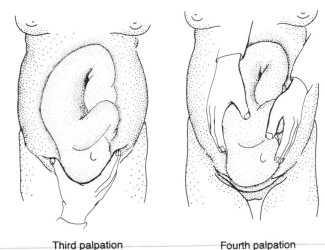

First palpation   Second palpation

Third palpation   Fourth palpation

FIGURE 16–4. Leopold's maneuvers for fetal position. (From Burroughs, A. [1992]. *Maternity nursing: An introductory text*, 6th ed., p. 93. Philadelphia: W. B. Saunders.)

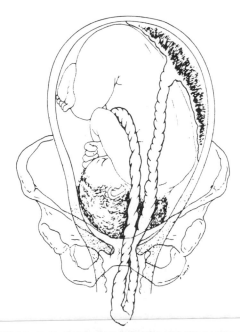

FIGURE 16–5. Prolapsed umbilical cord. (From Burroughs, A. [1992]. *Maternity nursing: An introductory text*, 6th ed., p. 410. Philadelphia: W. B. Saunders.)

(b) Call physician immediately

(c) Give oxygen

14. Monitor maternal vital signs
    a. Supine hypotensive syndrome
       (1) Pressure of enlarged uterus on vena cava
       (2) Decreased blood pressure and pulse, pallor, clammy skin
       (3) Place client in left lateral position to prevent or relieve
15. Treat nausea and vomiting with ice chips and deep breathing
16. Provide pain relief
    a. General comfort measures
    b. Encourage use of Lamaze or other breathing techniques
    c. Medicate as needed
17. Assist with breathing techniques
    a. Assess techniques learned prenatally
    b. Have client rest between contractions
    c. If hyperventilating, use paper bag for increasing CO_2
    d. Relieve significant other in coaching role
    e. Praise client and significant other for progress
18. Maintain physical safety
    a. Allow up only if membranes intact
    b. Keep side rails up
    c. Provide bedpan as needed

B. Second stage
    1. Transfer to delivery room when dilation of 8 to 9 cm for multigravidas and full dilation and perineal bulging with primigravidas
       a. Place in stirrups carefully or optimal position as decided by client and physician
       b. Use appropriate sterile technique
    2. Prepare perineal area
    3. Monitor FHR every 5 minutes
    4. Palpate fundus for contractions
    5. Monitor maternal blood pressure
    6. Encourage client to push with contractions
       a. Instruct client to take two breaths, hold, and bear down while slowly releasing air through open glottis
       b. Legs spread and knees slightly flexed
       c. Use short, rapid breaths to avoid pushing between contractions
    7. Allow coach to assist as possible
       a. Reassure client of progress
       b. Position mirror so delivery can be seen
       c. Provide frequent praise
    8. Note time of delivery
    9. Provide immediate care of newborn (see Chapter 18, Care of the Neonate)

10. Place newborn on mother's abdomen, allowing mother and significant other to touch and explore newborn
11. Cut umbilical cord

C. Third stage
    1. Assess for placental separation
       a. Uterus rises in abdomen, firm and contracting
       b. Changes to globular shape
       c. Sudden gush of blood
       d. Cord lengthens
    2. Schultze's mechanism: placenta presents by shiny fetal surface
    3. Duncan's mechanism: placenta turns to show dark roughened maternal surface
    4. Inspect for intactness of placenta
    5. Palpate for firm, contracted uterus
    6. Administer oxytocic drugs as ordered (see Table 16-5)
    7. Monitor maternal vital signs, especially blood pressure, for excessive blood loss
    8. Administer antilactation agents as ordered
    9. Send cord blood to laboratory if mother is O-positive or Rh-negative
    10. Continue allowing mother and significant other to see newborn; as soon as stable, allow further exploration and touching
    11. Initiate breast feeding, if able

D. Fourth stage
    1. Transfer to recovery room when stable
    2. Monitor vital signs every 15 minutes, including fundal height, position, and consistency
    3. Assess lochia
    4. Check perineum for pain, redness, swelling
    5. Palpate bladder for distention; measure output
    6. Perform peri care front to back; teach mother
    7. Promote comfort for afterpains and perineum
    8. See Chapter 17, Postpartum Care, for further information

V. Evaluation
   A. Client monitored properly throughout labor and delivery
   B. Client and fetus safely complete first stage of labor
   C. Client delivers healthy infant
   D. Client completes third phase of labor with expulsion of placenta
   E. Client bonds with infant
   F. Client completes recovery period without complications

NURSING PROCESS APPLIED TO PROBLEMS WITH LABOR AND DELIVERY

Dystocia

I. Assessment
- A. Definition: difficult labor and/or delivery because of problems with one of the "five P's"
- B. Incidence
  1. About 5% of pregnancies, especially primigravida
- C. Types
  1. Passenger: problems with fetal gestational age, size, attitude, presentation, and position; number of fetuses or placental type; sufficiency; and site of insertion
     - a. Abnormal position, persistent OP (about 25% of pregnancies)
     - b. Malpresentation
       - (1) Shoulder, face, or brow
       - (2) Breech
         - (a) Frank: thighs flexed on hips, knees extended
         - (b) Complete: thighs and knees flexed
         - (c) Footling: foot or feet extend below buttocks
         - (d) Incomplete: knees extended below buttocks
     - c. Multiple pregnancy
     - d. Abnormal fetal size
       - (1) Fetus more than 4000 g may be too large to pass through birth canal
       - (2) Fetal head less malleable as fetal head increases
       - (3) Hydrocephalus: abnormal accumulation of cerebrospinal fluid in ventricles of brain leading to enlargement of cranium; incidence, about one in 2000
  2. Passageway: problems with configuration and diameters of maternal pelvis, distensibility of lower uterine segment, cervical dilation, capacity for distention of vaginal canal and introitus
     - a. Cephalopelvic disproportion: discrepancy between size of fetal head and birth canal
     - b. Pelvic contractions
       - (1) Inlet
       - (2) Midpelvis
       - (3) Outlet
       - (4) Combination
  3. Powers: primary—duration, intensity, and frequency of contraction; secondary—bearing down effort
     - a. Hypotonic uterine contraction
       - (1) Decrease in frequency and intensity
       - (2) Uterine muscle weakness
       - (3) Tension not synchronous
       - (4) Contracture and fetal malposition one possible cause
       - (5) Overdistention of uterus with multiple births possible cause
     - b. Hypertonic uterine contractions
       - (1) Usually occurs before 4-cm dilation
       - (2) Increased muscle tonus
       - (3) Pain out of proportion to intensity and effectiveness of contractions without further dilation
       - (4) Contractions increase in frequency but uncoordinated
       - (5) Problem in latent phase
  4. Person/psychosocial responses: maternal position, previous experience, readiness, education and preparation, culture/ethnicity, support systems, and environment all may affect progress
  5. Prolonged labor, partogram (Fig. 16-6)
     - a. Lasting more than 18 hours
     - b. May result from any of above causes
     - c. Progress in first or second stage slowed
     - d. Latent phase may be prolonged: 20 hours or more in nulliparas or 14 hours or more in multiparas
     - e. Protracted active-phase dilation: cervical dilation less than 1.2 cm per hour in nulliparas or less than 1.5 cm in multiparas
     - f. Arrest of active phase: no progress for more than 2 to 4 hours
     - g. Prolonged deceleration phase: more than 3 hours in nulliparas or more than 1 hour in multiparas
     - h. Protracted descent: more than 1 cm per hour in nulliparas or more than 2 cm per hour in multiparas
     - i. Arrest of descent: no progress for 1 hour or more in nulliparas or 30 minutes or more in multiparas
- D. Clinical manifestations
  1. False versus true labor
  2. Presentation of fetus
  3. Meconium staining of fetus
  4. Anxiety
  5. No progression of labor
- E. Diagnostic examinations
  1. Vaginal examination, pelvimetry, ultrasound
  2. Diagnosis of type of dystocia

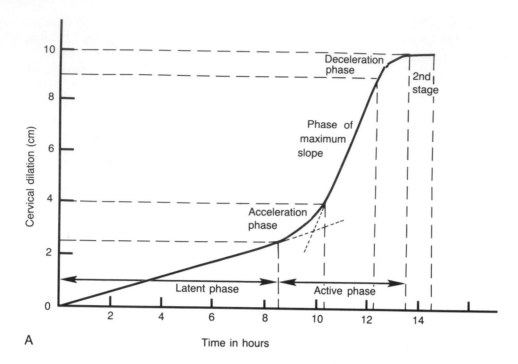

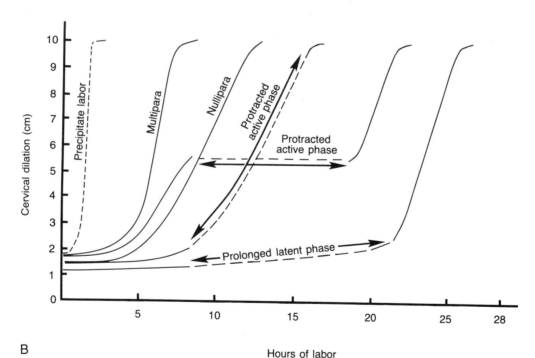

FIGURE 16–6. Partogram. (A) Normal labor. (B) Arrest of descent in active phase of labor.

3. Leopold's maneuver to determine position (see Fig. 16-4)
4. Plot client's labor against normal partogram

F. Complications
  1. Maternal exhaustion
  2. Infection
  3. Traumatic operative delivery
  4. Fetal injury or death

G. Medical management
  1. Sedation for hypertonicity
  2. Stimulation of labor for hypotonicity
H. Surgical management: cesarean section
II. Analysis
  A. Pain related to patient's inability to relax secondary to hypertonic uterine dysfunction
  B. Anxiety related to prolonged labor dysfunction

C. Knowledge deficit related to lack of understanding regarding labor dysfunction

III. Planning/goals, expected outcomes
A. Client will be monitored for early signs of dystocia
B. Client will have dystocia treated
C. Client will not be anxious during labor and delivery
D. Client will safely deliver healthy infant

IV. Implementation
A. Monitor uterine contractions
B. Assist with pelvic examination, measurements, ultrasounds, and other procedures
C. Assess FHR after physician ruptures membranes
D. Check for prolapse of cord after rupture of membranes
1. If prolapse occurs, place client in Trendelenburg's or knee-chest position to minimize pressure on cord
2. Give oxygen
3. Notify physician
4. Prepare for emergency cesarean section
E. Administer prophylactic antibiotics to prevent infection
F. Provide for rest and IV fluids for client
G. Administer oxytocin as ordered (see Table 16-5)
1. Follow hospital protocol
2. Physician must be available throughout procedure
3. Give only if actual hypotonic dysfunction, never if hypertonic dysfunction suspected
4. Assess that client in true labor, dilated at least 3 cm
5. Assess that no actual mechanical obstructions or uterine overdistention present or multiple fetuses
6. Administer only if
a. Fetus in good condition
b. Client usually less than 35 and less than para v
c. No history of cesarean births
7. Use infusion pump
8. Monitor vital signs, IV drip rate carefully and frequently
9. Continue to observe fetal monitor for contractions
10. Position client in left lateral position to reduce pressure on vena cava and aorta to increase uterine blood flow
11. Discontinue drip if uterine tetany or fetal distress occurs
12. Administer oxygen if fetal distress occurs
H. Provide comfort as with normal delivery
I. Assess client's fatigue and pain: administer sedatives and pain medications as ordered

J. Provide emotional support as needed
K. Assist with anesthesia for hypertonic contractions
L. Prepare client for vaginal delivery or cesarean section

V. Evaluation
A. Client's dystocia is diagnosed early
B. Client's dystocia is treated successfully
C. Client's anxiety during labor and delivery is minimized
D. Client delivers healthy infant

Precipitate Labor and Delivery

I. Assessment
A. Definition: labor that lasts less than 3 hours
B. Predisposing/precipitating factor: multiparity
C. Clinical manifestations
1. Tetanic-like contractions
2. Rapid labor and delivery
D. Complications
1. If birth canal not readily distensible
a. Uterine rupture
b. Severe lacerations of birth canal
2. Hypotonic uterus postdelivery with hemorrhage
3. Fetal hypoxia from decreased placental perfusion secondary to tetanic contractions
E. Surgical management
1. Episiotomy
2. Delivery

II. Analysis
A. Pain related to the rapid progress of labor
B. Ineffective individual coping related to rapid progress of labor and precipitous birth
C. High risk for injury related to rapid fetal descent

III. Planning/goals, expected outcomes
A. Client will not suffer from complications of precipitate delivery such as lacerations or postpartum bleeding
B. Client will deliver healthy infant

IV. Implementation
A. Stay with client at all times
B. Provide emotional support; keep client calm
C. Encourage mother to pant between contractions
D. Rupture membranes when head crowns if not already ruptured
E. Do not try to keep fetus from being delivered
F. Use gentle pressure to fetal head upward toward vagina to prevent damage to fetal head and vaginal lacerations
G. Deliver fetus between contractions, checking for cord around neck
H. Use restitution to deliver posterior shoulder

I. Use gentle downward pressure to move anterior shoulder under pubic symphysis

J. Use upward pressure for delivery of posterior shoulder

K. Clear infant's mouth; dry and cover infant to keep warm

L. If outside hospital and materials available, clamp cord in two places and cut between with clean knife or scissors; leave clamped

M. Allow placenta to separate naturally

N. Place infant on mother's abdomen or breast to induce uterine contractions

O. Institute measures as described in fourth stage of labor

V. Evaluation

A. Client does not suffer from complications of precipitate delivery such as lacerations or postpartum bleeding

B. Client delivers healthy infant

Preterm Labor

I. Assessment

A. Definition: labor occurring after 20th week but before 37th

B. Predisposing/precipitating factors

1. Maternal problems
   a. Trauma
   b. Abdominal surgery
   c. Preeclampsia
   d. Uterine abnormalities
   e. Cervical incompetence
   f. Sepsis
   g. Diabetes
   h. Renal or cardiovascular disease
   i. Premature rupture of membranes
   j. Smoking

2. Placental disorders
   a. Placental separation
   b. Extrachorial placenta

3. Fetal abnormalities
   a. Infections

b. Multiple pregnancies
c. Hydramnios
d. Congenital adrenal hyperplasia

4. Unknown causes

C. Complications

1. Fetal death, if infant delivered with low birth weight
2. From 35 weeks on, good chance of survival

D. Indications

1. Maternal complications requiring delivery of preterm infant
   a. Placental separation with uncontrolled hemorrhage
   b. Severe eclampsia or preeclampsia
   c. Uncontrolled renal or cardiovascular disease
   d. Premature rupture of membranes
   e. Chorioamnionitis

E. Medical management: administration of ritodrine to stop labor (Table 16-3)

II. Analysis

A. Knowledge deficit related to preterm labor causes and treatment regimen
B. Fear related to premature delivery
C. Ineffective individual coping related to inability to perform expected roles

III. Planning/goals, expected outcomes

A. Client's preterm labor will be controlled until at least 35 weeks
B. Client will deliver healthy infant

IV. Implementation

A. Maintain bedrest, quiet environment, lateral recumbent position
B. Administer tokolytic agents as ordered to suppress labor
   1. Vasodilan
   2. Ritodrine
   3. Terbutaline
   4. Magnesium sulfate
      a. Assess effects of drugs on labor and fetus

TABLE 16–3 Beta-Receptor Antagonist

Example	Action	Use	Common Side Effects	Nursing Implications
Ritodrine hydrochloride (Yutopar)	Drugs that have an antagonistic effect on beta-2–adrenergic receptors such as those in uterine smooth muscle	Management of preterm labor in suitable patients; contraindicated under 20 weeks' gestation	Dose-related alterations in maternal and fetal heart rates and maternal blood pressure; palpitations, tremors, nausea and vomiting, headache, erythema, malaise	Check maternal vital signs and monitor fetus; monitor uterine contractions; run as IV piggyback; use IV infusion pump; monitor potassium levels; teach patient use of oral form; keep in left lateral position during IV administration

b. Monitor for side effects of various drugs, especially reflexes, cardiovascular disorders, and respirations
c. Have antidote (calcium gluconate) available
C. Maintain adequate hydration
D. Use steroids to prevent respiratory distress syndrome in preterm infants if administered 24 to 48 hours before delivery
E. Prepare for delivery if labor cannot be stopped or if maternal complications indicate

V. Evaluation
A. Client's preterm labor is controlled
B. Client delivers healthy infant

Induction of Labor

I. Assessment
A. Definition: deliberate initiation of uterine contractions
B. Predisposing/precipitating factors—indications for induction
1. Pregnancy-induced hypertension
2. Uncontrolled diabetes
3. Postterm pregnancy
4. History of precipitous labor
5. Placental insufficiency
6. Premature rupture of membranes
C. Indications for assessing appropriateness for induction
1. Bishop's scale (Table 16-4)
a. Dilation of cervix
b. Effacement
c. Station
d. Cervical consistency
e. Fetal position
2. Cervix thinning and beginning to dilate
D. Contraindications
1. Cephalopelvic disproportion
2. Fetal distress
3. Previous cesarean section

TABLE 16–4 Bishop's Scale for Assessing Candidates for Induction of Labor

Assessment	Score*			
	0	1	2	3
Dilation (cm)	0	1–2	3–4	5–6
Effacement (%)	0–30	40 50	60–70	80
Station (cm)	−3	−2	−1	+1
Cervical consistency	Firm	Medium	Soft	
Fetal position	Posterior	Midline	Anterior	

Score _____

* Parous women induced at score of 5; nulliparous at score of 7.

4. Overdistended uterus
5. Grand multiparity (more than iv)
E. Medical management
1. Prostaglandin gel to cervix
2. Oxytocin
3. Artificial rupture of membranes

II. Analysis
A. Knowledge deficit related to procedure for induction of labor
B. High risk for altered tissue profusion (placental) related to oxytoxic uterine hyperstimulation
C. Pain related to uterine contractions

III. Planning/goals, expected outcomes
A. Client will have labor induced safely
B. Client will enter and maintain normal pattern of labor
C. Client will deliver healthy infant

IV. Implementation
A. Use Bishop's scale to assess induction potential
B. Apply fetal monitoring
C. Assist with application of prostaglandin gel to help soften cervix
D. Administer oxytocin as ordered (Table 16-5)
E. Continue to reassure client and inform her of progress of labor
F. Monitor closely for signs of fetal or maternal distress
G. Prepare for delivery of fetus

V. Evaluation
A. Client's labor safely induced
B. Client enters and maintains normal pattern of labor
C. Client delivers healthy infant

Rupture of Uterus

I. Assessment
A. Definition: rupture of uterus from stress of labor
B. Incidence: rare complication
C. Predisposing/precipitating factors
1. Prior uterine surgery or cesarean section
2. Oxytocin causing tetanic contractions
3. Labor that is not progressing
4. Hypertonic contractions
5. Fetal abnormalities
6. Faulty use of forceps
D. Complications
1. Hysterectomy
2. Maternal death
3. Fetal death
E. Clinical manifestations
1. Sudden onset of sharp, stabbing abdominal pain during labor

TABLE 16–5 Oxytocin (Pitocin)

Action	Side Effects	Nursing Implications
Stimulatory effect on the smooth muscle of the uterus; used to initiate or augment uterine contractions in the first or second stage of labor	Labor: hyperstimulation of the uterus; tetany and uterine rupture; rapid labor and birth; fetal distress and trauma from rapid delivery	Assess fetal heart rate, maternal vital signs, intake and output, uterine contraction frequency, duration, and resting tone
After delivery, the drug stimulates uterine contraction to prevent postpartum hemorrhage	After delivery: Water intoxication	Increase Pitocin drip according to hospital protocol and uterine response; piggyback oxytocin per secondary IV line; discontinue infusion if contractions exceed 60 seconds in duration, fetal distress presents, frequency of contractions is more than every 2 minutes, or insufficient relaxation of the uterus between contractions is noted

2. Manifestations of shock such as tachycardia, hypotension, and cold clammy skin
3. Cessation of uterine contractions
4. Rigidity of abdomen with internal bleeding
5. Palpation of hard uterine mass aside from fetus

  F. Surgical management
    1. Surgery to remove fetus
    2. Possible hysterectomy

II. Analysis
  A. Altered tissue perfusion related to excessive blood loss secondary to uterine rupture
  B. Pain related to uterine muscle rupture
  C. Fear related to birth outcome

III. Planning/goals, expected outcomes
  A. Client will not develop uterine rupture
  B. Client will have rupture diagnosed
  C. Client will have hemorrhage successfully treated
  D. Client will deliver healthy infant

IV. Implementation
  A. Assess client closely for development of hypertonic contractions
  B. Prepare client for emergency surgery
  C. Provide emotional support for client and family
  D. Monitor maternal and fetal vital signs closely
  E. Prepare client for possibility of emergency hysterectomy

V. Evaluation
  A. Client's uterus does not rupture
  B. Client's rupture is diagnosed early
  C. Client's hemorrhage is successfully treated
  D. Client delivers healthy infant

POST-TEST Labor and Delivery

1. Which of the following is the desired outcome of the second stage of labor?
  ① The client will be fully dilated
  ② The fetal head will be fully engaged
  ③ The client will deliver a healthy infant
  ④ The client will safely deliver the placenta

2. Which of the following is a typical manifestation of the third stage of labor?
  ① Increased bloody show rises
  ② Uterus assumes globular shape
  ③ Rectal pressure increases
  ④ Perineum bulges

3. Your client is a 25-year-old primigravida who is attached to a fetal monitor. The baseline FHR is 145 to 150 beats per minute. You notice that the FHR slows every time the client has a contraction and then returns to normal at the end of the contraction. This is best described as a:
  ① Type 1 deceleration
  ② Type 2 deceleration
  ③ Type 3 deceleration
  ④ Fetal distress

4. The treatment for the above alteration is to:
  ① Do nothing; this is a transient phenomenon
  ② Prepare for an emergency cesarean section
  ③ Reposition the client on her side
  ④ Prepare the client for impending vaginal delivery

5. Ann, a 26-year-old multigravida, is complaining of severe pain during the first stage of labor. Which of the following measures would treat the pain without interfering with the labor?
  ① Tranquilizers to calm her down
  ② Amnesiacs
  ③ Paracervical block
  ④ Pudendal block

6. Part of your initial assessment on a client

admitted in labor is to perform Leopold's maneuver to determine:

1. Contractions
2. Fetal position
3. FHR
4. Presence of fetal distress

7. Your client's membranes rupture spontaneously and in checking, you note that the umbilical cord has prolapsed. Which of the following is the priority nursing action for this situation?

1. Call the physician
2. Administer oxygen
3. Turn the mother to her side
4. Place the mother in Trendelenburg's position

8. Which of the following is the correct nursing intervention to help the client to push during delivery?

1. Instruct the client to take two breaths, hold, and bear down between contractions
2. Turn the client to her side and instruct her to use short breaths
3. Instruct the client to take two breaths, hold, and bear down with contractions
4. Encourage the client not to bear down since it may result in tears

9. Your client is suffering from dystocia in the form of hypotonic uterine contractions. Which of the following is a manifestation of the hypotonic contractions?

1. Increased frequency and intensity of contractions
2. Nonsynchronous uterine tension
3. Increased muscle tonus
4. Pain out of proportion to contractions

10. Which of the following is a clinical manifestation of prolonged labor?

1. Latent phase 8 hours in a primigravida
2. Active phase of 2 hours in a multipara
3. Dilation of 1 cm per hour in a multipara
4. Descent of less than 2 cm per hour in a multipara

11. Which of the following is an indication for the use of oxytocin for your client in labor?

1. Prolapse of the cord
2. History of previous cesarean section more than 5 years ago
3. Cervical dilation less than 3 cm
4. Hypotonic uterine contractions

12. Which of the following is an indication for stopping labor in a preterm mother?

1. Placental separation with hemorrhage
2. Severe eclampsia
3. Preterm contractions
4. Chorioamnionitis

13. Ritodrine is often used to treat preterm labor. Which of the following is a side effect of this drug?

1. Palpitations
2. Anorexia
3. Hyperkalemia
4. Constipation

14. Which of the following is an indication for induction of labor?

1. Persistant late decelerations
2. Uncontrolled diabetes
3. Hypertonic uterine contractions
4. Fetal bradycardia

15. Which of the following is a predisposing factor for rupture of the uterus?

1. Maternal age of less than 15
2. Hypotonic contractions
3. Primigravida
4. Cephalopelvic disproportion

POST-TEST Answers and Rationales

1. ③ The end of the second stage of labor is delivery of the fetus. The desired outcome is that the infant delivered is healthy. 3, IV. Labor and Delivery.

2. ② The uterus assumes a globular shape in the third stage of labor. Other options are typical of late first-stage labor. 1 & 2, IV. Labor and Delivery.

3. ① A Type 1 deceleration, known as early deceleration, is normal and is caused by pressure of the fetal head during contractions. Type 2 decelerations are late and indicate fetal hypoxia and decreased uteroplacental perfusion. Type 3 decelerations are variable and may indicate umbilical cord compression. 2, IV. Labor and Delivery.

4. ① Since this is a transient phenomenon caused by pressure of the fetal head, no action is needed. Choices 2 and 3 are actions for Types 2 and 3 decelerations. Choice 4 is inappropriate. 4, IV. Labor and Delivery.

5. ③ A paracervical block is a method of relieving pain without interfering with the progression of labor. Tranquilizers are not effective for pain, and amnesiacs are not used much anymore. A pudendal block is commonly used in the second stage of labor. 4, IV. Labor and Delivery.

6. ② Leopold's maneuver is performed to determine fetal position. It is done by palpation of the fundus for fetal parts to determine the position for delivery. 4, IV. Labor and Delivery.

7. ④ When the cord prolapses, it is an emergency because the blood flow to the fetus is disrupted. The priority action is to relieve the pressure on the cord, which can be done by placing the mother in Trendelenburg's. The nurse should also notify the physician and administer oxygen, but the priority action is the Trendelenburg's. 4, IV. Labor and Delivery.

8. ③ The client should bear down only during contractions, not between contractions. The client can push, so choice 4 is incorrect and choice 2 is ineffective. 4, IV. Labor and Delivery.

9. ② Hypotonic contractions are characterized by nonsynchronous uterine tension. The other options listed are symptoms of a hypertonic uterus. 1 & 2, IV. Labor and Delivery.

10. ④ Descent of less than 2 cm per hour in a multipara indicates a prolonged labor pattern. The remainder of the options are normal findings. 1 & 2, IV. Labor and Delivery.

11. ④ The only indication for oxytocin in the listed options is hypotonic uterine contractions. The other options are contraindicated for the use of oxytocin. 2, IV. Labor and Delivery.

12. ③ Preterm contractions are a symptom of preterm labor and may be controlled with ritodrine. The other options are indications for termination of the pregnancy. 2, IV. Labor and Delivery.

13. ① Palpitations are a common side effect of ritodrine administration. 1 & 2, IV. Labor and Delivery.

14. ② Uncontrolled diabetes is an indication for induction of labor. Other options are contraindications. 1 & 2, IV. Labor and Delivery.

15. ④ Cephalopelvic disproportion is a predisposing factor for rupture of the uterus. 1 & 2, IV. Labor and Delivery.

PRE-TEST Operative Procedures in Obstetrics

1. Which of the following is a characteristic of a mediolateral episiotomy?
   ① Effective and easily repaired
   ② Less painful
   ② Minimizes risk of extension to rectum
   ④ Less blood loss

2. Nursing care of an episiotomy would include which of the following during the first 4 hours?
   ① Using an ice pack
   ② Avoiding the use of analgesic sprays
   ③ Applying a heat lamp TID as ordered
   ④ Administering a sitz bath, especially after a bowel movement

3. Which of the following is a maternal predisposing factor for the use of forceps for delivery?
   ① Hypotonic dystocia
   ② Fetal tachycardia
   ③ Inability to push
   ④ Prolapse of the cord

4. Which of the following is a prerequisite to the use of forceps in delivery of a fetus?
   ① Cephalopelvic disproportion
   ② Fetal weight less than 7 lb
   ③ Engaged head
   ④ Occiput anterior position

5. Which of the following is likely to cause postpartum rectal incontinence and continued rectal problems?
   ① First-degree lacerations
   ② Second-degree lacerations
   ③ Third-degree lacerations
   ④ Mediolateral episiotomies

6. Which of the following complications is more likely to occur postpartum when the client has had a cesarean section rather than a normal vaginal delivery?
   ① Abdominal distention
   ② Uterine bleeding
   ③ Thrombophlebitis
   ④ Lochia rubra

PRE-TEST Answers and Rationales

1. ③ Mediolateral episiotomy minimizes the risk of extension to the rectum. Other options are considered advantages of a medial episiotomy. 1, IV. Operative Procedures.

2. ① Use of an ice pack in the immediately postpartum period minimizes the pain and edema to the area. Other options are appropriate later in the recovery period. 4, IV. Operative Procedures.

3. ③ Forceps are used when there is an inability to push. The other options are not considered indications. 1, IV. Operative Procedures.

4. ③ The fetal head must be engaged before application of forceps. Cephlopelvic

disproportion is a contraindication. 1, IV. Operative Procedures.

5. ③ Third-degree lacerations extend into the rectum through the sphincter, which results in problems with incontinence and healing. The scarring may cause long-term problems that may require further treatment to repair. 1 & 2, IV. Operative Procedures.

6. ① Abdominal distention is more likely to occur after abdominal surgery such as a cesarean section since the bowel must be moved to reach the uterus. This bowel manipulation results in abdominal distention. The other options occur in both cesarean section and normal vaginal delivery. 5, IV. Operative Procedures.

NURSING PROCESS APPLIED TO OPERATIVE PROCEDURES IN OBSTETRICS

Episiotomy

I. Assessment
   A. Definition: incision made into perineum to enlarge vaginal outlet and facilitate delivery
   B. Indications/purposes
      1. Large infant
      2. Rapid labor without enough time for stretching of perineum
      3. Malpresentation of fetus
      4. Narrow pubic arch and constricted outlet
      5. Prevents tearing of perineum
      6. Minimizes prolonged or severe stretching of muscles supporting bladder and rectum
      7. Reduces duration of second stage
      8. Enlarges vagina in case manipulation is needed
   C. Opposition to episiotomy
      1. Kegel exercises can work just as well both prenatally and postpartum
      2. Lacerations can occur even with episiotomy
      3. Pain from episiotomy distracts mother from infant interaction
   D. Types
      1. Median
         a. Most commonly used
         b. Effective and easily repaired
         c. Usually less painful
         d. Can result in third- or fourth-degree laceration into rectum
      2. Mediolateral (right or left)
         a. Minimizes risk of extension into rectum
         b. Greater blood loss
         c. More difficult to repair
         d. Healing more painful
   E. Clinical manifestations: (after episiotomy)
      1. REEDA method:
         a. *R*edness
         b. *E*dema
         c. *E*cchymosis
         d. *D*ischarge
         e. *A*pproximation
      2. Hematomas
      3. Pain
II. Analysis
   A. Pain related to effects of surgical episiotomy
   B. Knowledge deficit related to postdelivery episiotomy care
III. Planning/goals, expected outcomes
   A. Client will properly care for episiotomy
   B. Client will have episiotomy pain relieved
   C. Client will have episiotomy heal without complications
IV. Implementation
   A. Check episiotomy site for REEDA
   B. Institute measures to relieve pain
      1. Ice pack first 24 hours
      2. Sitz bath
      3. Heat lamp TID as ordered

4. Apply analgesic spray or ointment as ordered
C. Provide peri care using clean technique
D. Teach client proper care of incision
   1. Dry from front to back
   2. Blot area rather than wiping it
   3. Shower rather than tub bath
   4. Apply peri pad without touching inside surface
   5. Report any bleeding or discharge to physician
V. Evaluation
   A. Client cares for episiotomy properly
   B. Client's episiotomy pain relieved
   C. Client's episiotomy heals without complications

Forceps Delivery

I. Assessment
   A. Definition: two double-crossed, spoon-like articulated blades that are used to assist in delivery of fetal head
   B. Predisposing/precipitating factors
      1. Maternal
         a. Shorten second stage in dystocia
         b. Expulsive efforts deficient
         c. Cannot push because of cardiac decompensation or other risk
      2. Fetal
         a. Fetal distress close to delivery
         b. Arrested descent
         c. Difficult presentation
   C. Prerequisites to forceps delivery
      1. Fully dilated cervix
      2. Engaged head
      3. Vertex or face presentation
      4. Absence of cephalopelvic disproportion
      5. Empty bladder and bowel
   D. Types
      1. High forceps
         a. Biparietal dimension of vertex above ischial spine
         b. Not allowed in most institutions
      2. Midforceps
         a. Vertex at ischial tuberosities
         b. May be difficult delivery
      3. Low forceps
         a. Vertex distending introitus
         b. Use to control and guide head
         c. Should be easy delivery
   E. Complications
      1. Perineal lacerations
         a. First-degree laceration: fourchette, perineal skin, vaginal mucosa
         b. Second-degree laceration: skin, mucous membrane, muscles of perineal body
         c. Third-degree laceration: above plus rectal sphincter
         d. Fourth-degree laceration: above plus tear into lumen of rectum
      2. Damage to facial nerve of fetus from pressure with unilateral temporary paralysis
      3. Fetal death with high forceps or even midforceps
      4. Postpartal hemorrhage with midforceps
      5. Cystocele, rectocele, or uterine prolapse later in life
II. Analysis
   A. High risk for fetal/maternal injury related to forceps delivery
   B. Fear related to maternal/fetal risk of injury related to forceps delivery
III. Planning/goals, expected outcomes
   A. Client will be free from injury following forceps delivery
   B. Infant will be free from injury following forceps delivery
IV. Implementation
   A. Assist physician with correct forceps
   B. Reassure client and explain need for forceps
   C. Monitor mother and fetus during delivery
   D. Check infant and mother after delivery for any possible injury
   E. Assist with repair of any lacerations
V. Evaluation
   A. Client free from injury following forceps delivery
   B. Infant free from injury following forceps delivery

Vacuum Extraction

I. Assessment
   A. Definition: delivery of fetus in vertex presentation with use of cup suction applied to fetal scalp for traction; adds traction to involuntary and voluntary efforts; more physiological than forceps
   B. Predisposing/precipitating factors: same as for forceps delivery
   C. Complications
      1. Cephalotrauma, cerebral trauma, or fetal head tissue necrosis
      2. Trauma to vagina and cervix
      3. Postpartum hemorrhage
II. Analysis
   A. High risk for fetal/maternal injury related to vacuum delivery
   B. Fear related to maternal/fetal risk of injury related to vacuum delivery

III. Planning/goals, expected outcomes
  A. Client will be free from injury following vacuum delivery
  B. Infant will be free from injury following vacuum delivery
IV. Implementation
  A. Explain procedure to client
  B. Continue monitoring fetus and mother
  C. Pump suction apparatus per protocol or physician's orders
  D. Assess infant for cerebral trauma
V. Evaluation
  A. Client free from injury following vacuum delivery
  B. Infant free from injury following vacuum delivery

Cesarean Delivery

I. Assessment
  A. Definition: delivery of fetus through transabdominal incision of uterus
  B. Indications
    1. Past cesarean deliveries or uterine surgery
    2. Cephalopelvic disproportion
    3. Severe maternal disease: eclampsia, diabetes, cardiac disease
    4. Placenta previa or abruptio placentae
    5. Dystocia
    6. Pelvic tumors or trauma
    7. Maternal venereal disease such as herpes
    8. Fetal distress
    9. Prolapsed cord
    10. Multiple fetuses
    11. Fetal abnormalities, hydrocephalus
    12. Malpresentation
  C. Types
    1. Classic: vertical incision of skin and uterus
      a. Simple, rapid
      b. Good for anterior placenta previa
    2. Low cervical
      a. Pfannenstiel of skin with vertical incision of uterus
      b. Pfannenstiel of skin and low horizontal incision of uterus
  D. Complications (see Chapter 6, Surgical Intervention)
II. Analysis
  A. Knowledge deficit related to cesarean birth
  B. Impaired gas exchange related to shallow breathing from incisional pain
  C. Pain related to surgical incision and uterine involution
  D. High risk for infection related to surgical incision
III. Planning/goals, expected outcomes

A. Client will have need for cesarean delivery diagnosed early
B. Client will be physically and emotionally prepared for surgery
C. Client will deliver healthy infant
D. Client will recover from surgery without complication
IV. Implementation
  A. Preoperative
    1. If planned, prepare client, as discussed in Chapter 6
    2. If emergency, quickly explain need and procedure to client
    3. Obtain signed informed consent
    4. Make sure that usual preoperative diagnostic tests are done plus Rh factor
    5. Insert IV line and Foley catheter
    6. Prep abdomen as ordered
    7. Monitor client and fetus continuously for vital signs and signs of labor
    8. Provide emotional support
    9. Administer preoperative medications as ordered
  B. Postoperative
    1. Assess vital signs every 15 minutes until stable
    2. Encourage coughing and deep breathing
    3. Allow mother-infant interaction as soon as possible
    4. Monitor for signs of bleeding, both abdominal and vaginal
    5. Palpate position and consistency of fundus
    6. Continue postoperative care as described in Chapter 6, Surgical Intervention
V. Evaluation
  A. Client's need for cesarean delivery diagnosed early
  B. Client physically and emotionally prepared for surgery
  C. Client delivers healthy infant
  D. Client recovers from surgery without complication

POST-TEST Operative Procedures in Obstetrics

Lynn Graham, age 38, is admitted in the 39th week for a planned cesarean delivery because of total placenta previa.

---

1. Which of the following physician orders should the nurse question?
   ① Implement continuous FHR monitoring

   ② Insert Foley catheter
   ③ Monitor for uterine contractions
   ④ Check for cervical dilation/effacement

2. The chief potential problem for this fetus is:
   ① High risk for impaired gas exchange related to impaired circulation
   ② Alteration in nutrition: less than required nutrients
   ③ High risk for infection related to cesarean birth
   ④ High risk for injury related to placental placement

3. A primary goal before Lynn's delivery is:
   ① Client is free from undetected complications
   ② Client and significant other are together during preparation and surgery
   ③ Client expresses her fears and concerns
   ④ Client is well hydrated before delivery

4. A spinal anesthesia is administered, and the client appears relaxed. Immediately afterward, the blood pressure changes from 120/88 to 100/70 mm Hg and FHR drops from 144 to 118. What is the probable reason for this change?
   ① Adverse response to regional anesthetic
   ② Pressure on aorta and vena cava while supine
   ③ Poor oxygenation due to placenta previa
   ④ Anxiety about the cesarean delivery

5. What is the appropriate intervention for the above problem at this time?
   ① Elevate the feet and legs
   ② Administer oxygen by mask
   ③ Increase the IV infusion rate
   ④ Turn the client slightly to the left

6. A 7-lb daughter is delivered several minutes later. Apgar score is 9 and 10. Which of the following assessments would receive a score of 1 at the initial scoring?
   ① Heart rate of 128
   ② Loud cry
   ③ Blue feet
   ④ Flexed body

7. The total blood loss during delivery is 700 mL. The couple prefer to avoid a transfusion if possible. Based on her history and intrapartal situation, which of the following recovery room assessments is critical in addition to observing lochia?
   ① Blood pressure
   ② Pulse rate
   ③ Temperature
   ④ Level of consciousness

8. In assessing physiological adaptation to the postpartum period, which of the following statements made by the client indicates that she is able to be transferred to her regular room?
   ① "I have a little pain in the incision."
   ② "I'd like to sleep in my own room now."
   ③ "I am thirsty and would like my lips sponged."
   ④ "I feel my legs again as I move them."

9. The physician orders 1000 mL of Ringer's lactate at 124 mL/hr with Pitocin 10 units added to the IV line. The drip factor is 10 gtt/mL. Select the appropriate rate of infusion.
   ① 17 gtt per minute
   ② 21 gtt per minute
   ③ 27 gtt per minute
   ④ 31 gtt per minute

POST-TEST Answers and Rationales

1. ④ A pelvic examination to determine cervical dilation/effacement is contraindicated with suspected placenta previa so the nurse would question this order. 1, IV. Placenta Previa.

2. ④ The greatest danger to the fetus is from delivery of the placenta before the birth. This in turn leads to anoxia and fetal death unless immediate cesarean birth is performed. 2, IV. Placenta Previa.

3. ① During preparation for surgery, it is essential to observe for signs of bleeding or labor contractions. The other goals are part of the preparation for every woman and are not specific to this problem. 3, IV. Placenta Previa.

4. ② Hypotension and fetal bradycardia frequently follow administration of spinal anesthesia due to the pressure on the aorta and vena cava. 2, IV. Cesarean Section.

5. ④ This implementation is appropriate for any pregnant client who experiences a blood pressure drop; it is suggested for each woman throughout the pregnancy. 4, IV. Cesarean Section.

6. ③ Cyanosis of hands or feet results in a score of 1 of a possible 2. Other assessments are indications of normal adaptation to extrauterine life. 1, IV. Post-Cesarean Section.

7. ② Of the assessments suggested, pulse rate changes immediately in shock related to hemorrhage. Blood pressure often adapts on shock, and temperature and level of consciousness could be late signs. 1, IV. Post-Cesarean Section.

8. ④ When leg sensation and mobility return and the client is stable, she may be transferred out of the recovery room. 5, IV. Post-Cesarean Section.

9. ② 124 mL/60 min × 10 gtt/mL = 21 drops per minute. 4, IV. Post-Cesarean Section.

17

Postpartum Period

PRE-TEST Postpartum Period

Lisa Daley, age 37, delivered her fifth son 3 hours ago in the birthing room.

1. Which of the following data shared at morning report indicates a potential problem?
   ① The fundus is firm, just above the umbilicus
   ② The client is complaining about uterine cramps
   ③ The episiotomy is swollen with a small bruise
   ④ The vital signs are temperature 98°F, pulse 68, and respirations 20

2. Lisa's blood type is O-negative, and the baby is O-positive. RhoGam is ordered before discharge after results of the Coombs' test are known. What information is essential before giving the RhoGam?
   ① Isoimmunization has occurred
   ② RhoGam was given after the last birth
   ③ No antibodies are present
   ④ There are no known allergies

3. Lisa is concerned about how her other children, ages 2, 3, 5, and 15, will accept the baby. Which response shows an understanding of her feelings?
   ① "Things will be difficult in the first weeks."
   ② "Their reactions will depend on how you prepared them."
   ③ "Let's talk about what concerns you."

   ④ "Sometimes it's better to avoid worrying too much."

4. The client, who bottle-fed her older children, has many questions about breast-feeding. What approach is most helpful initially?
   ① Assess her knowledge and be available during feedings
   ② Use pamphlets and films as a first step in teaching
   ③ Introduce her to a successful breast-feeding mother
   ④ Tell her the reasons why breast-feeding is beneficial

5. Before discharge, Lisa discusses family planning. Which statement indicates that she needs further teaching?
   ① "I'll start to take oral contraceptives immediately."
   ② "If I want to use a diaphragm, I'll need to be checked first."
   ③ "We'll avoid intercourse when cervical mucus is stretchable."
   ④ "I will not rely on breast-feeding as contraception."

6. As the newborn is prepared for discharge, the father asks about care of the umbilical cord stump. Which of the following is the most appropriate response?
   ① "Apply an antibiotic ointment to the area daily."
   ② "Apply alcohol to the cord and base with each diaper change."
   ③ "Let the baby soak in the bath until the cord falls off."
   ④ "No special care is needed. The cord will heal in a week."

NURSING PROCESS APPLIED TO THE CLIENT DURING THE POSTPARTUM PERIOD

Physiology of the Puerperium

I. Assessment
   A. Definition: postpartum period (puerperium) starts immediately after delivery and is completed when reproductive tract returns to normal nonpregnant state (usually defined as 6 weeks)
   B. Uterus
      1. Involution: rapid diminution in size of uterus as it returns to nonpregnant state
         a. Weight of uterus decreases from 2 lb to 2 oz
         b. Endometrium regenerates
         c. Fundus steadily descends into pelvis; fundal height decreases about one fingerbreadth (1 cm) per day; by 10 days postpartum, cannot be palpated abdominally
      2. Lochia: discharge from uterus that consists of blood from vessels of placental site and debris from decidua
         a. Rubra: delivery day to day 3, bright red
         b. Serosa: days 4 to 10, brownish pink
         c. Alba: days 10 to 14, white
         d. Normally has fleshy odor
         e. Decreases daily in amount
         f. Increases with ambulation
      3. Afterbirth pains: contractions of uterus
         a. More common in multiparas
         b. More common in breast-feeding mothers
         c. More common in clients treated with oxytocic drugs
         d. More common in clients who had overdistended uterus during pregnancy
   C. Cervix and vagina
      1. Cervical involution
         a. After 1 week, muscle begins to regenerate
         b. External os remains wider in nonparous women
         c. Internal os closed after 1 week
      2. Vagina
         a. Vaginal distention decreases, although muscle tone never restored completely to pregravid state
         b. Vaginal rugae begin to reappear around third week
         c. Lacerations or episiotomy suture line gradually heal
   D. Ovarian function and menstruation
      1. Ovarian function depends on rapidity with which pituitary function restored
      2. Menstrual flow resumes within 8 weeks in non–breast-feeding mothers
      3. Menstrual flow usually resumes within 3 to 4 months in breast-feeding mothers; breast-feeding mothers may experience amenorrhea during entire period of lactation
      4. Women may ovulate without menstruating, so breast-feeding should not be considered form of birth control

E. Breasts
1. Little change in breasts during first 2 days postpartum
2. Breasts continue to secrete colostrum as during pregnancy
3. Decrease of estrogen and progesterone levels after delivery stimulate increased prolactin level, which promotes breast milk production
4. Breasts become distended with milk on third day
5. Breast-feeding will relieve engorgement
6. Engorgement 48 to 72 hours in non–breast-feeding mothers

F. Urinary tract
1. May have urinary retention due to loss of elasticity and tone and loss of sensation from trauma, drugs, anesthesia, loss of privacy
2. Diuresis: usually begins within first 12 hours after delivery
3. Kidney function returns to normal rapidly

G. Gastrointestinal tract
1. Women usually very hungry after delivery
2. Constipation can occur because of decreased muscle tone in intestines and perineal tenderness
3. Hemorrhoids common, generally subside

H. Vascular system
1. WBCs increase during labor and early postpartum period and then return to normal in a few days
2. Hemoglobin and RBCs decrease; hematocrit usually returns to normal in 1 week
3. Elevated fibrinogen levels during first week postpartum; may contribute to thrombophlebitis
4. Blood volume usually back to prenatal level by third week

I. Vital signs
1. Temperature may be elevated to 100.4°F (38°C) during first 24 hours without pathology
2. Bradycardia common during first week; range, 50 to 70
3. Blood pressure remains unchanged

II. Analysis
A. Knowledge deficit related to postpartum involutional changes and self-care behavior
B. Pain related to uterine involution and perineal trauma
C. Constipation related to decreased bowel tone, hormonal effects of pregnancy, and decreased activity level

III. Planning/goals, expected outcomes
A. Client will resume nonpregnant physiological function
B. Client will maintain satisfactory comfort level
C. Client will have opportunity to rest
D. Client will state an understanding of the involutional process and will facilitate process where indicated
E. Client will verbalize an understanding of nutritional requirements during the postpartum period

IV. Implementation
A. Assessments of involution
1. Check height, consistency, and location of fundus
2. Monitor vital signs
3. Check color, amount, and odor of lochia
4. Check breasts for engorgement
5. Maintain I & O as ordered
6. Check perineum for swelling or discoloration
7. Check episiotomy for healing
8. Monitor bowel status
9. Assess bonding with infant
10. Assess emotional status
11. Encourage ambulation
12. Check dressing of cesarean birth client
13. Administer RhoGam as ordered within 72 hours postpartum to Rh-negative client who is not sensitized

B. Comfort measures
1. Afterpains
a. Result of intermittent uterine contractions postdelivery
b. Encourage ambulation; makes uterine contractions more effective, less painful
c. Encourage frequent voiding
d. If client experiencing extreme discomfort with breast-feeding, administer analgesic 30 minutes before feeding
2. Perineal discomfort
a. Apply ice pack during first 24 hours to reduce swelling
b. After first 24 hours, use warmth (sitz baths or perineal light)
3. Discomfort from episiotomy
a. Teach client to administer perineal care after each voiding
b. Encourage use of analgesic spray such as Dermoplast
c. Encourage use of Tucks (witch hazel compresses); keep in refrigerator for increased analgesic effect
d. Administer analgesic only after other measures unsuccessful

4. Breast discomfort from engorgement
   a. Encourage wearing of supporting bra at all times, even while sleeping
   b. Use ice packs if not breast-feeding
   c. Use warm soaks before feeding for breast-feeding mother
   d. Administer analgesic if comfort measures not effective
5. Postoperative pain from cesarean section: managed same as postoperative pain from any abdominal surgery

C. Provide for rest
1. Arrange care to provide rest periods between feedings and visiting hours
2. Encourage client to take naps

D. Promote return to prepregnant state
1. Teach client appropriate exercises for postpartum period
2. Discuss client's schedule at home, and stress importance of adequate rest
3. Stress importance of 6-week checkup

E. Provide nutritional counseling
1. Discuss caloric intake: about 3000 calories if breast-feeding, about 2300 calories if not breast-feeding
2. Review basic four food groups
3. Encourage nutritious snacks and increased fluids
4. Advise lactating mothers to increase amount of protein, calcium, iron, phosphorus, and vitamins

V. Evaluation
A. Client resumes nonpregnant physiological function
B. Client maintains satisfactory comfort level
C. Client is rested
D. Client facilitates process of involution
E. Client's nutritional status is adequate

Emotional Reactions During Puerperium

I. Assessment
A. Rubin's postpartum phases
1. Taking-in (first 2 to 3 days)
   a. Mother's primary needs are her own—sleep, food
   b. Mother usually quite talkative, focusing on labor and delivery experience
   c. Important for nurse to listen and help mother interpret events to make them more meaningful; not optimum time to teach baby care
2. Taking-hold phase (third day to 2 weeks—varies with each individual)
   a. More in control; begins to take hold of task of "mothering"
   b. Important time for teaching; nurse must provide ego support because mother very sensitive about "doing things right"
3. Letting-go phase
   a. Mother may feel deep loss over separation of baby from part of body and may grieve over loss
   b. Mother may be caught in dependent-independent role, wanting to feel safe and secure yet wanting to make decisions; teenage mothers need special consideration because of conflicts taking place within them as part of adolescence
   c. Postpartum blues
      (1) May feel upset and depressed at times
      (2) Reaction varies with individual
      (3) Condition caused by physiological and emotional stress
      (4) Verbalization should be encouraged
      (5) Blues may progress to postpartum depression if unresolved
   d. Parenting
      (1) Readiness: client must be physically comfortable and emotionally ready
      (2) Skills need to be taught: feeding, bathing, dressing, growth and development, health considerations, safety measures
   e. Bonding/attachment
      (1) Better if facilitated early in puerperium (delivery room if possible)
      (2) Bonding process should be continuous

II. Analysis
A. Family coping: potential for growth related to birth experience
B. Knowledge deficit related to care of infant

III. Planning/goals, expected outcomes
A. Client will successfully adapt to parental role
B. Client will reach emotional equilibrium
C. Client will attach to newborn
D. Client will demonstrate competence in caring for newborn

IV. Implementation
A. Promote optimum parent-infant interactions during early postpartum period
1. Allow periods of time for both mother and significant other to be alone with infant
2. Allow parents to hold infant in delivery

room and recovery room; provide rooming-in and privacy

3. Encourage parents to make eye contact with infant
4. Encourage parents to explore infant
5. Compare baby's likenesses to and differences from other family members

B. Plan nursing care to reduce maternal fatigue and anxiety so that time with infant is pleasurable
C. Provide role model for parents
D. Support mother in infant care activities and use these opportunities to promote self-esteem
E. Demonstrate infant care skills as necessary
   1. Offer opportunity for mother to bathe infant in hospital
   2. Review and assess feeding technique
   3. Answer questions about newborn care, behavior, and basic needs
F. Review approaches to managing sibling rivalry—extra attention and special times needed for other children
G. Explain to parents that it is normal at this time to feel fatigued, tense, insecure, and sometimes depressed
H. Explain to parents that it is normal to feel overwhelmed with new roles and infant care; emphasize resources and written information for early discharge
I. Counsel client on discharge instructions
   1. Work—avoid heavy lifting for at least 3 weeks
   2. Rest—plan at least one rest period per day
   3. Hygiene—cleanse perineum from front to back; no douching until return for postpartum checkup
   4. Coitus—safe as soon as lochia has returned to alba and episiotomy is healed (about 3 weeks)
   5. Contraception—should begin after delivery or with initiation of coitus
   6. Follow-up—schedule at 4 to 6 weeks; report any signs of chills, fever, increased lochia, depressed feeling to physician/midwife immediately

V. Evaluation
   A. Client appears relaxed and secure in interactions with infant and new parental role
   B. Client does not appear unduly depressed or anxious
   C. Client exhibits bonding behaviors such as gazing at, cuddling, talking to, and fondling infant
   D. Client plans time away from infant

E. Client demonstrates increasing levels of competence in carrying out tasks of newborn care

Breast-Feeding

I. Assessment
   A. Establishment of lactation
      1. Colostrum secreted during first 2 to 3 days postpartum
      2. Prolactin released from anterior pituitary gland
      3. Oxytocin (released from posterior pituitary) causes let-down reflex
II. Analysis: effective breast-feeding related to basic breast-feeding knowledge
III. Planning/goals, expected outcome
   A. Client will position infant to breast to promote successful latch-on response
   B. Client will report regular and sustained sucking at the breast (8 to 10 times every 24 hours)
   C. Infant will appear content after feedings and demonstrate adequate weight gain
IV. Implementation
   A. Put baby to breast as soon as mother's and baby's condition stable—on delivery table if possible
   B. Stay with client each time she nurses until she feels secure or confident with baby and feelings
   C. Client education
      1. General principles
         a. Uterine cramping may occur first days after delivery while nursing, when oxytocin stimulation causes uterus to contract
         b. Use general hygiene and wash the breast once daily; do not use soap as it tends to remove natural oils and increase chances of cracking
         c. Nipple-rolling exercise should be done, particularly if nipple flattened
         d. Bra should be well-fitted and supporting
         e. Breasts may leak between feedings or during coitus; place breast pad in bra
         f. Calories should be increased to 3000 per day, including 1½ quarts of milk and 1000 mL additional fluids
         g. Baby's stools will be light yellow, watery, and frequent
         h. At 1 month, baby will nurse 15 to 20 minutes on each breast
         i. Medications should be avoided unless prescribed

j. Gas-producing foods should be avoided
k. Birth control pills should not be taken
2. Schedule
   a. Initially, infant should be put to breast as soon as possible after delivery
   b. If unable to nurse infant, initiate breast pump as soon as client can tolerate
   c. Gradually increase time on each breast with subsequent feedings
   d. Baby will develop own feeding schedule
3. Procedure for mother
   a. Wash hands and assume comfortable position
   b. Start with breast last feeding ended with (baby sucks more vigorously at the beginning of feeding)
   c. Stroke baby's cheek with nipple to stimulate rooting
   d. Guide nipple and surrounding areola into baby's mouth
   e. Gently press breast away from baby's nose
   f. After baby has nursed, release suction by depressing infant's chin or inserting clean finger into baby's mouth
   g. Burp baby after first breast
   h. Repeat procedure on second breast until the baby stops nursing
   i. Burp baby again
4. Problems and solutions
   a. Engorgement
      (1) Breast-feed frequently
      (2) Apply warm packs before feeding
      (3) Apply ice packs between feedings
   b. Retracted nipples
      (1) Do nipple rolling before feeding
      (2) Wear breast shield at beginning of feeding, which will act as a vacuum when baby sucks and will pull nipple out; then remove shield
   c. Cracked nipples
      (1) Lubricate with A & D ointment after feeding
      (2) Expose nipples to air for 10 to 20 minutes after each feeding
      (3) Rotate position of baby for each feeding
   d. Inadequate milk, manifested by baby's hunger as baby grows
      (1) Increase frequency of feedings to increase milk supply
      (2) Revert to longer intervals once supply increases
V. Evaluation
   A. Client successfully breast-feeds
   B. Client appears relaxed and comfortable while breast-feeding
   C. Client expresses satisfaction with ability to breast-feed
   D. Infant gaining weight and appears satisfied between feedings

Family Planning

I. Assessment
   A. Types of contraceptives (Table 17-1)
   B. Ineffective methods of family planning
      1. Coitus interruptus: withdrawal of penis before ejaculation
      2. Breast-feeding
II. Analysis: knowledge deficit related to proper use of chosen contraceptive method
III. Planning/goals, expected outcomes
   A. Client will be knowledgeable in methods of family planning
   B. Client will understand sexual adjustment that occurs after childbirth
IV. Implementation
   A. Review methods of family planning
   B. Discuss sexual adjustment: explain that sexual relations may be resumed as soon as healing takes place, bleeding stops, and client feels comfortable with it
   C. Warn that fatigue and hormonal changes may influence desires
   D. Tell couple that altered body image may affect satisfaction
   E. If client plans to use birth control measures, instruct her to begin as soon as she resumes coitus
   F. Client should consult physician before resuming use of birth control pills, diaphragm (must be refitted), or IUD
V. Evaluation
   A. Client knowledgeable concerning methods of family planning
   B. Client understands sexual adjustment that occurs after childbirth

Disorders During Puerperium

Postpartum Hemorrhage
I. Assessment
   A. Definition: bleeding of 500 mL or more following delivery
   B. Incidence

TABLE 17-1 Family Planning Measures

Type	Action	Teaching Implications
Natural family planning	Avoidance of coitus during fertile period	Daily body temperature recording plots time of ovulation; usually 14 days before next menses; abstinence recommended from day 6 through day 14 for an average 28-day cycle; cervical mucus becomes stretchable at ovulation; Spinnbarkeit (cervical mucus method)
Oral contraception	Inhibits ovulation; alters cervical mucus	Pill must be taken according to schedule; teach patient to report side effects; headaches, edema, hypertension, amenorrhea, breakthrough bleeding
Spermicides (creams, jelly, suppositories)	Destroys sperm or neutralizes vaginal secretions	Effectiveness increases when used with a condom; report any local tissue irritation
Long-acting progestin implants (Norplant)	Inhibits ovulation	Six Silastic capsules containing a progestin are implanted in the patient's arm; side effects include spotting, irregular bleeding, amenorrhea, weight gain, headache, depression; effective for up to 5 years
Diaphragm	Barrier method	Inserted before coitus with spermicidal cream or jelly placed around rim and in the dome; must be professionally fitted and rechecked after childbirth, weight gain, or loss of 15 lb; necessary to leave in place for 6 to 8 hours after coitus; side effects: urinary tract infections
Condom	Barrier method	Sheath placed over the erect penis before intercourse to collect semen; affords some protection against sexually transmitted diseases; side effects: perineal or vaginal irritation
Surgical sterilization (vasectomy/tubal ligation)	Permanent interruption of reproductive capacity	Even though procedures are theoretically reversible, permanency should be stressed before this procedure; vasectomy: ligation of the vas deferens; pain and swelling at the incision site during the first week is common; takes 4 to 6 weeks and 6 to 36 ejaculations to clear sperm from vas deferens; follow-up semen count necessary; tubal ligation: interruption of tubal patency by coagulation, ligation, or banding; complications include hemorrhage, infection, bowel perforation

1. Early: one in 200 births within first 24 hours after birth
2. Late: one in 1000 births between second day and sixth week
C. Predisposing/precipitating factors
    1. Uterine atony: most common cause
    2. Lacerations
    3. Retained placental fragments
D. Clinical manifestations
    1. Copious amount of vaginal bleeding with or without bright or dark red clots
    2. Boggy uterus, indicating uterine atony
    3. Manifestations of maternal shock
        a. Rapid pulse
        b. Pale, clammy skin
        c. Diaphoresis
        d. Restlessness
E. Complication: leading cause of maternal mortality, 25% of all maternal deaths from hemorrhagic complications
II. Analysis
    A. Fluid volume deficit related to postpartum hemorrhage secondary to uterine atony
    B. High risk for altered tissue perfusion related to excess lochia
    C. Anxiety related to change in health status
III. Planning/goals, expected outcomes
    A. Client will be monitored for signs of hemorrhage and shock
    B. Client will safely receive blood volume replacement as indicated
    C. Client will not experience uncontrollable anxiety
IV. Implementation
    A. Remain with client
    B. Assess and estimate blood loss—pad count
    C. Massage fundus, being careful not to over-massage
    D. Notify physician if hemorrhage occurs
    E. Check vital signs and fundus every 5 to 15 minutes
    F. Monitor I & O
    G. Monitor fluid replacement and oxytocin administration
    H. Observe for blood reactions if transfused
    I. Assess level of consciousness

J. Maintain asepsis since hemorrhage predisposes to infection

K. Monitor hemoglobin and hematocrit levels

L. Explain situation carefully to client and family to help allay anxiety

M. Return client to delivery room or to surgery for removal of placental tissue or to repair laceration

N. Teach client signs and symptoms of possible late hemorrhage

O. Counsel client to increase iron in diet; iron supplements and Imferon may be ordered

P. Arrange for follow-up care

V. Evaluation

A. Client free from hemorrhage

B. Client verbalizes manifestations of hemorrhage

C. Client's high anxiety level alleviated

Subinvolution

I. Assessment

A. Definition: condition that exists when normal involution of puerperal uterus retarded

B. Predisposing/precipitating factors

1. Poor uterine tone

2. Retained placenta

3. Endometritis

4. Fibroids or tumors

5. Displacement of uterus

C. Clinical manifestations

1. Enlarged, boggy, tender uterus

2. Profuse, prolonged lochia rubra

3. Backache

4. Pelvic discomfort

5. Dragging sensation

II. Analysis

A. Fluid volume deficit related to prolonged lochia secondary to uterine subinvolution

B. High risk for infection related to altered involution of the uterus

C. Anxiety related to alteration in health status

III. Planning/goals, expected outcomes

A. Client will demonstrate normal involution of puerperal uterus

B. Client will not demonstrate unusual anxiety

IV. Implementation

A. Administer Methergine or ergotrate as ordered (see Table 15–4)

B. Administer antibiotics as ordered to prevent infection

C. Explain condition and treatment to client

D. Encourage ambulation

V. Evaluation

A. Uterus decreases in size and descends into pelvis

B. Bleeding is controlled and loss of blood is minimized

C. Infection is prevented

D. Client's anxiety is allayed

Postpartum Infection

I. Assessment

A. Definition: any infection of reproductive organs that occurs within 28 days of delivery or abortion

B. Etiology

1. Bacterial causative agents

2. *Escherichia coli*

3. Mixed aerobic/anaerobic infection

C. Predisposing/precipitating factors

1. Weakened resistance due to prolonged labor and dehydration

2. Traumatic delivery

3. Excessive vaginal examinations during labor

4. Premature rupture of membranes

5. Excessive blood loss

6. Anemia

7. Intrautcrine manipulation

8. Retained placental fragments

D. Clinical manifestations

1. Temperature more than 101°F (38.3°C), chills

2. Foul-smelling lochia

3. Abdominal tenderness, pelvic pain

4. Dysuria, burning on urination

5. Tachycardia

6. Increased WBCs

7. Malaise, anorexia

8. Delayed involution

E. Complication: one of three leading causes of maternal mortality

II. Analysis

A. High risk for infection related to trauma associated with childbirth

B. High risk for social isolation related to precautions necessary to protect baby and others from exposure to infectious organisms

III. Planning/goals, expected outcomes

A. Client will be monitored for early clinical manifestations of local or systemic infection

B. Client's mother-baby relationship will be supported throughout treatment process

IV. Implementation

A. Administer antibiotics according to organism, as ordered

B. Maintain asepsis (isolate from baby)

C. Monitor temperature every 2 to 4 hours

D. Monitor IV therapy

E. Maintain bedrest

F. Monitor vital signs every 4 hours

G. Monitor I & O

1. Force fluids 3000 to 4000 mL, if not contraindicated

2. Encourage frequent voiding
H. Make client as comfortable as possible
   1. Keep warmed if chilled
   2. Position for comfort
   3. Use heat and cold as indicated to relieve localized pain
   4. Administer analgesics as needed
I. Provide restful environment; client usually anxious, exhausted, and very uncomfortable
J. Monitor laboratory studies with blood and urine
K. Provide nutritious high-calorie, high-protein diet
L. Place client in Fowler's or semi-Fowler's position
M. Position as ordered to promote drainage
N. Explain all procedures
O. Keep client informed about condition of newborn
P. Encourage client to express feelings about separation from infant
Q. Teach good perineal hygiene techniques and encourage handwashing
V. Evaluation
A. Client shows evidence of response to treatment for infection
B. Complications do not develop
C. Client-baby relationship maintained

Mastitis

I. Assessment
A. Definition: inflammation of breast as result of infection; mainly seen in breast-feeding mothers, 2 to 3 weeks after delivery
B. Etiology/incidence
   1. Bacteria causative agents
   2. Occurs in about 1% of women who have recently delivered
C. Predisposing/precipitating factors
   1. Nipple fissure
   2. Erosion of areola
   3. Milk stasis or overdistention
D. Clinical manifestations
   1. Breast lobe may appear hard, red, painful, and tender
   2. Engorgement
   3. Elevated temperature, chills
   4. Tachycardia
E. Complication: condition generally preventable; prompt and appropriate treatment with antibiotic therapy significantly decreases maternal morbidity
II. Analysis
A. Pain related to infectious process
B. High risk for infection related to nipple fissure, milk status, or overdistention

C. High risk for ineffective breast-feeding due to interruption of breast-feeding
III. Planning/goals, expected outcomes
A. Client will not experience undetected mastitis
B. Client will re-establish normal lactation pattern
C. Client will not develop complications such as breast abscess
IV. Implementation
A. Administer antibiotics as ordered
B. Promote comfort of client
   1. Support breasts with supportive brassiere
   2. Apply heat or cold as indicated
   3. Administer analgesics as ordered
C. Maintain lactation in breast-feeding mothers
   1. Regular nursing of infant (controversial, will vary with physician)
   2. Manual expression of breast milk or use of breast pump every 4 hours
D. Offer emotional support
E. If indicated, prepare client for incision and drainage of abscess
F. Teach good handwashing and breast hygiene
V. Evaluation
A. Client shows evidence of response to treatment for infection
B. Client re-establishes normal lactation pattern
C. Client does not develop breast abscess

Cystitis

I. Assessment
A. Definition: infection of bladder
B. Etiology/incidence
   1. Coliform bacteria
   2. Occurs in 5% of postpartum women
C. Predisposing/precipitating factors
   1. Trauma to bladder during delivery
   2. Catheterization during and/or after labor
   3. Temporary loss of bladder tone
D. Clinical manifestations
   1. Urinary frequency, urgency, or retention
   2. Dysuria, nocturia, tenderness
   3. Hematuria
   4. Fever, chills
   5. Abnormal urinalysis
E. Diagnostic examination: urine culture
II. Analysis
A. High risk for urinary retention related to edema and pain associated with infectious process
B. Knowledge deficit related to treatment regimen, self-care behaviors to avoid infections
III. Planning/goals, expected outcomes: client will be free from clinical manifestations of cystitis
IV. Implementation

A. Observe client closely postpartum for full bladder or residual urine
  1. Palpate bladder for distention
  2. Palpate fundus; full bladder displaces fundus upward and to sides
B. Obtain urine specimens for microscopic examination
C. Institute measures to help client void
D. Insert catheter, as ordered, using sterile technique
E. Force fluids to 3000 mL per day
F. Administer medications as ordered; may give systemic antibiotics
G. Provide emotional support
H. Teach prevention
  1. Good perineal hygiene
  2. Good handwashing
  3. Frequent and complete emptying of bladder
V. Evaluation: client does not experience clinical manifestations of cystitis

Hematoma

I. Assessment
A. Definition: collection of blood, often on external genitalia, as result of injury to blood vessel during spontaneous or forceps delivery
B. Incidence: occurs once in every 500 to 1000 deliveries
C. Predisposing/precipitating factors
  1. Prolonged pressure of fetal head on vaginal mucosa
  2. Forceps delivery
D. Clinical manifestations
  1. Complaints of severe perineal pain or rectal pressure
  2. Visible large mass at introitus or labia majora
  3. Bruising
  4. Pain on palpation
  5. Inability to void because of pressure of hematoma on urethra
  6. Clinical manifestations of shock in presence of well-contracted uterus and no visible vaginal bleeding
II. Analysis
A. Pain related to edema secondary to hematoma formation
B. Anxiety related to altered health status
III. Planning/goals, expected outcomes: client will be comfortable as hematoma resolves
IV. Implementation
A. Carefully examine hematoma and monitor to detect any enlargement
B. Notify physician of presence of hematoma

C. Promote general comfort
  1. Apply cold or heat to site as ordered
  2. Administer analgesics as ordered
D. Prepare client for surgery, if indicated, to evacuate hematoma
E. Continuously assess for vaginal bleeding postpartum
V. Evaluation
A. Client's hematoma resolves
B. Client's comfort level maintained

Thrombophlebitis

I. Assessment
A. Definition: vascular occlusion of vessels of pelvis or lower extremities
B. Etiology: results from infection, circulatory stasis, and increased postdelivery coagulability of blood
C. Predisposing/precipitating factors
  1. Maternal age of more than 30
  2. Multiparity
  3. Operative delivery
  4. Obesity
  5. Previous history of thrombophlebitis or thromboembolic disease
  6. Women on estrogen for suppression of lactation
  7. Bedrest
D. Clinical manifestations
  1. Discomfort in abdomen and pelvis
  2. Tenderness localized on one side of the pelvis
  3. Edema and pain in affected leg
  4. Chills and fever
E. Complication: pulmonary embolism
II. Analysis
A. Altered peripheral tissue perfusion related to impaired circulation
B. Anxiety related to altered health status
III. Planning/goals, expected outcomes
A. Client will be free from clinical manifestations of thrombophlebitis
B. Client will not suffer from undetected pulmonary embolus
C. Client will not suffer from unnecessary anxiety
IV. Implementation
A. Assess lower extremities for edema, tenderness, varices, and increased skin temperature
B. Evaluate legs for Homan's sign by extending the legs with knees slightly flexed and dorsiflexing the foot; if pain is reported, notify physician
C. Teach self-care measures to prevent thrombophlebitis
  1. Early ambulation

2. Avoid pressure behind the knees
3. Avoid crossing the legs
D. Maintain bedrest after clot present
E. Apply warm compresses, as ordered, for 15 to 20 minutes
F. Elevate affected leg
G. Apply bed cradle; keep bedclothes off leg
H. Never massage leg, and teach client not to do so
I. Apply antiembolic stockings to prevent clot formation and teach client proper use; apply to unaffected leg only if clot occurs
J. Administer heparin as ordered
K. Monitor for manifestations of pulmonary embolism
L. Allow client to express fears and concerns
M. Teach client to watch for manifestations of excessive bleeding

IV. Evaluation
A. Client's thrombophlebitis resolves
B. Client does not develop pulmonary embolism
C. Client's anxiety is allayed

Pulmonary Embolus

I. Assessment
A. Definition: passage of thrombus, often originating in one of uterine or other pelvic veins, into lung, where it disrupts circulation of blood
B. Incidence: usually seen at end of first week postpartum
C. Predisposing/precipitating factors
1. Infection
2. Hemorrhage
3. Thrombosis
D. Clinical manifestations
1. Sudden, intense chest pain
2. Severe dyspnea
3. Apprehension
4. Irregular, thready pulse
5. Pallor or cyanosis
6. Hemoptysis
7. Syncope
8. Shock
E. Complication: death
F. Prognosis: maternal mortality high with large or undetected clots

II. Analysis
A. Impaired gas exchange related to obstructive process
B. Pain related to obstructive process
C. Fear related to dyspnea and chest pain
D. Knowledge deficit related to disease process and treatment regimen

III. Planning/goals, expected outcomes
A. Client will demonstrate arterial blood gases within normal limits within 24 hours

B. Client's anxiety level will be maintained at appropriate level

IV. Implementation
A. Administer oxygen as ordered
B. Provide basic critical care to combat shock
1. Flat in bed
2. Monitor vital signs frequently
3. Keep warm
4. Increase IV fluids
C. Administer anticoagulants as prescribed by physician
D. Know that streptokinase may be given to dissolve clots
E. Give emotional support to client and family

V. Evaluation
A. Client's pulmonary embolus resolves
B. Client's anxiety is allayed

Postpartum Psychosis

I. Assessment
A. Definition: psychosis occurring within 4 to 6 weeks after delivery
B. Predisposing/precipitating factors
1. Approximately 33% of women probably had mental illness before pregnancy
2. Stresses of pregnancy, delivery, and new responsibilities of parenthood
C. Clinical manifestations
1. Clouding of consciousness
2. Depression, withdrawal
3. Hostility
4. Fear and suspiciousness
5. Feelings of inadequacy
6. Hallucinations

II. Analysis
A. Anxiety related to perceived loss of control; inappropriate behavior
B. Defensive coping related to impaired perception of reality, self-destructive behavior
C. Ineffective family coping related to effects of acute illness in family member

III. Planning/goals, expected outcomes: client will experience less anxiety and hostility

IV. Implementation
A. Have client state her perception of current situation and reasons for anxiety and hostility
B. Have client describe how she might cope with current situation
C. Explore potential resources client/family might use to reduce stresses
D. Administer psychotropic drugs as prescribed
E. Make referrals to appropriate health team members and/or agencies to increase resources available to client/family
F. Teach client/family parenting skills, giving positive feedback as much as possible

V. Evaluation: client demonstrates less anxiety and hostility

POST-TEST Postpartum Period

Terri Hastings, age 15, delivered a baby girl 1 hour ago. She held her infant daughter and appeared joyful at her alertness. As the initial newborn assessments are made, the mother asks many questions about the baby's condition.

1. Which of the following delivery room observations is abnormal?
   1. Severe molding of the head
   2. Cyanosis of hands and feet
   3. Irregular abdominal respirations
   4. Temperature of 35°C (95°F)
2. Baby girl Hastings is later assessed by the nurse, who determines that the infant is small for gestational age on the Ballard scale. A factor contributing to intrauterine growth retardation is:
   1. Maternal weight gain of more than 30 lb
   2. Multiparity
   3. Prolonged labor
   4. Sickle cell anemia
3. In observing an adolescent parent with her first child, which behavior would warrant further assessment by the nurse?
   1. Talking on the telephone while feeding the child
   2. Has many teenage friends as visitors
   3. Asks questions about cord care
   4. States she plans on returning to school in 3 months
4. Which question focuses on gathering data about the young mother's mastery of her developmental tasks?
   1. "What is your relationship with the baby's father?"
   2. "How do you feel about your parents' interest in the baby?"
   3. "Tell me how you feel about yourself as a young woman."
   4. "Do you feel that you can give love to an infant?"
5. Which of the following is an appropriate short-term goal for this young mother?
   1. She will be aware of the developmental needs of childhood
   2. She will feed, nurture, and provide care for her newborn
   3. She will resolve social problems within her family
   4. She will delay another pregnancy for 1 year

6. At the time of discharge, much time is spent reinforcing teaching of self-care and infant care. Which statement made by Terri indicates that further teaching is necessary?
   1. "If I need to, I'll use nonfat dry milk for feedings."
   2. "I'll hold and love the baby even when she doesn't cry."
   3. "After feeding, I'll put her to sleep on her tummy."
   4. "Until the cord is dry, I'll give her a sponge bath."

Maria Dobson, a diabetic, is admitted for termination of pregnancy in the 37th week when pelvic examination shows cervical softening and effacement. The physician and couple have agreed on labor induction.

7. The primary reason that a gestational diabetic is delivered early is to:
   1. Prevent problems that may result from placental insufficiency
   2. Reduce maternal stress during the second stage of labor
   3. Eliminate fetal hyperglycemia in the immediate newborn period
   4. Control maternal glucose/insulin balance in intrapartum
8. During the labor induction, which assessment is critical?
   1. Monitoring contractions and rest phase
   2. Observing maternal pain and relaxation
   3. Measuring I & O
   4. Noting blood pressure and pulse
9. After a 10-hour labor, a 9-lb son is delivered to Maria. Parents and newborn enjoy early contact, and breast-feeding is initiated. Which of the following assessments of the newborn indicates a need for immediate intervention?
   1. Respirations are 30
   2. Dextrostick (glucose) is 25
   3. Hematocrit is 48
   4. Coombs' test is negative
10. Baby and mother are discharged after 24 hours of hospitalization. Both appear to be in good health. Which statement made by Maria shows that discharge teaching was effective?
    1. "We'll bring the baby for his PKU test tomorrow."
    2. "Both the baby and I probably will always be diabetic."
    3. "Breast-feeding will help space the next pregnancy."
    4. "I'll start active exercise again right away."

POST-TEST Answers and Rationales

1. ④ This low body temperature places the newborn at risk for cold stress and respiratory distress. 1 & 2, IV. Intrapartal Care.

2. ④ While common causes of intrauterine growth retardation are many, only choice 4 is a correct response. The other choices are not risk factors for intrauterine growth retardation. 2, IV. Intrauterine Growth Retardation.

3. ① Lack of attention to newborn cues and feeding behavior warrants further assessments by the nurse. The other behaviors are normal observations of a teenage mother. 1, IV. Adolescent Pregnancy.

4. ③ The developmental task for this client is identity (Erikson). Choice 3 focuses on feelings of a sense of self, while choice 1 suggests intimacy and choices 2 and 4 suggest generativity. 4, IV. Normal Growth and Development.

5. ② A short-term goal that is appropriate for the newborn period focuses on immediate needs. 3, IV. Postpartal Care.

6. ① Whole milk products are avoided in the first year of life because the newborn cannot digest them. All other responses show learning has occurred. 5, IV. Postpartal Care.

7. ① Early delivery reduces infant mortality and morbidity rates related to large birth size and to placental oxygenation alterations. Choice 2 is incorrect. Because the newborn often experiences hypoglycemia, Choice 3 is not true. Choice 4 is unrelated to early delivery. 2, IV. Prenatal, Diabetes.

8. ① While caring for a woman induced with Pitocin, careful assessment of contraction frequency and intensity, rest phases, and fetal heart rate response are critical. The other responses are part of basic care for all laboring women. 2, IV. Intrapartal Care.

9. ② The low blood sugar indicates a need for further assessment and for possible early feeding of the newborn to prevent brain damage caused by hypoglycemia. All other assessments are normal. 1 & 2, IV. Postpartum, Diabetes.

10. ① Early discharge may prevent collection of the laboratory test, which must follow sufficient feeding to be accurate. The other responses are incorrect. 5, IV. Postpartal Care.

18

The Newborn

PRE-TEST Care of the Newborn

1. Baby James, 6 lb 1 oz, was just delivered after a long labor. His initial Apgar is 8. Which of the following nursing interventions would you perform first?
   ① Place infant under a warmer and dry him
   ② Administer blow-by oxygen
   ③ Assess heart rate
   ④ Footprint infant

2. Baby James is in the newborn nursery. In assessing his eyes and vision, which of the following would be an ABNORMAL finding?
   ① Crossed eyes
   ② Absent blink reflex
   ③ Positive red reflex
   ④ Edema of the eyelids

3. Which of the following would be an ABNORMAL finding when the nurse assesses James's cardiovascular system?
   ① Heart rate of 154
   ② Irregular heartbeats
   ③ Acrocyanosis of the extremities
   ④ Circumoral cyanosis

4. James is breathing with 10- to 15-second periods of apnea. The nurse knows that this means:
   ① Nothing, it is normal
   ② Impending respiratory distress
   ③ James will eventually develop asthma
   ④ James may be developing a respiratory infection

5. When the nurse is assessing James's renal system, which of the following would be considered an ABNORMAL assessment?
   ① Urine specific gravity 1.008
   ② First void after first 24 hours
   ③ Voiding up to 20 times a day
   ④ "Brick dust"–colored urine with the first void

6. Which of the following is INAPPROPRIATE in the care of an infant with hyperbilirubinemia?
   ① Withhold fluids during treatment
   ② Maintain neutral temperature
   ③ Administer phototherapy
   ④ Assist with exchange transfusions if needed

Mrs. S., gravida i para i, has just delivered a 7 lb 3 oz baby girl after a 10-hour labor. The baby was delivered vaginally with no complications.

---

7. To assess this newborn's immediate adaptation to extrauterine life, the nurse should perform which of the following tests?
   ① Apgar
   ② Silverman
   ③ Ballard/Dubowitz
   ④ Brazelton

8. To avoid heat loss by evaporation, the nurse should:
   ① Keep the baby away from drafts
   ② Avoid placing the baby on a cold surface
   ③ Dry the baby immediately after delivery
   ④ Pad the scale before weighing the baby

9. To prevent abnormal bleeding in the newborn, the nurse should:
   ① Wrap the baby in double blankets; pad the sides of the crib
   ② Feed the baby an iron-based formula
   ③ Administer vitamin K
   ④ Give cryoprecipitate

10. The newborn's first stool is:
    ① Yellow and loose
    ② Yellow and seedy
    ③ Thick and greenish-black
    ④ Loose and green

11. To rule out PKU, the nurse should test the baby:
    ① Immediately after delivery
    ② Before the first feeding
    ③ Two hours after the first feeding
    ④ Two to 3 hours after birth

PRE-TEST Answers and Rationales

1. ① The immediate concern is to prevent heat loss. Blow-by oxygen is not needed with this Apgar. Heart rate is assessed once baby is dry and under the warmer. Footprinting is done after initial assessment. 4, IV. Care of the Newborn.

2. ② The blink reflex is a protective reflex that is present at birth. The other choices are all normal assessments. 1, IV. Care of the Newborn.

3. ④ Circumoral cyanosis is an ominous sign of severe hypoxia and is not a normal finding. The other choices are normal assessment findings in the newborn. 1, IV. Care of the Newborn.

4. ① Short periods of apnea are normal in the newborn, and no action is needed. 1, IV. Care of the Newborn.

5. ② It is normal for the first voiding to be within the first 24 hours, not after it. The other assessment findings are normal in the newborn. 1, IV. Care of the Newborn.

6. ① It is important that the newborn be adequately hydrated to help prevent further complications from hyperbilirubinemia. The other choices are correct actions when caring for the newborn with hyperbilirubinemia. 4, IV. Care of the High-Risk Newborn.

7. ① The Apgar is a scoring method by which the newborn's adaptation to extrauterine life can be measured. The other tests are developmental in nature. 1 & 4, IV. Care of the Newborn.

8. ③ Evaporation occurs when there is heat loss through water evaporation, so drying the neonate helps prevent this. The other choices list ways to prevent cooling but not from evaporation. 4, IV. Care of the Newborn.

9. ③ The newborn is deficient in prothrombin, one of the clotting factors produced by the liver. Vitamin K is necessary in the production of prothrombin, so the newborn needs it to improve clotting ability. 4, IV. Care of the Newborn.

10. ③ The first stool is meconium and is thick and tarry. After this, the stools are brownish-green and then yellow and seedy in formula-fed infants and soft and yellow in breast-fed infants. 1, IV. Care of the Newborn.

11. ③ The PKU tests for the presence of phenylketonuria, which indicates whether the newborn is able to metabolize phenylalanine. If this deficiency is not discovered, brain damage and mental retardation can result. The test cannot be done until after the newborn is fed to see if the metabolism is functioning correctly. 4, IV. Care of the Newborn.

NURSING PROCESS APPLIED TO CARE OF THE NEWBORN

Care of the Newborn During Initial Period of Adaptation to Extrauterine Life

I. Assessment
  A. Physiological adaptations
    1. Initiation of respirations: ability to establish independent respirations
    2. Apgar score: method of assessing ability to adapt to extrauterine life
      a. Heart rate
      b. Respirations
      c. Muscle tone
      d. Reflex irritability
      e. Color
    3. Condition of cord
      a. Number of vessels: two arteries, one vein
      b. Bleeding
      c. Drainage
    4. Temperature stability: ability to maintain body temperature within normal range; immature temperature regulatory mechanism
      a. Brown fat at neck, between scapulae and behind sternum
      b. Inability to shiver or sweat
      c. Heat loss due to evaporation, radiation, conduction, convection
    5. Accurate identification
      a. Footprint infant

b. Fingerprint mother

c. Identification bracelets

6. Emergency conditions: problems requiring immediate intervention

  a. Low Apgar score indicative of cardiopulmonary problems

  b. Absence of spontaneous respirations

  c. Asphyxia

  d. Apnea

  e. Central nervous system (CNS) depression

  f. Hypoglycemia

B. Behavioral adaptations

1. First period of reactivity: 15 to 20 minutes of alert awareness and activity

2. Second period of reactivity: infant may have increased heart rate, gagging, choking, and regurgitation

3. Maternal-infant bonding

II. Analysis

A. High risk for ineffective airway clearance related to retained secretions

B. High risk for hypothermia related to environmental conditions, immature regulatory system

C. High risk for ineffective breathing pattern related to effects of delivery

D. Altered family process related to developmental transition

III. Planning/goals, expected outcomes

A. Physiological

1. Infant will establish regular, nonlabored respirations

2. Infant's Apgar score at 1 minute and at 5 minutes will be 7 or more

3. Infant's cord will be intact and have two arteries and one vein

4. Infant's temperature will remain stable

5. Infant will be properly identified by printing and name bracelets

6. Neonate's complications will be identified and treated

B. Behavioral

1. Infant will respond to mother during first period of reactivity

2. Mother-infant bonding will be initiated

IV. Implementation

A. Physiological

1. Observe or assist with initiation of respirations

  a. Assist with suctioning as needed

  b. Position infant on side or abdomen

  c. Take vital signs

  d. Note nasal flaring, grunting, retractions, see-saw respirations

  e. Note cry

2. Administer Apgar scoring test

  a. Perform and record Apgar score at 1 minute and at 5 minutes

  b. Assess each of five items to be scored and assign value of 0 to 2 (low to high) for each item

  c. Provide emergency care to those newborns with low Apgar scores

3. Observe condition of cord

  a. Count three vessels—two arteries and one vein

  b. Check for intact cord

  c. Note any bleeding or drainage

4. Maintain temperature stability

  a. Dry infant's skin and hair with warm towels

  b. Wrap baby in warm blankets or place on mother's abdomen and cover with warm blanket

  c. Place under warmer if examinations or treatments are needed or required

  d. Take axillary temperature

  e. Observe for signs of hypothermia or hyperthermia

  f. Postpone newborn's bath until temperature stabilizes

5. Ensure newborn's proper identification

  a. Footprint infant and fingerprint mother on identification sheet

  b. Place matching identification bracelets on mother and infant

6. Identify and react to emergency conditions

  a. Low Apgar score

    (1) Score of 4 to 6

      (a) Suction

      (b) Dry quickly

      (c) Maintain warmth

      (d) Ventilate 30 to 50 times a minute until heart rate above 100, color is pink, and spontaneous respirations begin

      (e) Provide oxygen

    (2) Score of 0 to 4

      (a) Clear airway

      (b) Insert endotracheal tube

      (c) "Bag" infant if necessary

      (d) Ventilate with 100% oxygen at 40 to 60 breaths per minute

      (e) Initiate full CPR at 1 : 5 ratio

      (f) Maintain body temperature

      (g) Direct someone to support parents

  b. Asphyxia

    (1) Suction

    (2) Ventilate

    (3) Provide oxygen

  c. Apnea

(1) Stimulate baby

(2) Maintain airway

(3) Ventilate

(4) Assist physician with intubation as needed

d. CNS depression

(1) Note manifestations of lethargy, jitteriness, high-pitched cry, seizures

(2) Note respiratory depression

(3) Observe body posture for hypotonia

(4) Administer naloxone (Narcan) as ordered

e. Hypoglycemia

(1) Note jitteriness and lethargy

(2) Obtain blood sample for Dextrostix

(3) Administer glucose as ordered

f. Sepsis

(1) Observe for manifestations of group B streptococcal infection

(a) Pallor

(b) Tachypnea

(c) Tachycardia

(d) Jaundice

(e) Apnea

(f) Decreased activity level

(g) Poor feeding

(h) Abdominal distention

(2) Check maternal history for premature rupture of membranes

(3) Assist physician in obtaining necessary cultures

(4) Administer antibiotics as ordered

B. Behavioral

1. Note first 15 to 20 minutes of intense interest in surroundings, open eyes, and strong suck

2. Keep infant with mother to facilitate bonding

3. Put infant to mother's breast if breast-feeding is planned

V. Evaluation

A. Physiological

1. Infant's respirations between 30 and 60, unlabored

2. Infant adapts to extrauterine life as seen by Apgar score of 7 or more

3. Infant suffers no cord-related complications

4. Infant's body temperature remains between 36.5°C and 37.5°C (97.7°F and 99.5°F)

5. No misidentification occurs

6. Emergency interventions are successful

B. Behavioral

1. Infant establishes eye contact with mother during the first period of reactivity

2. Infant attaches and sucks at mother's breast

Ongoing Care of the Newborn

Physical Examination

I. Assessment

A. Normal physical measurements

1. Body measurements

a. Length: 45 to 55 cm (18 to 22 in.)

b. Weight: 2500 to 4300 g (5.5 to 9.5 lb)

c. Head circumference: 33 to 35.5 cm (13 to 14 in.)

d. Chest circumference: 30 to 33 cm (12 to 13 in.); should be equal to or 2 to 3 cm less than head circumference

2. Vital sign measurements

a. Heart rate: 120 to 160 (apical)

b. Respirations: 30 to 60

c. Temperature: 36.5 to 37.5°C (97.7 to 99.5°F)

d. Blood pressure: 60/40 to 80/50 mm Hg

B. Posture

1. Arms and legs flexed

2. Chin flexed on upper chest

3. Sporadic movements that are well coordinated

4. Degree of hypotonicity or hypertonicity, indicative of CNS damage

C. Skin

1. Pinkish-red (light-skinned infant) to pinkish-brown or pinkish-yellow (dark-skinned infant)

2. Vernix caseosa

3. Lanugo

4. Acrocyanosis due to compromised peripheral circulation

5. Harlequin appearance of blanching on one side and paling on the other may occur

6. Mottled appearance in response to cold

7. Milia

8. Dry, peeling skin

9. Observe forceps marks

10. Ecchymoses and petechiae due to trauma of birth

11. Birthmarks

a. Telangiectatic nevi or stork bites

b. Port-wine stains

c. Cavernous hemangiomas

d. Strawberry hemangiomas

e. Mongolian spots

12. Erythema toxicum or newborn rash

13. Postmature syndrome: dry, cracking, leathery skin; scant to absent vernix

caseosa; absent lanugo; meconium-stained nails and skin

D. Head
1. 25% of body length (cephalocaudal development)
2. Bones of skull not fused; overlapping allows for passage through birth canal
3. Palpable sutures; sutures (connective tissue between the skull bones)
4. Fontanelles: unossified membranous tissue at junction of sutures
   a. Anterior fontanelle: soft, flat, diamond-shaped, 3 to 4 cm wide by 2 to 3 cm long; closes between 12 and 18 months
   b. Posterior fontanelle: triangular, 0.5 to 1 cm wide, located between occipital and parietal bones; closes between birth and 2 months of age
5. Molding: asymmetry of head due to pressure in birth canal; disappears in about 72 hours
6. Masses resulting from birth trauma
   a. Caput succedaneum: edema of soft tissue over bone; subsides within few days
   b. Cephalohematoma: swelling caused by bleeding into area between bone and its periosteum; usually absorbed within 6 weeks with no treatment
7. Head lag: common when pulling infant to sitting position; when prone, infant should be able to lift head slightly and turn from side to side

E. Eyes
1. Slate gray (light skin) or brown-gray (dark skin) in color
2. Symmetrical
3. Clear
4. Blink reflex present
5. Eyes cross due to weak extraocular muscles
6. Able to track and fixate momentarily
7. Red reflex present
8. Pupils equal, round, react to light by accommodation (PERRLA)
9. Eyelids often edematous
10. Preferential focus on bright colors, patterns, animated facial expressions

F. Ears
1. Symmetrical
2. Firm cartilage with recoil
3. Auricular skin tags
4. Pinna should be on or above line drawn from canthus of eye

G. Nose
1. Flat, broad, in center of face

2. Obligatory nose breathing
3. Occasional sneezing

H. Mouth
1. Pink, moist gums
2. Sucking pads inside cheeks
3. Soft and hard palate intact
4. Epstein's pearls (small, white cysts) may be present on hard palate
5. Uvula in midline
6. Tongue moves freely, is symmetrical, has short frenulum
7. Sucking and crying movements symmetrical
8. Able to swallow

I. Neck
1. Short and thick
2. Head held in midline
3. Raises head momentarily when prone
4. Good range of motion (ROM), able to flex and extend
5. Trachea in midline

J. Chest
1. Appears circular since anteroposterior and lateral diameters are about equal
2. Respirations diaphragmatic
3. Bronchial sounds on auscultation
4. Nipples prominent, often edematous
5. Milky secretion (witch's milk) common
6. Supernumerary nipples may be present

K. Abdomen
1. Round and protruding due to weak muscles
2. Umbilical hernia possible
3. Bowel sounds present

L. Spine
1. Straight
2. Posture flexed

M. Extremities
1. Flexed
2. Full ROM
3. Movements symmetrical
4. Fists clenched
5. Fingers and toes should be 10 each in number and separate (check for polydactyly or syndactyly)
6. Legs bowed
7. Creases on soles of feet
8. Pulses palpable (radial, brachial, femoral)
9. Observe for fractures (especially clavicle) or dislocations (hip)

N. Genitalia—female
1. Labia edematous, clitoris enlarged
2. Smegma present (thick white mucus discharge
3. Pseudomenstruation possible (blood-tinged mucus)

4. Hymen tag may be visible
5. Check for ambiguous genitalia
O. Genitalia—male
   1. Prepuce (foreskin) covers glans penis
   2. Scrotum edematous
   3. Meatus at tip of penis
   4. Testes descended but may retract on cold stress
   5. Check for inguinal hernia or hydrocele
   6. Check for ambiguous genitalia
P. Anus
   1. Anal opening patent
   2. No fissures
   3. Pilonidal dimple, if present, does not continue on into sinus tract
II. Analysis: high risk for altered growth and development related to effects of birth defect or injury
III. Planning/goals, expected outcomes
   A. Normal and abnormal physical parameters will be identified
   B. Physical findings will serve as a baseline for nursing interventions
IV. Implementation
   A. Keep infant warm during examination
   B. Begin with general observations and proceed to detailed findings
   C. Perform assessment maneuvers that are least disturbing to infant first
   D. Record all abnormal findings
   E. Initiate nursing interventions for abnormal findings
V. Evaluation
   A. Normal and abnormal parameters are identified
   B. Appropriate nursing interventions are instituted

Cardiovascular System

I. Assessment
   A. General considerations
      1. With clamping of umbilical cord, blood flow through placenta ceases, ductus venosus no longer functional
      2. Initial respirations cause pulmonary arteries to dilate
      3. Increased blood flow to lungs decreases pressure in right chambers of heart
      4. Blood flowing from lungs through pulmonary veins back to left atrium increases pressure on left side of heart
      5. Left-side heart pressure exceeds right-side pressure
      6. Ductus arteriosus and foramen ovale close functionally
      7. Small capillaries are immature and slow to dilate and constrict
   B. Observations
      1. Heart rate: 120 to 160
      2. Rhythm: irregular heartbeats or sinus arrythmia normal
      3. Point of maximum impact (PMI) between third and fourth intercostal spaces
      4. Loud, short, high-pitched sounds; functional murmurs common
      5. Hemoglobin, hematocrit, RBCs count elevated
      6. Acrocyanosis due to immaturity of small capillaries
      7. Ability to suck and swallow entire feeding
      8. Abnormal observations
         a. Cyanosis
         b. Persistent machinery murmurs
         c. Tachycardia and tachypnea on feeding
         d. Bleeding from the cord
II. Analysis
   A. High risk for decreased cardiac output related to structural abnnormalities, congenital defects
   B. Altered peripheral tissue perfusion related to hypothermia
III. Planning/goals, expected outcomes
   A. Infant will adapt to extrauterine circulation
   B. Infant's color will be pink with only transient acrocyanosis
   C. Heart rate will be 120 to 160
IV. Implementation
   A. Take apical heart rate for 1 full minute
   B. Listen for murmurs
   C. Look for cyanosis
   D. Blanch skin on trunk and extremities to assess circulation
   E. Palpate pulses
   F. Document inability to feed without distress
   G. Keep infant warm
   H. Observe cord stump for bleeding
V. Evaluation
   A. Infant's heart rate is 120 to 160
   B. Infant experiences no distress in adaptation to extrauterine circulation

Respiratory System

I. Assessment
   A. General considerations
      1. Respirations initiated by various stimuli
         a. Chemical: decreased oxygen and increased carbon dioxide
         b. Sensory: light, noise, handling
         c. Thermal: cold
         d. Mechanical: forces of labor
      2. Infant must be able to establish negative intrathoracic pressure for air to enter lungs

3. Surfactant facilitates lung expansion and contraction by lowering surface tension
4. Inhaled oxygen causes pulmonary vessels to dilate and pulmonary vascular resistance to decrease

B. Observations
1. Lung sounds loud and clear
2. Periodic breathing (apnea less than 15 seconds)
3. Increased mucus secretions
4. Weak muscles inhibiting coughing
5. Diaphragmatic breathing
6. Obligatory nose breathing
7. Trachea short and narrow
8. Tongue thick; may impede breathing
9. Abnormal observations
   a. Increased effort: grunting, nasal flaring, retractions
   b. Cyanosis
   c. Excessive mucus secretions or vomitus

II. Analysis
A. Ineffective airway clearance related to retained mucous secretions, inability to cough
B. High risk for ineffective breathing pattern related to decreased surfactant production
C. High risk for impaired gas exchange related to decreased lung expansion

III. Planning/goals, expected outcomes
A. Infant's respirations will begin spontaneously
B. Infant will have adequate oxygenation and gas exchange
C. Infant will be able to handle secretions and maintain clear, patent airway
D. Respirations will be 30 to 60 per minute

IV. Implementation
A. Position baby on side
B. Suction as needed to maintain patent airway
   1. Bulb syringe: for upper airway suctioning, compress bulb before insertion
   2. DeLee or French catheter for deeper suctioning
C. Observe for respiratory distress
   1. Nasal flaring
   2. Increasingly severe retractions
   3. Grunting
D. Maintain neutral temperature
E. Observe for manifestations of hypoxemia
   1. Cyanosis
   2. Bradycardia
   3. Low body temperature
   4. Periods of apnea lasting longer than 15 seconds
   5. Administer oxygen per hood if necessary

V. Evaluation
A. Infant able to maintain adequate oxygenation

B. Infant's respirations between 30 and 60 per minute and not labored

Hepatic System

I. Assessment
A. General considerations
   1. Inability to conjugate bilirubin
      a. Increased RBC breakdown produces indirect bilirubin
      b. Glucuronyl transferase converts indirect to direct bilirubin but due to immaturity and large numbers of RBCs cannot conjugate all of the indirect bilirubin
      c. Jaundice appears in about 50% of all newborns
      d. Normal or physiological jaundice (bilirubin 4 to 12.5 mg/dL appears after first 24 hours in full-term babies and after the first 48 hours in premature babies
      e. Physiological jaundice peaks about fifth day of life
   2. Blood coagulation
      a. Coagulation factors synthesized in liver dependent on vitamin K, which is not synthesized until there are some intestinal bacteria
      b. Newborn at risk for hemorrhagic disorders
   3. Liver stores iron passed from mother for 5 to 6 months
   4. Glycogen storage occurs in liver
B. Observations
   1. Inability to conjugate bilirubin
      a. Observe for jaundice in sclera, palms, soles, and gums
      b. Assess bilirubin levels
      c. Note age of infant at appearance of jaundice (onset before 24 hours indicative of hemolytic disorder; later onset may indicate sepsis or milk jaundice)
      d. Observe for passage of meconium; bilirubin present in meconium and subsequent stools
   2. Blood coagulation; assess for any hemorrhagic episodes
   3. Iron stores
      a. Assess mother's hemoglobin
      b. Assess infant's gestational age; premature babies more prone to deficient iron stores
   4. Glycogen stores; observe normal glucose level

II. Analysis: high risk for injury related to hypoglycemia, bleeding, high bilirubin levels

III. Planning/goals, expected outcomes
  A. Infant's jaundice will subside with minimal intervention
  B. Infant will have no bleeding episodes
  C. Infant's iron stores will be adequate
  D. Infant will have no hypoglycemic episodes
IV. Implementation
  A. Inability to conjugate bilirubin
    1. Feed early
    2. Watch for meconium passage and subsequent stools
    3. Prevent chilling; hypothermia can cause acidosis, which interferes with bilirubin excretion
    4. Monitor serum bilirubin levels
    5. For babies with breast milk jaundice, feed every 2 hours and temporarily suspend breast-feeding for 48 hours if bilirubin levels exceed 15 to 20 mg/dL
  B. Blood coagulation
    1. Handle carefully
    2. Monitor any bleeding episodes
    3. Administer one dose of vitamin K (Aquamephyton, 1 mg IM in the vastus lateralis muscle) to aid in coagulation
  C. Iron stores
    1. Check mother's hemoglobin to assess her ability to pass iron on to fetus
    2. Note infant's gestational age
    3. Check infant's hemoglobin level
  D. Glycogen storage
    1. Check blood glucose level
    2. Observe for hypoglycemia
V. Evaluation
  A. Infant's bilirubin level remains below 12.5 mg/dL and subsides in about 10 to 30 days
  B. Infant has no bleeding episodes
  C. Infant's iron stores are adequate
  D. Infant maintains normal blood sugar levels

Renal System
I. Assessment
  A. General considerations
    1. Immature kidneys unable to concentrate urine
    2. More fluid in extracellular spaces
    3. Limited ability to regulate sodium
    4. Weight loss of 5 to 15% during first week due to voiding and limited intake
  B. Observations
    1. Low specific gravity (1.008 normal)
    2. First void within 24 hours
    3. First void may be "brick dust" colored due to uric acid crystals
    4. Frequent voidings—up to 20 times per day, 150 mL/kg/day

II. Analysis: high risk for fluid volume deficit related to effects of immaturity of renal system
III. Planning/goals, expected outcomes
  A. Infant will take feedings
  B. Infant's hydration status will be adequate
IV. Implementation
  A. Feed infant
  B. Monitor I & O; weigh diapers
  C. Measure specific gravity
  D. Assess for manifestations of dehydration:
    1. Dry mucous membranes
    2. Sunken eyeballs
    3. Poor skin turgor
    4. Sunken fontanelles
  E. Weigh infant daily
V. Evaluation
  A. Infant is feeding well
  B. Infant is well hydrated
  C. Infant voiding 30 to 60 mL during the first 48 hours

Immune System
I. Assessment
  A. General considerations
    1. Elevated WBCs but poor response to infection
    2. Decreased inflammatory response
    3. Passive immunity via the placenta (IgG)
    4. Passive immunity from colostrum (IgA)
    5. Elevations in IgM indicate infection in utero
    6. Possible exposure to gonorrhea or *Chlamydia trachomatis* in birth canal, which might cause ophthalmia neonatorum
    7. Possible exposure to hepatitis B or HIV
  B. Observations
    1. Elevations in temperature
    2. Intact skin with good turgor
    3. Manifestations of localized swelling, redness, drainage
    4. Look for manifestations of purulent drainage from eyes
    5. Assess cord for drainage, odor
    6. If circumcised, assess for manifestations of drainage or bleeding
    7. Observe for manifestations of sepsis
II. Analysis
  A. High risk for infection related to inadequate immune response
  B. Altered skin integrity related to effects of immaturity
III. Planning/goals, expected outcome
  A. Infant will not be exposed to infection
  B. Infant will contract no infections
IV. Implementation
  A. Use aseptic technique when caring for infant

1. Aseptic scrub
2. Gowns
3. Crib bed equipped with individual supplies
4. Infection-free staff caring for infant
B. Observe any cracks or openings in skin
C. Observe universal precautions when handling infant
D. Monitor temperature
E. Administer eye medication to prevent ophthalmia neonatorum
   1. Erythromycin (0.5%) ophthalmic ointment or drops
   2. Tetracycline (1%) ophthalmic ointment or drops
   3. Silver nitrate (1%) solution (not favored choice because it causes severe conjunctivitis and is effective only against gonorrhea)
F. Provide cord care
   1. Apply topical triple dye or bacitracin ointment initially
   2. Keep cord clean and dry by wiping with alcohol
   3. Assess for odor, swelling, discharge
   4. Teach mother how to perform cord care
G. Provide circumcision care
   1. Properly restrain infant during procedure to reduce chance of complications
   2. Apply Vaseline gauze to penis
   3. Observe for manifestations of swelling, infection, or bleeding
   4. Observe for urinary retention
   5. Teach mother care of circumcision site
V. Evaluation
A. Infant's cord dries and falls off in about 2 weeks
B. Circumcised penis heals without infection or complication
C. Infant develops no infections

Metabolic System

I. Assessment
A. General considerations
   1. Able to digest simple carbohydrates
   2. Unable to digest fats due to lack of lipase
   3. Proteins may be only partially broken down, so may serve as antigens and provoke allergic reaction
   4. Small stomach capacity (about 90 mL) and rapid peristalsis (bowel emptying time 2½ to 3 hours)
B. Observations
   1. Ability to root, suck, swallow
   2. Look for excessive drooling
   3. First stool, meconium, appears within 24 hours; thick, tarry

4. Transition stool brownish green and less thick
5. Subsequent stools yellow and seedy in formula-fed babies, soft and yellow in breast-fed babies
6. Number of stools varies; some babies have stool with each feeding

II. Analysis
A. High risk for altered nutrition: less than body requirements related to knowledge deficit of caretaker
B. High risk for ineffective breast-feeding related to anxiety, ambivalence, knowledge deficit of mother, poor infant sucking reflex

III. Planning/goals, expected outcomes
A. Infant will be able to coordinate sucking and swallowing
B. Infant will retain and digest feedings
C. Infant will develop normal stool pattern

IV. Implementation
A. Feed small amount of water
   1. Observe feeding reflexes—rooting, sucking, swallowing, extrusion
   2. Rule out esophageal atresia
B. Assist mother with breast-feeding or formula-feeding
C. Provide caloric needs of 120 cal/kg/day (50 to 55 cal/lb/day)
D. Bubble baby during and after feeding
E. Assess regurgitations, vomiting
F. Position infant on right side or abdomen after feeding
G. Observe passage of meconium
H. Observe normal stool
   1. Soft, yellow for breast-fed infants
   2. Seedy, yellow for formula-fed infants
I. Perform PKU test before discharge or as outpatient; after sufficient caloric intake

V. Evaluation
A. Infant takes, retains, and digests feedings
B. Infant passes meconium stool in first 24 hours

Neurological System

I. Assessment
A. General considerations
   1. Head size proportionally larger than adult's due to cephalocaudal development
   2. Myelinization of nerve fibers incomplete, so primitive reflexes are present
   3. Fontanelles open to allow for brain growth
B. Observations
   1. Loud, lusty cry, not high-pitched
   2. Fontanelles soft, flat
   3. Head circumference slightly larger than chest circumference
   4. Transient tremors and startles common
   5. Body posture neither rigid nor hypotonic

6. Movements are symmetrical
7. Normal infant reflexes present

II. Analysis: high risk for altered sensory perception, related to effects of neurological deficit

III. Planning/goals, expected outcomes
   A. Infant will exhibit normal body posture and movement
   B. Normal infant reflexes will be present

IV. Implementation
   A. Measure and graph head circumference in relation to chest circumference and length
   B. Assess infant's movements, noting symmetry, posture, and abnormal movements
   C. Test newborn's reflexes
   D. Note lethargy
   E. Assess pitch of cry
   F. Observe jitteriness, marked tremors, seizures
   G. Assess abnormal-size or bulging anterior fontanelle

V. Evaluation
   A. Infant has normal, flexed posture and sporadic, well-coordinated movements
   B. Infant shows normal responses when reflexes are stimulated

Thermal Regulatory System

I. Assessment
   A. General considerations
      1. Neonates have larger surface area in relation to weight than adults
      2. Newborns have less adipose tissue
      3. Newborns do not shiver to produce heat
      4. Heat conserved through muscular activity, increased basal metabolic rate (BMR), and vasoconstriction
      5. Newborns have brown fat deposits, which produce heat
      6. Heat dissipated through vasodilation
      7. Prolonged cold stress depletes brown fat and glycogen stores
      8. Newborns lose heat through
         a. Evaporation
         b. Radiation
         c. Convection
         d. Conduction
   B. Observations
      1. Temperature
      2. Areas of brown fat in neck, thorax, and axilla and between scapulae
      3. Clinical manifestations of hypoglycemia: jitteriness, lethargy, irregular respirations, vomiting

II. Analysis: ineffective thermoregulation related to effects of immaturity

III. Planning/goals, expected outcomes
   A. Infant's heat loss will be minimized
   B. Infant's temperature will stabilize between 36.5°C and 37.5°C (97.9°F to 99.5°F)

IV. Implementation
   A. Prevent heat loss due to evaporation by keeping infant dry and well wrapped
   B. Prevent heat loss due to radiation by keeping infant away from cold objects, outside walls
   C. Prevent heat loss due to convection by shielding infant from drafts
   D. Prevent heat loss due to conduction by performing all treatments on a warm, padded surface
   E. Keep temperature in room warm
   F. Take temperature every 4 hours

V. Evaluation
   A. Infant suffers no cold stress
   B. Infant's temperature is 36.5°C to 37.5°C (97.9°F to 99.5°F)

Gestational Age

I. Assessment
   A. Assess infant according to Ballard or Dubowitz scale
   B. Identify newborn's gestational age
      1. Premature: less than 37 weeks' gestation
      2. Mature: 38 to 42 weeks' gestation
      3. Postmature: more than 42 weeks' gestation
   C. Determine infant's gestational size
      1. Small-for-gestational-age (SGA): less than 10th percentile for age
      2. Appropriate-for-gestational-age (AGA): between 10th and 90th percentiles for age
      3. Large-for-gestational-age (LGA): more than 90th percentile for age

II. Analysis: high risk for altered growth and development related to physical disabilities

III. Planning/goals, expected outcomes
   A. Infant's gestational age will be identified
   B. Infant's size in relation to age will be established

IV. Implementation
   A. Perform examination and score infant from 0 to 2 (low to high) on each of five items on the scale
   B. Use total score from scale to arrive at estimated age
   C. Use estimated age to categorize infant
      1. Preterm: less than 37 weeks' gestation
      2. Full-term: 38 to 42 weeks' gestation
      3. Postterm: more than 42 weeks' gestation
   D. Determine size (length, weight, head circumference) and categorize infant
      1. SGA: less than 10th percentile for age
      2. AGA: between 10th and 90th percentiles for age
      3. LGA: more than 90th percentile for age

E. Provide for immediate needs
  1. Preterm infant
    a. Respiratory distress
      (1) Stimulate respirations
      (2) Suction
      (3) Ventilate
    b. Hypoglycemia
      (1) Dextrostix assessment of blood sugar
      (2) Give glucose
    c. Fluid volume deficits: hypotension
    d. Nutritional problems
      (1) Special formulas
      (2) Special nipples
      (3) Tube feedings
      (4) Hyperalimentation
  2. Postterm infant
    a. Hypoglycemia (see above)
    b. Hypoxia
      (1) Stimulate
      (2) Ventilate
      (3) Oxygen
    c. Meconium aspiration
      (1) Suction
      (2) Clear airway
      (3) Pneumothorax secondary to meconium aspiration—chest tubes
  3. SGA infant
    a. Asphyxia
      (1) Stimulate
      (2) Suction
      (3) Ventilate
      (4) Oxygen
    b. Hypoglycemia
    c. Meconium aspiration
    d. Heat loss
      (1) Dry
      (2) Put in isolette or under warmer
  4. LGA infant
    a. Hypoglycemia
    b. Birth trauma due to size
V. Evaluation
  A. Infant's gestational age established
  B. Problems associated with size and maturity are anticipated and appropriate interventions are instituted

Behavioral Assessment
I. Assessment
  A. Examine and score newborn according to Brazelton Neonatal Behavioral Assessment Scale
  B. Assess
    1. First period of reactivity
    2. Period of inactivity
    3. Second period of reactivity
II. Analysis: high risk for altered parenting related to lack of knowledge, role identity, appropriate response of infant to environment
III. Planning/goals, expected outcomes
  A. Newborn's behavioral patterns and responses will be identified
  B. Newborn's unique behavior will be shared with and validated by parents
IV. Implementation
  A. Perform Brazelton assessment 3 days after birth
  B. Help parents identify their newborn's behavior pattern and responses, noting stimuli that calm or upset infant
  C. Help parents identify their own cues that calm or upset infant
V. Evaluation
  A. Behavior patterns and responses of infant identified
  B. Parents plan ways to respond to their infant's interactions

Parent Teaching
I. Assessment
  A. Identify common concerns of parents
    1. Feeding
    2. Bathing
    3. Clothing
    4. Cord care
    5. Care of circumcision
  B. Identify needs for anticipatory guidance
    1. Safety needs
    2. Follow-up care
II. Analysis: knowledge deficit of newborn care related to new role demands
III. Planning/goals, expected outcomes
  A. Parents will be able to provide care for their infant with comfort
  B. Infant's safety needs will be met
IV. Implementation
  A. Common concerns
    1. Feeding
      a. Formula feeding
        (1) Identify formula selected by parent
        (2) Review directions for mixing appropriate amounts of water
        (3) Teach sterilization techniques if water supply located in areas where purification process is questionable
        (4) Remind mother not to heat bottle of formula in microwave oven
        (5) Teach mother that formula sufficient diet for first 4 to 6 months
        (6) Assess mother's ability to burp infant and handle spitting up
      b. Breast-feeding

(1) Assess infant's ability to attach to mother's breast and suck

(2) Treat engorgement

(3) Teach mother how to pump her breasts and proper way to store breast milk

(4) Teach mother that breast milk sufficient diet for first 4 to 6 months

(5) Give mother telephone number of local organizations that offer support to breast-feeding mothers

2. Bathing
   a. Bathe in warm room, before feeding
   b. Have all equipment within reach
   c. Clean eyes from inner canthus outward
   d. Proceed from cleanest area to dirtiest
   e. Special care should be taken to clean under folds of neck, underarms, groin, and genitals
   f. Make bathtime enjoyable for both infant and mother

3. Clothing
   a. Assess with mother diaper and clothing needs
   b. Infant's head should be covered in cold weather to prevent heat loss

4. Cord care
   a. Clean with alcohol
   b. Keep diaper folded below cord
   c. Sponge bath until cord falls off
   d. Cord should fall off within 2 weeks

5. Care of circumcision
   a. Wash penis after voiding
   b. Observe for drainage, odor

B. Anticipatory guidance
   1. Safety needs
      a. Help mother select appropriate carseat
      b. Teach mother not to tie bibs, pacifiers, and so on around infant's neck
      c. Teach mother not to leave baby alone on a high surface
      d. Teach mother not to prop bottles
      e. Instruct mother to position infant on right side after feeding
   2. Follow-up care
      a. Make sure mother knows that she needs to return with infant for 6-week checkup
      b. Give mother telephone number she can call if she needs help (usually clinic or pediatrician)
      c. Give mother names and telephone numbers of other resources as needed
   3. Integration of newborn into family
      a. Identify ages of siblings
      b. Help mother plan ways to include siblings in newborn's care
      c. Help mother prepare for sibling rivalry

V. Evaluation
   A. Parents are comfortable in providing care for their baby
   B. Parents understand safety needs for this age infant
   C. Mother keeps follow-up appointments
   D. No injury occurs to infant

NURSING PROCESS APPLIED TO CARE OF THE HIGH-RISK NEWBORN

Identification of the High-Risk Newborn

I. Assessment
   A. Maternal history
      1. Age
      2. Parity
      3. Past pregnancy outcomes
      4. Nutritional status
      5. Alcohol, drug consumption
      6. Infections during pregnancy (cytomegalovirus [CMV], sexually transmitted diseases [STDs], toxoplasmosis, hepatitis, AIDS)
      7. Chronic illness (diabetes, renal disease, hypertension, cardiac disorders, sickle cell anemia)
      8. Prenatal care
      9. Genetic counseling
   B. Labor and delivery
      1. Dystocia
      2. Breech presentation
      3. Abnormal separation of placenta
      4. Cord complications
      5. Precipitous or difficult delivery
      6. Asphyxia
   C. Newborn
      1. Adaptation to extrauterine environment
      2. Gestational age and size
      3. Maintenance of adequate respirations
      4. Stabilization of body temperature
      5. Fluid/electrolyte and acid/base balance
      6. Complications that require immediate intervention
   D. Parents' coping abilities

II. Analysis
   A. High risk for altered growth and development related to effects of immaturity, physical disabilities, sensorimotor deficits
   B. High risk for altered parenting related to special care requirements, physical or mental handicaps

III. Planning/goals, expected outcomes
   A. Infants at significant risk will be identified
   B. Infant's complications will be identified and supportive measures instituted

C. Parents will be supported as they adjust to trauma of high-risk infant

IV. Implementation
  A. Take thorough maternal history
  B. Appraise abnormalities in labor and delivery process
  C. Perform Apgar scoring test, gestational assessment, and Silverman-Anderson test
  D. Appraise ability to initiate and sustain adequate respirations
  E. Keep newborn warm by using isolette or overhead heater
  F. Monitor blood gases
  G. Maintain IV line
  H. Administer medications as needed
  I. Prepare for transfer to high-risk center if appropriate
  J. Support parents

V. Evaluation
  A. Infant's risk factors are successfully identified
  B. Infant's problems are correctly identified and newborn responds to interventions
  C. Parents receive support and begin to bond with baby

Newborn With Respiratory Distress Syndrome (RDS)

I. Assessment
  A. Definition: serious lung disorder caused by immaturity and inability to produce surfactant

  B. Incidence: leading cause of death among premature infants; twice as common in males
  C. Predisposing/precipitating factors
    1. Prematurity
    2. Fetal asphyxia
    3. Birth trauma
    4. Infants of mothers who are diabetic or had placental bleeding
  D. Clinical manifestations
    1. Increasing dyspnea over first 6 hours
      a. Tachypnea
      b. Increasingly severe retractions
      c. Nasal flaring
      d. Expiratory grunting
      e. Inspiratory rales
      f. Shallow respirations
      g. Cyanosis
      h. Blood gases; Pao_2 below 40 mm Hg
    2. Need for ventilatory support
    3. Acidosis—respiratory and metabolic
    4. Nutrition/hydration needs
    5. Heat loss
    6. Fatigue

  7. Skin condition
  E. Mother/infant bonding

II. Analysis
  A. Impaired gas exchange related to inadequate expansion and contraction of lungs
  B. High risk for altered nutrition: less than body requirements related to impaired sucking and swallowing
  C. Altered family process related to situational crisis
  D. Anticipatory grieving, related to actual loss of idealized child, potential loss of infant

III. Planning/goals, expected outcomes
  A. Infant's respiratory efforts will be supported
  B. Infant will be able to maintain acid/base balance
  C. Infant's nutritional and hydration needs will be met
  D. Infant will maintain body temperature of approximately 36.5°C (97.9°F)
  E. Mother/infant bonding will be initiated
  F. Complications will be recognized and treated

IV. Implementation
  A. Perform Apgar, gestational age assessment, and Silverman-Anderson test to determine baseline for newborn
  B. Take vital signs
  C. Look for clinical manifestations of increasing respiratory distress
    1. Tachypnea: more than 60, may rise to 100 per minute
    2. Shallow respirations
    3. Increasingly severe retractions, particularly sternal
    4. Nasal flaring
    5. Expiratory grunt
    6. Inspiratory rales
    7. Cyanosis
    8. Hypotonic infant
  D. Support respirations
    1. Oxygen by hood or cannula
    2. Ventilation, using positive pressure
      a. Continuous positive air pressure (CPAP)
      b. Positive end-expiratory pressure (PEEP)
      c. Continuous positive-pressure ventilation (CPPV)
    3. Percussion and vibration: use padded small plastic cup or small oxygen mask for percussion; use electric toothbrush for vibration
    4. Suction every 2 hours or more often as necessary
    5. Position newborn on side or back with neck slightly extended
  E. Monitor oxygen saturation levels

1. Blood gases from umbilical artery: replace blood if infant becomes compromised
2. Transcutaneous measurement: noninvasive, no blood loss

F. Respiratory acidosis: IV sodium bicarbonate

G. Provide nutrition—120 cal/kg/day
   1. Nasogastric feedings
   2. Total parenteral nutrition (TPN) via peripheral or central line

H. Support bonding
   1. Encourage parents to look at and touch infant in early stage
   2. Help parents identify with infant
   3. Encourage mother to pump breasts for future breast-feeding if she so desires
   4. Encourage as much participation in infant's care as condition allows

I. Identify complications and initiate nursing interventions
   1. Bronchopulmonary dysplasia
      a. Identify lung tissue fibrosis caused by prematurity and respirator
      b. Prepare parents for short to long period of oxygen dependency (per nasal cannula)
   2. Retinopathy of prematurity
      a. Monitor blood gases so oxygen administered to newborn at lowest possible concentration to maintain adequate arterial oxygenation
      b. Schedule any premature infant who required oxygen support for eye examination before discharge
      c. Prophylactic administration of vitamin E
   3. Intraventricular hemorrhage
      a. Observe for clinical manifestations of increased intracranial pressure (ICP): bulging fontanelle, separated sutures
      b. Institute measures that prevent increases in ICP: suction only when necessary, elevate head 30 degrees
   4. Necrotizing enterocolitis
      a. Observe for abdominal distention, vomiting of residual feeding, occult blood in stools
      b. Begin TPN to rest gastrointestinal tract

V. Evaluation
   A. Infant maintains adequate oxygenation
   B. Infant's acidosis reversed, and acid-base balance stable
   C. Infant's nutritional needs are met
   D. Infant's temperature about 36.5°C (97.9°F)
   E. Parents interact with infant
   F. Complications are identified and interventions are responded to

Newborn With Hyperbilirubinemia

I. Assessment
   A. Definition: serum levels of unconjugated bilirubin more than 12 mg/dL in full-term infant, lower in premature infants
   B. Risk factors
      1. Rh incompatibility
      2. ABO incompatibility
      3. Sepsis
      4. RDS
      5. Diabetic mother
   C. Clinical manifestations
      1. Jaundice, particularly visible in sclera, palms, soles, and mucous membranes
      2. Elevated serum bilirubin levels
      3. Elevated direct Coombs, indicating maternal sensitization
      4. Kernicterus: bilirubin crosses over into central nervous system causing brain damage; occurs when bilirubin levels approach 20 mg/dL
         a. Early manifestations: lethargy, hypotonia, diminished reflexes
         b. Later manifestations: hyperflexia, spasticity

II. Analysis
   A. Altered sensory/perception related to diminished visual stimulation
   B. High risk for injury related to high levels of bilirubin

III. Planning/goals, expected outcomes
   A. Infant's bilirubin levels will lower in response to therapy
   B. Infant will not develop kernicterus

IV. Implementation
   A. Note presence of jaundice
   B. Monitor serum bilirubin and direct Coombs levels
   C. Hydrate infant
   D. Maintain neutral temperature
   E. Administer phototherapy
      1. Place infant under lamp with eyes and genitals covered
      2. Turn infant every 2 hours
      3. Increase hydration by 25%
      4. Monitor for loose, green stools
      5. Check eyes frequently for drainage
      6. Discontinue phototherapy, unwrap eyes, and hold for feedings
      7. Stroke and talk to infant
   F. Assist with exchange transfusion if needed

V. Evaluation
   A. Bilirubin levels fall in response to treatment
   B. Kernicterus prevented

The Addicted Newborn

I. Assessment
  A. Definition: newborn who has become passively addicted to drugs that have passed through placenta
  B. Risk factor: drug-abusing mother
  C. Clinical manifestations
    1. Neurological: hypertonic, irritable, jittery, high-pitched cry, hyperactivity, sleep disturbances, possible seizures
    2. Respiratory: tachypnea, tachycardia
    3. Gastrointestinal: vomiting, diarrhea, poor feeding, elevated temperature, sweating

II. Analysis
  A. Altered sensory perception related to chemical alteration caused by CNS drugs
  B. High risk for injury related to maternal drug use

III. Planning/goals, expected outcomes
  A. Infant will respond to quiet environment
  B. Infant will maintain adequate nutritional status
  C. Infant's mother will be involved in care

IV. Implementation
  A. Swaddle infant
  B. Put in quiet room and reduce stimulation
  C. Check vital signs
  D. Seizure precautions
  E. Measure I & O
  F. Allow longer period for feeding
  G. IV hydration if appropriate
  H. Protect skin from constant rubbing from hyperactive jitters
  I. Allow mother to ventilate feelings of anxiety and guilt
  J. Refer mother for treatment of drug problem

V. Evaluation
  A. Infant's withdrawal symptoms decline in quiet environment
  B. Infant's nutritional status not compromised
  C. Mother cares for infant

Newborn of Diabetic Mother

I. Assessment
  A. Definition: infant born to insulin-dependent or gestational diabetic mother
  B. Incidence: approximately one to two pregnancies per 100 and increasing
  C. Predisposing/precipitating factors: abnormal glucose metabolism causes large amounts of glucose to cross placenta, stimulating increased insulin production by fetus
  D. Clinical manifestations
    1. Hypoglycemia
      a. Blood glucose levels less than 30 mg/dL during first 3 days in full-term infant
      b. Blood glucose levels less than 20 mg/dL in premature infant
      c. Infant appears lethargic and jittery
      d. Irregular respirations
    2. Hypocalcemia: irregular respirations, edema, manifestations of hypoglycemia
    3. Birth size and maturity
      a. LGA infants predisposed to birth trauma and injury
      b. Prematurity predisposes infant to RDS
    4. Polycythemia
      a. Assess plethora
      b. Monitor hematocrit
    5. Hyperbilirubinemia
    6. Congenital anomalies

II. Analysis
  A. High risk for injury related to effects of hypoglycemia
  B. Altered growth and development related to maternal hyperglycemia

III. Planning/goals, expected outcomes
  A. Blood glucose will stabilize
  B. Calcium levels will be normal
  C. Infant will sustain no birth injuries or injuries will be identified
  D. Blood glucose levels will be in normal range
  E. Infant will sustain adequate oxygenation
  F. Infant will have associated anomalies identified and appropriate interventions will be taken
  G. Mother will cope with anxiety and will be able to establish emotional contact with infant

IV. Implementation
  A. Monitor blood glucose with Dextrostix; repeat as needed
  B. Feed early, 10% glucose water, breast milk, or formula
  C. Administer IV glucose if necessary
  D. Look for tremors, seizures, apnea, acidosis
  E. Give calcium gluconate IV if necessary to prevent tetany from calcium deficits
  F. Inspect infant for birth injuries
    1. Neurological damage such as paralysis of facial, phrenic, or brachial nerves; head trauma
    2. Orthopedic damages such as fractures of clavicle
    3. Bruises, abrasions, contusions
  G. Monitor hematocrit
    1. Perform heel stick hematocrit
    2. Feed baby
    3. Administer IV fluids as needed
    4. Assist with exchange transfusions if necessary
  H. Identify and treat hyperbilirubinemia
  I. Appraise clinical manifestations of RDS and initiate support systems as needed

J. Observe and treat associated anomalies
  1. Neurological: neural tube deformities, hydrocephalus
  2. Cardiac defects
K. Support parental attachment and coping
  1. Explain all treatments and procedures
  2. Encourage as much physical contact and caretaking as physical condition allows
V. Evaluation
  A. Blood glucose stabilizes within normal physiological range
  B. No hypocalcemia develops
  C. No birth injuries are sustained
  D. Normal respirations are sustained, RDS is identified and treated early
  E. Hematocrit and bilirubin levels remain within normal range
  F. Anomalies are identified early and appropriate interventions are initiated
  G. Parents understand infant's needs and are able to assume care on discharge

POST-TEST Care of the Newborn

Baby Susan is a 9 lb 2 oz infant born to a diabetic mother. She was delivered by cesarean section 12 hours ago. Her Apgar scores in the delivery room were 7 and 9.

1. You notice that Susan is lethargic and jittery and has irregular respirations. After checking the glucose level, the nurse should:
   1. Feed the infant glucose water (10%)
   2. Administer insulin subcutaneously
   3. Give oxygen
   4. Administer phenobarbital IM
2. Ten hours later, Susan develops tetany. Which of the following medications will you most likely give IV?
   1. Glucose
   2. Insulin
   3. Calcium gluconate
   4. Valium
3. Jaundice that appears after the first 48 hours of a newborn's life usually indicates:
   1. Rh or ABO incompatibility
   2. Normal physiological adaptation
   3. Breast-milk intolerance
   4. Liver abnormality
4. Expiratory grunting is:
   1. Normal in the newborn
   2. A sign of respiratory distress
   3. Common in babies of Rh-negative mothers
   4. Transitory in most instances

Baby Simon is a 9 lb 8 oz infant born at 43 weeks' gestation. He was delivered vaginally 10 hours ago. His Apgar scores were 7 and 8.

5. Simon's physical characteristics include:
   1. Cracked, peeling skin and scant vernix caseosa
   2. Abundant lanugo and thin, transparent skin
   3. Yellow-stained skin and abundant subcutaneous fat
   4. Ruddy complexion and flaccid extremities
6. Simon's gestational age puts him at risk for:
   1. Juvenile-onset diabetes
   2. Meconium aspiration syndrome
   3. Hemolytic anemia
   4. Hyperthermia
7. Baby Sarah, 7 lb 8 oz, was born today. She is in the newborn nursery, and you are caring for her cord. Which of the following nursing interventions is appropriate when caring for the umbilical cord?
   1. Apply a Vaseline gauze dressing over the site
   2. Apply a simple dry dressing over the site
   3. Clean the site vigorously with soap and water every day
   4. Apply topical triple dye or bacitracin ointment initially
8. Bowel transit time in the newborn is about:
   1. 1 to 1½ hours
   2. 2½ to 3 hours
   3. 1½ to 2 hours
   4. 3 to 3½ hours
9. The newborn infant needs approximately how many calories per day?
   1. 50 cal/kg/day
   2. 75 cal/kg/day
   3. 120 cal/kg/day
   4. 150 cal/kg/day
10. The newborn infant exhibits a number of reflexes at birth. Which of the following is NOT present at birth?
    1. Parachute reflex
    2. Moro reflex
    3. Sucking reflex
    4. Extrusion reflex
11. Which of the following is NOT a risk factor for RDS?
    1. Prematurity
    2. Maternal diabetes
    3. Birth trauma
    4. Postterm birth

POST-TEST Answers and Rationales

1. ① The infant of a diabetic mother is often hypoglycemic after birth, which means that the infant needs glucose. Choice 2 would increase the problem and choices 3 and 4 are inappropriate. 4, IV. Care of the High-Risk Newborn.

2. ③ Calcium gluconate is often needed to replace low calcium. Hypocalcemia causes tetany. 4, IV. Care of the High-Risk Newborn.

3. ② Jaundice is normal in more than half of all newborns after the first 48 hours of life. If it occurs before this time, it might well be a sign of Rh incompatibility or liver disorders. 1, IV. Care of the Newborn.

4. ② Grunting may indicate respiratory distress in the newborn. The infant may require suctioning or oxygen. 2, IV. Care of the Newborn.

5. ① Skin is often cracked and peeling with scant vernix caseosa in the postterm infant. There is extra subcutaneous fat. The other choices are incorrect. 1, II. Care of the Newborn.

6. ② The amniotic fluid often contains meconium at term, and since the infant is in utero longer, there is a greater chance of aspiration of the meconium. 1 & 2, IV. Care of the Newborn.

7. ④ The cord needs to dry and should be open to the air. An antibiotic ointment is applied initially, and then the cord cleaned with alcohol daily. The baby should receive sponge baths until the cord drops off. 4, IV. Care of the Newborn.

8. ② Normal bowel transit time in the newborn is about 2½ to 3 hours. 1, IV. Care of the Newborn.

9. ③ The normal newborn needs about 120 cal/kg/day or 50 cal/lb/day to grow normally. 1, II & IV. Care of the Newborn.

10. ① The parachute reflex appears at about 7 to 9 months and remains indefinitely. The other reflexes listed are reflexes that are present at birth and disappear later. 1, IV. Care of the Newborn.

11. ④ The postterm infant is not at special risk for RDS. The other choices listed are risk factors for RDS. 1, IV. Care of the High-Risk Newborn.

BIBLIOGRAPHY

Beachy, P., and Deacon, J. (1992). *NAACOG core curriculum for neonatal intensive care nursing.* Philadelphia: W. B. Saunders.

Bloom, R., and Cropley, C. (1987). *Textbook of neonatal resuscitation.* Dallas, TX: The American Heart Association.

Bobak, I., and Jensen, M. (1991). *Essentials of maternity nursing,* 3rd ed. St. Louis: C. V. Mosby.

Bobak, I., and Jensen, M. (1993). *Maternity and gynecologic care,* 5th ed. St. Louis: C. V. Mosby.

Clancy, G., Anand, K., and Lally, P. (1992). Neonatal pain management. *Critical Care Nursing Clinics of North America* 4 (3), 527–535.

Donaher-Wagner, B., and Braun, D. (1992). Infant cardiopulmonary resuscitation for expectant and new parents. *Maternal Child Nursing* 17 (1), 27–29.

Edgehouse, L., and Radzyminski, S. (1990). A device for supplemental breast feeding. *Maternal Child Nursing* 15 (1), 34–35.

Fuller, R. (1992). Group B streptococcal infection in the newborn. *Critical Care Nursing Clinics of North America* 4 (3), 487–493.

Grobman, D., and Foley, M. (1992). Surfactant replacement therapy in newborns with hyaline membrane disease. *Critical Care Nursing Clinics of North America* 4 (3), 515–520.

Jackson, C., and Saunders, R. (1993). *Child health nursing.* Philadelphia: J. B. Lippincott.

Jorgensen, K. (1992). The drug-exposed infant. *Critical Care Nursing Clinics of North America* 4 (3), 481–485.

Korones, S. (1986). *High risk newborn infants: The basis for intensive nursing care,* 4th ed. St. Louis: C. V. Mosby.

Ladewig, P., London, M., and Olds, S. (1990). *Essentials of maternal-newborn nursing,* 2nd ed. Redwood City, CA: Addison-Wesley.

Long, C. (1992). Teaching parents infant CPR—Lecture or audio-visual tape? *Maternal Child Nursing* 17 (1), 30–32.

Mattson, S., and Smith, J. (1992). *NAACOG core curriculum for maternal-newborn nursing.* Philadelphia: W. B. Saunders.

May, K., and Mahlmeister, L. (1990). *Comprehensive maternity nursing: Nursing process and the childbearing family,* 2nd ed. Philadelphia: J. B. Lippincott.

Mott, S., Fazekas, N., and James, S. (1990). *Nursing care of children and families: A holistic approach,* 2nd ed. Menlo Park, CA: Addison-Wesley.

Pillitteri, A. (1992). *Maternal and child health nursing.* Philadelphia: J. B. Lippincott.

Reeder, S., and Martin, L. (1991). *Maternity nursing,* 17th ed. Philadelphia: J. B. Lippincott.

Ross, T., and Dickason, E. (1992). Nurses' alert: vertical transmission of HIV and HBV. *Maternal Child Nursing* 17 (4), 192–195.

Rubin, R. (1961). Basic maternal behavior. *Nursing Outlook* (November): 683–686.

Schuler, K. (1979). When a pregnant woman is a diabetic: antepartal care. *American Journal of Nursing* (March): 448–450.

Schuler, K., Wimberly, D., Rancilio, N., and Vogel, M. (1979). When a pregnant women is a diabetic: a case study. *American Journal of Nursing* (March): 446–448.

Taptich, B., Iyer, P., and Bernocchi-Losey, D. (1990). *Nursing diagnosis and care planning.* Philadelphia: W. B. Saunders.

Whaley, L., and Wong, D. (1991). *Nursing care of infants and children,* 4th ed. St. Louis: C. V. Mosby.

UNIT V

The Mental Health Client

19

Treatment Modalities

PRE-TEST Therapeutic Modalities

1. In the second session of a therapeutic group, a member talks for 15 minutes about the cold winter weather and the possibility of a snowstorm during the coming week. This behavior is an example of which of the following characteristics?
   ① Attempt to provide structure for the group
   ② An attempt to act as leader of the group
   ③ A need to maintain interaction at a superficial level
   ④ A need to express dependence

2. Sally is a nurse on an acute inpatient psychiatric unit. She has been assigned to Joe, who was admitted the previous day. As Sally accompanies Joe to the interview room, he asks, "So what is going to happen now?" Sally's best response at this time would be
   ① "We can talk about anything you would like. Pick a topic that really interests you. Are you at all interested in sports or would you rather talk about something else?"
   ② "I will be meeting with you each day for 1 half hour to talk about problems that caused you to come to the hospital and issues you want to work on while you are here."
   ③ "What do you think is going to happen now?"
   ④ "You seem anxious. Why are you feeling that way?"

3. For the past 2 weeks, Joe has met with her at 10:00 A.M. each day, as he had agreed, for their one-on-one sessions. Today, it is 10:30 A.M., and Joe has not come. When Sally finds Joe asleep in the day room, he says he is tired of their meetings and would rather spend the time sleeping. Which of the following assessments is most correct?
   ① Joe needs extra sleep; it is important to consider his physiological need
   ② Joe is bored with Sally and needs to be assigned a different primary nurse
   ③ Joe is displaying antisocial behavior that must be brought to the attention of his psychiatrist
   ④ Joe is displaying resistance, a common occurrence during the working phase of the nurse-client relationship

4. Your assigned client comes to you in tears and says, "She was so terrible to me. She shouldn't treat me that way." Your best initial response would be
   ① "Who was terrible to you?"
   ② "What were your feelings when she was terrible to you?"
   ③ "Please describe what happened."
   ④ "What do you mean by 'terrible'?"

5. As the nurse approaches a client for their one-on-one session, she remarks, "You seem concerned about many things. What would you like to talk about today?" This broad opening statement by the nurse is intended to
   ① Encourage the client to delve into past experiences
   ② Introduce a topic of conversation
   ③ Encourage the client to set the focus of the interaction
   ④ Orient the client to reality

THERAPEUTIC COMMUNICATION AS PART OF THE NURSING PROCESS

I. Assessment and analysis (collect data and make inquiries)
   A. Definition: communication is a multidimensional reciprocal complex interaction by which information is exchanged, views are shared, and emotions are expressed between two human beings; encouraged by the nurse, based on trust, and goal directed
      1. Critical components of communication
         a. Sender (encoder): person or object intent on relaying message
         b. Message: what sender wishes to send, what is actually sent, and what receiver understands or perceives
         c. Receiver (decoder): person or object getting message or doing the listening (reciprocal behavior of receiver validates that message received)
         d. Feedback: receiver validates the message received
   B. Use therapeutic communication to effectively gather data and encourage clients to share; when meaning analyzed, it leads to formulation of nursing diagnosis
   C. Characteristics of therapeutic communication
      1. Client centered: nurse's activities and conversation designed to meet client's needs; sensitivity, comfort, and individuality of client take precedence
      2. Always goal directed, depending on stage of relationship
      3. Authenticity; health care providers work in accord with their own attitudes, beliefs, and values
      4. Self-disclosure by client; facilitated interactions kept confidential except when need to share with other health care providers
      5. Acceptance of client at present level of functioning

NURSING PROCESS APPLIED TO MENTAL HEALTH

I. Assessment: collection of data about the health status of the client in all dimensions
   A. Physical assessment
      1. Genetic data are assessed for evidence of client risk factors
      2. Physiological processes are assessed through history and physical examination
   B. Mental status examination
      1. Level of awareness and orientation
         a. Confusion: disorientation to time, place, and/or person
         b. Clouding of consciousness: slight-to-moderate disturbance in perception or thought
         c. Coma: loss of consciousness
      2. Appearance and behavior

a. Client appearance in relation to age
b. Type and amount of client behavior
3. Speech and communication
    a. Type and amount of client speech
    b. Volume of speech
4. Mood or affect
    a. Range of mood
    b. Depth of mood
    c. Appropriateness of mood to situation
5. Thought processes
    a. Clarity: coherent, confused, or incoherent
    b. Content: presence of delusions, obsessions, phobias, grandiosity, ideas of influence, ideas of reference, preoccupations
    c. Flow: thought blocking, loose associations, tangentiality, perseveration
    d. Memory: recent, remote, presence of confabulation
6. Perception
    a. Hallucinations: client experiences sensations that do not exist in reality
    b. Illusions: client distorts actual stimuli (a tree limb scratching the window is misinterpreted as a dead aunt speaking to him/her)
    c. Depersonalization: a feeling of unreality about oneself
7. Suicidal, assaultive, or elopement potential
8. Insight
    a. Insight into illness: client understanding of illness and need for treatment
    b. Judgment: ability to formulate a socially appropriate plan of action
    c. Capacity for abstract thought: ability to think conceptually or to plan for the future
II. Analysis of data base leads to nursing diagnosis
    A. Nursing diagnosis: NANDA approved, based on a synthesis of all data
    B. Psychiatric diagnosis: identified according to DSM-III-R guidelines, using a multiaxial approach to classification
III. Planning: establishment of goals for client from collaboration among the nurse, client, family members, and health care team
    A. Goals are mutually agreed on
    B. Once goals are achieved, they are revised so that the client assumes greater responsibility
    C. Short-term and long-term goals are formulated and refined as necessary
IV. Implementation: intervention in areas of disruption and disability
    A. Interventions to validate reality
    B. Interventions to reinforce positive behavior/coping mechanisms

C. Interventions to promote appropriate socialization
V. Evaluation: exploration of client reactions (thoughts and feelings) to plan of care to determine progress and/or attainment of goals

NURSE-CLIENT RELATIONSHIP

I. Definition: an interpersonal process intended to support the client as client evaluates needs, solves problems, shares thoughts and feelings, and acquires new coping skills
    A. Preinteraction phase
        1. Nurse explores personal beliefs and feelings
        2. Nurse examines personal strengths and weaknesses
        3. Nurse prepares for first interaction with client
    B. Orientation/initial phase
        1. Negotiation of purpose of the relationship; what will be worked on, expectations, boundaries
            a. Duration of sessions and relationship
            b. Place and time of meetings
            c. Issue of confidentiality
            d. Mutual goals that are realistic and achievable
        2. Nurse gathers information through observation and interviewing skills
            a. Assessment of data leads to formulation of nursing diagnosis
            b. Data used for nursing input to client treatment plan
        3. Formulation of contract agreement between nurse and client about plan of care
    C. Working phase
        1. Description and clarification of client problems
        2. Prioritization of problems; focus on most important problems first
        3. In-depth exploration of client issues
        4. Client begins to devise new methods of coping
        5. Client begins to express thoughts and feelings (self-disclosure)
        6. Client rehearses new patterns of behavior
        7. Empathy and rapport develop between nurse and client
        8. Nurse might encounter setbacks from client resistance, testing, lack of trust
    D. Termination phase
        1. Separation issues
            a. Client might avoid interactions
            b. Client might attempt to extend interactions

c. Client might regress to earlier behaviors

d. Client might display anger, sadness

2. Termination work should begin early in the nurse-client relationship

3. Progress summarized; degree of goal attainment is evaluated

4. Feedback is given by nurse

5. Nurse and client share feelings about the relationship and separation

6. Referral is made to support services

II. Therapeutic communication (Table 19-1)

   A. Focusing

   B. Interpreting

   C. Confronting

TABLE 19–1 Techniques of Therapeutic Communication

Technique	Rationale	Example
Use of broad opening statements	To encourage the client to set the focus of the conversation	"What would you like to talk about?"
Use of general leads	To encourage the client to continue; to indicate the client is being heard	"It sounds like your wife means a lot to you." "Go on." Nurse nods.
Reflection	To repeat part of what the client has said so client can consider and expand on statement	Client: "I was afraid to see my father again." Nurse: "You were afraid to see your father again."
Sharing an observation	To focus on a client's emotional state; to share an observation about a client's behavior	"I notice you begin pacing and shaking when you talk about your family."
Acknowledgment of feelings	To let the client know the client's feelings are understood and accepted; to encourage the further expression of feelings	"It must be devastating to learn your job has been eliminated."
Selective reflection	To emphasize the importance of a particular topic; nurse selects the most important idea out of many the client has stated	Client: "I'm mad at my husband because he always plays cards, and drinks, and never listens to me." Nurse: "You are angry your husband never listens to you?"
Use of silence	To slow the pace of the conversation and/or allow the client time to collect his or her thoughts	
Giving information	To provide the client with specific information	Nurse: "We will be having group therapy sessions daily."

D. Summarizing

E. Limit setting

F. Positive reinforcement

G. Active/cathartic listening

   1. Active hearing with understanding

   2. Beginning of dialogue

   3. Nurse earns client's respect and trust

   4. Focused on content and feeling of communication, "hears" words not uttered, sees clenched hands, understands silence

H. Use questioning

   1. Open-ended to encourage free expression on range of responses: "tell me about . . . ," "describe . . . ," used profitably at beginning of interview

   2. Closed: can be answered with one word; used when specific information needed; could be useful at close of interview when bits of information needed

  I. Give general leads

  J. Use silence as appropriate

III. Nontherapeutic communication (Table 19-2)

   A. Halo effect: generalizing groups of clients rather than rating each client individually

   B. Stereotyping: ascribing qualities to individuals that are typical of group

   C. Recording errors: result when too much time occurs between interview and documentation

   D. Countertransference: conscious or unconscious reaction to or identification with client; confuse clients with persons who are important in own life

   E. Egocentrism

   F. Denial

   G. Resistance

   H. Listening only to words

MILIEU THERAPY

I. Definition: structuring client environment for therapeutic purposes of enhancement of client self-esteem, facilitation of open communication, promotion of individual responsibility, cultivation of democratic environment, reduction of distance between staff and clients, control of deviant behavior, and promotion of social learning

II. Characteristics of therapeutic milieu

   A. Distribution of power: use of community meetings/client government to make decisions, air community issues, and solve community problems

   B. Open communication among staff members, among clients, and between staff and clients

   C. Consistency among staff members in approaches to clients

   D. Interdisciplinary team approach to client care

TABLE 19–2 Blocks to Therapeutic Communication

Technique	Rationale	Example
Use of reassurance	Conveys to client that nurse feels client is worrying needlessly or is not interested in his or her problems	"Everything will be all right."
Giving advice	Nurse imposes personal opinions on the client; undermines client's ability to make own decisions	"I think you should ___."
Giving approval	Nurse conveys judgment of client's behavior	"That's the right thing to do."
Requesting an explanation	Places the client on the defensive by making client defend his or her action	"Why did you do that?" "Why do you feel that way?"
Agreeing with the client	Nurse interjects own opinions; may prevent client from freely expressing himself or herself	"I agree with you. You are right about that."
Expressing disapproval	Placing a negative judgment on client's behavior	"You should stop feeling that way."
Belittling client feelings	Denies the importance of client's feelings	"That is nothing to worry about."
Defending	Implies client has no right to voice negative opinions	"The staff are all good and really care about you."
Making stereotypical comments	Nurse directs the conversation away from topics causing personal discomfort	"Every cloud has a silver lining."
Changing the subject	Superficial communication	"That reminds me of when. . . ."

E. Community and family involvement
F. Limit-setting by staff: limits set on client behavior that is deviant, destructive, disorganized, and/or dependent
G. Adaptation of environment to meet client needs
　1. Provide for client orientation
　2. Provide pleasant surroundings; furniture arranged to promote interaction
III. Role of the nurse
　A. Provide input into unit design
　B. Model appropriate behavior/open communication for clients
　C. Encourage client involvement in unit activities to enhance self-esteem
　D. Participate in conflict resolution between clients and staff members
　E. Set appropriate, consistent limits on deviant client behaviors

F. Function as a member of interdisciplinary team providing input on plan for client care and reporting on client progress

FAMILY THERAPY

I. Definition: modality focused on treatment of dysfunction in family system
　A. Characteristics
　　1. Entire family is viewed as "client"
　　2. Therapy focused on processes among family members that support and perpetuate symptoms
　　3. Family members are sufficiently oriented to reality to participate actively in therapy sessions
II. Role of the nurse
　A. Assessment of family communication patterns, secrets, rules/norms, anxieties, and hopes for future
　B. Intervention
　　1. Discussion of problems, stressors, and symptoms that led family to seek treatment
　　2. Discussion of role of each family member in maintaining problem
　　3. Discussion of effect of problem on each family member
　　4. Facilitation of trust and open communication among family members
　　5. Support of family members as they develop new coping mechanisms
　　6. Encouragement of family members to become more self-reliant
　C. Evaluation
　　1. Involve family in evaluation of goal attainment
　　2. Refer family to support services

GROUP THERAPY

I. Definition: two or more clients have frequent interactions with therapist to change maladaptive coping methods of individual members or to provide support
II. Characteristics
　A. Group process: continual interaction among group members
　B. Curative factors: elements of group process that help individual members
　　1. Instillation of hope: seeing progress in other members is encouraging
　　2. Universality: clients realize others have similar problems
　　3. Altruism: helping other members increases each client's self-esteem

4. Imitative behavior: leaders and clients act as role models
5. Interpersonal learning: clients learn to relate more effectively to others in group and to significant others in their lives
C. Stages in group development
  1. Orientation phase: involves anxiety, superficial sharing of information, establishment of group rules
  2. Working phase: involves members confronting each other and eventual conflict resolution
  3. Termination: may occur by scheduled termination, abrupt departure of group member, or group decision that its work has been accomplished
III. Role of the nurse
A. Select and orient new group members
B. Guide early stages of group development
C. Focus on present
D. Protect members from scapegoating by other group members
E. Serve as role model and supporter of change
F. Limit monopolizing, circumstantiality, and disclosure of delusional material
G. Promote interaction by reflecting what has been said, seeking reactions of group members, and summarizing

ELECTROCONVULSIVE THERAPY (ECT)

I. Definition: artificial induction of grand mal seizure by passing an electric current through electrodes applied to one or both temples
II. Characteristics
A. Client anesthetized, and seizure lessened by administration of a muscle relaxant
B. Number of treatments determined by severity of client's symptoms and client's response to treatment
C. ECT effective in treatment of clients with certain types of depression and schizophrenia
D. Contraindications include physical disorders such as brain tumors and weakness of lumbosacral spine; these should be ruled out in advance of treatments
III. Role of the nurse
A. Provide opportunity for client expression of feelings, anxieties
B. Nursing responsibilities similar to those involved in surgical procedures
C. Provide patient education and respond to questions
D. After treatment, assess client for increase in confusion or memory loss (indications that course of treatment should be discontinued)

E. Allay client anxieties about temporary memory loss following treatment

LEGAL ASPECTS OF PSYCHIATRIC NURSING

I. State laws
A. Each state has mental health code regulating treatment of persons who are mentally ill
  1. States vary in rights granted to mentally ill persons
  2. State laws govern how and when certain client rights may be withdrawn
B. Legal terms
  1. Voluntary commitment: mentally ill client voluntarily enters hospital for treatment
    a. Client can be discharged from hospital when she or he decides to leave
    b. In most states, while hospitalized, client can refuse treatment
  2. Involuntary commitment: mentally ill client involuntarily hospitalized, often on emergency basis, under state statutory conditions
    a. In most states, client must be not only mentally ill but also harmful to self, harmful to others, or unable to meet basic needs
    b. Client loses right to sign self out of hospital
    c. In some states, involuntary clients cannot refuse treatment

POST-TEST Therapeutic Modalities

1. In a therapeutic group, Jane, a group member, states that another member is cold and rejecting. Sam, the other group member, responds, "You just don't understand me. For that matter, you don't understand any of us." During which stage of group development would this interaction be most likely to occur?
   ① The orientation phase
   ② The working phase
   ③ The termination phase
   ④ The group process phase
2. Jane continues by stating that she feels the other group members do not understand her. Which of the following statements by the nurse would best facilitate group process?
   ① "Who else in the group feels this way?"
   ② "Who else in the group has something they would like to share?"
   ③ "Jane, are these feelings related to something that happened in your childhood?"
   ④ "Tell us more about your feelings, Jane. When did they start?"

3. In a mental status examination, asking a client to interpret a saying such as, "Don't cry over spilled milk," is done to assess which of the following?
   ① Capacity for abstract thought
   ② Insight into illness
   ③ General knowledge
   ④ Judgment

4. You are accompanying a newly admitted client to your unit from the emergency department. He had been brought to the hospital by his niece, who said she found him wandering in his yard, talking to himself. The client states, "All you nurses have keys . . . Florida Keys . . . it's hot there . . . hot and cold running water. . . ." This is an example of which of the following?
   ① Loose associations
   ② Thought blocking
   ③ An obsession
   ④ A phobia

5. Which of the following characteristics differentiates therapeutic communication from communication that is of a social nature?
   ① Involvement of the nurse and client
   ② Goal directedness
   ③ Clarity and conciseness
   ④ Confidentiality

POST-TEST Answers and Rationales

1. ② The working phase of group development is a conflictual phase during which clients often voice disagreement and openly confront each other. 1, III. Group Therapy.

2. ① This intervention continues with the theme of a feeling of not being understood but encourages other members to join in the discussion. Choices 3 and 4 focus on only one member. Choice 2 belittles the feeling by changing the subject. 4, III. Group Therapy.

3. ① Asking the client to interpret a saying assesses the client's ability to abstract a larger meaning from the words presented. 1, III. Mental Status Examination

4. ① Loose associations are loosely connected thoughts that do not proceed logically toward a goal. Thought blocking is an interruption in thought processes. An obsession is a recurrent thought. A phobia is an intense, unrealistic fear. 1, III. Mental Status Examination.

5. ② Therapeutic communication is goal directed. Both types of communication can involve the other three choices. 1, III. Communication.

20

Behavioral Disorders

PRE-TEST Behavioral Disorders

1. An appropriate intervention for a client experiencing anxiety at the level of panic is:
   1. Place the client alone in a seclusion room
   2. Ask the client for a detailed explanation of events leading to hospitalization
   3. Communicate with the client using simple words and short phrases
   4. Increase environmental stimuli

2. The most appropriate nursing diagnosis for a 23-year-old female college student who is engaged to be married and comes to the student health center frequently with panic attacks would be:
   1. Altered perception related to psychotic process
   2. Altered nutrition: more than body requirements related to environmental stress
   3. Altered thought processes related to separation anxiety
   4. Ineffective individual coping related to high levels of anxiety

3. Common causes of anxiety do NOT include which of the following?
   1. Nonspecific threats to self
   2. Defenses that are not working well
   3. Fear of failure
   4. Threat to the biological integrity

4. Which of the following goals is appropriate for the client suffering from severe anxiety?
   1. The client will be relieved of all anxiety
   2. The client will avoid panic attacks
   3. The client will enter into psychotherapy
   4. The client will develop no further anxiety

5. Which of the following is NOT a characteristic of a phobia?
   1. Anxiety is attributed to an external source
   2. Displacement keeps the source of anxiety out of the consciousness
   3. The condition can be helped by insight-oriented therapy
   4. Secondary gains may be very important to client

6. Julie has been diagnosed as having panic attacks associated with agoraphobia. The nurse assigned to care for Julie realizes the client will avoid:
   1. Cold environments
   2. People who are strangers to her
   3. Standing in line
   4. Riding in elevators

7. Which of the following is useful in helping clients overcome a phobia?
   1. Place clients in phobic situations to desensitize them
   2. Point out adaptive coping mechanisms and reinforce them
   3. Help clients to avoid anxiety-producing situations
   4. Avoid the use of tranquilizers in treatment

8. Bulimia is best defined as:
   1. A pathological disorder of binging and vomiting
   2. An eating disorder associated with vomiting
   3. A disorder of unknown cause associated with starving oneself
   4. A phobic disorder of fear of obesity

9. The typical bulimic is:
   1. A middle-aged woman
   2. An obese African-American woman
   3. A 21-year-old college graduate
   4. An 18-year-old man

10. Other disorders likely to develop in the bulimic include all of the following EXCEPT:
    1. Hyperkalemia
    2. Dental erosion
    3. Gastric ulcers
    4. Rectal bleeding

11. Which of the following might be a cause of death in the bulimic client?
    1. Hypernatremia and congestive heart failure
    2. Hypokalemia and cardiac arrhythmias and arrest
    3. Metabolic acidosis and renal failure
    4. Hyponatremia and circulatory collapse

12. Joe has been admitted to the hospital six times in the past year for "work-ups," including an exploratory laporotomy, to diagnose his persistent abdominal pain. Because members of the health care team have not been able to "cure" him, they might consider the diagnosis:
    1. Somatoform disorder
    2. Hypochondriasis
    3. Anxiety disorder
    4. Somatic delusions

13. Cindy is an 18-year-old, weighing 80 lb, who is admitted to an inpatient adolescent program with a diagnosis of anorexia. Cindy has probably refrained from eating because she:
    1. Feels better when she is not eating
    2. Views herself as obese
    3. Experiences pain when she eats
    4. Wants her mother's constant attention

14. When the nurse interviews Cindy's parents, they are most likely to describe their daughter as:
    1. Constantly in trouble with the law
    2. Isolative and introverted
    3. Dependable and obedient
    4. Impulsive and unpredictable

15. Sam, a 55-year-old depressed client, attempted suicide after his job of 30 years had been phased out. He says to the nurse, "My wife says I should just stay home and not look for another job." The nurse's best initial response would be:
    1. "Do you always let your wife make major decisions for you?"
    2. "What will your neighbors say if you stay home without work?"
    3. "What are your thoughts about this?"
    4. "It seems your wife's opinion really concerns you."

16. An antidepressant medication, amitriptyline (Elavil), has been prescribed for Sam. A common side effect of the medication is:
    1. Diarrhea
    2. Anticholinergic effects
    3. Urinary frequency
    4. Cholinergic effects

Susan Blum, a 30-year-old divorced mother of two preschool children, has been a patient in a psychiatric hospital for 3 weeks. She has a habit of washing her hands repeatedly for long periods of time. Her hands are chapped and raw-looking. She is a registered nurse.

---

17. The most basic function of ritualistic behavior such as Susan's handwashing is to:
    1. Reduce the probability of infection
    2. Occupy the mind with seemingly purposeful activity
    3. Relieve one's anxiety
    4. Manipulate one's environment

18. Which statement is generally true of a client such as Susan who exhibits ritualistic behavior?
    1. If the client can be made to understand that the behavior is unreasonable, she will stop it
    2. The frequency of performance of the ritual is unrelated to the degree of anxiety
    3. The client may be aware that the ritual is illogical but is helpless to stop it
    4. The client is likely to be aware that she is performing the ritual

19. One night the nurse interrupts Susan's ritual and attempts to escort her to bed. Susan slaps the nurse. The most probable reason for Susan's behavior is:
    1. She dislikes the nurse as a person
    2. She resents regulations such as bedtime
    3. Ritualistic behavior is usually accompanied by overt aggression
    4. Because the ritual was interrupted, she experienced excessive anxiety

20. Susan later approaches the nurse and says, "I'm sorry I slapped you. I don't know what made me do it." Which reply by the nurse would be most appropriate?
    1. "I've already forgotten all about it. Tell me about your plans for today."
    2. "It's not pleasant to be slapped. Let's talk about how you felt."
    3. "I'm glad you realize it and are sorry about it."
    4. "You really surprised me. I didn't expect it."

Ann Hopkins is a 19-year-old who has been repeatedly hospitalized because of chronic mental illness. During each hospitalization, medications are used to stabilize her, and she is discharged. She then stops her medications and must be readmitted.

---

21. When developing a care plan for Ann, which of the following should be considered?
    1. The natural rebelliousness of this age group
    2. The number of staff available to work with her
    3. The availability of a young staff member to work with her
    4. The community resources available to her after discharge

22. The defense mechanism Ann is probably using to help her deal with her unrealized expectations is:
    1. Rationalization
    2. Repression
    3. Projection
    4. Denial

23. A structured routine is planned for Ann's inpatient care. Which of the following outcomes would indicate the plan is working?
    1. Ann asks to stay in bed instead of attending the community meeting
    2. With frequent prompts from staff, Ann attends occupational therapy

③ Ann takes a shower without being reminded
④ Ann asks for help eating her breakfast cereal

24. Which of the following can be said of a defense mechanism?
① It operates on a conscious level
② It can be controlled by client
③ It is part of normal ego maintenance
④ It is viewed as a psychosis

25. If John is angry at his boss and comes home and yells at his wife, he is using the defense mechanism of:
① Distortion
② Reaction formation
③ Suppression
④ Displacement

26. Chuck is a very ungainly youth who is poor at sports, so he focuses all his energies on his studies. This is an example of the defense mechanism of:
① Compensation
② Conversion
③ Projection
④ Rationalization

27. John has been unfaithful to his wife, but he tells all his friends that his wife is having an affair with another man. This is an example of what defense mechanism?
① Conversion
② Projection
③ Regression
④ Rationalization

PRE-TEST Answers and Rationales

1. ③ Communication should be at a level the client can comprehend in his state of anxiety. The client may have difficulty communicating with the nurse and should therefore not be asked for detailed explanations. The client should not be left alone. Stimuli should be decreased. 4, III. Anxiety Disorders.

2. ④ Anxiety appears to be interfering with the client's functioning ability. No symptoms of psychosis are noted. 2, III. Anxiety Disorders.

3. ③ Fear of failure is rarely a cause of anxiety because it is a conscious act. The other choices refer to common causes of anxiety. 1, III. Anxiety.

4. ② Helping the client limit the anxiety attack and avoid panic attacks is one of the major goals of treatment for anxiety attacks. One will never eliminate all anxiety from life and psychotherapy is not necessary for most anxious clients unless real phobias develop. 3, III. Anxiety.

5. ③ A phobia cannot be treated by insight-oriented therapy. Desensitization is the most common form of therapy. The other choices are common characteristics associated with phobias. 1, III. Phobias.

6. ③ Clients with agoraphobia fear open spaces and situations in which they feel vulnerable. 1, III. Anxiety Disorders.

7. ② When attempting to help a client overcome a phobia, the nurse should help the client recognize and strengthen any adaptive coping mechanisms that the client develops. Clients cannot be placed directly into situations that confront the phobia, but they must be helped to gradually face anxiety-producing situations. Tranquilizers are commonly used to help control the anxiety a client is feeling. 4, III. Phobias.

8. ① Bulimia is a pathological condition where the client eats massive amounts of food and then purges by either vomiting or using excessive laxatives. It is not a simple eating disorder, nor is it a phobia. Anorexia is an eating disorder associated with starving oneself. 1, III. Eating Disorders.

9. ③ The typical bulimic is a well-educated young woman. Caucasians are more prone to the condition than African Americans.

The client is usually of normal weight or slightly overweight. 1, III. Eating Disorders.

10. ① With the vomiting and especially with the diarrhea from laxative overuse, potassium is lost, resulting in hypokalemia. The other choices are common disorders associated with bulimia. 2, III. Eating Disorders.

11. ② The diarrhea and vomiting lead to hypokalemia, which predisposes cardiac irritability and possible arrest. This may be the cause of death in these clients. The other choices are unlikely. 2, III. Eating Disorders.

12. ① Somatoform disorder features recurrent somatic complaints for which medical attention has been sought but that apparently are not caused by any physical disorder. Hypochondriasis involves interpretation of a physical sensation as abnormal. A somatic delusion is the false belief a change has occurred in a body part. 1, III. Somatoform Disorders.

13. ② Anorexia nervosa is characterized by an alteration in body image. Symptoms are not attention-seeking in nature. 1, III. Eating Disorders.

14. ③ The client with anorexia nervosa is thought to be a product of a family that is rigid and seeks perfection. The client uses the symptoms to assert control in an area of her life. 1, III. Eating Disorders.

15. ③ Use of reflection encourages the depressed client to assume responsibility rather than remaining dependent. 4, III. Affective Disorders.

16. ② Elavil produces anticholinergic effects such as dry mouth and urinary hesitancy. Constipation is also a side effect of Elavil. 4, III. Affective Disorders.

17. ③ Ritualistic behavior is a coping mechanism for reducing anxiety. The other answers do not address the basic function of ritualistic behavior. 2, III. Obsessive-Compulsive.

18. ③ Because ritualistic behavior helps reduce anxiety, the client becomes aware that it is illogical but cannot stop it. This is the only method the client has for reducing anxiety. 1, III. Obsessive-Compulsive.

19. ④ If a person is forced to stop their ritualistic behavior, their anxiety will rise. This can cause excessive anxiety where the person actually feels they must fight or flee. 2, III. Obsessive-Compulsive.

20. ② This statement acknowledges the nurse's honest response to the situation and also indicates that the nurse is willing to continue therapeutic discussion with the client. 4, III. Obsessive-Compulsive.

21. ① At this age, natural rebelliousness is a major consideration that must be taken into account when caring for a client. A young staff member will not necessarily be best, and the number of staff is not important unless there are none available. Although community resources are important, the client must be willing to use them after discharge for them to matter. 3, III. Chronic Mental Illness.

22. ① Rationalization will help to soften the failure associated with the expectations the client is unable to meet. It is important to support this defense mechanism since failure can further impair the client's ego and lead to further setbacks. 2, III. Chronic Mental Illness.

23. ③ Choice 1 indicates withdrawal and an attempt to avoid participation. The other choices may indicate limited improvement. 1, III. Chronic Mental Illness.

24. ③ A defense mechanism is a part of the normal ego maintenance that protects the self from trauma. It operates on an unconscious level and is not controlled by the client. It is normal and not viewed as a psychosis. 1, III. Defense Mechanisms.

25. ④ The description is of displacement—moving anger from the correct object to a safer object. The other choices refer to other defense mechanisms. 2, III. Defense Mechanisms.

26. ① When individuals are unable to excel in one area, they often overcompensate by focusing all their energies in another area. The other choices refer to other defense mechanisms. 2, III. Defense Mechanisms.

27. ② Attributing your feelings or behaviors to others is known as projection. The other choices refer to other defense mechanisms. 2, III. Defense Mechanisms.

NURSING PROCESS APPLIED TO CLIENTS WITH BEHAVIORAL DISORDERS

Anxiety Disorders

I. Assessment
  A. Definition: a normal function; a diffuse feeling of dread, apprehension, or unexplained discomfort; a subjectively painful warning of impending danger that motivates individuals to take corrective action to relieve unpleasant feeling (if discomfort arises from identifiable external threat, it is called fear)
  B. Degrees of anxiety
    1. Mild anxiety
      a. Increased perceptual field, alertness, and potential for growth
      b. Acts as motivating force to bring about change
      c. Uncomfortable, but manageable
    2. Moderate anxiety
      a. Perceptual field decreases, alertness increases
      b. Concentration becomes more difficult
      c. Irrelevant tasks are shut out
      d. Increased physical and psychological discomfort
    3. Severe anxiety
      a. Decreased perceptual field
      b. Inability to problem solve
      c. Focus on one detail
      d. Extreme physical and psychological discomfort
      e. Vital signs increased
    4. Panic state
      a. Disintegration of personality organization and coping ability
      b. Inability to communicate or to problem solve
      c. Feeling of dread or of losing control
  C. Anxiety common to most disorders in which client experiences emotional discomfort and/or has psychiatric diagnosis
    1. Coping mechanisms used to decrease anxiety
    2. Overuse of these coping mechanisms may lead to symptom formation
    3. Use of defense mechanisms (Table 20-1)
  D. Characteristics
    1. Subjective feeling of physical and psychological discomfort

TABLE 20–1 Defense Mechanisms

Type	Definition	Example
Compensation	Real or imagined inadequacy alleviated by substituting another goal to maintain self-respect and gain the approval of others	Uncoordinated boy compensates for his lack of sports ability by focusing on his studies
Conversion	Feelings become unbearable and rechanneled somatically into a physical symptom	Woman sees her child killed and suddenly goes blind
Denial	Painful or anxiety-inducing aspects of reality are rejected as they actually are, thus eliminating need for anxiety	Alcoholic denies problem by saying he is a social drinker who can stop anytime
Displacement	Occurs when feelings distorted, separated from original object, transferred toward less threatening object	Man, angry with boss, takes it out on wife at home
Identification	Behavior, qualities, and attributes of someone admired are imitated until they become actual part of individual	Young boy dresses like his favorite sports hero
Introjection	Conflicting feelings, values, and attitudes of another person are assimilated so that they are no longer an external threat	Candidate professes agreement with every special interest group so no one will be against him
Isolation	Certain feelings and ideas set apart from others; emotional and intellectual content separated	Nurse known for humanistic qualities will not let child visit ill grandmother in hospital because it is against rules
Projection	Attributing undesirable feelings to other people or objects when these feelings become unacceptable to oneself	Man who hates boss tells everyone that boss has it in for him
Rationalization	Unacceptable feeling or responses justified or excused with logical reasons	Girl fails math test and blames English teacher who gave assignment due at same time
Reaction formation	Unresolved conflicts between feelings or impulses alleviated by reinforcing one feeling while repressing another, thereby disguising true feelings from self	Child who is angry at mother over affection shown new baby shows extra affection to baby
Regression	Person adopts behavior patterns characteristic of an earlier, less stressful time of development	Hospitalized adult regresses under stress of cancer diagnosis
Repression	Unwanted feelings unconsciously kept from awareness	Woman forgets date of sister's birthday because she has always hated her
Suppression	Unwanted feelings consciously kept out of awareness	Student failing high school refuses counseling and says she will make an appointment next week
Sublimation	Substituting socially acceptable behavior for unacceptable impulses	Childless couple treats pet dog like child, showering it with love and affection
Undoing	Negative actions negated by positive actions	Mother brings dinner to child after punishing child for misdeeds

2. In mild degrees, anxiety is normal experience
3. When mild, anxiety motivates person to take constructive action
4. When severe, can interfere with activities of daily living (ADLs) and requires outside intervention
5. Unrelated to any specific object

E. Incidence
  1. Affects everyone in mild-to-moderate degree
  2. May affect 5% of population in severe-to-panic form

F. Etiology/theories
  1. Response to unresolved, unconscious conflict or threat of repressed drives to invade consciousness (psychodynamic)
  2. Individual did not receive unconditional love and nurturing required as a child; attempts to "earn" love, resulting in a fragile ego and fear of disapproval throughout life (interpersonal)
  3. Inherited potential for vulnerability in locus ceruleus and other sites in the brain (biological)

  4. Response to stressors/trauma (environmental)

G. Predisposing/precipitating factors
  1. Threat to self-concept
  2. Threat to biological integrity
  3. Individual's defenses are not working well
  4. Common elements are fear of exposure and loss of control
  5. Tasks of earlier stages of development were unresolved

H. Clinical manifestations
  1. Panic disorder
    a. Sudden, intense, and discrete periods of extreme fear
    b. Accompanied by dyspnea, palpitations, chest pain, choking sensations, dizziness, derealization, paresthesias, hot and cold flashes, sweating, faintness, trembling or shaking
    c. Fear of impending doom
    d. Nonpurposeful activity, such as pacing, wringing hands
    e. Lack of ability to fight or take flight; therefore feeling trapped and helpless
  2. Generalized anxiety disorder

a. Manifested by steady, continuous, and persistent anxiety symptoms (at least 6 months' duration)

b. Motor tension, autonomic hyperactivity

c. Apprehension, dread, vigilance

II. Analysis

A. Anxiety related to continuous sense of dread

B. Knowledge deficit related to symptoms of anxiety and panic disorders

C. Ineffective individual coping related to inability to control anxiety and prevent panic attacks

III. Planning/goals, expected outcomes

A. Client will develop an open, trusting relationship with mental health professional

B. Client will recognize symptoms of onset of anxiety and intervene before reaching panic

C. Client will learn and use alternative methods of coping with anxiety

IV. Implementation

A. Examine context in which manifestations occur

B. Reassure client of safety and security

C. Provide surroundings low in stimuli

D. Administer tranquilizing medication (Table 20-2)

E. Help client develop insight

F. Encourage client to talk about traumatic experience under nonthreatening conditions

G. Use clear, simple words to communicate

H. Actively listen to feelings and concerns

I. Be aware of own feelings and behavior and their impact on client

J. Reinforce effective and constructive coping

K. Teach alternative methods of coping—for example, assertion training, behavior modification

L. Provide physical outlets for anxiety, such as mild exercise, crying, or simple, structured activity

V. Evaluation

A. Client's anxiety decreases to level where problem solving can be accomplished

B. Client verbalizes signs/symptoms of escalating anxiety

C. Client uses techniques for interrupting progression of anxiety

D. Client expresses concerns and unmet needs assertively

Phobias

I. Assessment

A. Definition: intense irrational fear of a specific external object or situation, which may interfere with normal function of person

B. Common types

1. Agoraphobia: fear of being alone or in public open spaces from which escape would be difficult

2. Claustrophobia: fear of enclosed places

3. Social phobia: fear of possibly embarrassing situations

C. Characteristics

1. Client attributes anxiety to external sources

2. Client uses displacement and symbolization to keep original source of anxiety out of conscious awareness

3. Fear of object or situation is intense and irrational

4. Client is resistant to most insight-oriented therapy (style is avoidance)

5. Client cannot explain fear but feels powerless to control it

D. Incidence

1. May affect 8% of population

2. Occurs frequently in childhood (generally disappears without treatment)

E. Etiology

1. Anxiety precipitates stimulus

2. Individual attributes anxiety to external sources and becomes phobic

F. Clinical manifestations

1. Panic attack experienced when client exposed to phobic stimulus (see Clinical Manifestations of Panic)

2. Refusal to leave home alone or to eat, speak, or perform in public

3. Refusal to expose self to specific object or situation

4. Apprehension

5. Fight or flight behaviors

G. Complications: focusing only on phobia may lead to lack of awareness of frequently associated problems, such as depression, chronic anxiety, sexual problems

II. Analysis

A. Anxiety related to unacknowledged conflicts

B. Ineffective individual coping related to avoidance of anxiety-producing stimuli (objects or situations)

C. Fear related to specific environmental stimuli

III. Planning/goals, expected outcomes

A. Client will verbalize decreased anxiety when exposed to phobic stimulus

B. Client will identify and discuss fear

C. Client will demonstrate less avoidance of phobic stimulus

D. Client will accept and participate in treatment to reduce phobic responses

TABLE 20–2 Sedatives-Hypnotics

Class	Example	Daily Dosage	Action	Use	Common Side Effects	Nursing Implications
Antipsychotic medications	Chlorpromazine (Thorazine) Thioridizine (Mellaril) Trifluoperazine (Stelazine) Fluphenazine (Prolixin) Perphenazine (Trilafon) Halperidol (Haldol)	100-1200 mg 200-800 mg 2-20 mg 2-20 mg 8-64 mg 4-100 mg	Block receptors in brain to dopamine and norepinephrine; depress areas of brain that control activity and aggression	Psychotic reactions, schizophrenia, hyperactivity in children, nausea and vomiting, sedation, agitation, severe anxiety, bipolar disorders	Laryngospasms, dyspnea, extrapyramidal syndrome, agranulocytosis, jaundice, photosensitivity, orthostatic hypotension, tachycardia, decreased libido, sedation, constipation, dry mouth, blurred vision, neuroleptic malignant syndrome, tardive dyskinesia	Avoid other CNS depressants; monitor mood and affect; monitor for development of extrapyramidal symptoms; monitor for liver function changes such as jaundice; monitor for early signs of blood dyscrasias; monitor blood pressure for hypertension and orthostatic changes; watch for constipation; do not open capsules; do not give with antacids; teach about orthostatic changes; avoid sunshine
Antianxiety medications	Diazepam (Valium) Chlordiazepoxide (Librium) Oxazepam (Serax) Alprazolam (Xanax) Loraxapam (Ativan) Temazepam (Restoril)	5-40 mg 15-100 mg 30-120 mg 1-4 mg 2-6 mg 15-30 mg	Act selectively as presynaptic inhibitors of neural pathways throughout CNS; have similar activities to CNS depressants but more selective	To treat anxiety, pre-op sedation, status epilepticus, acute alcohol withdrawal syndrome, mild muscle relaxant	Confusion, headache, agitation, oversedation, drowsiness, constipation, decreased libido, urinary retention, hypersensitivity, lethargy, blurred vision; may be habit-forming, withdrawal syndrome with prolonged use	Withdraw drugs slowly; not safe for use in pregnancy; watch for changes in liver function; monitor for development of paradoxical excitement; assess mood and affect; avoid use with alcohol or CNS depressants; food and antacids decrease absorption; avoid overuse and abuse; use carefully in clients with renal or hepatic failure or glaucoma; give with food; do not mix parenteral solution with any other drug
Barbiturates	Secobarbital (Seconol) Pentobarbital	90-200 mg	Reversibly depress activity of all excitable tissues; CNS particularly sensitive; sleep induced has decreased REM time	Sedation, sleeplessness, anticonvulsant (phenobarbital), general anesthesia adjunct	Drowsiness, lethargy, headache, depression, hangover, hypersensitivity, blood dyscrasias, rapid development of tolerance	Warn client about potential drug interactions, especially other CNS depressants; use other means to promote sleep; avoid overuse or dependence; monitor for overdose; rapid withdrawal could cause death

IV. Implementation
  A. Initially, avoid exposing client to feared object or situation
  B. Encourage client to discuss phobic response
  C. Assist client with desensitization (gradual exposure to phobic stimulus)
  D. Help client develop coping mechanisms to effectively confront phobic stimulus
  E. Help client relabel anxiety-producing aspects of phobic situation and change negative statements about self
  F. Administer imipramine (Tofranil) (tricyclic antidepressant drug of choice for agoraphobia)
  G. Administer antianxiety drugs, tranquilizers (see Table 20-2)
  H. Encourage client to identify life situations that generate anxiety and conflict
  I. Listen to and positively reinforce client's experiences of participation with treatment
V. Evaluation
  A. Client free of disabling fear when exposed to phobic situation or object
  B. Client verbalizes ways to avoid phobic situation or object with minimal change in lifestyle
  C. Client demonstrates adaptive coping techniques that may be used to maintain anxiety to tolerable level
  D. Client participates in treatment

Obsessive-Compulsive Disorder

I. Assessment
  A. Definition
    1. Obsessions: involuntary, recurring thoughts that cannot be ignored or eliminated
    2. Compulsions: recurring drives to perform seemingly purposeless activity
  B. Characteristics
    1. Obsesssions/compulsions serve to prevent or neutralize anxiety
    2. Panic-level anxiety may result if an attempt is made to curtail or interrupt client's thoughts or activities
    3. Client attempts to feel more secure through attempts to control environment and self
    4. Client's anxiety increases as change increases
  C. Etiology/incidence: may affect 0.05% of population
  D. Predisposing/precipitating factors
    1. Excessive anxiety
    2. Inability to control thoughts and impulses in effective manner
    3. Repetitive patterns of behavior
    4. Unresolved conflict from earlier stages of development
  E. Clinical manifestations
    1. Recurrent thoughts of contamination, violence, or self-doubt
    2. Persistent behavior of ritualistic nature in response to anxiety produced by rituals
    3. Strong need for control
    4. Client strives for perfection
    5. Excessive concentration on details
    6. Lack of spontaneity
    7. Obsessions and rituals are time consuming and interfere with daily activities
    8. Difficulty with decision making
    9. When severe, worries border on delusions
    10. Client realizes that behavior is excessive and irrational but feels compelled to continue
II. Analysis
  A. Anxiety related to unmet needs for safety and security
  B. Altered thought processes related to severe anxiety
  C. Self-care deficit: total, related to ritualistic behavior
  D. Ineffective individual coping related to inability to directly express anxiety
  E. Ineffective family coping: disabling, related to time-consuming client rituals
III. Planning/goals, expected outcomes
  A. Client will cope effectively in ADL without resorting to obsessive-compulsive behaviors
  B. Client will accept limits on repetitive acts and participate in alternative adaptive activities
IV. Implementation
  A. Develop affirming, dependable relationship
  B. Make careful assessment of total health needs
  C. Determine types of situations that precipitate anxiety and ritualistic behavior
  D. Avoid verbalizing disapproval of behavior
  E. Allow time for rituals; unhurried attitude
  F. Support client to explore meaning and purpose of behavior
  G. Establish reasonable time limits for completing rituals
  H. Gradually enable client to increase activities and decrease ritualistic behaviors
  I. Provide positive reinforcement for nonritualistic behavior
  J. Teach client to recognize and anticipate situations that precipitate obsessive thoughts and/or ritualistic behaviors
  K. Teach thought-stopping techniques, relaxation techniques, constructive activity, and exercise to interrupt thoughts and behavior patterns

L. Develop plan for decreasing interference of rituals in ADLs

M. Plan therapeutic interactions for time after ritual has been completed

V. Evaluation

A. Client verbalizes clinical manifestations of increasing activities to manage anxiety

B. Client interrupts obsessive thoughts and refrains from compulsive behaviors in response to stress

C. Client has increased feelings of self-worth

D. Client participates in ritualistic behavior fewer times and is involved in other activities

Dissociative Disorder: Multiple Personality (Hysterical Neurosis, Dissociative Type)

I. Assessment:

A. Definition: existence of two or more distinct personalities within the client, each with a distinct way of relating to the environment and to self

B. Etiology

1. Client blocks off part of life from consciousness during periods of intolerable stress

2. Stressful emotion becomes separate entity as individual "splits" from it and mentally drifts into fantasy state

3. Transition from one identity to another becomes method of dealing with stressful situations

C. Predisposing/precipitating factors

1. Client has often experienced severe abuse in early childhood

2. Threat to physical integrity/self-concept is so severe that the client copes with painful emotions by dissociating from them

3. Severe level of repressed anxiety

D. Characteristics

1. Client experiences two or more distinct personalities that interfere with goal-directed activity

2. Transition from one personality to another suddenly and often associated with psychosocial stress

E. Clinical manifestations

1. Impaired recall of specific incidents and/or client's past life or identity

2. Assumption of additional identities that may or may not be aware of the other identities

3. Feeling of unreality; detachment from stressful situation/reality

4. Accompanied by dizziness, depression, obsessive ruminations, anxiety, fear of going insane, and disturbance in subjective sense of time

5. Responsiveness to environment diminished or inappropriate (client believes he or she is being taken over by another person)

II. Analysis

A. Ineffective individual coping related to severe anxiety, alterations in consciousness

B. Personal identity disturbance related to repression of personal history

C. Anxiety related to situational stressors

III. Planning/goals, expected outcomes

A. Client will demonstrate ability to cope with stress without dissociation

B. Client will recover deficits in memory

C. Client will understand existence of multiple personalities within self and recognize stressful situations that precipitate transition from one to another

D. Client will express intentions to seek long-term care for disorder

IV. Implementation

A. Provide security and freedom from harm by being with client

B. Assist client in identifying stressor that precipitates severe anxiety

C. Help client to define more adaptive coping strategies; offer alternatives to be tried

D. Provide reinforcement for attempts to change

E. Identify community resources for support

V. Evaluation

A. Client demonstrates alternative techniques in coping with stress to prevent dissociation

B. Client identifies and verbalizes relationship between severe anxiety and dissociative response

C. Client recalls all events of past life

D. Client recognizes existence and purpose of more than one personality

E. Client verbalizes intent to seek long-term outpatient treatment

Somatoform Disorders

I. Assessment

A. Definition: history of multiple physiological complaints that have no organic basis

B. Etiology

1. Unresolved, unconscious conflict

2. Psychosocial stressors, including fear of responsibility

3. Dependent personality traits

4. Depressed mood state

5. Negative self-concept

6. Exposure to persons with actual physical symptoms

C. Predisposing/precipitating factors

1. Client's feelings and emotional needs involving conflicts are expressed physiologically

2. Development of physical manifestations helps client cope with stress of emotions

3. Symptom formation protects client from conscious awareness of repressed, unresolved conflict

D. Characteristics

1. Client often seeks medical attention for somatic manifestations

2. Client has no insight into the origin of manifestations or the purpose they serve

E. Clinical manifestations

1. Preoccupation with bodily functions

2. History of continually seeking medical treatment

3. Expresses frustration when informed there is no physiological basis for manifestations

4. Denies relationship between physical manifestations and psychological conflicts/stressors

5. Demonstrates dramatic behavior when describing physical manifestations

6. Avoids certain activities as result of physical manifestations

II. Analysis

A. Ineffective individual coping related to unmet dependency needs, inability to deal effectively with conflict

B. Anxiety related to unresolved conflicts

C. Chronic pain related to recurrent somatic complaints, depression

III. Planning/goals, expected outcomes

A. Client will verbalize a significant decrease in physical manifestations

B. Client will demonstrate a significant decrease in anxiety in absence of physical manifestations

C. Client will verbalize relationship between physical manifestations and stress/unresolved conflict

D. Client will accept laboratory tests and diagnostic criteria as valid

IV. Implementation

A. Review all laboratory and diagnostic results with client in language at client's level of comprehension

B. Acknowledge that although manifestations are real to client, no organic pathology has been found

C. Encourage client to discuss anxieties rather than focusing on physical manifestations

D. Redirect when client focuses on physical manifestations

E. Help client to determine relationship between stressful life events and the onset of physical manifestations

F. Assist client to develop alternative methods of coping such as assertive communication and relaxation techniques

G. Praise client for use of adaptive coping mechanisms rather than reliance on physical manifestations

V. Evaluation

A. Client refrains from discussion of physical manifestations with staff or family

B. Client demonstrates absence of physical manifestations

C. Client functions independently and assertively

Eating Disorders

Bulimia

I. Assessment

A. Definition

1. Pathological clinical syndrome of binge eating (rapid consumption of large amount of food in discrete period of time, usually less than 2 hours) followed by self-induced vomiting

2. May be form of affective disorder

B. Etiology

1. Unknown

2. Assume multifactorial cause

C. Incidence

1. Typical bulimic is Caucasian woman of average weight or slightly overweight for height

2. Single, in late teens to mid-20s (average age 18 years)

D. Predisposing/precipitating factors

1. After several diets, client becomes aware of vomiting or laxatives as means of weight control

2. Prolonged restrictive dieting and difficulty in handling emotions

E. Clinical manifestations

1. 75% have significant depressive manifestations and self-deprecating thoughts following binges

2. Overeating and self-induced vomiting ("purging") usually secretive or solitary events

3. Binge eating may occur from once weekly to one or more times daily

4. Binge lasts approximately 1 hour 15 min-

utes and can add up to more than 3400 calories before terminated; may last as long as 8 hours and add up to 11,500 to 50,000 calories

5. Dental erosion from gastric acid, parotid swelling, subtle physical changes
6. Stomach ulcers, involuntary vomiting, sore throats, rectal bleeding common
7. Bulemic is aware that eating pattern is abnormal
8. Lowered serum potassium; myocardial contractility and fatal arrhythmias or cardiac arrest may develop (most common cause of death for bulimics)
9. Overriding feelings of guilt, shame, and self-contempt follow binges
10. Fear of loss of control and of not being able to stop eating voluntarily

F. Diagnostic examinations
1. In-depth history
2. Physical examination (menstrual history, and hormonal imbalance, diet history, and routine examinations for dental erosions and parotid swelling)

II. Analysis
A. Altered nutrition: less than body requirements related to self-induced vomiting
B. Ineffective individual coping related to compulsive behavior regarding food intake
C. Self-esteem disturbance related to feelings of worthlessness, inadequacy, or guilt

III. Planning/goals, expected outcomes
A. Client will verbalize increased sense of self-esteem
B. Client will identify non–food-related methods for dealing with stress
C. Client will verbalize importance of adequate nutrition

IV. Implementation
A. Administer antidepressant (especially monoamine oxidase [MAO] inhibitors) as ordered (Table 20-3)
B. Help client determine daily diet that is adequate and nutritious
C. Help client develop ways of relieving stress that are not related to eating
D. Set limits on client's eating habits (e.g., food portions should be weighed; client should eat at dining room table at designated meal time)
E. Refer client to Overeaters Anonymous as a source of empathy and support
F. Family approaches may be helpful
G. Make appropriate referrals

V. Evaluation
A. Client ceases to binge and purge
B. Self-esteem is increased

C. Family is supportive and understands client's dilemma
D. Client demonstrates alternative ways of dealing with stress

Anorexia nervosa
I. Assessment
A. Definition: symptom complex with compulsive resistance to eating, intense fear of becoming obese, disturbed body image, with weight loss of at least 25% of original body weight in absence of physical illness
B. Incidence
1. Primarily females (90 to 95%)
2. Increasing in United States and affluent countries
C. Etiology
1. Unknown
2. Theories
a. Family interaction model: overprotection, rigidity, lack of personal boundaries and independence, ambivalent feelings toward mother; focus on anorexia to avoid interpersonal conflicts and conflict resolution
b. Behavioral: attention gained by rejecting food; client learns to manipulate to gratify needs
c. Psychoanalytical: regression to oral or anal stage of development to avoid adolescent sexuality and independence
d. Medical: possible dysfunction of hypothalamus, increased catecholamine activity, and/or genetic predisposition
D. Predisposing/precipitating factors
1. Major life change (e.g., moving away from home, first sexual encounter)
2. Parent-child role reversal
3. Client has conflicts with issues of identity, separation from family, and independence
E. Clinical manifestations
1. Resistance to treatment (client does not know how to accept help)
2. Denial that there is sickness or a weight problem
3. Feelings of loneliness, isolation; client tired of working so hard to achieve perfection; may want help for these difficulties
4. Client has difficulty accepting nurturance (has little experience with it)
5. Weight loss
6. Amenorrhea
7. Constipation
8. Hyperactivity
9. Hypotension
10. Bradycardia

TABLE 20–3 Antidepressants

Class	Example	Daily Dosage	Action	Use	Common Side Effects	Nursing Implications
Tricyclic antidepressants	Amitriptyline (Elavil),	100-300 mg	Increases norepinephrine and/or serotonin levels in CNS by blocking their reuptake by presynaptic neurons	Depression, agitated depression, also used to treat childhood enuresis	Orthostatic hypotension, hypertension, arrhythmias, headache, sedation early in use, dry mouth, constipation, fine tremors, abnormal liver function, urinary retention, lethargy, fatigue, blurred vision	Use carefully in clients with cardiac disease, seizures, urinary problems, BPH, pregnancy or lactation, hyperthyroidism, and narrow-angle glaucoma; do not give with MAO inhibitors; monitor blood pressure, hemopoetic system; monitor liver function; withdraw drug gradually; increase fiber and fluid in diet; provide oral hygiene; monitor mood and affect; use alcohol with care; response takes 2 weeks; teach to avoid orthostatic changes; reduced dosage in treatment of elderly clients
	Desipramine (Norpramin)	100-300 mg				
	Nortriptyline (Aventyl, Pamelor)	75-150 mg				
	Imipramine (Tofranil)	100-300 mg				
	Dexeoin (Sinequan, Adapin)	25-300 mg				
MAO inhibitors	Phenelzine (Nardil)	15-75 mg	Psychomotor stimulation; block oxidative deamination of naturally occurring monoamines (epinephrine, norepinephrine, and serotonin) leading to CNS stimulation; effect lasts for weeks	To treat depression, some phobia-anxiety states, some use in narcolepsy	Interactions with food and drugs, especially those containing tyramine, leading to overdose and hypertensive crisis; orthostatic hypotension; dry mouth; constipation; hesitancy; confusion, especially in elderly; delayed ejaculation; jaundice; leukopenia; anorexia; insomnia; headache	Teach food and drugs to be avoided—aged cheese, sour cream, beer, wine (especially chianti), yogurt, yeasts, pickled herring, aged meats, meat tenderizers, chicken livers, chocolate and caffeine; teach methods to avoid orthostatic hypotension; warn about delayed initial response and prolonged effect after discontinuing drugs; teach about side effects; monitor mood and affect; should be taken only as prescribed; do not give at bedtime; monitor for hypertensive crisis; avoid over the counter cold medications, allergy medications, and diet preparations
	Isocarboxazid (Marplan)	10-30 mg				
	Tranylcypromine (Parnate)	10-30 mg				

11. Hypothermia
12. Hyperkeratosis of skin (overgrowth of horny layer of epidermis)
13. Secondary sexual organ atrophy
14. Leukopenia
15. Hypoglycemia
16. Reduced metabolism and hormonal functioning
17. Normal thyroid and adrenal cortical functioning

F. Diagnostic examinations: nursing responsibilities
   1. Weigh and calculate percentage of normal body weight lost
   2. Assess eating patterns (amount and type of food taken and time and place foods eaten)
   3. Determine if food is forced, if there is vomiting
   4. Assess presence of anemia, hypotension, or amenorrhea
   5. Assess relationship with parents, friends, and others

G. Complications
   1. 5 to 21% die from malnutrition
   2. Recurrent infections
   3. Electrolyte imbalance resulting in cardiac disorders
   4. Prone to suicide

II. Analysis
   A. Altered nutrition: less than body requirements related to inadequate food intake, self-induced vomiting
   B. Body image disturbance related to morbid fear of obesity
   C. Self-esteem disturbance related to perceived loss of control in some area of life
   D. Ineffective family coping related to issues of control

III. Planning/goals, expected outcomes
   A. Client will have electrolyte and nutritional balances restored
   B. Client will learn to nurture self and to accept nurturance from others
   C. Client will gain weight appropriate for height and age
   D. Client will establish nutritionally adequate eating pattern
   E. Client will possess realistic body image (realistic attitudes and perceptions about own body size, needs, and function)
   F. Client will participate in care plan and demonstrate effective coping with ADLs
   G. Family/significant others will know client needs positive reinforcement for weight gain, not food eaten
   H. Client will make follow-up appointments and knows who to call for emergency

IV. Implementation
   A. Hospitalize for intravenous or oral feedings, tube feedings, if ordered
   B. Provide caring and nurturance when possible
   C. Use empathic listening
   D. Grant or restrict privileges based on weight gain (or loss) as means of limit setting
   E. Use behavioral contract to enforce limits on client eating (specific mealtime, activity time)
   F. Provide education (especially concerning normal growth and development and normal nutrition)
   G. Use mutual planning (control issues, needs to accept responsibility for self without guilt and ambivalence)
   H. Provide surveillance during meals and 30 minutes to 1 hour afterward
   I. Weigh client three times weekly at same time of day and in same clothing
   J. Provide good skin care
   K. Provide opportunities for staff to ventilate feelings about manipulative and self-destructive behavior

V. Evaluation
   A. Client verbalizes feelings of anger and ineffectuality
   B. Client regains and maintains electrolyte and nutritional balances adequate for growth and development
   C. Client cooperates in treatment plan and expresses feelings reflecting realistic body image
   D. Family participates in treatment plan
   E. Client comes for follow-up appointments

Affective Disorders (Mood Disorders)

I. Definition: variety of states and syndromes that include extremes in affect of mood; states may be combined or alone and have varying degrees of severity and duration, from normal to pathological and from mild to psychotic

II. Types
   A. Depressive disorders
      1. Major depression: depression so severe that client loses contact with reality, develops symptoms of psychosis, and might be at risk for suicide
         a. Major depression, single episode: one-time occurrence of major depression
         b. Major depression, recurrent: repeated episodes of major depression
      2. Dysthymic disorder: chronic depressive mood characterized by lack of pleasure in

ADL, impairment in social skills, and bodily complaints

B. Bipolar disorders: disorders characterized by high and low moods with periods of effective functioning in between
1. Bipolar, mixed: rapidly alternating episodes of depression and mania (elation); must have had at least one episode of mania
2. Bipolar, depressed: in current episode, client displaying symptoms of major depression
3. Bipolar, manic: in current episode, client displaying symptoms of mania with elated, expansive, or irritable mood
4. Cyclothymic disorder: repeated episodes of abnormally elevated and abnormally depressed moods occurring over time

Depression

I. Assessment
A. Definition: mood state characterized by feelings of sadness, guilt, and low self-esteem, often related to real or perceived losses
B. Incidence
1. Most frequently occurring emotional illness
2. Only 20 to 25% of those afflicted seek treatment
3. 40% recover without treatment
C. Etiology
1. Medical disorders: endocrine diseases (hypothyroidism, Addison's disease), neurological (brain tumors, Parkinson's disease), cancer, alcoholism, side effects of some drugs (antihypertensive medications such as reserpine)
2. Biochemical causes: chemical alterations in neurotransmitters; decreased levels of norepinephrine and serotonin
3. Genetic: family history of depression appears to increase susceptibility
4. Existential: accumulated losses such as rejection, marital discord, economic difficulties, situational losses, and lack of social support
5. Learning theory: history of "learned helplessness" (believing one has no control over life situations)
6. Psychological: rage and hostility are turned inward against one's self
D. Predisposing/precipitating factors
1. Significant loss: relationships; change in body image, status, or prestige or self-assurance and confidence; physical illness resulting in loss

2. Decreased self-esteem due to lack of love, respect, or approval
3. Success: too much expected by self or others
4. Negative view of self
5. Family interaction: high expectations and little approval of self
E. Clinical manifestations
1. Depression
a. Depressed feelings (worthlessness, hopelessness, helplessness)
b. Frequent crying spells
c. Limited interactions; withdrawals
d. Sleep disturbance: early morning waking or difficulty falling asleep
e. Appetite and weight change
f. Affect flat, sad
g. Lack of energy for normal activity (poor personal hygiene)
h. Physical complaints
i. Poor problem-solving skills
j. Lack of meaning in life
k. Lack of interest in sex
l. Confusion, disorientation
m. Feelings of guilt
n. Suicidal thoughts
o. Difficulty concentrating
2. Dysthymic disorder (manifestations for at least 2 years)
a. Depressed mood
b. No pleasure in ADLs
c. Impairment in social skills
d. Somatic complaints
e. No psychotic manifestations
F. Medical management
1. Electroconvulsive therapy (ECT) (see Chapter 19)
2. Antidepressant medication (see Table 20-2)
a. MAO inhibitors
b. Tricyclic antidepressants
II. Analysis
A. High risk for violence: self-directed related to hopelessness
B. Chronic low self-esteem related to feelings of worthlessness
C. Dysfunctional grieving related to multiple losses
D. Hopelessness related to feelings of despair
E. Sleep pattern disturbance related to internal stressors
F. Altered nutrition: less than body requirements related to internal stressors
III. Planning/goals, expected outcomes
A. Client will not harm self

B. Client will experience feelings of increased self-worth

C. Client will verbalize improved mood

D. Client will have adequate sleep and nutrition

E. Client will be increasingly involved in activities

IV. Implementation

A. Safety

1. "No suicide contract" with client

2. Close, unobtrusive observation

3. Teach side effects of medications

B. Hygiene

1. Help clients with ADLs when necessary

2. Observe for illness or infection

C. Rest and activity

1. Allow additional time for activities

2. Plan simple, structured activities

3. Provide assistance when necessary

4. Provide opportunities for rest

D. Nutrition and elimination

1. Monitor body weight

2. Modify food intake by increasing fiber and fluids to prevent constipation

3. Provide small meals high in protein and carbohydrates

E. Psychosocial

1. Provide empathy in presence and listening

2. Maintain calm, serious approach

3. Encourage client to verbalize anger and other negative feelings

4. Encourage client to discuss losses

5. Aid client in resolution of grief

V. Evaluation

A. Client does not harm self

B. Client experiences feelings of increased worth

C. Client verbalizes improved mood

D. Client's sleep and nutrition return to adequate levels

E. Client becomes increasingly involved in activities

Mania

I. Assessment

A. Definition: denial of loss with temporary restoration of self-esteem

1. Types

a. Hypomania: mild-to-moderate levels

b. Delirious mania: most severe level

B. Incidence

1. Occurrence among relatives of afflicted individuals higher than in general population

2. Overall two times more common in women than in men

3. First episode of bipolar disorder, manic phase, occurs before age 30

C. Etiology

1. Genetic

a. Family history of bipolar disorder appears to predispose one to development of the disorder

b. Dominant X-linked factor suspected in transmission of disorder

2. Biochemical: elation and euphoria appear to be caused by excess norepinephrine in brain

3. Psychosocial: development of self-concept disrupted, giving way to uncontrollable impulsive behavior of mania

D. Predisposing/precipitating factors

1. History of unrealistic expectations for success imposed by self or others

2. History of many profound losses

E. Clinical manifestations

1. Euphoria, excitement

2. Hyperactivity, disruptive behavior

3. Rapid, "pressured" speech

4. Irritability, sarcasm, anger, aggression

5. Superficial interpersonal relationships

6. Psychotic thought, including flight of ideas and delusions of grandeur

7. Meager appetite, infrequent pauses to eat

8. Sleep disturbances with resulting fatigue

9. Poor judgment and impulsive behavior as demonstrated by spending sprees, inappropriate dress (bright colors, excessive make-up and jewelry), and sexual indiscretion

10. Distractibility and short attention span

11. Constant motor activity

12. Lack of regard for rules or limits set by staff

F. Medical management (Table 20-4)

1. Lithium carbonate

2. Antipsychotic medications: used to assist in control of agitation or psychotic manifestations

II. Analysis

A. High risk for violence: directed at others related to anger

B. High risk for injury related to hyperactivity and expansive mood

C. Altered nutrition: less than body requirements related to increased activity

D. Disturbed sleep pattern related to hyperactivity

E. Altered thought processes related to low self-esteem

F. Ineffective individual coping related to overuse of defense mechanisms

III. Planning/goals, expected outcomes

A. Client will not injure self or others

TABLE 20–4 Antimanics

Example	Daily Dosage	Action	Use	Common Side Effects	Nursing Implications
Lithium carbonate (Lithane, Eskalith, Litholoid, Carbolith)	Acute mania 1800-2400 mg Maintenance 300-1200 mg Therapeutic range 0.6-1.2 mEq/L Toxic range 2.0 mEq/L or higher	Naturally occurring salt; exact mechanism unknown; enhance uptake of biogenic amines in brain, thus lowering levels in body; may alter sodium metabolism within nerve and muscle cells	To treat and prevent mania, hypomania, and bipolar disorders	Tremors, headache, impaired memory, lethargy, fatigue, ECG changes, hypothyroidism, anorexia, nausea, diarrhea, polyuria, leukocytosis, muscle weakness, confusion	Assess mood and affect; monitor for toxicity with blood levels (convulsions, ataxia, persistent nausea and vomiting, severe diarrhea and death); give with food or milk; take drugs as ordered; monitor CBC, electrolytes, and ECG; teach client side effects; maintain balanced fluid intake (2000-3000 mL) and salt intake; teach importance of monitoring blood levels regularly

B. Client accepts limits set by staff

C. Client will consume adequate daily calories to maintain body weight within 10% of ideal body weight

D. Client will sleep 6 to 8 hours each night

E. Client will be able to sit and converse in one-to-one and group situations

F. Client will identify an escalation in behavior and will interrupt process

G. Client will handle anger constructively

H. Client will demonstrate decreased activity

I. Client will demonstrate decreased impulsivity

IV. Implementation

  A. Safety: monitor client for suicidal gestures and other behavior potentially harmful to self or others

  B. Hygiene
    1. When necessary, assist with ADLs
    2. Observe for symptoms of infection or illness

  C. Rest and activity
    1. Provide calm environment, free of distractions
    2. Provide constructive activities as outlets for excess energy (e.g., aerobic exercises or writing journal)
    3. Decrease stimulation before bedtime
    4. Protect client from exhaustion

  D. Nutrition and elimination
    1. Provide client with nutritious "finger foods" high in proteins and carbohydrates
    2. Monitor food and fluid intake

  E. Psychosocial
    1. Use nondefensive response to client criticism and anger
    2. Set limits on manipulative behavior

    3. Encourage client to discuss past losses
    4. Promote appropriate socialization
    5. Teach client to identify stressors and to manage these appropriately

V. Evaluation

  A. Client asks staff to help control behavior when necessary

  B. Client behaves in accord with rules and limits set by staff

  C. Client verbalizes anger and chooses appropriate alternative behaviors to cope with anger

  D. Client no longer exhibits hyperactive behavior

  E. Client demonstrates appropriate behavior in social situations

  F. Client no longer exhibits signs of physical agitation or behavior potentially injurious to self or others

Organic Mental Disorders

I. Assessment

  A. Definition: psychiatric conditions caused by neurophysiological, neurochemical, or structural alterations of the brain
    1. Acute: temporary; reversible with no residual effects
    2. Chronic: irreversible; progressive; mild-to-severe symptoms

  B. Classifications
    1. Delirium: acute, with rapid onset; characterized by clouded sensorium; client appears sick or bewildered
    2. Dementia: chronic, with slow onset; characterized by confusion and impaired function that develop gradually over time

C. Etiology
 1. Delirium: brain trauma; brain infections (encephalitis, meningitis); systemic infections with fever; drugs (psychoactive substance, prescribed medications); withdrawal from drugs, head injuries
 2. Dementia: Alzheimer's disease, Huntington's chorea, intracranial neoplasm
D. Incidence
 1. Delirium occurs more often in children, in adults over age 60, and in persons with a history of delirium, brain damage, or substance abuse
 2. Dementia is most often seen in persons over age 65
E. Predisposing factor: higher incidence in families with a history of dementia
F. Clinical manifestations
 1. Delirium
  a. Confusion, disorientation, inability to test reality
  b. Slowed thought processes; inability to reason or problem solve
  c. Incoherent speech
  d. Dream-like state
  e. Misperception of stimuli
  f. Manifestations often more pronounced at night or in early morning ("sundowner's syndrome")
  g. Emotional disturbances such as fear, anxiety, depression, anger, apathy, euphoria
 2. Dementia
  a. Impairment of short-term and long-term memory
  b. Impairment of intellectual functioning, judgment, reasoning, abstract thought
  c. Personality changes that interfere with socialization, work, and relationships
  d. Wandering; becoming lost
  e. Aphasia and apraxia may also occur
II. Analysis
A. Altered thought process related to confusion/dementia
B. High risk for injury related to confusion
C. Self-care deficits related to dementia
III. Planning/goals, expected outcomes
A. Client will not be injured
B. Client will attain optimal adaptive functioning within own limitations
C. Family will understand client situation and know where to find support or resources
IV. Implementation
A. Safety

 1. Provide anticipatory planning and safe, routine, printed schedule
 2. Introduce changes slowly
 3. Add visual cues to setting, such as clocks, calendars, orientation boards
B. Hygiene
 1. Add visual cues
 2. Check hearing aids and eyeglasses for effective function
C. Rest and activity
 1. Restrict intrusive or diagnostic procedures
 2. To promote sensory stimulation, expose patient to bright colors, textures, foods/flavors, and noncompetitive activities, such as movement therapy
 3. Promote rest and continuity of personnel
D. Nutrition and elimination: use behavior-modification techniques
E. Self-esteem and affiliation
 1. Reduce expectations to those that can be accomplished
 2. Give consistent, immediate praise for any degree of success
 3. Establish relationships that convey value of client
 4. Teach behavior-modification techniques to family, if appropriate
 5. Inform family about support groups and appropriate community resources
V. Evaluation
A. Client remains free from injury
B. Client attains optimal adaptive level of functioning
C. Family knows that support and referral are available

Schizophrenia
I. Assessment
A. Definition: disintegrative life pattern characterized by thinking disorder, withdrawal from reality, bizarre regressive behavior, poor communication, impaired interpersonal relationships, and changes in affect
 1. Types
  a. Catatonic
   (1) Stuporous state: mute, immobile, waxy flexibility, may retain urine and feces
   (2) Excited state: assaultive, aggressive, hyperactive, agitated
  b. Disorganized: incoherence, regressive behavior, loose associations
  c. Paranoid: delusions of persecution and grandeur

d. Undifferentiated: variety of manifestations found in other types

e. Residual: eccentric in behavior, social withdrawal, inappropriate affect

f. Schizoaffective: characteristics of schizophrenia in addition to change in mood; depression or elation

B. Etiology/incidence

1. Onset of prodromal or active phase of illness before age 45

2. First episode occurs in adolescence or young adulthood

3. Affects approximately 1% of total population

4. Most prevalent of major psychoses

5. Increased incidence in lower social class

6. No single cause

  a. Biological: excessive dopamine

  b. Psychological: disrupted family communication or relationships

C. Prognosis: 25% recover completely

D. Precipitating factors

1. Environmental stress

2. May be precipitated by experience of loss, separation, or use of drugs

E. Clinical manifestations

1. The four A's

  a. Associative looseness: lack of organized thought or logical progression of thought

  b. Flat affect: limited emotional tone

  c. Ambivalence: conflicting feelings about the same object or person

  d. Autism: highly personal and illogical withdrawal from the real world

2. Thought processes

  a. Blocking: breaks in the progression of thought

  b. Delusion: fixed belief, improbable in nature, and not influenced by reason or contrary experience

    (1) Delusion of persecution: "The mob is trying to kill me."

    (2) Delusion of grandeur: "I have the power to cause earthquakes."

    (3) Somatic elusion: "My heart has turned to stone."

    (4) Thought broadcasting: belief client's thoughts are being transmitted to others

    (5) Thought insertion: belief others can put thoughts into the client's mind

    (6) Thought withdrawal: belief that others can remove thoughts from the client's mind

    (7) Ideas of reference: belief that other persons or media messages (from newspapers, radio, etc.) refer directly to the client

    (8) Ideas of influence: belief the client's ideas are controlled by an outside force

3. Perception

  a. Hallucination: perceptual disorder involving any of the five senses that occurs in the absence of external stimuli

  b. Illusion: sensory misinterpretation of actual environmental stimuli

4. Speech

  a. Echolalia: repetition of words addressed to the client by others

  b. Flight of ideas: continuous flow or rapid speech with frequent change of topic

  c. Neologisms: words invented by the client that have personal meaning but cannot be understood by others

  d. Circumstantiality: frequent interruptions in speech for elaboration on unimportant details

  e. Perseveration: frequent repetition of the same word, phrase, idea, or symbol

5. Dysfunctional behavior

  a. Grimacing

  b. Negativism

  c. Anergia: state of inaction

  d. Suggestibility

  e. Poor hygiene

  f. Lack of social manners

  g. Social withdrawal

  h. Anhedonia: lack of ability to experience pleasure

6. Affect

  a. Blunted affect

  b. Inappropriate affect

II. Analysis

A. Altered thought process related to unmet needs

B. Altered perception related to high levels of anxiety

C. Chronic low self-esteem related to reduced social functioning level

D. Social isolation related to lack of trust

E. Impaired verbal communication related to psychiatric process

F. Ineffective family coping: disabling related to dysfunctional patterns

III. Planning/goals, expected outcomes

A. Client will demonstrate improved hygiene and grooming

B. Client will be physically safe (regarding environment, effect of drugs)

C. Client will maintain adequate nutrition and fluid and electrolyte balances

D. Client will develop trusting relationships with staff members (increased social interaction)

E. Client will demonstrate social skills in group and individual settings

F. Client will identify and test reality (dismiss internal voice or hallucinations)

G. Client will communicate more easily with family members

H. Client will increase decision making and develop ability to be self-supporting

IV. Implementation

A. Establish therapeutic relationship (understand, support, guide, be consistent, show acceptance)

B. Administer medication; monitor for side effects

C. Teach and support client adherence to prescribed medications

D. Interpret and reinforce reality to client

E. Support client's feelings and accept client's right to feel them, no matter how illogical

F. Support client in setting own goals

G. Help client explore new ways to express feelings

H. Work with family to continue facilitation of client's expression of feelings after discharge

I. Look for patterns or themes in client's verbalization

J. Observe and discuss ambivalence as normal state of being in all persons

K. Discuss with client how behavior affects and is viewed by others; how inappropriate behavior may alienate others

L. Be clear and concrete in statements

M. Tell client what you do and do not understand

N. Have client name fact that is causing anxiety and connect it with hallucination

O. Tell client you do not hear or see hallucinations or illusions and acknowledge client's anxiety

P. Walk with or talk to client

Q. If client hearing voices, ask what is going on at time and what the voices do for client

R. Focus on immediate environment and do not give status or recognition to voices

S. Avoid arguing with patient about delusional thoughts

V. Evaluation

A. Client does self-care for hygiene

B. Client does not injure self, has adequate rest, and does not experience side effects of drugs

C. Client maintains food and fluid intake adequately

D. Client develops relationship with staff member and begins interaction with others

E. Client does not pay attention to hallucinations; increases relationships with people

F. Client behaves appropriately in group and individual settings

G. Client increases adaptive communication with family members

H. Client makes some successful decisions, locates a healthy living space, and has plan to be self-supporting

Delusional (Paranoid) Disorder

I. Assessment

A. Definition: nonbizarre delusions of grandeur, persecution, jealousy, or somatic delusions involving situations that occur in real life; hallucinations are not prominent

B. Etiology

1. Onset occurs most often in mid or late adult life

2. Fear of loss of autonomy or loss of control

3. Crisis—developmental or situational

4. Possible genetic involvement

5. Parents may have been rigid, demanding, and perfectionistic, engendering rage, poor self-concept, and lack of trust in the individual

6. Organic dysfunction (dementia) or toxic state (substance abuse) might be related

7. Projection is the primary defense mechanism used

C. Clinical manifestations

1. Extreme suspicion

2. Expectations of trickery or harm

3. Guardedness or secretiveness

4. Hypercritical of others

5. Jealousy

6. Withdrawal from others

7. Overconcerned with hidden motives and special meanings

8. Clear, logical, persistent delusional system; may have only one area of fixed delusions

9. Develops paranoid community of "they" as source of danger

10. Severe anxiety; inability to relax

11. Expresses feelings of inadequacy, worthlessness

12. May display assaultive/violent behavior

II. Analysis

A. High risk for violence: directed at others related to perceived threats of danger

B. Altered thought processes related to excessive use of projection

C. Chronic low self-esteem related to lack of positive feedback

D. Social isolation related to mistrust of others

E. Powerlessness related to feelings of inadequacy

III. Planning/goals, expected outcomes

    A. Client will re-establish appropriate communication and feedback with staff member

    B. Client will verbalize increased self-esteem and decreased anxiety

    C. Client will increase verbal and nonverbal messages that are clear and consistent

    D. Client will express anger without aggression

IV. Implementation

    A. Protect client and others by observing closely, yet respect privacy

    B. Convey that you do not perceive reality in same way that the client does, but you are willing to listen, learn, and offer feedback

    C. Foster trust, follow through on commitments to lessen feelings of guilt and rejection

    D. Use several brief contacts rather than one prolonged one to minimize anxiety

    E. Respect privacy and preferences to increase cooperation

    F. Use consistency in approach

    G. Be as honest and open as possible to avoid misinterpretation and to increase trust

    H. Avoid power struggles; accept superior, sarcastic behavior calmly

    I. Avoid logic and reasoning

    J. Use simple, clear language and avoid physical contact

    K. Acknowledge fears and direct attention to other activities

    L. Let client fix own meals, eat out of original containers

    M. Offer noncompetitive solitary tasks that require some degree of concentration (jigsaw puzzles, crosswords, ceramics)

    N. Give concrete tasks to increase relatedness to reality

    O. Focus on the "here and now"

V. Evaluation

    A. Client establishes basic trust level as evidenced by willingness to confide in staff member

    B. Client participates in ADLs

    C. Client makes appropriate appraisals of situations and people

    D. Client gives up delusion; expresses feelings of anxiety

    E. Client improves social and mutual relationships by communicating feelings, needs, wants

    F. Family states that they are more comfortable with client

Personality Disorders

General Information

I. Definition: group behaviors or characteristics manifested by long-term patterns of maladaptive responses to stress

II. Types

    A. Paranoid personality: suspicious, fearful of attack, shy, aggressive, mistrusting

    B. Schizoid: withdrawn; restricted emotions

    C. Histrionic (hysterical) personality: dramatic displays of emotion, seduction, provocation, egocentric

    D. Obsessive-compulsive personality: orderly, obstinate, constrictive, rigid, perfectionistic, indecisive, restricted affection

    E. Passive-aggressive personality: resistant to performance in social and occupational settings by procrastination, forgetfulness, and inefficiency; covertly hostile, forgetful, obstructive, and inefficient

    F. Schizotypal personality: oddities of thought perception, speech, and behavior but not intense or often enough to be categorized as schizophrenia

    G. Narcissistic personality: grandiose sense of self-importance; preoccupation with fantasies of success, power, brilliance; exploitation of others

    H. Avoidant personality: social withdrawal as result of extreme sensitivity to rejection

    I. Dependent personality: allows others to assume responsibility for life because of inability to function independently; seeks constant reassurance, approval, or praise

Borderline Personality Disorder

I. Assessment

    A. Definition: personality disorder in which there is pervasive instability of mood, self-concept, and relationships

    B. Characteristics

        1. Client initially defending against abandonment and depression; needs assurance

        2. Splitting: primary defense mechanism for borderlines; inability to integrate negative and positive aspects of self and others

        3. Anger helps defend against closeness

        4. Intolerance of being alone

        5. Deep fear of abandonment when acting independently

        6. Inability to achieve boundaries of self (identity diffusion)

        7. Overuse of primary defenses (projection, denial, dissociation)

        8. Poor impulse control

        9. Acting out, manipulative behavior

10. May require hospitalization for transient psychotic symptoms
C. Etiology
   1. Basis of disorder established by age 3½
   2. Client must be 18 years or older for diagnosis
   3. More frequently diagnosed in women than in men
D. Predisposing/precipitating factors
   1. Mother feels threatened by increasing autonomy of child and withdraws emotional support or rewards clinging, dependent behavior
   2. Stress brings on alteration of behavior
E. Clinical manifestations
   1. Attempts to manipulate
   2. Pattern of unstable and intense interpersonal relationships (extremes of overidealization and evaluation)
   3. Impulsivity or unpredictability in at least two self-damaging areas (spending, sex, gambling, substance abuse, shoplifting, or overacting due to primitive thinking)
   4. Mood instability; usually lasts only a few hours, rarely more than three days and then returns to normal
   5. Inappropriate, intense anger; displays of temper, recurrent physical fights
   6. Recurrent suicidal threats, gestures, or behavior, or self-mutilating behavior
   7. Persistent identity disturbance; uncertainty regarding self-image, sexual orientation, long-term goals or career choice, and type of friends or values to have
   8. Chronic feelings of boredom or emptiness
   9. Alternating clinging and distancing behavior
   10. See in others attitudes not seen in self (projection)
   11. Feelings of depersonalization
   12. Poor reality testing
   13. Inability to control anger
II. Analysis
A. Personal identity disturbance related to overuse of splitting; unmet dependency needs
B. High risk for violence: self-directed related to impulsive, self-mutilating behavior
C. High risk for violence: directed at others related to intense/inappropriate expression of anger
D. Ineffective individual coping related to impulsive, self-destructive behavior
E. Impaired social interaction related to intense anger
III. Planning/goals, expected outcomes
A. Client will not harm self or others

B. Client will control impulses and will develop mature level of dependence and healthy and realistic coping behavior
C. Client will increase self-esteem, will accept own separateness and wholeness, and will relate well with others
D. Client will use therapeutic experiences as way to build trust
E. Client will be able to identify true source of angry feelings, own them, and express them socially
F. Client will not cling or distance self in interactions with others
IV. Implementation
A. Consistent approaches to patient by all staff members
   1. Encourage staff to discuss client's behavior and their responses
   2. Set firm limits without being punitive
B. Enable client to integrate good and bad images of people through consistent, nonexploitative relationships
C. Encourage self-monitored behavior-modification groups
D. Recommend marital and family therapy to help family separate and grow to autonomy
E. Give positive reinforcement for independent behaviors
F. Use psychotropic medications temporarily for psychotic-like episodes
   1. MAO inhibitors: clients with behavior on psychotic border (see Table 20-2)
   2. Lithium carbonate and phenothiazines: clients with core borderline syndrome for anxiety and depression (see Table 20-3)
   3. Antidepressants: adaptive, defended ''as if'' person, bland and superficial (see Table 20-2)
   4. Imipramine: border neurosis, child-like and clinging (see Table 20-2)
V. Evaluation
A. Client feels less anxiety and has no need for aggression or self-harm
B. Client verbalizes awareness of community support systems that can help when coping unsuccessful
C. Client does not manifest manifestations of depersonalization
D. Client interprets environment realistically
E. Client verbalizes how anger and acting out are related to maladaptive grieving
F. Client not using clinging and distancing behavior
G. Client understands use of clinging and distancing behaviors in failure of past relationships

Antisocial Personality Disorder

I. Assessment
A. Definition: chronic pattern of behavior since childhood that violates rights of others, yet client may appear pleasant and charming; an impulsive seeking of immediate gratification without feeling guilt and inability to learn from experience (sociopathic or psychopathic lay terms)
B. Characteristics
1. Pattern of behavior begins before age 15
2. Seldom seek treatment for the personality disorder
3. Inconsistent, neglectful parenting or parent with antisocial personality
4. Inadequate learning and control during childhood leads to client seeking instant gratification
C. Incidence
1. 5 to 15% of adult population; higher in socially deprived areas
2. 40% of prison population sociopathic or antisocial personality but this group responsible for 80 to 90% of crimes
3. More commonly diagnosed in men
D. Predisposing/precipitating factors (theoretical)
1. Client and parents display excessive EEG abnormalities, suggesting genetic involvement (biological)
2. Absence of parental discipline, extreme poverty, removal from home, not having parents of both sexes, erratic and inconsistent methods of discipline, never suffering consequences of own behavior, maternal deprivation (family dynamics)
3. Learned behavior within client's subculture (cultural)
E. Clinical manifestations
1. Exhibits patterns acceptable to self but creating conflict with others
2. Lack of guilt, remorse, or anxiety
3. Frequent violation of law, mores, and customs (lack of superego requires immediate gratification of needs)
4. Extreme impulsivity, repeated lying; inability to tolerate frustration
5. Difficulty in developing work behaviors and intimate relationship behaviors; unable to sustain either
6. Capacity to perpetuate interpersonal problems and to annoy others
7. Defense mechanisms commonly used: fantasy, isolation, dissociation, projection, somatization, splitting, and passive-aggressive behavior
8. Extremely low self-esteem, yet presents self as powerful
9. Irresponsible and antisocial behavior before age 15
10. Unable to function as responsible parent
11. Poor judgment and lack of long-range planning
12. Failure to honor financial responsibilities
13. Lack of concern for other people or own safety; reckless driving and driving while intoxicated

II. Analysis
A. High risk for violence: directed at others related to aggression
B. Ineffective individual coping related to inadequate coping methods
C. Impaired social interaction related to lack of empathy; inability to sustain long-term relationships
D. Disturbed self-esteem related to lack of positive feedback

III. Planning/goals, expected outcomes
A. Client will not harm others
B. Client will be able to delay gratification of own desires and follow rules and regulations
C. Client will verbalize positive perception of self
D. Client will develop one nonmanipulative relationship with another individual

IV. Implementation
A. Convey message to client that it is not client but behavior that is unacceptable
B. Maintain low-level stimuli and calm attitude to avoid increased agitation and provoking aggressive behavior
C. Observe behavior frequently without appearing watchful and suspicious
D. Remove all dangerous objects from environment
E. Assist client in identifying true object of anger
F. Encourage verbalization of hostile feelings
G. Explore alternative ways (e.g., physical exercise) of coping with frustration
H. Present show of strength if necessary to control client behavior (e.g., use restraints as protection)
I. Use tranquilizer medications with caution due to susceptibility to addictions
J. Demand accountability of client following an infraction in a matter-of-fact way
K. Use explanations that are concise, concrete, clear, with minimal risk of misinterpretation ("You'll be expected to . . .")
L. Give positive affirmation for acceptable behavior

V. Evaluation
  A. Client redirects hostility into socially acceptable behaviors
  B. Client discusses angry feelings and verbalizes appropriate ways to handle frustration
  C. Client follows rules and regulations
  D. Client verbally identifies which of own behaviors not acceptable
  E. Client respects others' rights by delaying own gratification
  F. Client does not manipulate others, considers their rights
  G. Client has satisfactory relationship with one other person and is able to identify reasons this was not possible in past

Psychoactive Substance Disorder

I. Assessment
  A. Definition: impairment in social and occupational functions related to regular use of specific substances that are intended to alter mood behavior (Table 20-5)
    1. Intoxication: specific clinical manifestations, unique to a drug or chemical, that occur following intake of the substance; may include relaxation, drowsiness, anxiety, euphoria. Behavioral changes occur because of the action of the drug or chemical on the central nervous system
    2. Abuse: excessive, harmful use of drugs that could lead to medical, social, and legal problems
    3. Dependence
      a. Physical: altered physiological state produced by drug
      b. Psychological: client needs drug to function with or without physical dependence
    4. Tolerance: a progressive need for more of the abused drug or chemical to achieve the desired effect
    5. Withdrawal: specific clinical manifestations that occur when intake of abused drug or chemical is decreased markedly or stopped abruptly
  B. Etiology (suggested hypotheses)
    1. Genetic predisposition is possible
    2. Environmental influences: acceptance/encouragement of use by culture
    3. Problems with family relationships
    4. Individual personality traits
      a. Learning theory: reflex response to stress

TABLE 20–5 Psychoactive Substance Disorder

Substance	Characteristic Effects	Characteristics of Overdose	Characteristics of Withdrawal	Nursing Implications
Alcohol	Emotional lability, reduced inhibition, reduced alertness, poor judgment	Aggression, loss of consciousness	Tremors, seizures, alcoholic hallucinosis, delirium tremens	Follow medication regimen for detoxification; chlordiazepoxide (Librium) to prevent DTs
Narcotics (heroin, morphine, codeine, opium)	Produce analgesia, relaxation, and euphoria; slurred speech; drowsiness; constricted pupils	Convulsions, coma, respiratory and circulatory depression	Muscle aches, nausea and vomiting, fever, sweating, runny nose, abdominal cramping, gooseflesh	Narcotic antagonist such as naloxone (Narcan) for narcotic overdose; withdrawal managed with rest and nutritional therapy
Depressants (barbiturate, antianxiety, and hypnotic medications)	Relief of anxiety, relaxation, drowsiness, slurred speech, euphoria, impaired judgment	Shallow respirations, clammy skin, dilated pupils, weak and rapid pulse, coma, possible death	Tremors, insomnia, nausea and vomiting, diaphoresis, seizures, tachycardia, elevated blood pressure	Substitution therapy may be instituted to decrease withdrawal symptoms; monitor vital signs, especially respiratory status
Stimulants (amphetamines, cocaine)	Psychomotor agitation, elation, hypervigilance, grandiosity, tachycardia dilated pupils, restlessness, insomnia	Increase in body temperature, hallucinations, seizures, possible death due to cardiac arrhythmias or cerebrovascular accident	Fatigue, depressed mood, irritability, anxiety, restlessness, drowsiness (residual psychological craving for drug)	Stabilization of vital signs; help client with psychological dependence; treat paranoid symptoms, if present
Hallucinogens (LSD, PCP)	Illusions, hallucinations, dilated pupils, elevated vital signs, anxiety, paranoid ideation, depression	Longer, more intense "trip"; psychosis; panic	Possible psychological dependence with fear, apprehension, or panic on withdrawal	Offer support during a "trip", observe for psychotic behaviors; flashbacks may occur

b. Personality trait theory: qualities within person that presumably predispose to alcohol dependence (fearful, inferior, dependent, self-destructive, orally fixated, low tolerance for frustration); this theory has little support
C. Incidence
1. Top three drugs seen in emergency clients: diazepam (Valium), alcohol, and heroin
2. Alcohol
a. Alcoholism affects approximately 10 million people in United States
b. Some consider alcoholism number 1 health problem (it is fourth largest national health problem)
c. 50% of hospital beds occupied with clients who have alcohol-related conditions
3. Drugs
a. Marijuana most frequently used illicit drug
b. 1 to 3 million heroin addicts
D. Predisposing/precipitating factors
1. Social pressures
2. Drug pattern beginning with alcohol, progressing to marijuana, followed by illicit drug use
3. Personality
a. Underlying self-doubts and passivity covered up by dominant and critical behavior
b. Rebellious attitude toward authority
c. Use of escapist defense mechanisms
d. Lack of close and lasting relationships
e. Marked narcissistic trends
E. Clinical manifestations: dependent on extent of abuse, drug of choice, and physical problems
1. Certain drug required to maintain functioning (usually with barbiturates, amphetamines, opiates, and alcohol)
2. Tolerance developed, requiring increased doses
3. Physical dependence; withdrawal symptoms experienced if drug is stopped or dosage is decreased
4. Psychological dependence; feeling it is impossible to get along without drug
F. Complications
1. Alcohol
a. Gastritis, chronic diarrhea, nutritional deficiencies
b. Disorders of neurological and cardiac systems
c. Pancreatitis, fatty liver, cirrhosis, hypoglycemia, hepatitis

d. Withdrawal symptoms become progressively more intense and life-threatening
(1) Stage 1: mild tremors, nausea, nervousness, tachycardia, increased blood pressure, diaphoresis (as early as 8 hours after cessation)
(2) Stage 2: gross tremors, hyperactivity, insomnia, anorexia, weakness, disorientation, illusions, nightmares, beginning of auditory and visual hallucinations
(3) Stage 3: 12 to 48 hours after cessation; all of Stages 1 and 2 plus severe hallucinations and grand mal seizures
(4) Stage 4: 3 to 5 days after cessation; delirium tremens (DTs), confusion, severe psychomotor activity, agitation, sleepiness, hallucinations, uncontrolled and unexplained tachycardia; can be life-threatening
e. Organic brain syndrome (confusion, especially time, place, and dwelling on imaginary past) Wernicke's syndrome/Korsakoff's syndrome (poor vision, memory loss, confusion, and sometimes coma)
f. Family disruption
2. Drugs
a. Infections, AIDS from use of contaminated needles and syringes, hepatitis
b. Erosion of nasal septum from cocaine "snorting"
c. Family disruption and social problems
d. Cross addiction: one drug suppresses manifestations of dependency from different drug and maintains dependent state
II. Analysis
A. High risk for violence: self-directed related to substance abuse and depression
B. High risk for violence: directed at others related to confusion/aggressive impulses related to acute intoxication
C. Chronic low self-esteem related to chronic dependence on chemicals/drugs
D. Powerlessness related to psychological dependence on/craving for abused substance
E. Impaired adjustment related to chronic dependence on chemicals/drugs
F. Ineffective individual coping related to denial of substance dependency
III. Planning/goals, expected outcomes
A. Client will experience gradual withdrawal or

detoxification from substance (alcohol or drugs) with minimal physical problems

   B. Client's physical problems will be minimized

   C. Client will have reduced feelings of panic during withdrawal

   D. Client will identify substance abuse as a problem

   E. Client will discuss and develop more effective coping mechanisms

   F. Client will discuss how to live without chemicals

   G. Client will seek out and accept support of others and accept limits set on behavior

   H. Client will have rehabilitation needs related to drug abuse and pattern of abuse met

   I. Client will assume responsibility for own behavior

IV. Implementation

   A. Stay with client until acute effects of drug wear off, giving verbal reassurance and reality orientation to reduce panic

   B. Provide adequate daily fluid intake (avoiding excessive coffee or tea) and frequent small feedings

   C. Administer antianxiety drugs (diazepam and chlordiazepoxide) or methadone (opiate user) to minimize withdrawal, and antacids for gastritis

   D. Involve client in meal planning, vitamin and nutritional therapy

   E. Keep client ambulatory during day

   F. Encourage and support client in accepting chemical dependency and its consequences in client's life (confrontation regarding blaming, defensiveness, and avoidance of responsibility and manipulative behavior)

   G. Discuss with client how to handle (without chemical) anticipated painful events of life

   H. Discuss with client that life without chemicals major loss; help client plan ways of adjusting to loss

   I. Design and hold lecture sessions for clients and families to better understand chemical dependency and how families can be "enablers"

   J. Provide opportunities to decrease social isolation and improve social skills (group counseling sessions and friendly conversation)

   K. Put client and family in contact with Alcoholics Anonymous, Al-Anon, Alateen when total abstinence is primary goal or with other mental health groups related to drug of choice (self-help group led by ex-addicts)

   L. Administer deterrents for follow-up treatment such as disulfiram (Antabuse), which causes toxic reaction if alcohol taken (Table 20-6)

V. Evaluation

   A. Client withdraws from chemical without preventable complications

   B. Client recognizes and accepts chemical dependency

   C. Client understands and participates daily in balanced program of food, fluid intake, exercise, rest, and recreation

   D. Client develops effective coping mechanisms

TABLE 20–6 Drugs Used to Treat Alcoholism

Example	Daily Dosage	Action	Use	Common Side Effects	Nursing Implications
Disulfiram (Antabuse)	250 mg	Enzyme inhibitor; antioxidant that blocks oxidative metabolism of alcohol and acetaldehyde; with alcohol ingestion, level of acetaldehyde rises sharply, producing very unpleasant side effects	Deter use of alcohol in management of alcohol dependence	Drowsiness, headache, depression, impotence; disulfiram reaction—flushing, throbbing headache, dyspnea, nausea and vomiting, diaphoresis, palpitations, hypotension, tachypnea, blurred vision, syncope, slurred speech	Ensure that client and family fully informed of therapy; avoid alcohol ingestion including sauces, cough syrup, and so on; monitor client closely to ensure compliance with drug taking; wear Medic-Alert tag; warn that sensitivity to alcohol increases with use; monitor blood pressure and ECG when started and periodically Teaching: any ingestion of alcohol up to 2 weeks after last dose can cause disulfiram reaction; therefore, avoid cough syrups and elixirs as well as external use of alcohol products, such as lotions and after shave

for life stresses and adapts to life without
drugs and/or alcohol

E. Client, family, or significant other belongs to
support group to strengthen new behavior
and increase socialization in drug-free environment

F. Client aware of drugs and their antagonistic,
addictive, or cross-tolerance interactions

POST-TEST Behavioral Disorders

1. Which of the following problems is associated
with severe anxiety?
① Problem solving is prevented
② Discomfort is diminished
③ The perceptual field is increased
④ Alertness is increased

2. The psychotic client often is given
antipsychotic medications to control the level
of anxiety. When a client is taking a major
tranquilizer such as chlorpromazine
(Thorazine), which of the following clinical
manifestations should be reported to the
physician?
① Dry mouth
② Drowsiness
③ Orthostatic hypotension
④ Pseudoparkinsonism

3. Your client is placed on diazepam (Valium) to
treat anxiety. Which of the following should
be included in your teaching?
① Take the drug with milk or food to
decrease nausea
② If you are drowsy, stop taking the drug
③ Do not use alcohol while on the drug
④ The drug can be given during the last
trimester of pregnancy

4. Important information that a nurse should
include in the care of clients on amitriptyline
(Elavil) includes teaching them:
① To take the drug in the morning for
maximal effect
② That the drug does not affect blood
pressure
③ To stop the drug immediately if blurred
vision occurs
④ That response to the drug takes about 2
weeks

5. When a client is placed on an MAO inhibitor
such as phenelzine (Nardil), which of the
following should be included in the teaching?
① Take the drug at bedtime only
② Stand up slowly to avoid hypotension
③ Stop the drug if diarrhea occurs
④ That the drug will take effect immediately

6. When clients are on MAO inhibitors, they
must avoid foods high in tyramine. Which of
the following foods should be avoided?
① Yogurt and sour cream
② Milk and cottage cheese
③ Cream cheese and decaffeinated coffee
④ Tea and fresh meats

7. The nurse would base care of the anorexic
client on all EXCEPT which of the following
beliefs:
① The client focuses on anorexia to avoid
interpersonal conflicts and conflict
resolution
② The client rejects food as a method of
getting attention
③ The client has a perfectionist attitude
with fear of failure
④ The client has regressed to avoid
adolescent sexuality and independence

8. Which of the following physical manifestations
is common in the client with anorexia
nervosa?
① Diaphoresis
② Tachycardia
③ Hypertension
④ Amenorrhea

9. Which order for an anorexic client should the
nurse question?
① Administer blenderized tube feedings as
ordered
② Weigh client at least daily
③ Allow client privacy during mealtime
④ Monitor client for self-destructive
tendencies

10. Borderline personality disorders are
characterized by ''splitting.'' Splitting is best
defined as the:
① Development of more than one
personality
② Fear of open spaces
③ View of people and objects as parts,
either good or bad
④ Intolerance of being isolated

11. Clinical manifestations of a borderline
personality would NOT include:
① Inappropriate, intense anger and temper
② Absence of suicidal behavior
③ Impulsivity and unpredictability
④ Chronic feelings of boredom and
emptiness

12. Which of the following is the most important
intervention in helping clients with borderline
personalities?
① Engage in early family therapy
② Encourage self-motivation
③ Avoid long-term day hospital care
④ Avoid use of tranquilizers

13. Your client is involved in alcohol abuse and is started on disulfiram (Antabuse). Which of the following is a common side effect of Antabuse?
    ① Elation
    ② Bradycardia
    ③ Depression
    ④ Hypertension

14. When a client is started on Antabuse, it is important for the nurse to teach the client to:
    ① Avoid most cough syrups
    ② Take the drug with milk
    ③ Withhold the drug if side effects occur
    ④ Take drug only if drinking is planned

Susan Blum, a 30-year-old divorced mother of two preschool children, has been a patient in a psychiatric hospital for 3 weeks. She has a habit of washing her hands repeatedly for long periods of time. Her hands are chapped and raw looking. She is a registered nurse.

---

15. Susan is experiencing an acute anxiety attack. The nurse is going to give a mild sedative as prescribed. Which of the following statements made by the nurse indicates the best understanding of the client?
    ① "Susan, as a nurse, you understand the benefit of this medication."
    ② "Susan, this should help you feel more comfortable."
    ③ "Susan, this medication is to help you feel less anxious. Your anxiety is causing your symptoms."
    ④ "Susan, I know you feel nervous. This medication will help you feel more relaxed and comfortable."

16. A new nurse introduced herself to Susan and asks her name. Susan responds, "I'm an obsessive-compulsive neurotic. I have had psychoanalysis for 10 years. What do you think you can do for me?" The nursing response that would be most helpful is:
    ① "Who was your analyst?"
    ② "You seem to feel hopeless."
    ③ "I need to know you better, Susan."
    ④ "Can we talk about that, Susan?"

17. Susan responds by saying, "You make me angry. None of you understand what my real problem is." Your best reply would be:
    ① "I know what your problem is. You're an obsessive-compulsive personality."
    ② "If I've upset you, I'll return later."

③ "You have a right to be upset when people don't seem to understand."
④ "That's a common thought. I understand. Let's talk about this."

18. Diazepam (Valium) has been prescribed for Susan. You have just completed your health care teaching with Susan about the effects of Valium. What statement on Susan's part would indicate she needs further health teaching about Valium?
    ① "I'm so glad this drug won't affect my driving ability."
    ② "I'm so glad I can eat dairy products while I'm taking this."
    ③ "I'm so glad no blood tests are necessary while I'm taking this."
    ④ "I'm so glad I'll only have to take this until I learn to be less anxious."

Fred Smith is an 18-year-old with a long history of antisocial behavior and drug use. He has been sent to the hospital for a psychiatric evaluation after breaking into a doctor's office to steal drugs.

---

19. Fred's early development probably was characterized by his:
    ① Kindness and spirituality
    ② Excellence in school
    ③ History of enuresis
    ④ Truancy and running away from home

20. Which of the following would be an appropriate approach to use with Fred?
    ① Allow him choices whenever possible to build responsibility
    ② Allow him passes and freedom quickly to assess his response
    ③ Provide for structured care with no deviations
    ④ Avoid confronting his acting-out behavior

21. When might Fred be expected to begin to exhibit socially acceptable behavior?
    ① Never; such clients rarely revert to normal behavior
    ② After about age 40, for unknown reasons
    ③ After going to jail for one of his crimes
    ④ When the correct therapist works with him

22. Mary is a 45-year-old woman in the hospital for major surgery. She has been very demanding of attention and seems to cry all the time without reason. This is an example of the use of what defense mechanism?
    ① Denial

② Projection
③ Conversion
④ Regression

23. Jane is a college student who has just failed a math test. She is blaming her failure on the teacher, who she says wrote an unfair test. This is an example of the use of which of the following defense mechanisms?
① Rationalization
② Conversion
③ Denial
④ Compensation

24. You have noticed that your childless friends have begun to treat their pet dog as if it were their child. This is an example of:
① Reaction formation
② Introjection
③ Sublimation
④ Identification

25. A woman who hates her sister goes out of her way to be nice to her. This is an example of which defense mechanism?
① Condensation
② Repression
③ Regression
④ Transference

POST-TEST Answers and Rationales

1. ① A client who is severely anxious is unable to solve even minor problems or make simple decisions. Discomfort is usually increased, and the perceptual field and alertness decrease. 1, III. Anxiety.

2. ④ One of the major side effects is the development of extrapyramidal symptoms. The most common of these are pseudoparkinsonian symptoms such as drooling, rigidity, and shuffling gait. If this develops, the physician should be notified since nonphenothiazine tranquilizers can be substituted. The other choices are common side effects that do not require physician interventions. 4, III. Anxiety.

3. ③ When a client is on a drug such as Valium, the use of any other central nervous system depressant is contraindicated. There is no need to take the drug with food or milk. The drug usually causes drowsiness and the client should be warned of this, but it does not require that the drug be stopped. The drug has not been shown to be safe at any time during pregnancy. 4, III. Anxiety.

4. ④ Elavil has a delayed response time until the blood levels are high enough. The client should be warned that the drug will not take effect immediately and not to become discouraged. The drug should never be stopped immediately. Because the drug causes drowsiness, it should be given at bedtime. The drug may cause an increase in blood pressure. 4, III. Eating Disorders.

5. ② Nardil can cause orthostatic hypotension, so the client should stand up slowly and be taught other ways to prevent orthostatic changes. The drug is given in divided doses, not at bedtime, and it does not start working immediately. The drug may cause diarrhea, but this is not a reason to stop it. 4, III. Eating Disorders.

6. ① Foods high in tyramine are yogurt, sour cream, aged meats, caffeine, and many other foods. They should be avoided when a client is on MAO inhibitors. The other choices include foods that are not limited with this drug. 4, III. Eating Disorders.

7. ③ Anorexic clients are not perfectionists although they do have an unrealistic body image. The other three choices are correct theories for the development of anorexia. 1, III. Eating Disorders.

8. ④ The typical anorexic client ceases to have menses. This is further reinforcement of the desire to avoid adolescent sexuality. The anorexic may also exhibit bradycardia and hypotension. 1, III. Eating Disorders.

9. ③ You must stay with the anorexic client during meals to ensure that the food is being eaten. The client is not above hiding food or pretending to eat. The client may be self-destructive. It is important to weigh the client each day at the same time and in the same clothes and to administer tube feedings as ordered. 4, III. Eating Disorders.

10. ③ Splitting occurs when a client views people and objects as parts, either good or bad. The client has only one personality, does not fear open space, and does not fear isolation. 1, III. Personality Disorders.

11. ② A borderline personality is often suicidal, with inappropriate, intense anger and chronic feelings of boredom and emptiness. 2, III. Personality Disorders.

12. ① Early family therapy is the most important intervention to treat a borderline personality since the cause is often poor family dynamics. Tranquilizers and day hospital care also are treatments. Self-motivation is ineffective because of the nature of the disorder. 4, III. Personality Disorders.

13. ③ Depression is a side effect of Antabuse, along with tachycardia. Hypertension only occurs if alcohol is ingested, otherwise hypotension is more common. 2, III. Personality Disorders.

14. ① Most cough syrups contain an alcohol base, so they cannot be taken with Antabuse. It is not necessary to take the drug with food. The drug is taken to help the client to stop drinking. It should be taken every day without fail. 4, III. Personality Disorders.

15. ② In talking to someone who is acutely anxious, keep your statements brief and to the point. The client's anxiety level prohibits them from understanding very much. 4, III. Obsessive-Compulsive Disorder.

16. ③ In the initial phase of the relationship, it is too soon to discuss feelings, as done in choice 2. Choice 4 leads to a yes or no

answer and does not further the discussion. Choice 1 is irrelevant. Choice 3 is best because it is appropriate for this phase of the relationship. 1, III. Obsessive-Compulsive Disorder.

17. ③ This reply acknowledges Susan's feelings. Choices 1 and 2 do not acknowledge her feelings. Choice 4 trivializes Susan's feelings by making them common. 4, III. Obsessive-Compulsive Disorder.

18. ① Susan obviously does not understand the effects of Valium, which would definitely impair her driving ability. 5, III. Obsessive-Compulsive Disorder.

19. ④ The client having problems with substance abuse and antisocial behavior often gives a history of rebelliousness and of never having behaved in socially acceptable ways. 1, III. Substance Abuse.

20. ③ It is important that the client be given a structured environment with no deviation from the accepted plan of care. These clients are often extremely manipulative and will use any instance of change as a sign of possible weakness and use it in a manipulative manner. 3, III. Substance Abuse.

21. ② Studies have shown that this type of behavior pattern often seems to burn out around age 40, with the client reverting to a more socially acceptable behavior pattern. None of the other options are appropriate. 5, III. Substance Abuse.

22. ④ A client who is faced with a very stressful situation often retreats to a more comfortable level of development temporarily. The other options refer to other defense mechanisms. 2, III. Defense Mechanisms.

23. ① Rationalization refers to blaming others for problems of one's own making rather than accepting the consequences of one's own actions. The other options refer to other defense mechanisms. 2, III. Defense Mechanisms.

24. ③ When a person is unable to have needs met in one way, they often meet those needs in secondary ways. Transferring the affection one would give a child to another object or person is an example of this. The other options refer to other defense mechanisms. 2, III. Defense Mechanisms.

25. ② Feelings that are unacceptable to the individual on a conscious level are often hidden from the self by overemphasizing the opposite feelings. The other options refer to other defense mechanisms. 2, III. Defense Mechanisms.

21

Crisis Intervention

PRE-TEST Crisis Intervention

1. A crisis that is acute but temporary and due to an external source best describes what type of crisis?
   1. Transitional
   2. Developmental
   3. Dispositional
   4. Traumatic
2. Your client is in a state of crisis. Which of the following is an appropriate nursing intervention for early in the crisis state?
   1. Ask the client to evaluate the situation
   2. Encourage the client to express feelings and emotions related to the crisis
   3. Encourage the client to begin the development of insight into response
   4. Require the client to be actively involved in the establishment of goals
3. Which of the following is appropriate in considering successful grieving?
   1. Restitution should occur within 6 months
   2. Shock and disbelief may last for months
   3. Preoccupation with the image of the loss is abnormal
   4. Awareness develops within weeks or months
4. Which of the following is a characteristic of morbid grief as opposed to normal grief?
   1. Avoidance of contact with others
   2. Feelings of guilt
   3. Feelings of hostility
   4. Somatic distress
5. Which of the following is an appropriate nursing intervention for the client who is grieving?
   1. Sedate the client to avoid a focus on the grief
   2. Allow the client to retreat from reality
   3. Allow the client to talk about feelings, even if negative
   4. Allow the client to avoid usual roles and responsibilities as long as possible

PRE-TEST Answers and Rationales

1. ③ A dispositional crisis is one that is acute, temporary, and due to an external source. The other types of crisis are defined in the text. 2, III. Crisis Intervention.
2. ② It is important for a client to express feelings and emotions related to a crisis to lessen anxiety. Insight is not possible at this early stage, and the client is unable to evaluate the situation. During the crisis, the client is unable to be involved in establishing goals. 4, III. Crisis Intervention.
3. ④ A sense of awareness develops gradually as grief begins to resolve. Shock and disbelief last only a few hours or days, and restitution may take up to 1 year. Preoccupation with the image of the lost one is very normal. 1, III. Crisis Intervention.
4. ① Avoidance of others is a characteristic of morbid grief. The other choices contain characteristics of normal grief. 1, III. Crisis Intervention.
5. ③ It is important for the client to be allowed to talk about all feelings, positive and negative. The client must ventilate to begin to work through feelings of grief. The client should never be sedated, should not retreat from reality, and should not avoid normal roles and responsibilities. 4, III. Crisis Intervention.

NURSING PROCESS APPLIED TO CLIENTS DURING CRISIS

Crisis

I. Assessment
  A. Definition: human response to situations perceived as health threats or problems, when customary problem-solving or decision-making methods are no longer adequate; state of psychological disequilibrium
  B. Characteristics
    1. Internal, subjective experience
    2. Self-limiting (lasts few days to weeks, with or without treatment)
    3. May be opportunity for growth (expansion of coping skills, turning point in life)
    4. Duration is usually less than 6 to 8 weeks
    5. Client amenable to change because crisis is intolerable (motivation high)
  C. Types
    1. Developmental crisis: results from a predictable life change, such as marriage, childbirth, retirement
    2. Situational crisis: results from a sudden, unanticipated change in life events, such as illness, unemployment, or natural disaster
  D. Predisposing/precipitating factors
    1. Frustration caused by impediments to goal attainment
    2. Usual coping measures tried and failed
    3. Chronic life stress
    4. Hazardous event
  E. Clinical manifestations
    1. Fight or flight response, conflicted, helpless/hopeless, dysfunctional behavior
    2. Difficulty in thinking clearly (indecisive, apathetic, unresponsive)
    3. Severe or panic anxiety behavior
    4. Disequilibrium or disorganization
    5. Energy directed toward relieving emotional distress (client may ruminate, perform motor activity, or become enraged at situation)
    6. Survivors of crisis may experience transformation of values; heightened awareness of life and in more control of life events
    7. Blaming others, avoiding responsibility (childish incompetence)
    8. Inability to carry out activities of daily living
    9. Increased dependence on others
    10. Increased somatic complaints due to emotional distress
  F. Phases of crisis
    1. Client perceives a threat that causes an increase in anxiety; attempts to cope with usual coping strategies
    2. Anxiety intensifies if strategies do not work
    3. Client mobilizes resources
      a. Most likely to seek help at this point
      b. May try new methods of coping
    4. Intense anxiety with disorganization of cognitive, emotional, and behavioral functions

II. Analysis
   A. Ineffective individual coping related to crisis, inadequate support systems
   B. Disturbed self-esteem related to inadequate coping mechanisms
   C. Impaired social interaction related to disorganization
   D. Anxiety related to ineffective coping mechanisms
III. Planning/goals, expected outcomes
   A. Client will seek help (problem solve) and search for alternative behaviors and effective coping mechanisms
   B. Client will avoid having serious psychiatric problems as aftermath of crisis
   C. Client will return to at least previous level of coping (job/roles) with realistic view of what has occurred
   D. Client will express feelings of decreased hopelessness and helplessness and regain degree of control over life
IV. Implementation/crisis intervention
   A. Assess suicidal or homicidal potential
   B. Assess client's coping skills
   C. Encourage open expression of feelings related to crisis
   D. Acknowledge client's emotional response
   E. Establish nurse/client relationship; nurse assumes active, directive role
   F. Clarify that relationship is time limited
   G. Explore meaning of crisis to client
   H. Help client realize others have had similar experiences (universality of experiences)
   I. Use problem-solving approaches to help client develop new, effective coping mechanisms
   J. Encourage client to use support systems
   K. As sessions continue, decrease role of nurse and increase responsibility of client
   L. Reinforce new coping mechanisms learned
   M. Provide anticipatory guidance
V. Evaluation
   A. Client verbalizes several options useful to cope with stress
   B. Client identifies community resource to use if faced with another hazardous situation
   C. Client has adequate support from family, friends, and job
   D. Client adequately expresses what occurred and feelings experienced at time
   E. Client returns to previous or better level of coping

Grief and Grieving

I. Assessment
   A. Definition: response to loss, usually of loved person through death or separation; may also follow loss of anything, tangible or intangible, that is highly valued; actual or anticipated
      1. Sexual role identity
      2. Self-concept of body image
      3. Nurturing, loss of significant other
   B. Types
      1. Normal
      2. Morbid
   C. Predisposing/precipitating factors
      1. Loss and separation
      2. Degree and duration depend on various factors
         a. Amount of support lost object provided
         b. Degree of ambivalence toward lost object
         c. Amount of preparation beforehand
         d. Extent that loss alters client's life
         e. Available support systems (social support)
         f. Previous losses reawakened
         g. Multiple losses
   D. Clinical manifestations
      1. Successful grieving stages
         a. Shock and disbelief (1 to 7 days)
         b. Developing awareness (weeks to several months)
         c. Restitution (1 year or more)
      2. Usually completed within year following death if all three stages experienced
      3. Normal grief
         a. Somatic distress
         b. Preoccupation with image of loss
         c. Feelings of guilt
         d. Feelings of hostility
         e. Loss of patterns of conduct
      4. Morbid grief
         a. Avoiding contact with others
         b. Increased interpersonal distance
         c. Deliberately excluding from thinking process all references to deceased
         d. Delayed reaction
         e. Distorted reaction
         f. Crying, restlessness, dependency, erratic behavior
         g. Depression
II. Analysis
   A. Impaired adjustment related to inability to accept loss
   B. Anxiety related to perceived threat to self-concept
   C. Ineffective individual coping related to feelings of guilt
   D. Dysfunctional grieving related to inability to accept loss
   E. Hopelessness related to perceived loss of control

III. Planning/goals, expected outcomes
  A. Client will go through grieving process adaptively
  B. Client will be able to verbally express awareness of the loss and its impact
  C. Client will be able to talk about positive and negative aspects of loss and make future plans
IV. Implementation
  A. Help client move along continuum of three stages (shock and disbelief, developing awareness, restitution)
  B. Reinforce reality
  C. Use emphatic listening to keep client talking about feelings; do not challenge statements
  D. Give sedation only if it will not subvert grieving process
  E. Prepare client for return to usual roles and responsibilities
  F. Provide resources for follow-up
V. Evaluation
  A. Client copes with loss by completing each stage of grief and mourning process
  B. Client expresses sadness over loss but also plans for future
  C. Client verbalizes how losses usually coped with and what situational supports most effective

Violence

Acting Out/Aggression
I. Assessment
  A. Definitions
    1. Violence: any physical, verbal, or symbolic behavior in pursuit of own interests that is destructive to self, others, or property
      a. Directed toward self (e.g., suicide)
      b. Directed toward others (e.g., murder, rape, abuse)
    2. Acting out: verbal and nonverbal aggressive/angry behavior that stops short of violence
    3. Aggression: state of inner tension causing discomfort and energizing person to overcome environment, using nonadaptive verbal or physical action
  B. Etiology (theoretical)
    1. Violent response to feelings of impotence and helplessness in face of perceived threat
    2. Learned and perpetuated by attitudes; rationalizations supported by subculture
  C. Predisposing/precipitating factors
    1. Increase of anxiety and stress, resulting in decreased reasoning ability where client responds more to isolated stimuli and less to content of situation

    2. May be perpetuated by hospital, social structure (e.g., coercion, regimentation, and invasion of personal space)
II. Analysis
  A. High risk for injury related to intense anger
  B. High risk for violence: directed at others, related to anger, delusional thought
  C. Ineffective individual coping related to poor impulse control
III. Planning/goals, expected outcomes
  A. Client will cease any violent behavior
  B. Client will cope with aggressive impulses by learning new coping alternatives (identifying and expressing feelings)
  C. Client will tolerate physical restraints
  D. Client will have increased ability to control aggressive impulses
IV. Implementation
  A. Give client space and keep some distance
  B. Ask other clients to withdraw and leave area
  C. Observe client from a distance
  D. Move slowly and deliberately
  E. Identify feelings of anxiety
  F. Encourage verbalization rather than "acting out"
  G. Offer alternative behavior, such as use of punching bag
  H. Provide reassurance or support and set limits
  I. Before application of restraints or placing of client in seclusion, explain to client that you are concerned about behavior and you are going to help control it now so client will not hurt self or others
    1. Gather sufficient staff beforehand
    2. Obtain physician's order for restraint and/or seclusion
    3. Allow client to verbally express feelings
    4. Remove all potentially dangerous items
    5. Check client every 15 minutes and document
      a. Document offers of food, fluids, and bedpan
      b. Check vital signs as needed
      c. Do passive range of motion (one extremity at a time) at least every 2 hours
  J. Remove restraints or seclusion when acute agitation subsides; at least two staff members should participate in removal of client from restraints and/or seclusion
  K. Explore violent episode with client; identify why done at this time, and did it have "payoff" of lessened anxiety or relief of frustration
  L. Identify precipitating factors
  M. Validate appropriate responses to frustration
  N. Encourage family to understand client and help develop new coping behaviors

V. Evaluation
   A. Client and family identify verbally events and feelings that preceded violent episode
   B. Client develops at least one effective alternative coping behavior to deal with aggressive impulses
   C. Client able to appropriately express feelings, to respect personal integrity of others, and to utilize assertive communication skills

Potential Suicide
I. Assessment
   A. Definition: taking of one's own life violently and intentionally; visible sign that person wishes to escape intolerable situation and has run out of positive alternatives
   B. Incidence
      1. Highest incidence in adolescence and over age 45
      2. Three times more males than females commit suicide; females attempt more frequently than males
   C. Etiology
      1. Complex sociocultural factors; physiological or psychological stressors
      2. Extreme loneliness, depression
      3. Severely impaired self-concept
      4. Physiological disorders (toxic state, chemical withdrawal, chronic brain syndrome)
   D. Predisposing/precipitating factors
      1. Failure to externalize aggressive feelings and turning them on self
      2. Unsuccessful attempt to solve conflict
      3. Person experiencing delusions or hallucinations may respond to voices—for example, a command to kill self
      4. Poor self-concept; low impulse control
      5. Populations at risk: single, widowed, separated, and divorced people; in United States more prevalent in whites than nonwhites; high in migrants, foreign born, elderly, and those living alone
      6. Factors associated with risk of suicide: depression, delusional thought, defiance, stress, hallucinations, loss, isolation, internal conflicts
      7. Assessment of lethality
         a. Previous suicide attempts
         b. Has a detailed plan
         c. Has means or weapon available
         d. Has threatening hallucinations and/or delusions
         e. Lacks available support system
   E. Clinical manifestations
      1. Verbal or nonverbal clues of intent; leaves suicide note or states, "I won't see you again."
      2. Cry for help: "I can't take it anymore," "Take care of me."
      3. Giving away prized possessions, making will
      4. Situational clue, such as notification of terminal cancer or maturational events
      5. Sudden changes in behavior, such as depressed client suddenly becoming cheerful and energetic
II. Analysis
   A. High risk for violence: self-directed related to depressed mood, misperceptions of reality
   B. Chronic low self-esteem related to feelings of guilt, worthlessness
   C. Hopelessness related to feelings of worthlessness
III. Planning/goals, expected outcomes
   A. Client will not harm self
   B. Client will express feelings in a safe manner
   C. Client will achieve a realistic and positive self-image
   D. Client will identify community resources
   E. Client will develop new effective coping mechanisms
   F. Client will be free from suicidal ideation, thoughts, and feelings
IV. Implementation
   A. Observe client closely in a safe environment
   B. Develop a "no suicide" contract with client
   C. Convey acceptance; emphasize protective, not punitive, attitude, and permit verbal expression of anger and hostility
   D. Encourage support through therapeutic relationship and through network of family, friends, or community groups
   E. Prevent isolation
   F. Discuss coping mechanisms other than suicide to use when feeling unable to solve problems
V. Evaluation
   A. Client demonstrates that suicidal potential eliminated (free of suicidal ideation, thoughts, and feelings)
   B. Client demonstrates adequate coping skills in dealing with stress
      1. Maintains adequate role functioning
      2. Has appropriate mood
      3. Verbalizes hope for future
      4. Develops positive self-concept
      5. Establishes meaningful relationships with others
      6. Expresses feelings appropriately

Post-Traumatic Stress
I. Assessment
   A. Definition: clinical manifestations of severe

anxiety that occurs after one has experienced a traumatic event outside the range of usual human experience
  1. Acute: clinical manifestations begin within 6 months of traumatic event and do not last longer than 6 months; client will probably return to precrisis level of functioning
  2. Chronic: clinical manifestations last from 6 months to 1 year
  3. Delayed: clinical manifestations begin after latency period of 6 months or more
  B. Etiology: loss of self-esteem and loss of control in traumatic situation
  C. Predisposing factors: traumatic events such as rape, assault, abuse, combat, torture
  D. Clinical manifestations
    1. Depersonalization and dissociation
    2. Numbness, disbelief, and emotional shock (marked disinterest in significant events and/or feelings of estrangement)
    3. Multiple bruises (abuse)
    4. Depression, anxiety
    5. Reexperiencing of traumatic event
      a. Recurrent/intrusive recollections of event
      b. Recurrent dreams of event
      c. Feelings that event is recurring, caused by environmental or ideational stimulus
    6. At least two of the following manifestations:
      a. Hyperalertness
      b. Exaggerated startle
      c. Sleep disturbance
      d. Guilt about surviving
      e. Memory impairment
      f. Poor concentration
II. Analysis
  A. Post-traumatic response related to stressful event
  B. Anxiety related to current memory of past traumatic life event
  C. Ineffective individual coping related to inadequate coping methods
  D. Powerlessness related to feeling overwhelmed by symptoms of anxiety
III. Planning/goals, expected outcomes
  A. Client will be able to recount event and cope with associated feelings
  B. Client will resume involvement in daily activities
IV. Implementation
  A. Help identify and prioritize immediate concerns
  B. Desensitize client's memories of the event by gradual introduction of discussion of event

  C. Relaxation training to decrease anxiety
  D. Encourage client to talk about situation in own words to diffuse impact and get control over own thoughts
  E. Encourage gradual increase of involvement in pretrauma activities and discuss related feelings
  F. Acknowledge significance of event and appropriateness of feelings
  G. Encourage client to identify and vent feelings of sadness, guilt, loss, anger, or frustration
  H. Refer client to community resources, especially a support group for survivors of similar trauma
V. Evaluation
  A. Client describes event and discusses feelings it aroused
  B. Client deals with trauma realistically
  C. Client is free of clinical manifestations

POST-TEST Crisis Intervention

1. Verbal and nonverbal angry behavior short of violence best describes:
   ① Aggressive behavior
   ② Violent behavior
   ③ Passive behavior
   ④ Acting out behavior
2. Which of the following is appropriate for the client who is exhibiting acting out behavior?
   ① Give the client sufficient space and distance
   ② Do not restrain the client
   ③ Encourage client to act out anger and then move on
   ④ Encourage client to interact with others to diffuse anger
3. Which of the following is true concerning suicides?
   ① Men are more likely to attempt suicide
   ② Women are more likely to commit suicide
   ③ The highest frequencies are between ages 10 and 24
   ④ People who talk about suicide do not commit suicide
4. Your client is alluding to a desire to commit suicide. Which of the following is the most appropriate nursing intervention?
   ① Discourage the client from talking about it
   ② Engage the client in detailed distracting activity
   ③ Talk to the client about positive coping mechanisms
   ④ Ask the client specifically what he or she is considering

5. Which of the following is a characteristic of post-traumatic stress disorder?
   1. It is more severe with non-manmade stressors
   2. It rarely involves reliving the event
   3. It involves the loss of self-esteem and the loss of control
   4. It is characterized by intense focusing on the event

6. When assessing a client for post-traumatic stress disorder, the nurse would observe for which of the following behaviors?
   1. Hyperalertness and hypervigilance
   2. Poor concentration and guilt about surviving
   3. Excessive sleepiness and exaggerated startle
   4. Recurrent dreams of event and decreased alertness

POST-TEST Answers and Rationales

1. ④ A client who acts out is demonstrating angry behavior that stops just short of violence. The other choices are other types of angry behavior. 1, III. Crisis Intervention.

2. ① It is important that clients who are acting out be allowed to keep their behavior short of violence. Allowing them space and privacy should help them control their behavior. If a client becomes violent, restraints may be needed. Interacting with others and expressing the anger only serve to increase the risk of violence. 4, III. Crisis Intervention.

3. ③ Suicide is most common in young people between ages 10 and 24. Women attempt suicide more, but men commit suicide more. It is a myth that people who talk about suicide do not kill themselves. 1, III. Crisis Intervention.

4. ④ If a client is alluding to a desire to commit suicide, the nurse must ask the client specifically about what is being considered. The nurse should ask if the client has a specific plan in mind. Distracting the client is ineffective, and talking to the client about coping measures is inappropriate at this time. 4, III. Crisis Intervention.

5. ③ Post-traumatic stress involves the loss of control and self-esteem. The client feels as if the situation has taken over his or her life. It usually involves manmade stressors such as rape or accidents. The client relives the event but does not focus on it. 1, III. Crisis Intervention.

6. ② For post-traumatic stress to be diagnosed, at least two of the following symptoms must be present: hyperalertness, exaggerated startle, sleep disturbance, guilt about surviving, memory impairment, and poor concentration. 2, III. Crisis Intervention.

BIBLIOGRAPHY

Bauer, B. B. and Hill, S. S. (1986). *Essentials of mental health care: Planning and interventions*. Philadelphia: W. B. Saunders.

Birkhead, L. M. *Psychiatric mental health nursing: Therapeutic use of self*. Philadelphia: J. B. Lippincott.

Cook, J. S. and Fonntaine, K. L. (1991). *Essentials of mental health nursing*, 2nd ed. Redwood City, Calif.: Addison-Wesley.

Deering, C. G. (1987). Developing a therapeutic alliance with the anorexia nervosa client. *Journal of Psychosocial Nursing* 25 (March).

Doenges, M. E., Townsend, M. C., and Moorhouse, M. F. (1989). *Psychiatric care plans: Guidelines for client care*. Philadelphia: F. A. Davis.

Fields, S. K. and Yurchuck, R., eds. (1985). *Psychiatric nursing review*. New Hyde Park, NY: Medical Examination Publishing.

Fortinash, K. M. and Holoday, P. A. (1991). *Psychiatric nursing care plans*. St. Louis: Mosby Year Book.

Gary, F. and Kavanagh, C. K. (1991). *Psychiatric mental health nursing*. Philadelphia: J. B. Lippincott.

McFarland, G. K. and Thomas, M. D. (1991). *Psychiatric mental health nursing: Application of the nursing process*. Philadelphia: J. B. Lippincott.

McFarland, G. and Wasli, E. (1986). *Nursing diagnoses and process in psychiatric and mental health nursing*. Philadelphia: J. B. Lippincott.

Neal, M. C., et al. (1985). *Nursing care planning guides for psychiatric and mental health care*, 2nd ed. Baltimore, Md.: Williams & Wilkins.

Parquette, M., Neal, M., and Rodemich, C. (1991). *Psychiatric nursing diagnosis and care plans for DSM-III-R*. Boston: Jones and Bartlett.

Pasquali, E. A., Arnold, H. M., and DeBasio, N. (1989). *Mental health nursing: A wholistic approach*, 3rd ed. St. Louis: Mosby Year Book.

Rawlins, R. P., Williams, S. R., and Beck, C. K. (1991). *Mental health-psychiatric nursing*. St. Louis: Mosby Year Book.

Riley, J. W. (1988). *Nursing care planning guides for mental health*. Baltimore, Md.: Williams & Wilkins.

Rozendal, N. A. and Fallon, P. M. (1978). *Psychiatric nursing: Pretest self-assessment and review*. Wallingford, Mass.: Pretest Service.

Stuart, G. and Sundeen, S. J. (1991). *Principles and practice of psychiatric nursing*, 4th ed. St. Louis: Mosby Year Book.

Townsend, M. C. (1988). *Nursing diagnosis in psychiatric nursing*. Philadelphia: F. A. Davis.

Wilson, H. S. and Kneisl, C. R. (1992). *Psychiatric nursing*, 4th ed. Redwood City, Calif.: Addison-Wesley.

UNIT VI

Practice
Test

Practice Test

1. Your client asks you about the recommended check-ups for cancer prevention. Which of the following is NO LONGER recommended by the American Cancer Society for early detection of cancer?
   ① Monthly breast self-examination and a mammogram for women over 50
   ② Yearly testing of stools for fecal occult blood for clients over 50
   ③ Digital rectal examination for men over 40
   ④ Annual sputum analysis and yearly chest x-ray for smokers

2. Which client is at the greatest risk for cervical cancer?
   ① Ms. A., who had an early onset of menstruation and suffered malnutrition
   ② Ms. B., who had two children before the age of 20
   ③ Ms. C., who had frequent sexual relations with multiple partners
   ④ Ms. D., who has abstained from sexual intercourse and is obese

3. Your client has been a heavy smoker and a heavy drinker for years. This client is at greatest risk for:
   ① Lung cancer
   ② Laryngeal cancer
   ③ Stomach cancer
   ④ Oral cancer

4. Breast self-examination is especially important for a woman who:
   ① Is over 50 and had children before the age of 20
   ② Has very large breasts and breast fed her children
   ③ Has a history of fibrocystic disease and is under 40
   ④ Has no children and has an aunt with breast cancer

Mrs. South has been diagnosed with cervical cancer and is to have an internal radium implant in for the next 48 hours.

---

5. The nurse should anticipate that Mrs. South is at greatest risk for which of the following problems while the implant is in place?
   ① Fear and isolation
   ② Nausea and vomiting
   ③ Vaginal bleeding
   ④ Pain from the implant

6. Which of the following actions will help protect the nurse from undue exposure to the radiation while caring for Mrs. South?
   ① Care for the patient no more than 10 minutes per day
   ② Wear a lead apron when giving direct care
   ③ Stand at the head of the bed whenever possible while giving care
   ④ Ask a family member to be present and to assist with care

7. Which action by the nurse will help ensure that Mrs. South's internal organs receive no more than the prescribed dose of radiation?
   ① Encourage the client to turn side to side every 2 hours
   ② Elevate the head of the bed for meals
   ③ Administer laxatives as ordered to prevent constipation
   ④ Carefully maintain the patency of the urinary catheter

8. When it is time for the implant to be removed, the nurse is responsible for:
   ① Noting the time of removal of Mrs. South's kardex
   ② Assisting the surgeon with the removal
   ③ Removing the implant and placing it in a lead container
   ④ Nothing: this is not a nursing responsibility

9. After removal of the implant, the nurse should teach Mrs. South to:
   ① Avoid all pregnant women for 6 weeks
   ② Limit her exposure to children to 30 minutes a day
   ③ Not sleep in the same bed as her husband for 1 month
   ④ Abstain from sexual intercourse for 6 weeks

10. The nurse provides Mrs. South with information on expected outcomes following removal of the implant. Which of the following outcomes would NOT be normal and would require that Mrs. South call the physician?
    ① Moderate constipation
    ② Brown, foul-smelling vaginal drainage
    ③ Urinary incontinence without the urge to void
    ④ Slightly blood-tinged urine

Mr. Coates, 55 years old, is receiving outpatient radiation therapy to his oral cavity and neck for laryngeal cancer.

---

11. Which statement about side effects of external radiation is correct?
    ① They are generalized to all body systems

② They are localized to the area treated

③ They are minimal with single-dose therapy

④ They are serious and potentially life-threatening

12. Nursing care of the skin over the site of Mr. Coates' radiation therapy should include:

① Daily cleansing with soap and water

② Applying of commercial lotion to prevent drying

③ Avoiding tight collars

④ Preventing any water from coming in contact with his neck

13. Which of the following side effects is Mr. Coates most likely to develop?

① Stomatitis

② Alopecia

③ Thrombocytopenia

④ Leukopenia

14. What is the most appropriate nursing intervention to treat this side effect?

① Avoid intramuscular injections

② Place the client in reverse isolation

③ Encourage the client to wear a wig or scarf

④ Administer xylocaine gargle before oral care

15. Mr. Jones has been experiencing angina. The physician orders a coronary vasodilator. The nurse should instruct him that which of the following is a common side effect of coronary vasodilators?

① Loss of appetite

② Increased urine output

③ Headache

④ Increased blood pressure

Mrs. Walter is a 50-year-old type I insulin-dependent diabetic who has been a diabetic for a number of years, and her condition is well controlled by insulin.

---

16. Recently, Mrs. Walter has been having marital difficulties that leave her emotionally upset. As a result of this stress, it is possible that she will exhibit:

① An insulin reaction more readily than usual

② Increased blood sugar levels

③ A need for less daily insulin

④ A need for more carbohydrates

17. The stress Mrs. Walter is experiencing leads to an increased production of glucocorticoid, which would tend to:

① Decrease the production of fatty acids and lower the blood sugar

② Increase the secretion of insulin and lower the blood sugar

③ Increase the need for insulin and raise the blood sugar

④ Increase the production of fatty acids and raise the blood sugar

18. Mrs. Walter is receiving 40 units of regular insulin at 7:30 a.m. daily. Based on this information, what is the most likely time for her to experience an insulin reaction?

① 9 a.m.

② 11 a.m.

③ 3:30 p.m.

④ 11 p.m.

19. If Mrs. Walter had been receiving NPH insulin instead at 7:30 a.m., what will be the most likely time for the reaction to occur?

① 8 a.m.

② 12 noon

③ 4 p.m.

④ 12 midnight

20. What characteristic symptom of insulin shock should alert the nurse to an early insulin reaction?

① Diaphoresis

② Drowsiness

③ Severe thirst

④ Coma

21. Which of the following is a priority goal of the nurse's discharge teaching for Mary, who had an ileostomy to treat ulcerative colitis?

① Mary understands stoma irrigation

② Mary obtains psychological counseling

③ Mary can care for the skin around the stoma

④ Mary knows that she must restrict fluids

22. Mary must know the problems occurring after her ileostomy that would require her to notify the physician. Which of the following is an important clinical manifestation of this complication?

① Three to four diarrheal or liquid stools for 3 days

② Daily fecal output greater than 1500 mL for 3 days

③ Intolerance to high-residue foods

④ A decrease in the size of her stoma within 2 months of surgery

---

Mr. Lake, a 65-year-old salesman, is admitted with a diagnosis of possible cancer of the colon.

---

23. Which diagnostic examination is most helpful in diagnosing cancer of colon?
    ① Barium enema
    ② Stool examination for fecal occult blood
    ③ CEA level
    ④ Colonoscopy and biopsy

24. What early clinical manifestation most likely led Mr. Lake to suspect colon cancer?
    ① Rectal bleeding and pain
    ② Change in bowel habits
    ③ Persistent nausea and vomiting
    ④ Clay-colored stools

Sara Miller is an obese, 40-year-old mother of four who is admitted with a history of chronic cholecystitis.

---

25. Mrs. Miller is ordered to receive vitamin K preoperatively. What is the purpose of this medication?
    ① To improve the digestion of fats
    ② To promote the healing of tissues
    ③ To help eliminate bile
    ④ To facilitate blood clotting

26. After surgery, the nurse places Mrs. Miller in semi-Fowler's position. What is the rationale for this position?
    ① To prevent aspiration
    ② To facilitate breathing
    ③ To decrease strain on the incision line
    ④ To reduce nausea

27. Mrs. Miller has a T-tube in place after surgery. What is the purpose of the T-tube?
    ① To remove bile leaking from the incision
    ② To provide a means of wound irrigation
    ③ To drain bile from the common bile duct
    ④ To prevent rupture of the inflamed gallbladder

28. Mrs. Miller is likely to develop jaundice preoperatively. What clinical manifestations of jaundice should the nurse assess for?
    ① Ascites
    ② Dermatitis
    ③ Icteric sclera
    ④ Dark-colored stools

Lin Sun Park, 29 years old, is admitted in active labor. Membranes are leaking clear amniotic fluid. Ultrasound examination determines that the fetus is about 38 weeks. There is no history of prenatal care. The family has been in the United States for just a few months, and speak little English. While Mrs. Park is very quiet, she appears afraid and tense.

---

29. What is the most important thing the nurse can do to meet Mrs. Park's emotional needs at the time of admission to the labor and delivery unit?
    ① Ask her husband or mother to remain with her
    ② Assign one nurse to provide consistent care
    ③ Contact social service to locate an interpreter
    ④ Allow her the privacy preferred in her culture

30. Because no prenatal records are available, the resident physician orders each of the following tests to be done. Which data are most important as a basis for management of care during the intrapartal course?
    ① Complete blood count
    ② Cervical culture and sensitivity
    ③ Blood type and Rh
    ④ ELISA serology

31. When the results of the above tests are received, which should the nurse immediately share with the physician?
    ① Hematocrit, 36; hemoglobin, 10
    ② Culture: no growth in 12 hours
    ③ Type A negative blood
    ④ Serology: HB_sAB positive

32. Analysis of the implications of the serology indicates that Mrs. Park has:
    ① Acute hepatitis A infection
    ② Recent exposure to hepatitis B
    ③ Active, acute hepatitis C
    ④ Immune response to hepatitis B

After a difficult transitional labor, Mrs. Park delivers a 6-pound male infant. The parents are delighted with the baby. The interpreter asks if the mother can hold the baby after the initial assessment. She reports that this is the couple's second child, but the first baby died in infancy. Both parents appear very worried.

---

33. Based on the history and this information, which of the following is an appropriate nursing goal for the Park family?
    ① Mother will initiate bottle feeding within 12 hours
    ② Mother will visit newborn frequently in the nursery
    ③ Parents will have carly and frequent contact with newborn
    ④ Parents will be knowledgeable of feeding techniques

34. Which of the following dinner menus, if selected by Mrs. Park, would show that she understands her basic nutritional needs?
    ① Chicken, rice, noodles, banana, tea
    ② Shrimp, rice, vegetables, apple, tea
    ③ Fish, rice, cheese, orange slices, tea
    ④ Pork, rice, beans, pear, tea

35. At the time of discharge, the nurse, interpreter, and family review health care for mother and the newborn. Emphasis is on hygiene and nutrition. Which of the following nursing observations indicates that further teaching is needed?
    ① Mother washes her hands before feeding the newborn
    ② The baby's diaper is changed when soiled
    ③ Mother feeds the newborn every 3 to 4 hours
    ④ Baby is given honey on a pacifier between feedings

36. While preparing to return home, Ms. Park complains of pain in her right calf. Which of the following is the appropriate first nursing action?
    ① Ask the family to return to the clinic tomorrow
    ② Massage the calf and assess pain relief
    ③ Apply warm moist compresses to the leg
    ④ Notify the physician immediately

37. The physician determines that the calf pain is a muscle spasm. Homan's sign is negative. Each of the following suggestions from the nurse is appropriate for a postpartum mother. Which is most important in the prevention of thrombus formation?
    ① "Rest as much as possible at home."
    ② "Increase the fluids in your diet."
    ③ "Walk about the home frequently."
    ④ "Avoid stair climbing or active exercise."

Mr. Green, 78 years old, is complaining of dizziness and lightheadedness and is admitted to the emergency room. His diagnosis is bradycardia. Atropine sulfate is administered intravenously.

---

38. What is the definition of bradycardia?
    ① Impaired impulse conduction through the atrioventricular node
    ② A heart rate greater than 100 beats per minute
    ③ An irregular heart rate
    ④ A heart rate less than 60 beats per minute

39. Which of the following is the most appropriate nursing diagnosis for Mr. Green?
    ① Decreased cardiac output
    ② Fluid volume deficit
    ③ Altered health maintenance
    ④ Ineffective breathing pattern

40. Atropine sulfate is contraindicated for clients with which of the following conditions?
    ① Congestive heart failure
    ② Diabetes mellitus
    ③ Glaucoma
    ④ Parkinson's disease

41. Mr. Green is scheduled for a pacemaker insertion. The pacemaker will assume the function of what part of the heart?
    ① Atrioventricular node
    ② Bundle of His
    ③ Right and left bundle branches
    ④ Sinoatrial node

42. A permanent-demand pacemaker is inserted. What is the nurse's emphasis when teaching Mr. Green about the pacemaker?
    ① To explain that the pacemaker will initiate an impulse continuously at a preset rate
    ② To explain that the pacemaker electrode is positioned in the left atrium
    ③ To take his own pulse daily and call the physician if it is below a specific rate
    ④ To instruct him to avoid taking tranquilizers

Mr. Jones has a colostomy as a result of surgery for low sigmoid colon cancer.

---

43. Which is the most important aspect of nursing care immediately after Mr. Jones' surgery?
    ① Checking for incisional infection
    ② Teaching the client colostomy care
    ③ Assessing the placement of the permanent colostomy appliance
    ④ Checking the color, size, and patency of the stoma

44. Which psychosocial manifestation should the nurse anticipate that Mr. Jones will experience within the first week after surgery?
    ① A change in body image
    ② A change in social role
    ③ Guilt feelings due to cancer
    ④ Regression

Mr. Jones is receiving chemotherapy because his cancer has widespread metastases.

45. Mr. Jones has developed leukopenia. The nurse knows that as a result he is most susceptible to:
    1. Infection
    2. Bleeding
    3. Hyperuricemia
    4. Septicemia

46. Mr. Jones has carpopedal spasms, numbness around his mouth, and difficulty talking. Which side effect of chemotherapy is he experiencing?
    1. Neurotoxicity
    2. Leukopenia
    3. Hyperuricemia
    4. Hypocalcemia

47. Mr. Jones tells the nurse that he has problems with balance and feels uncoordinated. This alerts the nurse to the possibility of neurotoxicity. Which of the following is the most appropriate nursing diagnosis for Mr. Jones?
    1. Pain
    2. Altered tissue perfusion
    3. High risk for injury
    4. Altered thought process

The staff at the child health clinic held a screening program for lead poisoning in an inner city community. Amanda Pace, 30 months old, is found to have an elevated blood lead level. She has been irritable lately and has a poor appetite. She is admitted to the pediatric unit of the local hospital for further treatment.

48. Which of the following is most likely to cause lead poisoning in children of Amanda's age group?
    1. Eating vegetables sprayed with insecticide
    2. Playing with toys decorated with lead-based paint
    3. Eating paint and plaster chips
    4. Inhaling chemical fumes

49. The initial nursing assessment reveals that Amanda tires easily, has a poor appetite, is pale and irritable. These data indicate that Amanda has which of the following sequela of lead poisoning?
    1. Encephalopathy
    2. Renal colic
    3. Peripheral neuritis
    4. Anemia

50. Amanda is in the playroom with three other toddlers. The nurse provides blocks for the group to play with. Which of the following best describes the play of a group of toddlers?
    1. The group builds a house together
    2. Each child tries to build his or her own block tower
    3. The children are uninterested in the blocks
    4. One child builds a tower while the other children watch

Art Riley, 45 years old, is admitted for the fifth time to a chemical dependency unit. In the past, he has signed himself out before completing his treatment. He is known to be abusive to his wife and family, and usually blames them for his return to drinking. His wife has stated that if he does not complete treatment this time, she is going through with a divorce. On this admission, Art is actively involved with a treatment based on the Alcoholics Anonymous format.

51. Art tells the nurse that he no longer has a drinking problem. The nurse realizes that Art is using which of the following defense mechanisms?
    1. Projection
    2. Reaction formation
    3. Denial
    4. Sublimation

52. The nurse knows that it is important to increase Art's fluid consumption during detoxification for the alcohol abuse. What is the reason for this?
    1. Fluids help clear alcohol from the body
    2. Alcohol is a diuretic, and fluids help prevent dehydration
    3. Fluids prevent the constipating effect of alcohol
    4. Fluids help prevent cirrhosis

53. The nurse knows that withdrawal from alcohol may cause delirium tremors (DTs). For which of the following symptoms of DTs will the nurse observe Art?
    1. Hyperthermia, catatonia, convulsions, tremors
    2. Hypotension, increased agitation, hallucinations

③ Hypertension, diaphoresis, tachycardia, delusions

④ Hypotension, visual hallucinations, tremors

54. Which of the following medications is most commonly used to control the symptoms of alcohol withdrawal?
① Phenobarbital
② Amitriptyline (Elavil)
③ Lithium carbonate
④ Chlorpromazine (Thorazine)

Gene Ray, 76 years old, has experienced leg cramps for several years. He recently began to have severe headaches, syncope, and short memory lapses. He is admitted to the hospital with a diagnosis of atherosclerosis/arteriosclerosis.

---

55. The nurse knows that which of the following is the most accurate test for diagnosing atherosclerosis?
① Serum cholesterol level
② Prothrombin time
③ Arteriogram
④ Doppler study

56. Mr. Ray's latest clinical manifestations may indicate that the condition has progressed. The nurse knows that which of the following are likely to be occurring with Mr. Ray?
① Pulmonary dysfunction
② Coronary occlusion
③ Cerebral involvement
④ Impending renal failure

57. The physician orders a low-fat diet. Mr. Ray says that he always has bacon, scrambled eggs, and toast for breakfast. The nurse suggests that which of the following would be a better breakfast?
① Poached egg and fresh fruit
② Cooked cereal and orange juice
③ Pancakes and 2% milk
④ French toast and coffee

58. During the initial assessment of Mr. Ray's lower extremities, which objective assessments might the nurse expect to find?
① Moist, warm skin and regular pulses
② Edema, pain when touched, and bounding pulses
③ Tingling, numbness, and slowed pulses
④ Pale, cool skin and diminished pulses

59. Which of the following medical conditions is a direct result of alcohol comsumption in the absence of adequate thiamine?

① Pick's syndrome
② Alzheimer's disease
③ Wernicke's syndrome
④ Wilson's disease

60. Your client has had a hemorrhoidectomy. Which of the following is most effective for the relief of postoperative pain?
① Tylenol #3
② A sitz bath
③ Laxatives
④ Stool softeners

61. Abrupt withdrawal of which of the following drugs can cause death?
① Heroin
② Cocaine
③ Barbiturates
④ Morphine

62. Mr. Adams is a 55-year-old businessman whose children have all just left home and whose parents are still alive and healthy Which of the following is a reasonable developmental goal for Mr. Adams?
① The client will accept retirement
② The client will establish a modified role relationship with his wife
③ The client will accept a dependent relationship with his children
④ The client will assume a caretaker role for his parents

63. Mrs. Wilson is 80 years old and healthy. Given the normal aging changes that occur within the musculoskeletal system, which of the following is a reasonably expectation for Mrs. Wilson?
① The client will maintain bedrest
② The client will be unable to ambulate without assistance
③ The client will be protected against falls
④ The client will be able to maintain all normal activities

64. Your client has an order for an IV of lactated Ringer's solution, 1000 mL to run from 10 a.m. until 7 p.m. The drip factor is 15 drops/min. What rate should the IV run?
① 12 gtts/min
② 14 gtts/min
③ 21 gtts/min
④ 28 gtts/min

Mr. Jackson is a 45-year-old executive who is admitted to the coronary care unit with a diagnosis of acute myocardial infarction. Mr. Jackson has a history of smoking and is overweight. His father died at age 40 from a heart attack.

---

65. During the night, Mr. Jackson is found to be restless and diaphoretic. Which of the following is an appropriate nursing intervention?
    ① Call his family to come to the hospital to provide emotional support
    ② Turn the alarms on low and decrease the number of times the client's sleep is interrupted
    ③ Assess the client's blood pressure and heart rate
    ④ Call the physician for an order for sedation

66. Mr. Jackson develops recurrent chest pain. Nitroglycerine IV is ordered. What is the goal of this treatment?
    ① To promote diuresis
    ② To increase the force of contraction of the myocardium
    ③ To produce an analgesic effect
    ④ To cause vasodilatation and decrease oxygen demand

67. Cardiac catheterization with coronary angiography is scheduled for Mr. Jackson. What is the goal of this procedure?
    ① To evaluate the client's exercise tolerance
    ② To study the client's conduction system
    ③ To evaluate coronary blood flow
    ④ To determine the effectiveness of various vasodilators

68. Which of the following nursing diagnosis is most appropriate for Mr. Jackson postcardiac catheterization?
    ① Pain
    ② Activity intolerance
    ③ High risk for altered tissue perfusion: peripheral
    ④ High risk for ineffective breathing pattern

Shawna Hutchins, 29, is an African-American primigravida with a history of sickle cell anemia. At the first antepartal visit, she asks about the potential problems the pregnancy may cause.

---

69. Which of the following statements should the nurse make to Ms. Hutchins about her condition?
    ① "Pregnancy should be avoided in women with this disease."
    ② "Adequate iron intake will prevent serious problems."
    ③ "Regular prenatal care is critical to detect abnormalities."

④ "Your condition will probably not be affected by pregnancy."

70. The nurse understands that the pathophysiology of sickle cell crisis involves:
    ① Altered metabolism and dehydration
    ② Tissue hypoxia and vascular occlusion
    ③ Increased bilirubin levels and hypertension
    ④ Decreased clotting factors and white cell increase

71. The nurse instructs Ms. Hutchins on specific clinical manifestations to be reported immediately. Which of the following problems is most likely to lead to sickle cell crisis?
    ① Slight weight loss
    ② Fatigue after mild exercise
    ③ Perspiring in a warm room
    ④ Recurrence of chronic UTI

72. Which of the following is NOT an appropriate nursing diagnosis for high-risk problems related to sickled hemoglobin during pregnancy?
    ① High risk for altered tissue perfusion: peripheral
    ② High risk for infection
    ③ Altered gas exchange
    ④ Altered nutrition: more than required

Mrs. Anderson, a 78-year-old widow, is admitted with a possible fractured hip. She was found on the floor by a neighbor.

---

73. Which of the following best describes the appearance of the leg with a fractured hip?
    ① Shortened, adducted, and internally rotated
    ② Shortened, abducted, and internally rotated
    ③ Shortened, adducted, and externally rotated
    ④ Shortened, abducted, and externally rotated

74. Prior to surgery, Mrs. Anderson will be maintained in Buck's traction. What is the main goal in use of Buck's traction?
    ① To reduce the fracture
    ② To decrease muscle spasms
    ③ To maintain complete bedrest
    ④ To set the fracture

75. Which of the following nursing assessments is the most important when caring for a client in Buck's traction?
    ① Assess skin under the Buck's boot every 8 hours

② Check the pin sites at least daily

③ Check the area around the hip where the traction is applied daily

④ Verify that the weights of at least 25 pounds are freely hanging

76. Which of the following would be an appropriate nursing diagnosis for Mrs. Anderson?

① High risk for altered thought process

② Urinary incontinence

③ Noncompliance

④ High risk for altered cardiac output

77. Which of the following best describes a comminuted fracture?

① Bone is broken into two parts that do not separate

② Bone partly bent and partly broken

③ Bone shattered into two or more fragments

④ Bone broken into two parts with complete separation

78. Which of the following is NOT a common cause of fractures?

① Osteoporosis

② Diabetes

③ Steroid therapy

④ Breast cancer

79. There are five stages of bone healing. Which of the following best describes the callus formation stage?

① New bone enters area, forming woven bone and beginning to knit the ends

② Blood clots and forms hematoma between broken ends of bone

③ Granulation tissue forms, which becomes firm and links the two fragments of bone

④ Mature cells formed, callus formed, tissue resembles normal bone

80. Which of the following is a closed reduction of a fracture?

① An Austin Moore hip prosthesis for a fractured hip

② Application of pins and screws to a fractured ankle followed by a cast

③ Manipulation of a Colles fracture after anesthesia and application of a cast

④ Insertion of rods into a fractured humerus under anesthesia

81. Which of the following is the priority nursing assessment that must be made on every fracture, open or closed?

① Circulation and sensation distal to the fracture

② Amount of swelling around the fracture site

③ Degree of bone healing that has occurred

④ Amount of pain that the fracture and healing are causing

82. Mr. Silverman suffered a fractured femur yesterday, which was treated by an open reduction. Today he is complaining of shortness of breath, chest pain, and he has petechiae across his chest. Which of the following is the most likely cause of his problem?

① Pulmonary embolus

② Fat embolus

③ Myocardial infarction

④ Anxiety attack

83. Although they are similar in many ways, rheumatoid arthritis differs from osteoarthritis in that rheumatoid arthritis is:

① Systemic

② Progressive

③ Degenerative

④ Chronic

84. In hepatic coma, dietary proteins are eliminated and lactulose administered to decrease the amounts of ammonia produced by the intestine. Which of the following is a likely outcome of the lactulose administration?

① Urinary frequency

② Diarrhea

③ Nausea and vomiting

④ Dizziness

85. Which of the following diets is recommended for the client with hepatitis A?

① High protein, high carbohydrate

② Low protein, low carbohydrate

③ High protein, low calorie

④ Low protein, high carbohydrate

Mrs. Love has cirrhosis and is exhibiting ascites. She has nonbleeding esophageal varices.

---

86. A low-sodium diet is prescribed for Mrs. Love because of her ascites. Which of the following meals, if chosen by Mrs. Love, would demonstrate that she understands her diet?

① Baked chicken with barbecue sauce and sauerkraut

② A bacon, lettuce, and tomato sandwich garnished with olives

③ A ham and cheese sandwich

④ A roast beef sandwich with fresh green beans

87. If blood is unable to flow through a necrotic liver, blood is forced to take collateral routes. This will NOT result in:
    ① Esophageal varices
    ② Hemorrhoids
    ③ Prominent veins across the abdomen
    ④ Rectal bleeding

Ricky Rome, 6 months old, has spastic cerebral palsy involving all extremities. He also has a history of grand mal seizures. He is admitted to the pediatric unit accompanied by his parents, with a diagnosis of bronchopneumonia.

---

88. All of the following data are elicited by the nurse who obtains Ricky's admission history. Which of the following information is essential to planning his nursing care?
    ① Activities of daily living
    ② Immunizations received
    ③ Family history of illnesses
    ④ Reactions to previous hospitalizations

89. Ricky was admitted with a diagnosis of bronchopneumonia. Because of this problem, which of the following is the most appropriate nursing diagnosis for Ricky?
    ① Ineffective breathing pattern
    ② Altered nutrition: less than required
    ③ Hypothermia
    ④ Fluid volume deficit

90. Ricky has a grand mal seizure. Of the following nursing interventions, which should receive the highest priority when a seizure occurs?
    ① Loosen the child's clothing and protect him from injury by padding the crib
    ② Maintain a patent airway by turning the child's head to the side and suctioning him if necessary
    ③ Remain with the child and administer anticonvulsant medications as ordered by the physician
    ④ Describe and record events before the onset of the seizure, during the seizure, and after the seizure

91. Mrs. Rome observes the nurse administering postural drainage to Ricky and then suctioning him. She asks the nurse why Ricky must have these treatments. The nurse replies:
    ① "Postural drainage and suctioning help Ricky breathe easier by removing retained secretions from his respiratory tract."

    ② "I am doing these procedures because Ricky's muscles are weak and he is unable to expectorate mucus."
    ③ "These procedures must be done to clear Ricky's respiratory passages so that he will be able to drink adequate fluids."
    ④ "Postural drainage and suctioning are done every hour to prevent Ricky from aspirating excessive mucus."

92. Ricky is on a pureed diet. While feeding him, the nurse observes that he has trouble eating. The probable cause of his feeding difficulty is:
    ① Lack of control of the muscles used in sucking and swallowing
    ② Delayed eruption of the lateral and central incisors
    ③ Inability to relax completely during meal time
    ④ Loss of appetite due to activity intolerance from the bronchopneumonia

93. Mrs. Rome discusses Ricky's progress with the nurse. She states, "Ricky is not progressing. I'm going to take him to another doctor who will take better care of him and help him get well." The nurse interprets Mrs. Rome's remark as an indication of:
    ① Anger at the health care team
    ② Nonacceptance of Ricky's condition
    ③ Guilt feelings about Ricky's birth
    ④ A lack of understanding of cerebral palsy

Sam O'Malley, 55 years old, has been admitted to the hospital. During the past month, he has become increasingly agitated and hyperexcitable with an increase in verbal and physical activity. He is also suffering from insomnia and has rapid speech patterns. He has been on a buying spree during this time but just gives it all away. He was admitted 5 years ago for similar problems.

---

94. Considering all of Mr. O'Malley's manifestations, which of the following best describes it?
    ① Panic attacks
    ② Paranoid behavior
    ③ Schizophrenia
    ④ Manic episode

95. When Mr. O'Malley is admitted, he is extremely agitated. Which of the following is a useful nursing intervention during this time?

① Place him in a quiet area separate from other clients

② Encourage him to organize some physical activity

③ Establish firm, set rules for his behavior

④ Include him in group activities

96. Which of the following explanations would describe the problem behind Mr. O'Malley's behavior?

① The client is unable to develop close relationships

② The client exhibits an overwhelming desire for approval

③ He is attempting to increase his self-esteem

④ He is angry with others and this diffuses it

97. Which of the following coping mechanisms is Mr. O'Malley probably using?

① Projection

② Sublimation

③ Regression

④ Conversion

98. Mr. O'Malley is feeling many aggressive fantasies. He channels this aggression into playing football. This is an example of which of the following defense mechanisms?

① Identification

② Sublimation

③ Projection

④ Reaction formation

Mary, 18 years old, is an above-average student. She recently began college at a large, highly competitive university. She became withdrawn, which resulted in failing grades. One day, her roommate found her sitting on her bed, staring and unresponsive. After 24 hours, she was admitted to a psychiatric unit by her parents.

---

99. A nurse observes that Mary remains in one area most of the day and moves her arms and legs only when someone moves them for her. This behavior is an example of:

① Negativism

② Waxy flexibility

③ Echopraxia

④ Decreased consciousness

100. For several days, Mary avoids her one-to-one nurse. She stays in the bathroom or lies in bed, feigning sleep. The nurse recognizes that this behavior indicates:

① A rejection of the nurse

② A negative transference toward the nurse

③ Coping behavior on Mary's part

④ Mary's unwillingness to seek help

101. As the nurse is getting ready for a group session in the day room, Mary picks up the ashtray and offers it to the nurse. Which of the following is this action a sign of?

① Reality testing

② Improvement

③ Regression

④ Anxiety

102. A student nurse asks for direction in how to respond when Mary talks about hearing voices. The nurse replies that the student should tell Mary to:

① Ignore the voices

② Discuss what she is hearing

③ Describe the voices in detail

④ Discuss the voices with her doctor

103. Mary expresses the belief that the FBI is out to kill her. In caring for her safety, the nurse should primarily recognize that Mary will:

① Probably see the nurse and doctors as protectors

② Interpret the hospital routine as anxiety producing

③ React impulsively out of fear for her life

④ Correct her thinking after the doctor has spoken to her

104. Which of the following goals is most realistic for Mary in the short term?

① Mary will go for a walk with the two others

② Mary will trust both friends and strangers

③ Mary will no longer fear for her life

④ Mary will take part in a play with her group

Mr. Allen, 60 years old, has a 5-year history of emphysema. He is admitted to the hospital with pneumonia and a chief complaint of shortness of breath and congestion

---

105. Which of the following possible nursing diagnoses is most important in meeting Mr. Allen's basic health needs?

① Altered nutrition: less than required related to inability to swallow

② Ineffective individual coping related to chronic illness

③ Impaired gas exchange related to chronic lung disease

④ Altered tissue perfusion related to congestive heart failure

106. Because of his current breathing problem, Mr. Allen is also likely to have problems with:
    1. Loss of consciousness
    2. Dehydration
    3. Fatigue
    4. Dementia

107. Which of the following nursing observations would indicate that Mr. Allen's problems are resolving?
    1. He sleeps through the night without nocturia
    2. He sits at the bedside for meals without distress
    3. He resumes normal bowel habits
    4. He ambulates the length of the hall without dyspnea

Mary Black, a 55-year-old mother of three, is admitted with a diagnosis of chronic lymphocytic leukemia, which has possibly become acute. She is in acute distress and seriously ill.

---

108. Because Mrs. Black's WBC is 20,000 mm³, the nurse should expect her to demonstrate:
    1. Enlargement of the lymph nodes
    2. Decreased resistance to infections
    3. Increased risk of phlebitis
    4. Increased clotting activity

109. The nurse observes that Mrs. Black is often irritable and difficult to please. Which of the following is the best explanation?
    1. She is probably a chronic worrier
    2. This is typical behavior for a person her age who has been hospitalized
    3. This is a common response to chronic, potentially terminal illnesses
    4. She has not accepted her illness and needs spiritual guidance

110. Considering her diagnosis of chronic lymphocytic leukemia, which of the following nursing diagnoses would be most appropriate for Mrs. Black?
    1. Altered thought process
    2. Pain
    3. Potential for infection
    4. Ineffective airway clearance

Mr. Mart, 68 years old, is admitted with a diagnosis of congestive heart failure. He has had this condition for 5 years. Over the last 2 days, Mr. Mart has been experiencing increased edema of the ankles and lower extremities.

---

111. Based on Mr. Mart's symptoms, the nurse knows that his heart failure is probably:
    1. Right-sided
    2. Left-sided
    3. Complete
    4. Cor pulmonale

112. Mr. Mart is placed on a low-sodium diet to help control the edema. He is hungry at bedtime. Which of the following snacks would be best?
    1. An apple and two Graham crackers
    2. A dish of ice cream
    3. A glass of milk and a slice of cheese
    4. Several slices of salami and crackers

113. Mr. Mart is to be placed on medication to strengthen contractions of his heart and decrease his edema. Which of the following is the most likely combination of drugs?
    1. Lasix and Pronestyl
    2. Isuprel and digoxin
    3. Digoxin and Diuril
    4. Lasix and Diuril

114. If Mr. Mart is given a thiazide diuretic, which of the following electrolyte imbalances could occur and predispose Mr. Mart to drug toxicity?
    1. Hyponatremia
    2. Hypercalcemia
    3. Hypophosphatemia
    4. Hypokalemia

115. Daily weights are to be done for Mr. Mart. The purpose of this nursing activity is to evaluate the client's:
    1. Fluid balance
    2. Nitrogen balance
    3. Blood volume
    4. Appetite

116. Mr. Mart suddenly exhibits respiratory distress with frothy sputum, severe pulmonary congestion, and symptoms of left-sided heart failure. Which of the following conditions should the nurse immediately suspect?
    1. A pulmonary embolus
    2. Right-sided heart failure
    3. Pulmonary edema
    4. Cor pulmonale

Mr. Parker, 49 years old, has been diagnosed with hypertension.

---

117. Hypertension can be described as a disease that:
    ① Can be controlled with treatment
    ② Can be cured
    ③ Often disappears without treatment
    ④ Is usually fatal

118. It is not unusual for a client with hypertension like Mr. Parker to stop taking his prescribed medication. A common reason for this is that Mr. Parker:
    ① Did not receive adequate instruction
    ② Cannot afford the medications
    ③ Finds taking the medications too bothersome
    ④ Doesn't feel bad, so he denies the disease

119. The treatment for hypertension is usually directed at:
    ① Lowering the blood pressure to below normal levels
    ② Repairing the damaged blood vessels
    ③ Increasing the urine output
    ④ Preventing further damage to the blood vessels

Mr. Baker has been receiving IV heparin. The IV is a mixture of 10,000 units in 1000 mL. The physician wants the client to receive 80 units per hour.

---

120. How many mL per hour should the nurse administer?
    ① 8 mL/hr
    ② 12 mL/hr
    ③ 16 mL/hr
    ④ 20 mL/hr

121. The IV has a minidrip attached to it. How many drops per minute should the nurse run the IV?
    ① 8 gtts/min
    ② 12 gtts/min
    ③ 16 gtts/min
    ④ 20 gtts/min

Thomas Farrel, 62 years old, underwent a transurethral resection (TUR) of the prostate this morning. He has a constant bladder irrigation (CBI) running. He is complaining of severe bladder spasms.

---

122. Which of the following is the highest priority nursing intervention?
    ① Medicate the client with Demerol 50 mg as ordered
    ② Slow the rate of the CBI
    ③ Speed up the rate of the CBI
    ④ Check the patency of the catheter

123. Which of the following medications would best relieve Mr. Farrel's bladder spasms and pain?
    ① Demerol
    ② Prostigmine
    ③ Pro-Banthine
    ④ Pyridium

124. Which of the following statements, if made by Mr. Farrel, indicates that he understands the outcome of his surgery?
    ① "I may have to have this surgery again in a few years."
    ② "I won't have to worry about birth control anymore."
    ③ "I'm upset that I will be impotent, but I guess I'll adjust."
    ④ "I know how to change the dressing daily."

Mary has experienced pregnancy-induced hypertension at 35 weeks gestation and has come to the antepartal testing unit for a nonstress test.

---

125. The nurse explains the test to Mary. The nurse knows that which of the following statements about a nonstress test is accurate?
    ① It is an invasive test which predicts 1 week of further intrauterine safety for the fetus
    ② It is a noninvasive test of fetal–placental reserve
    ③ It is considered positive if there are no late decelerations
    ④ It is considered reactive if there are no fetal heart tones

126. An L/S ratio is ordered for Mary. The nurse knows that the purpose of this test is to:
    ① Determine fetal lung maturity
    ② Estimate maternal–fetal estriol production
    ③ Determine fetal gender
    ④ Test the intrauterine fetal–placental circulation

127. A stress test (oxytocin challenge test) to determine fetal well-being is done. To evaluate the results of this test, the nurse should know that it is considered:
① Negative if no fetal heart rate accelerations occur with accompanying fetal movements
② Nonreactive if there are no late decelerations in more than half of the uterine contractions
③ Positive if the late decelerations occur in more than half of the uterine contractions
④ Reactive if the fetal heart rate accelerates with accompanying fetal movement

128. A biophysical profile (fetal biophysical profile) is conducted with a resulting score of 10. The nurse should know that these data indicate that:
① Immediate delivery by a cesarean section is necessary
② Mary should have a retest in 1 week
③ No further testing is necessary for Mary
④ Induction of labor within 48 hours is indicated

Mary has experienced contractions throughout the night and comes to the clinic for evaluation in the early morning.

---

129. The nurse should know that false labor contractions differ from true labor contractions in which of the following ways?
① They will be intensified by walking about
② They will be confined to the low back
③ They do not increase in intensity or frequency
④ They result in cervical effacement and dilation

Mr. Andrews, 48 years old, is admitted to the hospital with a diagnosis of acute gastroenteritis. He has had nausea, vomiting, and diarrhea for the last 48 hours.

---

130. Which of the following is the most important initial nursing assessment for Mr. Andrews?
① His knowledge of the upcoming diagnostic examinations
② His fluid and electrolyte balance
③ The presence of a viral infection
④ His ability to withstand the stress of hospitalization

131. Which of the following is the most important aspect of the nurse's ongoing assessment of Mr. Andrews?
① Vital signs
② Respiratory rate and breath sounds
③ Level of consciousness
④ Character and frequency of stools

132. Which of the following is another important assessment of Mr. Andrews?
① Total intake and output from all sources
② Ability to sleep through the night
③ Rate and amount of his IV fluids
④ Prior eating and elimination habits

133. Which of the following is a measurable nursing goal for discharge?
① Mr. Andrews will have less frequent stools
② Mr. Andrews will have diarrhea controlled and no recurrence
③ Mr. Andrews will have no more than one stool per day
④ Mr. Andrews will return to his normal bowel pattern

134. Once the nausea has resolved, which of the following would be an appropriate intervention to meet the goal for Mr. Andrews?
① Allow food and fluids as desired
② Limit all fluids until diarrhea disappears
③ Provide liberal amounts of fluid and a bland diet
④ Provide unlimited quantities of milk and fruit juice

135. The nurse discovers that Mr. Andrews has been admitted three times before for the same problem. As a result of this information, the nurse understands that an important nursing assessment would be which of the following?
① His usual bowel habits
② Whether other family members have the same symptoms
③ His usual eating pattern
④ Who in the family does the cooking

136. Medication dosages are often based on kilograms of body weight. In order to administer the proper dose of medication, the nurse knows that a 106-pound woman weighs about:
① 36 Kg
② 42 Kg
③ 48 Kg
④ 52 Kg

137. The physician orders gentamycin (Garamycin) for Andy Burns, a teenager with a severe wound infection. Which of the following should the nurse do before administering this medication?
    1. Obtain a culture of the wound
    2. Check for an allergy to penicillin
    3. Check the client's temperature
    4. Assure that the client's stomach is empty

Allen Morris, 22 years old, has been complaining of fatigue, thirst, and excessive urination. He is admitted to be worked-up for possible diabetes mellitus.

---

138. One of the first tests the physician orders is a glucose tolerance test. The nurse knows that preparation for this requires the client to:
    1. Fast for 24 hours prior
    2. Have only water for 12 hours
    3. Eat 100 g of glucose 2 hours before the test
    4. Eat no carbohydrates for 24 hours
139. Allen is diagnosed as having type I diabetes mellitus. The nurse knows that diabetes is best defined as:
    1. An absence of insulin in the system
    2. Failure of the body to successfully utilize glucose
    3. A complex condition related to the control of carbohydrate metabolism
    4. A disease affecting the pancreas, causing a lack of insulin
140. The physician decides to control Allen's condition with diet, exercise, and medication. Which of the following is the best description of the diabetic diet?
    1. It provides a well-balanced meal using an exchange list
    2. It severely limits carbohydrates but allows fats and protein
    3. It limits the intake of carbohydrates slightly
    4. It helps the client lose excess weight
141. The nurse should teach Allen that diabetics are much more prone to cardiovascular disease than nondiabetics because:
    1. Diabetics have difficulty metabolizing fats and proteins, with the end products of these accumulating in the vessels
    2. Diabetics are usually overweight, increasing the workload on the heart and blood vessels
    3. Most diabetics are elderly persons who are more likely to have degenerative cardiovascular disease
    4. Atherosclerotic changes occur in the blood vessels because of the high levels of glucose and fat with poor control
142. The nurse knows that an exercise regimen would be helpful for Allen for which of the following reasons?
    1. Exercise increases the rate of insulin secretion
    2. Exercise lowers the blood sugar level
    3. Exercise helps prevent obesity
    4. Exercise helps insulin circulate in the body
143. The nurse teaches Allen proper foot care and methods of maintaining and improving circulation to the lower extremities for which of the following reasons?
    1. Diabetics are more prone to gangrene if they develop foot infections
    2. Diabetics have no resistance to infection and can develop septicemia
    3. Diabetics have a chronically low white blood cell count, making them prone to infection
    4. Diabetics have a lowered resistance to infection and thrombocytopenia

---

Mrs. Matts, 56 years old, has a deficiency of parathormone.

---

144. For which of the following problems should the nurse monitor Mrs. Matts?
    1. Muscular weakness and somnolence
    2. Increased blood sugar
    3. Muscle twitching and spasms
    4. Renal calculi
145. The symptoms of parathormone deficiency are caused because parathormone regulates:
    1. Acid–base balance
    2. Potassium secretion
    3. Thyroid metabolism
    4. Calcium metabolism

Mrs. Lewis, 49 years old, has developed Cushing's syndrome.

---

146. The nurse should be aware that Cushing's syndrome is often associated with which of the following?
    ① Steroid therapy
    ② Adrenal atrophy
    ③ Hyperthyroidism
    ④ Decreased ACTH secretion

147. Nursing care for Mrs. Lewis would include which of the following?
    ① Giving a high-carbohydrate, low-protein diet
    ② Teaching the client the signs of hypoglycemia
    ③ Teaching the client to avoid infections
    ④ Maintaining the client on bedrest

148. Which of the following would NOT be a realistic goal for the client on steroid therapy?
    ① The client will not develop a gastric ulcer
    ② The client will not develop symptoms of Cushing's syndrome
    ③ The client will not develop an infection
    ④ The client will not develop hyperglycemia

Mrs. Klein, 42 years old, has just delivered her second child by cesarean section.

---

149. A nursing mother often does not return to menstruation for several months after delivery or until she discontinues breast feeding. Because of this, which of the following is it appropriate for the nurse to teach Mrs. Klein?
    ① As long as she is breast feeding, her estrogen levels will not return to normal levels
    ② Ovulation is not suppressed and pregnancy is possible even though she is breast feeding
    ③ The uterus will not return to a normal size while she is breast feeding
    ④ If she does not begin to menstruate in 3 months, she should stop breast feeding

150. The nurse notes that on the day after delivery, the lochia has a foul smell. Which of the following is the most appropriate nursing intervention?
    ① Report immediately to the physician that the client may have an infection
    ② Do nothing; this is normal during the first few days after delivery

③ Begin vaginal irrigations to decrease the odor and increase client comfort
④ Use tampons rather than perineal pads for the next few days

151. When administering an enema to Mrs. Klein postpartum, the nurse should:
    ① Use a small catheter
    ② Administer no more than 100 mL of solution
    ③ Be careful not to irritate the perineum when inserting the catheter
    ④ Encourage the client to administer her own so she will learn how to do so at home

152. Which of the following nursing interventions would decrease the incidence of postpartum thrombophlebitis in Mrs. Klein?
    ① Early ambulation
    ② Immobilization and elevation of the lower extremities
    ③ Administration of mild anticoagulants
    ④ Breast feeding the newborn

153. Which of the following nursing assessments is critical to detecting potential problems resulting from the use of Pitocin following delivery?
    ① Urinary output
    ② Uterine contractions
    ③ Temperature
    ④ Reflex responses

154. At the time of Mrs. Klein's discharge, a repeat CBC is taken. The results are hematocrit, 28%; hemoglobin, 7 g. The physician orders Imferon (iron-dextran) to be administered by Z-track. The nurse understands that which of the following is NOT a potential adverse reaction to this medication?
    ① Staining of the skin
    ② Thrombophlebitis
    ③ Pain at the site
    ④ Anaphylaxis

155. Discharge teaching for Mrs. Klein includes emphasis on an increase in dietary sources of iron. Which lunch menu, if selected by Mrs. Klein, indicates she understands the basic four food groups and sources of iron?
    ① Chef's salad, whole wheat toast, milk, an apple
    ② Liver sausage sandwich on rye, tomato, milk, apricots
    ③ Chicken vegetable soup, lettuce wedge, milk, a banana
    ④ Tacos, coleslaw, milk, sherbet

156. Which of the following would be an important goal for the client with lupus?

① The client will exercise several hours per day

② The client will not develop altered tissue perfusion

③ The client will not develop undetected hemorrhage

④ The client will not develop wrist deformities

Ms. Smith, 32 years old, has lymphosarcoma. She has enlarged lymph nodes in her neck, cervical, and parasternal regions. She is being treated with external radiation therapy. She is having some skin irritation from the radiation.

---

157. Which of the following is included in the nursing care of the irritated area?
    ① Applying oil-based cream three times a day
    ② Washing the area with soap and water twice a day
    ③ Exposing the area to a sun lamp daily
    ④ Protecting the area from injury

158. Which of the following is NOT a side effect of radiation therapy treatments in Ms. Smith?
    ① Esophagitis
    ② Proctitis
    ③ Laryngitis
    ④ Pericarditis

159. Massive destruction of cells results from radiation treatments. Which nursing assessments would be INAPPROPRIATE for Ms. Smith?
    ① Monitoring her CBC daily
    ② Checking urine volume and specific gravity daily
    ③ Measuring her abdominal girth daily
    ④ Monitoring levels of electrolytes and minerals weekly

Mr. Thompson, 76 years old, is a retired businessman who is admitted with a diagnosis of benign prostatic hypertrophy (BPH). He is scheduled for a transurethral resection (TUR). Postoperatively, he has a constant bladder irrigation (CBI) running.

---

160. Four hours after surgery, Mr. Thompson is complaining of bladder spasms. Which of the following is the most important assessment for the nurse to make?
    ① The time of his last pain shot
    ② The rate of flow of the CBI
    ③ The patency of the catheter
    ④ The urine output since surgery

161. Which of the following nursing actions is most likely to relieve Mr. Thompson's bladder spasms?
    ① Administer Demerol as ordered
    ② Administer Pro-Banthine as ordered
    ③ Stop the CBI
    ④ Increase the rate of the CBI

162. Which of the following statements, if made by Mr. Thompson, would indicate that he does NOT understand the outcome of his surgery?
    ① "I'll drink at least eight glasses of water a day."
    ② "I'll continue my perineal exercises every day until I regain bladder control."
    ③ "I won't do any heavy lifting for at least 6 weeks."
    ④ "I won't worry about developing the symptoms of BPH again."

163. Which of the following is the most common long-term outcome or complication of a TUR?
    ① Recurrent urinary infections
    ② Continued bladder spasms
    ③ Bladder neck strictures
    ④ Osteitis pubis

164. The nurse knows that which of the following prostate surgeries does NOT necessarily leave the client sterile?
    ① A transurethral resection
    ② A suprapubic prostatectomy
    ③ A retropubic prostatectomy
    ④ A perineal prostatectomy

Baby boy Sidney Brown, 6 days old, is admitted to the pediatric unit from the nursery with a diagnosis of Down's syndrome.

---

165. Which of the following problems should the nurse expect in caring for baby Brown?
    ① Excessive irritability when held
    ② High incidence of circulatory problems
    ③ Susceptibility to respiratory tract infections
    ④ Difficulty in hearing

166. Which clinical manifestation of Down's syndrome would be evident to the nursery nurse during the initial newborn assessment?
    ① Asymmetry of the gluteal folds
    ② Hypertonicity of the skeletal muscles
    ③ A rounded occiput
    ④ Simian creases on the palms and soles

167. Which of the following interventions is included in the special nursing care for Sidney?
    ① Frequent handling and rocking to keep him from crying
    ② Helping the parents learn to care for him
    ③ Teaching infant to nipple-feed
    ④ Preventing aspiration of formula by frequent burping

168. Which of the following is a common defect associated with Down's syndrome for which the nurse should assess Sidney?
    ① Deafness
    ② Congenital heart defects
    ③ Hydrocephaly
    ④ Muscular hypertonicity

169. Which of the following factors would probably be most significant for the nurse to assess when working with Mr. and Mrs. Brown?
    ① Their response to the reactions of family and friends to their infant
    ② Their ability to give physical care to their infant
    ③ Their ability to talk about changing plans they made for their infant
    ④ Their understanding of the factors causing Down's syndrome

170. As Sidney grows, his development lags and it is found that he is moderately retarded. Which of the following suggestions from the nurse would be most helpful to his parents?
    ① Offer challenging, competitive situations
    ② Offer simple, repetitive tasks
    ③ Concentrate on teaching detailed tasks
    ④ Offer complete directions at the beginning of the task to be accomplished

---

Tammy Sampson, 6 years old, has had numerous upper respiratory infections (URI). They have been complicated by middle ear infections. The pediatrician has recommended that she have her tonsils and adenoids removed.

---

171. During the admission procedure, the nurse obtains the following data. Which information should be communicated to the surgeon?

    ① Tammy's pulse is 92 and her respiratory rate is 24
    ② Tammy sometimes has difficulty swallowing
    ③ Tammy's upper right lateral incisor is loose
    ④ Tammy had an upper respiratory infection 2 weeks ago

172. The nurse plans to explain preoperative procedures, the operating room, the recovery room, and postoperative procedures to Tammy. Which of the following interventions should the nurse implement first?
    ① Explain the need for preoperative medications
    ② Tell Tammy that her parents will wait in her room
    ③ Describe the appearance of the recovery room and the operating room
    ④ Ask Tammy to tell her what she knows about the operation

173. Tammy is to receive atropine sulfate intramuscularly as a preoperative medication. Tammy weighs 50 pounds. What would be the correct dosage to administer to Tammy if the average adult dosage is 0.5 mg?
    ① 0.05 mg
    ② 0.1 mg
    ③ 0.2 mg
    ④ 0.3 mg

174. The nurse approaches Tammy to administer her preoperative medication. Tammy asks, "Is it going to hurt?" Which of the following replies by the nurse is most appropriate?
    ① "If you lie very still, it won't hurt."
    ② "Shots don't hurt brave boys and girls."
    ③ "Yes, but I'll stay with you until it stops."
    ④ "Yes, but only for a while."

175. Tammy arrives in the recovery room after surgery. In which of the following positions should the recovery room nurse position her?
    ① Semi-Fowler's position, with her head turned to the side
    ② Prone position, with the head of the bed slightly elevated
    ③ On her back, with her head turned to the right side
    ④ On her abdomen, with her head turned to the side

176. When Tammy returns to the pediatric unit, she is fully conscious. Which of the following fluids should the nurse offer to Tammy first?
    ① Cool water
    ② Cranberry juice
    ③ Milk
    ④ Orange juice

177. Discharge teaching for Tammy's parents should include information on when to seek medical

attention. The nurse should inform Tammy's parents that which of the following postoperative conditions merits such attention?
① Development of a heavy, dirty gray membrane over the tonsilar area
② Complaints of throat pain on the sixth postoperative day
③ Complaints of an earache without fever
④ Bleeding in the throat on the sixth postoperative day

178. Mr. Garcia has a lesion between the fifth and sixth cervical vertebrae. When testing his deep tendon reflexes, which of the following would the nurse expect to find?
① Abnormal brachioradialis reflex
② Abnormal patellar reflex
③ Absent Achilles tendon reflex
④ Positive plantar reflex

Mr. Anthes has had a recent cerebral vascular accident that has affected his seventh cranial nerve.

---

179. Which of the following symptoms should the nurse expect to result from dysfunction of the seventh cranial nerve?
① An absent gag reflex
② Unequal pupil size and response
③ Difficulty swallowing
④ Asymmetry of facial features

180. Which of the following tests would allow the nurse to assess whether Mr. Anthes' third, fourth and sixth cranial nerves were affected?
① Ask him to shut his eyes tightly
② Test his extraocular movements
③ Test his pupil response
④ Assess his visual fields

Mr. Franks, 67 years old, is scheduled for a CT scan to work-up his 3-month history of transient ischemic attacks (TIA).

---

181. He tells the nurse that he has a history of urticaria and pruritus following shrimp consumption. What effect will this information have on his proposed CT scan?
① It will not adversely affect the test
② The study will have to be canceled
③ Contrast media will not be used
④ An MRI will have to be done instead

182. Mr. Franks had a cerebral arteriogram done this morning. On return to his room, he is difficult to arouse, unable to speak, and unable to move his right hand. None of this was present before the test. As a result of this assessment, the nurse suspects that Mr. Franks is experiencing:
① A reaction to the anesthesia used
② An arterial occlusion
③ Hemorrhage at the insertion site
④ A local reaction to the dye

183. The goal of nursing care for a client undergoing an electroencephalogram is to:
① Facilitate the expression of fear
② Protect the client from CNS complications
③ Promote understanding of the invasive procedure
④ Prevent a reaction to the dye

184. Meniere's disease is a chronic disorder of the middle ear that is characterized by:
① Headache, tinnitus, visual changes, nausea, and vomiting
② Vertigo, hearing loss, and headache
③ Vertigo, tinnitus, hearing loss, nausea, and vomiting
④ Tinnitus, vertigo, and visual changes

Mrs. Jacks, 62 years old, visits the ophthalmology clinic with a diagnosis of wide-angle glaucoma.

---

185. The nursing care plan for Mrs. Jacks should be based on the nurse's knowledge that:
① Compliance with drug therapy is essential to prevent loss of vision
② Damage to the eye caused by glaucoma can be reversed in the early stages of the disease
③ With or without treatment, Mrs. Jacks will eventually lose peripheral vision
④ Mrs. Jacks will experience considerable pain until the optic nerve atrophies

186. Mrs. Jacks tells you she has heard that glaucoma may be a hereditary problem. She is concerned about her children, ages 45 and 33. Which of the following is the most appropriate response for the nurse to make?
① "There is no need for concern; glaucoma is not a hereditary disorder."
② "Your son should be evaluated, but only because he is over 40 years old."
③ "There may be a genetic factor with glaucoma and your children should be screened yearly."
④ "Are your children complaining of any eye problems?"

Mrs. Bailey, 45 years old and a mother of three, has been admitted with a diagnosis of chronic glomerulonephritis and impending renal failure.

187. Upon admission, the physician orders a blood urea nitrogen to be done. The nurse knows that the purpose of the test is to measure the amount of:
    ① Urine produced
    ② Nitrogenous wastes accumulating in the urine
    ③ Waste products accumulating in the blood
    ④ Amount of bacteria in the blood
188. Mrs. Bailey begins to suffer from some muscle twitching. Which of the following is the most important assessment for the nurse to make?
    ① Check for other neurological changes
    ② Assess the client's fluid intake
    ③ Check for circulatory changes
    ④ Assess her serum calcium level calcium
189. The nurse knows that the goal of treatment of chronic renal failure is to:
    ① Increase the urine output
    ② Prevent the loss of electrolytes
    ③ Increase the concentration of electrolytes in the urine
    ④ Reduce the workload on the kidneys

Sam, 19 years old, fractured his femur while skiing. He is placed in skeletal traction.

190. The nurse knows that the primary purpose of skeletal traction is to:
    ① Maintain the client on bedrest
    ② Prevent shifting of the bone fragments
    ③ Reduce and set the fracture
    ④ Relieve the painful muscle spasms
191. After the fracture has begun to heal, a long leg cast is applied. Sam complains that he is now having pain. Which of the following is the most important action for the nurse to take?
    ① Call the physician
    ② Medicate the client with the ordered analgesics
    ③ Elevate the casted leg
    ④ Check the circulation of the toes on the casted leg

Barb Long, 40 years old, is seen in the clinic with a severe exacerbation of rheumatoid arthritis.

192. Which of the following should the nurse recommend to Mrs. Long?
    ① Stay in bed until all symptoms subside
    ② Ride your bicycle daily to prevent contractures
    ③ Maintain a balance between rest and exercise
    ④ Exercise vigorously, followed by complete rest
193. If Mrs. Long is given a nonsteroidal anti-inflammatory medication, which of the following would the nurse teach her in order to avoid undue side effects?
    ① Take the medication only at bedtime
    ② Always take the medication with food
    ③ The medication should be taken before arising in the morning
    ④ Be sure to take it with at least three glasses of water
194. Which of the following types of arthritis is seen most commonly in the elderly?
    ① Acute rheumatoid arthritis
    ② Gouty arthritis
    ③ Osteoarthritis
    ④ Septic arthritis

Mr. Abdul, 66 years old, is a type I diabetic with peripheral vascular disease. He has just returned from an above-the-knee amputation.

195. Which of the following is the major goal of nursing care for Mr. Abdul?
    ① The client will not develop a flexion contracture
    ② The client will not develop phantom limb pain
    ③ The client will ambulate without canes within 1 month
    ④ The client will keep the stump straight 1 hour per day

Mrs. Arthur is receiving chemotherapeutic agents in the treatment of her cancer. She may suffer from numerous side effects, including leukopenia, thrombocytopenia, anemia, and gastrointestinal distress and bleeding.

196. The nurse knows that these side effects occur because:
    1. Chemotherapeutic agents are toxins
    2. Both normal and abnormal rapidly dividing cells are destroyed
    3. The dosages of chemotherapeutic agents are usually high in order to ensure cure
    4. Chemotherapeutic agents are lethal to all rapidly dividing cells

197. Nursing interventions for Mrs. Arthur, who is suffering from leukopenia secondary to chemotherapy, include:
    1. Advising her to avoid people with infections
    2. Avoiding administering injections
    3. Providing for periods of rest
    4. Administering antiemetics before meals

198. Nursing care for Mrs. Arthur while she is thrombocytopenic secondary to chemotherapy includes:
    1. Administering platelet transfusions as ordered
    2. Maintaining reverse isolation
    3. Providing for periods of controlled activity
    4. Administering xylocaine gargle before giving oral care

199. The most appropriate nursing diagnosis for Mrs. Arthur while she is suffering from anemia secondary to chemotherapy is:
    1. Pain
    2. Activity intolerance
    3. High risk for infection
    4. High risk for altered urinary elimination

200. Nursing care for Mrs. Arthur who is suffering from gastrointestinal distress secondary to chemotherapy would include:
    1. Protecting her from infection
    2. Avoiding sedatives
    3. Providing for periods of rest
    4. Administering antiemetics before meals

Mr. Carroll, aged 60, is admitted to the coronary care unit with a diagnosis of acute myocardial infarction. A CVP catheter has been inserted and the initial reading is 30 mm of H_2O.

201. What is the proper position for the tip of the CVP catheter?
    1. In the right atrium
    2. In the pulmonary artery
    3. In the right ventricle
    4. In the superior vena cava

202. When taking a CVP reading, in what position should the nurse place the client?
    1. Low Fowler's position
    2. High Fowler's position
    3. Supine
    4. Left lateral Sims' position

203. To measure the CVP, the nurse places the zero line of the manometer at what level?
    1. Angle of Louis
    2. Right atrium
    3. Carotid bifurcation
    4. Xiphoid process

Mary Jenkins, 27 years old, is a primigravida who suffered from a chlamydia infection early in pregnancy. She is now 41 weeks pregnant and has not experienced spontaneous labor. An induction of labor is planned for today.

204. The nurse knows that which of the following drugs is most commonly used to induce labor?
    1. Parlodel
    2. Phenergan
    3. Pitocin
    4. Premarin

205. Mary's induction has been started and she is now in the active phase of the first stage of labor. This phase is characterized by:
    1. Cervical dilation 1 to 3 cm; affect exhilarated and happy
    2. Cervical dilation 5 to 8 cm; affect concentration and introspection
    3. Cervical dilation 6 to 8 cm; affect alternating exhilaration and irritability
    4. Cervical dilation 8 to 10 cm; affect sudden mood change and irritability

206. Which of the following measurements is most important for the nurse in assessing the adequacy of Mary's pelvic measurements?
    1. Mid-pelvic capacity
    2. Direct conjugate
    3. Intertrochanteric diameter
    4. Depth of the true pelvis

207. Mary has developed bloody show. The nurse knows that this finding is primarily related to:
    1. Early placental separation
    2. Rupture of small cervical vessels
    3. Mild placenta previa
    4. Pressure of the uterus on the cervix

208. The nurse knows that the process by which Mary's cervix becomes thin and indistinct from the body of the uterus is called:
    1. Dilation
    2. Attitude
    3. Effacement
    4. Transition

209. Mary's pelvic examination notes that the fetus is at station −1. This indicates to the nurse that the presenting part of the fetus:
    1. Is visible on the perineum
    2. Has not yet entered the true pelvis
    3. Is above the ischial spines
    4. Is too large to fit through the opening into the true pelvis

210. In order to correctly assess the progress of Mary's labor, the nurse should time the frequency of Mary's contractions from the:
    1. End of one to the beginning of the next
    2. Beginning of one to the end of the next
    3. End of one to the end of the next
    4. Beginning of one to the beginning of the next

211. During transition, the nurse encourages Mary to practice breathing techniques to prevent her from:
    1. Bearing down
    2. Hyperventilating
    3. Losing control
    4. Needing medication

212. The nurse knows that the first stage of labor will be completed when Mary has:
    1. Delivered the baby
    2. Reached 10 cm dilation
    3. Pushed the baby down the birth canal
    4. Rectal pressure with contractions

213. Mary's labor monitor tracing has shown repeated mild variable decelerations. The nurse known that this finding is most often caused by which of the following?
    1. Cord compression
    2. Decreased cerebral blood flow
    3. Uteroplacental insufficiency
    4. Head compression

214. The nurse observes that Mary's fetus has developed a persistent mild bradycardia. This manifestation is most likely related to:
    1. Chorioamnionitis
    2. Beta-adrenergic drugs
    3. Immature fetal nervous system
    4. Maternal anxiety

215. Although the bradycardia persists, Mary's fetus continues to show beat-to-beat variability. The nurse knows that this manifestation indicates:
    1. A functional fetal autonomic nervous system
    2. The presence of a normal fetal sleep state
    3. Early fetal hypoxia
    4. A depressed fetal central nervous system

216. The nurse should know that, as a primigravida, Mary will most likely spend how long in the second stage of labor?
    1. 20 to 30 minutes
    2. 50 to 60 minutes
    3. 2 hours
    4. 3 hours

217. Which statement from Mary to the nurse, if made shortly after birth, would raise concern in the nurse that the normal bonding process was not beginning?
    1. "I do not plan to breast feed this baby."
    2. "It hurts when you massage my uterus."
    3. "We wanted a girl, not a boy."
    4. "Why is his head shaped like that?"

218. The third stage of labor has arrived for Mary. Which of the following nursing observations is NOT indicative of this fact?
    1. Palpation of the uterus to the right of the midline
    2. Absence of a cord pulse
    3. A spurt of blood from the vagina
    4. Extension of the cord outside the vagina

219. Mary complains of excruciating perineal pain the first hour after delivery. Which of the following should the nurse suspect?
    1. Uterine atony
    2. A hematoma
    3. A cervical laceration
    4. Retained placental fragments

220. During the fourth stage of labor, the nurse should assess the position of Mary's fundus at:
    1. 2 cm above the umbilicus
    2. To the right of the umbilicus
    3. 2 cm below the umbilicus
    4. At the level of the umbilicus

Mrs. Murphy, 75 years old, is admitted for a fractured hip. She had an open reduction and internal fixation yesterday.

---

221. Which of the following characteristics would lead the nurse to suspect that Mrs. Murphy is at risk for skin breakdown?
    1. She had an open reduction and internal fixation
    2. She was dehydrated before surgery
    3. She will be in bed until tomorrow
    4. She has a Foley catheter in place

222. While bathing Mrs. Murphy, the nurse notices a reddened area around her right shoulder. To prevent any further skin impairment, the nurse should:
  1. Place a rubber ring under her shoulder
  2. Rub the area vigorously with the fingertips
  3. Gently massage the area with lotion
  4. Keep her positioned only on her left side

223. Mrs. Murphy is also constipated. Because of her age and diagnosis, which of the following is the most appropriate nursing measure to treat constipation?
  1. Put her on the bedpan three times daily
  2. Administer milk of magnesia twice a day as ordered
  3. Administer enemas till clear as ordered
  4. Add prune juice and fiber to her diet

224. Mr. James had a partial gastrectomy for a bleeding ulcer. On the first postoperative day, the nurse should assist Mr. James out of bed and to a chair. The primary purpose of this nursing interventions is to prevent:
  1. Atelectasis
  2. Urinary retention
  3. Nausea and vomiting
  4. Constipation

225. When Mr. James is discharged, he will probably be placed on medication to prevent the recurrence of his ulcer. Which of the following medications is the physician most likely to order?
  1. ranitidine hydrochloride (Zantac)
  2. chlordiazepoxide hydrochloride (Librium)
  3. hyoscyamine sulfate and phenobarbital (Donnatal)
  4. diazepam (Valium)

226. Because Mr. James had a gastric resection and a partial gastrectomy, the nurse should teach him about several potential problems other than recurrence. If he developed symptoms of nausea, diaphoresis, and diarrhea about one half hour after eating, the most likely cause is:
  1. Pernicious anemia
  2. Pyloric obstruction
  3. Dumping syndrome
  4. Hyperemesis

227. The nurse knows that which of the following would NOT be considered a cause of ectopic pregnancy?
  1. Adhesions in the fallopian tubes
  2. Congenital abnormalities of the fallopian tubes
  3. A tumor outside the fallopian tube pressing on it
  4. Complete obstruction of the fallopian tubes

228. Martha has been told that she is Rh-negative, and she asks the nurse what the implications are for her and her fetus. The nurse would explain that a fetus is at the highest risk for Rh incompatibilities if the mother is Rh-negative and it is Martha's:
  1. First pregnancy with an Rh-positive fetus
  2. First pregnancy with an Rh-negative fetus
  3. Second pregnancy with an Rh-positive fetus and she received RhoGAM right after the first delivery
  4. Second pregnancy with an Rh-positive fetus and she received RhoGAM before second pregnancy

229. Which of the following is INCORRECT concerning a hydatidiform mole?
  1. It is a malignant neoplasm
  2. Vaginal bleeding is associated with its presence
  3. The uterus enlarges out of proportion for gestational age
  4. Transparent vesicles resembling grapes develop from the chorion

---

Mary Small, 39 years old, has had a class IV Pap smear. She is admitted for further diagnostic tests and possible surgery.

---

230. It is important for the nurse to be aware of risk factors for a disease so that the nurse can assist in educational and screening programs. The nurse understands that which of the following risk factors is highly associated with the development of cervical cancer?
  1. Low parity
  2. Upper socioeconomic group
  3. History of chronic cervical irritation
  4. Early menses, late menopause

231. Mrs. Small asks what a class IV Pap smear means. The nurse explains that it is which of the following?
  1. Highly suspicious of malignancy
  2. Probable malignancy
  3. Definitive for malignancy
  4. Tissue dysplasia

232. The nurse might expect Mary to exhibit which of the following symptoms?
  1. Irregular menses
  2. Increased menstrual flow
  3. Weight gain
  4. Postcoital bleeding

233. Multiple diagnostic tests are done on Mary to confirm the diagnosis of cervical cancer. Which of the following is NOT considered a specific diagnostic test for cervical cancer?
    1. A CT scan of the abdomen
    2. Schiller's test
    3. Colposcopic examination
    4. Conization for cytology

234. A goal of nursing care after the cervical radiation implant is in place is to keep it in the correct position. Which of the following nursing interventions is most likely to be effective in achieving this goal?
    1. Clamping and draining the Foley catheter at intervals
    2. Providing a high-residue diet
    3. Placing her on the bedpan at regular intervals
    4. Raising the head of the bed no more than 10 degrees

235. Which of the following would be a potential complication for the nurse to be aware of after Mary's hysterectomy since she had a preoperative radiation implant?
    1. Development of a vesicovaginal fistula
    2. Recurrence of vaginal bleeding
    3. Severe postoperative constipation
    4. Increased risk of wound infection

Ms. Abel, 25 years old, has a radium needle uterine implant for metastatic cervical cancer. She is in a private room and expressed no desire to have visitors.

---

236. Ms. Abel tells the nurse, "If only I could live my life over again." The best interpretation of this statement is that Ms. Abel is demonstrating:
    1. Suicidal thoughts and desires
    2. Depression
    3. Feelings of anger
    4. Bargaining

237. Which of the following is NOT an expected effect of Miss Abel's internal radiation?
    1. Foul-smelling vaginal discharge
    2. Abdominal cramps
    3. Nausea and vomiting
    4. Urine mixed with stools

Ms. Abel eventually develops acute carcinomatosis.

---

238. Which nursing observation is an early sign that Ms. Abel is developing septic shock?
    1. Warm, dry skin
    2. Hypertension
    3. Bradycardia
    4. Somnolence and coma

239. Ms. Abel developed syndrome of inappropriate antidiuretic hormone (SIADH). The nurse anticipates that her treatment will include which of the following medications?
    1. Glucagon and insulin
    2. Vasopressin
    3. Mannitol
    4. Imuran

240. The nurse also anticipates that nephrotoxicity can occur. Which of the following best assesses kidney function?
    1. Urine specific gravity
    2. Fluid intake
    3. Urinary pH
    4. Serum electrolytes

Amy Marsh, 42 years old, came to a medical clinical for a physical examination. Mrs. Marsh is a gravida 2, para 2, 5′2″ tall, and weighs 192 pounds. Her blood pressure is 180/100. She has had no serious illnesses, nor any family history of hypertension.

---

241. Which of the following would NOT be a predisposing factor to hypertension?
    1. Smoking
    2. Aerobic exercises
    3. Family history
    4. Obesity

242. Mrs. Marsh denies having headaches. Which of the following clinical manifestations of hypertension should the nurse assess Mrs. Marsh for?
    1. Blurred vision and ringing in the ears
    2. A slow pulse rate and anorexia
    3. Increased energy and dry skin
    4. Pallor and double vision

243. Which of the following would NOT be a potential complication for the client with cirrhosis?
    1. Portal hypertension
    2. Ascites
    3. Hepatic encephalopathy
    4. Hypervolemia

244. Mr. Aston has esophageal varices. Which of the following is the goal of vitamin K administration?

① Increase the prothrombin time to improve clotting
② Decrease serum ammonia levels
③ Reverse a prolonged prothrombin time
④ Decrease the platelet count

245. Which of the following is a laboratory test that can be used to diagnose the presence of the hepatitis B virus?
① Serum anti-HAV (IgM)
② Anti-HAV (IgG)
③ HIV antigen
④ HB$_s$AG

246. Which of the following would NOT be a contraindication for a liver biopsy?
① Prothrombin time of 12 seconds
② Massive ascites
③ An uncooperative client
④ Platelet count less than 30,000/mm^3

Clint Lane weighed 8 pounds at birth and had a complete cleft lip and palate. Mrs. Lane was quite alarmed by the appearance of her baby, and for some time she was unable to look at him without crying. After consulting with the pediatrician and plastic surgeon, Mr. and Mrs. Lane plan to have Clint's lip repaired when he is 4 weeks old.

---

247. Which of the following techniques is necessary for Clint before his lip and palate are repaired?
① Feed him in a flat position for ease of swallowing
② Feed him with a special spoon or straw
③ Offer small, frequent feedings so as not to tire him
④ Burp him frequently during feeding

248. In the recovery room, Clint suddenly becomes cyanotic. Which of the following is the first action the nurse should take?
① Call for assistance
② Administer oxygen
③ Suction the nasopharynx
④ Insert an oral airway

Mary Roberts is a secretary in a physician's office who has been calling in frequently. She complains of tiredness, sleepiness, and loss of appetite that has resulted in a 15-pound weight loss. Her employer told her that she might lose her job. She recently called her family and said good-bye. Her family, worried about her, brought her to the hospital.

---

249. The nurse knows that which of the following patterns best fits Ms. Roberts behavior?
① Withdrawal
② Depression
③ Antisocial behavior
④ Schizophrenia

250. In planning nursing care, which of the following techniques might be most helpful to the nurse?
① Being cheerful so that the client will be in a better mood
② Talking to her for short periods at scheduled intervals
③ Telling her that she is angry to help increase her insight
④ Helping her focus on others by sharing the nurse's problems with her

251. Which of the following is the major short-term goal in caring for Ms. Roberts?
① Client will not cause herself harm
② Client will not hurt any others
③ Client will interact with the group
④ Client will express her anger in a constructive way

252. Which of the following medications would help treat Ms. Roberts symptoms?
① Chloridiazepoxide (Librium)
② Amitriptyline (Elavil)
③ Lithium carbonate
④ Chlorpromazine (Thorazine)

253. Ms. Roberts becomes constipated. The nurse knows that a cause of constipation in clients like Ms. Roberts is:
① A desire to manipulate the nurse
② A need for more medication
③ Lack of another physical way to express emotion
④ Lack of activity and fluid intake

Sam Wilton, 65 years old, is admitted with coronary artery disease. He is scheduled for a cardiac catheterization.

---

254. Which of the following is the most important assessment for the nurse to make before the procedure?
① Verify if the client has been NPO since midnight
② Assess the pulses and temperature of his extremities
③ Ask whether the client has had chest pain in the last 24 hours
④ Determine if the client understands the procedure

255. Mr. Wilton returns from his cardiac catheter. Which of the following is a priority nursing action?
     ① Monitor the temperature and pulses distal to the insertion site
     ② Allow the client to walk around the room as soon as possible
     ③ Obtain a post-procedure ECG
     ④ Monitor the apical pulse hourly

256. Mr. Wilton is suffering from angina pectoris. He is started on sublingual nitroglycerine. Which of the following statements, if made by Mr. Wilton, indicates that he understands the action of this medication?
     ① "I'll take the medication if I have chest pain that is not relieved by rest."
     ② "I'll chew the tablet and then let it dissolve in my mouth."
     ③ "I'll only take one dose. If the pain doesn't stop, I'll call the doctor."
     ④ "I'll only take the medication while sitting or lying down."

257. Mr. Wilton is also started on Nitro-Dur patch daily. Which of the following assessments indicates that the medication is achieving the desired effect?
     ① Client's chest pain is relieved by nitroglycerine
     ② Client performs activities of daily living without chest pain
     ③ Client able to control pain with frequent nitroglycerine
     ④ Client tolerates minimal activity without pain

258. The nurse knows that the best time to perform postural drainage is which of the following?
     ① Before breakfast and dinner
     ② Right before visiting hours
     ③ Only during the night shift
     ④ After breakfast and lunch

259. The physician ordered Mr. Wiln, a client with COPD, to start on Theo-Dur, a bronchodilator. The nurse knows that the primary goal of this drug is to:
     ① Relax the diaphragm and intercostals to increase chest expansion
     ② Decrease contraction of the smooth muscles of the bronchi
     ③ Increase the contraction of the bronchi and alveoli
     ④ Decrease the amount of mucus secretions from the bronchi

260. The outcome of the disruption of closed chest drainage would be which of the following?
     ① Air will enter the thoracic cavity and collapse the lung
     ② Air will escape the thoracic cavity and expand the lung too rapidly

     ③ Water in the drainage bottle will flow into the pleural cavity
     ④ Hemorrhage will result

261. Which of the following is the goal of postoperative coughing and deep breathing exercises after a thoracotomy?
     ① It will be prohibited because of the severe pain
     ② It must be supervised by the surgeon only
     ③ It is needed for adequate ventilation in the unaffected lung
     ④ It will be done only if the client is not in too much pain

---

Mary Brennan, 24 years old, is a new client in the antepartal clinic. She has come for her first prenatal visit. She is a primigravida and has brought her husband with her today.

---

262. Mary reports that her home pregnancy test was positive. A positive pregnancy test is related to the presence of which of the following hormones?
     ① Chorionic gonadotropin
     ② Alpha fetoprotein
     ③ Lactogen
     ④ Estrogen

263. Which of the following goal statements by Mary would show that she understands the need for her daily iron requirement?
     ① "I will consume at least four glasses of milk daily."
     ② "I will add an extra source of red meat to my daily diet."
     ③ "I will take an iron supplement with a vitamin C source daily."
     ④ "I will include an extra source of fruits or vegetables in my daily diet."

264. Mary reports that her husband has exhibited weight gain, fatigue, and nausea throughout her pregnancy. The nurse knows that this phenomena is known as:
     ① Engrossment
     ② Couvade
     ③ Identification
     ④ Bonding

265. Which behavior, if exhibited by Mary, would illustrate the developmental task known as role transition?
     ① Participating in prepared childbirth classes
     ② Purchasing maternity clothes
     ③ Considering names for the new baby
     ④ Accepting the results of the positive pregnancy test

PRACTICE TEST Answers and Rationales

Legend: 1 to 5: Steps of the Nursing Process
I to IV: Areas of Client Needs

1. ④ All are recommended screening examinations except the sputum and chest x-ray, which were dropped because they did not improve early detection in these clients. 1, IV. Cancer.

2. ③ Risk factors for cervical cancer are anything that causes chronic cervical irritation. Choices 1, 2, and 4 are not irritants. 5, IV. Cervical Cancer.

3. ② This combination increases a person's risk for cancer of the larynx. Either factor alone may predispose the other options. 5, IV. Cancer.

4. ④ Family history is one of the highest risk factors for breast cancer. The other options contain low-risk factors. 5, IV. Breast Cancer.

5. ① While the implant is in place, she will be in a private room with staff and visitors only allowed in for limited periods. Also, the presence of an implant is usually very frightening for the client. The other options might be problems, but fear and isolation are usually the greatest problems. 3, II. Cervical Cancer.

6. ③ The important factors to remember when caring for a client with an implant are time, distance, and shielding. The nurse is most shielded by the client's body at the head of the bed. Care can be given for 15 to 30 minutes, a lead apron is not needed, and family visits are also limited. 4, I. Cervical Cancer.

7. ④ Bladder distention would move the bladder closer to the source of radiation. The client is kept on a low-residue diet so that the rectum is not moved closer to the implant. The other options would increase the movement of the implant. 2 & 4, I. Cervical Cancer.

8. ① It is the nurse's responsibility to note the time for the removal and to call the radiology department if it is not done on time. It is removed by the radiology department, not the surgeon. 4, II. Cervical Cancer.

9. ④ Because of the trauma to the vaginal and cervical mucosa caused by the radiation, all forms of irritation should be avoided for at least 6 weeks. The client is not radioactive. 4 & 5, IV. Cervical Cancer.

10. ③ The sudden development of urinary incontinence could indicate the presence of a vesicovaginal fistula, which often occurs spontaneously after radiation because of tissue breakdown between the bladder and vagina. The other options contain expected side effects of the therapy. 5, I & IV. Cervical Cancer.

11. ② Side effects from radiation are more likely to be localized to the area exposed, although some systemic effects may occur. Single-dose therapy would cause even more side effects, and the side effects are not life-threatening. 1, I & II. Radiation Therapy.

12. ③ The client should avoid any irritation of the irradiated skin that may increase the breakdown of the skin. Warm water and prescribed lotions can be used over the area. 4, IV. Radiation Therapy.

13. ① Stomatitis is the irritation of the mucous membranes caused by either radiation or chemotherapy. The other side effects are not associated with radiation of the head and neck. 1, I. Radiation Therapy.

14. ④ The mouth is very sore with stomatitis and local anesthesia must be administered before meals and mouth care. The other interventions treat side effects other than stomatitis. 4, I & II. Radiation Therapy.

15. ③ Coronary vasodilators also dilate other arteries, causing side effects, such as headache, orthostatic hypotension, and fainting. 2, III. CAD.

16. ② Stress causes the adrenals to secrete more cortisol, which leads to gluconeogenesis and insulin antagonism, raising the blood sugar. Because Mrs. Walter's blood sugar is high, she will not need less insulin or carbohydrates or suffer from hypoglycemia. 1, II. Diabetes Mellitus.

17. ③ Glucocorticoids raise the blood sugar and are also insulin antagonists. This increases the need for insulin. 2, II. Diabetes Mellitus.

18. ② The peak of regular insulin is about 4 hours; before lunch, the blood sugar would be at a low. The 9 a.m. reaction would occur only if the client took the

insulin and did not eat. By 3:30 p.m. or 11 p.m. the insulin would not be active. 3 & 5, I. Diabetes Mellitus.

19. ③ The peak for NPH insulin is about 8 hours, which means that the client's blood sugar would be lowest prior to dinner. At 8 a.m. or noon, it would not be effective enough to cause an insulin reaction. By midnight, the NPH should not be able to cause a reaction. 3 & 5, I. Diabetes.

20. ① Diaphoresis and a shaky feeling are early signs of hypoglycemia. Severe thirst is a sign of hyperglycemia, and drowsiness and coma are late symptoms of hypoglycemia. 3 & 5, I. Diabetes Mellitus.

21. ③ Care of the skin around the stoma is the most important aspect of care, because skin excoriation is a real risk and will lead to breakdown and further problems. Irrigation is not done with an ileostomy. Fluids should never be restricted, since dehydration could occur. There is no reason to assume that the client will need psychological counseling, unless some problems arise later. 3 & 5, I. Ulcerative Colitis/Ileostomy.

22. ② The client's stools always have a liquid consistency, and three to four stools a day is normal. The only way to determine diarrhea is the amount of drainage. The usual amount of drainage is 1200 mL per day. Some intolerance to high-residue foods is expected and the stoma always takes about 2 to 3 months to shrink down to its normal size. 1, II. Ulcerative Colitis/Ileostomy.

23. ④ The colonoscopy is used to visualize the lesion, and a biopsy of that lesion is the only accurate diagnostic test for colon cancer. A barium enema is very inaccurate and a CEA level is not diagnostic of cancer; it is a tumor marker. A positive stool for occult blood is suspicious but not diagnostic. 2, II. Colon Cancer.

24. ② A change in bowel habits is one of the major early symptoms of colon cancer. Rectal bleeding is an early symptom, but pain is not. Nausea and vomiting and clay colored stools are not associated with colon cancer. 2, II. Colon Cancer.

25. ④ Chronic cholecystitis may lead to a

decrease in normal bile secretion, limiting the absorption of fat-soluble vitamins, especially vitamin K. Vitamin K is essential for the production of prothrombin, an essential clotting factor. 4 & 5, I. Cholecystitis.

26. ② Semi-Fowler's position increases lung expansion after a cholecystectomy. The incision is high and may interfere with respiratory exchange. The other options would not be aided by this position. 4, II. Cholecystectomy.

27. ③ A T-tube is used after a common bile duct exploration to maintain patency of the duct until healing can occur. A T-tube should never be irrigated except by a physician if it is obstructed. The goal is bile drainage. 5, II. Cholecystectomy.

28. ③ Jaundice occurs when the common bile duct is obstructed with stones. Yellowish coloring around the eyes is a common symptom of jaundice. The stool would be clay colored, and pruritis is a late sign. Ascites is not directly associated with jaundice. 1, II. Obstructive Jaundice.

29. ③ Although family presence is important, because no one in the family speaks English well, the interpreter will provide explanations and support. 4, IV. Prenatal Care.

30. ④ All the laboratory reports are critical for the care of this client, but results of the serology may alter management for Mrs. Park and for others in contact with her body fluids. 1 & 3, IV. Prenatal Care.

31. ④ Prior exposure to hepatitis is evident. The physician must be notified immediately. It does not mean that the hepatitis is active. 3 & 4, IV. Prenatal Care.

32. ④ Prior exposure and immune response are evident; active disease is not. It is not determined when exposure occurred. 2, IV. Prenatal Care.

33. ③ Although Mrs. Park may be advised not to breast feed, the parents need frequent contact with their newborn so that bonding may occur. 3, IV. Postpartal Care.

34. ③ The selection of this menu includes sources of protein, calcium, vitamin C, carbohydrates, fats, and other needed vitamins and minerals. 5, IV. Postpartal Care.

35. ④ Each behavior except choice 4 shows that

the mother has learned hygiene and infant nutrition. Honey should not be given to infants, because it has been linked to the occurrence of botulism. 5, IV. Postpartal Care.

36. ④ Although the nurse can perform many independent functions, this situation needs immediate assessment by the physician. The client must be kept on bedrest until that time, because it might be a blood clot. 4, IV. Postpartal Care.

37. ③ Ambulation is suggested as a prevention of vascular complications following delivery. Although the remaining options are part of discharge teaching, they do not affect circulation. 4, IV. Postpartal Care.

38. ④ Bradycardia refers to a heart rate less than 60 beats per minute. Tachycardia is a heart rate greater than 100 beats per minute. 2, II. CAD.

39. ① A decreased heart rate leads to a decrease in cardiac output. The client might have a fluid volume excess, not a deficit. Health maintenance and breathing pattern should not be affected. 2, II. CAD.

40. ③ Atropine causes the pupil to dilate, narrowing the canal of Schlemm and leading to a rapid increase in intraocular pressure. This is very dangerous in clients with glaucoma and can lead to blindness. 1, II. CAD.

41. ④ The pacemaker of the heart is the sinoatrial node. The sinoatrial node demonstrates the highest degree of automaticity. 2, II. CAD.

42. ③ Pulse taking is important in order to assess for a malfunction. The client needs to learn to assess his own pulse rate. The other options are incorrect. 4, I & II. CAD.

43. ④ Immediate postoperative care of the colostomy client must include close observation of the stoma for possible circulatory impairment. Although the other observations may be made, this is the most significant observation. 1, II. Colostomies.

44. ① Changes in body image is a reality within the first week after a colostomy. Change in social role and regression are not expected, and guilt feelings about cancer is only a conjecture. 5, IV. Colostomies.

45. ① Clients with leukopenia are most susceptible to infections. Septicemia, which is a septic infection, may occur with or without leukopenia. Bleeding may occur due to thrombocytopenia or due to chemical toxicity on fragile blood vessels, whereas hyperuricemia may occur due to massive cell destruction due to cancer or due to effects of chemotherapeutic drugs or radiation therapy. 5, I & II. Chemotherapy.

46. ④ Hypocalcemic tetany is manifested by numbness around the mouth, laryngeal spasms, difficulty talking, carpopedal spasms. 1, II. Chemotherapy.

47. ③ Neurotoxicity of chemotherapy is manifested by sensory changes. The client will be at a higher risk for injury with this altered sensation. There is no change in circulation; and although the client may have paresthesias, pain is not severe. There is no alteration in the thought process. 2, II. Chemotherapy.

48. ③ Developmentally, both infants and toddlers place many nonfood substances in their mouths. The majority of cases of lead poisoning are caused by repeated ingestion of chips of interior or exterior lead-based paint. Older housing in disrepair is a major contributing factor to lead poisoning in young children. 1 & 2, I. Lead Poisoning.

49. ④ Lead interferes with the biosynthesis of heme, preventing the formation of hemoglobin. Reduction of the heme molecule in the red blood cell results in anemia. 2, II. Lead Poisoning.

50. ② Toddlers engage in parallel play. They play alongside, not with, others in their peer group. 1, IV. Lead Poisoning.

51. ③ Denial is a common defense mechanism to help the client overcome the feelings of guilt. The alcoholic is in a cycle of self-deception with increased guilt, usually leading to further drinking. 2, III. Substance Abuse.

52. ② Because alcohol is a diuretic, it is important that the client receive sufficient fluids to prevent dehydration. The client may need IVs, because he may be unable to keep sufficient fluids down. Fluids do not help clear the alcohol or prevent cirrhosis. Alcohol itself is not constipating. 3, III. Substance Abuse.

53. ③ The symptoms associated with alcohol withdrawal are hypertension, diaphoresis, tremors. tachycardia, delusions. hallucinations, and agitation. It is important for the nurse to recognize these symptoms early and prevent the client from injuring himself. 1 & 3, III. Substance Abuse.

54. ① Phenobarbital is now the drug of choice to control the symptoms of alcohol withdrawal. It sedates the client and helps to prevent problems such as convulsions. 5, III. Substance Abuse.

55. ③ An arteriogram allows the visualization of the inside of the artery. Serum cholesterol suggests that plaque may be present, but the only way it can be seen is through an arteriogram. A Doppler study would show turbulence, but not the cause; a prothrombin time looks at bleeding. 1, II. Atherosclerosis.

56. ③ The clinical manifestations he is exhibiting are of decreased cerebral blood flow. Cerebral hypoxia from the narrowing of cerebral arteries would produce these manifestations. The other problems are unrelated to his current status. 2, II. Atherosclerosis.

57. ② The diet he usually follows is very high in fat and cholesterol. Eggs are high in cholesterol. Cereal and juice would provide the lowest amounts of fat and cholesterol for his breakfast. 5, IV. Atherosclerosis.

58. ④ The clinical manifestations the nurse is observing are typical signs of peripheral vascular disease. When a client has atherosclerosis in one area of the body, it is likely present in other parts of the body also. 1, II. Peripheral Arterial Disease.

59. ③ Wernicke's syndrome is a degenerative neurological disorder associated with alcohol ingestion and thiamine deficiency. The other options are incorrect. 1 & 2, III. Substance Abuse.

60. ② A sitz bath is the most helpful treatment for the pain of a hemorrhoidectomy. A stool softener and some types of emollient laxative will help with the first bowel movement, but not with the pain in general. Tylenol #3 contains codeine, which will cause constipation and straining that will increase the pain. 5, H, I. Hemorrhoidectomy.

61. ③ Barbiturate withdrawal can precipitate convulsions, coma, and even death in severe cases. These drugs should be withdrawn slowly and under supervision. The other drugs are habit forming, but they do not cause death with abrupt withdrawal. 5, III. Substance Abuse.

62. ② During middle age, one of the major developmental tasks is establishing a new role with one's spouse. Often, the role has been one totally of family, and now the partners must redefine their role as couple again. They may be preparing for retirement, but not yet accepting it, nor are they ready for choices 3 or 4, which are more tasks of the elderly. 5, IV. Middle Age.

63. ③ One of the main risks of an older adult is falling which, with the normal osteoporosis, makes fractures a great problem. The elderly should not be on bedrest or dependent. Choice 4 is not practical for an 80 year old, because all activities may be unrealistic. 3, I. Elderly.

64. ④ The IV is to run 9 hours or 540 minutes. $1000/540 \times 15 = 15000/540 = 28$ gtts/min. The formula is mL over minutes times the drip factor. 4, I. IV Calculation.

65. ③ Further assessment is necessary. Restlessness and diaphoresis may be signs of decreased cardiac output and serious complications associated with myocardial infarction. 1, III. CAD.

66. ④ Nitroglycerine is a vasodilator. Venous return is decreased, which aids in reducing myocardial oxygen demand. 3, II. CAD.

67. ③ By injecting contrast dye into the coronary arteries, cardiac catheterization with angiography allows visualization of the coronary arteries and provides information on their patency. 3, II. CAD.

68. ③ After the cardiac catheterization, it is important to assess the circulation distal to the catheter insertion site. The risks are hemorrhage, hematoma formation, and thrombus formation, all of which may lead to altered tissue perfusion. Pain is not expected, nor is an ineffective breathing pattern. The client must be on bedrest for 12 to 24 hours, but activity intolerance should not result simply from this or the test itself. 2, II. CAD.

69. ③ This emphasis on routine care is correct. Although pregnancy was not suggested in the past for women with sickle cell disease, current practice is to monitor health closely. Iron has no impact on disease course. Choice 4 is false. 4, IV. Prenatal Care/Sickle Cell Disease.

70. ② This response combines two correct statements. Sickling leads to clumping of cells, which in turn results in tissue hypoxia and occlusion. Although jaundice occurs in crisis, hypertension is not usually present. Dehydration may cause a crisis, but is not a pathophysiologic change. White cell increase depends on concurrent infection. 1 & 2, IV. Prenatal Care/Sickle Cell Disease.

71. ④ Infections are the most frequent predisposing factor for sickle cell crisis, being associated with one third of sickle cell crises in adults. UTI is one of the infections most commonly seen in pregnant women with a history of the disease. The other options would not precipitate a crisis. 1 & 2, IV. Sickle Cell Disease.

72. ④ Altered nutrition: more than required is not related to the problems seen in hypoxia and occlusion. Fetus and mother are at risk during pregnancy. The other options are correct. 2, IV. Prenatal Care/Sickle Cell Disease.

73. ④ The typical look of a fractured hip is shortened, abducted, and externally rotated. 5, II. Fractured Hip.

74. ② Buck's traction is used to decrease pain by reducing muscle spasms. It is not a strong enough pull to set or reduce the fracture. The client in Buck's traction does not have to be on strict bedrest. 3, I. Fractured Hip.

75. ① There are no pin sites, and 25 pounds is much too great a pull. The area around the hip should be assessed, but it is more important to check the skin under the boot, because a shearing force is being applied to it. 1, I. Fractured Hip.

76. ① Considering her age and the unexpected nature of her hospitalization, it is not unusual for confusion to develop. If urinary incontinence or apparent noncompliance does develop, it is likely they are occurring secondary to confusion. There are no data to suggest

cardiac output would be decreased. 2, II. Fractured Hip.

77. ③ The definition of comminuted fracture is that it is fragmented. Choice 1 is the definition of an incomplete fracture; choice 2, a greenstick fracture; and choice 4, a complete fracture. 1, II. Fractures.

78. ② Diabetes does not directly cause fractures. The other options are common causes of fractures, all by osteoporosis. 5, II. Fractures.

79. ① By definition, callus formation is when new bone enters, forming woven bone to begin the process of knitting. The other options describe other stages of bone healing. 5, II. Fractures.

80. ③ A closed reduction involves reducing the fracture without surgery and setting it with a cast. The other options are all examples of open reduction, involving surgery. 2, II. Fractures.

81. ① Circulation and sensation are the priority assessments that must be made after any fracture because of the possibility of nerve or circulatory involvement. Swelling is an indirect assessment, because it might disrupt circulation. The degree of healing and pain are important, but not the priority assessments. 1, I. Fractures.

82. ② The complication possible with a fracture of a long bone is a fat embolus. The symptoms in the situation are those of a fat embolus. A pulmonary embolus, anxiety, and a myocardial infarction do not cause petechiae. 2, II. Fractures.

83. ① Rheumatoid arthritis is systemic and osteoarthritis is localized. Both are chronic and progressive. Osteoarthritis is degenerative; rheumatoid is not. 1, I. Rheumatoid Arthritis.

84. ② Lactulose is administered to decrease the amounts of ammonia, a cerebral toxin, produced in the intestine. A major source of ammonia is from the bacterial and enzymatic deamination of amino acids in the intestines. Lactulose acts by increasing peristalsis and decreasing bowel transit time, leading to diarrhea. 3 & 5, II. Hepatic Coma.

85. ① A high-protein, high-carbohydrate diet is the optimum diet to allow recovery of injured lever cells. Protein is decreased

only in liver disease, when the serum ammonia levels increase. 3, II. Hepatitis.

86. ④ A roast beef sandwich and green beans is the dietary selection with the least amount of dietary sodium. The other selections all contain at least one item high in sodium. 5, II. Ascites.

87. ④ Esophageal varices, hemorrhoids, and prominent veins across the abdomen are all examples of collateral circulation when blood flow is obstructed. Rectal bleeding is not caused by the increased resistance in the liver. Hemorrhoidal bleeding might occur, not rectal bleeding. 5, II. Cirrhosis.

88. ① When a child with cerebral palsy is hospitalized, routines utilized at home should be followed to provide continuity and therefore facilitate optimal development. 3, IV. Cerebral Palsy.

89. ① Decreased mobility over an extended period of time leads to stasis of secretions in the tracheobronchial tree and an ineffective breathing pattern. The unmoving secretions become an ideal medium for bacterial growth. 3, II. Cerebral Palsy.

90. ② The highest priority during a grand mal seizure is to maintain a patent airway. Accumulated secretions must be removed from the nasopharynx. 4, I. Cerebral Palsy/Seizures.

91. ① Postural drainage facilitates the removal of secretions from the lower lung segments into the main bronchi and trachea by gravity. The secretions are then removed by suctioning or coughing. 3, I & II. Cerebral Palsy/Pneumonia.

92. ① Children with cerebral palsy often have feeding difficulties due to poor sucking ability and persistent tongue thrust. He needs to sit up to promote swallowing. The other options are inappropriate. There is nothing to imply that he has lost his appetite. 5, I & II. Cerebral Palsy.

93. ② Parents of handicapped children experience a period of mourning for the normal child they were expecting. Denial of the child's condition is expressed by consulting a variety of physicians, one of whom, it is hoped, will change the child's diagnosis. 5, III. Cerebral Palsy.

94. ④ During the manic phase of manic depression, all the body systems speed

up, as described in the situation. 1 & 2, III. Manic/Depressive Behavior.

95. ① To protect the client, move him into a quiet environment away from others. This will help him regain some control and will not produce unneeded stimuli. Choices 2 and 3 would only increase his agitation, and setting limits will not help at this point. 4, III. Manic/Depressive Behavior.

96. ③ The client's behavior is an attempt on his part to build up his self-esteem and to prevent depression. That is what interferes with his other relationships and behavior. 1, III. Manic/Depressive Behavior.

97. ① The overactive client projects his feelings and anxieties outside of himself. The client directs his anger at things outside of himself. 2, III. Manic/Depressive Behavior.

98. ② Sublimation is a way to channel unacceptable desires into acceptable methods of expression. Instead of taking out his aggression in a destructive way, he sublimates the aggression to an acceptable form. 5, III. Manic/Depressive Behavior.

99. ② This is an example of waxy flexibility. She does not have a decreased level of consciousness. The others are simply incorrect. 1, III. Schizophrenia.

100. ③ This is Mary's way of avoiding contact with the nurse. Her method of coping is to withdraw and avoid contact. The other choices are incorrect interpretations of Mary's behavior. 2, III. Schizophrenia.

101. ② Mary's method of coping has been to withdraw and avoid communication with her nurse. This action on Mary's part of approaching the nurse and offering her something is a sign of improvement. She is able to cope in a less withdrawn manner. The other choices are not involved in this interaction. 5, III. Schizophrenia.

102. ② When a client is hearing voices, it is important to know what they are experiencing so that you can understand what is reality to them. The other choices are not appropriate because they either ignore her reality or make the voices seem real by directly talking about them. 3, III. Schizophrenia.

103. ③ The nurse's primary responsibility is to

provide for the safety of clients and others who are involved. The possibility of impulsive actions as a result of fear must be recognized. The other choices do not address this critical safety issue as specifically as choice 3 does. 3, III. Schizophrenia.

104. ① Social isolation is a real problem with schizophrenics. This goal is realistic in that it involves Mary with a small group at first. Choices 2, 3, and 4 are unrealistic at this time for Mary. 3, III. Schizophrenia.

105. ③ Oxygenation is always a priority in meeting the basic health needs. Nutrition and depression are less immediate concerns at this time, and there is no indication at this point that circulation is impaired. 2, II. Emphysema.

106. ③ Decreased oxygenation leads to fatigue. This symptom is always present in the hypoxic client. For loss of consciousness to occur, the client would have to be very hypoxic. Dehydration and dementia could occur, but are much less likely at this point in time for Mr. Allen. 2, I. Emphysema.

107. ④ One way to assess improvement in oxygenation is through increased ability to perform activities without increasing fatigue. The other options are not appropriate. Choice 1 would be more appropriate for the client whose dyspnea is due to CHF. 5, I. Emphysema.

108. ② The increase in the white blood cells, the leukocytes, in leukemia are misleading because most of them are immature and therefore ineffective. The client, therefore, has a lower resistance to infection. The lymph nodes may or may not be enlarged. If anything, there is a decrease in clotting because of the effect on the normal marrow. 5, II. Leukemia.

109. ③ It is not unusual for the leukemic client to seem irritable and short-tempered. The nurse should accept that this behavior is common in clients with chronic, potentially terminal illnesses. Her age is not a factor, and there are no data to support either choice 1 or 4. 5, III. Leukemia.

110. ③ The immature white blood cells common in leukemia are ineffective in fighting infection. There are no data to support the other choices. 2, II. Leukemia.

111. ① Right-sided heart failure is characterized by a back-up of pressure in the venous system, the periphery. Left-sided or complete heart failure would include pulmonary edema, and cor pulmonale is associated with COPD. 5, II. CHF.

112. ① Fresh fruits are very low in sodium, as are most fresh vegetables. The other snacks are high in sodium. 4, II. CHF.

113. ③ In order to both strengthen the contraction of his heart and decrease his edema, he will need a cardiac glycoside (digoxin) and a diuretic (Diuril). Pronestyl is an antidysrhythmic and not indicated in this situation. Although Isuprel would strengthen cardiac contraction, it would stimulate the sympathetic nervous system and add to the overload on the already stressed heart, and would not help with the edema. Lasix and Diuril are both diuretics and would not be used together. 2 & 5, I & II. CHF.

114. ④ Thiazide diuretics cause the loss of potassium. Although levels of all electrolytes are affected, the greatest affect is on potassium. Hypokalemia predisposes the client to digitalis toxicity. 5, I & II. CHF.

115. ① An indirect way to measure a client's fluid balance is to weigh him or her at the same time, on the same scale, in the same clothes daily. This measures excessive fluid loss or gain. Choice 3 is incorrect because the fluid retained when a client experiences CHF is at least partially interstitial fluid and would not be accounted for in blood volume alone. 5, II. CHF.

116. ③ Left-sided heart failure is characterized by an increased pressure in the pulmonary vasculature, leading to pulmonary edema. The other choices would not produce these symptoms. 2, II. CHF.

117. ① Hypertension is a lifelong problem that can be controlled with diet, medication, and other therapies. It is not curable; its symptoms, not the disease itself, disappear with treatment. It is fatal only if untreated. 2, II. Hypertension.

118. ④ There are few symptoms to hypertension itself, so clients do not perceive themselves as ill. Taking the medication is not bothersome, although the side effects may be. There are no data to support the other options. 5, I. Hypertension.

119. ④ The focus of the treatment in hypertension is to minimize the damage to the blood vessels. Because the disease has no early warning symptoms, some damage is often found at time of diagnosis. Choice 2 is an unreasonable expectation, and increasing the urine output is often a desired outcome when the client suffers from hypervolemia. Lowering the blood pressure below normal could result in inadequate circulation to vital organs. 5, I. Hypertension.

120. ① The heparin is in the concentration of 10 units/mL of IV fluid. To give the client 80 units per hour, the nurse would run in 8 mL of heparin solution. 4, I. IV Calculation.

121. ① With a minidrip, the mL/hr = gtts/min because the drip factor is 60. 4, I. IV Calculation.

122. ④ When the post-TUR client has bladder spasms, it often means that either there is excessive bleeding or the catheter is obstructed. Checking the patency of the catheter and the color of the drainage from the catheter are priority actions. Demerol would not help, and slowing the CBI would increase the risk of bleeding and clots. Increasing the rate might work if it was not obstructed. 4, I. TUR/ Prostate.

123. ③ Pro-Banthine is a smooth muscle relaxant and is the best drug for bladder spasms. Demerol is not very effective, Prostigmin is not appropriate, and Pyridium is used to treat UTIs. 4, II. TUR/Prostate.

124. ① A TUR cannot remove the entire prostate gland, so the gland will continue to hypertrophy and exhibit hyperplasia and may have to be removed again in later years. The client may or may not be sterile and should not be impotent. There is no dressing with a TUR. 5, I. TUR/ Prostate.

125. ② A nonstress test is a noninvasive test conducted with a fetal monitor and designed to determine the intrauterine safety of the fetus. This safety is a reflection of the amount of reserve the placenta contains, which will permit it to nourish and provide satisfactory amounts of oxygen to the fetus. It is considered reactive only if the fetal heart rate increases in response to its own movements. 2, I & IV. Pregnancy-Induced Hypertension.

126. ① An L/S ratio determines the relationship of two components of the fetal lung, lecithin and sphingomyelin, two components of the substance surfactant. The ratio of one to the other is reflective of the maturity of the fetal lung and is predictive of the fetus's chances of developing respiratory distress at birth. The test is conducted via amniocentesis. 1 & 3, I & IV. Prenatal Care.

127. ③ An oxytocin challenge test or stress test, also known as the oxytocin contraction stress test, is conducted by giving an intravenous infusion of oxytocin to the mother and evaluating the fetus's response to subsequent uterine contractions as plotted on a fetal monitor. The test is negative if there are no late decelerations and positive if there are late decelerations in more than one half of the contractions. 2, II & IV. Prenatal Care.

128. ② A biophysical profile score is an evaluation of fetal status conducted when the pregnancy is considered high risk. The first four parts are conducted by ultrasound, followed by a nonstress test. Two points are given for the following: fetal breathing movements, gross fetal body movements, fetal tone, quantitative of amniotic fluid measurement, and quality of the nonstress test. A perfect score is 10, which indicates a state of relative safety in the uterus for the fetus. However, this predictive measure requires that the mother be retested in 1 week to assure ongoing safety. 1 & 2, I & IV. Prenatal Care.

129. ③ False labor contractions diminish when walking, are irregular in nature, with discomfort usually experienced in the lower abdomen, are not concentrated in one part of the uterus, do not increase in intensity and frequency, and do not result in cervical effacement or dilation. 1 & 2, I & IV. Prenatal Care.

130. ② Because of the prolonged nausea and

vomiting, the most important area to assess is the fluid and electrolyte balance. This is the most potentially life-threatening complication. The other options are not vital to assess. 1, II. Gastroenteritis.

131. ④ Because his presenting symptom is diarrhea, the number and consistency of stools is the most important assessment for this client. His vital signs are important, but not the priority. There is no reason to assume the other options are important. 1, II. Gastroenteritis.

132. ① When clients experience nausea, vomiting, and diarrhea, fluid imbalance is one of the next most important assessments. The other options are not as high a priority. 1, II. Gastroenteritis.

133. ④ Goal setting is an important part of care planning. Goals should be specific and measurable and relate directly to the individual client. The most appropriate goal for him is to return to his normal bowel pattern. This will be less frequent, but may be more than one per day. Having the diarrhea controlled may not be enough. 3, I. Gastroenteritis.

134. ③ A bland diet will help prevent further nausea and the fluids are needed to replace those lost. Milk and fruit juice and unlimited fluids and food may increase the diarrhea. Withholding fluids is contraindicated. 4, II. Gastroenteritis.

135. ② Because this a recurrent problem, it would be helpful to know if anyone else in the family also had the problem. This could help to determine if something in the environment is contributing to the condition. The other options are not important. 1, II. Gastroenteritis.

136. ③ The conversion is 2.2 pounds per kilogram; 106/2.2 = 48. 4, II. Medication Administration.

137. ① If antibiotics are started before the culture is obtained, an accurate culture is impossible. Whenever possible, the culture should be obtained before the drugs are started. There is no cross-allergy between penicillins and "mycins." The medication is only given IV and therefore the client's intake of food is unimportant. It is not necessary to retake the temperature before administering it. 4, II. Infections.

138. ② The client must be NPO, except for water, for 12 hours, then is given a high-carbohydrate source and tested for glucose in the blood and urine. The other options are incorrect. 4, II. Diabetes Mellitus.

139. ③ Diabetes is a complex condition affecting carbohydrate metabolism. This is the best, most inclusive definition listed. The others may contain a part of it, but choice 3 is complete. 1, II. Diabetes Mellitus.

140. ① The diabetic diet is a well-balanced diet with controlled amounts of food in the various exchange categories. All food groups are distributed within the diet; although carbohydrates are controlled, they are not actually limited. The diet will help the client lose only the weight necessary, if he is overweight. 1, II. Diabetes Mellitus.

141. ④ With poor diabetic control, levels of fat and glucose are high and cause atherosclerosis. The diabetic client may also be overweight, but this is not the primary contributing factor. 1, II. Diabetes Mellitus.

142. ② Exercise acts to increase oxidation of carbohydrates without increases in insulin. The other options are incorrect. 5, I. Diabetes Mellitus.

143. ① Diabetics have a decrease in the microcirculation, especially of the lower extremities. If they suffer an injury, it is more likely to become gangrenous. Diabetics are not likely to become septic or bleed, because their circulation is so bad. They do not have a lower white blood cell count than normal. 3 & 5, I. Diabetes Mellitus.

144. ③ Parathormone controls calcium metabolism and a decrease leads to hypocalcemia, which can cause muscle tetany. Muscle weakness and calculi are associated with hypercalcemia, and choice 2 is unrelated. 4, II. Hypoparathyroidism.

145. ④ Parathormone controls carbohydrate metabolism. It is not responsible for any of the others. 2, II. Parathyroid Disorders.

146. ① Clients receiving steroids develop Cushing's syndrome from the excessive amounts of cortisone. Choices 2 and 4 are associated with low levels of cortisone,

and choice 3 is not related to cortisone levels. 1, II. Cushing's Syndrome.

147. ③ Steroids are immune suppressants and the client is more prone to infections. The client is more prone to hyperglycemia, so choices 1 and 2 are incorrect. The client should never be encouraged to remain on bedrest, because more complications are likely to occur. 4, II. Cushing's Syndrome.

148. ② It is impossible to prevent all the symptoms of Cushing's syndrome. Some of them may be controllable, but not all. The others are reasonable and important and goals for the client. 3, I. Cushing's Syndrome.

149. ② Although menstruation usually does not occur, ovulation may occur, so lactation is not a reliable method of contraception. Breast feeding helps return the uterus to its normal shape faster by stimulating the endogenous production of oxytocin, which maintains the uterus in a steady state of contraction. Estrogen levels are not affected by breast feeding. 2, IV. Postpartal Care.

150. ① Foul lochial odor, elevated temperature of 38.4°C (101°F) or more within 24 hours after delivery; malaise, and tachycardia are signs of puerperal infection caused by bacterial invasion of placental site or endometrium and should be reported to the physician so that antibiotics can be started. None of the other options properly address the problem. Tampons should never be used. 4, I & IV. Postpartal Care.

151. ③ It is important to be gentle because the episiotomy is easily irritated and hemorrhoids are quite common. A small catheter and 100 mL of fluid would make the enema less effective. There is no reason for the mother to do it herself, because she should not need it on a chronic basis. 4, IV. Postpartal Care.

152. ① Early ambulation is the most effective and safest way to prevent thrombophlebitis. Immobility increases the risk of thrombophlebitis, and breast feeding has no effect on the development of thrombophlebitis. Anticoagulants may cause postpartal hemorrhage. 4 & 5, I. Postpartal Care.

153. ① Pitocin is given following delivery to increase uterine muscle tone and promote uterine contraction. One adverse effect of the medication is an antidiuretic effect, which results in a decrease of free H_2O exchange in the kidneys, leading to a marked decrease in urine output. It is important, therefore, to closely monitor the urine output. It does not affect any of the other options. 2, II. Post C-Section.

154. ② Thrombophlebitis is not an adverse response to Imferon. The rest of the choices are possible reactions to Imferon. 4, II. Post C-Section.

155. ② This menu includes sufficient protein and iron to meet the woman's needs. The other options do not contain as much of both. 5, II & IV. Post C-Section.

156. ② The connective tissue is effected by lupus. Tissue perfusion can be altered, resulting in eventual amputations. It is an important goal to prevent this altered tissue perfusion as long as possible. Deformities are not common from the arthritis, and some degree of discomfort is inevitable. It is important for the client with lupus to rest rather than exercise, in order to prevent exacerbation of the disease. 3, I. Lupus.

157. ④ Irradiated skin is fragile and susceptible to injury. Protection from the sun and other irritants is necessary. Care of the skin, including washing it gently with warm water, patting it gently dry, and using lanolin or A&D ointment with physician's orders, to dry areas. 4, I. Radiation Therapy.

158. ② Proctitis, or inflammation of the rectum, should not occur in radiation treatment of lymphosarcoma. Usually, the cervical and thoracic regions are the sites of radiation therapy. Side effects may include pharyngitis, laryngitis, and tracheitis. 1, I. Radiation Therapy.

159. ③ There is no reason to assume that radiation would cause ascites; therefore, there is no need to measure abdominal girth. The other options are appropriate assessments. 1, I. Radiation Therapy.

160. ③ Bladder spasms have many causes, one of which is obstruction of the Foley catheter, usually with clots. The flow rate of the CBI is usually not a problem unless it is not running fast enough to prevent clots. The time of his last pain shot is

irrelevant. The urine output may suggest that the catheter is plugged; however, to be sure, the patency of the catheter should be checked. 1, I. Prostatectomy.

161. ② The best medication to treat bladder spasms is an antispasmodic such as Pro-Banthine. Changing the rate of the CBI might only serve to increase the spasms by increasing the clots, and Demerol is not as effective for spasms. 5, I. Prostatectomy.

162. ④ A TUR removes only part of the prostate gland, so what is left can continue to hypertrophy and exhibit hyperplasia. This may result in the recurrence of BPH and another TUR may be needed. The other options indicate correct understanding of the surgery. 5, I. Prostatectomy.

163. ③ Bladder neck strictures are common long-term problems of a TUR. Recurrent UTIs and spasms are unlikely, and osteitis pubis may be a problem after a retropubic prostatectomy. 5, I & IV. Prostatectomy.

164. ① A TUR does not remove the entire gland; therefore, the client may still be fertile. With all the other surgeries, the entire gland is removed, so sperm will die. Retrograde ejaculation is common after all but a TUR. A perineal prostatectomy may also cause impotence, so it is done only for prostatic cancer. 5, IV. Prostatectomy.

165. ③ Babies with Down's syndrome have decreased muscle tone, which compromises respiratory expansion as well as an adequate drainage of mucus, contributing to an increased susceptibility to upper respiratory tract infections. The other options have no applicability with Down's syndrome babies. 3, II. Down's Syndrome.

166. ④ Simian creases are the only symptom always observable. Other physical characteristics may suggest Down's syndrome, such as oblique palpebral fissures with abnormal epicanthal skin folds, excess posterior cervical skin, flat facial profile, hyperflexible joints, and muscle hypotonia. The other options contain characteristics not seen in babies with Down's syndrome. 1, II. Down's Syndrome.

167. ② The parents' response to the child may greatly influence decisions regarding future care. Learning about the child and Down's syndrome may help lessen their feelings of guilt. Choice 1 is usual care, and the other choices are not particularly appropriate for the Down's syndrome infant. 4, I. Down's Syndrome.

168. ② Babies with Down's syndrome have a high incidence of congenital heart disease, especially atrial defects. Their muscle tone is usually hypotonic, and their heads and trunks are of normal size. Deafness is more common from maternal rubella. 1, II. Down's Syndrome.

169. ③ When the parents can verbalize the need to change plans that they had made for their infant, it usually signifies they are beginning to face reality. Choices 1 and 2 might indicate some beginning acknowledgment, but choice 3 is more complete. Choice 4 could be seen as a way to intellectualize as opposed to true acceptance. 1 & 3, I. Down's Syndrome.

170. ② A child who is moderately retarded is unable to follow complicated procedures or remember detailed directions. Simple, repetitive tasks provide all the challenge needed. 4, II & IV. Down's Syndrome.

171. ③ Loose teeth are potential hazards during the anesthetic procedure. They may become dislodged and aspirated by the child. The vital signs are normal. Choices 2 and 4 are expected considering the diagnosis. 1, I & II. Tonsillectomy.

172. ④ The first step in the teaching/learning process is to determine the child's present knowledge. Further explanations are then planned accordingly. The other options could be implemented later. 1 & 4, I. Tonsillectomy.

173. ③ Dosage may be determined by the use of Clark's rule. Weight of child in pounds/ 150 pounds × average adult dose = child's dose; 50/150 × 0.5 = 0.167 or 0.2 mg. Many drug dosages are also now listed in mg/Kg. 4, I. Pediatric Medication Administration.

174. ③ Simple, truthful explanations of procedures provides a basis for establishing trust with the school-age child. The nurse should remain with Tammy after the procedure in order to encourage her to verbalize her feelings. Choice 4 does not reassure the child that

someone will be there. 4, I. Tonsillectomy.

175. ④ Before the child is fully awake, she should be placed on her abdomen with her head turned to the side to facilitate the drainage of secretions and to prevent aspiration. When alert, she may sit up, but should remain in bed for the remainder of the day. 4, I. Tonsillectomy.

176. ① Cool water or synthetic fruit juices are offered first. Red juices are avoided so that fresh blood in the emesis can be distinguished from ingested fluid. Citrus juices are avoided because they are irritating. Milk is not given because it coats the throat, causing the child to clear her throat often, which may lead to bleeding. No full liquids are given until clear liquids are retained. Soft foods such as cooked fruits, sherbet, soups, and mashed potatoes are started on day one as tolerated. Eating promotes healing because it increases the blood supply to the tissues. 2 & 4, I. Tonsillectomy.

177. ④ Bleeding from 5 to 10 days postoperatively is a complication of a tonsillectomy and adenoidectomy. This is the time when there is tissue sloughing as healing occurs. The manifestation noted is frequent swallowing and it requires immediate medical attention. Objectionable mouth odor and slight ear pain with a low-grade fever are common occurrences a few days postoperatively; however, persistent severe earache, fever, or cough necessitate medical attention. Most children are ready to resume normal activity within 1 to 2 weeks postoperatively. 1 & 4, I. Tonsillectomy.

178. ① Both the biceps and brachioradialis reflexes test the function of nerves at the level of the fifth and sixth cervical vertebra. The plantar, Achilles, and patellar tendon reflexes measure the function of nerves lower in the spinal cord. 1, II. Neurological Examination.

179. ④ Motor function of the face is controlled by the seventh cranial nerve. The other choices would occur if different cranial nerves were affected. 1, II. Neurological Examination.

180. ② Abnormal responses to extraocular movements will identify the muscles and cranial nerves III, IV, and VI. The other tests measure the function of different cranial nerves. 1, II. Neurological Examination.

181. ③ Iodine-based dyes are used for enhancement and allergies to shellfish indicate an allergy to iodine. The CT can still be done, but only without infusion. An MRI can be done with or without infusion. 2, I. CT Scans.

182. ② Spasm-occluded target vessels cause symptoms similar to those of a stroke. There are no data to assume the other choices have occurred. 2, II. Cerebral Angiography.

183. ① An EEG is a noninvasive test that frightens many clients because of the electrodes being attached to the skull. The client needs reassurance that the test does not produce a "shock" or "read the mind." There are no complications associated with this test. 3, IV. EEG.

184. ③ Headache and visual changes are not characteristic manifestations of Meniere's disease. Vertigo, hearing loss, tinnitus, nausea, and vomiting best describe the most frequent clinical manifestations of this disease. 1, II. Meniere's Disease.

185. ① Intraocular pressure must be decreased to halt the progression of glaucoma, one of the major causes of blindness, if left untreated. Miotics, timolol, and carbonic anhydrase inhibitors are drugs frequently used to treat glaucoma. If blindness occurs, it is irreversible. Glaucoma occurs without pain. 3, II. Glaucoma.

186. ③ Glaucoma has a strong hereditary tendency. Those with a family history of glaucoma should have intraocular pressure monitored yearly after the age of 30 instead of waiting until after 40, as with low-risk individuals. Clients should not wait until eye problems occur to be tested. 2 & 4, I. Glaucoma.

187. ③ Normally, the urea nitrogen is filtered out through the kidneys. With renal failure, it accumulates in the blood. The other options are incorrect. 2, II. Renal Failure.

188. ① As the toxic waste products build up in the blood, CNS changes can begin to occur. The nurse should monitor closely for neurological changes. Intake is irrelevant, as is the need for more calcium. Circulatory changes would not

produce this manifestation. 2, I & II. Renal Failure.

189. ④ The goal in chronic renal failure is to prevent acute failure and maintain whatever function is left. This is best done by minimizing stress and workload on the kidneys. Choices 1 and 2 are unrealistic goals, and the concentration of electrolytes in the urine is too high already. 3, I. Renal Failure.

190. ③ Skeletal traction actually reduces and sets fractures by direct pull on the bone. It does help prevent shifting of fragments and reduce muscle spasms, but these are not the primary purpose. 2, II. Skeletal Traction.

191. ④ The first action is to check the circulation in the toes. If it is impaired, the physician should be called. Choices 2 and 3 could make the situation worse. 1, II. Fractures/Casts.

192. ③ It is important for the arthritic client to balance rest and activity in order to maintain function and reduce deformity. The other activities would cause more problems. 3, I & II. Rheumatoid Arthritis.

193. ② Nonsteroidal anti-inflammatories cause gastrointestinal distress and possible gastrointestinal bleeding if taken on an empty stomach. Food helps to decrease this side effect. The other options are incorrect. 4, II. Rheumatoid Arthritis.

194. ③ Osteoarthritis is a result of the degeneration of the bones that occurs with aging. The others are not particularly common in the elderly. 2, IV. Osteoarthritis.

195. ① The major goal is that the client not develop a flexion contracture. Choices 2 and 3 are not realistic and choice 4 is not an adequate goal. 3, I. Amputations.

196. ② The side effects of chemotherapy and radiation therapy occur because both malignant and normal rapidly dividing cells are destroyed. The cells of the bone marrow and the mucous lining of the gastrointestinal tract are some of the most rapidly dividing cells in the body. 5, I. Chemotherapy.

197. ① A lowered white blood cell count increases the client's risk of contracting an infection. The other options are

treatment for other side effects of chemotherapy. 4, I & II. Chemotherapy.

198. ① A low platelet count predisposes the client to bleeding. If the client's count is below 30,000 or if the client is bleeding, platelet transfusions are considered. The other options relate to prevention of other side effects of chemotherapy. 4, I & II. Chemotherapy.

199. ② Red blood cells are also destroyed by chemotherapy, leaving the client anemic and fatigued. Activity intolerance is the most appropriate diagnosis for this client. The other options relate to other side effects of chemotherapy. 2, I & II. Chemotherapy.

200. ④ Gastrointestinal distress occurs because of destruction of the mucous membrane lining of the gastrointestinal tract, which often leads to nausea, vomiting, diarrhea, and anorexia. Antiemetics before meals may help the client to eat. The other options relate to other side effects of chemotherapy. 4, I & II. Chemotherapy.

201. ① The CVP catheter tip should be located in the right atrium. The other options are incorrect. 2, II. CAD.

202. ③ The client should be lying supine when a CVP reading is taken. The other options are incorrect. 4, II. CAD.

203. ② The level of the right atrium should be estimated and marked. It is approximately halfway up the chest when the client is supine. All CVP readings should be taken at this level. 4, II. CAD.

204. ③ The drug used to induce labor contractions is synthetic oxytocin, known as Pitocin. Parlodel is used to suppress lactation; Phenergan is used as an anti-anxiety agent during labor, and Premarin is used as estrogen replacement therapy for menopausal women. 4, II & IV. Labor and Delivery.

205. ② The first stage of labor is divided into three phases: the first is latent or early, characterized by cervical dilation of up to 4 cm and a maternal affect of excitement. The middle phase is known as the active phase and is characterized by dilation of from 5 to 8 cm, with the maternal affect of concentration and introspection. The third phase is called transition and is characterized by dilation of 8 to 10 cm and an affect of sudden mood change,

irritability, and out-of-control behavior. 2, I & IV. Labor and Delivery.

206. ② The most important pelvic measurement is the direct conjugate, the measurement from bottom of the pubic bone to the sacral promontory. From this measurement, the true conjugate can be estimated. The true conjugate is the smallest diameter through which the fetus must pass; therefore, its adequacy is crucial. It represents the distance from the top of the pubic bone to the sacral promontory. This measurement cannot be calculated digitally, but must be estimated by subtracting 1.5 cm from the diagonal conjugate. 1, II & IV. Labor and Delivery.

207. ② Bloody show is the result of rupture of small blood vessels in the cervix, which occurs as the cervix dilates and effaces. It is unrelated to placenta previa, placenta abruptio, or uterine pressure. 1 & 2, II & IV. Labor and Delivery.

208. ③ The definition of effacement is thinning of the cervix, wherein the muscles of the uterus pull the cervix up into the body of the uterus, making the cervix an indistinct entity. Dilation refers to cervical opening, attitude to fetal posture, and transition to the last phase of the first stage of labor. 2, II & IV. Labor and Delivery.

209. ③ Station refers to the relationship of the biparietal diameter of the fetal head to the ischial spines of the mother. When this diameter reaches the ischial spine, the station is known as zero. A minus station refers to how many centimeters above the spine the diameter is located, with a −3 being unengaged or not yet entered into the true pelvis. The presenting part of the fetus is visible on the perineum at a +3. A −1 indicates that the fetus is 1 cm above the ischial spines. 5, IV. Labor and Delivery.

210. ④ The correct method to timing the frequency of contractions is from the beginning of one contraction to the beginning of the next. When the contraction ends is only of concern when the nurse needs to know the duration of the contraction, not frequency. 1, II & IV. Labor and Delivery.

211. ① Breathing techniques are used during transition to prevent the mother from bearing down before her cervix is completely dilated. A pant, pant, blow exercise will ensure her sufficient oxygen, while blowing will prevent her from bearing down too soon. Hyperventilation can be prevented by slow breathing or breathing into a paper bag. Although breathing techniques are helpful in all phases of labor, they cannot prevent a woman from temporary loss of control and are never meant to keep a client from using all of the tools available, including using medication appropriately to accomplish a satisfactory childbirth. 2, I & IV. Labor and Delivery.

212. ② The first stage of labor is defined as beginning with the onset of true uterine contractions and ending with complete dilation and effacement of the cervix. Delivery of the baby, pushing the baby down the birth canal, and feeling of rectal pressure are events that are concerned with the second stage of labor. 5, II & IV. Labor and Delivery.

213. ① Mild variable decelerations are evidence of cord compression. Uteroplacental insufficiency is related to the development of late decelerations. Head compression is related to the development of early decelerations. Decreased cerebral blood flow cannot be documented. 2 & 5, I & IV. Labor and Delivery.

214. ② Persistent, mild fetal bradycardia is most likely related to the use of beta-adrenergic drugs, the presence of fetal cardiac anomalies, or the use of some regional anesthetics. It may also be idiopathic in nature. The presence of chorioamnionitis, an immature fetus, or maternal anxiety will produce fetal tachycardia. 2 & 5, II & IV. Labor and Delivery.

215. ① Beat-to-beat fetal heart variability refers to the satisfactory functioning of the autonomic nervous system. The sympathetic portion is responsible for acceleration, the parasympathetic portion for deceleration. This is important because one can then infer that the central nervous system is intact if the autonomic nervous system is intact. 2 & 5, I & IV. Labor and Delivery.

216. ② The second stage of labor for a primigravida is about 1 hour; for a multipara, as little as several minutes. When the second stage of labor lasts 2 to 3 hours, it is prolonged and may be indicative of cephalopelvic disproportion or fetal malposition. In this case, the woman should be evaluated to determine whether she will, indeed, be able to deliver vaginally or whether a cesarean birth may be needed. 1, I & IV. Labor and Delivery.

217. ③ When a woman verbalizes her displeasure with the newborn's gender, the nurse should be concerned enough to continue to evaluate the relationship formation between mother and newborn. Maternal responses that are normal may be that she does not wish to breast feed at the time of birth. Many women experience significant and appropriate discomfort with the vaginal examination that follows the delivery procedure. Nearly every mother asks questions about her infant's bluish color and molding of the head. 1 & 5, III & IV. Labor and Delivery.

218. ① Signs of placental separation are contractions and elevation of the uterus, absence of the cord pulse, a spurt of blood from the vagina, and a lengthening of the cord outside the vagina. The uterus does not move to the right of the midline at this time. 1 & 5, II & IV. Labor and Delivery.

219. ② A mother's complaint of excruciating perineal pain following birth is frequently related to the development of a perineal hematoma. The pain results when the perineal tissue is saturated with blood, causing a great deal of stretching and pressure. There is no discomfort associated with uterine atony, cervical laceration, or retained placental fragments. 1 & 5, E, I & IV. Labor and Delivery.

220. ④ The fourth stage of labor is the first 1 to 4 hours following birth, when the fundus should be contracted at the umbilicus. On the second day the nurse will find the fundus below the umbilicus. When it is located to the right or above the umbilicus, the bladder should be assessed to determine whether it is full. 1 & 5, I & IV. Labor and Delivery.

221. ② Adequate hydration helps prevent tissue breakdown. The other choices would not necessarily lead to skin breakdown. Choice 4 is likely to prevent it, because she will not be incontinent. 2, II. Immobility.

222. ③ Gentle massage with lotion will help to restore circulation without causing tissue trauma. A rubber ring increases stasis, and vigorous rubbing could cause more trauma. Keeping her on only her left side will just cause breakdown there. 4, I. Immobility.

223. ④ Constipation is associated with decreased mobility and with the decreased peristalsis of age. It is better to treat it with dietary measures rather than medications if at all possible. Putting her on the bedpan could worsen the constipation. Using a commode that permits natural position would help. 4, II. Immobility.

224. ① Atelectasis is the most common early postoperative problem in clients with high abdominal incisions and general anesthesia. In order to facilitate lung expansion, the client needs to be moved and ambulated. Choices 2 and 4 may be helped by ambulation, but they are not the primary reason it is done. It will have no affect on nausea and vomiting. 5, I. Gastrectomy.

225. ① Zantac, an H_2 histamine receptor antagonist, blocks the release of gastric acid, thereby preventing the recurrence of ulcers. It is very effective, and no other medications are needed. The other medications are inappropriate. 5, II. Gastric Ulcers.

226. ③ Dumping syndrome is a physiological problem associated with too rapid movement of food through the remaining stomach. When this undigested hypertonic mass reaches the intestine, fluids are drawn to dilute it, which results in hypotension. This is known as dumping syndrome. Pernicious anemia is the inability to absorb vitamin B_{12}. This is a complication of gastric resection, but these are not the symptoms of it, nor would it occur immediately postoperatively. Hyperemesis or pyloric obstruction would have vomiting as the major symptom. 5, I & II. Gastric Resection/Dumping Syndrome.

227. ④ If the tubes are completely obstructed, fertilization cannot occur anywhere. The other options could all result in an ectopic pregnancy. 5, IV. Ectopic Pregnancy.

228. ④ RhoGAM must be given within 72 hours after delivery in Rh-incompatible births so that the mother does not produce antibodies. Receiving it later makes it ineffective, which means the fetus is at greater risk. 5, IV. Rh Incompatibility.

229. ① A hydatidiform mole is considered a benign tumor, but follow-up for the development of malignancy is always recommended. The other options contain characteristics of the mole. 1 & 5, IV. Hydatidiform Mole.

230. ③ Risk factors for cervical cancer include high parity, low socioeconomic group, and history of chronic cervical irritation. Early menses and late menopause are risk factors for breast cancer. 1 & 5, IV. Cervical Cancer.

231. ① A class IV Pap smear is highly suspicious for malignancy. A class V smear is probable for malignancy, and a class III is tissue dysplasia. Definitive for malignancy would require a biopsy. 2 & 5, II & IV. Cervical Cancer.

232. ④ Postcoital bleeding is a common symptom of cervical cancer. Irregular menses and increased menstrual flow are more common with uterine cancer. Weight loss is another symptom of cervical cancer. 1, IV. Cervical Cancer.

233. ① A CT scan of the abdomen would be a general test for possible spread of cervical cancer. The other tests are common diagnostic tests associated with the diagnosis of cervical cancer. 5, II & IV. Cervical Cancer.

234. ④ Once the cervical radiation implant is in place, keeping it in the exact measured position without disruption is the primary goal of care. In order to accomplish this, the head of the bed should be only slightly raised. The other options all could potentially cause the implant to shift. 3, I & IV. Cervical Cancer.

235. ① Because of the exposure to radiation preoperatively, the client's tissues will not heal as well and may be prone to breakdown. If there is excessive irritation, a fistula might occur. None of the other options are more likely after this surgery than any other. Some vaginal bleeding is expected. 5, II & IV. Cervical Cancer.

236. ④ Bargaining is the most correct response. The client's statement does not reflect any of the other options. 5, II. Cervical Cancer.

237. ④ The presence of urine mixed with stool after removal of intracavital radiation device from the cervix or uterus indicates a rectovaginal/vesicovaginal fistula. Nausea and vomiting, abdominal cramps, and foul-smelling vaginal discharge are expected effects of the radiation implant. 5, I. Cervical Cancer.

238. ① Warm, dry skin are initial clinical manifestations of septic shock. Bradycardia and coma are very late symptoms of shock, and hypertension is not a manifestation of shock. 1, II. Carcinomatosis.

239. ③ Osmotic diuretics such as mannitol are given to clients with SIADH to rid the body of the excessive fluids that are being retained. The other medications are not used to treat SIADH. 3, II. Carcinomatosis.

240. ① Kidney function is reflected through the urine specific gravity. Fluid intake indirectly determines output but not renal function directly unless it is very low. Serum electrolytes only vaguely and indirectly reflect renal function. Urinary pH would not provide any useful information on nephrotoxicity. 1 & 5, II. Carcinomatosis.

241. ② Aerobic exercises are appropriate cardiovascular exercises that actually improve cardiovascular function, not cause hypertension. The others are predisposing factors for hypertension. 1 & 5, II. Hypertension.

242. ① With severely increased blood pressure, blurred vision and tinnitus are common problems. The other clinical manifestations listed would not occur with hypertension. 1, II. Hypertension.

243. ④ Portal hypertension, ascites, and hepatic encephalopathy are all potential complications of cirrhosis. Hypervolemia is not, because the excessive fluid is interstitial, not intravascular. 5, II. Cirrhosis.

244. ③ Vitamin K may be administered to promote hepatic formation of active prothrombin, lowering the prothrombin time. A low time means normal clotting. It will not affect the platelet count or serum ammonia level. 3, I & II. Cirrhosis.

245. ④ The presence of HB$_s$Ag-hepatitis B surface antigen usually indicates hepatitis B. The others relate to hepatitis A or HIV. 2, II. Hepatitis.

246. ① Thrombocytopenia (platelet count below 30,000/mm^3), massive ascites, and an uncooperative client are all contraindications for a liver biopsy. A prothrombin time of 12 seconds is normal, and therefore not a contraindication for the procedure. 1, I & II. Liver Biopsy.

247. ④ Frequent burping is necessary, because he tends to swallow large amounts of air. He must be fed upright to make swallowing easier and reduce the chance of aspiration. Straws or special spoons are not to be used, because he is not to form a vacuum seal and they may injure his mouth. 1, I & IV. Cleft Lip and Palate.

248. ③ Clearing the airway with gentle suction first to make sure that it is free of mechanical obstruction is the priority. Inserting an airway or administering oxygen would not be helpful if secretions are blocking the airway. There is no need for the nurse to call for assistance. 4, II. Cleft Lip and Palate.

249. ② Sadness, loss of appetite, insomnia, and weight loss are all symptoms of depression. Saying good-bye in light of the depression may mean a thought of suicide. 1 & 2, III. Suicidal Behavior.

250. ② When working with depressed clients, it is better to establish contact, to give structure to the client's day. This can become a lifeline that the client can look forward to. None of the other responses are effective when dealing with depressed clients. 3, III. Suicidal Behavior.

251. ① Depressed clients use introjection to turn their anger inward so that it is no longer an external threat. They internalize everything and are the greatest threat to themselves. They are of no harm to others and are unable to interact with groups at this point. It is also unrealistic at this point to hope that her anger is constructive. 3, III. Suicidal Behavior.

252. ② Tricyclic antidepressants are the drugs of choice to treat depression. The other drugs are tranquilizers that might further depress the client. 1 & 2, III. Suicidal Behavior.

253. ④ All body systems slow down when the client is depressed. The poor diet is also contributing to the constipation. None of the other responses are correct. 1, II. Suicidal Behavior.

254. ② When the client is scheduled for an arteriogram, it is vital that the pulses and temperature distal to the insertion site be assessed prior to the procedure. The other assessments are important, but not the priority. 1, I. Cardiac Catheterization.

255. ① Post-test, the priority again is monitoring the pulses and temperature distal to the insertion site. The client should be on bedrest for 24 hours post-test and the insertion site closely monitored for a hematoma or bleeding. ECGs and the apical pulse are not important assessments at this time. 1, I. Cardiac Catheterization.

256. ④ Nitroglycerine is a vasodilator and could cause orthostatic hypotension; so for safety, the client should only take it while lying or sitting down. The other options indicate the need for more teaching about this drug. 5, IV. Cardiac Medications.

257. ② Nitro-Dur is used to prevent angina so that the client can perform the normal activities of daily living without chest pain. The other options are not reasonable outcomes, because they do not indicate the patch is effective. 5, I & II. Cardiac Medications.

258. ① The coughing following postural drainage is excessive and could trigger vomiting if done after meals. It should be done before meals, and it should be accompanied by good oral hygiene so that the client can eat. 2 & 4, II. COPD.

259. ② The action of Theo-Dur, a bronchodilator, is to relax the bronchial smooth muscles, opening the airways and making breathing easier. 3, II. COPD.

260. ① If the closed drainage system is disrupted, the pleura loses the negative pressure and the lung collapses. None of the other options would occur. 3 & 5, I & II. Closed Water-Seal Drainage.

261. ③ The unaffected lung is very prone to underinflation, atelectasis, and infection. Coughing and deep breathing exercises are vital to a normal return of respiratory function. The client will be in severe pain, and so must be medicated before coughing and deep breathing is done. 3 & 5, II. Thoracotomy.

262. ① Chorionic gonadotropin is a placental hormone which, when present, indicates the presence of pregnancy. Progesterone and lactogen are present during pregnancy but are unrelated to the reading of a pregnancy test. Alpha fetoprotein is abnormal during pregnancy. 2, IV. Prenatal Care.

263. ③ Iron needs during pregnancy can most readily be met by taking iron supplements. Milk contains virtually no iron; an extra source of red meat does not contain sufficient iron, nor does an extra source of fruits or vegetables. 3 & 5, II & IV. Prenatal Care.

264. ② When the expectant mother's partner develops symptoms similar to hers, the phenomenon is called *couvade* or *mitleiden*. Engrossment, identification, and bonding are terms that refer to the parent's relationship with the newborn. 1 & 2, IV. Prenatal Care.

265. ① Role transition is the last developmental task with which the expectant mother must deal. At this time, she exhibits behaviors that will prepare her to change her role from pregnant woman to new mother. Attending childbirth classes will prepare her to successfully accomplish this transition. The other behaviors listed are seen in the tasks called fetal embodiment, fetal distinction, and acceptance of the pregnancy. 1 & 2, III & IV. Prenatal Care.

BREAKDOWN OF TEST QUESTIONS BY NURSING PROCESS AND AREA OF CLIENT NEEDS

Assessment	Analysis	Planning	Implement	Evaluate
Pretest	Pretest	Pretest	Pretest	Pretest
1, 2, 5, 6, 10, 15, 16, 17, 30, 31, 33, 34, 36, 43, 47, 48, 51, 53, 54, 55, 58, 69, 70, 76, 78, 80, 81, 84, 88, 90, 92	3, 4, 12, 13, 14, 15, 19, 22, 25, 26, 50, 52, 68, 75, 83, 89	3, 7, 11, 21, 24, 32, 37, 38, 39, 40, 41, 47, 48, 59, 67, 74, 77, 82, 86, 91	8, 9, 10, 13, 14, 18, 19, 20, 22, 23, 25, 26, 27, 28, 29, 35, 42, 44, 45, 46, 49, 53, 57, 60, 62, 65, 66, 71, 72, 73, 79, 87	23, 35, 37, 39, 56, 61, 75, 89, 93
Practice Test	Practice Test	Practice Test	Practice Test	Practice Test
1, 11, 13, 16, 22, 28, 30, 40, 43, 46, 48, 50, 53, 55, 58, 59, 65, 70, 71, 75, 77, 81, 83, 94, 96, 99, 126, 128, 129, 130, 131, 132, 135, 139, 140, 141, 146, 158, 159, 160, 166, 168, 169, 171, 172, 177, 178, 179, 180, 184, 191, 206, 207, 210, 216, 217, 218, 219, 220, 229, 230, 232, 238, 240, 241, 242, 246, 247, 249, 252, 253, 254, 255, 264, 265	7, 15, 17, 23, 24, 38, 39, 41, 47, 48, 49, 51, 56, 59, 68, 70, 71, 72, 76, 80, 82, 94, 97, 100, 105, 106, 110, 113, 116, 117, 125, 127, 128, 129, 145, 149, 153, 176, 181, 182, 186, 187, 188, 190, 193, 199, 201, 207, 208, 211, 213, 214, 215, 221, 231, 249, 258, 262, 264, 265	5, 18, 19, 20, 21, 30, 33, 52, 53, 63, 66, 67, 74, 84, 85, 88, 89, 91, 102, 103, 104, 126, 133, 143, 148, 156, 165, 169, 183, 185, 189, 192, 195, 234, 239, 244, 250, 251, 259, 260, 261, 263	6, 7, 8, 9, 12, 14, 25, 26, 29, 31, 36, 37, 42, 64, 69, 90, 95, 112, 120, 121, 122, 123, 134, 136, 137, 138, 144, 147, 150, 151, 152, 154, 157, 167, 170, 172, 173, 174, 175, 176, 177, 186, 192, 197, 198, 200, 202, 203, 222, 223, 248, 258	2, 3, 4, 9, 10, 18, 19, 20, 21, 25, 27, 34, 35, 44, 45, 54, 57, 60, 61, 62, 73, 78, 79, 84, 86, 87, 92, 93, 98, 101, 107, 108, 109, 111, 113, 114, 115, 118, 119, 124, 142, 143, 152, 155, 161, 162, 163, 164, 196, 209, 214, 215, 217, 218, 219, 220, 224, 225, 226, 227, 228, 229, 230, 231, 233, 235, 236, 237, 240, 241, 243, 256, 257, 260, 261, 263

Safe, Effective Care	Physiological Integrity	Psychological Integrity	Health Promotion and Maintanence
Pretest	Pretest	Pretest	Pretest
3, 4, 5, 7, 8, 9, 10, 11, 12, 13, 14, 16, 18, 19, 20, 22, 23, 24, 25, 26, 28, 29, 30, 33, 37, 38, 39, 40, 41, 42, 46, 47, 49, 50, 52, 57, 60, 62, 63, 64, 67, 85, 86, 87, 91	1, 2, 14, 15, 17, 21, 27, 30, 31, 32, 34, 35, 36, 44, 45, 51, 52, 53, 54, 55, 58, 61, 62, 64, 66, 76, 78, 80, 81, 83, 84, 87, 88, 89	43, 71, 82, 90, 92, 93	6, 42, 48, 56, 59, 65, 68, 69, 70, 72, 73, 74, 75, 77, 79, 82
Practice Test	Practice Test	Practice Test	Practice Test
6, 7, 10, 11, 13, 14, 18, 19, 20, 21, 25, 42, 45, 48, 60, 63, 64, 74, 75, 81, 83, 90, 91, 92, 106, 107, 113, 114, 118, 119, 120, 121, 122, 124, 125, 126, 128, 129, 133, 142, 143, 148, 150, 152, 156, 157, 158, 159, 160, 161, 162, 163, 167, 169, 171, 172, 173, 174, 175, 176, 177, 181, 186, 188, 189, 192, 195, 196, 197, 198, 199, 200, 205, 211, 213, 215, 216, 219, 220, 222, 224, 226, 234, 237, 244, 246, 247, 254, 255, 257, 260	5, 8, 11, 14, 16, 17, 22, 23, 24, 26, 27, 28, 38, 39, 40, 41, 42, 43, 45, 46, 47, 49, 55, 56, 58, 65, 66, 67, 68, 73, 76, 77, 78, 79, 80, 82, 84, 85, 86, 87, 89, 91, 92, 105, 108, 110, 111, 112, 113, 114, 115, 116, 117, 123, 127, 130, 131, 132, 134, 135, 136, 137, 138, 139, 140, 141, 144, 145, 146, 147, 153, 154, 155, 165, 166, 168, 170, 171, 178, 179, 180, 182, 184, 185, 187, 188, 190, 191, 192, 193, 197, 198, 199, 200, 201, 202, 203, 204, 206, 207, 208, 210, 212, 214, 218, 221, 223, 225, 226, 231, 233, 235, 236, 238, 239, 240, 241, 242, 243, 244, 245, 246, 248, 253, 257, 258, 259, 260, 261, 263	15, 51, 53, 54, 61, 93, 94, 95, 96, 97, 98, 99, 100, 101, 102, 103, 104, 109, 217, 249, 250, 251, 252, 265	1, 2, 3, 4, 9, 10, 12, 29, 30, 31, 32, 33, 34, 35, 36, 37, 44, 50, 59, 62, 69, 70, 71, 72, 88, 125, 126, 127, 128, 129, 149, 150, 151, 155, 163, 164, 170, 183, 194, 205, 206, 207, 208, 209, 210, 211, 212, 213, 214, 215, 216, 217, 218, 219, 220, 227, 228, 229, 230, 231, 232, 233, 234, 235, 247, 256, 262, 263, 264, 265

Appendix

State Boards of Nursing

Alabama
Alabama Board of Nursing
RSA Plaza, Suite 250
770 Washington Avenue
Montgomery, Alabama 36130
205/242-4060

Alaska**
Alaska Board of Nursing Licensing
Department of Commerce
& Economic Development
Division of Occupational Licensing
PO Box 110806
Juneau, Alaska 99811-0806
907/561-2878

Arizona
Arizona Board of Nursing
2001 W. Camelback Road, Suite 350
Phoenix, Arizona 85015
602/255-5092

Arkansas
Arkansas State Board of Nursing
University Tower Building
1123 South University Avenue, Suite 800
Little Rock, Arkansas 72204
501/686-2700

California*
California Board of Registered Nursing
PO Box 944210
400 R Street, Suite 4030
Sacramento, California 95814
916/322-3350

AS OF SEPTEMBER, 1991:
* Mandatory Continuing Education—required for all
R.N.s for license renewal.
** Mandatory C.E. in special situations (e.g., nurse
practitioners, not actively employed) to activate a li-
cense.

Colorado*
Colorado Board of Nursing
1560 Broadway, Suite 670
Denver, Colorado 80202
303/894-2430

Connecticut
Department of Health Services
Connecticut Board of
Examiners for Nursing
150 Washington Street
Hartford, Connecticut 06106
203/566-1041

Delaware**
Delaware Board of Nursing
Margaret O'Neill Building
Federal & Court Streets
PO Box 1401
Dover, Delaware 19903
302/739-4522

District of Columbia**
District of Columbia Board of Nursing
614 H Street, NW, Room 112
PO Box 37200
Washington, DC 20001
202/727-7461

Florida*
Florida State Board of Nursing
111 Coastline Drive East, Suite 516
Jacksonville, Florida 32202
904/359-6331

Georgia
Georgia Board of Nursing,
Registered Nurses
166 Pryor Street, SW, Suite 400
Atlanta, Georgia 30303
404/656-3943

Guam
Guam Board of Nurse Examiners
PO Box 2816
Agana, Guam 96910
671/477-8766 or 8517

Hawaii
Board of Nursing, State of Hawaii
PO Box 3469
Honolulu, Hawaii 96801
808/548-3086

Idaho**
Idaho Board of Nursing
2800 North 8th Street, Suite 210
Boise, Idaho 83720
208/334-3110

Illinois
Illinois Department of
   Professional Regulation
320 West Washington Street, 3rd Floor
Springfield, Illinois 62786
217/785-0800

Indiana
Indiana State Board of Nursing
Health Professions Service Bureau
402 West Washington Street, Room 041
Indianapolis, Indiana 46204
317/232-2960

Iowa*
Iowa Board of Nursing
1223 East Court
Des Moines, Iowa 50319
515/281-3255

Kansas*
Kansas Board of Nursing
Landon State Office Building
900 SW Jackson, Room 551
Topeka, Kansas 66612-1256
913/296-4929

Kentucky*
Kentucky State Board of Nursing
4010 Dupont Circle, Suite 430
Louisville, Kentucky 40207
502/897-5143

AS OF SEPTEMBER, 1991:
* Mandatory Continuing Education—required for all
R.N.s for license renewal.
** Mandatory C.E. in special situations (e.g., nurse
practitioners, not actively employed) to activate a li-
cense.

Louisiana*
Louisiana State Board of Nursing
150 Baronne Street, Room 912
New Orleans, Louisiana 70112
504/568-5464

Maine
Maine State Board of Nursing
State House Station #158
Augusta, Maine 04333-0158
207/624-5275

Maryland
Maryland State Board of Nursing
Metro Executive Center
4201 Patterson Avenue
Baltimore, Maryland 21215-2299
410/764-4747

Massachusetts*
Massachusetts Board of
   Registration in Nursing
100 Cambridge Street, Suite 1519
Boston, Massachusetts 02202
617/727-9961

Michigan
Michigan Board of Nursing
PO Box 30018
Lansing, Michigan 48909
517/373-1600

Minnesota*
Minnesota Board of Nursing
2700 University Avenue West, Suite 108
St. Paul, Minnesota 55114
612/642-0567

Mississippi**
Mississippi Board of Nursing
239 North Lamar, Suite 401
Jackson, Mississippi 39201
601/359-6170

Missouri
Missouri State Board of Nursing
3605 Missouri Boulevard
Box 656
Jefferson City, Missouri 65102
314/751-0681

Montana
Montana State Board of Nursing
Department of Commerce
Arcade Building, Lower Level
111 North Jackson
Helena, Montana 59620-2071
406/444-4279

Nebraska*
Nebraska Board of Nursing
State House Station, Box 95007
Lincoln, Nebraska, 68509
402/471-2115

Nevada*
Nevada State Board of Nursing
1281 Terminal Way, Suite 116
Reno, Nevada 89502
702/786-2778

New Hampshire**
New Hampshire Board of Nursing
Division of Public Health Services
Health and Welfare Building
6 Hazen Drive
Concord, New Hampshire 03301-2657
603/271-2323

New Jersey
New Jersey Board of Nursing
1100 Raymond Boulevard, Room 508
Newark, New Jersey 07101
201/648-2490

New Mexico*
New Mexico Board of Nursing
4253 Montgomery NE, Suite 130
Albuquerque, New Mexico 87109
505/841-8340

New York**
New York State Board for Nursing
State Education Department
Cultural Education Center
Albany, New York 12230
518/474-3843

AS OF SEPTEMBER, 1991:
* Mandatory Continuing Education—required for all R.N.s for license renewal.
** Mandatory C.E. in special situations (e.g., nurse practitioners, not actively employed) to activate a license.

North Carolina
North Carolina Board of Nursing
PO Box 2129
Raleigh, North Carolina 27602-2129
919/782-3211

North Dakota
North Dakota Board of Nursing
919 South 7th Street, Suite 504
Bismarck, North Dakota 58504-5881
701/224-2974

Ohio
Ohio Board of Nursing
77 South High Street, 17th Floor
Columbus, Ohio 43266-0316
614/466-3947

Oklahoma
Oklahoma Board of Nursing Registration
  and Nursing Education
2915 North Classen Boulevard, Suite 524
Oklahoma City, Oklahoma 73106
405/525-2076

Oregon**
Oregon State Board of Nursing
10445 SW Canyon Road, Suite 200
Beaverton, Oregon 97005
503/644-2767

Pennsylvania
Pennsylvania State Board of Nursing
PO Box 2649
Harrisburg, Pennsylvania 17105
717/783-7142

Puerto Rico
Colegio de Professionales de la
  Enfermeria de Puerto Rico
Board of Nurse Examiners
Call Box 10200
Santurce, Puerto Rico 00908
809/725-8161

Rhode Island
Rhode Island Board of Nursing
  Registration & Nursing Education
Cannon Health Building, Room 104
75 Davis Street
Providence, Rhode Island 02908
401/277-2827

South Carolina
State Board of Nursing for South Carolina
220 Executive Center Drive, Suite 220
Columbia, South Carolina 29210
803/731-1648

South Dakota
South Dakota Board of Nursing
3307 South Lincoln Avenue
Sioux Falls, South Dakota 57105-5224
605/335-2977

Tennessee
Tennessee State Board of Nursing
283 Plus Park Boulevard
Nashville, Tennessee 37247-1010
615/367-6232

Texas
Board of Nurse Examiners for the
    State of Texas
9101 Burnet Road, Suite 104
Austin, Texas 78758
512/835-4880

Utah
Utah State Board of Nursing
Division of Occupational and
    Professional Licensing
Heber M. Wells Building, 4th Floor
160 East 300 Street, PO Box 45802
Salt Lake City, Utah 84145-0801
801/530-6736

Vermont
Vermont State Board of Nursing
109 State Street
Montpelier, Vermont 05602
802/828-2396

Virgin Islands
Virgin Islands Board of Nurse Licensor
Kongens Gade #3
PO Box 4247
St. Thomas, Virgin Islands 000803
809/776-7397

Virginia
Virginia State Board of Nursing
1601 Rolling Hills Drive
Richmond, Virginia 23229
804/662-9909

Washington
Washington State Board of Nursing
Division of Professional Licensing
PO Box 47864
Olympia, Washington 98504-7864
206/753-2206

West Virginia
West Virginia Board of Examiners for
    Registered Nurses
Room 309, Embleton Building
922 Quarrier Street
Charleston, West Virginia 25301
304/348-3596

Wisconsin
Wisconsin Board of Nursing
PO Box 8935, Room 174
Madison, Wisconsin 53708-8935
608/266-0145

Wyoming
Wyoming State Board of Nursing
Barrett Building, 2nd Floor
2301 Central Avenue
Cheyenne, Wyoming 82002
307/777-7601

Provincial Canadian Registering/Licensing Boards

Canadian Nurse Association
50 The Driveway
Ottawa, Ontario K2P 1E2
613/237-2133

Alberta Association of Registered Nurses
11620—168th Street
Edmonton, Alberta T5M 4A6
403/451-0043

Association of Nurses of Prince Edward Island
17 Pownal Street, Box 1838
Charlottetown, Prince Edward Island C1A 7N5
902/368-3764

Association of Registered Nurses of Newfoundland
55 Military Road
PO Box 6116
St. John's, Newfoundland A1C 5X8
709/753-6040

College of Nurses of Ontario
101 Davenport Road
Toronto, Ontario M5R 3P1
416/928-0900

Manitoba Association of Registered Nurses
647 Broadway Avenue
Winnipeg, Manitoba R3C 0X2
204/774-3477

Northwest Territories Registered Nurses Association
PO Box 2757
Yellowknife, Northwest Territories X1A 2R1
403/873-2745

Nurses Association of New Brunswick
165 Regent Street
Fredericton, New Brunswick E3B 3W5
506/458-8731

Order of Nurses of Québec
4200 ouest, boulevard Dorchester
Montréal, Québec H3Z 1V4
514/935-2501

Registered Nurses Association of British Columbia
2855 Arbutus Street
Vancouver, British Columbia V6J 3Y8
604/736-7331

Registered Nurses Association of Nova Scotia
Suite 104, 120 Eileen Stubbs Avenue
Dartmouth, Nova Scotia B3B 1Y1
902/468-9744

Saskatchewan Registered Nurses Association
2066 Retallack Street
Regina, Saskatchewan S4T 2K2
306/757-4643

Yukon Nurses Society
PO Box 5371
Whitehorse, Yukon Y1A 4Z2
403/667-4062

INDEX

Note: Page numbers in *italics* refer to illustrations; page numbers followed by t refer to tables.